Life stage group	Potassium (g/d)	Chloride (g/d)	Calcium (mg/d)	Phosphorus (mg/d)	Magnesium (mg/d)	Iron (mg/d)	Zinc (mg/d)	Selenium (µg/d)	Iodine (µg/d)	Copper (µg/d)	Manganese (mg/d)	Fluoride (mg/d)	Chromium (µg/d)	Molybdenum (µg/d)	Water (L/d)[8]
Infants															
0-6 mo	0.4*	0.18*	210*	100*	30*	0.27*	2*	15*	110*	200*	0.003*	0.01*	0.2*	2*	0.7*
7-12 mo	0.7*	0.57*	270*	275*	75*	11	3*	20*	130*	220*	0.6*	0.5*	5.5*	3*	0.8*
Children															
1-3 y	3.0*	1.5*	500*	460	80	7	3	20	90	340	1.2*	0.7*	11*	17	1.3*
4-8 y	3.8*	1.9*	800*	500	130	10	5	30	90	440	1.5*	1*	15*	22	1.7*
Males															
9-13 y	4.5*	2.3*	1,300*	1,250	240	8	8	40	120	700	1.9*	2*	25*	34	2.4*
14-18 y	4.7*	2.3*	1,300*	1,250	410	11	11	55	150	890	2.2*	3*	35*	43	3.3*
19-30 y	4.7*	2.3*	1,000*	700	400	8	11	55	150	900	2.3*	4*	35*	45	3.7*
31-50 y	4.7*	2.3*	1,000*	700	420	8	11	55	150	900	2.3*	4*	35*	45	3.7*
51-70 y	4.7*	2.0*	1,200*	700	420	8	11	55	150	900	2.3*	4*	30*	45	3.7*
>70 y	4.7*	1.8*	1,200*	700	420	8	11	55	150	900	2.3*	4*	30*	45	3.7*
Females															
9-13 y	4.5*	2.3*	1,300*	1,250	240	8	8	40	120	700	1.6*	2*	21*	34	2.1*
14-18 y	4.7*	2.3*	1,300*	1,250	360	15	9	55	150	890	1.6*	3*	24*	43	2.3*
19-30 y	4.7*	2.3*	1,000*	700	310	18	8	55	150	900	1.8*	3*	25*	45	2.7*
31-50 y	4.7*	2.3*	1,000*	700	320	18	8	55	150	900	1.8*	3*	25*	45	2.7*
51-70 y	4.7*	2.0*	1,200*	700	320	8	8	55	150	900	1.8*	3*	20*	45	2.7*
>70 y	4.7*	1.8*	1,200*	700	320	8	8	55	150	900	1.8*	3*	20*	45	2.7*
Pregnancy															
≤18 y	4.7*	2.3*	1,300*	1,250	400	27	12	60	220	1,000	2.0*	3*	29*	50	3.0*
19-30 y	4.7*	2.3*	1,000*	700	350	27	11	60	220	1,000	2.0*	3*	30*	50	3.0*
31-50 y	4.7*	2.3*	1,000*	700	360	27	11	60	220	1,000	2.0*	3*	30*	50	3.0*
Lactation															
≤18 y	5.1*	2.3	1,300*	1,250	360	10	13	70	290	1,300	2.6*	3*	44*	50	3.8*
19-30 y	5.1*	2.3	1,000*	700	310	9	12	70	290	1,300	2.6*	3*	45*	50	3.8*
31-50 y	5.1*	2.3	1,000*	700	320	9	12	70	290	1,300	2.6*	3*	45*	50	3.8*

[8]The AI for water represents total water from drinking water, beverages, and moisture from food.

Sources: Data compiled from *Dietary Reference Intakes for Calcium, Phosphorus, Magnesium, Vitamin D, and Fluoride.* Washington, DC: National Academies Press; 1997. *Dietary Reference Intakes for Thiamin, Riboflavin, Niacin, Vitamin B₆, Folate, Vitamin B₁₂, Pantothenic Acid, Biotin, and Choline.* Washington, DC: National Academies Press; 1998. *Dietary Reference Intakes for Vitamin C, Vitamin E, Selenium, and Carotenoids.* Washington, DC: National Academies Press; 2000. *Dietary Reference Intakes for Vitamin A, Vitamin K, Arsenic, Boron, Chromium, Copper, Iodine, Iron, Manganese, Molybdenum, Nickel, Silicon, Vanadium, and Zinc.* Washington, DC: National Academies Press; 2001. *Dietary Reference Intakes for Water, Potassium, Sodium, Chloride, and Sulfate.* Food and Nutrition Board. Washington, DC: National Academies Press; 2004. These reports may be accessed via http://nap.edu. Reprinted with permission by the National Academy of Sciences, courtesy of the National Academies Press, Washington, DC.

Tolerable Upper Intake Levels (UL[1])

Life stage group	Vitamin A[2] (µg/d)	Vitamin D (µg/d)	Vitamin E[3,4] (mg/d)	Niacin[4] (mg/d)	Vitamin B$_6$ (mg/d)	Folate[4] (µg/d)	Vitamin C (mg/d)	Choline (g/d)	Calcium (g/d)	Phosphorus (g/d)	Magnesium[5] (mg/d)	Sodium (g/d)
Infants												
0-6 mo	600	25	ND[7]	ND	ND	ND	ND	ND	ND	ND	ND	ND
7-12 mo	600	25	ND	ND	ND	ND	ND	ND	ND	ND	ND	ND
Children												
1-3 y	600	50	200	10	30	300	400	1.0	2.5	3	65	1.5
4-8 y	900	50	300	15	40	400	650	1.0	2.5	3	110	1.9
Males, females												
9-13 y	1,700	50	600	20	60	600	1,200	2.0	2.5	4	350	2.2
14-18 y	2,800	50	800	30	80	800	1,800	3.0	2.5	4	350	2.3
19-70 y	3,000	50	1,000	35	100	1,000	2,000	3.5	2.5	4	350	2.3
>70 y	3,000	50	1,000	35	100	1,000	2,000	3.5	2.5	3	350	2.3
Pregnancy												
≤18 y	2,800	50	800	30	80	800	1,800	3.0	2.5	3.5	350	2.3
19-50 y	3,000	50	1,000	35	100	1,000	2,000	3.5	2.5	3.5	350	2.3
Lactation												
≤18 y	2,800	50	800	30	80	800	1,800	3.0	2.5	4	350	2.3
19-50 y	3,000	50	1,000	35	100	1,000	2,000	3.5	2.5	4	350	2.3

Life stage group	Iron (mg/d)	Zinc (mg/d)	Selenium (µg/d)	Iodine (µg/d)	Copper (µg/d)	Manganese (mg/d)	Fluoride (mg/d)	Molybdenum (µg/d)	Boron (mg/d)	Nickel (mg/d)	Vanadium[6] (mg/d)	Chloride (g/d)
Infants												
0-6 mo	40	4	45	ND	ND	ND	0.7	ND	ND	ND	ND	ND
7-12 mo	40	5	60	ND	ND	ND	0.9	ND	ND	ND	ND	ND
Children												
1-3 y	40	7	90	200	1,000	2	1.3	300	3	0.2	ND	2.3
4-8 y	40	12	150	300	3,000	3	2.2	600	6	0.3	ND	2.9
Males, females												
9-13 y	40	23	280	600	5,000	6	10	1,100	11	0.6	ND	3.4
14-18 y	45	34	400	900	8,000	9	10	1,700	17	1.0	ND	3.6
19-70 y	45	40	400	1,100	10,000	11	10	2,000	20	1.0	1.8	3.6
>70 y	45	40	400	1,100	10,000	11	10	2,000	20	1.0	1.8	3.6
Pregnancy												
≤18 y	45	34	400	900	8,000	9	10	1,700	17	1.0	ND	3.6
19-50 y	45	40	400	1,100	10,000	11	10	2,000	20	1.0	ND	3.6
Lactation												
≤18 y	45	34	400	900	8,000	9	10	1,700	17	1.0	ND	3.6
19-50 y	45	40	400	1,100	10,000	11	10	2,000	20	1.0	ND	3.6

[1]UL = The maximum level of daily nutrient intake that is likely to pose no risk of adverse effects. Unless otherwise specified, the UL represents total intake from food, water, and supplements. Due to lack of suitable data, ULs could not be established for vitamin K, thiamin, riboflavin, vitamin B$_{12}$, pantothenic acid, biotin, or carotenoids. In the absence of ULs, extra caution may be warranted in consuming levels above recommended intakes.

[2]As preformed vitamin A (retinol) only.

[3]As α-tocopherol; applies to any form of supplemental α-tocopherol.

[4]The ULs for vitamin E, niacin, and folate apply to synthetic forms obtained from supplements, fortified foods, or a combination of the two.

[5]The ULs for magnesium represent intake from a pharmacological agent only and do not include intake from food and water.

[6]Although vanadium in food has not been shown to cause adverse effects in humans, there is no justification for adding vanadium to food and vanadium supplements should be used with caution. The UL is based on adverse effects in laboratory animals and these data could be used to set a UL for adults but not children or adolescents.

[7]ND = Not determinable due to lack of data on adverse effects in this age group and concern with regard to lack of ability to handle excess amounts. Source of intake should be from food only to prevent high levels of intake.

Sources: Data compiled from *Dietary Reference Intakes for Calcium, Phosphorus, Magnesium, Vitamin D, and Fluoride.* Washington, DC: National Academies Press; 1997. *Dietary Reference Intakes for Thiamin, Riboflavin, Niacin, Vitamin B$_6$, Folate, Vitamin B$_{12}$, Pantothenic Acid, Biotin, and Choline.* Washington, DC: National Academies Press; 1998. *Dietary Reference Intakes for Vitamin C, Vitamin E, Selenium, and Carotenoids.* Washington, DC: National Academies Press; 2000. Institute of Medicine, Food and Nutrition Board. *Dietary Reference Intakes for Vitamin A, Vitamin K, Arsenic, Boron, Chromium, Copper, Iron, Manganese, Molybdenum, Nickel, Silicon, Vanadium, and Zinc.* Washington, DC: National Academy Press, 2001. *Dietary Reference Intakes for Water, Potassium, Sodium, Chloride, and Sulfate.* Washington, DC: National Academies Press; 2004. These reports may be accessed via http://nap.edu. Reprinted with permission by the National Academy of Sciences, courtesy of the National Academies Press, Washington, DC.

Nutrition

Third Edition

Paul Insel
Stanford University

R. Elaine Turner
University of Florida

Don Ross
California Institute of Human Nutrition

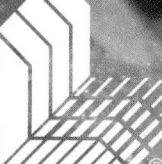

AMERICAN DIETETIC ASSOCIATION

JONES AND BARTLETT PUBLISHERS

Sudbury, Massachusetts

BOSTON   TORONTO   LONDON   SINGAPORE

World Headquarters
Jones and Bartlett Publishers
40 Tall Pine Drive
Sudbury, MA 01776
978-443-5000
info@jbpub.com
www.jbpub.com

Jones and Bartlett Publishers Canada
6339 Ormindale Way
Mississauga, Ontario L5V 1J2
CANADA

Jones and Bartlett Publishers International
Barb House, Barb Mews
London W6 7PA
UK

Jones and Bartlett's books and products are available through most bookstores and online booksellers. To contact Jones and Bartlett Publishers directly, call 800-832-0034, fax 978-443-8000, or visit our website, www.jbpub.com.

Substantial discounts on bulk quantities of Jones and Bartlett's publications are available to corporations, professional associations, and other qualified organizations. For details and specific discount information, contact the special sales department at Jones and Bartlett via the above contact information or send an email to specialsales@jbpub.com.

Production Credits

Chief Executive Officer: Clayton Jones
Chief Operating Officer: Don W. Jones, Jr.
President, Higher Education and Professional Publishing: Robert W. Holland, Jr.
V.P., Design and Production: Anne Spencer
V.P., Manufacturing and Inventory Control: Therese Connell
V.P., Sales and Marketing: William J. Kane
Acquisitions Editor: Jacqueline Mark-Geraci
Senior Production Editor: Julie Champagne Bolduc
Associate Editor: Patrice M. Andrews
Editorial Assistant: Amy L. Flagg
Production Assistant: Jennifer M. Ryan
Marketing Manager: Wendy Thayer
Composition: Graphic World, Inc.
Cover Design: Anne Spencer
Cover Image: © Dianne Maire/ShutterStock, Inc.
Printing and Binding: Courier
Cover Printing: Lehigh Press

Library of Congress Cataloging-in-Publication Data
Insel, Paul M.
    Nutrition / Paul Insel, R. Elaine Turner, Don Ross. -- 3rd ed.
       p. cm.
    Includes index.
    ISBN-13: 978-0-7637-4252-2 (alk. paper)
    ISBN-10: 0-7637-4252-X
    1. Nutrition. I. Turner, R. Elaine. II. Ross, Don. III. Title.
    QP141.I63 2007
    612.3--dc22
                                            2006101683

6048

Printed in the United States of America
11 10 09 08 07   10 9 8 7 6 5 4 3 2 1

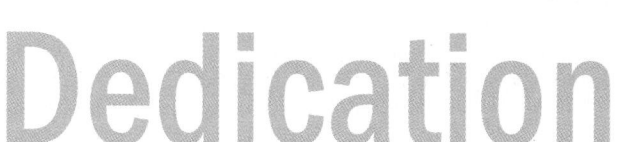

Dedication

To Sis and Lenore with love

*To Allen, Mitchell, and Ted for their
love, patience, and understanding*

*To Donna and Mackinnon for their
sustenance of love, support, and patience*

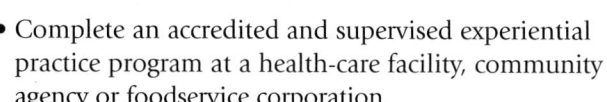

The material in this book has been favorably reviewed by the American Dietetic Association.

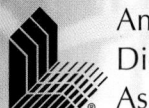

American Dietetic Association
120 South Riverside Plaza
Suite 2000
Chicago, IL 60606
(800) 877-1600

www.eatright.org

With nearly 65,000 members, the American Dietetic Association is the nation's largest organization of food and nutrition professionals.

ADA was founded in Cleveland, Ohio, in 1917 by a visionary group of women, led by ADA's first president, Lulu C. Graves, and co-founder Lenna F. Cooper, who were dedicated to helping the government conserve food and improve the American public's health and nutrition during World War I.

Members

Approximately 75 percent of ADA's members are registered dietitians (RDs) and four percent are dietetic technicians, registered (DTRs). Other ADA members include clinical and community dietetics professionals, consultants, food-service managers, educators, researchers, dietetic technicians, and students.

ADA members represent a wide range of practice areas and special interests, including public health; sports nutrition; medical nutrition therapy; nutrition counseling for weight control, cholesterol reduction, diabetes, heart and kidney disease, and many other health concerns; foodservice management in business, hospitals, restaurants, long-term care facilities, and education systems; education of other health-care professionals; and scientific research. Members can also join 29 special interest or dietetic practice groups.

What is a registered dietitian?

A registered dietitian is a food and nutrition expert who has met the minimum academic and professional requirements to qualify for the credential "RD." In addition to RD credentialing, many states have laws that regulate the licensure or credentialing of dietitians and nutrition practitioners. Frequently these state requirements are met through the same education and training required to become an RD.

Registered dietitians must:

• Complete at least a bachelor's degree and course work approved by ADA's Commission on Accreditation for Dietetics Education.

• Complete an accredited and supervised experiential practice program at a health-care facility, community agency or foodservice corporation.
• Pass a national examination administered by the Commission on Dietetic Registration.
• Complete continuing professional educational requirements to maintain registration.

What is a dietetic technician, registered?

Dietetic technicians, registered (DTRs), often working in partnership with registered dietitians, screen, evaluate and educate patients; provide guidance in prevention of diseases such as diabetes and obesity; and monitor the progress of a patient or client. DTRs provide expert assistance in hospices, home health-care programs, day-care centers, foodservice operations, government, and community programs such as Meals on Wheels.

Dietetic technicians, registered must:

• Complete at least a two-year associate's degree in an approved dietetics technology program from an accredited U.S. college or university.
• Complete a minimum of 450 hours of supervised practice experience in community programs, health care and foodservice facilities.
• Pass a nationwide examination and continuing education courses throughout their careers.

Commission on Dietetic Registration

The Commission on Dietetic Registration, the credentialing agency for ADA, awards credentials at entry, fellow, and specialty levels to individuals who have met its standards for competency to practice in the profession, including successful completion of its national certification examination and recertification by continuing professional education and/or examination.

Start thinking now about a career in dietetics

Within the field of dietetics, you can choose to be either a registered dietitian (RD) or a dietetic technician, registered (DTR). Whichever option you choose, you'll share your knowledge of food and nutrition to help people make healthful food choices.

Scholarship information

The American Dietetic Association Foundation (ADAF) offers scholarships to encourage eligible students to enter the field of dietetics. Once you are enrolled in a college dietetics program accredited by the Commission on Accreditation for Dietetics Education you may be eligible for an ADAF scholarship.

Brief Contents

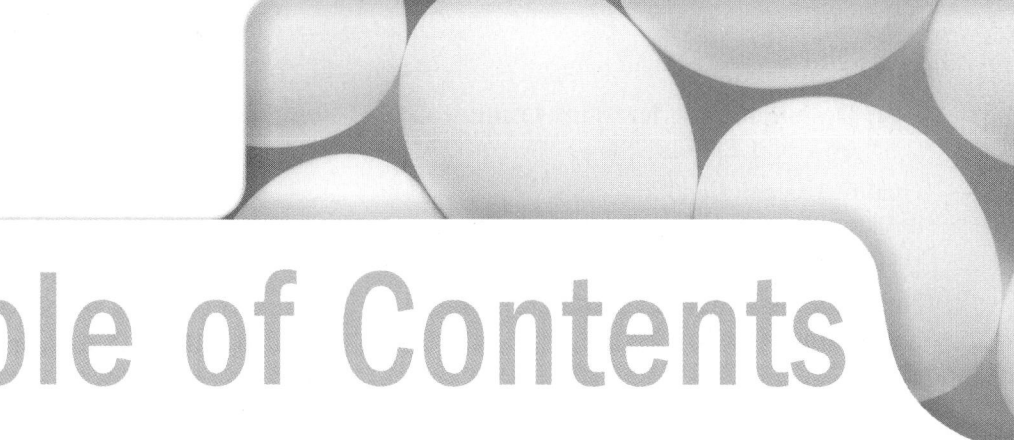

Table of Contents

Chapter 11
Water and Major Minerals 456

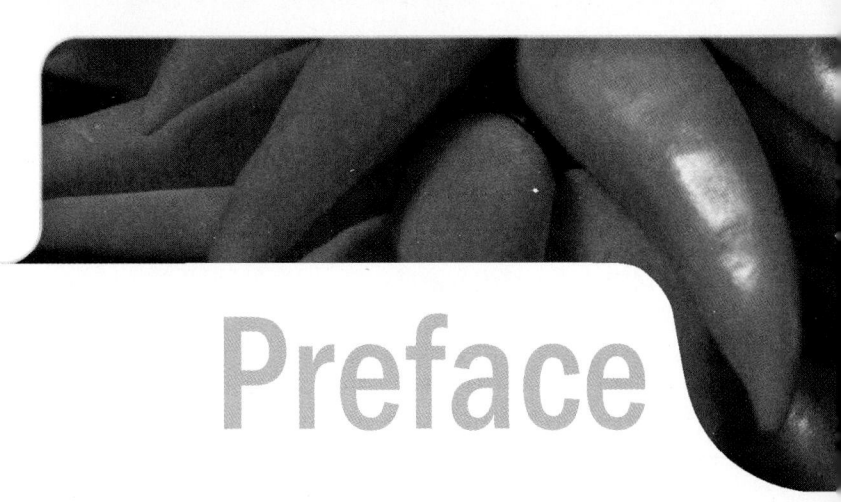

Preface

*B*ecause changes in nutrition-related information occur so rapidly, and because we are committed to providing comprehensive, current, and accurate information on the most pressing issues, we have prepared this third edition of *Nutrition*. The overall content, organization, and features remain, but within this framework, key topics and issues have been updated with the most recent information available. Our goals in writing this book can be stated simply:

- To present scientifically based, accurate, up-to-date information in an accessible format
- To involve students in taking responsibility for their nutrition, health, and well-being
- To instill a sense of competence and personal power in students

The first of these goals means making expert knowledge about nutrition available to the individual. *Nutrition* brings scientifically based, accurate, up-to-date information to students about topics and issues that concern them—a balanced diet, nutritional supplements, weight management, exercise, and a multitude of others. Current, complete, and straightforward coverage is balanced with "user-friendly" features designed to make the text appealing.

Our second goal is to involve students in taking responsibility for their nutrition and health. To encourage students to think about the material they're reading and how it relates to their own lives, *Nutrition* uses innovative pedagogy and unique interactive features. We invite students to examine the issues and to analyze their nutrition-related behaviors.

Perhaps our third goal in writing *Nutrition* is the most important: stimulate a sense of competence and personal power in the students who read the book. Everyone has the ability to monitor, understand, and affect his or her own nutritional behaviors.

2005 Dietary Guidelines for Americans

The sixth edition of *Dietary Guidelines for Americans* places stronger emphasis on reducing calorie consumption and increasing physical activity. Eating a healthy balance of nutritious foods continues as a central point in the *Dietary Guidelines*, but balancing nutrients is not enough for health. Total calories also count, especially as more Americans are gaining weight. Because almost two-thirds of Americans are overweight or obese, and more than half get too little physical activity, the *2005 Dietary Guidelines* place a stronger emphasis on calorie control and physical activity. The report identifies several key recommendations. As you read the chapters, look for these recommendations highlighted in the margins.

USDA MyPyramid

MyPyramid, which replaces the Food Guide Pyramid introduced in 1992, is part of an overall food guidance system that emphasizes the need for a more individualized approach to improving diet and lifestyle. MyPyramid incorporates recommendations from the *2005 Dietary Guidelines for Americans* and uses interactive technology found on http://www.MyPyramid.gov. These interactive activities allow individuals to obtain a more personalized recommendation on their daily calorie level based on the *2005 Dietary Guidelines for Americans*. It also allows individuals to find general food guidance and suggestions for making smart choices from each food group. Concepts from MyPyramid and the *Dietary Guidelines* are carried throughout the book and fully integrated into the chapter text. MyPyramid intake recommendations are summarized in Appendix C.

Trans Fat Labeling

Nutrition delivers the tools for students to understand food labels, including the new *trans* fat information, and incorporate positive nutritional behaviors into their everyday lives. The *Dietary Guidelines for Americans* recommend reducing the intake of *trans* fats and saturated fats. The new United States labeling requirement for *trans* fat will provide a more complete picture of fat content in foods—allowing students and other consumers to choose foods low in *trans* fat, saturated fat, and cholesterol. The FDA estimates that *trans* fat labeling will prevent from 600 to 1,200 cases of coronary heart disease and 250 to 500 deaths each year.

Nutrition Science in Action

New to this edition is *Nutrition Science in Action*, an exciting feature that walks students through science experiments involving nutrition. Each *Nutrition Science in Action* presents observations and hypotheses, an experimental plan, and results, conclusions, and discussions that allow students to apply their knowledge of nutrition to real-life experiments outside of the classroom.

Position Statements

Also new to this edition are position statements from distinguished organizations such as the American Dietetic Association, the American College of Sports Medicine, and the American Heart Association that relate to the chapter topics under discussion. These position statements bolster the assertions made by the authors by showcasing concurrent opinions held by some of the leading organizations in nutrition and health.

Bioterrorism and the Food Supply

How safe is our food supply? In the aftermath of the terrorist attacks on the World Trade Center in September 2001 and the spread of anthrax through the mail, there is heightened concern over the vulnerability of our food supply to bioterrorism. *Nutrition* explores past attacks on U.S. and Canadian food supplies, points of vulnerability, and food safety strategies that students can use to help protect themselves.

These are just a sampling from a complete menu of updates throughout the book, including the latest DRIs, revised macronutrient chapters, the latest references, expanded coverage of diet and health, and more.

Accessible Science

Nutrition makes use of the latest in learning theory and balances the behavioral aspects of nutrition with an accessible approach to scientific concepts. You will find the book to be a comprehensive resource that communicates nutrition both graphically and personally.

Think About It questions at the beginning of each chapter present realistic nutrition-related situations and ask the students to consider how they would behave in such circumstances.

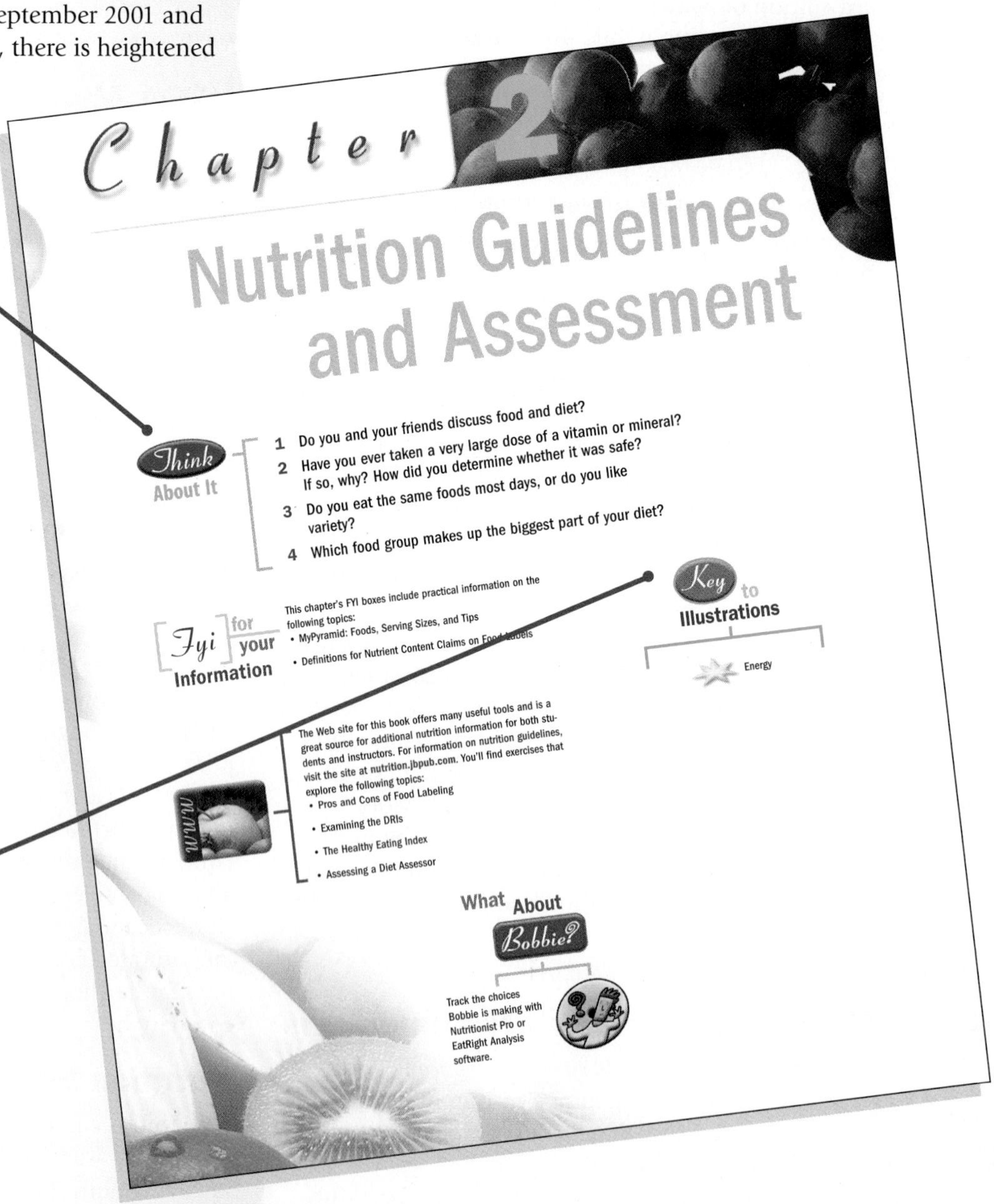

The **Key to Illustrations** at the beginning of each chapter identifies the icons students will encounter throughout the book. These *chemical icons* identify molecular components of nutrient molecules, making their construction and deconstruction visually and conceptually accessible.

Chapter **2**

Nutrition Guidelines and Assessment

Think About It

1 Do you and your friends discuss food and diet?
2 Have you ever taken a very large dose of a vitamin or mineral? If so, why? How did you determine whether it was safe?
3 Do you eat the same foods most days, or do you like variety?
4 Which food group makes up the biggest part of your diet?

[*Fyi*] for your Information

This chapter's FYI boxes include practical information on the following topics:
• MyPyramid: Foods, Serving Sizes, and Tips
• Definitions for Nutrient Content Claims on Food Labels

www

The Web site for this book offers many useful tools and is a great source for additional nutrition information for both students and instructors. For information on nutrition guidelines, visit the site at nutrition.jbpub.com. You'll find exercises that explore the following topics:
• Pros and Cons of Food Labeling
• Examining the DRIs
• The Healthy Eating Index
• Assessing a Diet Assessor

Key to Illustrations

✳ Energy

What About *Bobbie?*

Track the choices Bobbie is making with Nutritionist Pro or EatRight Analysis software.

We present technological concepts in an engaging, non-intimidating way with an appealing, step-wise, parallel development of text and annotated illustrations. Illustrations in all chapters use consistent representations. Each type of nutrient, for example, has a distinct color and shape. Icons of an amino acid, a protein, a triglyceride, and a glucose molecule represent "characters" in the nutrition story and are instantly recognizable as they appear throughout the book.

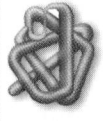
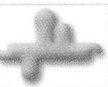

This textbook is unique in the field of nutrition and leads the way in depicting important biological and physiological phenomena, such as emulsification, glucose regulation, digestion and absorption, and fetal development. Extensive graphic presentations make nutrition and physiological principles come alive. The illustrations use pictures to teach and are part of a multimedia package that coordinates the text with illustrations and software. The EatRight Analysis and the Nutritionist Pro software programs are fully integrated ancillaries designed to help students track their diets, make choices, and hone their nutritional skills.

In addition to these strengths, the contents of this book have been technically reviewed by the American Dietetic Association, the nation's largest organization of food and nutrition professionals with nearly 65,000 members.

The Pedagogy

Nutrition focuses on teaching behavioral change, personal decision making, and up-to-date scientific concepts in a number of novel ways. This interactive approach of *Nutrition* addresses different learning styles, making it the ideal text to ensure mastery of key concepts. Beginning with Chapter 1, the material engages students in considering their own behavior in light of the knowledge they are gaining. The pedagogical aids that appear in most chapters include:

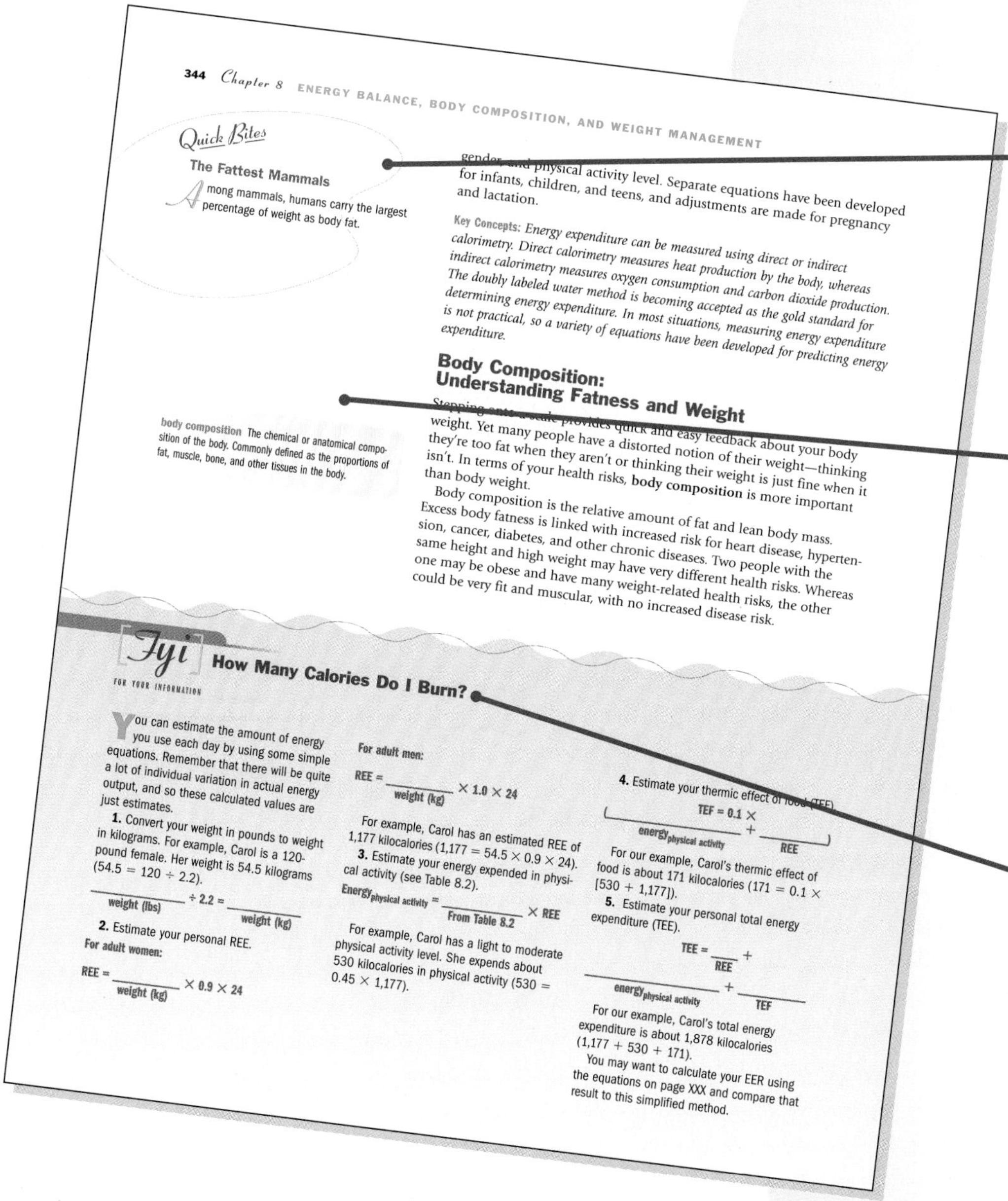

Quick Bites are sprinkled throughout the book. They offer fun facts about nutrition-related topics such as exotic foods, social customs, origins of phrases, folk remedies, medical history, and so on.

Key terms are in boldface type the first time they are mentioned. Their definitions also appear in the margins near the relevant textual discussion, making it easy for students to review material and items.

For Your Information offer more in-depth treatment of controversial and timely topics, such as unfounded claims about the effects of sugar, whether athletes need more protein, and usefulness of the glycemic index.

The following is reproduced from the sample textbook page shown:

344 *Chapter 8* ENERGY BALANCE, BODY COMPOSITION, AND WEIGHT MANAGEMENT

Quick Bites

The Fattest Mammals
Among mammals, humans carry the largest percentage of weight as body fat.

gender, and physical activity level. Separate equations have been developed for infants, children, and teens, and adjustments are made for pregnancy and lactation.

Key Concepts: *Energy expenditure can be measured using direct or indirect calorimetry. Direct calorimetry measures heat production by the body, whereas indirect calorimetry measures oxygen consumption and carbon dioxide production. The doubly labeled water method is becoming accepted as the gold standard for determining energy expenditure. In most situations, measuring energy expenditure is not practical, so a variety of equations have been developed for predicting energy expenditure.*

Body Composition: Understanding Fatness and Weight

Stepping onto a scale provides quick and easy feedback about your body weight. Yet many people have a distorted notion of their weight—thinking they're too fat when they aren't or thinking their weight is just fine when it isn't. In terms of your health risks, **body composition** is more important than body weight.

Body composition is the relative amount of fat and lean body mass. Excess body fatness is linked with increased risk for heart disease, hypertension, cancer, diabetes, and other chronic diseases. Two people with the same height and high weight may have very different health risks. Whereas one may be obese and have many weight-related health risks, the other could be very fit and muscular, with no increased disease risk.

body composition The chemical or anatomical composition of the body. Commonly defined as the proportions of fat, muscle, bone, and other tissues in the body.

Fyi
FOR YOUR INFORMATION **How Many Calories Do I Burn?**

You can estimate the amount of energy you use each day by using some simple equations. Remember that there will be quite a lot of individual variation in actual energy output, and so these calculated values are just estimates.

1. Convert your weight in pounds to weight in kilograms. For example, Carol is a 120-pound female. Her weight is 54.5 kilograms (54.5 = 120 ÷ 2.2).

$$\frac{}{\text{weight (lbs)}} \div 2.2 = \frac{}{\text{weight (kg)}}$$

2. Estimate your personal REE.
For adult women:

$$REE = \frac{}{\text{weight (kg)}} \times 0.9 \times 24$$

For adult men:

$$REE = \frac{}{\text{weight (kg)}} \times 1.0 \times 24$$

For example, Carol has an estimated REE of 1,177 kilocalories (1,177 = 54.5 × 0.9 × 24).
3. Estimate your energy expended in physical activity (see Table 8.2).

$$Energy_{physical\ activity} = \frac{}{\text{From Table 8.2}} \times REE$$

For example, Carol has a light to moderate physical activity level. She expends about 530 kilocalories in physical activity (530 = 0.45 × 1,177).

4. Estimate your thermic effect of food (TEF)

$$TEF = 0.1 \times \left(\frac{}{energy_{physical\ activity}} + \frac{}{REE} \right)$$

For our example, Carol's thermic effect of food is about 171 kilocalories (171 = 0.1 × [530 + 1,177]).
5. Estimate your personal total energy expenditure (TEE).

$$TEE = \frac{}{REE} + \frac{}{energy_{physical\ activity}} + \frac{}{TEF}$$

For our example, Carol's total energy expenditure is about 1,878 kilocalories (1,177 + 530 + 171).
You may want to calculate your EER using the equations on page XXX and compare that result to this simplified method.

Key Concepts summarize previous text and highlight important information.

Label to Table helps students apply their new decision-making skills at the supermarket. It walks students through the various types of information that appear on food labels, including government-mandated terminology, misleading advertising phrases, and amounts of ingredients.

If the diet contains high amounts of fiber, some people, such as young children and the elderly, may become full before meeting their energy and nutrient needs. Because of a limited stomach capacity, they must be careful that their fiber intake does not interfere with their ability to consume adequate energy and nutrients.

Due to the bulky nature of fibers, excess consumption is likely to be self-limiting. Although a high fiber intake may cause occasional adverse gastrointestinal symptoms, serious chronic adverse effects have not been observed. As part of an overall healthy diet, a high intake of fiber will not produce significant deleterious effects in healthy people. Therefore, a Tolerable Upper Intake Level (UL) is not set for fiber.

Key Concepts: High sugar intake promotes dental caries and can contribute to nutrient deficiencies by replacing more nutritious foods in the diet. High intake of foods rich in dietary fiber offers many health benefits, including reduced risk of obesity, type 2 diabetes, cardiovascular disease, and gastrointestinal disorders. Increase fiber intake gradually while drinking plenty of fluids; children and the elderly with small appetites should take care that their energy needs are still met. The DRIs do not contain a UL for fiber.

Quick Bites

Fierce Fiber and Flatulence

The Jerusalem artichoke surpasses even dry beans in its capacity for facilitating flatulence. This artichoke contains large amounts of nondigestible carbohydrate. After passing through the small intestine undigested, the fiber is attacked by gas-generating bacteria in the colon.

Label [to] Table

This label highlights all the carbohydrate-related information you can find on a food label. Look at the center of the Nutrition Facts label and you'll see the Total Carbohydrates along with two of the carbohydrate "subgroups": Dietary Fiber and Sugars. Recall that carbohydrates are classified into simple carbohydrates and the two complex carbohydrates starch and fiber.

Using this food label you can determine all three of these components. There are 19 total grams of carbohydrate with 14 grams coming from sugars and 0 grams from fiber. This means the remaining 5 grams must be from starch, which is not required to be listed separately on the label. Without even knowing what food this label represents, you can decipher that it contains a high proportion of sugar (14 of the 19 grams) and is probably sweet. If this is a fruit juice, that level of sugar would be expected; but if this is cereal, you'd be getting a lot more sugar than complex carbohydrates, and probably not be making the best choice!

Do you see the 6% listed to the right of "Total Carbohydrates"? This doesn't mean that the food item contains 6% of its calories from carbohydrate. Instead, it refers to the daily allotment (or Daily Value) of carbohydrates listed at the bottom of the label. There you can see that a person consuming 2,000 kcalories per day should consume 300 grams of carbohydrates each day. This product contributes 19 grams per serving, which is just 6% of the Daily Value of 300 grams per day. Note that the % Daily Value for fiber is 0% because this food item lacks fiber.

The last highlighted section on this label, at the bottom of some Nutrition Facts labels, is the number of calories in a gram of carbohydrate. Recall that carbohydrates contain 4 kilocalories per gram. Armed with this information and the product's calorie information, can you calculate the percentage of calories that come from carbohydrate?

Here's how:

$$19 \text{ g carbohydrate} \times 4 \text{ kcal per g} = 76 \text{ carbohydrate kcal}$$

$$76 \text{ carbohydrate kcal} \div 154 \text{ total kcal} = 0.49 \text{ or } 49\% \text{ carbohydrate kcal}$$

Nutrition Facts

Serving Size: 1 cup (248g)
Servings Per Container: 4

Amount Per Serving

Calories 154 Calories from fat 35

	% Daily Value*
Total Fat 4g	6%
Saturated Fat 2.5g	12%
Trans Fat 0.5g	
Cholesterol 20mg	7%
Sodium 170mg	7%
Total Carbohydrate 19g	6%
Dietary Fiber 0g	0%
Sugars 14g	
Protein 11g	

Vitamin A 4%	•	Vitamin C 6%	
Calcium 40%	•	Iron 0%	

* Percent Daily Values are based on a 2,000 calorie diet. Your daily values may be higher or lower depending on your calorie needs:

		Calories:	2,000	2,500
Total Fat	Less Than		65g	80g
Sat Fat	Less Than		20g	25g
Cholesterol	Less Than		300mg	300mg
Sodium	Less Than		2,400mg	2,400mg
Total Carbohydrate			300g	375g
Dietary Fiber			25g	30g

Calories per gram:
Fat 9 • Carbohydrate 4 • Protein 4

The **Learning Portfolio** at the end of each chapter collects, in one place, all aspects of nutrition information students need to solidify their understanding of the material. The various formats will appeal to students according to their individual learning and studying styles.

Key Terms lists all new vocabulary alphabetically with the page number of the first appearance. This arrangement allows students to review any term they do not recall and turn immediately to the definition and discussion of it in the chapter. This approach also promotes the acquisition of knowledge, not simply memorization.

Study Points is a bulleted list that summarizes the content of each chapter with a synopsis of each major topic. The points are in the order in which they appear in the chapter, so related concepts flow together.

LEARNING *Portfolio*

LEARNING PORTFOLIO **27**

c h a p t e r **1**

Key **Terms**

	page
amino acids	14
antioxidant	13
calorie	16
carbohydrate	14
case control study	19
circulation	14
clinical trials	19
control group	19
correlations	19
double-blind study	19
energy	21
epidemiology	16
essential nutrients	18
experimental group	11
experiments	19
flavor	19
hormones	5
hypotheses	14
inorganic	18
kilocalories (kcal) [KILL-oh-kal-oh-rees]	13
legumes	16
lipids	14
	14

	page
macrominerals	15
macronutrients	13
microminerals	15
micronutrients	13
minerals	15
neophobia	4
nutrients	11
nutrigenomics	19
nutrition	4
organic	13
peer review	23
phytochemicals	13
pica	7
placebo	20
placebo effect	21
proteins	14
social facilitation	8
trace minerals	15
triglycerides	14
umami [ooh-MA-mee]	5
vitamins	14

Study **Points**

➤ Most people make food choices for reasons other than nutrient value.

➤ Taste and texture are the two most important factors that influence food choices.

➤ In all cultures, eating is the primary way of maintaining social relationships.

➤ Although Americans know about healthful food choices, their eating habits do not always reflect this knowledge.

➤ Food is a mixture of chemicals. Essential chemicals in food are called nutrients.

➤ Carbohydrates, lipids, proteins, vitamins, minerals, and water are the six classes of nutrients found in food.

➤ Nutrients have three general functions in the body: They serve as energy sources, structural components, and regulators of metabolic processes.

➤ Vitamins regulate body processes such as energy metabolism, blood clotting, and calcium balance.

➤ Minerals contribute to body structures and to regulating processes such as fluid balance.

➤ Water is the most important nutrient in the body. We can survive much longer without the other nutrients than we can without water.

➤ Energy in foods and the body is measured in kilocalories. Carbohydrates, fats, and proteins are sources of energy.

➤ Carbohydrate and protein have a potential energy value of 4 kilocalories per gram, and fat provides 9 kilocalories per gram.

➤ Scientific studies are the cornerstone of nutrition. The scientific method uses observation and inquiry to test hypotheses.

➤ Research designs used to test hypotheses include epidemiological, animal, cell culture, and human studies.

➤ Double-blind, placebo-controlled clinical trials are considered the "gold standard" of nutrition studies.

➤ Information in the public media is not always an accurate or complete representation of the current state of the science on a particular topic.

Study Questions encourage students to probe deeper into the chapter content, making connections and gaining new insights. Although these questions can be used for pop quizzes, they will also help students to review, especially students who study by writing out material. They can check their work by looking at the **Answers to Study Questions** included in the back of the book and on the *Nutrition* Web site http://nutrition.jbpub.com.

What About Bobbie? tracks the eating habits and health-related decisions of a typical college student so that students can apply the material they have learned in the chapter to a typical situation. Following the individual case of Bobbie takes students from the general concepts to the specific application of new information. As a complement to this textual feature, the Nutritionist Pro or EatRight Analysis software programs allow students to track the various choices Bobbie makes, as well as their own food choices.

Try This activities are for curious students who like to experiment. These suggestions for hands-on activities encourage students to put theory into practice. It will especially help students whose major learning style is experimental.

The **Learning Portfolio** (continued)

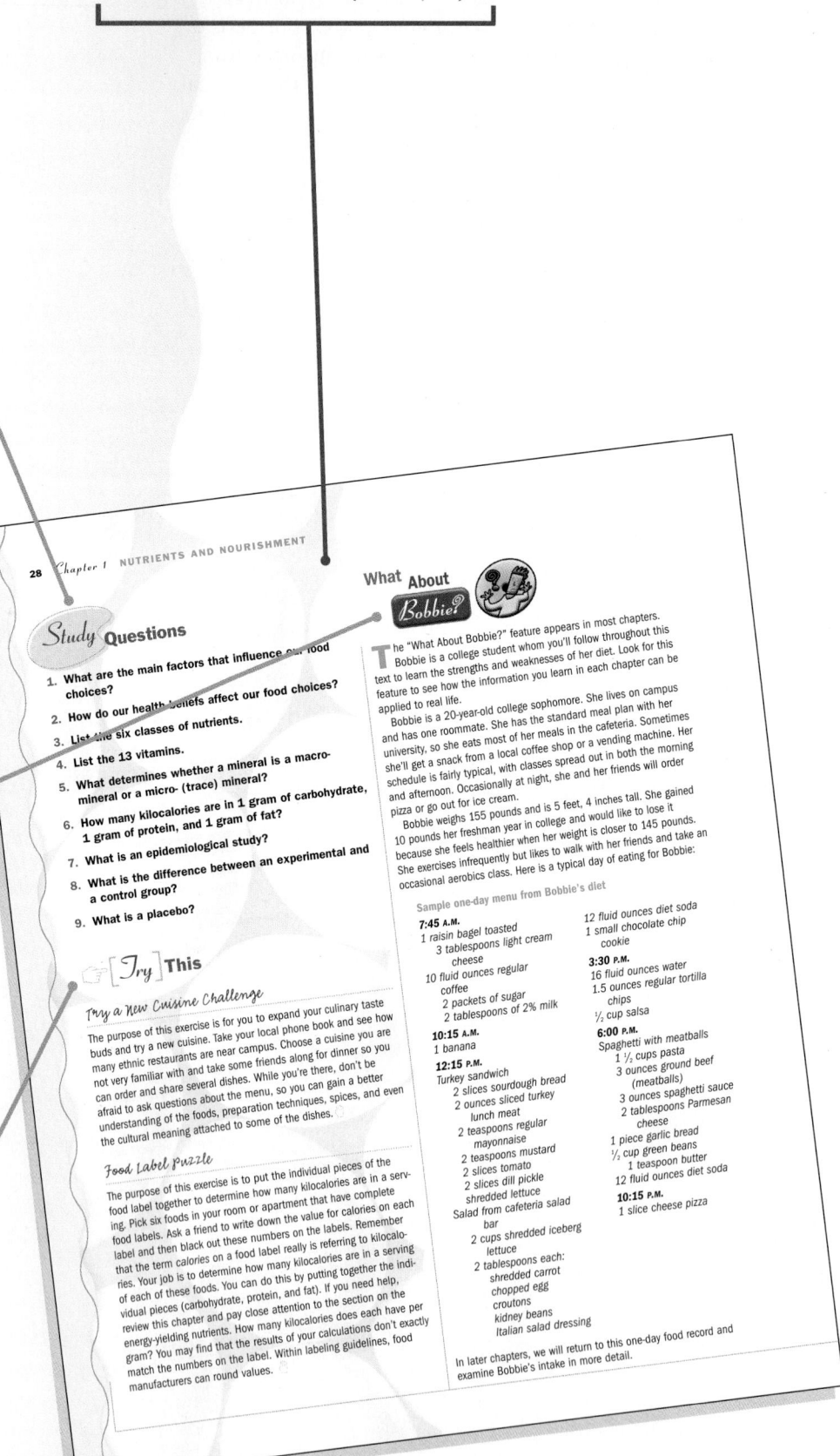

28 *Chapter 1* NUTRIENTS AND NOURISHMENT

Study **Questions**

1. What are the main factors that influence our food choices?
2. How do our health beliefs affect our food choices?
3. List the six classes of nutrients.
4. List the 13 vitamins.
5. What determines whether a mineral is a macro-mineral or a micro- (trace) mineral?
6. How many kilocalories are in 1 gram of carbohydrate, 1 gram of protein, and 1 gram of fat?
7. What is an epidemiological study?
8. What is the difference between an experimental and a control group?
9. What is a placebo?

Try **This**

Try a New Cuisine Challenge

The purpose of this exercise is for you to expand your culinary taste buds and try a new cuisine. Take your local phone book and see how many ethnic restaurants are near campus. Choose a cuisine you are not very familiar with and take some friends along for dinner so you can order and share several dishes. While you're there, don't be afraid to ask questions about the menu, preparation techniques, spices, and even the cultural meaning attached to some of the dishes.

Food Label Puzzle

The purpose of this exercise is to put the individual pieces of the food label together to determine how many kilocalories are in a serving. Pick six foods in your room or apartment that have complete food labels. Ask a friend to write down the value for calories on each label and then black out these numbers on the labels. Remember that the term calories on a food label really is referring to kilocalories. Your job is to determine how many kilocalories are in a serving of each of these foods. You can do this by putting together the individual pieces (carbohydrate, protein, and fat). If you need help, review this chapter and pay close attention to the section on energy-yielding nutrients. How many kilocalories does each have per gram? You may find that the results of your calculations don't exactly match the numbers on the label. Within labeling guidelines, food manufacturers can round values.

What About Bobbie?

The "What About Bobbie?" feature appears in most chapters. Bobbie is a college student whom you'll follow throughout this text to learn the strengths and weaknesses of her diet. Look for this feature to see how the information you learn in each chapter can be applied to real life.

Bobbie is a 20-year-old college sophomore. She lives on campus and has one roommate. She has the standard meal plan with her university, so she eats most of her meals in the cafeteria. Sometimes she'll get a snack from a local coffee shop or a vending machine. Her schedule is fairly typical, with classes spread out in both the morning and afternoon. Occasionally at night, she and her friends will order pizza or go out for ice cream.

Bobbie weighs 155 pounds and is 5 feet, 4 inches tall. She gained 10 pounds her freshman year in college and would like to lose it because she feels healthier when her weight is closer to 145 pounds. She exercises infrequently but likes to walk with her friends and take an occasional aerobics class. Here is a typical day of eating for Bobbie:

Sample one-day menu from Bobbie's diet

7:45 A.M.
1 raisin bagel toasted
3 tablespoons light cream cheese
10 fluid ounces regular coffee
2 packets of sugar
2 tablespoons of 2% milk

10:15 A.M.
1 banana

12:15 P.M.
Turkey sandwich
2 slices sourdough bread
2 ounces sliced turkey lunch meat
2 teaspoons regular mayonnaise
2 teaspoons mustard
2 slices tomato
2 slices dill pickle
shredded lettuce
Salad from cafeteria salad bar
2 cups shredded iceberg lettuce
2 tablespoons each:
shredded carrot
chopped egg
croutons
kidney beans
Italian salad dressing

12 fluid ounces diet soda
1 small chocolate chip cookie

3:30 P.M.
16 fluid ounces water
1.5 ounces regular tortilla chips
½ cup salsa

6:00 P.M.
Spaghetti with meatballs
1 ½ cups pasta
3 ounces ground beef (meatballs)
3 ounces spaghetti sauce
2 tablespoons Parmesan cheese
1 piece garlic bread
½ cup green beans
1 teaspoon butter
12 fluid ounces diet soda

10:15 P.M.
1 slice cheese pizza

In later chapters, we will return to this one-day food record and examine Bobbie's intake in more detail.

The Integrated Learning and Teaching Package

Integrating the text and ancillaries is crucial to deriving their full benefit. Based on feedback from instructors and students, Jones and Bartlett Publishers offers the following supplements.

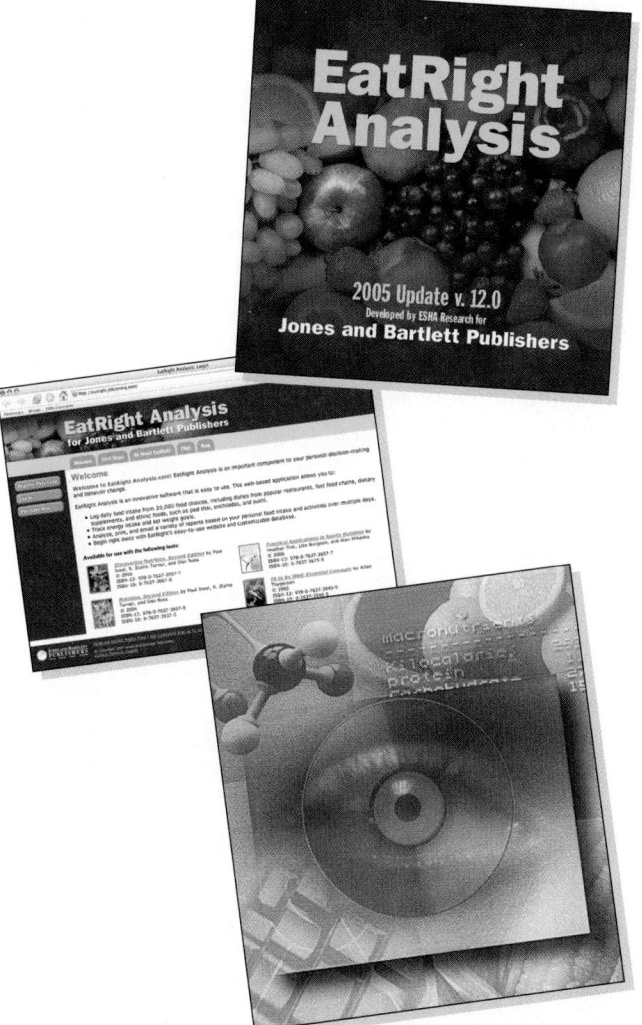

Contact your Publisher's Representative for discount package opportunities.

Diet analysis software is an important component of the behavioral change and personal decision-making focus of a nutrition course. Both **EatRight Analysis**, developed by ESHA Research, and **Nutritionist Pro**, created by Axxya Systems, provide software that enables students to analyze their diets by calculating their nutrient intake and comparing it to recommended intake levels. EatRight Analysis offers dietary software on CD-ROM and online at http://EatRight.jbpub.com. With this new online tool, you and your students can access personal records from any computer with Internet access. Through a variety of reports, students learn to make better choices regarding their diet and activity habits.

The **Instructor's ToolKit CD-ROM** is a comprehensive teaching resource available to adopters of the book. It includes:

- PowerPoint Lecture Presentation Slides
- Image Bank: Provides art that can be imported into PowerPoints, tests, or used to create transparencies
- Instructor's Manual: Includes chapter outlines and strategies for teaching difficult concepts
- Computerized TestBank
- Table Bank: Provides tables that can be imported into PowerPoints, tests, or used to create transparencies

The resources on the Instructor's ToolKit CD-ROM have been formatted so that instructors can integrate them into many popular online course management systems. Consult the CD-ROM packaging booklet for more information on this feature. Please feel free to contact Jones and Bartlett technical support with questions.

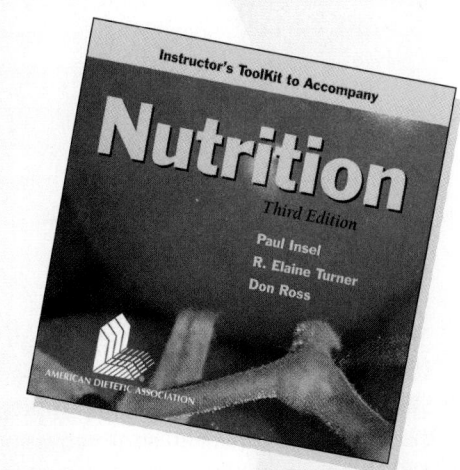

Contact your Publisher's Representative at **http://health.jbpub.com**.

The **Instructor's Manual** is a comprehensive teaching resource available to adopters of the book. It includes chapter outlines, strategies for teaching difficult concepts, and a Test Bank.

Contact your Publisher's Representative at **http://health.jbpub.com**.

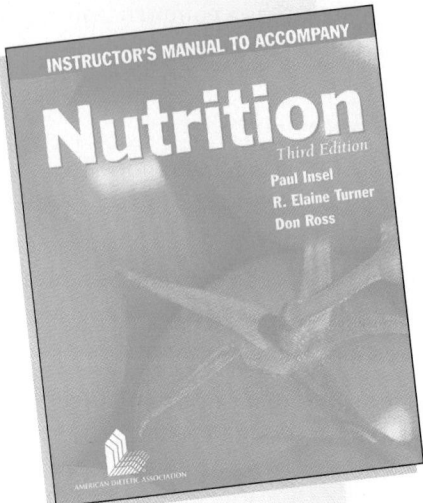

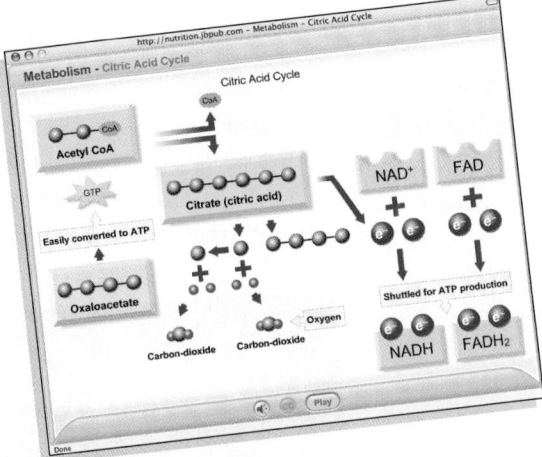

Nutrition Science Animations   These new scientifically based animations give nutrition students an accurate, accessible explanation of the major scientific concepts and physiological principles presented in *Nutrition*. More than thirty of the most difficult processes are graphically presented in an interactive, easy-to-understand format. These Nutrition Science Animations, available at http://nutrition.jbpub .com/animations, complement online courses, classroom lectures, and independent studying. Access is free and does not require a password. The Nutrition Science Animations are also available on CD-ROM (ISBN-13: 978-0-7637-4497-7 / ISBN-10: 0-7637-4497-2).

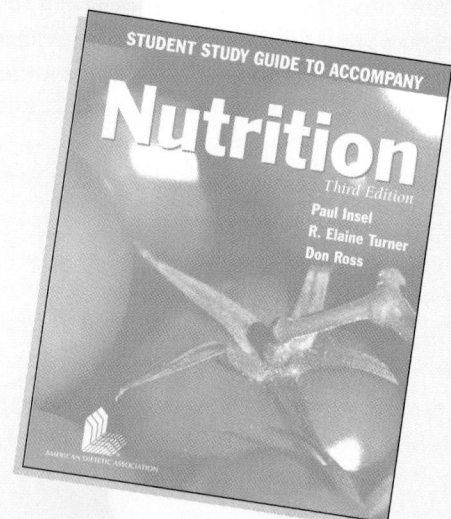

Contact your Publisher's Representative for discount package opportunities.

The **Student Study Guide to Accompany Nutrition** provides a powerful learning tool to students using *Nutrition*. The Student Study Guide follows the chapter topics and offers fill-in-the-blank questions and summaries so that students can test themselves. Also included are exercises for students to gain familiarity with the key terms in each chapter and tips for making assessments of their own dietary habits. The Student Study Guide is available with every new text at no additional cost to your students.

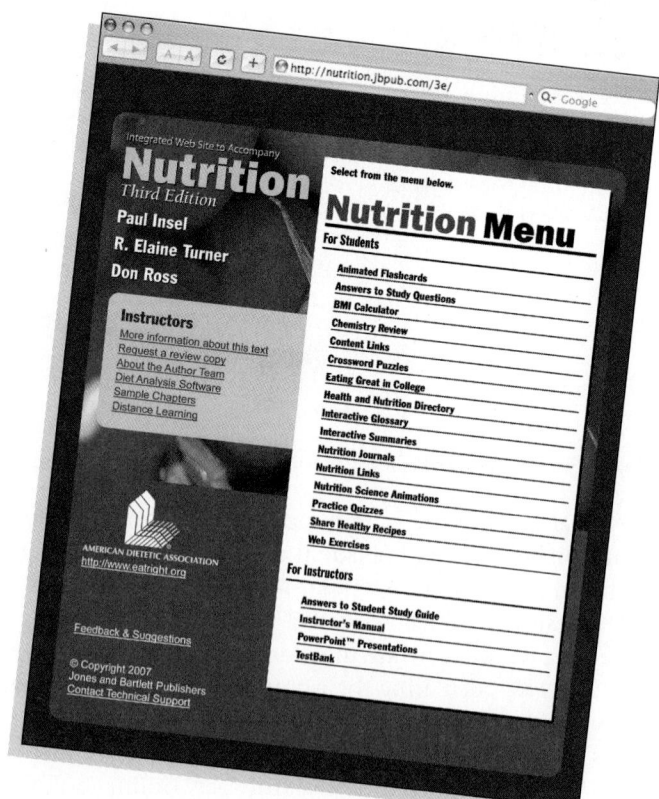

The **Web site** for *Nutrition*, **http://nutrition.jbpub.com**, offers students and instructors an unprecedented degree of integration between the text and the online world through many useful study tools, activities, and supplementary health information.

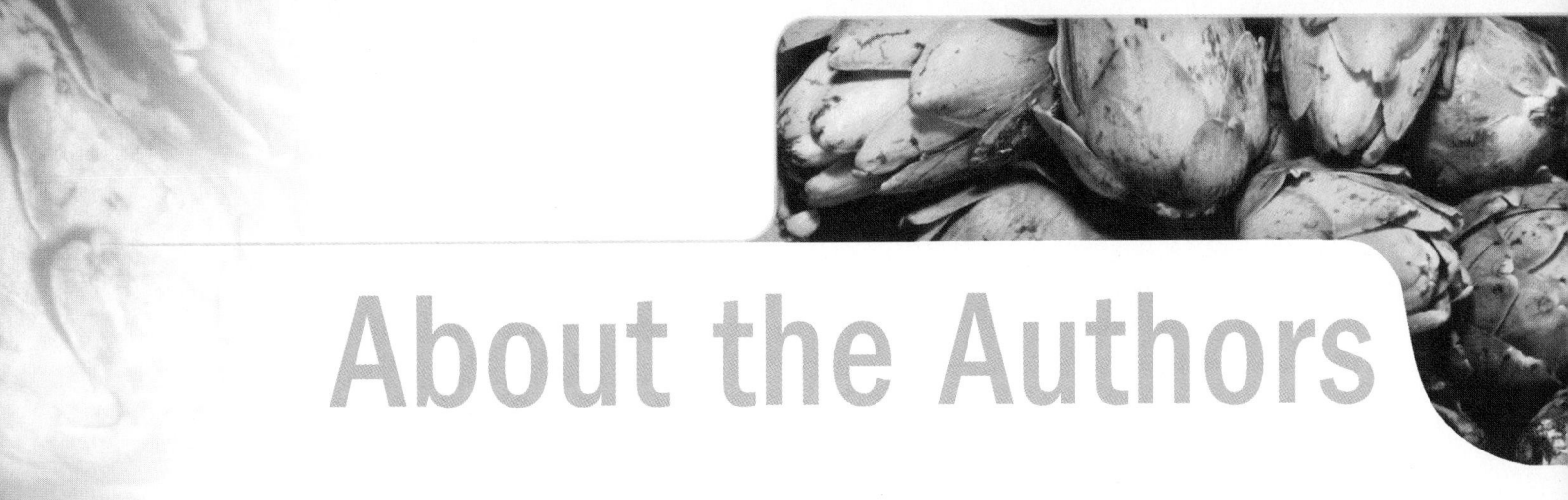

About the Authors

The *Nutrition* author team represents a culmination of years of teaching and research in psychology and nutrition science. The combined experience of the authors yields a balanced presentation of both the science of nutrition and the components of behavioral change.

Dr. Paul Insel is Adjunct Clinical Associate Professor of Psychiatry and Behavioral Sciences at Stanford University (Stanford, California). In addition to being the principal investigator on several nutrition projects for the National Institutes of Health (NIH), he is the senior author of the seminal text in health education and has co-authored several best-selling nutrition books.

Dr. R. Elaine Turner is a Registered Dietitian, Associate Professor in the Food Science and Human Nutrition Department, and Associate Dean for the College of Agricultural and Life Sciences at the University of Florida (Gainesville, Florida). Dr. Turner has been teaching courses in introductory and life-cycle nutrition for more than 20 years. Her interests include nutrition labeling and dietary supplement regulations, computer applications in nutrition and education, maternal and infant nutrition, and consumer issues. Dr. Turner was named Undergraduate Teacher of the Year, 2000–2001, for the College of Agricultural and Life Sciences, and in 2004, was recognized with a National Award for Excellence in College and University Teaching in the Food and Agricultural Sciences by the USDA.

Don Ross is director of the California Institute of Human Nutrition (Redwood City, California). For more than 20 years he has co-authored multiple textbooks and created educational materials about health and nutrition for consumers, professionals, and college students. He has special expertise in communicating complicated physiological processes with easily understood graphical presentations. The National Institutes of Health selected his Travels with Cholesterol for distribution to consumers. His multi-disciplinary focus brings together the fields of psychology, nutrition, biochemistry, biology, and medicine.

Contributors

The following people contributed to this project:

Janine T. Baer, PhD, RD
University of Dayton
Chapter 13 Sports Nutrition
Chapter 15 Life Cycle: Maternal and Infant Nutrition

Toni Bloom, MS, RD, CDE
San Jose State University
Pedagogy

Boyce W. Burge, PhD
California Institute of Human Nutrition
Chapter 17 Food Safety and Technology

Eileen G. Ford, MS, RD
Drexel University
Chapter 15 Life Cycle: Maternal and Infant Nutrition

Ellen B. Fung, PhD, RD
University of Pennsylvania
Chapter 12 Trace Minerals

Michael I. Goran, PhD
University of Southern California
Chapter 8 Energy Balance, Body Composition, and
Weight Management

Nancy J. Gustafson, MS, RD, FADA
Director, Sawyer County Aging Unit, WI
Chapter 4 Carbohydrates
Chapter 6 Proteins and Amino Acids

Rita H. Herskovitz, MS
University of Pennsylvania
Chapter 12 Trace Minerals

Nancy I. Kemp, MD
University of California, San Francisco
Chapter 11 Water and Major Minerals

Sarah Harding Laidlaw, MS, RD, MPA
Editor, Nutrition in Complementary Care, *DPG 18*
Chapter 16 Life Cycle: From Childhood through
Adulthood

Rick D. Mattes, MPH, PhD, RD
Purdue University
Chapter 1 Nutrients and Nourishment

Maye Musk, MS, RD
Past President of the Consulting Dietitians of Canada
Chapter 18 World View of Nutrition

Joyce D. Nash, PhD
Chapter 8 Energy Balance, Body Composition, and
Weight Management

Rachel Stern, MS, RD, CNS
North Jersey Community Research Initiative
Chapter 5 Lipids
Spotlight on Alcohol
Chapter 18 World View of Nutrition

Lisa Stollman, MA, RD, CDE, CDN
State University of New York, Stony Brook
Chapter 3 Digestion and Absorption

Barbara Sutherland, PhD
University of California, Davis
Chapter 7 Metabolism

Debra M. Vinci, PhD, RD, CD
Appalachian State University
Chapter 13 Sports Nutrition

Stella L. Volpe, PhD, RD, FACSM
University of Massachusetts
Chapter 8 Energy Balance, Body Composition, and
Weight Management

The authors also would like to acknowledge the valuable
contributions of:

C.J. Nieves
Coordinator of Nutrition Education Programs
University of Florida

Reviewers

Namanjeet Ahluwalia, PhD
Pennsylvania State University

Nancy K. Amy, PhD
University of California-Berkeley

R. James Barnard, PhD
University of California, Los Angeles

Susan I. Barr, PhD, RDN
University of British Columbia

Richard C. Baybutt, PhD
Kansas State University

Beverly A. Benes, PhD, RD
University of Nebraska-Lincoln

Marion Birdsall, PhD, RD
University of Pennsylvania

Melanie Tracy Burns, PhD, RD
Eastern Illinois University

N. Joanne Caid, PhD
California State University, Fresno

Beverly E. Conway, MS
Williston State College

Jane B. Dennis, PhD, RD
Tarleton State University

Holly A. Dieken, PhD, MS, BS, RD
University of Tennessee-Chattanooga

Betty J. Forbes, RD, LD
West Virginia University

Debra K. Goodwin, PhD, RD
Jacksonville State University

Margaret Gunther, PhD
Palomar Community College

Shelley R. Hancock, MS, RD, LD
University of Alabama

Donna V. Handley, MS, RD
University of Rhode Island

Jeffrey Harris, DrPH, MPH, CNS, RD
West Chester University

Nancy Gordon Harris, MS, RD, LDN
East Carolina University

Diana Himmel, RDH, MS
Tunxis Community College

Michael Jenkins
Kent State University

Simon Jenkins, DPhil
University of Bath

Mary Beth Kavanagh MS, RD, LD
Case Western Reserve University

Zaheer Ali Kirmani, PhD, RD, LD
Sam Houston State University

Anda Lam, MS, RD
Pasadena City College

Samantha R. Logan, DrPH, RD
University of Massachusetts

Mary-Pat Maciolek, MBA, RD
Middlesex County College

Patricia Z. Marincic, PhD, RD, LD, CLE
College of Saint Benedict/Saint John's University

Melissa J. Martilotta, MS, RD
Pennsylvania State University

Keith R. Martin, PhD
Pennsylvania State University

Glen F. McNeil, MS, RD/LD
Fort Hays State University

Mark S. Meskin, PhD, RD
California State Polytechnic University-Pomona

Kristin Moline MS, Ed.
Lourdes College

Katherine O. Musgrave, MS, RD, CAS
University of Maine-Orono

Deborah Myers, MS, RD, LD
Bluffton University

J. Dirk Nelson, PhD
Missouri Southern State College

Anne O'Donnell, MS, MPH, RD
Santa Rosa Junior College

Rebecca S. Pobocik, PhD, RD
Bowling Green State University

Alayne Ronnenberg, ScD
University of Massachusetts Amherst

Susan T. Saylor, RD, EdD
Shelton State University

Brian Luke Seaward, PhD
Paramount Wellness Institute

Mohammad R. Shayesteh, PhD, RD, LD
Youngstown State University

LuAnn Soliah, PhD, RD
Baylor University

Bernice Gales Spurlock, PhD
Hinds Community College

James H. Swain, PhD, RD, LD
Case Western Reserve University

Joy E. Swanson, PhD
Cornell University

Priya Venkatesan MS, RD, CLE
Pasadena City College

Janelle Walter, PhD
Baylor University

Shahla M. Wunderlich, PhD
Montclair State University

Joseph J Zielinski, MPH, RD
SUNY Brockport

Nancy Zwick MED, RD, LD
Northern Kentucky University

Acknowledgments

We would like to thank the following people for their hard work and dedication. They have helped make this new edition a reality. Thank you Cindy Kogut for a thorough and careful copyedit; to Julie Bolduc of Jones and Bartlett for shepherding the manuscript through to completion; and to Denise DeLancey, Chris Lane, and the team at Graphic World for making this book look so great. We would also like to thank Jacqueline Mark-Geraci, Patrice Andrews, Wendy Thayer, Amy Flagg, and Jen Ryan for giving us help and direction when we needed it.

Thanks also to Virginia Bragg of Utah State University, Anda Lam of Pasadena City College, Betty Forbes of West Virginia University, Marion Birdsall of the University of Pennsylvania, Pamela Fletcher of Albuquerque Technical Vocational Institute, Jeffrey Harris of West Chester University, Janet Anderson of Utah State University, and R. James Barnard of the University of California-Los Angeles for their insightful reviews of the previous edition.

Thanks also to Anne Spencer, Philip Regan, Dawn Mahon Priest, and Kristin Ohlin for spending countless hours on the nutrition media packaging.

Finally, the authors would also like to thank Jessica Clines for creating and updating the Student Study Guide, Instructor's Manual, and PowerPoint Presentations and Kristen Carnavale for updating the Web content and TestBank.

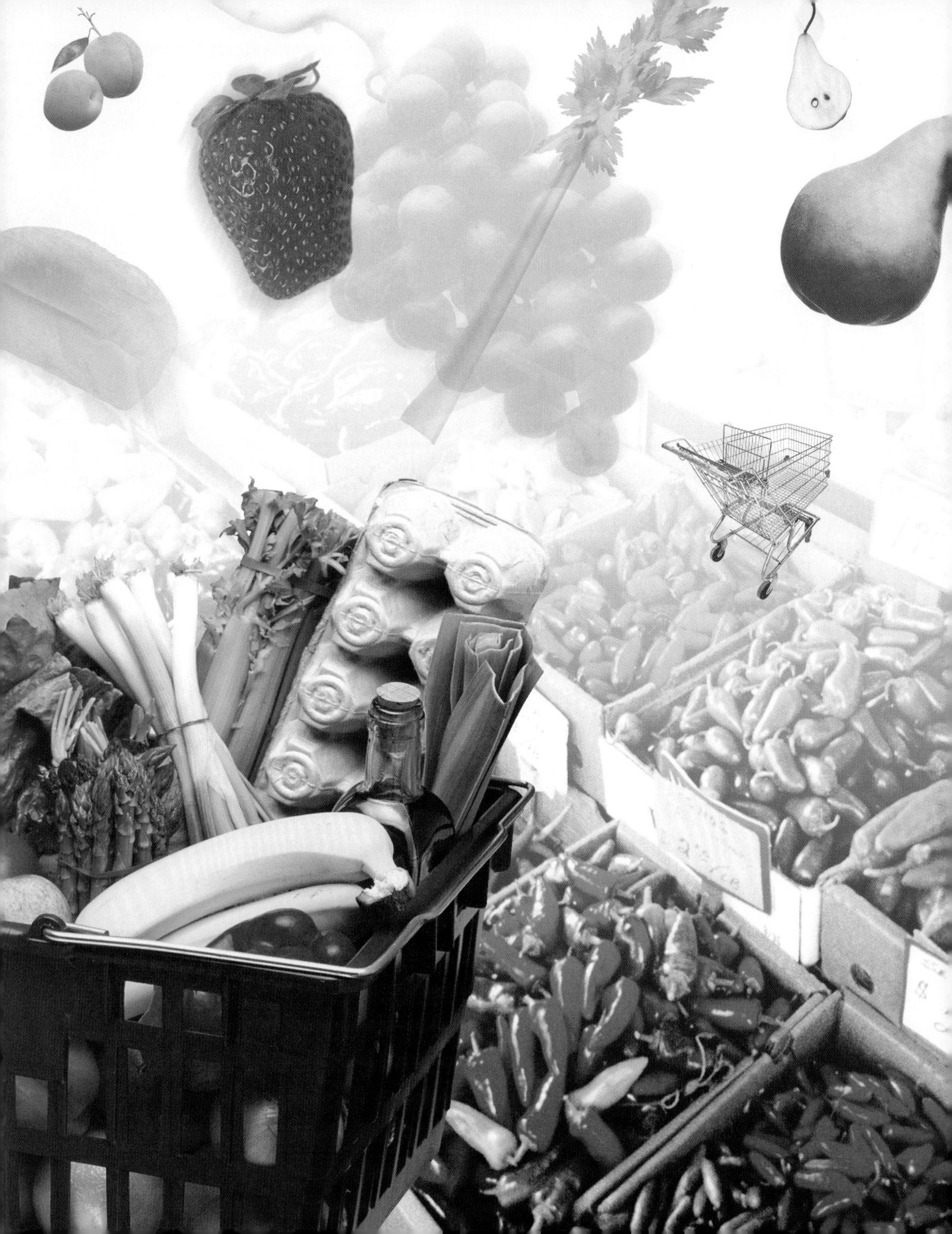

Chapter

Nutrients and Nourishment

Think About It

1 How many different foods have you eaten in the last 24 hours? The last week?

2 Do you have a preference for sweets? Chocolate? Ice cream? If so, where do you think it comes from?

3 What do you think is driving the popularity of vitamins and other supplements?

4 Where do you get the majority of your information about nutrition?

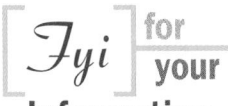

Fyi for your Information

This chapter's FYI boxes include practical information on the following topics:

- Are Nutrigenomics in Your Future?
- Evaluating Information on the Internet

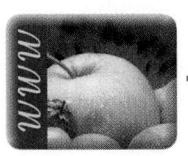

The Web site for this book offers many useful tools and is a great source for additional nutrition information for both students and instructors. For information on nutrients and nourishment, visit the site at **nutrition.jbpub.com**. You'll find exercises that explore the following topics:

- The French Diet (*bon appetit!*)
- Why Are the Jains Vegetarians?
- Taste and Smell Disorders
- What Do You Eat?
- Ethnic Foods

What About Bobbie?

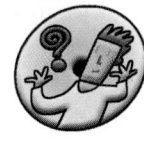

Track the choices Bobbie is making with Nutritionist Pro or EatRight Analysis software.

Key to Illustrations

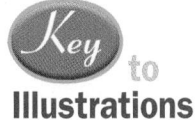 Carbohydrates

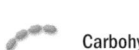 Energy

 Minerals

 Phospholipids

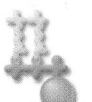 Proteins

 Sterols

 Triglycerides

 Vitamins

 Water

nutrition The science of foods and their components (nutrients and other substances), including the relationships to health and disease (actions, interactions, and balances); processes within the body (ingestion, digestion, absorption, transport, functions, and disposal of end products); and the social, economic, cultural, and psychological implications of eating.

neophobia A dislike for anything new or unfamiliar.

A group of friends goes out for pizza every Thursday night. A college freshman greets his girlfriend with a box of chocolates. A 5-year-old imitates her parents after they salt their food. A firefighter who is asked to explain why hot dogs are his favorite food says it has something to do with going to baseball games with his father. A professor recently recruited from a Chinese university feels dissatisfied unless she eats a bowl of rice daily. A parent punishes a misbehaving child by withholding dessert. What do these people have in common? They are all using food for something other than its nutrient value. Can you think of a holiday that is not celebrated with food? For most of us, food is more than a collection of nutrients. While many of the foods people choose are nourishing and contribute to good health, the same, of course, may be true of the foods we reject.

The science of **nutrition** helps us improve our food choices by identifying the amounts of nutrients we need, the best food sources of those nutrients, and the other components in foods that may be helpful or harmful. Learning about nutrition will help us make better choices and not only improve our health but also reduce our risk of disease and increase our longevity. Keep in mind, though, that no matter how much you know about nutrition, you are still likely to choose some foods simply for their taste or just because they make you feel good.

Why Do We Eat the Way We Do?

Do you "eat to live" or "live to eat"? For most of us, the first is certainly true—you *must* eat to live. But there may be times when our *enjoyment* of food is more important to us than the nourishment we get from it. Factors such as age, sex, genetic makeup, occupation, lifestyle, and family and cultural background affect our daily food choices. We use food to project a desired image, forge relationships, express friendship, show creativity, and disclose our feelings. We cope with anxiety or stress by eating or not eating; we reward ourselves with food for a good grade or a job well done; or, in extreme cases, we punish failures by denying ourselves the benefit and comfort of eating.

Food preferences begin early in life and then change as we interact with parents, friends, and peers. Further experiences with different people, places, and situations often—but not always—cause us to expand or change our preferences. Taste and texture are the two most important things that influence our food choices; next are cost and convenience.[1] What we eat reveals much about who we are.

Age is a factor in food preferences. Young children prefer sweet or familiar foods; babies and toddlers are generally willing to try new things. (See **Figure 1.1**.) Experimental evidence suggests infants exposed to a variety of flavors are even more likely to accept novel foods.[2] Preschoolers typically go through a period of food **neophobia** (a dislike for anything new or unfamiliar), school-aged children tend to accept a wider array of foods, and teenagers are strongly influenced by the preferences and habits of their

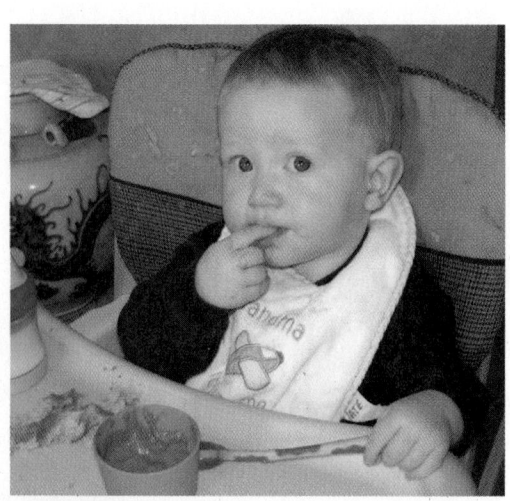

Figure 1.1 **Adventures in eating.** Babies and toddlers are generally willing to try new things.

peers. If you track the kinds of foods you have eaten in the past year, you might be surprised to discover how few basic foods your diet includes. By the time we reach adulthood, we have formed a core group of foods we prefer. Of this group, only about 100 basic items account for 75 percent of our food intake.

Like many aspects of human behavior, food choices are influenced by both inborn (biological) and environmental factors, and it's not always easy to separate them. However, we can look at food preferences in terms of the sensory properties of foods, cognitive factors that influence our choices, and environmental influences such as culture. Exploring each of these areas may help you understand why you prefer certain foods. (See **Figure 1.2**.)

Sensory Influences: Taste, Texture, and Smell

In making food choices, we are drawn to what appeals to our senses. People often refer to **flavor** as a collective experience that describes both taste and smell. Texture is also part of the picture.[3] You may prefer foods that have a crisp, chewy, or smooth texture. You may reject foods that feel grainy, slimy, or rubbery. Other sensory characteristics that affect food choice are color, moisture, and temperature.

We are familiar with the classic four tastes—sweet, sour, bitter, and salty—but studies show that there are more. One of these additional taste sensations is **umami**, which is a Japanese term for the taste produced by glutamate.[4] Glutamate is an amino acid (a building block of protein) that is found in monosodium glutamate (MSG). It gives food a distinctive meaty or savory taste. The way we experience different tastes can be affected by our genetic makeup. Researchers have identified a single gene that determines whether a person can taste a certain intensely bitter substance. This may help explain why some people love broccoli but others cannot bear the bitter taste.[5] (See Chapter 3, "Digestion and Absorption," for more information about taste and smell.)

flavor The collective experience that describes both taste and smell.

umami [ooh-MA-mee] A Japanese term that describes a delicious meaty or savory sensation. Chemically, this taste detects the presence of glutamate.

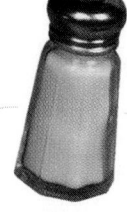

Quick Bites

Sweetness and Salt

*S*alt can do more than just make your food taste salty. Researchers at the Monell Chemical Senses Center demonstrated that salt also suppresses the bitter flavors in foods. When combined with chocolate, in a chocolate-covered pretzel, for example, salt blocks some of the bitter flavor, making the chocolate taste sweeter. This may explain why people in many cultures salt their fruit.

Environmental	Sensory	Cognitive
economic	flavor (taste and smell)	learned food habits
environment	texture	social factors
lifestyle	appearance	emotional needs
cultural beliefs and traditions		nutrition and health beliefs
religious beliefs and traditions		advertising

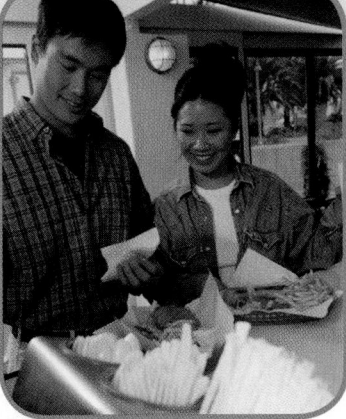

Health Status	Genetics
physical restrictions due to disease	taste sensitivity
declining taste sensitivity	preference for sweets
age and gender	avoidance of bitter
	possible "fat tooth"

Figure 1.2 **Factors that affect food choices.** We often select a food to eat automatically, without thought. But in fact, our choices are complex events involving the interactions of a multitude of factors.

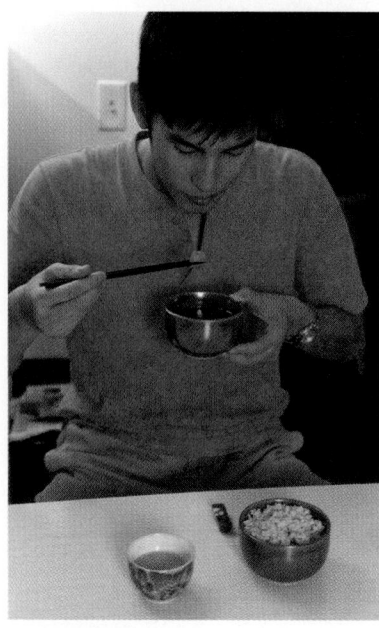 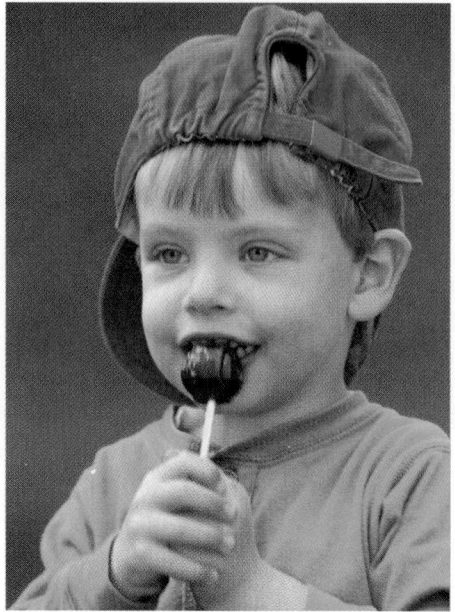 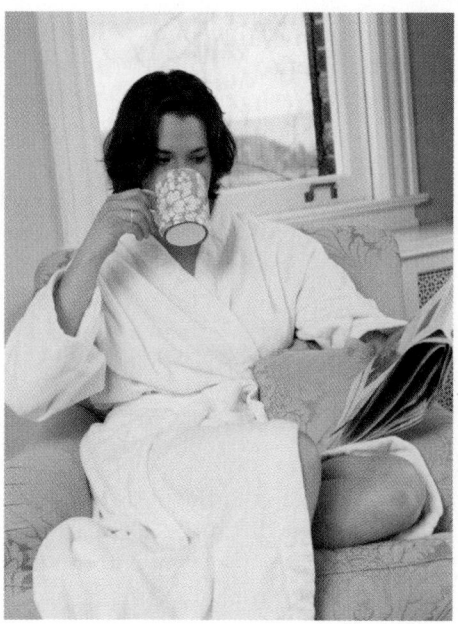

Figure 1.3 **Comfort foods.** Depending on your childhood food experiences, a bowl of traditional soup, a remembered sweet, or a mug of hot chocolate can provide comfort in times of stress.

Cognitive Influences

Along with our experiences, our thoughts and feelings about food influence decisions about what to eat and when. We call these factors *cognitive* influences because they affect our thinking and the decisions we make. Cognitive influences can affect many of our food habits, including eating routines, choices of comfort food, food avoidance and cravings, food buying behavior, and nutrition beliefs.

Day-to-Day Influences on Food Choices: Habits

Your eating and cooking habits are likely to reflect what you learned from your parents. We typically learn to eat three meals a day, at about the same times each day. Quite often we eat the same foods, particularly for breakfast (e.g., cereal and milk) and lunch (e.g., sandwiches). This routine makes life convenient, and we don't have to think much about when or what to eat. But we don't have to follow this routine! How would you feel about eating mashed potatoes for breakfast and cereal for dinner? Some people might get a stomachache just thinking about it, while others might enjoy the prospect of doing things differently. Look at your eating habits and see how often you make the same choices every single day.

Comfort and Discomfort Foods

Our desire for particular foods is often based on behavioral motives, even though we are not always aware of them. For some people, food becomes an emotional security blanket. Consuming our favorite foods can make us feel better, relieve stress, and allay anxiety. (See **Figure 1.3**.) Starting with the first days of life, food and affection are intertwined. Infants experience both physical and psychological satisfaction when eating. As we grow older, this experience is continually reinforced. For example, chicken soup and hot tea with honey are favorites when we feel under the weather because Mom and Dad fixed them especially for us. If we were rewarded for good behavior with a particular food (e.g., ice cream, candy, cookies), our positive feelings about that food may persist for a lifetime. The foods that we

---

Quick Bites

What Is an Ice Cream Headache?

After ingesting a cold substance quickly, such as when you take a big bite of ice cream, you may experience what is commonly known as an ice cream headache, or brain freeze. When cold substances touch the back part of the palate, blood vessels, including those that go to the brain, constrict (tighten), resulting in a sharp pain in the mid-frontal part of the brain. About one-third of the population experience this phenomenon.

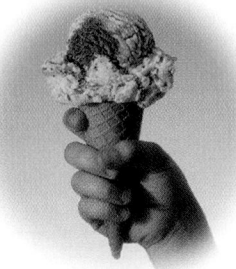

associate with positive childhood experiences often continue to generate secure and supportive feelings.

On the other hand, children who have negative associations with certain foods are unlikely to choose those foods as adults. Maybe you avoid a certain food because you *know* it will make you sick. Chances are that at some point in your childhood, you got sick soon after eating that food, and consequently the two events are linked forever. Repeated power struggles with your parents over a helping of broccoli or zucchini may have turned you away from eating those vegetables. Fortunately, these behaviors can be reversed. Psychologists have shown us that negative associations are easier to extinguish than positive ones. Thus, time and the knowledge that vegetables are beneficial may help us overcome negative associations.

Food Cravings

Chocolates for breakfast? Only if you are one of those people who can't survive more than one waking hour without a chocolate rush. Is the intense desire or craving for a particular food psychological or physiological? It's likely to be both, and these factors may interact to increase the intensity of the desire. Add ice cream to chocolate and you have the top two candidates on the food craver's agenda. The use of chocolate and ice cream as rewards in early childhood often sets the stage for later cravings.

Some people offer a nutritional explanation for food cravings: The body senses a nutrient deficit that triggers the desire for a food rich in that nutrient. Some claim that the practice of eating nonfood items such as dirt, clay, and laundry starch results from nutrient deficits. The craving for and consumption of such substances is called **pica** and is often associated with pregnancy. It has been suggested that iron deficiency drives the pregnant woman's craving so she seeks iron in any form. In some groups, family traditions and cultural acceptance of pica have made it an expected behavior during pregnancy. Although research has shown an association between lowered iron status and pica,[6] it has not shown conclusively whether pica is a cause or an effect of iron deficiency.[7]

Advertising and Promotion

It may not surprise you that some of the most popular food products are high-fat and high-sugar baked goods and alcoholic beverages. Aggressive and sometimes deceptive advertising programs can influence people to buy foods of poor nutritional quality. On the other hand, we are seeing more innovative and aggressive advertising from the commodity boards that promote milk, meat, cranberries, and other more nutrient-dense products.

Consumers make an estimated 70 percent of their food purchase decisions while shopping rather than before arriving at the market. Accurate nutritional information in the supermarket aisles can improve food choices.[8] Advertising like that in **Figure 1.4**, for example, can be helpful, especially to consumers whose diets need improvement. In the mid-1980s, Kellogg's launched a print and television ad campaign for All-Bran cereal to suggest that a high-fiber diet would reduce the risk of cancer. Not only did sales of All-Bran increase dramatically in the months that followed, but so did the sales of all high-fiber cereals.[9] When the oat bran craze first hit in the late 1980s, sales of oat bran products by the Quaker Oats Company increased 700 percent in one year.

The popularity of different diets drives changes in food products. Beginning in the late 1980s, low-fat diets became popular and were accompanied by an

pica The craving for and consumption of nonfood items like dirt, clay, or laundry starch.

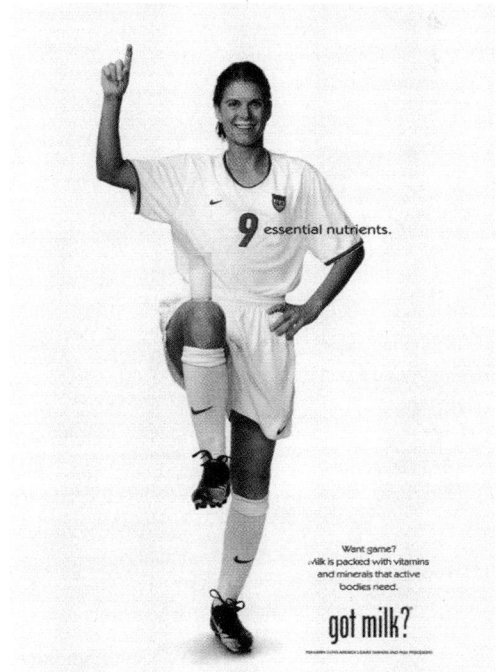

Figure 1.4 **Healthy advertising.** Got milk? is an example of a successful healthy advertising campaign.

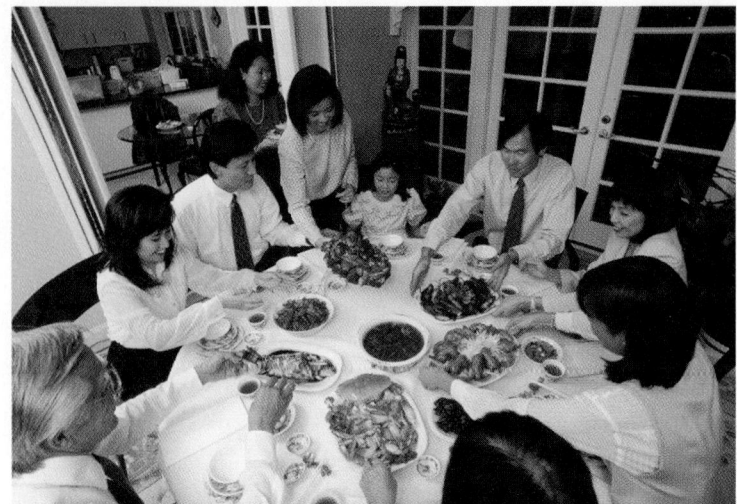

Figure 1.5 **Social facilitation.** Interactions with others can affect your eating behavior.

social facilitation Encouragement of the interactions between people.

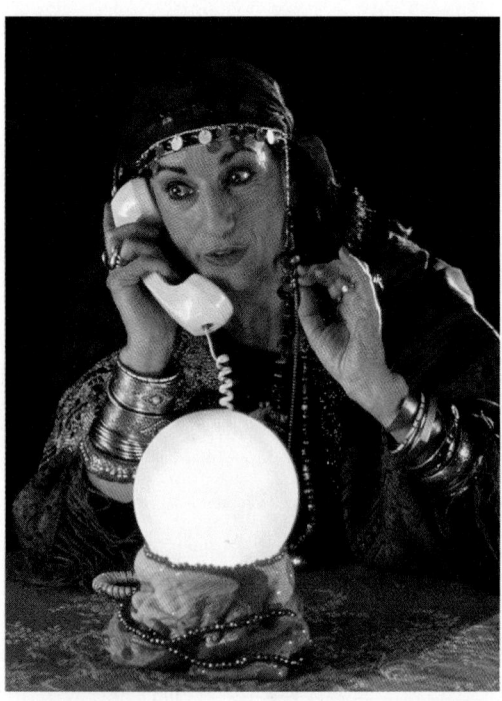

Figure 1.6 **Where do you get your nutrition information?** We are constantly bombarded by food messages. Which sources do you find most influential? Are they also the most reliable?

explosion of reduced-fat, low-fat, and fat-free products. In fact, between 1987 and 2004 over 35,000 such products were introduced.[10] When the "low-carb" diet swung back into popularity, so did low-carb or no-carb products—nearly 3,500 were introduced in 2003 and 2004 alone.

Social Factors

Social factors exert a powerful influence on food choice. By observing their parents, infants and children learn which foods and combinations of foods are appropriate to consume and under what circumstances. Perhaps even more influential, though, are the messages from peers about what to eat or how to eat.[11] Although food neophobia is common among young children, it can often be overcome when they see another child enjoying a food they have yet to sample. With age and increased social contact, children and teens are likely to increasingly adopt not only food preferences but also their peers' eccentric preparations. "Mark eats his sandwiches in triangles; that's the way I want mine!"

As **Figure 1.5** illustrates, eating is also a social event that brings together different people for a variety of purposes (e.g., religious or cultural celebrations, business meetings, and family dinners). Thanks to **social facilitation**, food intake increases because of the social climate surrounding its consumption.[12] Social pressures, however, can also restrict our food intake and selection. We might, for example, order nonmeat dishes when dining with a group of vegetarian friends.[13]

Nutrition and Health Beliefs

Information about food and nutrition is abundant. To whom do you turn for nutrition advice? (See **Figure 1.6**.) Why do some people ignore health information and indulge themselves with foods that may lead to health problems, whereas others take the same information and commit themselves to a healthful diet? To examine these questions, we must consider consumers' health beliefs, perceptions of their susceptibility to disease, and attitudes toward taking action to prevent or delay disease onset. For instance, if people feel vulnerable to disease and believe that dietary change will lead to positive results, they are more likely to pay attention to information about links between dietary choices, dietary fat, and risks for heart disease and cancer. A desire to lose weight can be a powerful force shaping decisions to accept or reject particular foods.[14] Information about nutrient content on food labels, along with health claims that describe links between food components and diseases, aids consumers who are trying to make positive choices.

Key Concepts: *Many factors influence our decisions about what to eat and when to eat. The four main factors are taste, texture, cost, and convenience. Habits, experiences, social factors, advertising, and knowledge of relationships between food and health also influence our food decisions.*

Environmental Influences

Your environment—where you live, how you live, who you live with—has a lot to do with what you choose to eat. People around us influence our food choices, and we prefer the foods we grew up eating. Environmental factors that influence our food choices include economics, lifestyle, culture, and religion.

Economic Factors

Cost is a major determinant of food choice. You may have "lobster tastes" but a "bologna budget." The types of foods purchased and the percentage of income used for food are affected by total income. Wealthier households spend only about 7 percent of their after-tax income on food, whereas low-income families spend nearly 25 percent of their income on food.[15] We often assume that wealthier households have more nutritious diets because they can afford to purchase higher-quality lean meats, more fish and seafood, and more fruits and vegetables. Analysis of fruit and vegetable expenditures shows that low-income households spend significantly less on fruits and vegetables; in any given week, nearly 20 percent of low-income households bought no fruits or vegetables.[16] This supports theories that limited finances shift food choices toward inexpensive high-fat, high-sugar choices.[17] But does a healthier diet necessarily cost more? A 2004 analysis by the U.S. Department of Agriculture found that consumers could eat three servings of fruits and four servings of vegetables daily for only 64 cents.[18]

Lifestyle

Another influential factor is lifestyle. Our fast-paced society has little time or patience for food preparation. Forty percent of our food dollars are spent away from home. Convenience foods, from frozen entrees to complete meals "in a box," saturate supermarket shelves. Current trends suggest that we're eating at home more often, but what we often eat there is store-bought ready-to-eat or heat-and-eat food. Only one-third of all main dishes in 2002 were made from scratch.[19]

Cultural Influences

One of the strongest influences on food preferences is tradition or cultural background. In all societies, no matter how simple or complex, eating is the primary way of initiating and maintaining human relationships. Sometimes these culturally acquired preferences can seem quite peculiar to those of a different culture. The college student who serves pickled herring to her friends may have learned to enjoy it from her Jewish parents, who introduced it to her as a child in comforting surroundings. Likewise, it is not uncommon for people of Mexican heritage to enjoy eating hot peppers, which were introduced to them early in life in highly gregarious social settings.

The Japanese boast the longest life spans in the world. Can we attribute their increased longevity to nutrition? In part, yes! Studies have shown that Japanese immigrants to the United States who have acquired Western tastes in food also have an increased incidence of heart disease and cancer. What do the Japanese eat? Rice, consumed with almost every meal, is an important food in Japan. Equally important in the Japanese diet is fish, which is consumed at more than 154 pounds per person per year (about 0.5 pound per person per day).

Rice also is an important staple in China. A traditional Chinese breakfast is a bowl of rice congee (rice gruel cooked with bits of meat) served with pickles or another salty side dish and tea. Lunch may be a bowl of noodle soup or may include soup, rice, and mixed dishes of vegetables and fish, meat, or poultry. Dinner, the main meal of the day, usually is a larger version of lunch. Meals are communal, with dishes placed in the center of the table and shared by all.

To a large extent, culture defines our attitudes. "One man's food is another man's poison." Look at **Figure 1.7**. How does the photo make you feel? Insects, maggots, and entrails are delicacies to some, whereas just

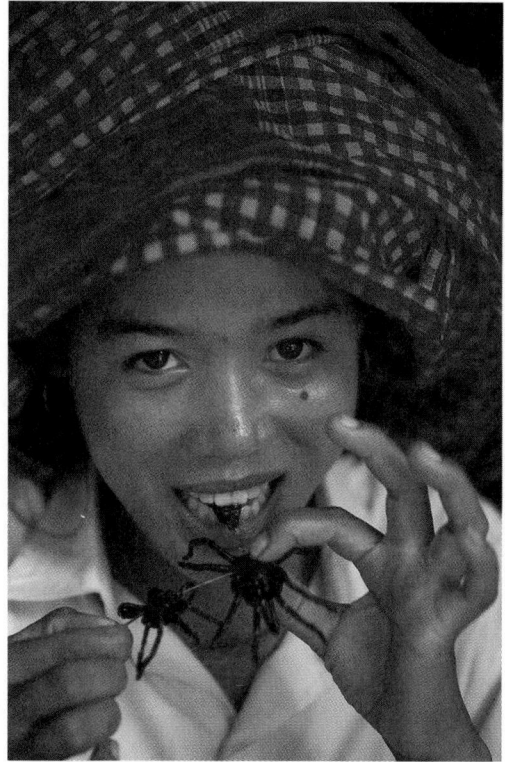

Figure 1.7 **Cultural influences.** What would you do if you were visiting this country? Would you be willing to try this delicacy?

Quick Bites

Nerve Poison for Dinner?

The puffer fish is a delicacy in Japan. Danger is part of its appeal; eating a puffer fish can be life threatening! The puffer fish contains a poison called tetrodotoxin (TTX), which blocks the transmission of nerve signals and can lead to death. Chefs who prepare the puffer fish must have special training and licenses to prepare the fish properly, so diners feel nothing more than a slight numbing feeling.

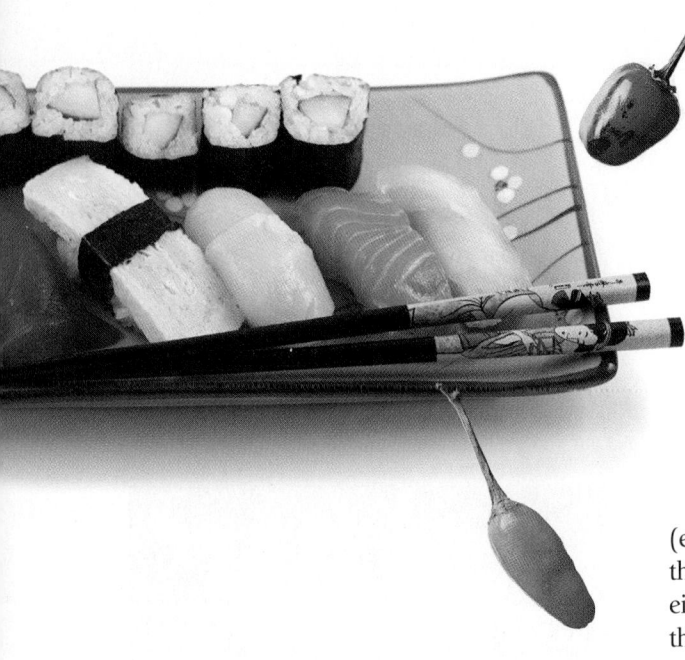

the thought of ingesting them is enough to make others retch. So powerful are cultural forces that if you were permitted only a single question to establish someone's food preferences, a good choice would be "What is your ethnic background?"[20]

Knowledge, beliefs, customs, and habits all are defining elements of human culture.[21] Although genetic characteristics tie people of ethnic groups together, culture is a learned behavior and consequently can be modified through education, experience, and social and political trends.[22]

In many cultures, food has symbolic meanings related to family traditions, social status, and even health.[23] Indeed, many folk remedies rely on food. Some of these have gained wide acceptance, such as the use of spices and herb teas for purposes ranging from allaying anxiety to preventing cancer and heart disease.[24] Traditional medical practices in many cultures follow the belief that nature is composed of two opposing forces (e.g., yin and yang in traditional Chinese medicine). It is typically believed that good health reflects a balance of the two opposing forces. Excesses in either direction cause illness, which then must be treated by giving foods of the opposite force. This idea of balance, accompanied by terms describing illnesses and foods as either "hot" or "cold," also is found in other Asian cultures, including India and the Philippines, and in Latin American cultures.

Just as cultural distinctions eventually blur when ethnic groups take part in the larger American culture, so do many of the unique expectations about the ability of certain foods to prevent disease, restore health among those with various afflictions, or enhance longevity. These beliefs are still apparent, however, in older, less assimilated groups. Food habits are among the last practices to change when an immigrant adapts to a new culture.[25]

Religion

Food is an important part of religious rites, symbols, and customs. Some religious rules apply to everyday eating, whereas others are concerned with special celebrations.

Christianity, Judaism, Hinduism, Buddhism, and Islam all have distinct dietary laws, but within each religion different interpretations of these laws give rise to variations in dietary practices. For example, Jewish dietary laws specify the foods that are "fit and proper," or *kosher*, to eat. To be kosher, meat must come from clean animals that chew their cud and have cloven hooves. Fish must have fins and scales. Pork, crustaceans and shellfish, and birds of prey are not acceptable. The Orthodox laws of Judaism prohibit eating meat and milk at the same meal or even preparing or serving them with the same dishes and utensils. Islam identifies acceptable foods as *halal* and has rules similar to those of Judaism for slaughtering animals. Islamic faith prohibits the consumption of pork, flesh of clawed animals, alcohol, and other intoxicating drugs. Intoxicating beverages are also prohibited in Buddhism.[26] The Church of Jesus Christ of Latter-Day Saints disapproves of coffee, tea, and alcoholic beverages. Most Hindus are vegetarians and do not eat eggs. The Jain religion (in India) forbids eating meat or animal products (milk, eggs, etc.) and anything grown in darkness (e.g., potato or garlic).

Religious rules may also define when and how often we eat. During the holy month of Ramadan, Muslims fast from dawn to sunset. They consume two meals per day, one before the sunrise and one after sunset.[27] Religious laws (e.g., the traditional Catholic practice of substituting fish for meat on Fridays during Lent) also define the types of foods eaten on specific occasions.[28]

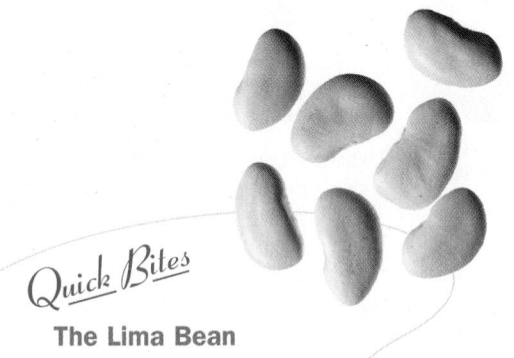

Quick Bites

The Lima Bean

The lima bean has been in cultivation in Peru since 6000 B.C.E. Not so coincidentally, Peru's capital is Lima.

Cultural Cuisine

Diet and culture affect each other. Each contributes to the identity of the other, and both help to define our values, preferences, and practices. As a result, neither is abandoned easily or quickly, even in the face of changing world events. Even so, the question arises: What impact will our increasing mobility have on food choice? Cultural interactions and exposure to various cuisines will undoubtedly increase. Will this ultimately lead to a heightened appreciation and preservation of different culinary practices or the formation of a single new hybrid cuisine?

Key Concepts: *The cultural environments in which people grow up have a major influence on what foods they prefer, what foods they consider edible, and what foods they eat in combination and at what time of day. Many factors work to define a group's culture: economics, geographic location, traditions, and religious beliefs. As people from other cultures immigrate to new lands, they adopt new behaviors consistent with their new homes. However, food habits are among the last to change.*

The American Diet

What, then, is a typical *American* diet? As a country influenced by the practices of both Native Americans and immigrants, there is no easy, single answer to this question. The U.S. diet is as diverse as Americans themselves. Many people around the world imagine that the American diet consists mainly of hamburgers, french fries, and cola drinks! Our fondness for fast food and the marketability of such restaurants overseas make them seem like icons of American culture. And many of the stereotypes are true. The most commonly consumed grain product in the United States is white bread, the favorite meat is beef, and the most frequently eaten vegetable is the potato, usually as french fries. Despite the variety available to us, the American diet is still heavy on meat and potatoes and light on fruits and whole grains. We also are eating more cereals, snack foods, soft drinks, and noncitrus juices than ever before.[29]

So, how healthful is the "American" diet? Although we are bombarded with information about health and nutrition, this doesn't necessarily translate into better food choices. People are not "natural nutritionists"; that is, they don't know instinctively which foods to choose for good health. The majority of the population has never taken a course in nutrition. They probably will never take the time to become well-informed consumers— not just of food, but also of information about food and nutrition. So it is probably not surprising when national surveys indicate that although Americans *know* that nutrition and food choices are important factors in health, few have made the recommended changes (e.g., eating less fat, sugar, and salt and more fruits and vegetables).[30]

You are in a position to gather more information than the average consumer. By taking this course in nutrition, you will be getting the full story: the nutrients we need for good health, the science behind the health messages, and the food choices it will take to implement them. Whether you use this information is up to you, but at least you will be a well-informed consumer!

Key Concepts: *"American" cuisine is truly a melting pot of cultural contributions to foods and tastes. Although Americans receive and believe many messages about the role of diet in good health, these beliefs do not always translate into better food choices.*

Quick Bites

America's Favorite Vegetables

When Americans eat vegetables, they are most likely to eat potatoes (especially french fries), tomatoes (usually part of tomato sauce or ketchup), onions, and iceberg lettuce.

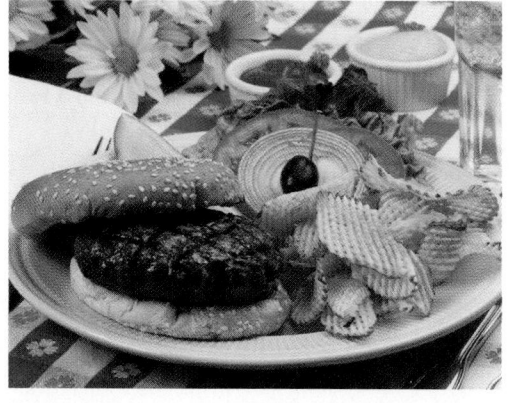

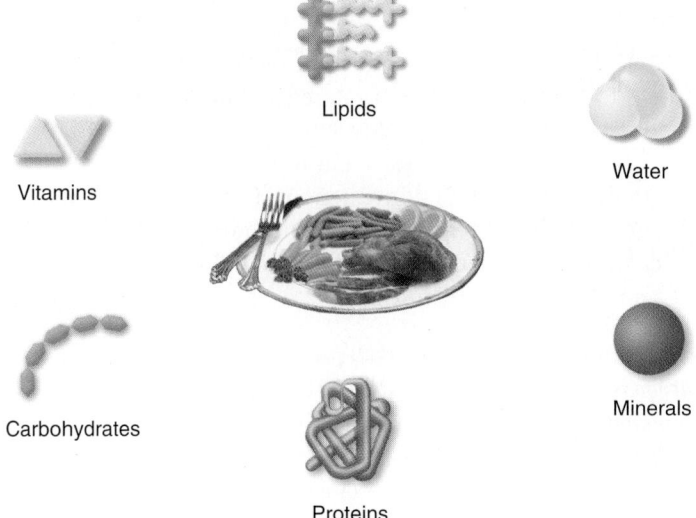

Lipids

Water

Vitamins

Carbohydrates

Minerals

Proteins

Figure 1.8 **The six classes of nutrients.** Water is our most important nutrient, and we cannot survive long without it. Because our bodies need large quantities of carbohydrate, protein, and fat, they are called macronutrients. Our bodies need comparatively small amounts of vitamins and minerals, so they are called micronutrients.

nutrients Any substances in food that the body can use to obtain energy, build tissues, or regulate functions.

essential nutrients Substances that must be obtained in the diet because the body either cannot make them or cannot make adequate amounts of them.

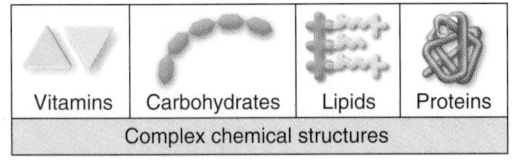

| Vitamins | Carbohydrates | Lipids | Proteins |

Complex chemical structures

Organic – contains carbon

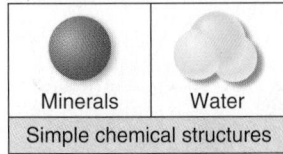

| Minerals | Water |

Simple chemical structures

Inorganic – no carbon

Introducing the Nutrients

Although we give food meaning through our culture and experience and make dietary decisions based on many factors, ultimately the reason for eating is to obtain nourishment—nutrition.

Just like your body, food is a mixture of chemicals, some of which are essential for normal body function. These essential chemicals are called **nutrients.** You need nutrients for normal growth and development, for maintaining cells and tissues, for fuel to do physical and metabolic work, and for regulating the hundreds of thousands of body processes that go on inside you every second of every day. Further, food must provide these nutrients; the body either cannot make these **essential nutrients** or cannot make enough of them. There are six classes of nutrients in food: *carbohydrates, lipids* (fats and oils), *proteins, vitamins, minerals,* and *water.* (See **Figure 1.8.**) The minimum diet for human growth, development, and maintenance must supply about 45 essential nutrients.

Definition of Nutrients

In studying nutrition, we focus on the functions of nutrients in the body so that we can see why they are important in the diet. However, to define a nutrient in technical terms, we focus on what happens in its absence. A nutrient is a chemical whose absence from the diet for a long enough time results in a specific change in health; we say that a person has a deficiency of that nutrient. A lack of vitamin C, for example, will eventually lead to scurvy. A diet with too little iron will result in iron-deficiency anemia. To complete the definition of a nutrient, it also must be true that putting the essential chemical back in the diet will reverse the change in health if done before permanent damage occurs. If taken early enough, supplements of vitamin A can reverse the effects of deficiency on the eyes. If not, prolonged vitamin A deficiency can cause permanent blindness.

Nutrients are not the only chemicals in food. Other substances add flavor and color, some contribute to texture, and others, such as caffeine, have physiological effects on the body. Some substances in food, such as fiber, have important health benefits (as you will discover in Chapter 3, "Digestion and Absorption") but do not fit the classic definition of a nutrient. One of the newest areas of research in nutrition is the area of **phytochemicals**. Although these "plant chemicals" are not nutrients, they have important health functions, such as **antioxidant** activity, which may reduce risk for heart disease or cancer.

The six classes of nutrients serve three general functions: They provide energy (fuel), regulate body processes, and contribute to body structures. (See **Figure 1.9**.) Although virtually all nutrients can be said to regulate body processes and many contribute to body structures, only protein, carbohydrate, and fat are sources of energy. Because the body needs large quantities of carbohydrate, protein, and fat, these are called **macronutrients**; the vitamins and minerals are **micronutrients** because the amounts the body needs are comparatively small.

In addition to their functions, there are several other key differences among the classes of nutrients. First, the chemical composition of nutrients varies widely. One way to divide the nutrient groups is based on whether the compounds contain the element carbon. Substances that contain carbon are **organic** substances; those that do not are **inorganic**. Carbohydrates, lipids, proteins, and vitamins are all organic; minerals and water are not. Structurally, nutrients can be very simple—minerals such as sodium are single elements, although we often consume them as larger compounds (e.g., sodium chloride, which is table salt). Water is also very simple in structure. The organic nutrients have more complex structures—the carbohydrates, lipids, and proteins we eat are made of smaller building blocks, and the vitamins are elaborately structured compounds.

It is rare for a food to contain just one nutrient. Meat is not just protein any more than bread is solely carbohydrate. Foods contain mixtures of nutrients, although in most cases, protein, fat, or carbohydrate dominates. So while bread is certainly rich in carbohydrates, it also contains some protein, a little fat, and many vitamins and minerals. If it's whole-grain bread

phytochemicals Substances in plants that may possess health-protective effects, even though they are not essential for life.

antioxidant A substance that combines with or otherwise neutralizes a free radical, thus preventing oxidative damage to cells and tissues.

macronutrients Nutrients, such as carbohydrate, fat, or protein, that are needed in relatively large amounts in the diet.

micronutrients Nutrients, such as vitamins and minerals, that are needed in relatively small amounts in the diet.

organic In chemistry, any compound that contains carbon, except carbon oxides (e.g., carbon dioxide), sulfides and metal carbonates (e.g., potassium carbonate). The term *organic* also is used to denote crops that are grown without synthetic fertilizers or chemicals.

inorganic Any substance that does not contain carbon, excepting certain simple carbon compounds such as carbon dioxide and monoxide. Common examples include table salt (sodium chloride) and baking soda (sodium bicarbonate).

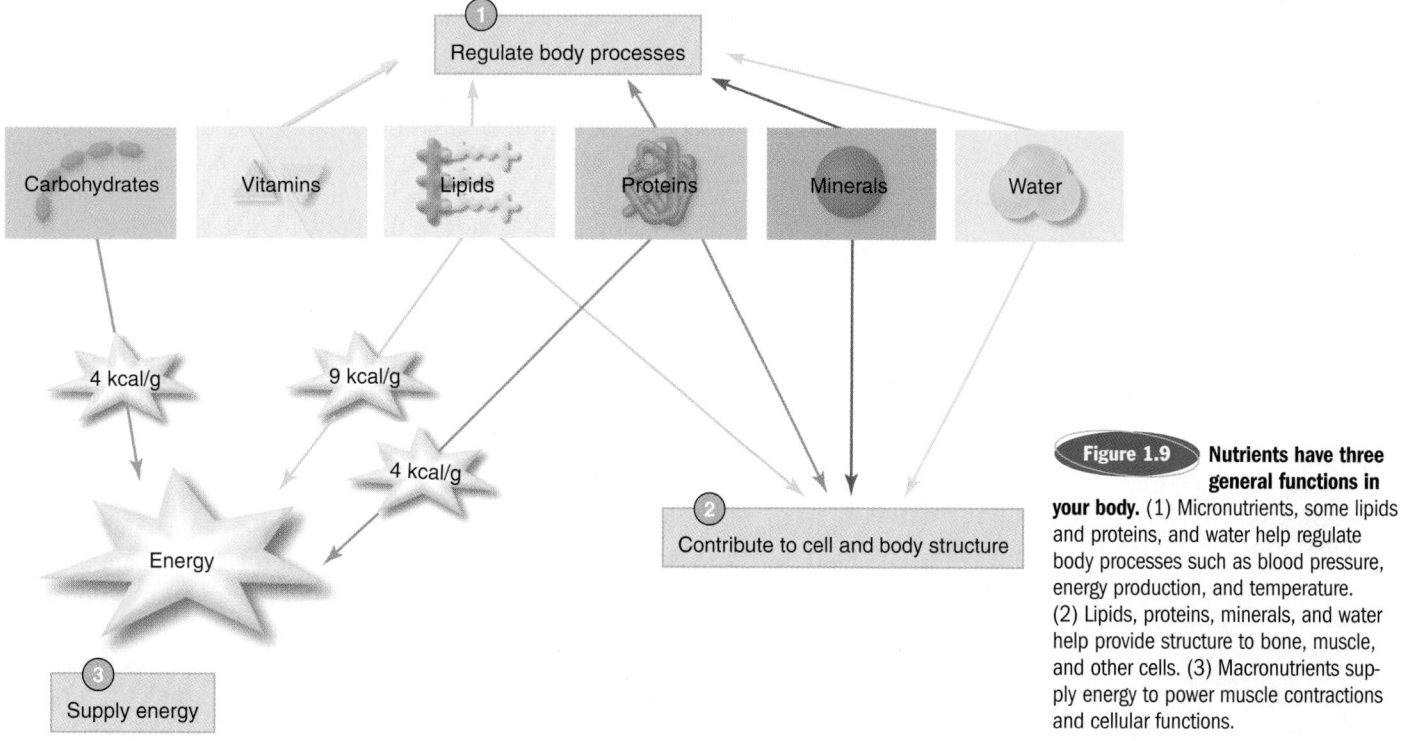

Figure 1.9 **Nutrients have three general functions in your body.** (1) Micronutrients, some lipids and proteins, and water help regulate body processes such as blood pressure, energy production, and temperature. (2) Lipids, proteins, minerals, and water help provide structure to bone, muscle, and other cells. (3) Macronutrients supply energy to power muscle contractions and cellular functions.

carbohydrate Compounds, including sugars, starches, and dietary fibers, that usually have the general chemical formula $(CH_2O)n$, where n represents the number of CH_2O units in the molecule. Carbohydrates are a major source of energy for body functions.

legumes A family of plants with edible seed pods, such as peas, beans, lentils, and soybeans; also called pulses.

circulation Movement of substances through the vessels of the cardiovascular or lymphatic system.

lipids A group of fat-soluble compounds that includes triglycerides, sterols, and phospholipids.

triglycerides Fats composed of three fatty acid chains linked to a glycerol molecule.

hormones Chemical messengers that are secreted into the blood by one tissue and act on cells in another part of the body.

proteins Large, complex compounds consisting of many amino acids connected in varying sequences and forming unique shapes.

amino acids Organic compounds that function as the building blocks of protein.

vitamins Organic compounds necessary for reproduction, growth, and maintenance of the body. Vitamins are required in miniscule amounts.

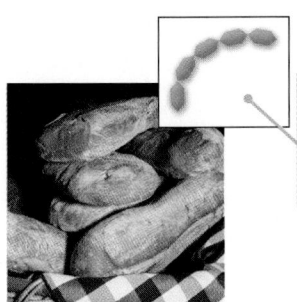

Whenever you see this icon, we'll be talking about **carbohydrates**

Provide:
Energy (4 kcal/g)

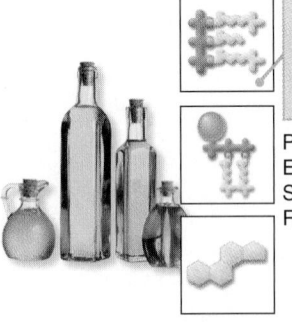

Whenever you see one of these 3 icons, we'll be talking about **lipids**

Provide:
Energy (9 kcal/g)
Structure
Regulation (hormones)

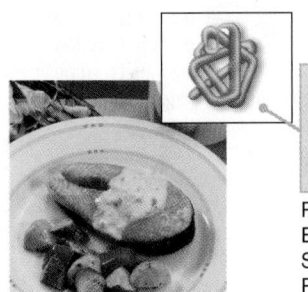

Whenever you see this icon, we'll be talking about **proteins**

Provide:
Energy (4 kcal/g)
Structure
Regulation

you're eating, you also get fiber, not technically a nutrient, but an important compound for good health nonetheless.

Key Concepts: *Nutrients are the essential chemicals in food that the body needs for normal functioning and good health; they must come from the diet because they either cannot be made in the body or cannot be made in sufficient quantities. Six classes of nutrients—carbohydrates, proteins, lipids, vitamins, minerals, and water—can be described by their composition or by their function in the body.*

Carbohydrates

The word **carbohydrate**, or literally "hydrate of carbon," tells you exactly what this nutrient is made of, if you think "water" when you hear the word *hydrate*. Carbohydrates are made of carbon, hydrogen, and oxygen, and are a major source of fuel for the body. Dietary carbohydrates are the starches and sugars found in grains, vegetables, **legumes** (dry beans and peas), and fruits. We also get carbohydrates from dairy products, but practically none from meats. Your body converts most dietary carbohydrates to glucose, a simple sugar compound. It is glucose that we find in **circulation**, providing a source of energy for cells and tissues.[31]

Lipids

The term **lipids** refers to substances we know as fats and oils, but also to fatlike substances in foods, such as cholesterol and phospholipids. Lipids are organic compounds and, like carbohydrates, contain carbon, hydrogen, and oxygen. Fats and oils—or, more correctly, **triglycerides**—are another major fuel source for the body. In addition, triglycerides, cholesterol, and phospholipids have other important functions: providing structure for body cells, carrying the fat-soluble vitamins (A, D, E, and K), and providing the starting material (cholesterol) for making many **hormones**. Dietary sources of lipids include the fats and oils we cook with or add to foods, the naturally occurring fats in meats and dairy products, and less obvious plant sources such as coconut, olives, and avocado.

Proteins

Proteins are organic compounds made of smaller building blocks called **amino acids**. Unlike carbohydrates and lipids, amino acids contain nitrogen as well as carbon, hydrogen, and oxygen. Some amino acids also contain the mineral sulfur. The amino acids that we get from dietary protein combine with the amino acids made in the body to make hundreds of different body proteins. Body proteins help build and maintain body structures and regulate body processes. Protein also can be used for energy.

Proteins are found in a variety of foods, but meats and dairy products are among the most concentrated sources. Grains, legumes, and vegetables all contribute protein to the diet, whereas fruits contribute negligible amounts.

Vitamins

Vitamins are organic compounds that contain carbon, hydrogen, and perhaps nitrogen, oxygen, phosphorus, sulfur, or other elements. Vitamins regulate body processes such as energy production, blood clotting, and calcium balance. Vitamins help to keep organs and tissues functioning and healthy. Because vitamins have such diverse functions, a lack of a particular vitamin can have widespread effects. Although the body does not break down vitamins to yield energy, vitamins have vital roles in the extraction of energy from carbohydrate, fat, and protein.

Vitamins are usually divided into two groups: fat-soluble and water-soluble. The four fat-soluble vitamins—A, D, E, and K—have very diverse roles. What they have in common is the way they are absorbed and transported in the body and the fact that they are more likely to be stored in larger quantities than the water-soluble vitamins. The water-soluble vitamins comprise vitamin C and eight B vitamins: thiamin (B_1), riboflavin (B_2), niacin (B_3), pyridoxine (B_6), cobalamin (B_{12}), folate, pantothenic acid, and biotin. Most of the B vitamins are involved in some way with the pathways for energy metabolism.

Vitamins are found in a wide variety of foods, not just fruits and vegetables—although these are important sources—but also meats, grains, legumes, dairy products, and even fats. Choosing a well-balanced diet usually makes vitamin supplements unnecessary. In fact, when taken in large doses, vitamin supplements—especially those containing vitamins A, D, B_6, or niacin—can be harmful.

Think About It
3

Minerals

Structurally, **minerals** are simple, inorganic substances. At least 16 minerals are essential to health; among them are sodium, chloride, potassium, calcium, phosphorus, and magnesium. Because the body needs these minerals in relatively large quantities compared with other minerals, they are often called **macrominerals**. The body needs the remaining minerals only in very small amounts. These **microminerals**, or **trace minerals**, include iron, zinc, copper, manganese, molybdenum, selenium, iodine, and fluoride. As with vitamins, the functions of minerals are diverse. Minerals can be found in structural roles (e.g., calcium, phosphorus, and fluoride in bones and teeth) as well as regulatory roles (e.g., control of fluid balance and regulation of muscle contraction).

Food sources of minerals are just as diverse. Although we often associate minerals with animal foods such as meats and milk, plant foods are important sources as well. Deficiencies of minerals, except iron and perhaps calcium, are uncommon. A balanced diet provides enough minerals for most people. However, individuals with iron-deficiency anemia may need iron supplements, and others may need calcium supplements if they cannot or will not drink milk or eat dairy products. As is true for vitamins, excessive intake of some minerals as supplements can be toxic.

Water

Next to the mineral elements, water is chemically the simplest nutrient. Water is also the most important nutrient! We can survive far longer without any of the other nutrients in the diet, indeed without food at all, than we can without water. Water has many roles in the body, including temperature control, lubrication of joints, and transportation of nutrients and wastes.

Because your body is nearly 60 percent water, regular fluid intake to maintain adequate hydration is important. Water is found not only in beverages but also in most food products. Fruits and vegetables in particular are high in water content. Through many chemical reactions, the body makes some of its own water, but this is only a fraction of the amount needed for normal function.

Key Concepts: *The body needs larger amounts of carbohydrates, lipids, and proteins (macronutrients) than vitamins and minerals (micronutrients). Carbohydrates, lipids, and proteins provide energy; proteins, vitamins, minerals, water, and some fatty acids regulate body processes; and proteins, lipids, minerals, and water add to body structure.*

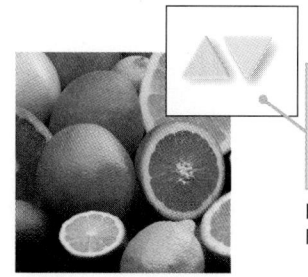

Whenever you see these icons, we'll be talking about **vitamins**

Provide:
Regulation

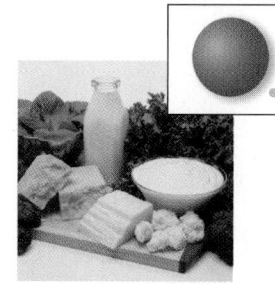

Whenever you see this icon, we'll be talking about **minerals**

Provide:
Structure
Regulation

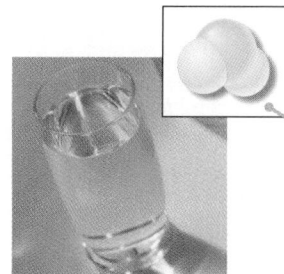

Whenever you see this icon, well be talking about **water**

Provides:
Structure
Regulation

minerals Inorganic compounds needed for growth and for regulation of body processes.

macrominerals Major minerals required in the diet and present in the body in large amounts compared with trace minerals.

microminerals See *trace minerals*.

trace minerals Trace minerals are present in the body and required in the diet in relatively small amounts compared with major minerals. Also known as microminerals.

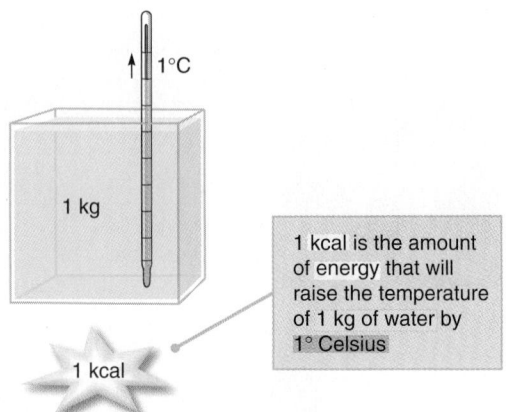

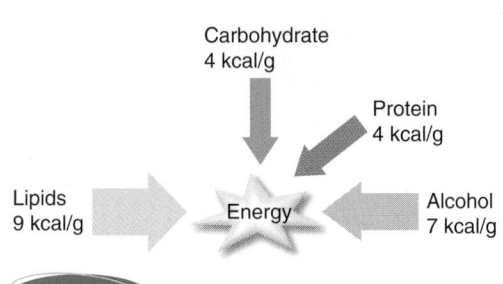

Figure 1.10 **Energy sources.** Carbohydrate, fat, protein, and alcohol provide different amounts of energy per gram.

energy The capacity to do work. The energy in food is chemical energy, which the body converts to mechanical, electrical, or heat energy.

kilocalories (kcal) [KILL-oh-kal-oh-rees] Units used to measure energy. Food energy is measured in kilocalories (1,000 calories = 1 kilocalorie).

calorie The general term for energy in food, used synonymously with the term *energy*. Often used instead of *kilocalorie* on food labels, in diet books, and in other sources of nutrition information.

Nutrients and Energy

One of the main reasons we eat food, and the nutrients it contains, is for **energy**. Every cellular reaction, every muscle movement, every nerve impulse requires energy. Three of the nutrient classes—carbohydrates, lipids (triglycerides only), and proteins—are energy sources. When we speak of the energy in foods, we are really talking about the *potential* energy that foods contain. Energy itself is not a food component.

Different scientific disciplines use different measures of energy. In nutrition, we discuss the potential energy in food, or the body's use of energy, in units of heat called **kilocalories** (1,000 calories). One kilocalorie (or kcal) is the amount of energy (heat) it would take to raise the temperature of 1 kilogram (kg) of water by 1 degree Celsius. For now, this may be an abstract concept, but as you learn more about nutrition, you will discover how much energy you likely need to fuel your daily activities. You will also learn about the amounts of potential energy in various foods.

Energy in Foods

Energy is available from foods because foods contain carbohydrate, fat, and protein. These nutrients can be broken down completely (metabolized) to yield energy in a form that cells can use. When completely metabolized in the body, carbohydrate and protein yield 4 kilocalories of energy for every gram (g) consumed; fat yields 9 kilocalories per gram; and alcohol contributes 7 kilocalories per gram. (See **Figure 1.10**.) Therefore, the energy available from a given food or from a total diet is reflected by the amount of each of these substances consumed. Because fat is a concentrated source of energy, adding or removing fat from the diet can have a big effect on available energy.

When Is a Kilocalorie a Calorie?

Many people inappropriately use the terms *calorie* and *kilocalorie* interchangeably. To clear up this confusing situation, you should use the term *calorie* as a general term for energy and *kilocalorie* as a specific measurement or unit of that energy. *Calories* is like referring to gas for a car, and *kilocalories* is like referring to gallons of fuel. When in doubt, substitute the word *energy* for *calories*. The following sentence illustrates the use of *kilocalorie* and *calorie*: Because fat contains 9 *kilocalories* per gram, more than double that of protein or carbohydrate, foods high in fat are rich in *calories* (energy).

You'll find that food labels, diet books, and other sources of nutrition information use the term *calorie*, not *kilocalorie*. Technically, the potential energy in foods is best measured in kilocalories; however, the term *calorie* has become familiar and commonplace.

How Can We Calculate the Energy Available from Foods?

To calculate the energy available from food, multiply the number of grams of fat, carbohydrate, and/or protein by 9, 4, and 4, respectively, and then add the results. For example, if we assume that one bagel plus 1.5 ounces of cream cheese contains 39 grams of carbohydrate, 10 grams of protein, and 16 grams of fat, we can determine the available energy from each component.

39 g carbohydrate × 4 kcal/g	=	**156 kcal**
10 g protein × 4 kcal/g	=	**40 kcal**
16 g fat × 9 kcal/g	=	**144 kcal**
Total	=	340 kcal

To calculate the *percentage* of calories each of these components contributes to the total, divide the individual results by the total, and then multiply by 100. For example, to determine the percentage of calories from fat in the previous example, divide the 144 fat kilocalories by the total of 340 kilocalories and then multiply by 100, as follows: $(144 \div 340) \times 100 = 42$ percent.

Be Food Smart: Calculate the Percentages of Calories in Food

Current health recommendations suggest limiting fat intake to 20 to 35 percent of *total* energy intake. You can monitor this for yourself in two ways. If you like counting fat grams, you can first determine your suggested maximum fat intake. For example, if you need to eat 2,000 kilocalories each day to maintain your current weight, at most 35 percent of those calories can come from fat.

2,000 kcal × 0.35	=	700 kcal from fat	
700 kcal from fat ÷ 9 kcal/g	=	77.8 g of fat	

Therefore, your maximum fat intake should be about 78 grams. You can check food labels to see how many fat grams you typically eat.

Another way to monitor your fat intake is to know the percentage of calories that come from fat in various foods. If the proportion of fat in each food choice throughout the day exceeds 35 percent of calories, then the day's total of fat will be too high as well. Some foods contain virtually no fat calories (e.g., fruits and vegetables), whereas others are nearly 100 percent fat calories (e.g., margarine, salad dressing). Being aware that a snack such as the bagel and cream cheese provides 42 percent of its calories from fat can help you select lower-fat foods at other times of the day.

Obesity: A Public Health Crisis

Americans and Canadians are getting fatter. Statistics show that more than half are overweight or obese, and that number has grown dramatically over the last decade, most alarmingly in children. Results from the 1999–2002 National Health and Nutrition Examination Survey (NHANES), using measured heights and weights, indicate that an estimated 65 percent of U.S. adults are either overweight or obese.[32]

This obesity epidemic poses a major threat to public health because of the clear association between obesity and a variety of chronic diseases, such as type 2 diabetes, heart disease, cancer, stroke, gallbladder disease, and hypertension. (See Chapter 8, "Energy Balance, Body Composition, and Weight Management.") However, standard public health measures (as seen in the war against tobacco) have not helped reduce the weight of North Americans. Many people prefer a sedentary lifestyle and have a dependence on fast food.

One of the national health objectives for the year 2010 is to reduce the prevalence of obesity among adults from 30 percent to less than 15 percent.[33] Research indicates, however, that the situation is worsening rather than improving. A number of factors influence overweight or obesity, including the following:

- *Behavior.* Eating too many calories while not getting enough physical activity.
- *Environment.* Home, work, school, or community can provide barriers to or opportunities for an active lifestyle.
- *Genetics.* Heredity plays a large role in determining how susceptible people are to overweight and obesity. Genes also influence how the body burns calories for energy or stores fat.

CALCULATING THE ENERGY
AVAILABLE FROM FOODS

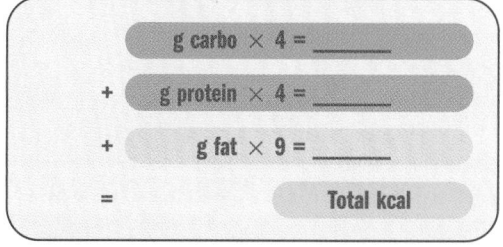

Example:
275 g carbohydrate × 4 kcal/g = 1,100 kcal

75 g protein × 4 kcal/g = 300 kcal

67 g fat × 9 kcal/g = 600 kcal (rounded from 603 kcal)

Total = 2,000 kcal

CALCULATING THE PERCENTAGE OF
KILOCALORIES FROM NUTRIENTS

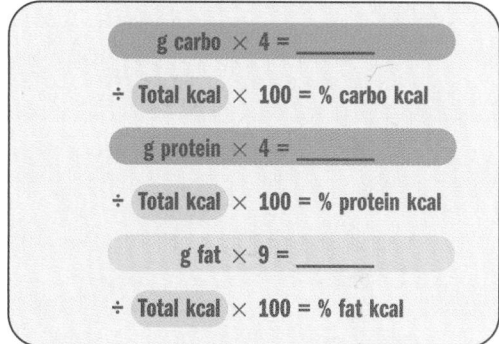

Example:
275 g carbohydrate × 4 = 1,100 kcal
1,100 kcal ÷ 2,000 kcal × 100 = 55% carbo kcal

75 g protein × 4 = 300 kcal
300 kcal ÷ 2,000 kcal × 100 = 15% protein kcal

67 g fat × 9 = 600 kcal (rounded from 603 kcal)
600 kcal ÷ 2,000 kcal × 100 = 30% fat kcal

Behavioral and environmental factors are the main contributors to overweight and obesity and provide the greatest opportunity for prevention and treatment.

The foods we choose do more than provide us with an adequate diet. The balance of energy sources can affect our risk of chronic disease. For example, high-fat diets have been linked to heart disease and cancer. Excess calories contribute to obesity, which also increases disease risk. Other nutrients, such as the minerals sodium, chloride, calcium, and magnesium, affect blood pressure, and lack of the vitamin folate prior to conception and in early pregnancy can cause serious birth defects. Nonnutrient components in the diet (e.g., phytochemicals) may have antioxidant or immune-enhancing properties that can keep us healthy. The choices we make can reduce our disease risk as well as provide energy and essential nutrients.

Key Concepts: *All cells and tissues need energy to keep the body functioning. Energy in foods and in the body is measured in kilocalories. The carbohydrates, lipids, and proteins in food are potential sources of energy, meaning that the body can extract energy from them. Triglycerides (fats) are the most concentrated source of energy, with 9 kilocalories per gram. Carbohydrates and proteins provide 4 kilocalories per gram, and alcohol has 7 kilocalories per gram.*

Applying the Scientific Process to Nutrition

Whether it's identifying essential nutrients, establishing recommended intake levels, or exploring the effects of vitamins on cancer risk, scientific studies are the cornerstone of nutrition. Although we may use creative, artistic talents to choose and serve a pleasing array of healthful foods, the fundamentals of nutrition are developed through the scientific process of observation and inquiry.

The scientific process enables researchers to test the validity of **hypotheses** that arise from observations of natural phenomena. For example, it was common knowledge in the eighteenth century that sailors on long voyages would likely develop scurvy (which we now know results from a deficiency of vitamin C). Scurvy had been recognized since ancient times, and its common symptoms—pinpoint skin hemorrhages, swollen and bleeding gums, joint pain, fatigue and lethargy, and psychological changes such as depression and hysteria—were well known. Native populations discovered plant foods that would cure this illness; among Native Americans these included cranberries in the Northeast and many tree extracts in other parts of the country. From observations such as this come questions that lead to hypotheses, or "educated guesses," about factors that might be responsible for the observed phenomenon. Scientists then test hypotheses using appropriate research designs. Poorly designed research produces useless results or false conclusions.

Epidemiological Studies

An epidemiological study compares disease rates among population groups and attempts to identify related conditions or behaviors such as diet and smoking habits. The observation that scurvy developed during prolonged time at sea is an example of one aspect of **epidemiology**. Another example is the association between dietary intakes of soy and breast cancer rates. While Japanese women have high dietary intakes of soy and low breast can-

hypotheses Scientists' "educated guesses" to explain phenomena.

epidemiology The science of determining the incidence and distribution of diseases in different populations.

cer rates, American women have comparatively low dietary intakes of soy and high breast cancer rates.

Epidemiological studies provide information about relationships but do not clarify cause and effect. The results of these studies show **correlations**— relationships between two factors. For example, with soy and breast cancer, epidemiological studies show only that populations with higher soy intake (e.g., Japanese women) have lower breast cancer rates; they do not establish that soy intake prevents breast cancer. However, epidemiological studies provide clues and insights that lead to animal and human studies that can further clarify diet and disease relationships.

Animal Studies

Animal studies can provide preliminary data that lead to human studies or can be used to study hypotheses that cannot be tested on humans. It was shown in the 1890s that feeding polished (refined) rice to chickens led to a disease similar to beriberi (thiamin-deficiency disease), whereas a diet of rice with the hull intact did not. It's important to keep in mind that although animal studies give scientists important information that furthers nutrition knowledge, the results of animal studies cannot be transferred directly to humans. Animal studies need to be followed with cell culture studies or human clinical studies to determine specific effects in humans.

Cell Culture Studies

Another way to study nutrition is to isolate specific types of cells and grow them in a laboratory. Scientists can then use these cells to study the effects of nutrients or other components on metabolic processes in the cell. An important area of nutrition research called **nutrigenomics** explores the effect of specific nutrients and other chemical compounds on gene expression. (See the FYI feature "Are Nutrigenomics in Your Future?") This area of molecular biology will help us to explain individual differences in chronic disease risk factors and may lead to designing diets based on an individual's genetic profile rather than on guidelines for the population in general.[34]

Human Studies

The **case control study** and clinical trials are the two primary types of **experiments** used to test hypotheses in humans. Case control studies are small-scale epidemiological studies in which one group of individuals who have a condition (e.g., breast cancer) are compared with a similar group of individuals who do not have the condition. Researchers then identify factors other than the disease in question, such as fruit and vegetable intake, that differ between the two groups. These factors provide researchers with clues about the cause, progression, and prevention of the disease. It is important that the two groups be matched as closely as possible for major characteristics such as age, gender, and race.

Clinical trials are controlled studies in which some type of intervention—a nutrient supplement, controlled diet, or exercise program—is used to determine its impact on certain health parameters. These studies include an **experimental group** (the people who are given the intervention) and a **control group** (similar people who are not treated). Scientists measure aspects of health or disease in each group and compare the results.

correlations Connections, co-occurring more frequently than can be explained by chance or coincidence, but without a proven cause.

nutrigenomics The study of how nutrition interacts with specific genes to influence a person's health.

case control study An investigation that uses a group of people with a particular condition, rather than a randomly selected population. These cases are compared with a control group of people who do not have the condition.

experiments Tests to examine the validity of a hypothesis.

clinical trials Studies that collect large amounts of data to evaluate the effectiveness of a treatment.

experimental group A set of people being studied to evaluate the effect of an event, substance, or technique.

control group A set of people used as a standard of comparison to the experimental group. The people in the control group have characteristics similar to those in the experimental group and are selected at random.

placebo An inactive substance that is outwardly indistinguishable from the active substance whose effects are being studied.

James Lind's experiments with sailors aboard the *Salisbury* in 1747 are considered to be the first dietary clinical trial. (See **Figure 1.11**.) His observation that oranges and lemons were the only dietary elements that seemed to cure scurvy was an important finding. However, it took more than 40 years before the British Navy began routinely giving all sailors citrus juice or fruit, such as lemons or limes—a practice that led to the nickname "limey" when referring to British sailors. It took nearly 200 years (until the 1930s) for scientists to isolate the compound we call vitamin C and show that it had antiscurvy activity.[35] The chemical name for vitamin C, ascorbic acid, comes from its role as an "antiscorbutic" (antiscurvy) compound.

There are several important elements in a modern clinical trial: random assignment to groups, use of placebos, and the double-blind method. Subjects are assigned randomly—as by the flip of a coin—to the experimental group or the control group. This reduces the risk of introducing bias into either group. People in the experimental group receive the treatment or specific protocol (e.g., consuming a certain nutrient at a specific level). People in the control group do not receive the treatment but usually receive a **placebo**. A placebo is an imitation treatment (such as a sugar pill) that looks the same as the experimental treatment but has no effect. The placebo is also important for reducing bias because subjects do not know if they are receiving the intervention and are less inclined to alter their responses or reported symptoms based on what they think should happen.

Fyi Are Nutrigenomics in Your Future?

FOR YOUR INFORMATION

Nutritional genomics, or *nutrigenomics*, is the study of how different foods can interact with particular genes to alter a person's risk of developing diseases such as type 2 diabetes, obesity, heart disease, and cancers.

Many of these diseases are especially common among minority populations. African American men, for example, have a 60 percent higher risk of being diagnosed with prostate cancer than do Caucasian men.[1] Half of all adult Pima Indians in the United States have type 2 diabetes, compared with 6.5 percent of adult Americans of Caucasian descent. Genetics, diet, economic and social conditions, culture, and behavior may all contribute to these differences.[2]

Thanks to human genomics research, we now know that all people share the vast majority of human genetic information. Indeed, any two individuals share 99.9 percent of their DNA sequence—or about 1 difference in every 1,000 base pairs. Similarly, all racial and ethnic groups share most genetic variations. The small differences that do exist are responsible for diverse human characteristics such as hair and skin colors, height and weight potential, and other "gene-based" variations such as susceptibility to disease. The incidence of disease or patterns of progression differ among different groups. Risk factors for common diseases such as obesity, coronary heart disease, diabetes, prostate cancer, and birth defects must take into account both genetic and environmental/behavioral/social factors. The science of nutrigenomics studies how genes, diet, and disease interact to create health disparities

for certain human populations that evolved from different geographic regions.

While diet can be a serious risk factor for a number of diseases, the exact effect of different components of food may depend on a person's genetic makeup. Thus, it is not a question of whether your genes are good or bad, but rather how they interact with your environment. A single-letter change in DNA in people from Scandinavia 10,000 years ago, for example, allows most Caucasian adults today to drink cow's milk without getting sick due to lactose intolerance.[3]

The nutrigenomics effort seeks to identify genes controlled by nutrients and other naturally occurring chemicals in food and to study how some of these genes can tip the balance between health and disease. Nutrients alter molecular processes such as DNA structure

When the members of neither the experimental nor the control groups know what treatment they are receiving, we say the subjects are "blinded" to the treatment. If a clinical trial is designed so neither the subjects nor the researchers collecting data are aware of the subjects' group assignments (experimental or control), the study is called a **double-blind study**. This reduces the possibility that researchers will see the results they want to see even if these results do not occur. In this case, another member of the research team holds the code for subject assignments and does not participate in the data collection. Double-blind, placebo-controlled clinical trials are considered the "gold standard" of nutrition studies. These studies can show clear cause-and-effect relationships, but often require large numbers of subjects and are expensive and time-consuming to conduct.

More on the Placebo Effect

Because the **placebo effect** can exert a powerful influence, research studies must take it into account. For example, when researchers tested the effectiveness of a medication in reducing binge eating among people with bulimia, they used a double-blind, placebo-controlled study to eliminate the placebo effect.[36] After a baseline number of binge-eating episodes was determined, 22 women with bulimia were given the medication or a placebo. After a period of time, the number of binge-eating episodes was reassessed. The study found a 78 percent reduction in binge-eating episodes among those

double-blind study A research study set up so that neither the subjects nor the investigators know which study group is receiving the placebo and which is receiving the active substance.

placebo effect A physical or emotional change that is not due to properties of an administered substance. The change reflects participants' expectations.

formation, gene expression, and metabolism, which in turn may alter disease initiation, development, or progression. Individual genetic variations can influence how nutrients are assimilated, metabolized, stored, and excreted by the body. Nutritional genomics will enable individuals to better manage their health and well-being by precisely matching their diets to their unique genetic makeup.

The conceptual basis for this new branch of genomic research can best be summarized by the following Five Tenets of Nutrigenomics:[4]

1. Under certain circumstances and in some individuals, diet can be a serious risk factor for a number of diseases.
2. Common dietary chemicals can act on the human genome, either directly or indirectly, to alter gene expression or structure.
3. The degree to which diet influences the balance between healthy and disease states may depend on an individual's particular genetic makeup.
4. Some diet-regulated genes (and their normal, common variants) are likely to play a role in the onset, incidence, progression, and/or severity of chronic diseases.
5. Dietary intervention based on knowledge of nutritional requirements, nutritional status, and genotype (i.e., "intelligent nutrition") can be used to prevent, mitigate, or cure chronic disease.

Personalized Nutrition

Just as pharmacogenomics has inspired the concept of "personalized medicine" and "designer drugs," the new field of nutrigenomics is opening the way for "personalized nutrition."[5] In other words, by understanding our nutritional needs, our nutritional status, and our genotype, nutrigenomics should enable people to better manage their health and well-being by precisely matching their diets with their unique genetic makeup. Stay tuned!

1 University of California–Davis. New center will probe links between diet, genes, and disease. Press release. January 21, 2003.

2 Ibid.

3 Enattah NS, et al. Identification of a variant associated with adult-type hypolactasia. *Nat Genet.* 2002;30(2): 233–237.

4 NCMHD Center of Excellence for Nutritional Genomics. What is nutrigenomics and how does it relate to me? University of California–Davis. http://nutrigenomics .ucdavis.edu. Accessed 11/20/06.

5 McCarthy JJ, Hilfiker R. The use of single-nucleotide polymorphism maps in pharmacogenomics. *Nat Biotechnol.* 2000;18(5):505–508.

1. Observation
Sailors on long voyages all became ill with scurvy.

2. Hypothesis
Lack of certain foods causes scurvy.

3. Experimentation
Experiment to test hypothesis.
Predicts that some dietary element will cure scurvy.

Key	Controlled variables
	Experimental variables
	Results
	Conclusions

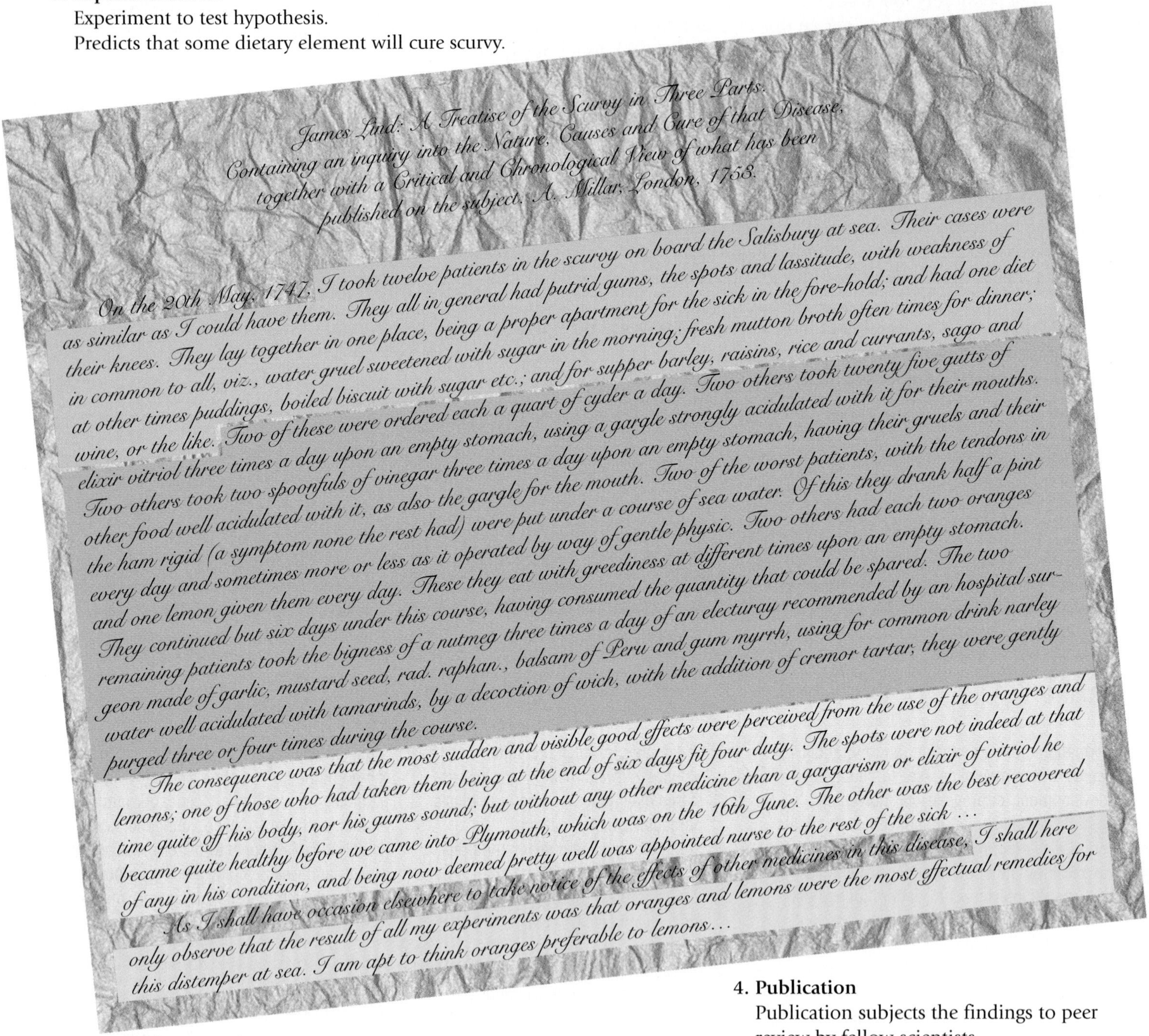

James Lind: A Treatise of the Scurvy in Three Parts. Containing an inquiry into the Nature, Causes and Cure of that Disease, together with a Critical and Chronological View of what has been published on the subject. A. Millar, London. 1753.

On the 20th May, 1747, I took twelve patients in the scurvy on board the Salisbury at sea. Their cases were as similar as I could have them. They all in general had putrid gums, the spots and lassitude, with weakness of their knees. They lay together in one place, being a proper apartment for the sick in the fore-hold; and had one diet in common to all, viz., water gruel sweetened with sugar in the morning; fresh mutton broth often times for dinner; at other times puddings, boiled biscuit with sugar etc.; and for supper barley, raisins, rice and currants, sago and wine, or the like. Two of these were ordered each a quart of cyder a day. Two others took twenty five gutts of elixir vitriol three times a day upon an empty stomach, using a gargle strongly acidulated with it for their mouths. Two others took two spoonfuls of vinegar three times a day upon an empty stomach, having their gruels and their other food well acidulated with it, as also the gargle for the mouth. Two of the worst patients, with the tendons in the ham rigid (a symptom none the rest had) were put under a course of sea water. Of this they drank half a pint every day and sometimes more or less as it operated by way of gentle physic. Two others had each two oranges and one lemon given them every day. These they eat with greediness at different times upon an empty stomach. They continued but six days under this course, having consumed the quantity that could be spared. The two remaining patients took the bigness of a nutmeg three times a day of an electuray recommended by an hospital surgeon made of garlic, mustard seed, rad. raphan., balsam of Peru and gum myrrh, using for common drink narley water well acidulated with tamarinds, by a decoction of wich, with the addition of cremor tartar, they were gently purged three or four times during the course.

The consequence was that the most sudden and visible good effects were perceived from the use of the oranges and lemons; one of those who had taken them being at the end of six days fit four duty. The spots were not indeed at that time quite off his body, nor his gums sound; but without any other medicine than a gargarism or elixir of vitriol he became quite healthy before we came into Plymouth, which was on the 16th June. The other was the best recovered of any in his condition, and being now deemed pretty well was appointed nurse to the rest of the sick …

As I shall have occasion elsewhere to take notice of the effects of other medicines in this disease, I shall here only observe that the result of all my experiments was that oranges and lemons were the most effectual remedies for this distemper at sea. I am apt to think oranges preferable to lemons…

4. Publication
Publication subjects the findings to peer review by fellow scientists.

5. More experiments
Further experiments replicate the findings and extend knowledge.

6. Theory
Scientists consolidate acquired knowledge into a theory that explains the observed phenomenon.

Figure 1.11 **The first clinical trial.** In 1758, physician James Lind reported the careful process of his clinical trial among British sailors afflicted with scurvy.

taking the medication and a 70 percent reduction in the placebo group. This showed that the *expectation* that the medication would be effective was nearly as effective as the medication itself. However, a review of placebo or no-treatment clinical trials concluded that placebos do not generally have significant effects in studies with objective outcomes, but may have small benefits in studies where the outcome measures were subjective, such as pain intensity.[37] Based on this information, the often-quoted value that one-third of patients show improvement after receiving a placebo is probably an overstatement.

Think About It 4

Key Concepts: *The scientific method is used to expand our nutrition knowledge. Hypotheses are formed from observations and are then tested by experiments. Epidemiological studies observe patterns in populations. Animal and cell culture studies can test effects of various treatments. For human studies, randomized, double-blind, placebo-controlled clinical trials are the best research tool for determining cause-and-effect relationships.*

From Research Study to Headline

What about the nutrition and health headlines we see in the newspapers, hear on TV, or read about on the Internet daily? Consumers are often confused by what they see as the "wishy-washiness" of scientists—for example, coffee is good, then coffee is bad. Margarine is better than butter—no wait, maybe butter is better after all. These contradictions, despite the confusion they cause, show us that nutrition is truly a science: dynamic, changing, and growing with each new finding.

Publication of Experimental Results

Once an experiment is complete, scientists publish the results in a scientific journal to communicate new information to other scientists. Generally, before articles are published in scientific journals, other scientists who have expert knowledge of the subject critically review them. **Peer review** ensures that only high-quality research findings are published. Peer-reviewed journals such as the *American Journal of Clinical Nutrition* and the *Journal of the American Dietetic Association* help nutritionists and dietitians keep up with current research.

peer review An appraisal of research against accepted standards by professionals in the field.

SCIENTISTS DISPUTE CLAIMS OF GINKGO BILOBA EFFECTIVENESS

There have been over four hundred scientific studies conducted on proprietary stand...

Schwabe Co. of Karlsruhe, Germa[ny]
producer of the proprietary extra[ct]
EGb 761. Ginkgo extract is a goo[d]
exa[...]
mu[...]
deli[...]
scie[...]
the[...]
for[...]

Researchers Link Caffeine and Cancer

Some Say Ginkgo Biloba Improves Memory

[C]ancer and Vitamin E Link Disputed

[...]es causing a multitude of other offenses [again]st human health, free radicals are the main [...]ts underlying cardiovascular disease. Growing [...] medical literature suggests that [...] [chol]esterol)

hardening of the arteries. Briefly, here's how it works: Excess free radicals in the bloodstream oxidize particles of LDL. Immune system cells in the arterial walls recognize the oxidized LDLs as toxic to the body and gobble them up. When the immune cells become overloaded with LDLs, they break down into pathological cells called foam cells. The foam [...]

Vitamin E Reduces Risk of Cancer

The walls recognize the risk of oxidized LDLs as toxic to the body and gobble them up. This vitamin has been shown to be instrumental in reducing some forms of cancer in certain patients. When the immune cel[...]

Vitamin E reduces the risk of LDL cholesterol being oxidized and therefore attaching to the cell wall. Because it is fat soluble, Vitamin E can get inside the LDL cholest[erol] molecule wh[...]

logical cells called foam cell[s]. The foam cells attach readil[y] the vessel wall and start the [p]rocess of hardening of [...]

Figure 1.12 **Sifting facts and fallacies.** From original research to the evening news, each step along the way introduces biases as information is summarized and restated. Whether on television, radio, the Internet, or in print, the best consumer information cites sources for reported facts.

As scientific information is made accessible to more and more people, less detail is provided and more opinion and sensationalism are introduced.

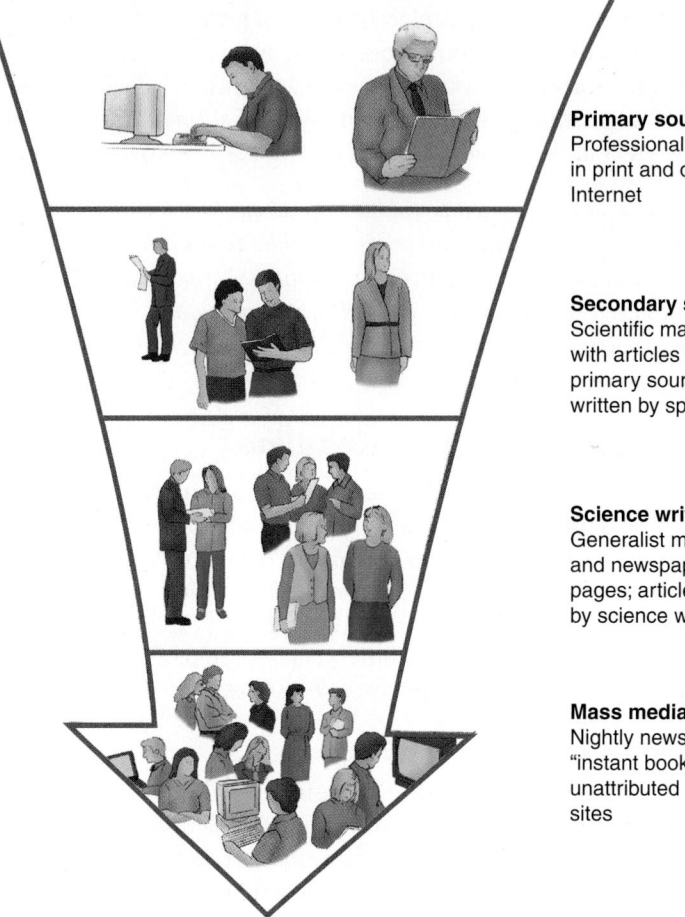

Primary sources: Professional journals in print and on the Internet

Secondary sources: Scientific magazines with articles based on primary source material written by specialists

Science writing: Generalist magazines and newspapers' science pages; articles written by science writers

Mass media: Nightly news bites "instant books," unattributed Internet sites

Each time that research findings are summarized and reported, some degree of opinion is introduced into the report. A large-scale clinical trial or a long-term observational report produces mountains of data. Researchers must decide, using their experience and judgment, which data-analysis methods to use and which results to summarize for peer-reviewed publication. The journalist who regularly scans scientific journals for potential headlines decides which studies will get media attention and then summarizes study results in nontechnical terms. A news article becomes a 30-second sound bite that often is far removed from the original data. In some cases, the study may be distorted, with its results misstated or overstated. (See **Figure 1.12**.)

Sorting Facts and Fallacies in the Media

People tend to believe what they hear repeatedly. Even when it has no basis in fact, a claim can seem credible if heard often enough. For example, do you believe that sugar makes kids hyperactive? There is no *scientific* evidence to support this claim!

The public is surrounded by messages from various media: TV, radio, newspapers, magazines, books, and the Internet. Because a large audience translates into high ratings or sales and subsequently high advertising rates, the media make money attracting viewers, listeners, and readers. To increase the number of viewers or listeners, media may sensationalize and oversimplify nutrition-related topics. This is particularly true of stories related to obesity, cancer, vitamins and minerals, and food safety. Although news stories may be based on reports in the scientific literature, the media may distort the facts through omission of details. (See the FYI feature "Evaluating Information on the Internet.")

As you learn about nutrition, you will undoubtedly be more aware not only of your eating and shopping habits but also of nutrition-related information in the media. As you see and hear reports, stop to think carefully about what you are hearing. Headlines and news reports often overstate the findings of a study. You may want to find the scientific article and read it for yourself. At first, reading journal articles will be difficult, but with experience (and growing nutrition knowledge) you will understand more of the information presented. Talk to your instructor for ideas about journal articles that might help you evaluate headlines. Two other things to keep in mind: One study does not provide all the answers to our nutrition questions; and if it sounds too good to be true, it probably is!

Your study of nutrition is just beginning. As you learn about the essential nutrients, their functions and food sources, be alert to your food choices and the factors that influence them. When the discussion turns to the role of diet in health, think about your preconceived ideas and evaluate your beliefs in the light of current scientific evidence. Keep an open mind, but also think critically. Most of all, remember that food is more than the nutrients it provides; it is part of the way we enjoy and celebrate life!

American Dietetic Association

Food and Nutrition Misinformation

It is the position of the American Dietetic Association that food and nutrition misinformation can have harmful effects on the health and economic status of consumers. Nationally credentialed dietetics professionals working in health care, academia, public health, nutrition communications, media, and the food industry and serving in policy-making/regulatory roles are uniquely qualified to advocate for and promote sound, science-based nutrition information to the public, function as primary nutrition educators to health professionals, and actively counter and correct food and nutrition misinformation.

J Am Diet Assoc. 2006;106:601–607.

Reprinted with permission.

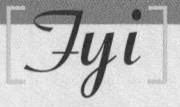

Evaluating Information on the Internet

FOR YOUR INFORMATION

Surfing the Web has made life easier in many ways. You can buy a car, check stock prices, search out sources for a paper you're writing, chat with like-minded people, and stay up to date on news or sports scores. Hundreds of Web sites are devoted to nutrition and health topics, and you may be asked to visit such sites as part of your course requirements. So, how do you evaluate the quality of information on the Web? Can you trust what you see?

First, it's important to remember that there are no rules for posting on the Internet. Anyone who has the equipment can set up a Web site and post any content he or she likes. Although the Health on the Net Foundation has set up a Code of Conduct for medical and health Web sites, following their eight principles is completely voluntary.[1]

Second, consider the source, if you can tell what it is! Many Web sites do not specify where the content came from, who is responsible for it, or how often it is updated. If the site lists the authors, what are their credentials? Who sponsors the site itself? Educational institutions (.edu), government agencies (.gov), and organizations (.org) generally have more credibility than commercial (.com) sites, where selling rather than educating may be the motive.[2] Identifying the purpose for a site can give you more clues about the validity of its content.

Third, when you see claims for nutrients, dietary supplements, or other products, and results of studies or other information, keep in mind the scientific method and the basics of sound science. Who did the study? What type of study was it? How many subjects? Was it double-blind? Were the results published in a peer-reviewed journal? Think critically about the content, look at other sources, and ask questions of experts before you accept information as truth. What is true of books, magazines, and newspapers also applies to the Internet: Just because it is in print or online doesn't mean it's true.

Finally, be on the lookout for "junk science"—sloppy methods, interpretations, and claims that lead to public misinformation. The Food and Nutrition Science Alliance (FANSA) is a coalition of four professional societies: the American Dietetic Association (ADA), the American Society for Clinical Nutrition (ASCN), the American Society for Nutritional Sciences (ASNS), and the Institute of Food Technologists (IFT). FANSA has developed the "10 Red Flags of Junk Science" to help consumers identify potential misinformation.[3] Use these red flags to evaluate Web sites.

The 10 Red Flags of Junk Science

1. Recommendations that promise a quick fix

2. Dire warnings of danger from a single product or regimen

3. Claims that sound too good to be true

4. Simplistic conclusions drawn from a single study

5. Recommendations based on a single study

6. Dramatic statements that are refuted by reputable scientific organizations

7. Lists of "good" and "bad" foods

8. Recommendations made to help sell a product

9. Recommendations based on studies published without peer review

10. Recommendations from studies that ignore differences among individuals or groups

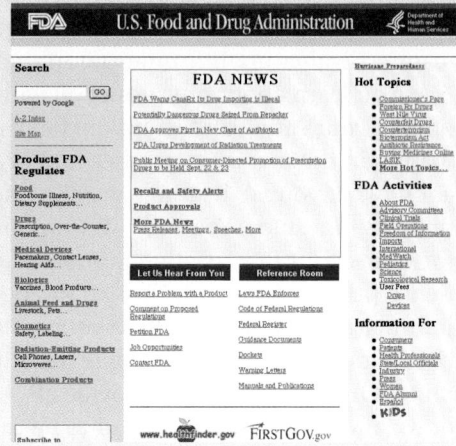

Use the Internet; it's fun and can be educational. Don't forget about the library, though; many scientific journals are not available online. Treat claims as "guilty until proven innocent"—in other words, don't accept what you read at face value until you have evaluated the science behind it. If it sounds too good to be true, it probably is!

Note: The American Dietetic Association provides reliable, objective food and nutrition information and provides links to other reliable Internet sources on the ADA Web site at http://www.eatright.org /cps/rde/xchg/ada/hs.xsl/nutrition_5420_ENU _HTML.htm. Accessed 5/17/06.

[1] Health on the Net Foundation. HON code of conduct. http://www.hon.ch/HONcode/Conduct.html. Accessed 5/17/06.

[2] The wheat from the chaff: sorting out nutrition information on the Internet. *J Am Diet Assoc.* 1998;98:1270–1272.

[3] Junk science: Scientists issue 10 red flags for consumers. http://www.eatright.org. Reprinted with permission from the American Dietetic Association. Accessed 11/20/06.

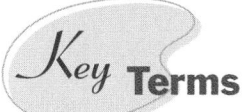

LEARNING *Portfolio* chapter 1

Key Terms

	page		page
amino acids	14	macrominerals	15
antioxidant	13	macronutrients	13
calorie	16	microminerals	15
carbohydrate	14	micronutrients	13
case control study	19	minerals	15
circulation	14	neophobia	4
clinical trials	19	nutrients	11
control group	19	nutrigenomics	19
correlations	19	nutrition	4
double-blind study	21	organic	13
energy	16	peer review	23
epidemiology	18	phytochemicals	13
essential nutrients	11	pica	7
experimental group	19	placebo	20
experiments	19	placebo effect	21
flavor	5	proteins	14
hormones	14	social facilitation	8
hypotheses	18	trace minerals	15
inorganic	13	triglycerides	14
kilocalories (kcal) [KILL-oh-kal-oh-rees]	16	umami [ooh-MA-mee]	5
legumes	14	vitamins	14
lipids	14		

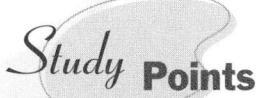

Study Points

- ➤ Most people make food choices for reasons other than nutrient value.

- ➤ Taste and texture are the two most important factors that influence food choices.

- ➤ In all cultures, eating is the primary way of maintaining social relationships.

- ➤ Although Americans know about healthful food choices, their eating habits do not always reflect this knowledge.

- ➤ Food is a mixture of chemicals. Essential chemicals in food are called nutrients.

- ➤ Carbohydrates, lipids, proteins, vitamins, minerals, and water are the six classes of nutrients found in food.

- ➤ Nutrients have three general functions in the body: They serve as energy sources, structural components, and regulators of metabolic processes.

- ➤ Vitamins regulate body processes such as energy metabolism, blood clotting, and calcium balance.

- ➤ Minerals contribute to body structures and to regulating processes such as fluid balance.

- ➤ Water is the most important nutrient in the body. We can survive much longer without the other nutrients than we can without water.

- ➤ Energy in foods and the body is measured in kilocalories. Carbohydrates, fats, and proteins are sources of energy.

- ➤ Carbohydrate and protein have a potential energy value of 4 kilocalories per gram, and fat provides 9 kilocalories per gram.

- ➤ Scientific studies are the cornerstone of nutrition. The scientific method uses observation and inquiry to test hypotheses.

- ➤ Research designs used to test hypotheses include epidemiological, animal, cell culture, and human studies.

- ➤ Double-blind, placebo-controlled clinical trials are considered the "gold standard" of nutrition studies.

- ➤ Information in the public media is not always an accurate or complete representation of the current state of the science on a particular topic.

Study Questions

1. **What are the main factors that influence our food choices?**

2. **How do our health beliefs affect our food choices?**

3. **List the six classes of nutrients.**

4. **List the 13 vitamins.**

5. **What determines whether a mineral is a macro-mineral or a micro- (trace) mineral?**

6. **How many kilocalories are in 1 gram of carbohydrate, 1 gram of protein, and 1 gram of fat?**

7. **What is an epidemiological study?**

8. **What is the difference between an experimental and a control group?**

9. **What is a placebo?**

☞ [*Try*] This

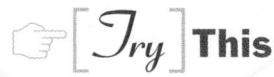

Try a New Cuisine Challenge

The purpose of this exercise is for you to expand your culinary taste buds and try a new cuisine. Take your local phone book and see how many ethnic restaurants are near campus. Choose a cuisine you are not very familiar with and take some friends along for dinner so you can order and share several dishes. While you're there, don't be afraid to ask questions about the menu, so you can gain a better understanding of the foods, preparation techniques, spices, and even the cultural meaning attached to some of the dishes.

Food Label Puzzle

The purpose of this exercise is to put the individual pieces of the food label together to determine how many kilocalories are in a serving. Pick six foods in your room or apartment that have complete food labels. Ask a friend to write down the value for calories on each label and then black out these numbers on the labels. Remember that the term *calories* on a food label really is referring to kilocalories. Your job is to determine how many kilocalories are in a serving of each of these foods. You can do this by putting together the individual pieces (carbohydrate, protein, and fat). If you need help, review this chapter and pay close attention to the section on the energy-yielding nutrients. How many kilocalories does each have per gram? You may find that the results of your calculations don't exactly match the numbers on the label. Within labeling guidelines, food manufacturers can round values.

What About *Bobbie?*

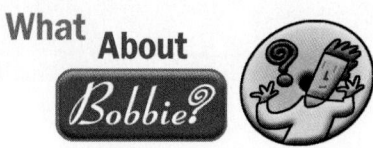

The "What About Bobbie?" feature appears in most chapters. Bobbie is a college student whom you'll follow throughout this text to learn the strengths and weaknesses of her diet. Look for this feature to see how the information you learn in each chapter can be applied to real life.

Bobbie is a 20-year-old college sophomore. She lives on campus and has one roommate. She has the standard meal plan with her university, so she eats most of her meals in the cafeteria. Sometimes she'll get a snack from a local coffee shop or a vending machine. Her schedule is fairly typical, with classes spread out in both the morning and afternoon. Occasionally at night, she and her friends will order pizza or go out for ice cream.

Bobbie weighs 155 pounds and is 5 feet, 4 inches tall. She gained 10 pounds her freshman year in college and would like to lose it because she feels healthier when her weight is closer to 145 pounds. She exercises infrequently but likes to walk with her friends and take an occasional aerobics class. Here is a typical day of eating for Bobbie:

Sample one-day menu from Bobbie's diet

7:45 A.M.
1 raisin bagel toasted
   3 tablespoons light cream cheese
10 fluid ounces regular coffee
   2 packets of sugar
   2 tablespoons of 2% milk

10:15 A.M.
1 banana

12:15 P.M.
Turkey sandwich
   2 slices sourdough bread
   2 ounces sliced turkey lunch meat
   2 teaspoons regular mayonnaise
   2 teaspoons mustard
   2 slices tomato
   2 slices dill pickle
   shredded lettuce
Salad from cafeteria salad bar
   2 cups shredded iceberg lettuce
   2 tablespoons each:
      shredded carrot
      chopped egg
      croutons
      kidney beans
      Italian salad dressing

12 fluid ounces diet soda
1 small chocolate chip cookie

3:30 P.M.
16 fluid ounces water
1.5 ounces regular tortilla chips
½ cup salsa

6:00 P.M.
Spaghetti with meatballs
   1 ½ cups pasta
   3 ounces ground beef (meatballs)
   3 ounces spaghetti sauce
   2 tablespoons Parmesan cheese
1 piece garlic bread
½ cup green beans
   1 teaspoon butter
12 fluid ounces diet soda

10:15 P.M.
1 slice cheese pizza

In later chapters, we will return to this one-day food record and examine Bobbie's intake in more detail.

References

1 Kennedy N. Learning to taste and food preferences begin in the early years of childhood. *San Francisco Chronicle.* January 12, 2005.

2 Gerrish CJ, Mennella JA. Flavor variety enhances food acceptance in formula-fed infants. *Am J Clin Nutr.* 2001;73(6):1080–1085.

3 Smith DV, Margolskee RF. Making sense of taste. *Scientific American.* 2001;284(3):32–39.

4 Yamaguchi S, Ninomiya K. Umami and food palatability. *J Nutr.* 2000;130:921S–926S.

5 Kim U, Jorgenson E, Coon H, et al. Positional cloning of the human quantitative trait locus underlying taste sensitivity to phenylthiocarbamide. *Science.* 2003;299;1221–1226.

6 Corbett RW, Ryan C, Weinrich SP. Pica in pregnancy: does it affect pregnancy outcome? *Am J Maternal/Child Nurs.* 2003;28:183–189.

7 Sandstead HH. Syndrome of iron deficiency anemia, hepatosplenomegaly, hypogonadism, dwarfism and geophagia. *J Trace Elements Exper Med.* 2001;14(2):145–155.

8 Ceonnell D, Goldberg JP, Folta SC. An intervention to increase fruit and vegetable consumption using audio communications: in-store public service announcements and audiotapes. *J Health Commun.* 2001;6(1):31–43.

9 Levy AS, Stokes RC. Effects of a health promotion advertising campaign on sales of ready-to-eat cereals. *Public Health Reports.* 1987;102(4):398–403.

10 Kuchler F. Golan E. Is there a role for government in reducing the prevalence of overweight and obesity? *Choices.* Fall 2004. http://www.choicesmagazine.org/2004-3/obesity/2004-3-03.htm. Accessed 5/17/06.

11 Birch LL. Development of food preferences. *Ann Rev Nutr.* 1999;19:41–62.

12 De Castro JM, Brewer ME. The amount eaten in meals by humans is a power function of the number of people present. *Physiol Behav.* 1991;51:121–125; and Patel KA, Schlundt DG. Impact of moods and social context on eating behavior. *Appetite.* 2001;36(2):111–118.

13 Dubois L, Girard M. Social position and nutrition: a gradient relationship in Canada and the USA. *Eur J Clin Nutr.* 2001;55(5):366–373.

14 Mooney K, Walbourn L. When college students reject food: not just a matter of taste. *Appetite.* 2001;36(1):41–50.

15 Drewnowski A, Spencer SE. Poverty and obesity: the role of energy density and energy costs. *Am J Clin Nutr.* 2004;79:6–16.

16 Blisard N, Stewart H, Jolliffe D. *Low-Income Households' Expenditures on Fruits and Vegetables.* Washington, DC: US Department of Agriculture, Economic Research Service, May 2004. Agricultural Economic Report, No. 833. http://www.ers.usda.gov/publications/AER833. Accessed 5/17/06.

17 Drewnowski A, Spencer SE. Op. cit.

18 Reed J, Frazão E, Itskowitz R. *How Much Do Americans Pay for Fruits and Vegetables?* Washington, DC: US Department of Agriculture, July 2004. Agriculture Information Bulletin, No. 790.

19 Sloan AE. What, when, and where Americans eat: 2003. *Food Tech.* 2003;57(8):48–66.

20 Rozin P. Human food intake choice: biological, psychological and cultural perspectives. *Eur J Clin. Nutr.* 2000;54(suppl 4):S1–S20.

21 Kittler PG, Sucher KP. *Food and Culture.* 4th ed. Belmont, CA: Wadsworth, 2004.

22 Fieldhouse P. *Food and Nutrition: Customs and Culture.* London: Chapman and Hall, 1996.

23 Zeman FJ, Ney DM. Cultural factors in nutrition care. In: Davis KM, ed. *Applications in Medical Nutrition Therapy.* Englewood Cliffs, NJ: Prentice-Hall, 1996:125–138.

24 Sloan AE. America's appetite '96: the top 10 trends to watch and work on. *Food Technology.* 1996;50:55–71.

25 Kittler PG, Sucher KP. Op. cit.

26 Zeman FJ, Ney DM. Op. cit.; Fieldhouse P. Op. cit.; and Kittler PG, Sucher KP. Op. cit.

27 Chiva M. Cultural aspects of meals and meal frequency. *Brit J Nutr.* 1997;77(suppl):S21–S28; and Zeman FJ, Ney DM. Op. cit.

28 Fieldhouse P. Op. cit.

29 Moshfegh A, Goldman J, Cleveland L. *What We Eat in America.* Washington, DC: US Department of Agriculture, Agricultural Research Service, 2005.

30 US Department of Agriculture, Center for Nutrition Policy and Promotion. Beliefs and attitudes of Americans toward their diet. *Nutrition Insights.* June 2000;19:1–2.

31 Lowell B. Regulation of energy expenditure. In: Tschoep M, ed. *Obesity.* http://www.endotext.org/obesity/index.htm. Accessed 6/6/06.

32 Hedley AA, Ogden CL, Johnson CL, et al. Overweight and obesity among US children, adolescents, and adults, 1999–2002. *JAMA* 2004;291:2847–2850.

33 US Department of Health and Human Services. *Healthy People 2010.* 2nd ed. Washington, DC: US Goverment Printing Office, November 2000. http://www.healthypeople.gov/. Accessed 5/17/06.

34 Kauwell GPA. Emerging concepts in nutrigenomics: a preview of what is to come. *Nutr Clin Pract.* 2005;20:75–87.

35 Johnston CS. Vitamin C. In: Bowman BA, RM Russell, eds. *Present Knowledge in Nutrition.* 8th ed. Washington DC: ILSI Press, 2001.

36 Alger SA, Schwalberg MD, Bigaouette JM, et al. Effect of a tricyclic antidepressant and opiate antagonist on binge-eating behavior in normal weight, bulimic, and obese binge-eating subjects. *Am J Clin Nutr.* 1991;53:865–871.

37 Hrobjartsson A, Gotzsche PC. Is the placebo powerless? An analysis of clinical trials comparing placebo with no treatment. *N Engl J Med.* 2001;344:1594–1602.

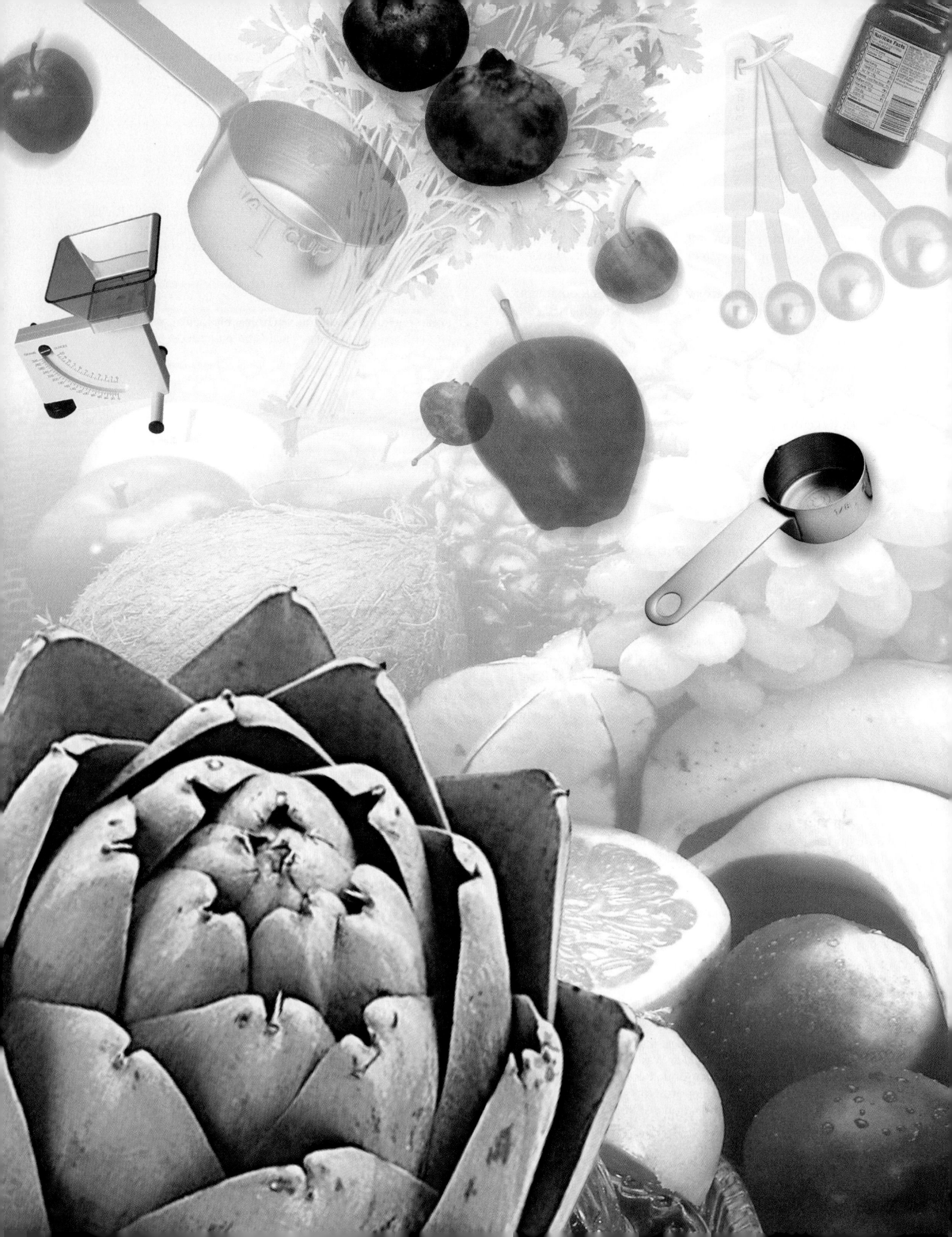

Chapter 2

Nutrition Guidelines and Assessment

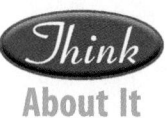 **Think About It**

1 Do you and your friends discuss food and diet?

2 Have you ever taken a very large dose of a vitamin or mineral? If so, why? How did you determine whether it was safe?

3 Do you eat the same foods most days, or do you like variety?

4 Which food group makes up the biggest part of your diet?

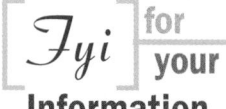 **Fyi for your Information**

This chapter's FYI boxes include practical information on the following topics:

- MyPyramid: Foods, Serving Sizes, and Tips

- Definitions for Nutrient Content Claims on Food Labels

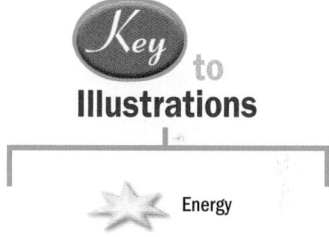 **Key to Illustrations**

Energy

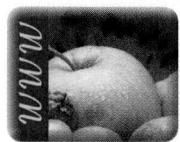

The Web site for this book offers many useful tools and is a great source for additional nutrition information for both students and instructors. For information on nutrition guidelines, visit the site at **nutrition.jbpub.com**. You'll find exercises that explore the following topics:

- Pros and Cons of Food Labeling

- Examining the DRIs

- The Healthy Eating Index

- Assessing a Diet Assessor

What About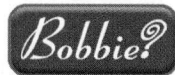

Track the choices Bobbie is making with Nutritionist Pro or EatRight Analysis software.

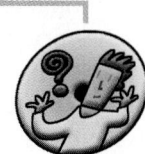

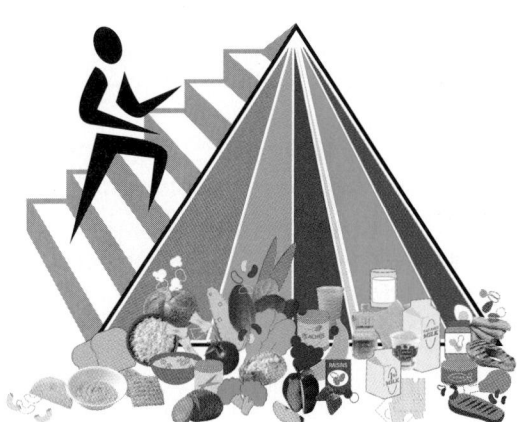

So, you want to be healthier—maybe that's why you are taking this course! You probably already know that a well-planned diet is one important element of being healthy. Although most of us know that the foods we choose have a major impact on our health, we aren't always certain about what choices to make. Choosing the right foods isn't made any easier when we are bombarded by headlines and advertisements: Eat less fat! Get more fiber in your diet! Moderation is the key! Build strong bones with calcium!

For many Americans, nutrition is simply a lot of hearsay, or maybe the latest slogan coined from last week's news headlines. Conversations about nutrition start off with *"They* say you should . . ." or "Now *they* think that . . ." Have you ever wondered who "they" are and why "they" are telling you what to eat or what not to eat?

It's no secret that a healthy population is a more productive population, so many of our nutrition guidelines come from the federal government's efforts to improve our overall health. Thus, the government is one "they." Many important elements of nutrition policy focus on relieving undernutrition in some population groups. To prevent widespread deficiencies, the government requires food manufacturers to add nutrients to certain foods: iodine to salt, vitamin D to milk, and thiamin, riboflavin, niacin, iron, and folic acid to enriched grains. Dietary standards such as the Dietary Reference Intakes make it easier to define adequate diets for large groups of people.

Overnutrition has led to changes in public policy as well. Health researchers have discovered links between diet and high blood pressure, cancer, and heart disease; as a result, nutritionists suggest that we reduce sodium and saturated fat intake. The public's need to know what is in the food supply has led to increased nutrition information on food labels. And public education efforts have resulted in the development of teaching tools such as MyPyramid.

New information about diet and health will continue to drive public policy. This chapter explores current dietary standards, guidelines, and diet-planning tools, as well as the measurements that evaluate nutritional health. While you're reading, think about your diet and how it measures up to current guidelines and standards.

Linking Nutrients, Foods, and Health

We all know that what we eat affects our health. Nutrition science has made many advances in identifying essential nutrients and the foods in which they are found. Eating foods with all the essential nutrients prevents nutritional deficiencies such as scurvy (vitamin C deficiency) or pellagra (deficiency of the B vitamin niacin). In the United States, few people suffer nutritional deficiencies as a result of dietary inadequacies. More often, Americans suffer from chronic diseases such as heart disease, cancer, hypertension, and diabetes—all linked to overconsumption and lifestyle choices. Your future health depends on today's lifestyle choices, including your food choices.

Think About It

1

Moderation, Variety, and Balance: Words to the Wise

Living in a high-tech world, we expect immediate solutions to long-term problems. It would be nice if we could avoid the consequences of overconsumption just by taking a pill, drinking a beverage, or getting a shot. But no magic food, nutrient, or drug exists. Instead, you have to rely on healthful foods, exercise, and lifestyle choices to reduce your risk of chronic disease. Even in the twenty-first century, we need to follow the same advice we have been hearing for decades: Healthful eating requires moderation, variety, and balance.

Moderation

Not too much or too little of anything—that's what moderation means. Moderation does *not* mean that you have to eliminate high-fat foods from your diet, but rather that you can occasionally include small amounts of them. Moderation also means not taking anything to extremes. You probably have heard that vitamin C has positive effects, but that doesn't mean huge doses of this essential nutrient are appropriate for you. It's important to remember that substances that are healthful in small amounts can sometimes be dangerous in large quantities. For example, the body needs zinc for hundreds of chemical reactions, including those that support normal growth, development, and immune function. Too much zinc, however, can cause deficiency of another essential mineral, copper, and can impair immune function.

Food guides and their graphics convey the message of moderation by showing suggested amounts of different food groups. Appearing in diverse shapes, food guides from other countries reflect their cultural contexts. Korea, for example, uses the shape of a pagoda. (See **Figure 2.1**.)

Variety

How many *different* foods do you eat on a daily basis? 10? 15? Would it surprise you that one of Japan's dietary guidelines suggests eating 30 different foods each day?[1] Now that's variety!

Variety means including lots of different foods in the diet: not just different food groups such as fruits, vegetables, and grains but also different foods from each group. Eating two bananas and three carrots each and every day may give you the minimum number of recommended daily servings for fruits and vegetables, but it doesn't add much variety.

Variety is important for a number of reasons. Eating a variety of fruits, for example, will provide a broader mix of vitamins, minerals, and phytochemicals than just including one or two fruits. Choosing a variety of protein sources, such as lean meat, fish, and legumes, will give you a different balance of fats and other nutrients than will always choosing hamburger or steak. Variety can add interest and excitement to your meals while preventing boredom with your diet. Perhaps most important, variety in your diet helps ensure that you get all the nutrients you need. Studies have shown that people who have varied diets take in more vitamin C and less sodium, sugar, and saturated fat.[2]

Balance

A healthful diet requires a balance of food groups, energy sources (carbohydrates, protein, and fat), and other nutrients. Your diet is balanced if you choose a variety of foods and eat a moderate amount. Your diet is balanced if the amount of energy (calories) you take in through what you eat equals the amount of energy you expend in daily activities and exercise.

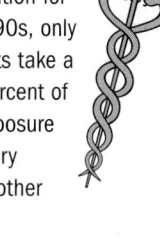
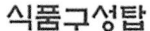

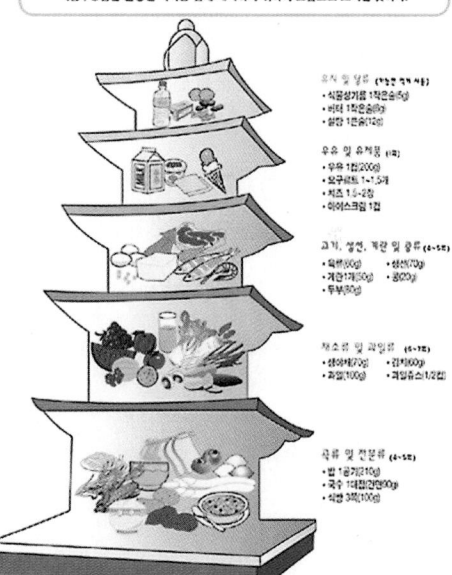

Figure 2.1 **Korean Dietary Guidelines.** Around the world, countries have adopted food guide presentations tailored to their individual cultures as well as physical needs. Both Korea and China use the pagoda shape for their food guides. The United States uses a pyramid and Canada uses a rainbow. Mexico and most European countries use a circular form.
Source: Painter J, Jee-Hyun R, Yeon-Kyung L. Comparison of international food guide pictorial representations. *J Am Diet Assoc.* 2002;102:483–489. © The American Dietetic Association. Reprinted with permission.

There is no magic diet, food, or supplement. Instead, your overall, long-term food choices can bring you the benefits of a healthful diet. Let's take a look at some general guidance for making those food choices.

Key Concepts: *Food and nutrient intake play a major role in health and risk of disease. For most Americans, overnutrition is more of a problem than undernutrition. The ideas of moderation, variety, and balance are important concepts in choosing a healthful diet.*

Dietary Guidelines

To help citizens improve their overall health, many countries have developed dietary guidelines—simple, easy-to-understand statements about food choices. Governments certainly have an interest in keeping their citizens healthier—a healthy population is more productive and puts less strain on health care resources. This section examines dietary guidelines for the United States and Canada.

Dietary Guidelines for Americans

In 1980 the **U.S. Department of Agriculture (USDA)** and the **U.S. Department of Health and Human Services (DHHS)** jointly released the first edition of the *Dietary Guidelines for Americans*. Revised guidelines have been released every five years as scientific information about links between diet and chronic disease is updated. The purpose of the *Dietary Guidelines for Americans* is to provide science-based advice to promote health and to reduce risk for chronic diseases through diet and physical activity.[3] The *Guidelines* are targeted to healthy Americans over the age of 2 years. Released in 2005, the most recent edition of the *Dietary Guidelines for Americans* (see **Figure 2.2**) offers key recommendations grouped under nine interrelated focus areas that are discussed in the following subsections. Taken together, these recommendations encourage Americans to eat fewer calories, be more active, and make wiser food choices.[4] You'll find additional recommendations for specific population groups highlighted in later chapters.

Adequate Nutrients Within Calorie Needs

One of the key elements of a healthful diet is selecting foods that will meet nutrient needs for growth and health while keeping calorie intake in line with calorie needs. By obtaining nutrients from foods rather than supplements, you also get the benefit of hundreds of phytochemicals and other naturally occurring substances that may reduce chronic disease risk.

Key Recommendations

- Consume a variety of nutrient-dense foods and beverages within and among the basic food groups while choosing foods that limit the intake of saturated and *trans* fats, cholesterol, added sugars, salt, and alcohol.

- Meet recommended intakes within energy needs by adopting a balanced eating pattern, such as the USDA Food Guide or the DASH Eating Plan.

Weight Management

Over the last 20 years, the prevalence of overweight and obesity has increased dramatically. Excess body fat is associated with increased risk for chronic diseases such as heart disease, cancer, high blood pressure, and dia-

U.S. Department of Agriculture (USDA) The government agency that monitors the production of eggs, poultry, and meat for adherence to standards of quality and wholesomeness. The USDA also provides public nutrition education, performs nutrition research, and administers the WIC program.

U.S. Department of Health and Human Services (DHHS) The principal federal agency responsible for protecting the health of all Americans and providing essential human services. The agency is especially concerned with those Americans who are least able to help themselves.

Dietary Guidelines for Americans The *Dietary Guidelines for Americans* are the foundation of federal nutrition policy and are developed by the U.S. Department of Agriculture (USDA) and the Department of Health and Human Services (DHHS). These science-based guidelines are intended to reduce the number of Americans who develop chronic diseases such as hypertension, diabetes, cardiovascular disease, obesity, and alcoholism.

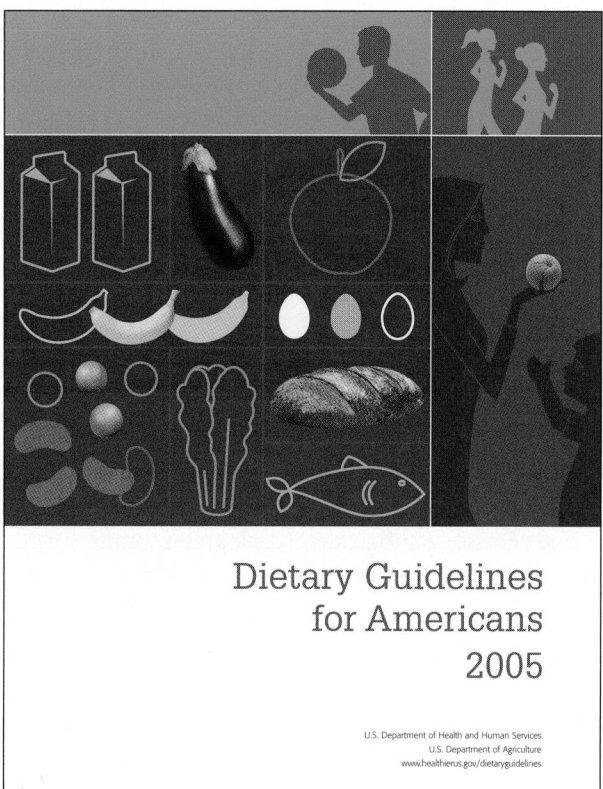

Dietary Guidelines
for Americans
2005

U.S. Department of Health and Human Services
U.S. Department of Agriculture
www.healthierus.gov/dietaryguidelines

Figure 2.2 ***Dietary Guidelines for Americans.*** A revised *Dietary Guidelines for Americans* was released in 2005.
Source: http://www.health.gov/dietaryguidelines/. Accessed 10/19/06.

betes. Ideally, adults should strive to achieve and maintain a weight that optimizes their health.

Key Recommendations

- To maintain body weight in a healthy range, balance calories from foods and beverages with calories expended.

- To prevent gradual weight gain over time, make small decreases in food and beverage calories and increase physical activity.

Physical Activity

Exercise is an important factor in weight control and overall fitness. Exercise can help lower chronic disease risk and improve emotional well-being. For disease risk reduction benefits, aim for at least 30 minutes of moderate-intensity activity on most days of the week. To prevent the gradual weight gain often associated with aging, more exercise is needed—60 minutes daily. Maintaining weight loss may require even more.

Key Recommendations

- Engage in regular physical activity and reduce sedentary activities to promote health, psychological well-being, and a healthy body weight.

- Achieve physical fitness by including cardiovascular conditioning, stretching exercises for flexibility, and resistance exercises or calisthenics for muscle strength and endurance.

Quick Bites

Do School Cafeterias Follow Nutrition Guidelines?

*C*hildhood obesity is on the rise, and high-fat school lunches may be part of the problem. Although the USDA mandated in 1995 that schools follow the *Dietary Guidelines for Americans* and reduce fat and salt in their cafeterias, many lunches still have too many calories from fat. In addition, according to a government study, children throw away 42 percent of cooked and 30 percent of raw vegetables. Every year, the government spends $7.9 billion on school lunches for more than 29 million children.

Food Groups to Encourage

Most Americans do not currently consume the recommended amounts of fruits, vegetables, whole grains, and fat-free or low-fat milk and milk products. In fact, according to one survey, only 23 percent of adults eat five or more servings of fruits and vegetables daily—about the same number that gets regular exercise![5]

Not only are these foods important sources of key nutrients, but also they contain other components, such as fiber and phytochemicals, that may help to reduce chronic disease risk.

Key Recommendations

- Consume a sufficient amount of fruits and vegetables while staying within energy needs. Two cups of fruit and 2½ cups of vegetables per day are recommended for a reference 2,000-calorie intake, with higher or lower amounts depending on the calorie level.

- Choose a variety of fruits and vegetables each day. In particular, select from all five vegetable subgroups (dark green, orange, legumes, starchy vegetables, and other vegetables) several times a week.

- Consume 3 or more ounce equivalents of whole-grain products per day, with the rest of the recommended grains coming from enriched or whole-grain products. In general, at least half the grains should come from whole grains.

- Consume 3 cups per day of fat-free or low-fat milk or equivalent milk products.

Fats

Although it is important to have some fat in the diet, high intake of saturated fats, *trans* fats, and cholesterol increases blood lipid levels, which, in turn, increase heart disease risk.

Key Recommendations

- Consume less than 10 percent of calories from saturated fatty acids and less than 300 milligrams per day of cholesterol, and keep *trans* fatty acid consumption as low as possible.

- Keep total fat intake between 20 to 35 percent of calories, with most fats coming from sources of polyunsaturated and monounsaturated fatty acids, such as fish, nuts, and vegetable oils.

- When selecting and preparing meat, poultry, dry beans, and milk or milk products, make choices that are lean, low-fat, or fat-free.

- Limit intake of fats and oils high in saturated or *trans* fatty acids or both, and choose products low in such fats and oils.

Carbohydrates

Carbohydrates are an important source of energy for the body, and high-carbohydrate foods often are also good sources of fiber. Diets rich in fiber can help lower chronic disease risk. High carbohydrate intake in the form of added sugar, however, can add excess calories to the diet without providing many nutrients.

Key Recommendations

- Choose fiber-rich fruits, vegetables, and whole grains often.

- Choose and prepare foods and beverages with little added sugars or caloric sweeteners, such as amounts suggested by the USDA Food Guide and the DASH Eating Plan.

American Dietetic Association

Total Diet Approach to Communicating Food and Nutrition Information

It is the position of the American Dietetic Association that all foods can fit in a healthful eating style. The ADA strives to communicate healthful eating messages to the public that emphasize the total diet, or overall pattern of food eaten, rather than any one food or meal. If consumed in moderation with appropriate portion size and combined with regular physical activity, all foods can fit into a healthful diet.

J Am Diet Assoc. 2002;102:100–108.
Reprinted with permission.

- Reduce the incidence of dental caries by practicing good oral hygiene and consuming sugar- and starch-containing foods and beverages less frequently.

Sodium and Potassium

High sodium intake (usually as sodium chloride, that is, table salt) is linked to high blood pressure. To reduce your risk of high blood pressure, eat less salt, eat more potassium, maintain a healthy weight, exercise regularly, and eat an overall healthful diet.

Key Recommendations

- Consume less than 2,300 milligrams of sodium per day (approximately 1 teaspoon of salt).
- Choose and prepare foods with little salt. At the same time, consume potassium-rich foods, such as fruits and vegetables.

Alcoholic Beverages

Alcohol may have beneficial effects on chronic disease risk when consumed in moderation. However, heavy alcohol consumption increases risk for liver disease, high blood pressure, and certain cancers. Some people should avoid alcohol completely.

Key Recommendations

- Those who choose to drink alcoholic beverages should do so sensibly and in moderation—defined as the consumption of up to one drink per day for women and up to two drinks per day for men.
- Some people should not consume alcoholic beverages: women of childbearing age who may become pregnant, pregnant and lactating women, people who cannot restrict their alcohol intake, people taking medications that can interact with alcohol, and those with specific medical conditions.
- People engaging in activities that require attention, skill, or coordination, such as driving or operating machinery, should avoid alcoholic beverages.

Food Safety

Proper food handling is an important way to avoid foodborne illnesses. It is estimated that about 76 million Americans become ill each year from harmful microorganisms in food.

Key Recommendations

- Clean your hands, food contact surfaces, and fruits and vegetables. Meat and poultry should not be washed or rinsed.
- Separate raw, cooked, and ready-to-eat foods while shopping, preparing, or storing foods.
- Cook foods to a safe temperature to kill microorganisms.
- Chill (refrigerate) perishable food promptly and defrost foods properly.
- Avoid raw (unpasteurized) milk or any products made from unpasteurized milk, raw or partially cooked eggs or foods containing raw eggs, raw or undercooked meat and poultry, unpasteurized juices, and raw sprouts.

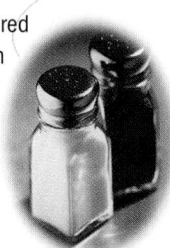

Quick Bites

Pass Up the Salt

We require only a few hundred milligrams of sodium each day, but this would be difficult to achieve given our current food supply, and would be unpalatable—so the guideline is to eat less sodium, but not down to the level of actual requirements.

Using the Guidelines

The *Dietary Guidelines for Americans* were written mainly for use by policy makers, health care providers, nutritionists, and nutrition educators. They form the foundation for federal nutrition policy and can be used in developing educational materials and designing nutrition-related government programs. They don't identify specific foods to consume or avoid, but instead give advice about the overall composition of the diet. Think about your diet and consider your overall food intake to determine whether it is consistent with the *Dietary Guidelines for Americans.* Choose more fruits, vegetables, and whole grains to make sure you are getting all the nutrients you need while lowering your intake of saturated fat, *trans* fat, and cholesterol. Eat fewer high-fat toppings and fried foods to help you balance energy intake and expenditure. Exercise regularly. Use the extra things—sugar, salt, and alcohol—in moderation. Drink water more often than soft drinks; and if you choose to drink alcohol at all, use caution.

Canada's Guidelines for Healthy Eating

Promoting healthy eating habits among Canadians has been a priority of Health Canada for many years. Health Canada is the federal department responsible for helping the people of Canada maintain and improve their health. In the 1980s, a high priority was given to developing a single set of dietary guidelines. The result of this effort was the 1990 *Nutrition Recommendations for Canadians.* This report updated the existing dietary standards and provided a scientific description of the characteristics of a healthy dietary pattern. Also published in 1990 was **Canada's Guidelines for Healthy Eating**, a set of five positive, action-oriented messages for healthy Canadians over the age of 2:[6]

- Enjoy a VARIETY of foods.
- Emphasize cereals, breads, other grain products, vegetables, and fruits.
- Choose lower-fat dairy products, leaner meats and foods prepared with little or no fat.
- Achieve and maintain a healthy body weight by enjoying regular physical activity and healthy eating.
- Limit salt, alcohol, and caffeine.

Dietary guidelines in the United States and Canada address similar issues—less fat; more fruits, vegetables and grains; less salt; and achieving healthy weights. In addition, both countries have developed graphic depictions of a healthful diet by showing the balance of food groups to be consumed each day. You can read about the USDA Food Guide Pyramid, its new MyPyramid, and *Canada's Food Guide to Healthy Eating* in the next section, "Food Groups and Food Guides." Canada's Guidelines for Healthy Eating is under review to bring recommendations in line with new knowledge of nutrient requirements and linkages between food patterns and risk of chronic disease.

Key Concepts: Dietary guidelines are statements based on current science that "guide" people toward more healthful choices. Both the United States and Canada have dietary guidelines that embody the basic principles of balance, variety, and moderation.

Food Groups and Food Guides

For many years, nutritionists and teachers have used **food groups** to illustrate the proper combination of foods in a healthful diet. Even young children can sort food into groups and fill a plate with foods from each group.

Nutrition Recommendations for Canadians A set of scientific statements that provide guidance to Canadians for a dietary pattern that will supply recommended amounts of all essential nutrients while reducing the risk of chronic disease.

Canada's Guidelines for Healthy Eating Key messages that are based on the 1990 *Nutrition Recommendations for Canadians* and provide positive, action-oriented, scientifically accurate eating advice to Canadians.

food groups Categories of similar foods, such as fruits or vegetables.

The foods within each group are similar because of their origins—fruits, for example, all come from the same part of different plants. But from a nutritional perspective, what fruits have in common is the balance of macronutrients and the similarities in micronutrient composition. Even so, the foods in one group may differ significantly in their vitamin and mineral profiles. Some fruits (e.g., citrus, strawberries, and kiwi) are rich in vitamin C, and others (e.g., apples and bananas) have very little. Here again, we can see the importance of variety, of not simply including different food groups but also choosing a variety of foods *within* each group.

A Brief History of Food Group Plans

In 1916, the USDA published its first daily food guide using food groups.[7] This initial guide stressed the importance of consuming enough fat and sugar, energy-rich foods to support daily activity. Because people performed more manual labor in those days, many people were simply not getting enough calories! Canada's Official Food Rules (1942) recommended a weekly serving of liver, heart, or kidney and regular doses of fish liver oils— good sources of vitamins A and D. Later food group plans, including the Basic Four that was popular from the 1950s through the 1970s, focused on fruits, vegetables, grains, dairy products, and meats and their substitutes.

The Basic Four food plan (dairy, meats, fruits and vegetables, and grains) was developed as a guide to a foundation diet; that is, it was intended to meet only a portion of the daily calorie and nutrient needs. The Basic Four was usually illustrated as either a circle or a square, with each group having an equal share. The implication was that people should consume equal amounts of food from each group. Nutrition science now tells us that those proportions give us a diet too high in fat and protein for our modern lifestyle, and not high enough in carbohydrates and fiber. After the development of the *Dietary Guidelines for Americans* in 1980, the USDA developed a new food guide that would promote overall health, and be consistent with the *Dietary Guidelines*. To bring this new food guide to the attention of consumers, there was a need for a memorable way to convey its key messages.[8] Consequently, in the late 1980s and early 1990s, both the USDA and Health Canada were working to develop a new graphic image for the food groups.

The USDA Food Guide Pyramid

In 1992 the USDA introduced the **Food Guide Pyramid** (see **Figure 2.3**) to visually represent the variety, moderation, and proportionality needed for a healthful diet.[9] The Pyramid was designed to illustrate the *Dietary Guidelines for Americans* in terms of food groups and recommended numbers of daily servings. The design of the Pyramid illustrated that plant foods (grains, fruits, and vegetables) were to make up the majority of daily food servings, and meat and meat alternates and dairy foods were to be consumed in smaller quantities. Fats, oils, and sweets at the tip of the Pyramid were recommended to be used sparingly. Just as with any form of dietary guidance, advances in science drive the need for change. So, in 2005, the USDA unveiled its new food guidance system: **MyPyramid** (see **Figure 2.4**).

MyPyramid

The USDA MyPyramid food guidance system is more than just a graphic. The system provides many options to help Americans make healthy food choices and be active every day. MyPyramid is based on both the *Dietary Guidelines for Americans* and the Dietary Reference Intakes, translating these

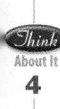

Think About It 4

Food Guide Pyramid A graphic representation of U.S. dietary guidelines; now replaced by MyPyramid.

MyPyramid An educational tool that translates the principles of the 2005 *Dietary Guidelines for Americans* and other nutritional standards to help consumers in making healthier food and physical activity choices.

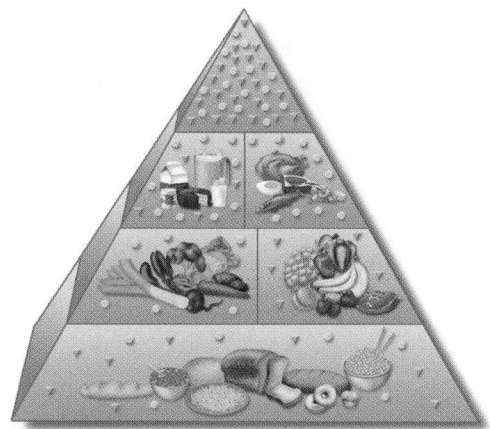

Figure 2.3 **Food Guide Pyramid.** The USDA's Food Guide Pyramid has been replaced by MyPyramid.
Source: U.S. Department of Agriculture. *The Food Guide Pyramid.* Home and Garden Bulletin, No. 252; August 1992, revised October 1996.

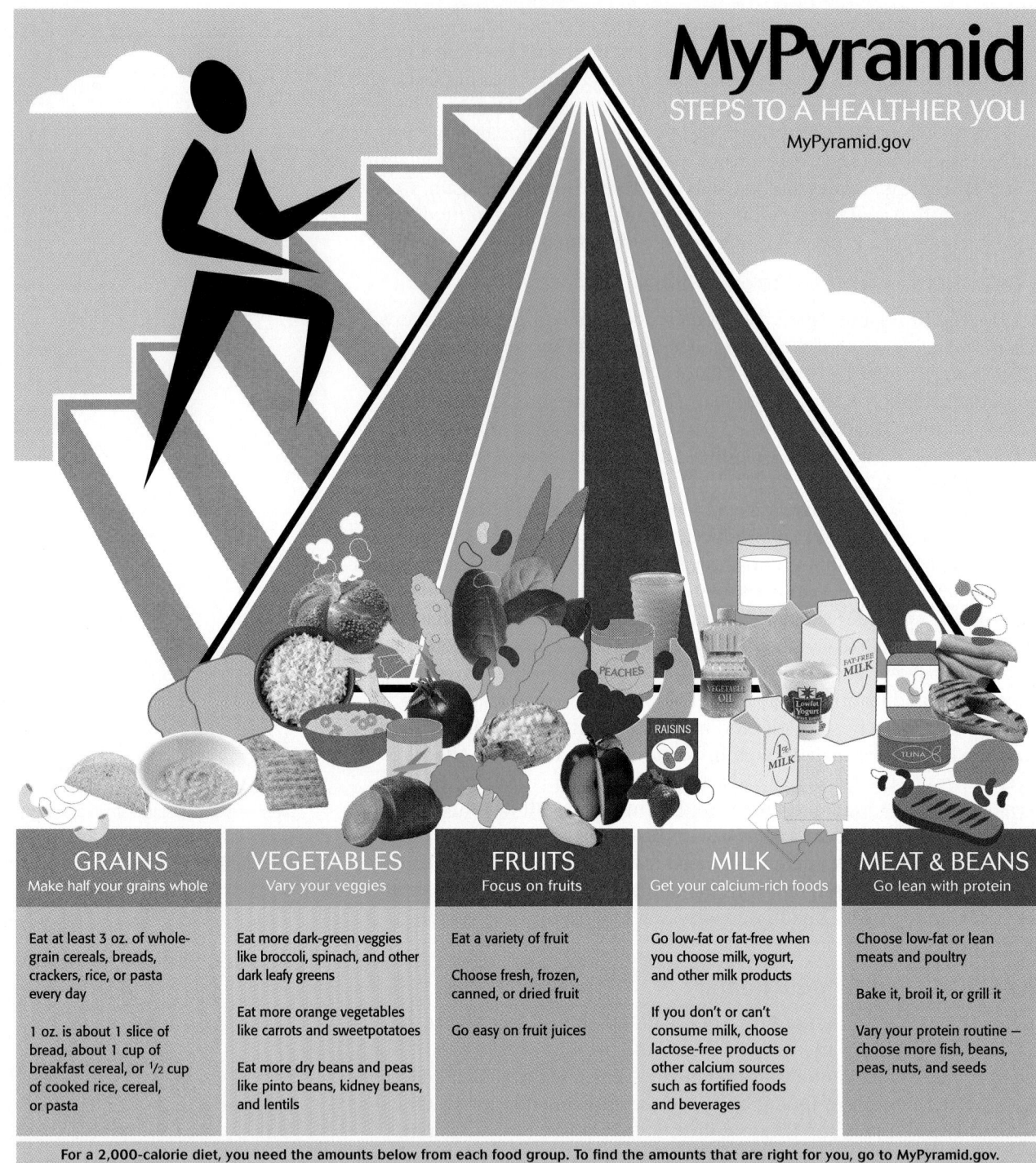

Figure 2.4 **MyPyramid.** Released in 2005, MyPyramid is an Internet-based educational tool that helps consumers implement the principles of the 2005 *Dietary Guidelines for Americans* and other nutritional standards. **Source:** www.MyPyramid.gov.

One size doesn't fit all

USDA's new MyPyramid symbolizes a personalized approach to healthy eating and physical activity. The symbol has been designed to be simple. It has been developed to remind consumers to make healthy food choices and to be active every day. The different parts of the symbol are described below.

Activity

Activity is represented by the steps and the person climbing them, as a reminder of the importance of daily physical activity.

Moderation

Moderation is represented by the narrowing of each food group from bottom to top. The wider base stands for foods with little or no solid fats or added sugars. These should be selected more often. The narrower top area stands for foods containing more added sugars and solid fats. The more active you are, the more of these foods can fit into your diet.

Personalization

Personalization is shown by the person on the steps, the slogan, and the URL. Find the kinds and amounts of food to eat each day at MyPyramid.gov.

Proportionality

Proportionality is shown by the different widths of the food group bands. The widths suggest how much food a person should choose from each group. The widths are just a general guide, not exact proportions. Check the Web site for how much is right for you.

Variety

Variety is symbolized by the 6 color bands representing the 5 food groups of the Pyramid and oils. This illustrates that foods from all groups are needed each day for good health.

Gradual Improvement

Gradual improvement is encouraged by the slogan. It suggests that individuals can benefit from taking small steps to improve their diet and lifestyle each day.

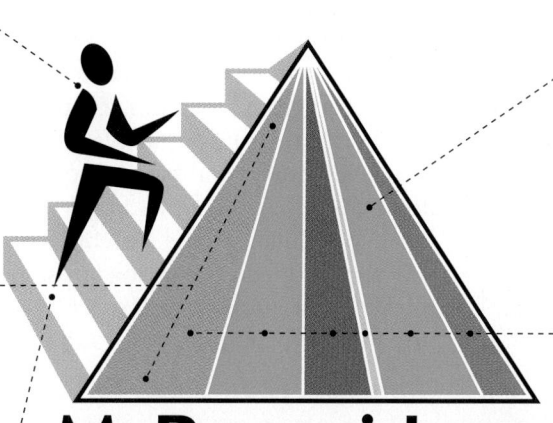

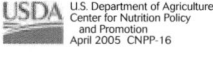

Figure 2.5 **One size doesn't fit all—anatomy of MyPyramid.** The USDA's MyPyramid symbolizes a personalized approach to healthy eating and physical activity. The symbol has been designed to remind consumers to make healthy food choices and be active every day. **Source:** www.MyPyramid.gov.

into a total diet that meets nutrient needs from food sources and that aims to moderate or limit dietary components often consumed in excess. The new MyPyramid symbol (see **Figure 2.5**) was designed to be a simple visual reminder to make healthy food choices and be physically active every day. More detailed information is available online at MyPyramid.gov.

MyPyramid illustrates six basic concepts:

- *Variety*, symbolized by the six color bands representing the five food groups of MyPyramid plus oils. Foods from all groups are needed each day for good health.
- *Moderation*, represented by the narrowing of each food group from bottom to top. The wider base stands for foods with little or no solid fats, added sugars, or caloric sweeteners. These should be selected more often to get the most nutrition from calories consumed.
- *Proportionality*, shown by the different widths of the food group bands. The widths suggest how much food a person should choose from each group.

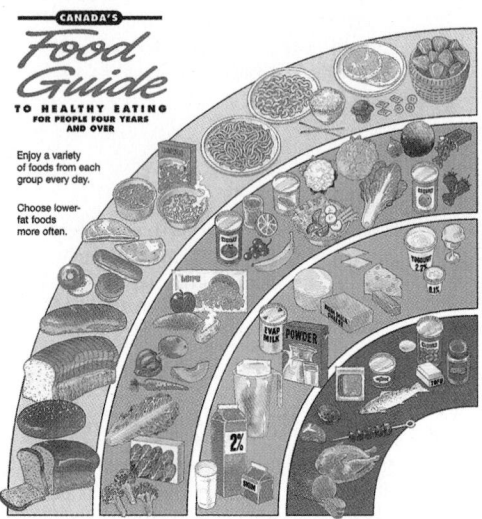

Grain Products	Vegetables and Fruit	Milk Products	Meat and Alternatives
Choose whole grain and enriched products more often.	Choose dark green and orange vegetables and orange fruit more often.	Choose lower-fat milk products more often.	Choose leaner meats, poultry and fish, as well as dried peas, beans and lentils more often.

Figure 2.6 **Canada's Food Guide to Healthy Eating.** The rainbow portion of *Canada's Food Guide* sorts food into groups from which people can make wise food choices. For the complete guide, see Appendix D.
Source: Health Canada. Using the *Food Guide.* http://www.hc-sc.gc.ca/fn-an/food-guide-aliment/ res/using_food_guide-servir_guide_alimentaire_e.html. Accessed 2/15/06. Reproduced with the permission of the Minister of Public Works and Government Services Canada.

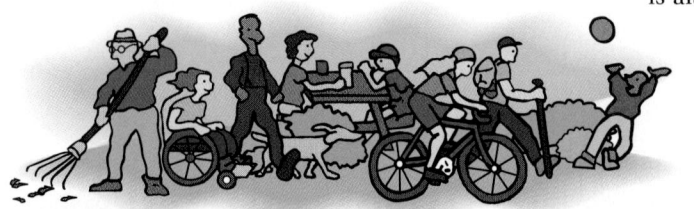

Figure 2.7 **Vitality.** Health Canada promotes the concept of vitality—enjoying eating well, being active, and feeling good about yourself.
Source: Health Canada. Using the *Food Guide.* http://www.hc-sc.gc.ca/fn-an/ food-guide-aliment/res/using_food_guide-servir_guide_alimentaire_e.html. Accessed 2/15/06. Reproduced with the permission of the Minister of Public Works and Government Services Canada.

- *Physical activity*, represented by the steps and the person climbing them, as a reminder of the importance of daily physical activity.
- *Gradual improvement*, encouraged by the slogan "Steps to a Healthier You." Individuals can benefit from taking small steps to improve their diet and lifestyle each day.
- *Personalization*, demonstrated by the MyPyramid Web site. There, you can get a personalized recommendation regarding the kinds and amounts of food to eat each day.

The MyPyramid.gov Web site provides more in-depth information for every food group, including examples of foods, recommended amounts, and everyday tips. You can also develop a customized MyPyramid Plan that gives a quick estimate of how much you should eat from the different food groups, or you can set up MyPyramid Tracker to compare a typical day's food intake to the current recommendations. See the FYI feature "MyPyramid: Foods, Serving Sizes, and Tips" later in this chapter for examples of foods and serving sizes for each of the groups. A complete set of food intake patterns can be found in Appendix C.

Canada's Food Guide to Healthy Eating

As science advanced and nutritional concerns changed, Canada's Official Food Rules evolved into **Canada's Food Guide to Healthy Eating** (see **Figure 2.6**). The *Food Guide* is based on the *Nutrition Recommendations for Canadians* and is a key educational tool for Canadians aged 4 years and over. The "rainbow" side of the *Food Guide* places foods into four groups: Grain Products, Vegetables and Fruits, Milk Products, and Meat and Alternatives. It also describes the kinds of foods to choose from each group. For example, under the Vegetables and Fruit group, the *Food Guide* suggests "Choose dark-green and orange vegetables and orange fruit more often." *Canada's Food Guide* illustrates that grains, vegetables, and fruits should be the major part of the diet, with milk products and meats in smaller amounts.

The "bar" side of the *Food Guide* (see Appendix D) shows how many daily servings are recommended from each group and gives examples of serving sizes. For milk products, recommendations are specific to each age group, and also for pregnant and breastfeeding women. In addition, the *Food Guide* acknowledges that "other foods" in moderation can be incorporated into a healthy diet. The *Food Guide* is currently undergoing revision.

Eating a healthful diet based on *Canada's Food Guide to Healthy Eating* is a cornerstone of Vitality, a concept that grew out of Health Canada's strategy to promote healthy weights. The three principles of Vitality—eating well, being active, and feeling good about yourself—aim to enhance people's physical, psychological, and social well-being. (See **Figure 2.7**.) Vitality is also concerned with creating environments in the community that support healthy choices.

Using MyPyramid or *Canada's Food Guide* in Diet Planning

Before you start using MyPyramid or *Canada's Food Guide* for diet planning, become familiar with the types of food in each group, the number of recommended servings, and the appropriate serving sizes. (For an intuitive guide to serving sizes, see **Table 2.1**.) Let's take fruits, for example. According to MyPyramid, a 2,000-calorie diet should include 2 cups of fruit each day.

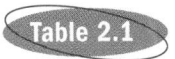 **Table 2.1** **Playing with Pyramid Portions**

Your favorite sports and games can help you visualize MyPyramid portion sizes.

GRAINS	1 cup dry cereal	2 ounce bagel	1/2 cup cooked cereal, rice, or pasta
	4 golf balls	1 hockey puck	tennis ball
VEGETABLES	1 cup of vegetables		
	1 baseball or 1 Rubik's cube		
FRUITS	1 large orange (equivalent of 1 cup of fruit)		
	1 softball		
OILS	1 teaspoon vegetable oil	1 Tablespoon salad dressing	
	1 die (11/16″ size)	1 jacks ball	
MILK	1 1/2 ounces of hard cheese	1/3 cup shredded cheese	
	6 dice (11/16″ size)	1 billiard ball or racquetball	
MEAT AND BEANS	3 ounces cooked meat	2 tablespoons hummus	
	1 deck of playing cards	1 ping pong ball	

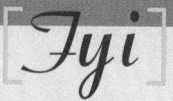
MyPyramid: Foods, Serving Sizes, and Tips
FOR YOUR INFORMATION

Grains	Amount Equal to 1 Ounce	Common Portions and Ounce Equivalents
Bagels	1 "mini" bagel	1 large bagel = 4 ounce equivalents
Biscuits	1 small (2″ diameter)	1 large (3″) = 2 ounce equivalents
Breads	1 regular slice	2 regular slices = 2 ounce equivalents
Bulgur	½ cup cooked	
Cornbread	1 small piece (2½″ × 1¼″ × 1¼″)	1 medium piece = 2 ounce equivalents
English muffin	½ muffin	1 muffin = 2 ounce equivalents
Muffins	1 small (2½″ diameter)	1 large (3½″ diameter) = 3 ounce equivalents
Oatmeal	½ cup cooked	
Pancakes	1 pancake (4½″ diameter)	3 pancakes (4½″ diameter) = 3 ounce equivalents
Popcorn	3 cups, popped	1 microwave bag, popped = 4 ounce equivalents
Ready-to-eat cereals	1 cup flakes; 1¼ cups puffed	
Rice	½ cup cooked (1 ounce dry)	1 cup cooked = 2 ounce equivalents
Pasta	½ cup cooked (1 ounce dry)	1 cup cooked = 2 ounce equivalents
Tortillas	1 small (6″ diameter)	1 large (12″ diameter) = 4 ounce equivalents

Tips: Make half your grains whole. Choose foods that name one of the following first on the label's ingredient list: brown rice, bulgur, graham flour, oatmeal, whole oats, whole rye, whole wheat, wild rice. Go easy on high-fat or sugary toppings.

Vegetables	Amount Equal to 1 Cup of Vegetables	Vegetables	Amount Equal to 1 Cup of Vegetables
Dark-Green Vegetables		**Starchy Vegetables**	
Spinach, romaine, collards, mustard greens, kale, other leafy greens	2 cups raw or 1 cup cooked	Corn	1 cup or 1 large ear (8″ to 9″ long)
		Green peas	1 cup
		White potatoes	1 cup diced or mashed
Broccoli	1 cup chopped or florets		1 medium potato, boiled or baked
Orange Vegetables		**Other Vegetables**	
Carrots	1 cup, raw or cooked	Bean sprouts	1 cup cooked
	2 medium whole	Green beans	1 cup cooked
	1 cup baby carrots (about 12)	Mushrooms	1 cup raw or cooked
Pumpkin, sweet potato, winter squash	1 cup, cooked	Tomatoes	1 large raw whole (3″)
Dry Beans and Peas			1 cup chopped, sliced, or cooked
Black, garbanzo, kidney, pinto, soy beans; black-eyed peas, split peas	1 cup whole or mashed, cooked		
Tofu	1 cup of ½″ cubes		

Tips: Vary your veggies. Eat more dark-green vegetables, more orange vegetables, more dry beans and peas. Buy fresh vegetables in season for best taste and lowest cost. Buy vegetables that are easy to prepare.

Fruit	Amount Equal to 1 Cup of Fruit	Milk	Amount Equal to 1 Cup of Milk
Apple	1 small	Milk	1 cup
Applesauce	1 cup	Yogurt	1 regular container (8 ounces)
Banana	1 large (8" to 9" long)	Cheese	1½ ounces hard cheese
Melon	1 cup diced or melon balls		⅓ cup shredded cheese
Grapes	1 cup whole; 32 seedless grapes		2 ounces processed cheese
Canned fruit or diced raw fruit	1 cup		2 cups cottage cheese
Orange or peach	1 large	Milk-based desserts	1 cup pudding made with milk
Strawberries	About 8 large berries		1 cup frozen yogurt
100% fruit juice	1 cup		
Avocado	½ avocado		

Tips: Focus on fruit. Eat a variety of fruit. Choose fresh, frozen, canned, or dried fruit. Go easy on juices. When choosing a juice, look for "100% juice" on the label.

Tips: Get your calcium-rich foods. Go low-fat or fat-free. If you don't or can't consume milk, choose lactose-free or other calcium sources such as calcium-fortified juices, cereals, breads, soy beverages, or rice beverages.

Meat and Beans	Amount Equal to 1 Ounce
Cooked lean beef, pork, ham	1 ounce
Cooked chicken or turkey, without skin	1 ounce
Cooked fish or shellfish	1 ounce

Common Portions and Ounce Equivalents

1 small steak = 3½ to 4 ounce equivalents
1 small lean hamburger = 2 to 3 ounce equivalents
1 small chicken breast half = 3 ounce equivalents
1 can tuna, drained = 3 to 4 ounce equivalents
1 salmon steak = 4 to 6 ounce equivalents
1 small trout = 3 ounce equivalents

Eggs	1 egg
Nuts and seeds	½ ounce of nuts (12 almonds, 24 pistachios, 7 walnut halves)
	½ ounce of seeds, roasted
	1 tablespoon of peanut butter
Dry beans and peas	¼ cup cooked dry beans or peas
	¼ cup baked beans, refried beans
	¼ cup tofu
	1 ounce tempeh
	2 tablespoons hummus

Tips: Go lean on protein. Choose low-fat or lean meats and poultry. Bake it, broil it, or grill it. Vary your choices, with more fish, beans, peas, nuts, and seeds.

Oils

Vegetable oils (canola, corn, cottonseed, olive, safflower, soybean, sunflower)
Nuts
Olives
Some fish
Avocados

Tips: Know your oils. Make most of your fat sources from fish, nuts, and vegetable oils. Limit solid fats such as butter, stick margarine, shortening, and lard.

Source: USDA. MyPyramid. http://www.MyPyramid.gov. Accessed 11/20/06.

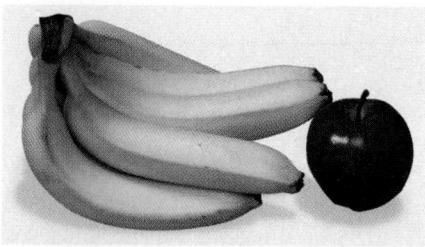

2–4 servings of fruit

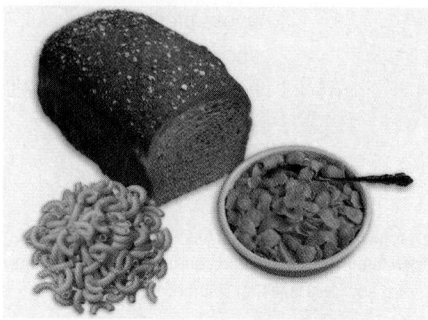

6–11 servings of bread, pasta, rice, and cereal

Exchange Lists for Meal Planning Lists of foods that in specified portions provide equivalent amounts of carbohydrate, fat, protein, and energy. Any food in an Exchange List can be substituted for any other without markedly affecting macronutrient intake.

Suppose you have 4 fluid ounces of orange juice for breakfast and half a banana on your cereal. Add an apple for an afternoon snack, and you have already had 2 cups!

Now let's try the grain group. Six ounce equivalents of grain (with half from whole grains) is recommended for 2,000 calories. A bowl (approximately 1 cup) of cornflakes cereal and a slice of whole-wheat toast for breakfast would be 2 ounces. A sandwich with two slices of whole-wheat bread for lunch adds 2 more. Add a cup of pasta with dinner, and you've got all 6 ounces! So, you see, it's not hard to meet the recommendations.

Table 2.2 shows the recommended amounts of food for three calorie-intake levels. This table will give you an idea of how MyPyramid varies with different energy needs. Keep in mind that what you may consider a serving may differ from the sizes defined in MyPyramid. Research shows that Americans' serving sizes for common foods such as pasta, cookies, cereal, soft drinks, and french fries have increased significantly.[10] Do large portions promote overeating and obesity? See the Nutrition Science in Action feature "Portion Distortion" for a scientific exploration related to this question.

Sometimes it's difficult to figure out how to account for foods that are mixtures of different groups—lasagna, casseroles, or pizza, for example. Try separating such foods into their ingredients (e.g., pizza contains crust, tomato sauce, cheese, and toppings, which might be meats or vegetables) to estimate the amounts. You should be able to come up with a reasonable approximation. All in all, MyPyramid and *Canada's Food Guide* are easy-to-use guidelines that can help you select a variety of foods.

Key Concepts: *MyPyramid is a complete food guidance system based on the* Dietary Guidelines for Americans *and Dietary Reference Intakes to help Americans make healthy food choices and remind them to be active every day. The interactive tools on the MyPyramid.gov Web site can help you monitor your food choices.*

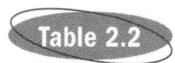 **Table 2.2** **MyPyramid Suggested Daily Amounts for Three Levels of Energy Intake**

	Energy Intake Level		
Food Group	*Low* (1,400 kcal)[a]	*Moderate* (2,000 kcal)[b]	*High* (2,800 kcal)[c]
Grains	5 oz eq	6 oz eq	10 oz eq
Vegetables	1½ cups	2½ cups	3½ cups
Fruits	1½ cups	2 cups	2½ cups
Milk	2 cups	3 cups	3 cups
Meat and beans	4 oz eq	5½ oz eq	7 oz eq
Oils	4 tsp	6 tsp	8 tsp

[a]1,400 kilocalories is about right for many young children.
[b]2,000 kilocalories is about right for teenaged girls, active women, and many sedentary men.
[c]2,800 kilocalories is about right for teenaged boys, and many active men.

Note: Your calorie needs may be higher or lower than those shown. Women may need more calories when they are pregnant or breastfeeding.

Source: Adapted from MyPyramid. http://mypyramid.gov. Accessed 2/15/06.

Canada's Food Guide to Healthy Eating *illustrates the* Nutrition Recommendations for Canadians. *These graphic tools show the appropriate balance of food groups in a healthful diet: more whole grains, vegetables, and fruits and less dairy, meat, and added fats and sugars.*

Exchange Lists

Another tool for diet planning that uses food groups is called the **Exchange Lists for Meal Planning**. Like MyPyramid, the Exchange Lists divide foods into groups. Diets can be planned by choosing a certain number of servings, or exchanges, from each group each day. The original purpose of the Exchange Lists was to help people with diabetes plan diets that would provide consistent levels of energy and carbohydrates—both are essential for dietary management of diabetes. For this reason, the foods are organized into groups or lists not only by the type of food (e.g., fruits or vegetables) but also by the amount of macronutrients (carbohydrate, protein, and fat) in each portion. The portions are defined so that each "exchange" has a similar composition. For example, 1 fruit exchange is ½ cup of orange juice or 17 small grapes or 1 medium apple or ½ cup of applesauce. All of these exchanges have approximately 60 kilocalories, 15 grams of carbohydrate, 0 grams of protein, and 0 grams of fat. In the Exchange Lists, starchy vegetables such as potatoes, corn, and peas are grouped with breads and cereals instead of with other vegetables because their balance of macronutrients is more like bread or pasta than carrots or tomatoes.

Figure 2.8 shows the amounts of carbohydrate, protein, fat, and kilocalories in one exchange from each group, along with a sample serving size. For a complete set of the Exchange Lists, see Appendix B or go to **nutrition.jbpub.com**.

Using the Exchange Lists in Diet Planning

In addition to their use by people with diabetes, Exchange Lists are used in many weight-control programs. Planning a diet using the Exchange Lists is done in much the same manner as using MyPyramid. The first step is to become very familiar with the components of each group, the variations in fat content for the dairy and meat lists, and ways that other foods may be included. Then, an individual diet plan can be used to select meals and snacks throughout the day. An exchange-based diet plan specifies the number of exchanges

Key

- Energy kilocalories
- Carbohydrate grams
- Protein grams
- Fat grams

	Energy	Carbohydrate	Protein	Fat	
Starch	80	15	3	<1	1 slice bread = ½ English muffin = ½ c. corn or peas = ⅓ c. pasta
Fruits	60	15	0	0	1 small apple = 17 small grapes = ½ c. orange juice = ½ c. applesauce
Fat-free and low-fat milk	90	12	8	0-3	1 cup fat-free or 1% milk = ⅔ c. plain fat-free yogurt
Reduced fat milk	120	12	8	5	1 cup 2% milk = ¾ c. plain low-fat yogurt
Whole milk	150	12	8	8	1 cup whole milk
Other	Varies	15	Varies	Varies	3 sm. sugar-free cookies = 2 Tbsp light syrup = ½ c. gelatin
Vegetables	25	5	2	0	1 c. raw salad greens = ½ c. cooked carrots = 1 lg. tomato
Very lean	35	0	7	0-1	1 oz chicken = 1 oz canned (water packed) tuna = ½ c. cooked beans = ¼ c. low-fat cottage cheese
Lean	55	0	7	3	1 oz beef tenderloin = 1 oz salmon = 1 oz roast pork
Medium fat	75	0	7	5	1 oz ground beef = 4 oz tofu = 1 egg
High fat	100	0	7	8	1 oz sausage = 1 oz cheese = 1 turkey hot dog
Fats	45	0	0	5	1 tsp butter = 8 large black olives = 1 slice bacon = 10 peanuts

Figure 2.8 **Exchange Lists for Meal Planning.** This is a widely used system for meal planning for people with diabetes. It is also helpful for people interested in healthy eating and weight control. See Appendix B for the complete Exchange Lists.
Source: American Diabetes Association and the American Dietetic Association. *Exchange Lists for Meal Planning.* Alexandria, VA: 2003.

NUTRITION SCIENCE IN ACTION

Portion Distortion

Observations: The increasing portion sizes of convenience food parallel the rising prevalence of obesity in the United States. Although large portions of food may contribute to excess energy intake and obesity, this link has not been well studied.

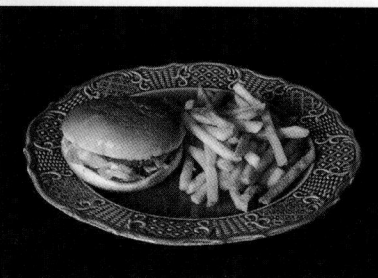
20 years ago

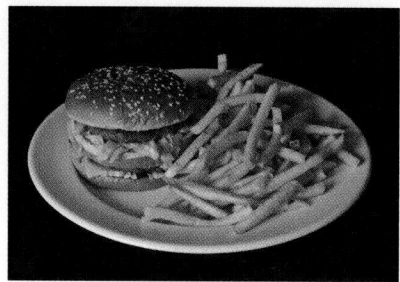
Today

Hypothesis: Larger portion sizes lead to greater energy intake.

Experimental Plan: Using posters and newspaper advertisements, recruit 51 male and female adult study participants, in good health and not currently dieting or trying to gain weight. On four separate days at least one week apart, have participants eat a lunch entrée of macaroni and cheese. At each lunch, offer each participant one of four portion sizes: 500, 600, 750, or 1,000 grams. Among participants, randomly vary the order of the four portion sizes.

Results: As the portion size of the lunch entrée increased, participants consumed significantly greater amounts. Participants consumed 30 percent more food and energy when presented with the largest portion than when presented with the smallest portion.

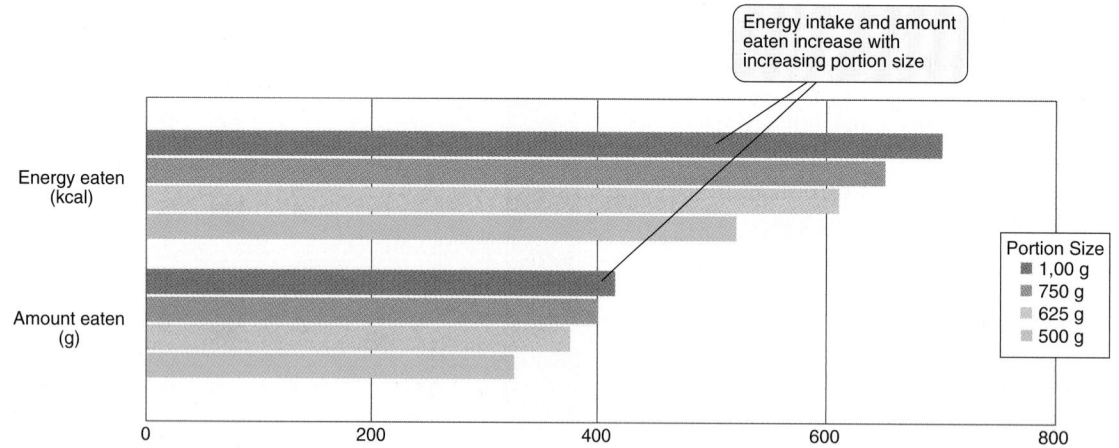

Energy intake and amount eaten increase with increasing portion size

Conclusion and Discussion: The results show that increasing the portion size of macaroni and cheese directly increases food intake by adults during a single meal. Additional research is needed to determine whether the effect persists over a longer period or whether people compensate for excess energy intake by reducing their intake at subsequent meals. Because portion sizes can be modified easily—either positively or negatively—portion sizes should be considered in efforts to prevent and treat obesity.

Source: Based on Rolls BJ, Morris EL, Roe LS. Portion size of food affects energy intake in normal-weight and overweight men and women. *Am J Clin Nutr.* 2002;76:1207–1213.

to be consumed from each group at each meal. For example, a 1,500-kilocalorie weight reduction diet plan might have the following meal pattern:

Breakfast:	2 starch, 1 fruit, 1 milk, 1 fat
Lunch:	3 meat, 2 starch, 1 fruit, 1 vegetable, 1 fat
Snack:	1 milk, 1 starch, 1 fat
Dinner:	2 meat, 1 starch, 2 vegetable, 2 fat
Snack:	2 starch, 1 fruit

Using this pattern and a complete set of the Exchange Lists, you could then plan out a day or week of menus. Here's one sample:

Breakfast:	$\frac{1}{2}$ cup orange juice, $\frac{3}{4}$ cup corn flakes, 1 cup 2% milk, 1 slice toast, 1 tsp margarine
Lunch:	3 oz cooked hamburger on bun, 1 tsp mayonnaise, $\frac{1}{2}$ cup baby carrots, 1 medium apple
Snack:	$\frac{3}{4}$ cup low-fat yogurt, $\frac{1}{2}$ bagel with 1 Tbsp cream cheese
Dinner:	2 oz cooked pork chop, $\frac{1}{2}$ cup rice with 1 tsp margarine, $\frac{1}{2}$ cup yellow squash and $\frac{1}{2}$ cup zucchini stir-fried in 1 tsp vegetable oil
Snack:	1 toasted English muffin, 1 medium pear

Key Concepts: *The Exchange Lists are a diet-planning tool that uses the idea of food groups, but defines groups specifically in terms of macronutrient (carbohydrate, fat, and protein) content. Individual diet plans can be developed for people who need to control energy or carbohydrate intake, such as for weight control or management of diabetes mellitus.*

Recommendations for Nutrient Intake: The DRIs

So far, the tools we have described (*Dietary Guidelines for Americans,* Canada's Guidelines for Healthy Eating, MyPyramid, *Canada's Food Guide,* and Exchange Lists) have dealt with whole foods and food groups rather than individual nutrient values; foods are what we think about in planning our daily meals and shopping lists. Sometimes, though, we need more specific information about our nutritional needs—a healthful diet is healthful because of the balance of *nutrients* it contains. Before we can choose foods that meet our needs for specific nutrients, we need to know how much of each nutrient we require daily. This is what **dietary standards** do—they define healthful diets in terms of specific amounts of the nutrients.

Understanding Dietary Standards

Dietary standards are sets of recommended intake values for nutrients. These standards tell us how much of each nutrient we should have in our diets. In the United States and Canada, the **Dietary Reference Intakes (DRIs)** are the current dietary standards.

Consider the following scenario. You are running a research center located in Antarctica and staffed by 60 people. Because they will not be able to leave the site to get meals, you must provide all of their food. You must keep the group adequately nourished; you certainly don't want anyone to become ill as a result of a nutrient deficiency. How would you (or the nutritionist you hire) start planning? How can you be sure to provide adequate amounts of the essential nutrients? The most important tool would be a set of dietary standards! Essentially the same scenario faces those who plan and provide food for groups of people in more routine circumstances—the

dietary standards Set of values for recommended intake of nutrients.

Dietary Reference Intakes (DRIs) A framework of dietary standards that includes Estimated Average Requirement (EAR), Recommended Dietary Allowance (RDA), Adequate Intake (AI), and Tolerable Upper Intake Level (UL).

Recommended Nutrient Intakes (RNIs) Canadian dietary standards that have been replaced by Dietary Reference Intakes.

Recommended Dietary Allowances (RDAs) The nutrient intake levels that meet the nutrient needs of almost all (97 to 98 percent) individuals in a life-stage and gender group.

Food and Nutrition Board A board within the Institute of Medicine of the National Academy of Sciences. It is responsible for assembling the group of nutrition scientists who review available scientific data to determine appropriate intake levels of the known essential nutrients.

Figure 2.9 **Dietary Reference Intakes.** The Dietary Reference Intakes are a set of dietary standards that include Estimated Average Requirement (EAR), Recommended Dietary Allowance (RDA), Adequate Intake (AI), and Tolerable Upper Intake Level (UL).

military, prisons, and even schools. To assess nutritional adequacy, diet planners can compare the nutrient composition of their food plans to recommended intake values.

A Brief History of Dietary Standards

Beginning in 1938, Health Canada published dietary standards called **Recommended Nutrient Intakes (RNIs)**. In the United States, the **Recommended Dietary Allowances (RDAs)** were first published in 1941. By the 1940s, nutrition scientists had been able to isolate and identify many of the nutrients in food. They were able to measure the amounts of these nutrients in foods and to recommend daily intake levels. These levels then became the first RNI and RDA values. Committees of scientists regularly reviewed the standards and published revised editions; for example, the tenth (and final) edition of RDAs was published in 1989.

In the mid-1990s, the **Food and Nutrition Board** of the National Academy of Sciences began a partnership with Health Canada to make fundamental changes in the approach to setting dietary standards and to replace the RDAs and RNIs. In 1997, the first set of DRIs was published for calcium, phosphorus, magnesium, vitamin D, and fluoride—nutrients that are important for bone health.

Dietary Reference Intakes

Since the inception of the RDAs and RNIs, we have learned more about the relationships between diet and chronic disease, and nutrient-deficiency diseases have become rare in the United States and Canada. The new DRIs reflect not just intake levels for dietary adequacy but also for optimal nutrition.

The DRIs are reference values for nutrient intakes to be used in assessing and planning diets for healthy people. (See **Figure 2.9**.) The Dietary Reference Intakes include four basic elements: Estimated Average Requirement (EAR), Recommended Dietary Allowance (RDA), Adequate Intake (AI), and Tolerable Upper Intake Level (UL). Underlying each of these values is the definition of a **requirement** as the "lowest continuing intake level of a nutrient that, for a specific indicator of adequacy, will maintain a defined level of nutriture in an individual."[11] In other words, a requirement is the smallest amount of a nutrient you should take in on a regular basis to remain healthy. In the DRI report on macronutrients, two other concepts were introduced: the Estimated Energy Requirement (EER) and the Acceptable Macronutrient Distribution Ranges (AMDRs).[12]

THE DRIs: DIETARY REFERENCE INTAKES

All DRI values refer to intakes averaged over time

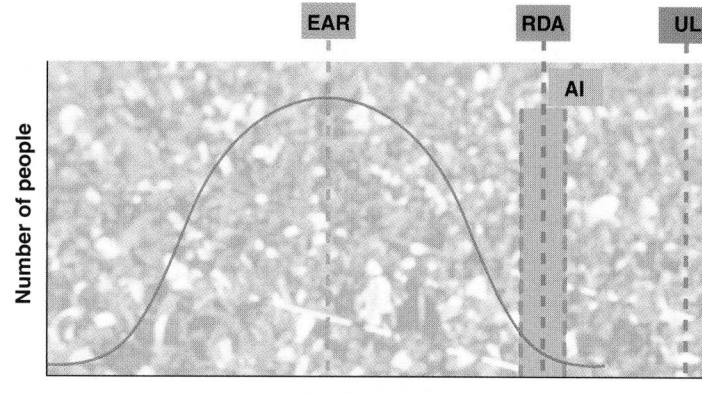

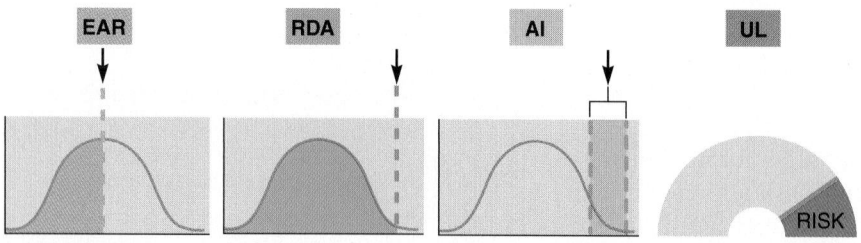

The **Estimated Average Requirement** is the nutrient intake level estimated to meet the need of 50% of the individuals in a life-stage and gender group.

The **Recommended Dietary Allowance** is the nutrient intake level that is sufficient to meet the need of 97–98% of the individuals in a life-stage and gender group. The RDA is calculated from the EAR.

Adequate Intake is based upon expert estimates of nutrient intake by a defined group of healthy people. These estimates are used when there is insufficient scientific evidence to establish an EAR. AI is not equivalent to RDA.

Tolerable Upper Intake Level is the maximum level of daily nutrient intake that poses little risk of adverse health effects to almost all of the individuals in a defined group. In most cases, supplements must be consumed to reach a UL.

Estimated Average Requirement

The **Estimated Average Requirement (EAR)** reflects the amount of a nutrient that would meet the needs of 50 percent of the people in a particular life-stage (age) and gender group. For each nutrient, this requirement is defined using a specific indicator of dietary adequacy. This indicator could be the level of the nutrient or one of its breakdown products in the blood, or the amount of an enzyme associated with that nutrient.[13] The EAR is used to set the RDA, and EAR values can also be used to assess dietary adequacy or plan diets for groups of people.

Recommended Dietary Allowance

The Recommended Dietary Allowance (RDA) is the daily intake level that meets the needs of most people (97 to 98 percent) in a life-stage and gender group. The RDA is set at two standard deviations above the EAR. A nutrient will not have an RDA value if there are not enough scientific data available to set an EAR value.

People can use the RDA value as a target or goal for dietary intake, and make comparisons between actual intake and RDA values. It is important to remember, however, that the RDAs do not define an *individual's* nutrient requirements. Your actual nutrient needs may be much lower than average, and therefore the RDA would be much more than you need. An analysis of your diet might show, for example, that you consume 45 percent of the RDA for a certain vitamin, but that might be adequate for your needs. Only specific laboratory or other tests can determine a person's true nutrient requirements and actual nutritional status. An intake that is consistently at or near the RDA level is highly likely to be meeting your needs.

requirement The lowest continuing intake level of a nutrient that prevents deficiency in an individual.

Estimated Average Requirement (EAR) The intake value that meets the estimated nutrient needs of 50 percent of individuals in a specific life-stage and gender group.

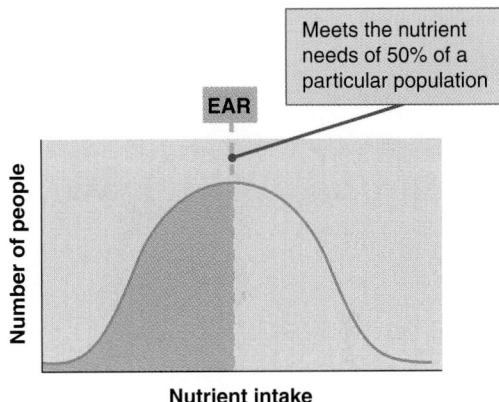

ESTIMATED AVERAGE REQUIREMENT

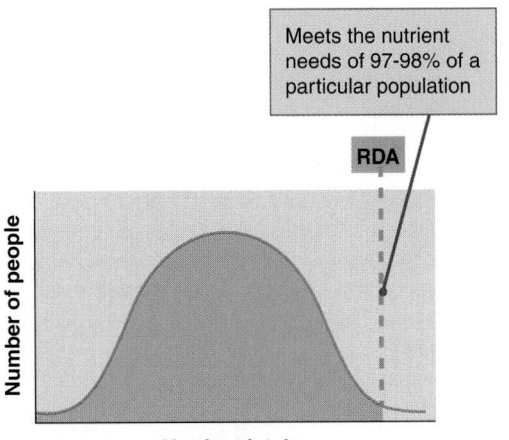

RECOMMENDED DIETARY ALLOWANCE

The RDA takes into account 97–98% of the population.

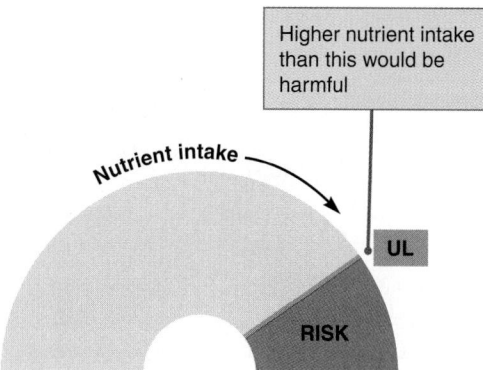

Target intake level of a nutrient based on people's estimated dietary intake

AI

Number of people

Nutrient intake

ADEQUATE INTAKE

Higher nutrient intake than this would be harmful

Nutrient intake

UL

RISK

TOLERABLE UPPER INTAKE LEVEL

Adequate Intake (AI) The nutrient intake that appears to sustain a defined nutritional state or some other indicator of health (e.g., growth rate or normal circulating nutrient values) in a specific population or subgroup. AI is used when there is insufficient scientific evidence to establish an EAR.

Tolerable Upper Intake Levels (ULs) The maximum levels of daily nutrient intakes that are unlikely to pose health risks to almost all of the individuals in the group for whom they are designed.

Estimated Energy Requirement (EER) Dietary energy intake that is predicted to maintain energy balance in a healthy adult of a defined age, gender, weight, height, and level of physical activity consistent with good health.

Acceptable Macronutrient Distribution Ranges (AMDRs) Range of intakes for a particular energy source that are associated with reduced risk of chronic disease while providing adequate intakes of essential nutrients.

Adequate Intake

If not enough scientific data are available to set an EAR level, a value called an **Adequate Intake (AI)** is determined instead. AI values are determined in part by observing healthy groups of people and estimating their dietary intake. All the current DRI values for infants are AI levels because there have been too few scientific studies to determine specific requirements in infants. Instead, AI values for infants are usually based on nutrient levels in human breast milk, a complete food for newborns and young infants. Values for older infants and children are extrapolated from human milk and from data on adults. For nutrients with AI instead of RDA values for all life-stage groups (e.g., calcium, vitamin D), more scientific research is needed to better define the nutrient requirements of population groups. AI values can be considered target intake levels for individuals.

Tolerable Upper Intake Level

Tolerable Upper Intake Levels (ULs) have been defined for many nutrients. Consumption of a nutrient in amounts higher than the UL could be harmful. The ULs have been developed partly in response to the growing interest in dietary supplements that contain large amounts of essential nutrients. The UL is *not* to be used as a target for intake, but rather should be a cautionary level for people who regularly take nutrient supplements.

Estimated Energy Requirement

The **Estimated Energy Requirement (EER)** is defined as the energy intake that is estimated to maintain energy balance in healthy, normal-weight individuals. It is determined using an equation that considers weight, height, age, and physical activity. Different equations are used for males and females and for different age groups. These equations are described in more detail in Chapter 8, "Energy Balance, Body Composition and Weight Management."

Acceptable Macronutrient Distribution Ranges

Acceptable Macronutrient Distribution Ranges (AMDRs) indicate the recommended balance of energy sources in a healthful diet. These values consider the amounts of macronutrients needed to provide adequate intake of essential nutrients while reducing the risk for chronic disease. The AMDRs are shown in **Table 2.3**.

Table 2.3	Acceptable Macronutrient Distribution Ranges for Adults
Fat	20–35
Carbohydrate	45–65
Protein	10–35
n-6 Polyunsaturated fatty acids	5–10
α-Linolenic acid	0.6–1.2

Note: All values are percentage of energy intake.
Source: Institute of Medicine, Food and Nutrition Board. *Dietary Reference Intakes for Energy, Carbohydrate, Fiber, Fat, Fatty Acids, Cholesterol, Protein, and Amino Acids.* Washington, DC: National Academy Press; 2005. Reprinted with permission.

Use of Dietary Standards

The most appropriate use of DRIs is to plan and evaluate diets for large groups of people. Remember the North Pole scenario at the beginning of this section? If you had planned menus and evaluated the nutrient composition of the foods that would be included and if the average nutrient levels of those daily menus met or exceeded the RDA/AI levels, you could be confident that your group would be adequately nourished. If you had a very large group—thousands of soldiers, for instance—the EAR would be a more appropriate guide.

Dietary standards are also used to make decisions about nutrition policy. The Special Supplemental Food Program for Women, Infants, and Children (WIC), for example, takes into account the DRIs as it provides food or vouchers for food. The goal of this federally funded supplemental feeding program is to improve the nutrient intake of low-income pregnant and breastfeeding women, their infants, and young children. The guidelines for school lunch and breakfast programs are also based on DRI values.

Often, we use dietary standards as comparison values for individual diets, something you may be doing in class. It can be interesting to see how your daily intake of a nutrient compares to the RDA or AI. However, an intake that is less than the RDA/AI doesn't necessarily mean deficiency; your individual requirement for a nutrient may be less than the RDA/AI value. You can use the RDA/AI values as targets for dietary intake, while avoiding nutrient intake that exceeds the UL.

Future of the DRIs

The Food and Nutrition Board continues to develop DRI values in an ongoing review and revision process. By 2005, all the essential nutrients had been included. Future reports will consider phytochemicals and other food components. In addition, the Food and Nutrition Board is partnering with the Food and Drug Administration to incorporate DRI values into nutrition labeling standards.

Key Concepts: *Dietary standards are levels of nutrient intake recommended for healthy people. These standards help the government set nutrition policy and also can be used to guide the planning and evaluation of diets for groups and individuals. The Dietary Reference Intakes are the dietary standards for the United States and Canada. These standards focus on maintaining optimal health and lowering the risks of chronic disease, rather than simply on dietary adequacy.*

Food Labels

Now that you understand diet-planning tools and dietary standards, let's focus on your use of these tools—for example, when making decisions at the grocery store. One of the most useful tools in planning a healthful diet is the **food label**.

Specific federal regulations control what can and cannot appear on a food label and what *must* appear on it. The **Food and Drug Administration (FDA)** is responsible for assuring that foods sold in the United States are safe, wholesome, and properly labeled. The Health Products and Food Branch of Health Canada has similar responsibilities. The FDA's jurisdiction does not include meat, meat products, poultry, or poultry products; the USDA regulates these foods.

food label Labels required by law on virtually all packaged foods with five requirements: (1) a statement of identity; (2) the net contents (by weight, volume, or measure) of the package; (3) the name and address of the manufacturer, packer, or distributor; (4) a list of ingredients; and (5) nutrition information.

Food and Drug Administration (FDA) The federal agency responsible for assuring that foods sold in the United States (except for eggs, poultry, and meat, which are monitored by the USDA) are safe, wholesome, and labeled properly. The FDA sets standards for the composition of some foods, inspects food plants, and monitors imported foods. The FDA is an agency of the Department of Health and Human Services (DHHS).

Nutrition Labeling and Education Act (NLEA) An amendment to the Food, Drug, and Cosmetic Act of 1938. The NLEA made major changes to the content and scope of the nutrition label and to other elements of food labels. Final regulations were published in 1993 and went into effect in 1994.

statement of identity Mandate that commercial food products display prominently the common or usual name of the product or identify the food with an "appropriately descriptive term."

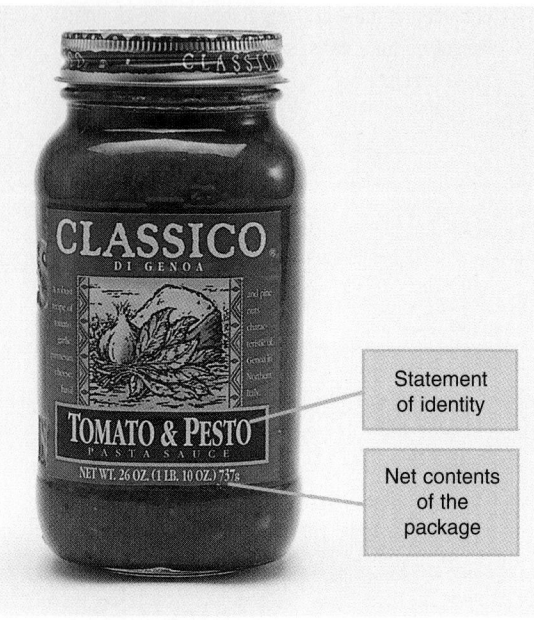

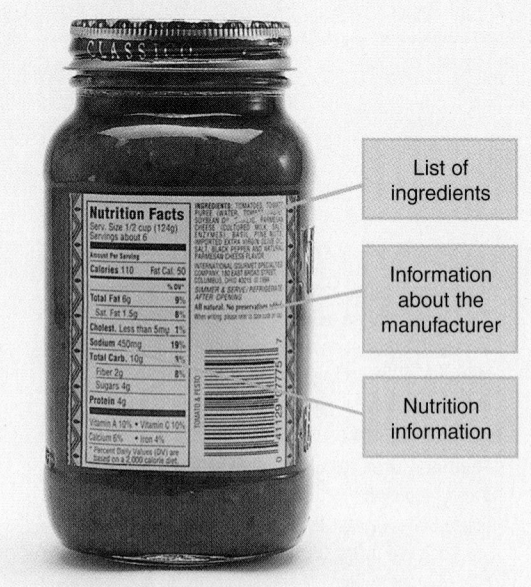

Figure 2.10 **The five mandatory requirements for food labels.** Federal regulations determine what can and cannot appear on food labels.

As information about the role of diet in chronic disease grew during the 1970s and 1980s, so did the demand for nutrition labels on all food products. As a result, in 1990 Congress passed the **Nutrition Labeling and Education Act (NLEA)**. Once the necessary regulations had been developed, new "Nutrition Facts" labels began appearing on foods in 1994. By 1997, 96.5 percent of food products had nutrition labels.[14] Voluntary nutrition labeling was introduced in Canada in 1988, and final regulations to make nutrition labeling mandatory were released in 2002. Canadian nutrition labels now are similar in format to U.S. nutrition labels.

Ingredients and Other Basic Information

The label on a food you buy today has been shaped by many sets of regulations. As **Figure 2.10** shows, food labels have five mandatory components:

1. A statement of identity
2. The net contents of the package
3. The name and address of the manufacturer, packer, or distributor
4. A list of ingredients
5. Nutrition information

The **statement of identity** requirement means that the product must prominently display the common or usual name of the product or identify the food with an "appropriately descriptive term." For example, it would be misleading to label a fruit beverage containing only 10 percent fruit juice as a "juice." The statement of net package contents must accurately reflect the quantity in terms of weight, volume, measure, or numerical count. Information about the manufacturer, packer, or distributor gives consumers a way to contact someone in case they have questions about the product. Ingredients must be listed by common or usual name, in descending order by weight; thus, the first ingredient listed is the primary ingredient in that food product. Let's compare two cereals:

Cereal A ingredients: Milled corn, sugar, salt, malt flavoring, high-fructose corn syrup

Cereal B ingredients: Sugar, yellow corn flour, rice flour, wheat flour, whole oat flour, partially hydrogenated vegetable oil (contains one or more of the following oils: canola, soybean, cottonseed), salt, cocoa, artificial flavor, corn syrup

In Cereal B, the first ingredient listed is sugar, which means this cereal contains more sugar by weight than any other ingredient. Cereal A's primary ingredient is milled corn. If we were to read the nutrition information, we would find that a one-cup serving of Cereal A contains 2 grams of sugars, whereas a similar amount of Cereal B contains 12 grams of sugars. Quite a difference!

As you probably have noticed, when the ingredient list includes the artificial sweetener aspartame, it also displays a warning statement. Also, preservatives and other additives in foods must be listed, along with an explanation of their function. Accurate and complete ingredient information is vital for people with food allergies who must avoid certain food components. As of January 2006, the labels of foods that contain any of the eight major food allergens (egg, wheat, peanuts, milk, tree nuts, soy, fish, and crustaceans) are required to include common names when listing these ingredients. For example, an ingredient list might show "albumen (egg)."

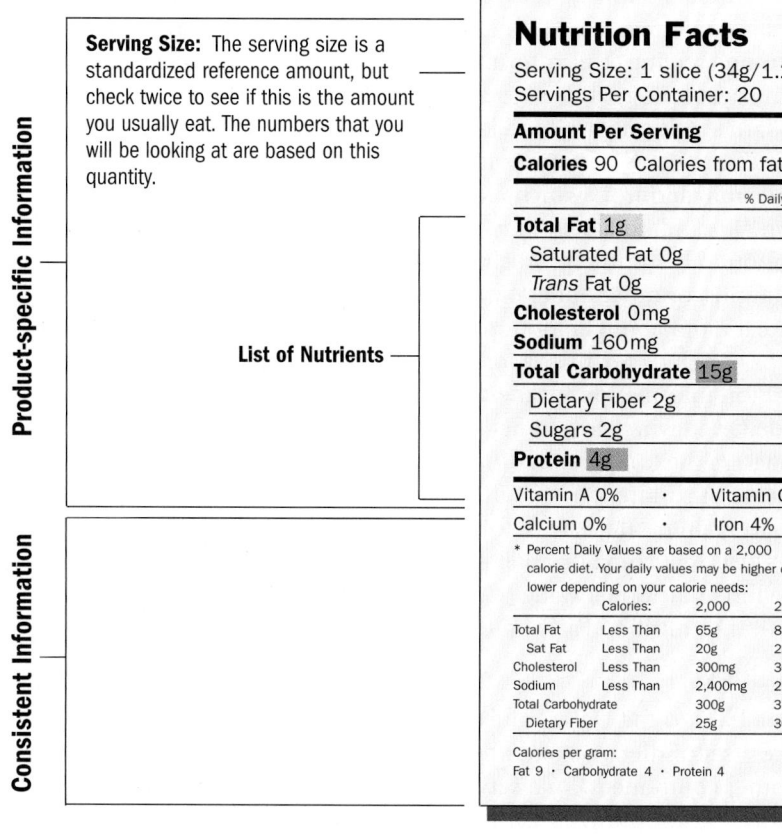

Serving Size: The serving size is a standardized reference amount, but check twice to see if this is the amount you usually eat. The numbers that you will be looking at are based on this quantity.

List of Nutrients

Product-specific Information

Consistent Information

Title

Calories Per Serving: Having the number of calories and the number of calories from fat next to each other makes it easy to see if a food is high in fat.

% Daily Values: These percentages are based on the values given below in the footnote for a 2,000-calorie diet. If your caloric intake is different, you will need to adjust these values appropriately.

Daily Values Footnote: Daily Values are shown for two caloric intake levels to emphasize the importance of evaluating your own diet to apply the information on the label.

Caloric Conversion Information: Handy reference values help you check the math on your own calculations!

Figure 2.11 **The Nutrition Facts panel.** Consumers can use the Nutrition Facts panel to compare the nutritional values of different products.

Nutrition Facts A portion of the food label that states the content of selected nutrients in a food in a standard way prescribed by the Food and Drug Administration. By law Nutrition Facts must appear on nearly all processed food products in the United States.

Nutrition Facts Panel

The **Nutrition Facts** panel contains the most important label information for the health-conscious consumer. The Food Marketing Institute's 2004 survey *Shopping for Health* indicated that 83 percent of shoppers regularly check the Nutrition Facts panel when buying a product for the first time, and 91 percent will make a purchasing decision based on nutrition information.[15] Although fat content is the most frequently sought piece of information, consumers are also looking for foods that are "low calorie," "whole grain," and "low salt/sodium." The Nutrition Facts panel not only is a source of information about the nutritional value of a food product but can also be used to compare similar products.

Let's take a closer look at the elements of the Nutrition Facts panel. It was designed so that the nutrition information would be easy to find on the label. The heading "Nutrition Facts" stands out clearly (see **Figure 2.11**). Just under the heading is information about the serving size and number of servings per container. It is important to note the serving size, because all of the nutrient information that follows is based on that amount of food, and the listed serving size may be different from what you usually eat. An 8-ounce bag of potato chips may be a small snack to a hungry college student, but according to the manufacturer the bag really contains eight servings! Serving sizes are standardized according to reference amounts developed by the FDA. Similar products (cereals, for instance) will have similar serving sizes (1 ounce).

The next part of the label shows the calories per serving and the calories that come from fat. This information reveals at a glance whether a food product is high or low in fat. If most of the calories in a product come from fat, it

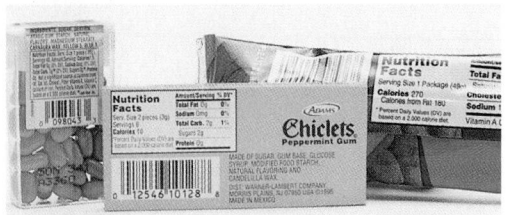

Figure 2.12 **Nutrition Facts on small packages.** When a product package has insufficient space to display a full Nutrition Facts panel, manufacturers may use an abbreviated version.

enrich The addition of vitamins and minerals lost or diminished during food processing, particularly the addition of thiamin, riboflavin, niacin, folic acid, and iron to grain products.

fortify Refers to the addition of vitamins or minerals that weren't originally present in a food.

Daily Values (DVs) A single set of nutrient intake standards developed by the Food and Drug Administration to represent the needs of the "typical" consumer, and used as standards for expressing nutrient content on food labels.

nutrient content claims These claims describe the level of a nutrient or dietary substance in the product, using terms such as *good source*, *high*, or *free*.

is a high-fat food. Following this is a list of the amounts of total fat, saturated fat, *trans* fat, cholesterol, sodium, total carbohydrate, dietary fiber, sugars, and protein in one serving. This information is given both in quantity (grams or milligrams per serving) and as a percentage of the Daily Value—a comparison standard specifically for food labels (this standard is described in the following section). Listed next are percentages of Daily Values for vitamins A and C, calcium, and iron, which are the only micronutrients that must appear on all standard labels. Manufacturers may choose to include information about other nutrients, such as potassium, polyunsaturated fat, additional vitamins, or other minerals, in the Nutrition Facts panel. However, if they make a claim about an optional component (e.g., "good source of vitamin E") or **enrich** or **fortify** the food, the manufacturers must include specific nutrition information for these added nutrients. This information must be included even when government regulations require enrichment or fortification, such as the fortification of milk with vitamin D to prevent rickets (a bone disease in children that results from vitamin D deficiency) and the fortification of grain products with folic acid to reduce the risk of birth defects. Food products that come in small packages (e.g., gum, candy, and tuna) or that have little nutritional value (e.g., diet soft drinks) can have abbreviated versions of the Nutrition Facts on the label, as **Figure 2.12** shows.

Daily Values

Let's come back to the Daily Values part of the label. The **Daily Values (DVs)** are a set of dietary standards used to compare the amount of a nutrient (or other component) in a serving of food to the amount recommended for daily consumption. This information lets consumers see at a glance how a food fits into their diets. Let's say you rely on your breakfast cereal as a major source of dietary fiber intake. Comparing two packages, as in **Figure 2.13**, you find that a serving of corn flakes cereal has 4 percent of the DV for dietary fiber, but choosing bran flakes cereal will give you 20 percent. You don't have to know anything about grams to see which has more! You can find a complete list of Daily Values inside the back cover of this text. Keep in mind that the Daily Values (which were established in 1993) may not exactly match the more recent DRI values, but in most cases, the differences are small.

Nutrient Content Claims

The NLEA and the associated FDA regulations allow food manufacturers to make **nutrient content claims** using a variety of descriptive terms on labels, such as *low fat* and *high fiber*. The FYI feature "Definitions for Nutrient Content Claims on Food Labels" contains a list of terms that may be used. The FDA has made an effort to make the terms meaningful, and the regulations have reduced the number of potentially misleading label statements. It would be misleading, for example, to print "cholesterol free" on a can of vegetable shortening—a food that is 100 percent fat and high in saturated and *trans* fatty acids (types of fat that raise blood cholesterol levels). This type of statement misleads consumers who associate "cholesterol free" with "heart healthy." Under the NLEA regulations, statements about low cholesterol content can be used only when the product is also low in saturated fat (less than 2 grams per serving). In addition to the content claims defined in the regulations, companies may submit to the FDA a notification of a new nutrient content claim based on "an authoritative statement from an appropriate scientific body of the United States Government or the National Academy of Sciences."[16] A nutrient content claim related to choline was

Nutrition Facts

| Serving Size: | | 1 Cup (28g/1.0 oz.) |
| Servings Per Container: | | About 18 |

Amount Per Serving	Cereal	with 1/2 cup Skim Milk
Calories	100	140
Fat Calories	0	0
% Daily Value		
Total Fat 0g	0%	0%
Saturated Fat 0g	0%	0%
Trans Fat 0g		
Cholesterol 0mg	0%	0%
Sodium 300mg	13%	15%
Potassium 25mg	1%	7%
Total Carbohydrate 24g	8%	10%
Dietary Fiber 1g	4%	4%
Sugars 2g		
Other Carbohydrates 21g		
Protein 2g		
Vitamin A	15%	20%
Vitamin C	25%	25%
Calcium	0%	15%
Iron	45%	45%
Vitamin D	10%	25%
Thiamin	25%	30%
Riboflavin	25%	35%
Niacin	25%	25%
Vitamin B$_6$	25%	25%
Folate	25%	25%
Vitamin B$_{12}$	25%	35%

Nutrition Facts

| Serving Size: | | 3/4 Cup (30g) |
| Servings Per Container: | | About 15 |

Amount Per Serving	Cereal	with 1/2 cup Skim Milk
Calories	100	140
Calories from fat	5	5
% Daily Value		
Total Fat 0.5g	1%	1%
Saturated Fat 0g	0%	0%
Trans Fat 0g		
Cholesterol 0mg	0%	0%
Sodium 210mg	9%	12%
Potassium 200mg	6%	11%
Total Carbohydrate 24g	8%	10%
Dietary Fiber 5g	20%	20%
Sugars 5g		
Other Carbohydrates 14g		
Protein 3g		
Vitamin A	15%	20%
Vitamin C	0%	2%
Calcium	0%	15%
Iron	45%	45%
Vitamin D	10%	25%
Thiamin	25%	30%
Riboflavin	25%	35%
Niacin	25%	25%
Vitamin B$_6$	25%	25%
Folate	25%	25%
Vitamin B$_{12}$	25%	35%

Figure 2.13 **Comparing cereals.** These cereal labels come from different types of breakfast cereal: corn-flakes cereal (left) and bran-flakes cereal (right). What might influence your decision to buy one over the other?

added in 2001 based on the AI levels for choline developed by the Food and Nutrition Board.[17]

Health Claims

With the passage of the NLEA, manufacturers also were allowed to add health claims to food labels. A **health claim** is a statement that links one or more dietary components to reduced risk of disease—such as a claim that calcium helps reduce the risk of osteoporosis. Before the NLEA was passed, products making such claims were considered drugs, not foods.

A health claim must be supported by scientifically valid evidence for it to be approved for use on a food label. Regulations require a finding of "significant scientific agreement" before the FDA may authorize a new health claim. In addition, there are specific criteria for the use of claims. For example, a high-fiber food that is also high in fat is not eligible for a health claim. So far, the FDA has approved the following health claims:

- *Calcium and osteoporosis:* Adequate calcium along with regular exercise may reduce the risk of osteoporosis.

- *Sodium and hypertension (high blood pressure):* Low-sodium diets may help lower blood pressure.

health claim Any statement that associates a food or a substance in a food with a disease or health-related condition. The FDA authorizes health claims.

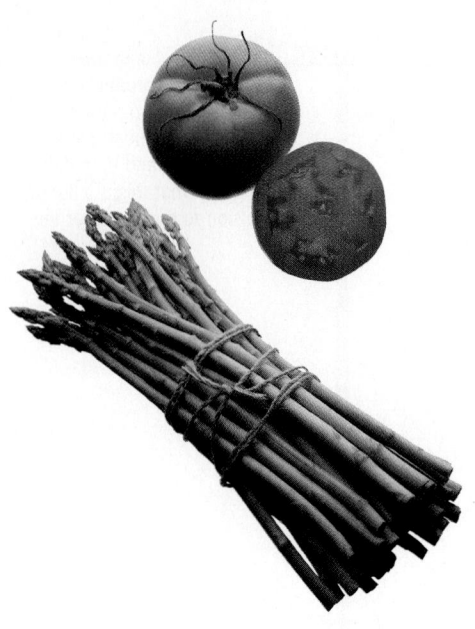

- *Dietary fat and cancer:* Low-fat diets may reduce the risk for some types of cancer.

- *Dietary saturated fat and cholesterol and risk of coronary heart disease (CHD):* Diets low in saturated fat and cholesterol may reduce risk for heart disease.

- *Fiber-containing grain products, fruits, and vegetables and cancer:* Diets low in fat and rich in high-fiber foods may reduce the risk of certain cancers.

- *Fruits, vegetables, and grain products that contain fiber, particularly pectins, gums, and mucilages, and risk of CHD:* Diets low in fat and rich in these types of fiber may reduce the risk of heart disease.

- *Fruits and vegetables and cancer:* Diets low in fat and rich in fruits and vegetables may reduce the risk of certain cancers.

- *Folate and neural tube defects:* Adequate folate intake prior to and early in pregnancy may reduce the risk of neural tube defects (a birth defect).

- *Dietary noncarcinogenic carbohydrate sweeteners and dental caries (cavities):* Foods sweetened with sugar alcohols do not promote tooth decay.

𝓕𝓎𝓲 Definitions for Nutrient Content Claims on Food Labels

FOR YOUR INFORMATION

Free: Food contains no amount (or trivial or "physiologically inconsequential" amounts). May be used with one or more of the following: fat, saturated fat, cholesterol, sodium, sugar, and calories. Synonyms include *without, no,* and *zero.*

Fat-free: *less than 0.5 g of fat per serving*

Saturated fat-free: *less than 0.5 g of saturated fat per serving, and less than 0.5 g of trans fatty acids per serving*

Cholesterol-free: *less than 2 mg of cholesterol and 2 g or less of saturated fat per serving*

Sodium-free: *less than 5 mg of sodium per serving*

Sugar-free: *less than 0.5 g of sugar per serving*

Calorie-free: *fewer than 5 calories per serving*

Low: Food can be eaten frequently without exceeding dietary guidelines for one or more of these components: fat, saturated fat, cholesterol, sodium, and calories. Synonyms include *little, few,* and *low source of.*

Low-fat: *3 g or less per serving*

Low-saturated fat: *1 g or less of saturated fat per serving; no more than 15 percent of calories from saturated fat*

Low-cholesterol: *20 mg or less and 2 g or less of saturated fat per serving*

Low-sodium: *140 mg or less per serving*

Very low sodium: *35 mg or less per serving*

Low-calorie: *40 calories or less per serving*

Lean and extra lean: Describe the fat content of meal and main dish products, seafood, and game meat products.

Lean: *less than 10 g fat, 4.5 g or less saturated fat, and less than 95 mg of cholesterol per serving and per 100 g*

Extra lean: *less than 5 g fat, less than 2 g saturated fat, and less than 95 mg of cholesterol per serving and per 100 g*

High: Food contains 20 percent or more of the Daily Value for a particular nutrient in a serving.

Good source: Food contains 10 to 19 percent of the Daily Value for a particular nutrient in one serving.

Reduced: Nutritionally altered product containing at least 25 percent less of a nutrient or of calories than the regular or reference product. (*Note:* A "reduced" claim can't be used if the reference product already meets the requirement for "low.")

Less: Food, whether altered or not, contains 25 percent less of a nutrient or of calories than the reference food. *Fewer* is an acceptable synonym.

- *Dietary fiber, such as that found in whole oats and psyllium seed husk, and CHD:* Diets low in fat and rich in these types of fiber can help reduce the risk of heart disease.

- *Soy protein and CHD:* Foods rich in soy protein as part of a low-fat diet may help reduce the risk of heart disease.

- *Plant sterol/stanol esters and CHD:* Diets low in saturated fat and cholesterol that contain significant amounts of these additives may reduce the risk of heart disease.

- *Whole-grain foods and CHD or cancer:* Diets high in whole-grain foods and other plant foods and low in total fat, saturated fat, and cholesterol may help reduce the risk of heart disease and certain cancers.

- *Potassium and high blood pressure/stroke:* Diets that contain good sources of potassium may reduce the risk of high blood pressure and stroke.

A new health claim may be proposed at any time, so this list will expand. As with nutrient content claims, food manufacturers may propose new health claims based on an authoritative statement from a scientific body.

Light: This descriptor can have two meanings:
1. A nutritionally altered product contains one-third fewer calories or half the fat of the reference food. If the reference food derives 50 percent or more of its calories from fat, the reduction must be 50 percent of the fat.
2. The sodium content of a low-calorie, low-fat food has been reduced by 50 percent. Also, *light in sodium* may be used on a food in which the sodium content has been reduced by at least 50 percent.

Note: The term *light* can still be used to describe such properties as texture and color as long as the label clearly explains its meaning (e.g., *light brown sugar* or *light and fluffy*).

More: A serving of food, whether altered or not, contains a nutrient that is at least 10 percent of the Daily Value more than the reference food. This also applies to *fortified*, *enriched*, and *added* claims, but in those cases, the food must be altered.

Healthy: A *healthy* food must be low in fat and saturated fat and contain limited amounts of cholesterol (less than 60 mg) and sodium (less than 360 mg for individual foods and less than 480 mg for meal-type products). In addition, a single-item food must provide at least 10 percent or more of one of the following: vitamins A or C, iron, calcium, protein, or fiber. A meal-type product, such as a frozen entrée or dinner, must provide 10 percent of two or more of these vitamins or minerals, or protein, or fiber, in addition to meeting the other criteria. Additional regulations allow the term *healthy* to be applied to raw, canned, or frozen fruits and vegetables and enriched grains even if the 10 percent nutrient content rule is not met. However, frozen or canned fruits or vegetables cannot contain ingredients that would change the nutrient profile.

Fresh: Food is raw, has never been frozen or heated, and contains no preservatives. *Fresh frozen, frozen fresh,* and *freshly frozen* can be used for foods that are quickly frozen while still fresh. Blanched foods also can be called fresh.

Percent fat-free: Food must be a low-fat or a fat-free product. In addition, the claim must reflect accurately the amount of nonfat ingredients in 100 g of food.

Implied claims: These are prohibited when they wrongfully imply that a food contains or does not contain a meaningful level of a nutrient. For example, a product cannot claim to be made with an ingredient known to be a source of fiber (such as "made with oat bran") unless the product contains enough of that ingredient (e.g., oat bran) to meet the definition for "good source" of fiber. As another example, a claim that a product contains "no tropical oils" is allowed, but only on foods that are "low" in saturated fat, because consumers have come to equate tropical oils with high levels of saturated fat.

Source: Food and Drug Administration, http://www.cfsan.fda.gov/~dms/lab-nutr.html. Accessed 2/15/06.

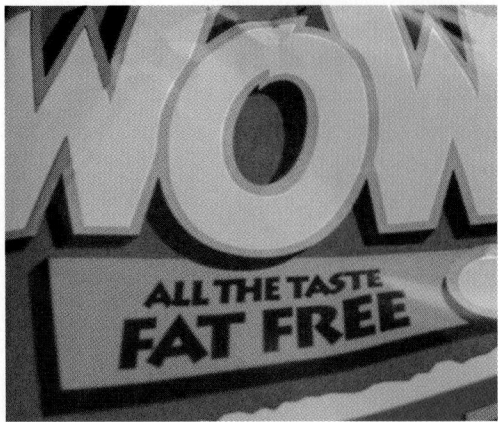 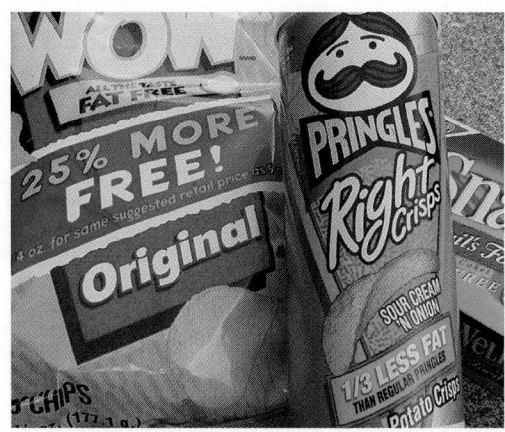

Qualified Health Claims

Through a new initiative called Consumer Health Information for Better Nutrition, the FDA hopes to facilitate the flow of information about sound dietary choices to consumers by allowing additional claims for foods and supplements. For many relationships between food components and the reduction of disease risk, the current scientific evidence is supportive but doesn't rise to the level of "significant scientific agreement" required for health claims. Consequently, the FDA will now allow manufacturers to submit for approval health claims for which the "weight of the evidence" supports the claimed relationship.[18] Such qualified health claims may also be made for dietary supplements.[19]

When a qualified health claim is approved, the allowed language and acceptable range of products is very specific. For example, the claim "Scientific evidence suggests but does not prove that eating 1.5 ounces per day of most nuts [such as name of specific nut] as part of a diet low in saturated fat and cholesterol may reduce the risk of heart disease. [See nutrition information for fat content.]" can appear on almonds, hazelnuts, peanuts, pecans, some pine nuts, pistachio nuts, and walnuts.

Structure/Function Claims

structure/function claims These statements may claim a benefit related to a nutrient-deficiency disease (like *vitamin C prevents scurvy*) or describe the role of a nutrient or dietary ingredient intended to affect a structure or function in humans; for example, *calcium helps build strong bones.*

Food labels also may contain **structure/function claims** that describe potential effects of a food, food component, or dietary supplement component on body structures or functions, such as bone health, muscle strength, and digestion. As long as the label does not claim to diagnose, cure, mitigate, treat, or prevent a disease, a manufacturer can claim that a product "helps promote immune health" or is an "energizer" if *some* evidence can be provided to support the claim. Currently, structure/function claims on foods must be related to the food's nutritive value. Many scientists are concerned about the lack of a consistent scientific standard for both health claims and structure/function claims. For more on structure/function claims, see the "Spotlight on Complementary and Alternative Nutrition."

Using Labels to Make Healthful Food Choices

nutrition assessment Measurement of the nutritional health of the body. It can include anthropometric measurements, biochemical tests, clinical observations, and dietary intake, as well as medical histories and socioeconomic factors.

What's the best way to start using the information on food labels to make food choices? Let's look at a couple of examples. Perhaps one of your goals is to add more iron to your diet. Compare the cereal labels in Figure 2.13.

Which cereal contains a higher percentage of the Daily Value for iron? How do they compare in terms of sugar content? What about vitamins and other minerals?

Maybe it's a frozen entrée you're after. Look at the two examples in **Figure 2.14**. Which is the best choice nutritionally? Are you sure? Sometimes the answer is not clear-cut. Product A is higher in sodium, whereas Product B has more saturated and *trans* fat. It would be important to know about the rest of your dietary intake before making a decision. Do you already have quite a bit of sodium in your diet, or are you likely to add salt at the table? Maybe you never salt your food, so a bit extra in your entrée is okay. If you know that your saturated fat intake is already a bit high, however, Product A might be a better choice. To make the best choice, you should know which substances are most important in terms of your own health risks. The label is there to help you make these types of food decisions.

Key Concepts: *Making food choices at the grocery store is your opportunity to implement the* Dietary Guidelines for Americans *and your MyPyramid-planned diet. The Nutrition Facts panel on most packaged foods contains not only the specific amounts of nutrients shown in grams or milligrams, but also comparisons between the amounts of nutrients in a food and the recommended intake values. These comparisons are reported as %DV (Daily Values). The %DV information can be used to compare two products or to see how individual foods contribute to the total diet.*

Nutrition Assessment: Determining Nutritional Health

In a nutritional sense, what does it mean to be healthy? Nutritional health is quite simply obtaining all of the nutrients in amounts needed to support body processes. We can measure nutritional health in a number of ways. Taken together, such measurements can give you much insight into your current and long-term well-being. The process of measuring nutritional health is usually termed **nutrition assessment**.

Nutrition assessment serves a variety of purposes. It may help evaluate nutrition-related risks that may jeopardize a person's current or future health. Nutrition assessment is a routine part of the nutritional care of hospitalized patients. In this setting, nutrition assessment not only identifies risks, but also measures the effectiveness of treatment. In public health, nutrition assessment helps to identify people in need of nutrition-related interventions and to monitor the effectiveness of intervention programs. Sometimes, assessments determine the nutritional health of an entire population—identifying health risks common in a population group so that specific policy measures can be developed to combat them.

The Continuum of Nutritional Status

Your nutritional status can be seen as a point along a continuum, with undernutrition and overnutrition at the extremes. Chronic undernutrition results in the development of nutritional deficiency diseases, as well as conditions of energy and protein malnutrition, and can lead to death. Unlike starvation, **undernutrition** is a condition in which *some* food is being consumed, but the intake is not nutritionally adequate. Although chronic undernutrition and associated deficiency diseases were common in the United States in the 1800s and early 1900s, today they are rare. Undernutrition now is most often associated with extreme poverty, alcoholism, illness, or some types of eating disorders.

Nutrition Facts

Serving Size: 1 Entree (240g)
Servings Per Container: 1

Amount Per Serving	
Calories 400 Calories from fat 150	
	% Daily Value*
Total Fat 16g	25%
Saturated Fat 2.5g	13%
Trans Fat 1g	
Cholesterol 10mg	3%
Sodium 780mg	33%
Total Carbohydrate 56g	19%
Dietary Fiber 2g	8%
Sugars 2g	
Protein 8g	

Vitamin A 2%	•	Vitamin C 4%
Calcium 6%	•	Iron 4%

Product A

Nutrition Facts

Serving Size: 1 package (269g)
Servings Per Container: 1

Amount Per Serving	
Calories 400 Calories from fat 140	
	% Daily Value*
Total Fat 16g	24%
Saturated Fat 6g	30%
Trans Fat 2g	
Cholesterol 40mg	14%
Sodium 690mg	29%
Total Carbohydrate 48g	16%
Dietary Fiber 2g	9%
Sugars 5g	
Protein 15g	

Vitamin A 10%	•	Vitamin C 8%
Calcium 20%	•	Iron 15%

Product B

Figure 2.14 **Comparing product labels.** Labels may look similar, but appearances can be deceptive. Compare the amounts of saturated fat and sodium in these two products.

undernutrition Poor health resulting from the depletion of nutrients due to inadequate nutrient intake over time. It is now most often associated with poverty, alcoholism, and some types of eating disorders.

Overnutrition is the chronic consumption of more than is necessary for good health. Specifically, overnutrition is the regular consumption of excess calories, fats, saturated fats, or cholesterol—all of which increase risk for chronic disease. Today, nutrition-related chronic diseases such as heart disease, cancer, stroke, and diabetes are among the 10 leading causes of death in the United States. All of these problems have been linked to dietary excess. (Remember that epidemiological [population] studies can show associations between various factors and diseases, but these correlations do not necessarily indicate cause and effect.)

Between these two extremes lies a region of good health. In 1988, the U.S. Surgeon General wrote, "for the two out of three adult Americans who do not smoke and do not drink excessively, one personal choice seems to influence long-term health prospects more than any other: what we eat."[20] Good food and lifestyle choices, a balanced diet, and regular exercise help to reduce the risk of chronic disease and delay its onset, keeping us in a region of good health for more of our lifetime.

Nutrition Assessment of Individuals

In health care settings, a registered dietitian or physician may do an individual nutrition assessment of a patient or client. Depending on the purpose of the nutrition assessment, the measures may be very comprehensive and detailed. A dietitian can then use this information to plan individualized nutrition counseling. Nutrition assessment measures are often repeated in order to assess the effectiveness of nutrition counseling or a change in diet.

Nutrition Assessment of Populations

Typically, nutrition assessment of populations is not as comprehensive as an assessment of an individual. One of the largest ongoing nationwide surveys of dietary intake and health status is the National Health and Nutrition Examination Survey (NHANES). The survey is unique in that it combines interviews and physical examinations.

The NHANES program began in the early 1960s and has been conducted as a series of surveys focusing on different population groups or health topics. In 1999, the survey became a continuous program to meet emerging needs with a changing focus on a variety of health and nutrition measurements.[21] Data from NHANES have told us a great deal about the nutritional status and dietary intake of our population. This information is released periodically as the *What We Eat in America* report.

Nutrition Assessment Methods

Just as there is not one measure of physical fitness, there is not just one indicator of nutritional health. Nutrients play many roles in the body, so measures of nutritional status must look at many factors. Often these factors are termed the **ABCDs of nutrition assessment**: anthropometric measurements, biochemical tests, clinical observations, and dietary intake. (See **Table 2.4**.)

Anthropometric Measurements

Anthropometric measurements are physical measurements of the body, such as height and weight, head circumference, girth measurement, or skinfold measurements.

Table 2.4	The ABCDs of Nutrition Assessment
Assessment Method	*Why It's Done*
Anthropometric measures	Measure growth in children; show changes in weight that can reflect diseases (e.g., cancer or thyroid problems); monitor progress in fat loss
Biochemical tests	Measure blood, urine, and feces for nutrients or metabolites that indicate infection or disease
Clinical observations	Assess change in skin color and health, hair texture, fingernail shape, etc.
Dietary intake	Evaluate diet for nutrient (e.g., fat, calcium, protein) or food (e.g., number of fruits and vegetables) intake

Height and Weight

To provide useful information, height and weight must be accurately measured. For infants and very young children, measurement of height is really measurement of recumbent length (that is, length when they are lying down). Careful measurement of length at each checkup gives a clear indication of a child's growth rate. Standard growth charts show how the child's growth compares to that of others of the same age and sex. For children 2 to 20 years old, charts illustrating growth are based on standing height, or stature. (See Appendix I.)

The standing height of older children and adults can be determined with a tape measure fixed to a wall and a sliding right-angle headboard for reading the measurement. Aging adults lose some height due to bone loss and curvature, so it is important to *measure* height and not simply rely on remembered values.

Weight is a critical measure in nutrition assessment. It is used to assess children's growth, predict energy expenditure and protein needs, and determine body mass index. Weight should be measured using a calibrated scale. For assessments that need a high degree of precision, subtract the weight of the clothing. Because many calculations and standards use metric measures of height and weight, it's important to be familiar with standard conversion factors.

For the anthropometric assessment of infants and young children, a third measurement is common: head circumference. This is measured using a flexible tape measure placed snugly around the head. Head circumference measures are compared to standard growth charts and are another useful indicator of normal growth and development, especially during rapid growth from birth to age 3.

Skinfolds

Skinfold measurements serve a variety of purposes. Because a significant amount of the body's fat stores is located right beneath the skin (subcutaneous fat), skinfold measurements at various sites around the body can give a good indication of body fatness. This information may be used to evaluate the physical fitness of an athlete or predict the risk of obesity-related disorders. Skinfold measurements are also useful in cases of illness; the maintenance of fat stores in a patient's body may be a valuable indicator of dietary adequacy. Skinfold measurements are done with special

> To convert inches to centimeters, multiply the number of inches by 2.54
>
> inches $\times$ 2.54 = centimeters

> To convert pounds to kilograms, divide the number of pounds by 2.2
>
> pounds $\div$ 2.2 = kilograms

skinfold measurements A method to estimate body fat by measuring with calipers the thickness of a fold of skin and subcutaneous fat.

Figure 2.15 **Skinfold measurements.** A significant amount of the body's fat stores lie just beneath the skin, so when done correctly skinfold measurements can provide an indication of body fatness. An inexperienced or careless measurer, however, can easily make large errors. Skinfold measurements usually work better for monitoring malnutrition than for identifying overweight and obesity. They also are widely used in large population studies.

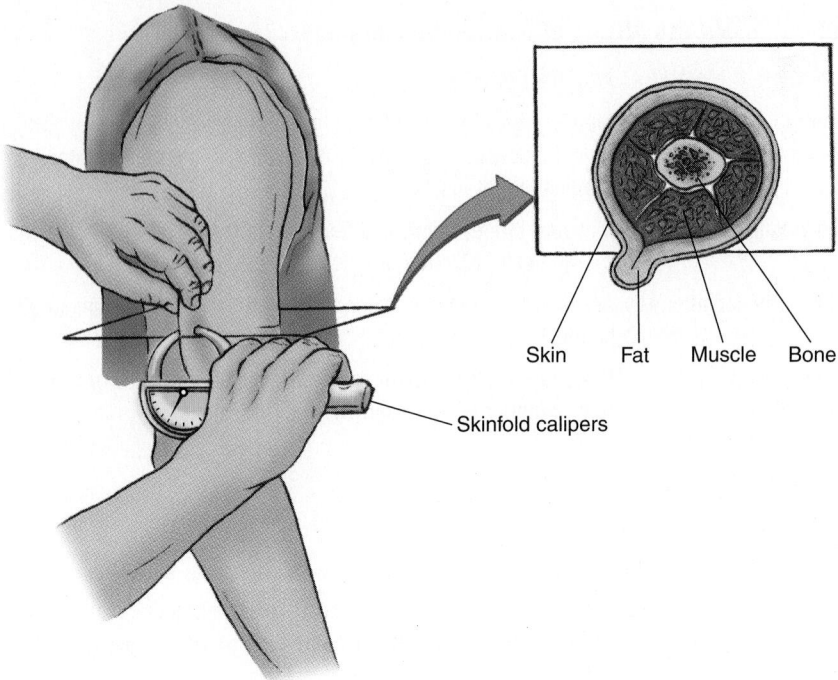

Skin   Fat   Muscle   Bone

Skinfold calipers

biochemical assessment Assessment by measuring a nutrient or its metabolite in one or more body fluids such as blood and urine or in feces. Also called laboratory assessment.

calipers (see **Figure 2.15**). For reliable measurements, training in the use of calipers is essential. Skinfold measurements can be used to estimate the percentage of body fat or can be compared to percentile tables for specific sex and age categories. Other methods for estimating body fat and body composition are discussed in Chapter 8, "Energy Balance, Body Composition, and Weight Management."

Biochemical Tests

Because of their relation to growth and body composition, anthropometric measurements give a broad picture of nutritional health—whether the diet contains enough calories and protein to maintain normal patterns of growth, normal body composition, and normal levels of lean body mass. However, anthropometric measures do not give specific information about *nutrients*. For that information, a variety of biochemical tests are useful.

Biochemical assessment measures a nutrient or metabolite (a related compound) in one or more body fluids, such as blood or urine, or in feces. For example, the concentration of albumin (an important transport protein) in the blood can be an indicator of the body's protein status. If little protein is eaten, the body produces smaller amounts of body proteins such as albumin.

Biochemical assessments may include measurements of a nutrient metabolite, a storage or transport compound, an enzyme that depends on a vitamin or mineral, or another indicator of the body's functioning in relation to a particular nutrient. These measures usually are a better indicator of nutritional status than directly measuring blood levels of nutrients such as vitamin A or calcium. The levels of nutrients excreted in the urine or feces also provide valuable information.

Clinical Observations

Clinical observations—the characteristics of health that can be seen during a physical exam—help to complete the picture of nutritional health. Although often nonspecific, clinical signs are clues to nutrient deficiency or excess that can be confirmed or ruled out by further testing. In a clinical nutrition examination, a clinician observes the hair, nails, skin, eyes, lips, mouth, bones, muscles, and joints. Specific findings, such as cracking at the corners of the mouth (suggestive of riboflavin, vitamin B$_6$, or niacin deficiency) or petechiae (small, pinpoint hemorrhages on the skin indicative of vitamin C deficiency), need to be followed by other assessments.

Dietary Intake

A picture of nutritional health would not be complete without information about dietary intake. Dietary information may confirm the lack or excess of a dietary component suggested by anthropometric, biochemical, or clinical evaluations.

There are a number of ways to collect dietary intake data. Each has strengths and weaknesses. It is important to match the method to the type and quantity of data needed. Remember, too, that the quality of information obtained about people's diets often relies heavily on people's memories, as well as their honesty in sharing those recollections. How well do you remember *everything* you ate yesterday?

Diet History

The most comprehensive form of dietary intake data collection is the **diet history**. In this method, a skilled interviewer finds out not only what the client has been eating in the recent past but also the client's long-term food consumption habits. The interviewer's questions may also address other risk factors for nutrition-related problems, such as economic issues.

Food Record

Food records, or diaries, provide detailed information about day-to-day eating habits. Typically, a person records all foods and beverages consumed during a defined period, usually three to seven consecutive days. Because food records are recorded concurrently with intake, they are less prone to inaccuracy from lapses in memory. Because the data are completely self-reported, however, food records will not be accurate if the person fails to record all items. To make food records more precise, the items in a meal can be weighed before consumption. Remaining portions are weighed at the end of the meal to determine exactly how much was eaten. **Weighed food records** are much more time-consuming to complete.

Food Frequency Questionnaire

A **food frequency questionnaire (FFQ)** asks how often the subject consumes specific foods or groups of foods, rather than what specific foods the subject consumes daily. A food frequency questionnaire may ask, for example, "How often do you drink a cup of milk?" with the response options of daily, weekly, monthly, and so on (see **Figure 2.16**). This information is used to estimate that person's average daily intake.

Although food frequency questionnaires do not require a trained interviewer and can be relatively quick to complete, there are disadvantages to this method of data collection. One problem is that it is often difficult

clinical observations Assessment by evaluating the characteristics of well-being that can be seen in a physical exam. Nonspecific, clinical observations can provide clues to nutrient deficiency or excess that can be confirmed or ruled out by biochemical testing.

diet history Record of food intake and eating behaviors that includes recent and long-term habits of food consumption. Done by a skilled interviewer, the diet history is the most comprehensive form of dietary intake data collection.

food records Detailed information about day-to-day eating habits; typically includes all foods and beverages consumed for a defined period, usually three to seven consecutive days.

weighed food records Detailed food records obtained by weighing foods before eating, and then weighing leftovers to determine the exact amount consumed.

food frequency questionnaire (FFQ) A questionnaire for nutrition assessment that asks how often the subject consumes specific foods or groups of foods, rather than what specific foods the subject consumes daily. Also called food frequency checklist.

to translate a person's response to how often they drink milk, or how many cups of milk they drink per week, into specific nutrient values without more detailed information. More important, food frequency questionnaires require a person to average, over a long period, foods that may be consumed erratically in portions that are sometimes large and sometimes small.

24-Hour Recall

24-hour dietary recall A form of dietary intake data collection. The interviewer takes the client through a recent 24-hour period (usually midnight to midnight) to determine what foods and beverages the client consumed.

The **24-hour dietary recall** is the simplest form of dietary intake data collection. In a 24-hour recall, the interviewer takes the client through a recent 24-hour period (usually midnight to midnight) to determine what foods and beverages the client consumed. To get a complete, accurate picture of the subject's diet, the interviewer must ask probing questions such as "Did you put anything on your toast?" but not leading questions such as "Did you put butter and jelly on your toast?" Comprehensive population surveys frequently use 24-hour recalls as the main method of data collection. Although a single 24-hour recall is not very useful for describing the nutrient content of an individual's overall diet (there's too much day-to-day variation), in large-scale studies it gives a reasonably accurate picture of the average nutrient intake of a population. Multiple dietary recalls also are useful for estimating the nutrient intake of individuals.

Methods of Evaluating Dietary Intake Data

Once the data are collected, the next step is to determine the nutrient content of the diet and evaluate that information in terms of dietary standards or other reference points. This is commonly done using nutrient analysis software. Computer programs remove the tedium of looking up foods in tables of nutrient composition; large databases allow for simple access to food composition, and the computer does the math automatically.

	Average Use During Past Year					
Food Item	**<1 serving per month**	**1–3 servings per month**	**1–4 servings per week**	**5–7 servings per week**	**2–4 servings per day**	**5+ servings per day**
Coffee					√	
Dark bread	√					
Ice cream				√		

	Your Serving Size				How Often?				
Food Item	**Medium Serving**	**S**	**M**	**L**	**Day**	**Week**	**Month**	**Year**	**Never**
Coffee	(1 cup)			√	2				
Dark bread	(1 slice)								√
Ice cream	(1/2 cup)		√			3			

Figure 2.16 **Examples of food frequency questionnaire formats.**
Source: Adapted from Lee RD, Nieman DC. *Nutritional Assessment.* 3rd ed. St. Louis: Mosby, 2002.

Comparison to Dietary Standards

It is possible to compare a person's nutrient intake to dietary standards such as the RDA or AI values. Although this will give a quantitative idea of dietary adequacy, it cannot be considered a definitive evaluation of a person's diet because we don't know that individual's specific nutrient requirements. The bottom line is that comparisons of individual diets to RDA or AI values should be interpreted with caution.[22]

Comparison to MyPyramid and the Dietary Guidelines for Americans

The MyPyramid system has several online tools for assessment of dietary intake. Individuals (or evaluators) can use the MyPyramid Tracker feature on the MyPyramid Web site to compare a typical day's intake to the MyPyramid groups and *Dietary Guidelines*. Although these evaluations usually are not specific, they give a general idea of whether the subject's diet is high or low in saturated fat, or whether the subject is eating enough fruits, vegetables, and whole grains.

Outcomes of Nutrition Assessment

When taken together, anthropometric measures, biochemical tests, clinical exams, and dietary evaluation, along with the individual's family history, socioeconomic situation, and other factors, give a complete picture of nutritional health. A client's assessment may lead to a recommendation for a diet change to reduce weight or blood cholesterol, the addition of a vitamin or mineral supplement to treat a deficiency, the identification of abnormal growth due to inadequate infant feeding, or simply the affirmation that dietary intake is adequate for current nutrition needs.

Key Concepts: *Nutrition assessment involves the collection of various types of data—anthropometric measurements, biochemical tests, clinical observations, and dietary intake—for a complete picture of one's nutritional health. Such data are compared to established standards to diagnose nutritional deficiencies, identify dietary inadequacies, or evaluate progress as a result of dietary changes.*

Label [to] **Table**   Nutrition Labels: Do They Help Us Choose a Healthful Diet?

The Nutrition Labeling and Education Act of 1990 (NLEA) changed food labeling and brought us the Nutrition Facts panel we see on food labels today. One of the NLEA's primary objectives was to help consumers select foods for a healthful diet. Labels were designed to be educational rather than merely informational. Thus, rather than just listing the amounts (e.g., grams and milligrams) for a product's nutrients, Daily Values were developed to make comparisons possible; terms such as *reduced, light, low,* and *free* were defined; and health claims for certain relationships between diet and disease were developed.

Now, nearly half of food labels have a nutrient content claim, and another 10 percent have either a health claim or structure/function claim.[1] These are dramatic changes from the informational labels of the 1970s and 1980s. But do they work? Do the additional information and new format encourage more healthful purchases? Policy makers had high hopes for what the changes to nutrition labels would bring. One study predicted four scenarios for behavior change resulting from implementation of the NLEA.[2] Over a period of 20 years, those changes in food choices could lead to a gain of 40,000 to 1.2 million life-years. The potential dollar value of such effects is staggering, ranging from $3 billion to more than $100 billion!

A study of adults found that nutrition labels *are* useful for people who want to lower the fat content of their diets—an important health goal for most Americans.[3] In this study, adults in Washington State were surveyed by telephone about their use of nutrition labels; their dietary habits as they relate to fat, fruit, and vegetable intake; health behaviors; and demographic characteristics. Women were more likely than men to read nutrition labels and to look at information on serving size, calories, and grams of fat; men were more likely to look at cholesterol information. People under age 35 were more likely to consider serving size, calories from fat, and grams of fat, whereas those 35 and older read cholesterol information more frequently.

Label use was associated with a lower intake of fat, but there was no relation between label use and fruit and vegetable intake. Regular reading of nutrition labels was associated with a reduction in fat intake of at least 5 percent. Although this is lower than the 13 percent figure used by the study that predicted the possible advantages of label use, this level of fat intake reduction would still have significant health benefits for the population as a whole.

A study of African American adults in North Carolina had similar findings.[4] Nutrition label use was more common among women, older individuals, and those with more than a high school education. Label users had lower fat intakes but also had higher fruit and vegetable intakes. Although teens are just as likely to read labels as adults, they don't necessarily use them to make healthier choices. Label use by male adolescents was associated with higher fat intake, whereas fat intake in teen girls didn't differ with label use.[5]

It appears that most label readers still focus on the numbers of grams, calories, or milligrams rather than the %DV. The Washington State study found that although 80 percent of the subjects read nutritional labels, only 39 percent of those label readers used the %DV for fat. It is possible that this information is not well understood by consumers and that the "E" in NLEA (Education) has not been effective or widespread enough to cause consumers to make full use of the information provided. Other surveys indicate that consumers are not clear on the definition of terms such as "low fat" or "cholesterol free."[6] Although these terms are strictly defined in the regulations, the average shopper is not aware of the definitions. In addition, consumers don't readily discriminate between package size and serving size of snack foods.[7]

If food labels are going to help the United States realize savings in health care costs, the average consumer needs to learn more about how to use the valuable information provided on food labels. As the studies have shown, those involved in health education need to focus on educating consumers about food label information. Otherwise, health claims and label statements will just be part of consumers' information overload, rather than a pathway to healthful food choices.

You will find the "Label to Table" feature near the end of most chapters. Use these features to sharpen your critical thinking skills and become an informed consumer who intelligently evaluates nutrition information found on food labels.

1 LeGault L, Brandt MB, McCabe N, et al. 2000–2001 Food Label and Package Survey: an update on prevalence of nutrition labeling and claims on processed, packaged foods. *J Am Diet Assoc.* 2004;104:952–958.

2 Zarkin GA, Dean N, Mauskopf JA, Williams R. Potential health benefits of nutrition label changes. *Am J Public Health.* 1993;83:717–724.

3 Neuhouser ML, Kristal AR, Patterson RE. Use of food nutrition labels is associated with lower fat intake. *J Am Diet Assoc.* 1999;99:45–53.

4 Satia JA, Galanko JA, Neuhouser ML. Food nutrition label use is associated with demographic, behavioral, and psychosocial factors and dietary intake among African Americans in North Carolina. *J Am Diet Assoc.* 2005;105:392–402.

5 Huang TT-K, Kaur H, McCarter KS, et al. Reading nutrition labels and fat consumption in adolescents. *J Adol Health.* 2004;35:399–401.

6 Resnick ML. *Proceedings of the Human Factors and Ergonomics Society 41st Annual Meeting.* 1997;395–399.

7 Pelletier AL, Chang WW, Delzell JE, McCall JW. Patients' understanding and use of snack food package nutrition labels. *J Am Board Fam Pract.* 2004;17:319–323.

LEARNING *Portfolio* chapter 2

Key Terms

Study Points

- Moderation, balance, and variety are general guiding principles for healthful diets.

- The *Dietary Guidelines for Americans* give consumers advice regarding general components of the diet.

- The MyPyramid is a graphic representation of a food guidance system that supports the principles of the *Dietary Guidelines for Americans.*

- Each food group in MyPyramid has a recommended daily amount based on calorie needs. Choose a variety of foods from each group to obtain all the nutrients.

- The Exchange Lists are a diet-planning tool most often used for diabetic or weight-control diets.

- Servings for each food in the Exchange Lists are grouped so that equal amounts of carbohydrate, fat, and protein are provided by each choice.

- Dietary standards are values for individual nutrients that reflect recommended intake levels. These values are used for planning and evaluating diets for groups and individuals.

- The Dietary Reference Intakes are the current dietary standards in the United States and Canada. The DRIs consist of several types of values: EAR, RDA, AI, UL, EER, and AMDR.

- Nutrition information on food labels can be used to select a more healthful diet.

- Label information not only provides the gram or milligram amounts of the nutrients present, but also gives a percentage of Daily Values so that the consumer can compare the amount in the food to the amount recommended for consumption each day.

- Nutrition information, label statements, and health claims are specifically defined by the regulations that were developed after passage of the Nutrition Labeling and Education Act of 1990.

- Nutrition assessment is a process of determining the overall health of a person as related to nutrition.

- Nutrition assessment involves four major factors: anthropometric measurements, biochemical tests, clinical observations, and dietary intake.

Study Questions

1. Define undernutrition and overnutrition.

2. What is the purpose of the *Dietary Guidelines for Americans*? List the nine focus areas of the 2005 Dietary Guidelines for Americans.

3. What are the recommended amounts for each of the food groups of MyPyramid for a 2,000-calorie diet?

4. Describe how the exchange system works and why people with diabetes might use it.

5. List and define the four main Dietary Reference Intake categories.

6. List the five mandatory components found on all food labels.

7. The standard Nutrition Facts panel shows information on which nutrients?

8. What is the purpose of the "% Daily Value" listed next to most nutrients on the label?

9. Define the three types of claims that may be found on food labels.

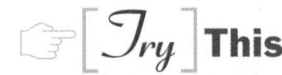

Try This

Are You a Pyramid Pleaser?

Keep a detailed food diary for three days. Make sure to include things you drink, along with the amounts (cups, ounces, tablespoons, etc.) of each food or beverage. How well do you think your intake matches the *Dietary Guidelines* and MyPyramid recommendations? To find out, go to MyPyramid.gov and click on MyPyramid Tracker, and then on Assess Your Food Intake. This feature allows you to do an online assessment of your food intake. Follow the directions to register and then enter your Personal Profile. Then click on Proceed to Food Intake and enter each food you ate for one day. Once you are done, you can click on Analyze Your Food Intake and see the comparisons to the *Dietary Guidelines* and MyPyramid. How did you do? From which groups did you tend to eat more than is recommended? Were there any groups for which you did not meet the recommendations? Was there a day-to-day variation in the number of servings you ate of each group? Use the results of this activity to plan ways you can improve your diet. You may want to visit this site frequently to monitor changes you are making in your food intake.

Grocery Store Scavenger Hunt

On your next trip to the grocery store, find a food item that has any number other than a "0" listed for the two vitamins and two minerals required to be listed on the food label %DV. It doesn't matter if you choose a cereal, soup, cracker, or snack item, as long as it has numbers other than "0" for all four items. Once you're home, review the Daily Values (inside the back cover) and calculate the number of milligrams of calcium, iron, and vitamin C found in each serving of your food. Next, take a look at vitamin A: How many International Units (IUs) does each serving of your product have? If you can calculate these, you should have a better understanding of % Daily Values.

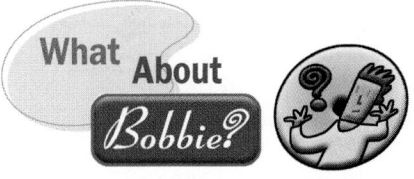

What About *Bobbie?*

Now that you have learned something about the recommendations for a healthful diet, how do you think Bobbie did? Review her one-day food record in Chapter 1. How closely does Bobbie's intake fit MyPyramid? Do you think she met most of the *Dietary Guidelines?* What about the RDA and AI values? Was her diet balanced enough to meet most of these recommendations?

The following table summarizes the results of a computerized nutrient analysis of Bobbie's diet. You may be completing a similar analysis of your own diet as part of your course requirements. In future chapters, you will explore many of these nutrients further and look at the foods in Bobbie's diet that contributed various nutrients. Keep in mind that this is only a one-day food record and may or may not represent her typical diet.

	Bobbie	RDA/AI	%RDA/AI
Calories	2,300	2,290*	100%
Carbohydrates	292 g	130 g	225%
Fiber	25 g	25 g	100%
Fat	86 g	—	—
Cholesterol	261 mg	—	—
Protein	96 g	46 g	209%
Vitamin A	493 mcg RAE	700 mcg RAE	70%
Vitamin D	0.5 mcg	5 mcg	10%
Vitamin E	9 mg	15 mg	60%
Thiamin	2.0 mg	1.1 mg	182%
Riboflavin	2.2 mg	1.1 mg	200%
Niacin	27.5 mg	14 mg	196%
Vitamin B$_6$	2.0 mg	1.3 mg	154%
Folate	650 mcg	400 mcg	163%
Vitamin B$_{12}$	3.7 mcg	2.4 mcg	154%
Vitamin C	42 mg	75 mg	56%
Pantothenic acid	3.7 mg	5 mg	74%
Sodium	4,820 mg	1,500 mg	321%
Potassium	2,890 mg	4,700 mg	61%
Calcium	710 mg	1,000 mg	71%
Phosphorus	1,230 mg	700 mg	176%
Magnesium	310 mg	310 mg	100%
Iron	20 mg	18 mg	111%
Zinc	12 mg	8 mg	125%
Copper	1,560 mcg	900 mcg	173%
Manganese	2.8 mg	1.8 mg	156%
Selenium	152 mcg	55 mcg	276%

*EER for 19-year-old female, 155 pounds, 5′4″, low active.

How do you think Bobbie's food choices fit with the *Dietary Guidelines for Americans* and MyPyramid? Can you classify all of Bobbie's foods into one of the MyPyramid groups? Some items, like the cheese pizza, have elements of more than one group. Others, like the dill pickle, don't seem to fit anywhere.

When Bobbie entered her food intake into MyPyramid Tracker, she got the following results:

As you can see, Bobbie's diet was low in Milk, Fruits, and Meat and Beans. She was high in the Grains group, but without much whole grain. Her fat intake was also a little high, as was sodium. It's probably not fair to evaluate just this single day of eating, though. We would need to know much more about Bobbie's usual diet and lifestyle before making specific recommendations.

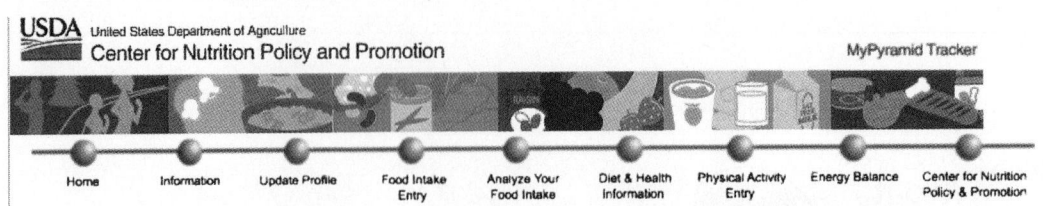

USDA United States Department of Agriculture
Center for Nutrition Policy and Promotion
MyPyramid Tracker

Home | Information | Update Profile | Food Intake Entry | Analyze Your Food Intake | Diet & Health Information | Physical Activity Entry | Energy Balance | Center for Nutrition Policy & Promotion

The 2005 Dietary Guidelines (DG) Recommendations for Bobbie

Dietary Guidelines Recommendations	Emoticon	Number of cup/oz. Equivalent Eaten	Number of cup/oz. Equivalent Recommended
Grain	☺	12.3 oz equivalent	6 oz equivalent
Vegetable	☺	5.8 cup equivalent	2.5 cup equivalent
Fruit	☹	1.3 cup equivalent	2 cup equivalent
Milk	☹	0.8 cup equivalent	3 cup equivalent
Meat and Beans	☹	4.1 oz equivalent	5.5 oz equivalent

Dietary Guidelines Recommendations	Emoticon	Amount Eaten	Recommendation or Goal
Total Fat	☹	36.4% of total calories	20% to 35%
Saturated Fat	☺	11.4% of total calories	less than 10%
Cholesterol	☺	254 mg	less than 300 mg
Sodium	☹	4,720 mg	less than 2,300 mg
Oils	*	*	*
Discretionary calories (solid fats, added sugars, and alcohol)	*	*	*

* Calculations for oils and discretionary calories from foods are under revision.

Comparison of Bobbie's Intake with MyPyramid Recommendations

Bobbie's Pyramid Stats

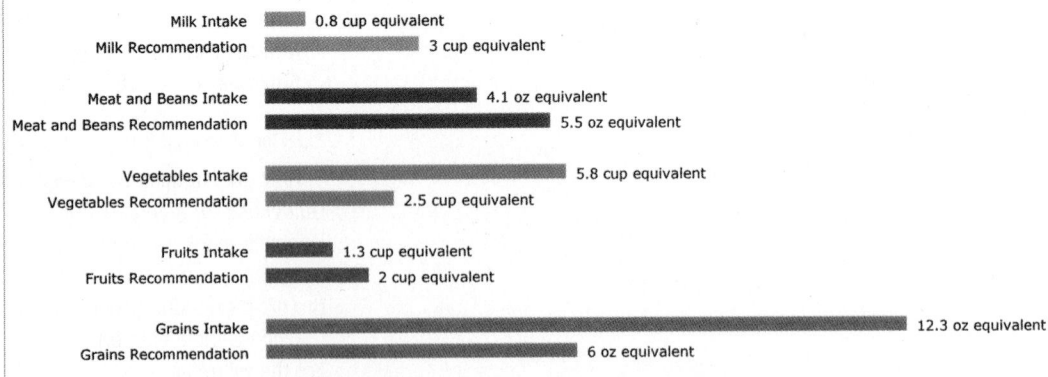

Milk Intake — 0.8 cup equivalent
Milk Recommendation — 3 cup equivalent

Meat and Beans Intake — 4.1 oz equivalent
Meat and Beans Recommendation — 5.5 oz equivalent

Vegetables Intake — 5.8 cup equivalent
Vegetables Recommendation — 2.5 cup equivalent

Fruits Intake — 1.3 cup equivalent
Fruits Recommendation — 2 cup equivalent

Grains Intake — 12.3 oz equivalent
Grains Recommendation — 6 oz equivalent

Pyramid Categories	Bobbies Percent of Recommendation
Milk	27%
Meat and Beans	75%
Vegetables	232%
Fruits	65%
Grains	205%

References

1 Uauy R. Hertrampf E, Dangour AD. Food-based dietary guidelines for healthier populations: international considerations. In: Shils ME, Shike M, Ross AC, Cabellero B, Cousins RJ, eds. *Modern Nutrition in Health and Disease.* 10th ed. Baltimore, MD: Lippincott Williams & Wilkins, 2006.

2 Drewnowski A, Henderson, SA, Driscoll A, Rolls BJ. The Dietary Variety Score: assessing diet quality in health young and older adults. *J Am Diet Assoc.* 1997;97:266–271.

3 US Department of Health and Human Services and US Department of Agriculture. *Dietary Guidelines for Americans, 2005.* 6th ed. Washington, DC: US Government Printing Office, 2005.

4 Ibid.

5 Centers for Disease Control and Prevention. *Behavior Risk Factor Surveillance System Survey Data.* http://apps.nccd.cdc.gov/brfss. Accessed 2/15/06.

6 Health Canada. Canada's guidelines for healthy eating. http://www.hc-sc.gc.ca/fn-an/nutrition/diet-guide-nutri/fg-ga-guide_e.html. Accessed 2/16/06.

7 Davis CA, Britten P, Myers EF. Past, present, and future of the Food Guide Pyramid. *J Am Diet Assoc.* 2001; 101:881–885.

8 US Department of Agriculture, Human Nutrition Information Service. *USDA's Food Guide: Background and Development.* Washington, DC: US Department of Agriculture, 1993. Miscellaneous publication no. 1514.

9 Dixon LB, Cronin FJ, Krebs-Smith SM. Let the Pyramid guide your food choices: capturing the total diet concept. *J Nutr.* 2001;131(suppl):461S–472S.

10 Smiciklas-Wright H, Mitchell DC, Mickle SJ, Goldman JD, Cook A. Foods commonly eaten in the United States, 1989–1991 and 1994–1996: are portion sizes changing? *J Am Diet Assoc.* 2003;103:41–47.

11 Institute of Medicine, Food and Nutrition Board. *Dietary Reference Intakes for Calcium, Phosphorus, Magnesium, Vitamin D, and Fluoride.* Washington, DC: National Academy Press, 1997; Institute of Medicine, Food and Nutrition Board. *Dietary Reference Intakes for Thiamin, Riboflavin, Niacin, Vitamin B-6, Folate, Vitamin B-12, Pantothenic Acid, Biotin, and Choline.* Washington, DC: National Academy Press, 1998; Institute of Medicine, Food and Nutrition Board. *Dietary Reference Intakes for Vitamin C, Vitamin E, Selenium, and Carotenoids.* Washington, DC: National Academy Press, 2000; Institute of Medicine, Food and Nutrition Board. *Dietary Reference Intakes for Vitamin A, Vitamin K, Arsenic, Boron, Chromium, Copper, Iodine, Iron, Molybdenum, Nickel, Silicon, Vanadium, and Zinc.* Washington, DC: National Academy Press, 2001.

12 Institute of Medicine, Food and Nutrition Board. *Dietary Reference Intakes for Energy, Carbohydrate, Fiber, Fat, Fatty Acids, Cholesterol, Protein, and Amino Acids.* Washington, DC: National Academy Press, 2005.

13 Yates AA, Schlicker SA, Suitor CW. Dietary Reference Intakes: the new basis for recommendations for calcium and related nutrients, B vitamins and choline. *J Am Diet Assoc.* 1998; 98:699–706.

14 Brecher SJ, Bender MM, Wilkening VL, et al. Status of nutrition labeling, health claims, and nutrient content claims for processed foods: 1997 food label and package survey. *J Am Diet Assoc.* 2000;100:1057–1062.

15 Food Marketing Institute. Shoppers demand healthier foods and more nutrition information from nation's supermarkets and manufacturers, according to "2004 Shopping for Health." FMI News; November 22, 2004. http://www.fmi.org/media/mediatext.cfm?id=684. Accessed 2/16/06.

16 US Food and Drug Administration. Guidance for industry: notification of a health claim or nutrient content claim based on an authoritative statement of a scientific body. http://www.cfsan.fda.gov/~dms/hclmguid.html. Accessed 2/16/06.

17 US Food and Drug Administration. Nutrient content claims notification for choline containing foods. http://www.cfsan.fda.gov/~dms/flcholin.html. Accessed 2/16/06.

18 Turner RE, Degnan FH, Archer DL. Label claims for foods and supplements: a review of the regulations. *Nutr Clin Pract.* 2005;20:21–32.

19 US Food and Drug Administration. *FDA's Consumer Health Information for Better Nutrition Initiative.* http://www.fda.gov/oc/nutritioninitiative/whitepaper.html. Accessed 2/16/06.

20 US Department of Health and Human Services. *The Surgeon General's Report on Nutrition and Health.* Washington DC: US Government Printing Office, 1988.

21 US Department of Health and Human Services. National Health and Nutrition Examination Survey, 2005–2006: overview. http://www.cdc.gov/nchs/data/nhanes/OverviewBrochureEnglish_May05.pdf Accessed 2/15/06.

22 Barr SI, Murphy SP, Poos MI. Interpreting and using the Dietary Reference Intakes in dietary assessment of individuals and groups. *J Am Diet Assoc.* 2002;102:780–788.

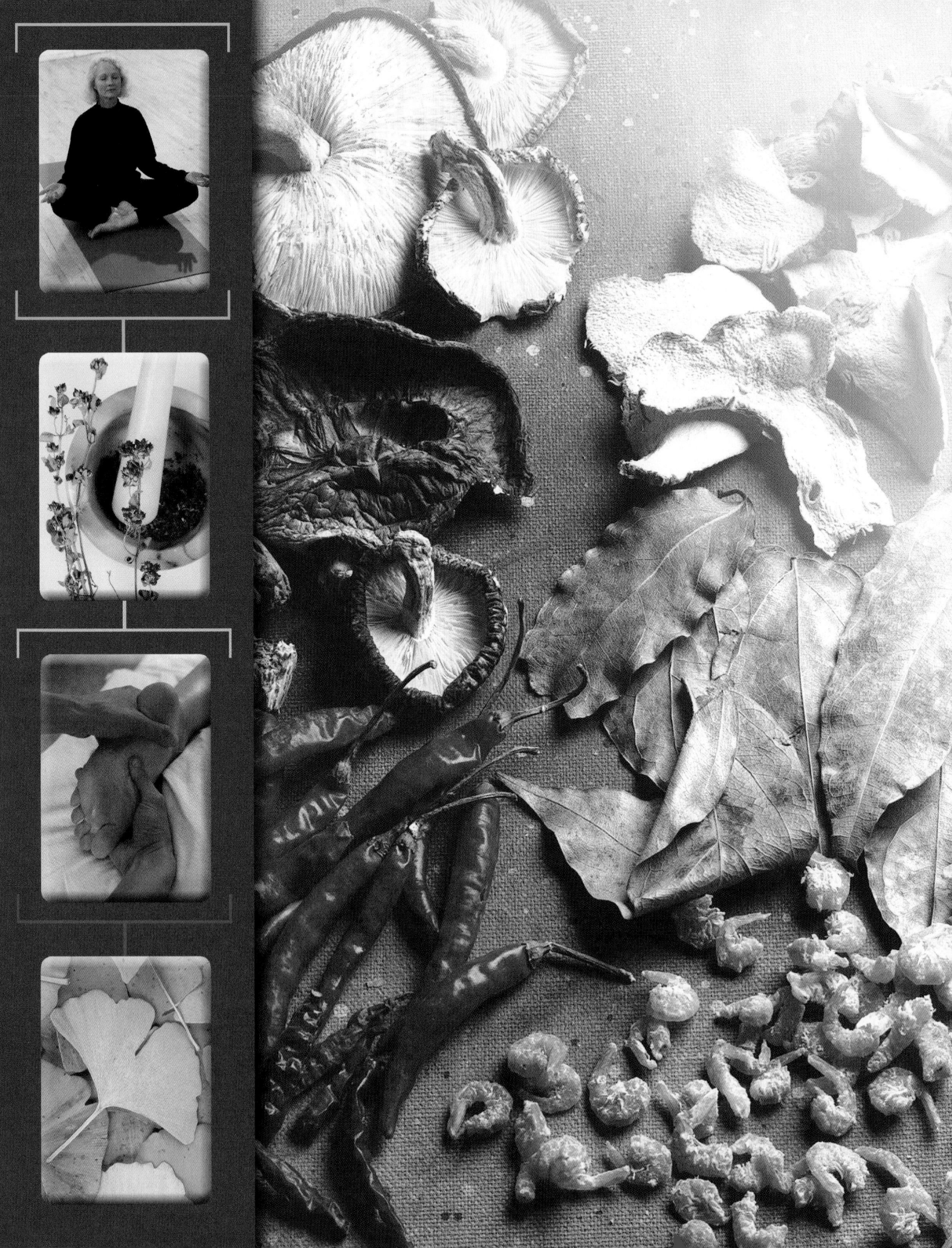

Spotlight on

Complementary and Alternative Nutrition

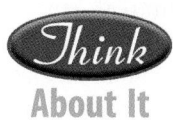

Think About It

1 When choosing food, what consideration do you give to health benefits beyond basic nutrition?

2 What are your feelings about the safety of high doses of vitamin and nutrient supplements?

3 Would you ask your physician before taking an herbal supplement?

4 If a friend told you about a new herbal extract that is guaranteed to tone muscles, would you try it?

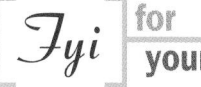

Fyi for your Information

This chapter's FYI boxes include practical information on the following topics:

• The Saccharin Story

• Shopping for Supplements

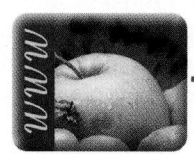

The Web site for this book offers many useful tools and is a great source for additional nutrition information for both students and instructors. For information on complementary and alternative nutrition, visit the site at nutrition.jbpub.com. You'll find exercises that explore the following topics:

• The ADA's Dietetics Practice Groups

• The ADA and Diets Versus Supplements

• Complementary and Alternative Therapies

• The Office of Dietary Supplements

isoflavones Plant chemicals that include genistein and daidzein and may have positive effects against cancer and heart disease. Also called phytoestrogens.

dietary supplements Products taken by mouth in tablet, capsule, powder, gelcap, or other nonfood form that contain one or more of the following: vitamins, minerals, amino acids, herbs, enzymes, metabolites, or concentrates.

complementary and alternative medicine (CAM) A broad range of healing philosophies, approaches, and therapies that include treatments and health care practices not taught widely in medical schools, not generally used in hospitals, and not usually reimbursed by medical insurance companies.

functional food A food that may provide a health benefit beyond basic nutrition.

lycopene One of a family of plant chemicals, the carotenoids. Others in this big family are alpha-carotene and beta-carotene.

Quick Bites

Take Out the Bad, Leave in the Good

*I*n Japan, the development of functional foods minimizes undesirable qualities as well as maximizes desirable food factors. This has led to the removal of allergens and the development of hypoallergenic foods.

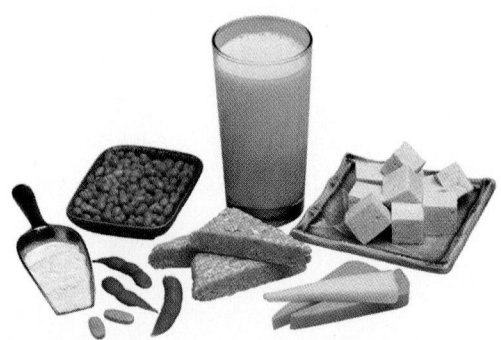

Figure SAN.1 **Tofu is rich in phytochemicals.** Soybeans contain phytochemicals called isoflavones. High intake of soy products is linked to a lower incidence of heart disease and cancer.

When she feels down, Jana takes the herb St. John's wort to help pull her out of the doldrums. Whenever she has the option, Sherina chooses calcium-fortified foods. Carlos swears by creatine in his muscle-building regimen. Jason tries a new energy bar with added ginkgo biloba, hoping it will improve his memory. Others in search of better health turn to massage therapy, magnets, macrobiotic diets, homeopathy, acupuncture, and many other practices.

Any trip to the grocery store will tell you that a new era in product development is here—one in which food products are more often touted for what they contain (e.g., soy **isoflavones**, vitamins and minerals, herbal ingredients) than for what they lack (e.g., fat, cholesterol). Beverages, energy bars, and teas marketed as foods sit side by side on the shelf with similar products labeled as **dietary supplements**. And the market for dietary supplements—which are much more than the simple vitamins and minerals our parents knew—continues to grow.

This Spotlight looks at functional foods, dietary supplements, and the role of nutrition in **complementary and alternative medicine (CAM)**. We will look at the claims made for products and therapies in terms of current scientific knowledge; we'll also consider regulatory and safety issues. Making decisions about nutrition and health requires consumers and professionals alike to stay informed and consult reliable sources before trying a new product or embarking on a new health regimen.

Functional Foods

What do garlic, tomato sauce, tofu, and oatmeal all have in common? They aren't in the same food group, nor do they have the same nutrient composition. Instead, all of these foods could be considered "functional foods." Although there is not yet a legal definition for the term, a **functional food** is widely considered to be a food or food component that provides a health benefit beyond basic nutrition.[1] Garlic contains sulfur compounds that may reduce heart disease risk, and tomato sauce is rich in **lycopene**, a compound that may reduce prostate cancer risk. The soy protein in tofu and the fiber in oatmeal are thought to help reduce the risk of heart disease. (See **Figure SAN.1**.) The functional food industry has grown rapidly since its birth in Japan in the late 1980s. In the United States, the functional food industry was predicted to grow from $20 billion per year in 2002 to $33 billion in 2006.[2]

All the functional foods mentioned previously get their health-promoting properties from naturally occurring compounds that are not considered nutrients but are called phytochemicals. Although the word *phytochemical* itself may sound futuristic, its meaning is simple: "plant chemical." It seems you can't pick up a health magazine these days without seeing an article about phytochemicals. But what do we really mean when we talk about phytochemicals, and why is there so much interest in these compounds?

Phytochemicals Make Foods Functional

A vitamin is a food substance essential for life. Phytochemicals, in contrast, are substances in plants that may promote good health, even though they are not essential for life. Phytochemicals are complex chemicals that vary

Think About It 1

from plant to plant. They include pigments, antioxidants, and thousands of compounds, many of which have been associated with protection from heart disease, hypertension, cancer, and diabetes. **Table SAN.1** lists many examples of phytochemicals and their potential benefits.

Plants contain phytochemicals in abundance because these substances are of benefit to the plant itself. For example, an orange has at least 170 distinct phytochemicals. Singly and together, these compounds help plants resist the attacks of bacteria and fungi, the ravages of free radicals, and high levels of ultraviolet light from the sun. When we eat these plants, the phytochemicals end up in our tissues and provide many of the same protections that plants enjoy.

Phytochemicals are part of the reason why the *Dietary Guidelines for Americans* recommends ample servings of fruits and vegetables each day. In the MyPyramid food system, 2 cups of fruits and 2½ cups of vegetables are recommended daily for someone eating 2,000 calories. Of course, fruits and vegetables are also naturally low in fat and calories and tend to be rich in fiber, potassium, and vitamins. In addition, studies show that groups of people who consume more fruits and vegetables tend to have lower rates of common chronic diseases.

Benefits of Phytochemicals

What are some of the specific benefits of phytochemicals? People who eat tomatoes and processed tomato products take in lycopene, which is associated with a decreased risk of chronic diseases such as cancer and cardiovascular diseases.[3] Scientists believe that the large consumption of soy products in Asian countries contributes to lower rates of cancers of the colon, prostate, uterus, and breast.[4] In fact, a study of over 3,000 Chinese women suggests that high soy intake during adolescence may reduce the risk of breast cancer in later life.[5] However, some have suggested that the biological effects of traditional Asian soy foods may differ from processed forms of soy or soy isoflavone supplements.[6] Also, the effect of soy differs in pre- and postmenopausal women, and soy supplements are not recommended for those with a history of breast cancer. The foods and herbs with the highest anticancer activity include garlic, soybeans, cabbage, ginger, and licorice, as well as the family of vegetables that includes celery, carrots, and parsley.

How do phytochemicals work to prevent chronic diseases? A number of phytochemicals, including those from soybeans and from the cabbage family, are able to modify estrogen metabolism or block the effect of estrogen on cell growth. Since levels of estrogen and other hormones are in turn closely linked to the development of breast, ovarian, and prostate tumors, it is apparent how phytochemicals might inhibit development of such cancers.

Other phytochemicals neutralize **free radicals**. Free radicals (active oxidants) are continually produced in our cells and over time can result in damage to DNA and important cell structures. We are exposed to free radicals in our environment as well as the free radicals produced in the body. Eventually, damage can promote both cancer and cell aging. Free radical oxidation of lipids contributes to heart disease risk. Many different plant chemicals, such as the pigments in grapes and red wine (see **Figure SAN.2**), are able to neutralize or reduce concentrations of free radicals, thus protecting us against the development of both cancer and heart disease.

Phytochemicals in fruits and vegetables have a number of other potential benefits. Lutein and zeaxanthin are carotenoids (plant pigments) found in dark-green leafy vegetables, corn, and egg yolks. Increased consumption of these compounds is associated with a lower incidence of age-related macular degeneration, the leading cause of blindness in older people.[7]

free radicals Short-lived, highly reactive chemicals often derived from oxygen-containing compounds, which can have detrimental effects on cells, especially DNA and cell membranes.

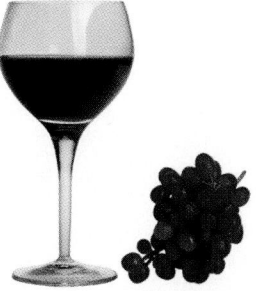

Figure SAN.2 **Grapes, red wine, and heart disease.** Grapes and red wine contain phytochemicals that appear to reduce the risk of heart disease. Studies show that moderate consumption of alcohol independently reduces heart disease risk.

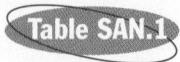 **Table SAN.1**   **Examples of Functional Components**

Class/Components	Source(s)[a]	Potential Benefit(s)
Carotenoids		
Beta-carotene	Carrots, various fruits	Neutralizes free radicals that may damage cells; bolsters cellular antioxidant defenses
Lutein, zeaxanthin	Kale, collards, spinach, corn, eggs, citrus	May contribute to maintenance of healthy vision
Lycopene	Tomatoes and processed tomato products	May contribute to maintenance of prostate health
Dietary (Functional and Total) Fiber		
Beta-glucan[b]	Oat bran, rolled oats, oat flour	May reduce risk of coronary heart disease (CHD)
Cellulose and mucilages	Wheat bran, psyllium seed husk	May contribute to maintenance of a healthy digestive tract
Gums and mucilages	Legumes, psyllium seed husk	May reduce risk of CHD
Whole grains[b]	Cereal grains	May reduce risk of CHD and cancer; may contribute to maintenance of healthy blood glucose levels
Fatty Acids		
Monounsaturated fatty acids (MUFAs)	Tree nuts	May reduce risk of CHD
Polyunsaturated fatty acids (PUFAs) & omega-3 fatty acids—ALA	Walnuts, flaxseed	May contribute to maintenance of mental and visual function
PUFAs—omega-3 fatty acids—DHA/EPA	Salmon, tuna, marine, and other fish oils	May reduce risk of CHD; may contribute to maintenance of mental and visual function
PUFAs—conjugated linoleic acid (CLA)	Beef and lamb; some cheese	May contribute to maintenance of desirable body composition and healthy immune function
Flavonoids		
Anthocyanidins	Berries, cherries, red grapes	Bolster cellular antioxidant defenses; may contribute to maintenance of brain function
Flavanols—catechins, epicatechins, procyanidins	Tea, cocoa, chocolate, apples, grapes	May contribute to maintenance of heart health
Flavanones	Citrus foods	Neutralize free radicals that may damage cells; bolster cellular antioxidant defenses
Flavonols	Onions, apples, tea, broccoli	Neutralize free radicals that may damage cells; bolster cellular antioxidant defenses
Proanthocyanidins	Cranberries, cocoa, apples, strawberries, grapes, wine, peanuts, cinnamon	May contribute to maintenance of urinary tract health and heart health
Isothiocyanates		
Sulphoraphane	Cauliflower, broccoli, broccoli sprouts, cabbage, kale, horseradish	May enhance detoxification of undesirable compounds and bolster cellular antioxidant defenses

Class/Components	Source(s)[a]	Potential Benefit(s)
Phenols		
Caffeic acid, ferulic acid	Apples, pears, citrus fruits, some vegetables	May bolster cellular antioxidant defenses; may contribute to maintenance of healthy vision and heart health
Plant Stanols/Sterols		
Free stanols/sterols[b]	Corn, soy, wheat, wood oils, fortified foods and beverages	May reduce risk of CHD
Stanol/sterol esters[b]	Fortified table spreads, stanol ester dietary supplements	May reduce risk of CHD
Polyols		
Sugar alcohols—xylitol, sorbitol, mannitol, lactitol[b]	Some chewing gums and other food applications	May reduce risk of dental caries
Prebiotics/Probiotics		
Inulin, fructo-oligosaccharides (FOS), poly-dextrose	Whole grains, onions, some fruits, garlic, honey, leeks, fortified foods and beverages	May improve gastrointestinal health; may improve calcium absorption
Lactobacilli, bifidobacteria	Yogurt, other dairy and nondairy applications	May improve gastrointestinal health and systemic immunity
Phytoestrogens		
Isoflavones—daidizein, genistein	Soybeans and soy-based foods	May contribute to maintenance of bone health, healthy brain, and immune function; for women, maintenance of menopausal health
Lignans	Flax, rye, some vegetables	May contribute to maintenance of heart health and healthy immune function
Soy Protein		
Soy protein[b]	Soybeans and soy-based foods	May reduce risk of CHD
Sulfides/Thiols		
Diallyl sulfide, allyl methyl trisulfide	Garlic, onions, leeks, scallions	May enhance detoxification of undesirable compounds; may contribute to maintenance of heart health and healthy immune system
Dithiolthiones	Cruciferous vegetables	Contribute to maintenance of healthy immune function

[a]Examples are not an all-inclusive list.

[b]FDA-approved health claim established for component.

Source: IFIC Foundation. Background on functional foods. February 2004. http://www.ific.org/nutrition/functional/upload/FuncFdsBackgrounder.pdf. Accessed 3/1/06. Reprinted with permission from the International Food Information Council Foundation, 2005.

American Dietetic Association

Functional Foods

It is the position of the American Dietetic Association (ADA) that functional foods, including whole foods and fortified, enriched, or enhanced foods, have a potentially beneficial effect on health when consumed as part of a varied diet on a regular basis, at effective levels. The Association supports research to define further the health benefits and risks of individual functional foods and their physiologically active components. Dietetics professionals will continue to work with the food industry, the government, the scientific community, and the media to ensure that the public has accurate information regarding this emerging area of food and nutrition science.

J Am Diet Assoc. 2004;104:814–826.
Reprinted with permission.

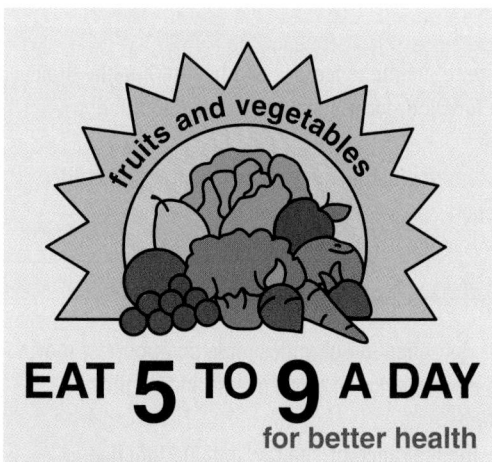

Figure SAN.3 **The national 5 to 9 a Day for Better Health program.** This program encourages Americans to eat five to nine servings of fruits and vegetables every day for better health. It was developed by the National Cancer Institute of the U.S. Department of Health and Human Services and the Produce for Better Health Foundation, a nonprofit consumer education foundation representing the fruit and vegetable industry and has expanded to include 10 partner organizations.

The phytochemicals in whole grains are generally similar to those found in fruits and vegetables and are also important in prevention of both cancer and heart disease. One class of grain phytochemicals, the terpenoids, produces a significant reduction in total and low-density lipoprotein (LDL) cholesterol levels, thus reducing the risk of heart disease. Before you reach for your next slice of bread, it is worth remembering that refined wheat, the source of white flour, has lost more than 99 percent of its phytochemical content, and only four vitamins and one mineral are added when refined grains are enriched.

Adding Phytochemicals to Your Diet

Since phytochemicals are so beneficial, why can't we just purify the important ones and add them to our diet as supplements, the way we put vitamins back into white flour after processing? The short answer is that we don't know enough about how phytochemicals function.

Many phytochemicals appear to act in concert, both fighting free radicals and blocking the negative effects of hormones. It is not surprising, then, that when a single pure phytochemical, such as beta-carotene, is given as a long-term supplement, only minor benefits are seen. In fact, some studies have shown no health benefits from such purified supplements, and have even found higher lung cancer rates in smokers taking beta-carotene supplements. Yet there is no doubt that consumption of plant foods containing multiple antioxidants is strongly associated with health benefits. The weight of evidence and experience strongly favors finding a place for more fruits and vegetables in the diet (see **Figure SAN.3**). The FDA allows the dietary guidance message "Diets rich in fruits and vegetables may reduce the risk of some types of cancer and other chronic diseases" on food labels along with the "5 to 9 A Day" logo. The advice of MyPyramid to "Make half your grains whole" will assure intake of disease-fighting phytochemicals found in grains.

Changing your diet to include more functional foods and fewer empty calories needn't be painful if you use your imagination. Sometimes you can have your pizza and eat it too. The next time you indulge, ask for a pizza with minimum cheese and maximum vegetables. Whole-wheat crust would be a plus. The combination of lycopene from tomato sauce, quercetin from onions, glucarates from green peppers, and carotenoids from basil and spinach can turn a potential nutritional train wreck into a phytochemical cornucopia.

Foods Enhanced with Functional Ingredients

Another type of functional food is one that gets its health-promoting properties from what has been added during processing. Calcium-fortified orange juice, breakfast cereals fortified with folic acid, yogurt with live active cultures, and margarines with added plant sterol and plant stanol esters are examples. Health properties come from added nutrients, bacteria, fiber, or other substances. There are also foods and beverages that contain herbal compounds like those sold in pill form as dietary supplements. As a result, there is a wide variety of products making an often confusing array of label statements and health claims.

Regulatory Issues for Functional Foods

The FDA defines foods as "articles used for food or drink, chewing gum, and articles used for components of any other such article."[8] Although this may sound a little confusing, a food is a product that we eat or drink, as well as all the components of that product. This definition distinguishes a food from a drug, which is a substance intended to diagnose, cure, mitigate, treat, or prevent disease. Foods also are distinct from dietary supplements, which are products intended to supplement the diet but which do not represent themselves as a conventional food, meal, or diet. You will learn more about dietary supplements later in this Spotlight.

Although some manufacturers have tried to market functional products as dietary supplements rather than foods to take advantage of broader allowances for label claims, the FDA's position is that conventional foods and beverages are subject to the regulations for food and not for dietary supplements. A substance added to a food for health benefits must still conform to FDA regulations for food **additives**.

Key Concepts: *Functional foods provide health benefits beyond basic nutrition. They get their health-promoting properties from naturally occurring compounds called phytochemicals. Phytochemicals are "plant chemicals" and include thousands of compounds, pigments, and natural antioxidants, many of which are associated with protection from heart disease, hypertension, cancer, and diabetes. Just like conventional foods, functional foods are subject to FDA regulations for claims and safety.*

Food Additives

Food additives work in many different ways to give us a safe, plentiful, varied, and relatively inexpensive food supply. Food additives can be either direct or indirect. **Direct additives** are added to a food for a specific reason. Aspartame, saccharin, and sucralose are direct food additives, used instead of sugar to sweeten food. Direct additives are identified in the ingredient list on the food label. **Indirect additives** are substances that unintentionally become part of the food in trace amounts—for example, chemicals from a food's packaging can become part of the food. The FDA evaluates both direct and indirect additives for safety.

Direct additives are used in foods for five main reasons:

1. *To maintain product consistency.* Emulsifiers give products such as peanut butter a consistent texture and prevent them from separating. Stabilizers and thickeners give ice cream a smooth, uniform texture. Anti-caking agents help substances such as salt to flow freely.

2. *To improve or maintain nutritional value.* Vitamins and minerals are added to many common foods such as milk, flour, cereal, and margarine to make up for elements likely to be lacking in a person's diet, replace those lost in processing, or improve shelf life.

3. *To keep the food appetizing and wholesome.* Preservatives help protect against mold, air, bacteria, fungi, or yeast, which all can cause food to spoil.

4. *To provide leavening or control acidity and alkalinity.* Leavening agents help cakes, biscuits, and other baked goods to rise during baking. Other additives modify the acidity and alkalinity of foods for flavor, taste, and color.

5. *To enhance flavor or give a desired color.* Many spices and added flavors enhance the taste of foods. Colors enhance the appearance of certain foods to make them more appealing or to meet consumer expectations.

Although most people think additives are complex chemicals with unfamiliar names, the three most common additives are sugar, salt, and corn syrup. These three, plus citric acid (found naturally in oranges and lemons), baking soda, vegetable colors, mustard, and pepper, account for more than 98 percent by weight of all food additives used in the United States and Canada.

additives Substances added to food to perform various functions, such as adding color or flavor, replacing sugar or fat, improving nutritional content, or improving texture or shelf life.

direct additives Substances added to foods for a specific purpose.

indirect additives Substances that become part of the food in trace amounts due to its packaging, storage, or other handling.

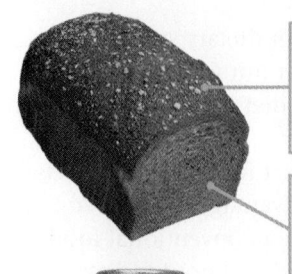

Maturing and bleaching agents such as bromates, peroxides, and ammonium chloride speed up the natural aging and whitening processes of milled flour, allowing it to be used more quickly for baking products.

Leavening agents such as yeast, baking powder, and baking soda produce carbon dioxide bubbles, which create a light texture in breads and cakes.

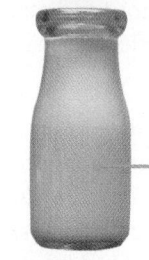

Vitamin D is added to milk to improve its nutritional quality. Many other vitamins and minerals are added to a variety of other foods.

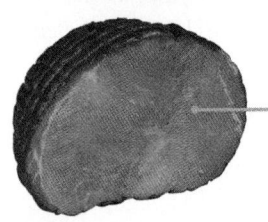

Curing and pickling agents such as nitrates and nitrites are added to bacon, ham, hot dogs, and other cured meats primarily to prevent the growth of *Clostridium botulinum*, the bacterium that causes botulism. Nitrates also give these meats their characteristic pink color. When consumed, nitrates are converted by the body to nitrosamines, which are carcinogenic. Other additives, such as vitamin C, inhibit this conversion.

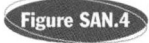

Figure SAN.4 **Common foods that contain additives.** Substances may be added to foods to improve texture, shelf life, nutritional quality, and safety.

Quick Bites

Early Food Laws

In 1202, King John of England proclaimed the first English food law, the Assize of Bread, which prohibited adulteration of bread with such ingredients as ground peas or beans.

color additive Any dye, pigment, or other substance that can impart color when added or applied to a food, drug, or cosmetic or to the human body.

Generally Recognized as Safe (GRAS) Refers to substances that are "generally recognized as safe" for consumption and can be added to foods by manufacturers without establishing their safety by rigorous experimental studies. Congress established the GRAS list in 1958.

Regulation by the FDA

Although food additives serve important functions (see **Figure SAN.4**), you might be skeptical about their safety. Additives fall into four regulatory categories: food additives, color additives, Generally Recognized as Safe substances, and prior-sanctioned substances. The FDA must approve a new food additive before it can be put on the market. The manufacturer must provide convincing research evidence that the additive not only performs its intended function but also is not harmful at expected consumption levels. Based on this and other scientific information, the FDA decides whether to approve the additive and determines the types of foods that may contain the additive, the quantities that can be used, and the way the substance will be identified on labels.

A **color additive** is any dye, pigment, or substance that can give color when added to a food, drug, or cosmetic or to the human body. Colors allowed for use in food are classified as either certified or exempt from certification. Certified colors are synthetic. The manufacturer and the FDA test each batch to ensure their purity. Certified colors added to a food must be listed on the food's ingredient list by common name. Colors exempt from certification include natural substances derived from vegetables, minerals, or animals. These colors also must be produced according to specifications that ensure purity.

A third type of additive falls under the category **Generally Recognized as Safe (GRAS)**. Congress first defined GRAS substances in 1958 when it passed the Food Additives Amendment to the Food, Drug, and Cosmetic Act. If a substance is classified as GRAS, experts generally consider it safe to use, either because it was safely used in food before 1958 or because there is published scientific evidence for its safety. Salt, sugar, spices, vitamins, and monosodium glutamate (MSG), along with several hundred other substances, are considered GRAS. Manufacturers themselves may assert that a food has GRAS status or petition the FDA to have a new food additive be considered GRAS. In either case, the manufacturer must have evidence of safety and a basis for concluding that this evidence is known and accepted by qualified experts.

If the FDA or USDA had determined that an additive was safe for use in a specific food before the 1958 legislation, then it is a **prior-sanctioned substance**, the fourth category of additives. Examples include sodium nitrite and potassium nitrite used to preserve luncheon meats.

Delaney Clause

Food additives and color additives cannot be approved if they cause cancer in humans or animals. This provision of the law is often referred to as the **Delaney Clause**, named for the congressman who sponsored it.

prior-sanctioned substance All substances that the FDA or the U.S. Department of Agriculture (USDA) had determined were safe for use in specific foods before passage of the 1958 Food Additives amendment are designated as prior-sanctioned substances. These substances are exempt from the food additive regulation process.

Delaney Clause The part of the 1960 Color Additives Amendment to the Federal Food, Drug, and Cosmetic Act that bars the FDA from approving any additives shown in laboratory tests to cause cancer.

The Saccharin Story

FOR YOUR INFORMATION

The granddaddy of all sugar substitutes is saccharin. Discovered in 1879, it was used during both world wars to sweeten foods, helping to compensate for sugar shortages and rationing. It is 300 times sweeter than sugar.

In 1907 an early attempt to ban saccharin was thwarted when President Theodore Roosevelt proclaimed the top safety official behind the effort to be "an idiot." Safety questions resurfaced in 1911 when a board of federal scientists called the artificial sweetener "an adulterant" that should not be used in foods. This same board later decided to limit saccharin just to products "intended for invalids," a restriction that was lifted after sugar shortages developed during World War I.

In 1958, when Congress passed the Food Additives Amendment to the Food, Drug, and Cosmetic Act, saccharin was one of the ingredients "generally recognized as safe," or GRAS. That same year the saccharin-based product Sweet 'N Low took the public by storm. Food and beverage companies scrambled to offer saccharin-sweetened products, which came to include the diet soda Tab and a plethora of gelatins, candies, and baked goods.

By the early 1970s, studies of rats who had been fed saccharin raised concerns about the sweetener's role in causing bladder cancer, but

scientists later suggested that impurities, not saccharin, may have caused the tumors. Then in 1977, a Canadian study looked specifically at the role of saccharin in test animals. Researchers fed rats high doses of saccharin equivalent to 5 percent of their diet. The results again showed that saccharin caused bladder cancer in rats.

Because the Delaney Clause prohibits the use of any food additive shown to cause cancer in animals or humans, the FDA proposed an immediate ban on saccharin. The FDA proposal prompted a public outcry, fueled in part by media reports that the test rats were fed the equivalent of as many as 800 diet sodas a day.[1] Congress responded by passing the Saccharin Study and Labeling Act, which placed a two-year moratorium on any ban of the sweetener while additional safety studies were conducted. Congress extended the moratorium several times over the years. The law also required that any foods containing saccharin must carry a label that reads "Use of this product may be hazardous to your health. This product contains saccharin, which has been determined to cause cancer in laboratory animals."

In May 2000, the National Toxicology Program (NTP) removed saccharin from its list

of possible human carcinogens. The NTP concluded that the types of tumors caused by saccharin in rats arose from a mechanism that is not relevant to humans. This ruling is in keeping with the opinion of other scientific bodies. The National Cancer Institute (NCI) states in its *Cancer Facts* that "epidemiological studies do not provide clear evidence" of a link between saccharin and human cancer. Regina Ziegler, Ph.D., an NCI epidemiologist, says, "Typical intakes of saccharin at normal levels for adults show no evidence of a public health problem."[2] Other health groups, including the American Medical Association, the American Cancer Society, and the American Dietetic Association, agree that saccharin use is acceptable. And in 2000, Congress repealed the warning label requirement for saccharin-containing foods.

Saccharin remains on the market and continues to have a fairly large appeal as a tabletop sweetener, particularly in restaurants, where it is available in single-serving packets under trade names such as Sweet 'N Low.

1 Henkel J. Sugar substitutes: Americans opt for sweetness and lite. *FDA Consumer*, Nov/Dec 1999.
2 Ibid.

Although the Delaney Clause sounds good in principle, it has become one of the most controversial food laws on the books. To determine a chemical's safety, researchers often administer massive doses to rodents. Many experts question whether an additive that causes cancer in laboratory animals at extremely high levels should be banned from use in foods at low levels. They argue that feeding animals large doses of a substance over their entire lifetimes may have little relevance to human consumption of trace amounts of that same substance.

For now, the Delaney Clause remains part of our food safety laws. Future scientific techniques might decrease reliance on animal testing and improve accuracy in predicting the effects of food additives on human health.

Additives in Functional Foods

Using additives to create functional foods raises questions of how much should be used and how much is safe. In addition, although there are guidelines for the use of vitamins and minerals in the fortification of food and for the use of approved food additives, little is known about what happens to many novel ingredients, such as botanical extracts, when they are put into a food.[9]

Because so many products with added herbal and other novel ingredients have appeared on the market, the FDA has been reminding manufacturers that food additives not GRAS require approval before being sold. Any food containing an unapproved food additive is considered adulterated and cannot legally be marketed in the United States.[10] Companies that have marketed foods containing herbal compounds that were not considered GRAS have received warning letters from the FDA.[11] These companies were warned that as formulated, the FDA considered the products to be adulterated.

Key Concepts: *Direct food additives are used for specific purposes. Indirect food additives become part of the food in trace amounts when the food comes in contact with the substance. Food additives are used for many reasons; these include improving product quality, maintaining freshness, and improving nutritional value. Unless a new additive meets the requirements to be considered GRAS or is a prior-sanctioned ingredient, the FDA demands that it undergo extensive testing to be proved safe and effective. The FDA is responsible for approving and regulating food additives. The Delaney Clause prohibits the approval of an additive if it is found to cause cancer in humans or animals.*

Claims for Functional Foods

In Chapter 2, "Nutrition Guidelines and Assessment," you learned about the wide variety of nutrient content and health claims allowed on food labels and the restrictions on the use of these claims. When a functional food meets the appropriate FDA guidelines, it may make a nutrient content claim or health claim on the label. For example, tofu containing at least 6.25 grams of soy protein per serving may make a health claim about the role of soy protein in reducing the risk of heart disease. However, research conducted since the approval of this health claim in 1999 has not supported more than a minimal role for soy protein or its isoflavones in reducing LDL cholesterol or other heart disease risk factors.[12] Oatmeal with an adequate amount of beta-glucan fiber can highlight its benefit in reducing risk of heart disease. One health claim applies to a functional food created through the addition of plant sterol or plant stanol esters to a vegetable

Quick Bites

Old Concept, New Frontier

Functional foods are a new frontier of nutrition and food science, but the idea has been around for centuries. Hippocrates, the father of modern medicine, proclaimed, "Let food be your medicine, and let your medicine be your food."

oil–based spread. The Benecol and Take Control product lines (spreads and salad dressings) contain these plant esters, which have been shown to reduce cholesterol levels when consumed daily in adequate amounts (see **Figure SAN.5**). Certain types of nuts (e.g., almonds, hazelnuts, peanuts, pecans, pistachio nuts, and walnuts) may make a qualified health claim on the label linking nut consumption with reduced risk of heart disease.

Structure/Function Claims for Functional Foods

Structure/function claims must be based on the food's nutritive value. An example is orange juice with added vitamin C, vitamin E, and zinc to "support your natural defenses." The term "nutritive value" is not clearly defined in the regulations, but so far no one has challenged this provision in court. So, at present, many manufacturers are making claims about non-nutrients in foods and their effects on body structure or function. For example, a cereal with added St. John's wort and kava kava extract is "accented with herbs to support emotional and mental balance," and a bottled tea is "infused with mind-enhancing ginkgo biloba and Panax ginseng." The FDA has sent warning letters to manufacturers of herbal-enhanced products charging that structure/function claims related to the herbal ingredients mislead consumers and may, if a specific disease is mentioned, make the product an unapproved drug.[13]

Key Concepts: *Under FDA guidelines, a functional food's label may have a nutrient content claim, health claim, or structure/function claim. A structure/function claim promotes a substance's effect on the structure or function of the body. For foods, the claimed effect must be based on the food's "nutritive value," a term without a clear regulatory definition. Currently, many manufacturers make structure/function claims about non-nutrients in foods.*

Strategies for Functional Food Use

So, should you go all out and fill your shopping cart with functional foods? Which ones would you buy? The best course of action is to stick with what scientists have agreed upon so far. First, fruits and vegetables promote health and reduce disease risk through a whole host of natural phytochemicals. Use the list of foods and phytochemicals in Table SAN.1 to enhance your shopping list with nature's functional foods. Second, consider nutrient-fortified products when a particular nutrient is lacking in your diet and you either don't like or can't eat good food sources of that nutrient. For example, if you are allergic to milk and dairy products, consider calcium-fortified orange juice as a nutritious way to get the calcium that you need. Third, *read, read, read* about functional foods, and not just what's on the Internet. Do your homework by looking at scientific articles—your instructor can help you find and interpret studies of functional food components. Finally, be critical of advertising and hype—if it sounds too good to be true, it probably is!

Dietary Supplements: Vitamins and Minerals

Dietary supplements contain various ingredients—vitamins, minerals, amino acids, herbals, glandular extracts, enzymes, and many others. The marketplace includes a wide variety of products claiming to do everything from enhancing immune function to improving mood. **Table SAN.2** lists many popular supplements, claims, and important cautions. Despite the enticing claims made for many non-nutrient supplements, scientific evidence of efficacy and long-term safety is still lacking.

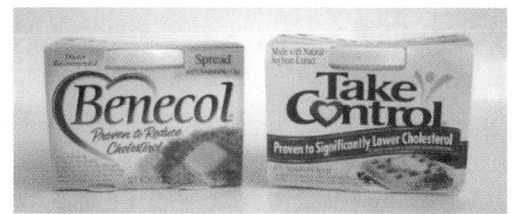

Figure SAN.5 **Some functional foods can make health claims.** Manufacturers have obtained approval from the FDA to make health claims for these margarine products.

American Dietetic Association

Fortification and Nutritional Supplements

It is the position of the American Dietetic Association (ADA) that the best nutritional strategy for promoting optimal health and reducing the risk of chronic disease is to wisely choose a wide variety of foods. Additional nutrients from fortified foods and/or supplements can help some people meet their nutritional needs as specified by science-based nutrition standards such as the Dietary Reference Intakes.

J Am Diet Assoc. 2005;105:1300–1311.
Reprinted with permission.

Table SAN.2   **Examples of Dietary Supplements and Their Claims**

Supplement	Claimed Benefits	Current Reasearch and Caveats
Beta-carotene	Prevents cancer and heart disease and boosts immunity	Diets rich in fruits and vegetables containing beta-carotene reduce heart disease and cancer risk. Supplements have not been shown to be beneficial. Taking supplements may increase lung cancer risk in smokers.
Chromium picolinate	Builds muscle, prevents and treats diabetes, promotes weight loss	No solid evidence that chromium picolinate performs as claimed or benefits healthy people. Links to diabetes need further study. Some evidence that it may harm cells.
Coenzyme Q_{10}	Cure-all; prevents and treats heart disease, treats Parkinson's disease, slows aging	May have value in preexisting heart disease, but benefits for healthy people are unproved.
Creatine	Improves athletic performance, helps burn fat	May enhance power and strength for some athletes, but is meaningless for casual exercisers and distance athletes. No evidence for weight-loss claims.
Echinacea	Cures colds, boosts immunity	Inconsistent evidence of benefit. Products on the market are unstandardized. Don't take if you have an immune-related disorder such as lupus or rheumatoid arthritis.
Ephedra (ma huang)	Weight loss, muscle building, improves athletic performance	Ephedra raises heart rate and blood pressure, and is dangerous for people with diabetes, high blood pressure, or heart disease. The FDA has prohibited sales of ephedra-containing supplements, although this ban was overturned.
Garlic	Lowers blood pressure and cholesterol, prevents stomach cancer	Some evidence that garlic reduces cholesterol.
Ginkgo biloba	Improves blood flow and circulatory disorders; prevents or cures absentmindedness, memory loss, and dementia	Limited benefits for some Alzheimer's patients. No proven benefit for others. Products on market are unstandardized.
Ginseng	Improves athletic performance, fights fatigue, cures cancer and heart disease	No evidence that ginseng has any beneficial effects. Many products on the market contain no ginseng.
Glucosamine and chondroitin sulfate	Reduces joint pain; halts, reverses, or cures arthritis	Some evidence of reduced pain, especially in people with moderate to severe knee pain, although more studies are needed. Does not reverse arthritis.
Melatonin	Promotes sleep, counters jet lag, slows aging, improves sex life, etc.	Studies are contradictory relative to sleep/jet lag. No evidence for antiaging or sex drive claims. No data on long-term safety.
Saw palmetto	Shrinks prostate, reduces symptoms of benign prostate hyperplasia	Limited evidence for improvement of urinary tract symptoms associated with prostate enlargement. No evidence for prevention of prostate cancer. May affect PSA test and diagnosis of prostate cancer.
St. John's wort	Alleviates depression	Studies in Europe suggest efficacy for mild depression. Clinical studies in the United States show no effect on major depression of moderate severity. Should not be taken with prescription antidepressants.

Sources: UC Berkeley Wellness Letter.com. *Wellness Guide to Dietary Supplements.* http://www.berkeleywellness.com/html/ds/dsSupplements.php. Accessed 5/15/06; and Sarubin Fragakis A. *The Health Professional's Guide to Popular Dietary Supplements.* 2nd ed. Chicago: American Dietetic Association, 2003.

"Should I take a vitamin (or mineral) supplement?" Apparently many people already have answered that question for themselves: Multivitamin/ mineral supplements and other single vitamin or mineral supplements are the most popular supplements, and are taken by a substantial percentage of Americans.[14] (See **Figure SAN.6**.) We will look at two levels of vitamin and mineral supplementation: (1) moderate doses that are in the range of the Daily Values (DVs) or levels you might eat in a nutrient-rich diet and (2) **megadoses**, or high levels that are typically multiples of the DVs and much greater amounts than diet alone could supply.

Moderate Supplementation

Health care practitioners often recommend moderate nutrient supplementation for people with elevated nutrient needs and people who may not always eat well enough.[15] Some examples include the following:

- *Pregnant and breastfeeding women.* Taking supplemental folic acid prior to and during pregnancy can reduce the incidence of birth defects. During pregnancy, it's hard to meet the increased needs for iron and other nutrients through diet alone. "Morning sickness" makes it even harder. When a woman breastfeeds, some of her nutrient needs are even higher than they were in pregnancy.

- *Women with heavy menstrual bleeding.* Women with high iron losses may need a supplement, but they should not take high doses of iron without a doctor's recommendation. Lab tests can show whether a woman gets enough blood-building nutrients or whether she needs supplements.

- *Children.* A supplement can help balance the diets of picky eaters or children on a food jag (eating only a few specific foods), and it can ease parental worries.

- *Infants.* If their access to sunlight is restricted, infants may need supplemental vitamin D. Doctors also may prescribe fluoride in areas where water is not fluoridated.

- *People with severe food restrictions, either self-imposed or prescribed.* Supplements may help people on a strict weight-loss diet, those who have eating disorders, those who have mental illnesses, and those who limit their eating because of social or emotional situations.

- *Strict vegetarians who abstain from animal foods and dairy products.* People who don't eat meat or dairy products may need supplemental vitamin B_{12} and perhaps calcium, zinc, iron, and other minerals.

- *Elders.* Because inadequate stomach acid (which is needed for normal absorption of vitamin B_{12}) is common among older people, elders may need extra vitamin B_{12}. When elders have limited exposure to the sun and their diets lack dairy products, they should take supplements of vitamin D, calcium, and possibly other nutrients to help maintain bone health.

Many people take nutrient supplements to ensure that they meet their nutritional needs. However, taking supplements to "fix" a poor diet is a bad idea. Foods provide not only nutrients but also fiber and other health-promoting phytochemicals. Whenever possible, meet your nutritional needs with food.

Many supplements contain multiple vitamins and minerals. If you are one of those who should take multivitamin/mineral supplements, look for brands that contain at least 20 vitamins and minerals, each no more than 150 percent of its Daily Value. (See **Figure SAN.7**.) For some minerals, even

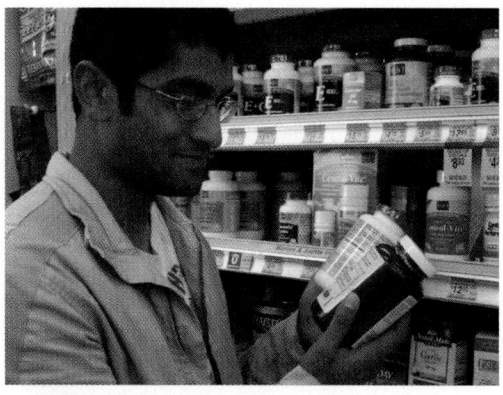

Figure SAN.6 **Popular dietary supplements.** Vitamin/mineral supplements remain the most widely used dietary supplements.

megadoses Doses of a nutrient that are 10 or more times the recommended amount.

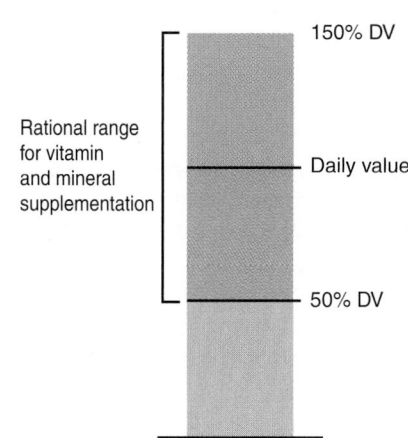

150% DV

Rational range for vitamin and mineral supplementation

Daily value

50% DV

Figure SAN.7 **Moderate supplementation.** Health care practitioners often recommend moderate nutrient supplementation for people with elevated nutrient needs and for people who have consistently poor diets.

50 percent of the DV in a tablet would make a multivitamin/mineral supplement too large to swallow, so people take these supplements separately. Although most products have appropriate nutrient levels, some formulas are irrational and unbalanced, with less than 10 percent of the Daily Value of some nutrients and more than 1,000 percent of others.

Key Concepts: *Vitamin and mineral supplements are popular; however, it is better to obtain nutrients from food. Some conditions and circumstances make it difficult to meet nutritional needs through food alone or to consume enough food to accommodate increases in nutrient needs. Multivitamin/mineral supplements should be well balanced, with doses no greater than about 150% DV of each nutrient.*

Megadoses in Conventional Medical Management

High doses of vitamins and minerals have become so much a part of treating certain illnesses that when physicians prescribe these nutrients, many see themselves as following standard medical practice rather than as practicing nutrition. Here are some situations in which physicians prescribe megadoses:

- When a medication dramatically depletes or destroys the stores or blocks the functions of vitamins or minerals, megadosing can overcome these effects. For example, folic acid and vitamin B_6 are used during long-term treatment with some tuberculosis drugs. B vitamins also may be prescribed along with seizure medications or medicines that block the metabolism of **nucleic acids**.[16]

- People with **malabsorption syndromes** often take large doses of nutrients to compensate for nutritive losses and to override intestinal barriers to absorption. Megadoses routinely are given to patients with colitis or cystic fibrosis, for example.

nucleic acids A family of more than 25,000 molecules found in chromosomes, nucleoli, mitochondria, and cytoplasm of cells.

malabsorption syndromes Conditions that result in imperfect, inadequate, or otherwise disordered gastrointestinal absorption.

Fyi Shopping for Supplements

FOR YOUR INFORMATION

Thinking about buying a dietary supplement? Before you do, ask yourself "Why do I need this supplement?" and "Is it suitable for me?" Think about your typical diet and what it may be lacking. Remember, the word *supplement* means just that—a product meant to supplement your food intake. A well-chosen supplement can be beneficial under some circumstances, especially if your diet is limited. However, if you're healthy and eat a good balance of healthful foods, supplements won't help you much.

It's a good idea to let your doctor know your supplement plans. Some supplements are contraindicated during pregnancy or lactation; others should not be used with certain chronic illnesses. Supplements sometimes interfere with the action of medicines. Some

slow blood clotting, which is a concern if surgery is planned.

To a great extent, you'll need to rely on your own understanding of diet and nutrition to make your selection. And you must rely on the supplement manufacturer for the product's safety, its purity and cleanliness, and the label's accuracy. If you're concerned about potential side effects or contraindications, you'll probably need to contact the manufacturer or distributor; you could also talk to your pharmacist or a registered dietitian.

Choose Quality

The FDA has proposed guidelines for good manufacturing practices by supplement manufacturers. Until standards are implemented, you can use tip-offs to judge a quality company—the kind you'd expect to have good quality

control procedures and to manufacture, store, and transport products safely and carefully.

A quality company will not promise miracles on its Web site, in catalogues, in commercials or advertisements, or in in-store promotions. Promises to make you smarter or thinner (unless you cut calories along with taking the supplement), to keep you young, to increase or decrease the size of various body parts, and so forth should raise a red flag. A quality company will not manipulate statistics or distort research findings in an attempt to mislead you.

A quality company will take care with its labels, print materials, and Web information. Misspelling of terms; confusion of milligrams, grams, and micrograms; and omission of

- Megadoses of vitamin B_{12} can overcome the malabsorption seen in pernicious anemia, a condition in which a key substance needed for vitamin B_{12} absorption is lacking. Ordinarily, an intricate series of steps during digestion prepares B_{12} for normal intestinal absorption; if there is malfunction during any of these steps, the vitamin is lost. Megadoses allow a small amount of the vitamin to diffuse across the intestine, thus overriding the normal mechanism and preventing deficiency.[17]

- A vitamin at megadose levels can have pharmacological activity—that is, it acts as a drug. Nicotinic acid (niacin) is the best example. At usual levels (around 10 or 20 mg), it functions as a vitamin, but at levels 50 or 100 times higher, it acts as a drug to lower blood lipid levels. Like any drug, though, it can have serious side effects.[18]

Benefits from high doses of other vitamins are not clear-cut. Researchers have tried prescribing B vitamins, including niacin, for emotional disturbances and mental illnesses; they work well when there's an underlying deficiency, but otherwise results have been mixed and often disappointing. Vitamin E has been tried for some neurological illnesses, to minimize complications of diabetes mellitus, and to reduce the risk of coronary artery disease. Megadoses of vitamin C cannot effectively prevent the common cold or treat cancer, but the vitamin may help prevent other conditions, such as cataracts.[19] Supplementation with vitamins B_6, B_{12}, and folic acid has been linked to reduced heart disease risk. However, an independent panel of medical experts has concluded that evidence is insufficient to recommend for or against the use of supplements of vitamins A, C, or E, multivitamins with folic acid, or combinations of antioxidants for the prevention of cancer or heart disease.[20]

American Heart Association

Dietary Supplements, Powders, and Other Formulas

The American Heart Association does not recommend using vitamin, mineral, or herbal supplements to treat or prevent heart disease and stroke. To avoid developing nutrient deficiencies, the AHA recommends eating a variety of foods including five or more servings of fruits and vegetables per day.

Reproduced with permission. www.americanheart.org.
© 2006, American Heart Association, Inc.

important or required information on labels are indicators of the manufacturer's carelessness or ignorance.

Confirm Supplement Ingredients

Use resources that analyze and confirm supplement content, dose, and purity. ConsumerLab.com (www.consumerlab.com) is one such service. Pharmaceutical researchers also report findings on supplement label accuracy; a search on Pub Med (www.nlm.nih.gov) can lead you to this information.

Look for the U.S. Pharmacopeia logo (USP verification mark) on supplement labels. The mark certifies that the USP has found the ingredients consistent with those stated on the label; that the supplement has been manufactured in a safe, sanitary, controlled facility; and that the product dissolves or disintegrates to release nutrients in the body. (However, the USP does not test the supplement's efficacy.)

Choose Freshness

Finding the freshest supplement is often easier if you shop in a retail store. Avoid dust-covered containers. Choose a store where turnover is likely to be quick. Supplements should be displayed away from direct sunlight, bright lights, or nearby heat sources, because heat ages many supplements. Expiration dates can also give you a clue regarding freshness.

Expect Accountability

How easily can you obtain information about the product? Look for a phone number on the label so you can call with questions or to report side effects. On Web sites, look for a domestic address and phone number, in addition to an e-mail contact. Does a knowledgeable company representative respond to your questions, or is the only person available one who reads a scripted response?

If you're shopping online but are uncertain the supplement is right for you, check the Web retailer's return policy. A Web retailer that also has a brick-and-mortar outlet near your locale may be preferable.

orthomolecular medicine The preventive or therapeutic use of high-dose vitamins to treat disease.

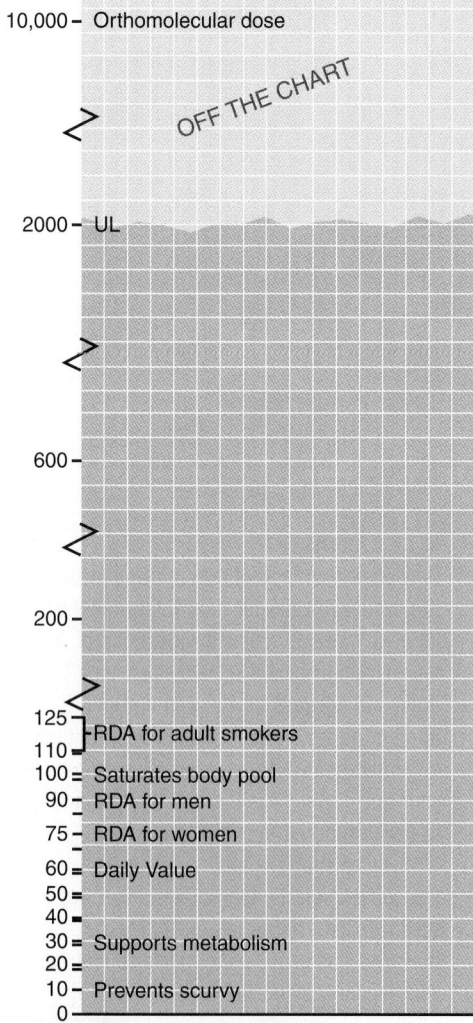

VITAMIN C

10,000 –	Orthomolecular dose
	OFF THE CHART
2000 –	UL
600 –	
200 –	
125 –	RDA for adult smokers
110 –	
100 –	Saturates body pool
90 –	RDA for men
75 –	RDA for women
60 –	Daily Value
50 –	
40 –	
30 –	Supports metabolism
20 –	
10 –	Prevents scurvy
0 –	

Figure SAN.8 **Megadose supplementation.**
Advocates of vitamin C megadoses endorse much higher intakes than recommended.

Megadosing Beyond Conventional Medicine: Orthomolecular Nutrition

In 1968 Linus Pauling, the best-known advocate of megadosing, coined the term **orthomolecular medicine**. To him, "orthomolecular" meant achieving the optimal nutrient levels in the body.[21] Few nutritionists argue with the importance of optimum nutrition. In fact, some nutritionists share Pauling's concerns that the typical diet is too refined to provide adequate nutrients and that intake equal to RDA values may not be high enough to achieve optimal body levels.

Most nutritionists would argue, however, with the high doses Pauling recommended to attain those optimal body levels and with the therapeutic value he and his followers attributed to those doses. Most notably, Pauling suggested in the early 1970s that an optimal daily intake of vitamin C was 2,000 milligrams, more than 30 times the Daily Value. (See **Figure SAN.8**.) Some advocates of vitamin C recommend even higher doses, relying on intravenous administration to avoid causing diarrhea. Dr. Pauling claimed megadoses of vitamin C prevented or cured the common cold. Although many researchers have attempted to confirm this theory, studies do not support the idea that vitamin C prevents colds. A few studies have found that colds were slightly less severe or less frequent in certain people, but most studies found no beneficial effect.[22] The most controversial claim for vitamin C was its purported ability to prevent and treat cancer. Well-controlled studies have now disproved this claim.[23]

Drawbacks of Megadoses

Megadose vitamins and minerals remain popular. But when taken without recommendation or prescription from a qualified health professional, they can cause problems. Since high doses of a nutrient can act as a drug, with a drug's risk of adverse side effects, people who choose to take megadoses should always check first with their doctors.

Excesses of some nutrients can create deficits of other nutrients. High doses of supplemental minerals, especially calcium, iron, zinc, and copper, can interfere with absorption of the others.[24] In general, it's riskier to megadose with minerals than with vitamins.

It's easy to reach toxic levels if you use high doses of the fat-soluble vitamins A and D. Vitamins E and K appear relatively safe, although at high doses vitamin E can interfere with the normal use of vitamin K and blood clotting. Megadosing with water-soluble vitamin B_6 at 50 to 100 times the DV can cause nerve damage. You may want to review the DRI tables for Tolerable Upper Intake Levels (ULs) for vitamins and minerals (see the inside of the back cover).

Megadoses often are recommended for sick people, but sick people may be least able to tolerate them. Supplemental iron is very hard on a sensitive digestive system, for example, and high doses of vitamin C can cause diarrhea. Although people who drink a lot of alcohol often are deficient in vitamin A, supplements not much greater than the DV produce undesirable liver changes in alcoholics.[25]

Megadoses can also interfere with medications and treatments. Although some people who take antiseizure medications also may need folic acid supplementation, too much folic acid can allow "breakthrough seizures." Vitamin K interferes with medication to control blood clotting and should be taken only under a doctor's direction. People undergoing surgery should describe their nutritional supplements to their doctor, because high-dose vitamin E, especially if accompanied by blood thinners such as ginkgo biloba, aspirin, or fish oil, can cause bleeding problems in the operating room. Antioxidant nutrients may counteract chemotherapy or radiation aimed at oxidative destruction of cancer cells.

Key Concepts: High doses (megadoses) of vitamins or minerals turn nutrients into drugs—chemicals with pharmacological activity. Although there may be medical reasons for prescribing high-dose supplements, they should be taken under a physician's supervision. Many claims for high-dose supplements, such as claims that vitamin C prevents cancer, are not supported by clinical studies.

Dietary Supplements: Natural Health Products

Supplementation with herbal and other "natural" products is a popular form of complementary medicine. (See **Figure SAN.9**.) The 1990s saw a dramatic rise in the popularity of dietary supplements. In a recent survey in the United States, 33 percent of adults use a dietary supplement containing an herbal or other natural product, and 65 percent take multivitamins/minerals.[26] Health Canada estimates that 71 percent of Canadians have consumed natural health products: herbals, vitamins and minerals, and homeopathic products.[27] **Herbal therapy (phytotherapy)** is nothing new, however. Most cultures have long traditions of using plants (and some animal products) to treat illness or sustain health. For centuries there were no other medicines. Even now, most of the world's people depend primarily on plants for medications; in some remote areas, modern medicines are just not obtainable.

In the Western world, the feeling that "natural" is better than "chemical" or "synthetic" has launched the expansion of the herbalism industry.[28] Herbalists reason that natural products are likely to contain a complex of healing ingredients, whereas a purified pharmaceutical product contains only one or two. They believe that when active ingredients are combined with many other plant components, their side effects may be blunted or neutralized. Using herbal medicine sounds simple and easy. But in fact herbalism calls for a great deal of skill. Traditional healers typically serve long apprenticeships and acquire a subjective "feel" for their therapies after much experience. They must learn to judge the safety and potency of individual plants, which vary from season to season, location to location, part of the plant, and age of the plant. They must know how to prepare the plant—whether to extract it and with what, or how to make it into a salve or an oral preparation. They must know how to blend it with other herbs and with other therapies. In traditional Chinese medicine, for example, a blend of herbs, sometimes 30 or more, can be used at once; the mixture usually is simmered in water and taken as a tea or "soup." Other herbal traditions use only one or two carefully chosen herbs at a time.

Traditional herbalists know their patients and individualize their herbal remedies accordingly. In the United States that includes knowing results of diagnostic testing; in other cultures it includes recognizing and understanding symptoms. But those who turn to the mass market for herbal supplements rarely receive such attention.

Helpful Herbs, Harmful Herbs

People who decide to use herbs instead of conventional medicines must choose their practitioners carefully. Herbalists must know their herbs, but they also must know when to tell patients to seek conventional care. People who use both an herbalist and a conventional doctor should tell both practitioners about the other and disclose all treatments.

Until recently, most research on herbs was published in obscure or foreign-language journals that were hard to locate or read. Traditional herbal medical

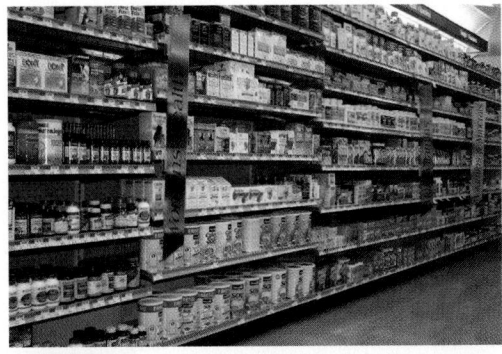

Figure SAN.9 **Use of herbal supplements is growing in popularity.** Use of herbal supplements grew nearly eightfold during the last decade.

herbal therapy The therapeutic use of herbs and other plants to promote health and treat disease. Also called phytotherapy.

phytotherapy See *herbal therapy.*

Quick Bites

Culinary Herbs Are Not Medicinal Herbs—Or Are They?

Herbs used in cooking are called *culinary herbs* to distinguish them from medicinal herbs. But culinary herbs are also rich in phytochemicals. Some examples are beta-carotene in paprika, the antioxidants in rosemary, the mild antibiotic allicin in garlic, and the mild antiviral curcumin in turmeric.

Think
About It
3

National Center for Complementary and Alternative Medicine (NCCAM) An NIH organization established to stimulate, develop, and support objective scientific research on complementary and alternative medicine for the benefit of the public.

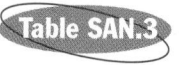

Table SAN.3 Claimed Benefits for Popular Herbal Supplements

Ginkgo biloba: combat cerebral vascular insufficiency

Ginseng (Asian): energy and mood improvement

Garlic: reduce cholesterol and blood pressure; has anticoagulant properties

Echinacea: stimulate the immune system prior to and during the cold and flu season

St. John's wort: treat mild to moderate depression

Saw palmetto: promote prostate health and treat benign prostatic hyperplasia

Cranberry: treat urinary tract irritations and infections

Valerian: a mild sedative and to treat insomnia

Kava: a tranquilizer and sedative

Milk thistle: detoxify the liver

Feverfew: relieve migraine headaches

practices are difficult to study in a controlled manner because they use plants to make teas or soups, a far cry from the purified extracts and herbal blends sold in a supermarket. Nevertheless, for some herbs, researchers have enough data to plan carefully controlled studies. The **National Center for Complementary and Alternative Medicine (NCCAM)** within the National Institutes of Health (NIH) funded a large study of St. John's wort, based on preliminary evidence that it fights mild depression and sleeplessness.[29] However, in that study, St. John's wort was no better than a placebo in treating moderately severe major depression.[30] Milk thistle may be helpful for liver disease, but more research is needed.[31] Ginkgo biloba appears to help blood circulation, and some evidence suggests it may help in treating Alzheimer's disease, although efficacy has not been established.[32] Short-term studies indicate that saw palmetto extract improves urinary tract function in men with benign prostate enlargement,[33] but a one-year supplementation study found no difference between saw palmetto and placebo.[34] Drinking cranberry juice discourages urinary tract infections by inhibiting harmful bacteria from sticking to the urinary tract's lining.[35]

The suggested benefits of other herbs are based not on scientific study, but on years of informal observation: mint helps indigestion; ginger helps nausea and motion sickness; lemon perks appetite; chamomile helps insomnia. (See **Table SAN.3** for popular supplements and claimed benefits.)

If you're considering using an herb, remember this important rule of thumb: Any herb that is strong enough to help you can be strong enough to hurt you. Like any medicine, herbs can have side effects, and herbs can be contraindicated. Ginkgo biloba is a blood thinner and has caused harmful bleeding in some people.[36] Just like any other new, unusual substance, herbs can cause sudden allergic reactions.

Herbs can interfere with standard medicines, and they can make people with underlying health problems quite sick.[37] For example, licorice extract—even as a flavoring in chewing tobacco—flushes potassium from the body, raises blood pressure, and can interfere with blood pressure medication.[38] (Most licorice candy is now flavored synthetically; naturally flavored licorice has little effect unless routinely eaten in large amounts.) The FDA has issued a public health advisory warning of interactions between St. John's wort and some prescription medications, including several used in the treatment of HIV/AIDS.[39] **Table SAN.4** lists some possible interactions of herbs and drugs.

Some herbs and herbalist treatments are downright dangerous. (See **Table SAN.5.**) Some hazardous therapies even use lead or arsenic, known poisons.[40] The herbs yohimbe, ephedra (ma huang), chaparral, and comfrey have been shown to be dangerous.[41] Senna, cascara, and rhubarb are powerful laxatives used in products described as "colon cleansers," "colon purifiers," or even "blood purifiers"; their overuse is as damaging as overuse of conventional laxatives. In fact, in November 2002 the FDA ruled that aloe and cascara sagrada are not GRAS and therefore can't be used in over-the-counter laxatives. In February 2004, the FDA issued a final rule prohibiting the sale of dietary supplements containing ephedra. Although this ban was overturned by a district court in 2005, it was upheld by the U.S. Tenth Circuit Court of Appeals in 2006. Health Canada requested a recall of similar products in 2002. Also in 2002, both Health Canada and the FDA issued advisories warning consumers not to use products containing kava due to European reports of liver toxicity.

Herbal blends marketed for specific conditions, such as "healthy bone formula" or "female blend," do not always make sense in light of current scientific knowledge. For example, pennyroyal and St. John's wort—herbs

Think About It

4

Table SAN.4 — Possible Herb–Drug Interactions

Herb	Drug	Interaction
Feverfew, garlic, ginger, ginkgo biloba, guarana, and pau d'Arco	Warfarin, aspirin	Increase anticoagulant effect by inhibiting platelet aggregation.
Alfalfa and ginseng	Warfarin	Decrease anticoagulant effect.
Ephedra (ma huang), ginseng, and guarana	Antihypertensive medications	Increase blood pressure and inhibit the activity of medications used to control blood pressure.
Hawthorn and horse chestnut	Digoxin, diuretics	Affect cardiac function and blood pressure. Should not be taken with digoxin and diuretics.
Aloe, senna (laxative), cascara, and licorice	Digoxin, diuretics	Cause electrolyte imbalance; true licorice increases blood pressure. Do not take with diuretics and digoxin.
Kava and valerian	Anxiolytics, narcotics, and alcohol	Increase sedative effects.
St. John's wort	Antidepressants, indinavir (Crixivan) and other protease inhibitors, cyclosporine	Should not be taken with prescription antidepressants. Risk of hypertensive crisis if taken with antidepressants. St. John's wort makes several prescription medications less effective. The herb speeds up activity in a key pathway responsible for breaking down these drugs in the body. When the medications are taken with St. John's wort, the end result is that blood levels of the drugs decrease because the body breaks them down faster.

Sources: Fugh-Berman A. Herb-drug interactions. *Lancet.* 2000;355:134–138, and Hu Z, Yang X, Ho PCL, et al. Herb-drug interactions: a literature review. *Drugs.* 2005;66:1239–1282.

that should not be used during pregnancy—have shown up in some "prenatal formulas." Also, a popular blend used to treat prostate cancer actually had hormonal (estrogenic) activity, which promotes growth of cancer cells.[42]

Quality control is a big issue in herbal medicines. Contaminants have caused acute illness and death.[43] A common problem is poorly standardized strength, or potency. There can be as much as a 17-fold difference in potency of the popular, over-the-counter St. John's wort supplements.[44] One analysis showed that the quantity of active ingredient in ginseng supplements varied from the amount stated on the label by as much as 200-fold.[45]

To correct these problems, the FDA proposed regulations in March 2003 to update the Current Good Manufacturing Practices (CGMPs) in the manufacturing, packing, and storage of dietary supplements. These regulations would establish standards to ensure that dietary supplements and dietary ingredients are not adulterated with contaminants or impurities, and are labeled accurately to reflect active and other ingredients.[46]

To guarantee quality, each step from field to market must be monitored carefully. However, monitoring the production of herbal supplements poses special challenges. Herbs are grown and harvested in far-flung, sometimes remote areas of the world. Extraction or preparation of the herbs may take place somewhere else. Mixing the herbs and putting them in capsules, tonics, or teas typically takes place in yet another location.

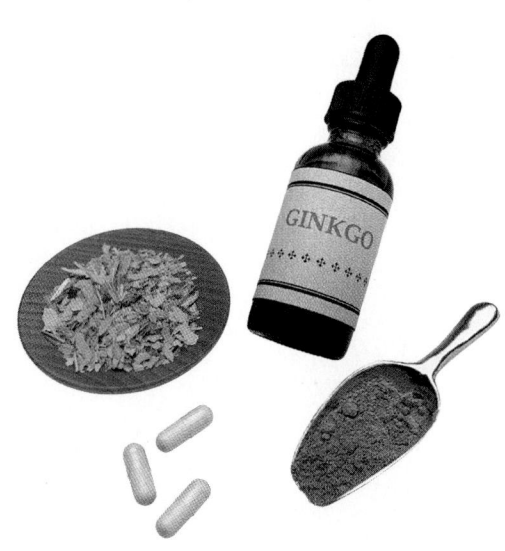

Other Dietary Supplements

The supplement market used to include only vitamins, minerals, and a handful of other products such as brewer's yeast and sea salt. Today there are hundreds more products, with new ones continuously popping up. Although some are useful, many are of dubious benefit.

Quick Bites

Office of Dietary Supplements

The Office of Dietary Supplements (ODS) is a Congressionally mandated office in the National Institutes of Health (NIH). The mission of ODS is to strengthen knowledge and understanding of dietary supplements by evaluating scientific information, stimulating and supporting research, disseminating research results, and educating the public to foster an enhanced quality of life and health for the U.S. population. The ODS Web site is http://ods.od.nih.gov.

Table SAN.5 — Potential Adverse Effects of Selected Herbs

Herb	Adverse Effects
Chamomile (tea)	Allergic reaction; digestive upset
Chaparral	Liver toxicity
Comfrey	Liver and kidney disease
Echinacea	Allergic reaction; stimulation of immune system: not for use by those with systemic/autoimmune diseases
Ephedra	Insomnia, headaches, nervousness, seizures, increased blood pressure, stroke, death
Ginkgo biloba	Inhibits blood clotting; do not take with aspirin, anticoagulants, vitamin E
Ginseng	Headaches, insomnia, diarrhea, heart palpitations, vaginal bleeding
Kava	Slowed reaction time; scaly dermatitis; liver damage
Licorice	Headaches, fluid retention, increased blood pressure, electrolyte imbalance, heart failure
Pau d'Arco	Severe nausea, vomiting; anemia; bleeding tendencies
Pennyroyal	Liver damage, convulsions, abortions, coma, death; oil is very toxic
St. John's wort	Adverse interactions with antidepressant and HIV/AIDS medications; possible photosensitivity
Senna	Laxative dependency, diarrhea, cramps, electrolyte disturbances
Valerian	Headache, excitability, insomnia

Sources: McGuffin M, Hobbs C, Upton R, Goldberg A. *American Herbal Products Association Botanical Safety Handbook.* Boca Raton, FL: CRC Press, 1997; Sarubin Fragakis A. *The Health Professional's Guide to Popular Dietary Supplements.* 2nd ed. Chicago: American Dietetic Association, 2003; and Foster S, Tyler VE. *Tyler's Honest Herbal: A Sensible Guide to the Use of Herbs and Related Remedies.* Binghamton, NY: Haworth Herbal Press, 1999.

bioflavonoids Naturally occurring plant chemicals, especially from citrus fruits, that reduce the permeability and fragility of capillaries.

Supplement categories now include protein powders, amino acids, carotenoids, **bioflavonoids**, digestive aids, fatty acid formulas and special fats, lecithin and phospholipids, probiotics, products from sharks and other sea animals, algae, metabolites such as coenzyme Q_{10} and nucleic acids, glandular extracts, garlic products, and fibers such as guar gum. Supplement producers also blend these products with herbs and nutrients, resulting in a countless array of individual and combination supplements sold today. In many cases, labeling and advertising claims go beyond current knowledge about these products.

Key Concepts: *Herbal products are among the many dietary supplements available today. Herbal medicine has a long history in many cultures. Although there is anecdotal support for the use of many herbal products, there is little scientific evidence to back it up. The FDA and manufacturers are working to set standards for the production and sale of herbal supplements. It is important to remember that any herb that is strong enough to help you can also be strong enough to hurt you. Before taking any supplements, it's a good idea to consult your health care practitioner.*

Dietary Supplements in the Marketplace

Although some dietary supplements have druglike actions (e.g., reducing cholesterol levels), government agencies regulate supplements differently from drugs. Manufacturers are allowed to make a wide variety of claims for product effects without having to provide scientific evidence to support those claims. The freedoms of speech and press prevail; in practical terms, almost anything goes. Promotional books, magazine articles, audio- and videotapes, lectures, staged interviews, and messages posted on Internet chat lines are all protected by the First Amendment, and their authors have the freedom to inform or to deceive. It's up to the listener or reader to distinguish fact from fiction. (See **Figure SAN.10**.)

The FTC and Supplement Advertising

The Federal Trade Commission (FTC) in the U.S. Department of Commerce is responsible for ensuring that advertisements and commercials are truthful and do not mislead. The agency depends on and encourages self-monitoring by the supplement industry. In pursuing companies that skirt the regulations, the FTC gives priority to cases that seriously put people's health and safety at risk or that affect sick and vulnerable consumers.[47] The FTC's Operation Cure-All targets false and unsubstantiated claims on the Internet.

The FDA and Supplement Regulation

The FDA has primary responsibility for regulating the labeling and content of dietary supplements, under the Federal Food, Drug, and Cosmetic Act as amended by the 1994 **Dietary Supplement Health and Education Act (DSHEA)**.[48] How do you know a product is a "dietary supplement"? Simple. DSHEA defines any product intended to supplement the diet as a dietary supplement and requires that the word *supplement* be clearly stated on the

Quick Bites

Pronouncing the Acronym

The Dietary Supplement Health and Education Act of 1994 is better known by its acronym DSHEA, pronounced "da-shay."

Dietary Supplement Health and Education Act (DSHEA) Legislation that regulates dietary supplements.

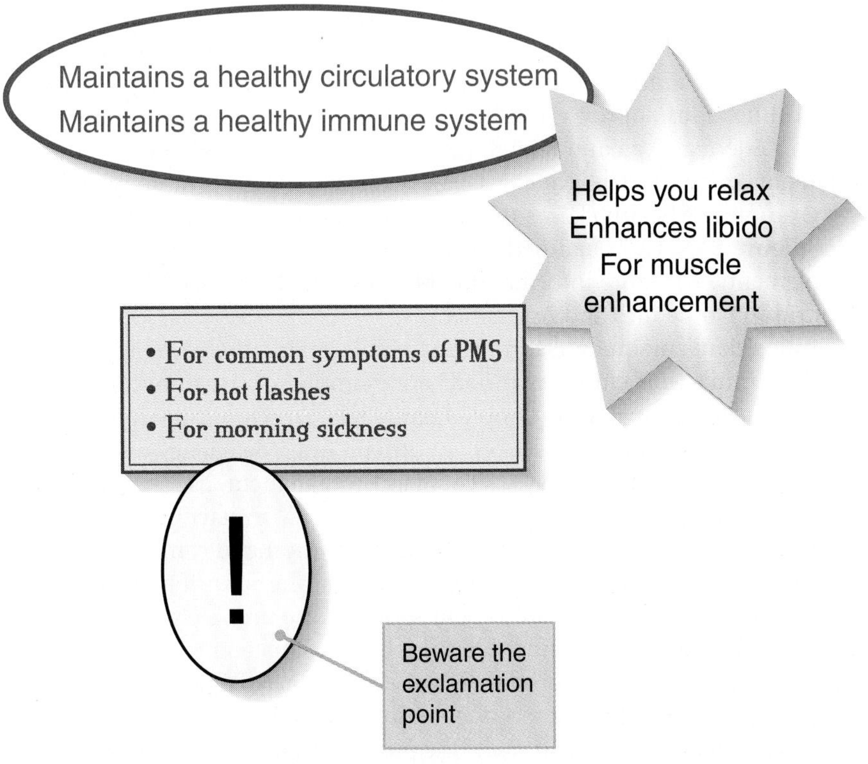

Figure SAN.10 **Dietary supplement label claims.** Although claims such as these appear on dietary supplement labels, they do not have to be approved by the FDA. All should be viewed with skepticism.

Maintains a healthy circulatory system
Maintains a healthy immune system

Helps you relax
Enhances libido
For muscle
enhancement

- For common symptoms of PMS
- For hot flashes
- For morning sickness

!

Beware the exclamation point

label. Dietary supplements include vitamins, minerals, herbs, and amino acids as well as other substances such as enzymes, organ tissues, metabolites, extracts, or concentrates.

Dietary supplements are *not* drugs. A drug is intended to diagnose, cure, mitigate, treat, or prevent disease. Before marketing, drugs must undergo extensive studies of effectiveness, safety, interactions with other substances, and dosing. The FDA gives formal premarket approval to a drug and monitors its safety after the drug is on the market. If a drug is subsequently shown to be dangerous, the FDA can act quickly to have it removed from the market. None of this is true for dietary supplements.

Dietary supplements and their ingredients also are *not* food additives, which are subject to premarket approval. For new ingredients in dietary supplements, the manufacturer finds information (usually not scientific proof) to show the substance is safe if used as directed and submits this information to the FDA 75 days before the supplement is first marketed. However, formal approval by the FDA is not required. A new dietary supplement that contains ingredients already in use does not require such advance notification. Unlike pharmaceutical manufacturers, who must prove the safety and efficacy of their products before they sell them, supplement manufacturers can market their products without the FDA's approval. To restrict sale and use of a dietary supplement, the FDA must prove that it isn't safe after it is on the market, a process that can take years.

Supplement Labels

Like food labels, supplement labels have mandatory and optional information. All labels on dietary supplements must include ingredient information and a **Supplement Facts** panel.[49] You'll notice in **Figure SAN.11** that the format is similar to the Nutrition Facts on food labels. However, a Supplement Facts panel can include substances for which no Daily Value has been established. In combination products, any nutrients with Daily Values are listed first, followed by other dietary ingredients. Herbal ingredients must list the plant part, such as root or leaf.

Supplement labels, like food labels, may contain health claims, structure/function claims, and nutrient content claims. However, only a few of the health claims approved for foods are appropriate for dietary supplements. "Adequate calcium may reduce risk of osteoporosis" and "adequate folate intake by women reduces risk of neural tube defects in newborns" are examples of health claims that could appear on supplement labels. (See **Figure SAN.12**.) Qualified health claims may also apply to dietary supplements. For more information about health claims, see Chapter 2, "Nutrition Guidelines and Assessment."

"Antioxidants maintain cell integrity," "fiber maintains bowel regularity," and "St. John's wort enhances mood" are examples of structure/function claims that might appear on supplement labels. Structure/function claims also may describe the link between a nutrient and a deficiency disease (such as vitamin C and scurvy), as long as the statement also mentions the prevalence of the disease in the United States. Manufacturers can use structure/function claims without FDA authorization and can base their claims on their own review and interpretation of the scientific literature.

Structure/function claims are easy to spot because they are accompanied by the disclaimer "This statement has not been evaluated by the Food and Drug Administration. This product is not intended to diagnose, treat, cure, or prevent any disease." There is often a fine line between structure/function claims and claims that would make the product an unauthorized drug. For

Supplement Facts Content information that must appear on all dietary supplements.

example, the claim "promotes urinary tract health" on a bottle of cranberry extract capsules would be allowable, whereas "prevents urinary tract infections" would not. A dietary supplement with a label claiming to cure or treat a specific condition is considered an unapproved drug.

Nutrient content claims must be consistent with the definitions approved for foods. With few exceptions, nutrient content claims can be made only for a nutrient or dietary substance that has an established Daily Value.

Serving Size is the manufacturer's suggested serving expressed in the appropriate unit (tablet, capsule, softgel, packet, teaspoonful).

Each Tablet Contains heads the listing of dietary ingredients contained in the supplement.

Each dietary ingredient is followed by the quantity in a serving. For proprietary blends, the total weight of the blend is listed, with components listed in descending order by weight.

Dietary ingredients that have no Daily Value are listed below this line.

Botanical supplements must list the part of plant present and its common name (Latin name if common name not listed in *Herbs of Commerce*).

%DV indicates the percentage of the Daily Value of each nutrient that a serving provides.

An **asterisk** under %DV indicates that a Daily Value is not established for that ingredient.

Supplement Facts

Serving Size 1 Tablet

Each Tablet Contains		%DV
Vitamin A	5,000 IU	100%
50% as Beta-Carotene		
Vitamin C	90 mg	150%
Vitamin D	400 IU	100%
Vitamin E	45 IU	150%
Thiamin	1.5 mg	100%
Riboflavin	1.7 mg	100%
Niacin	20 mg	100%
Vitamin B_6	2 mg	100%
Folate	400 mcg	100%
Vitamin B_{12}	6 mcg	100%
Calcium	100 mg	10%
Iron	18 mg	100%
Iodine	150 mcg	100%
Magnesium	100 mg	25%
Zinc	15 mg	100%

Ginseng Root		
(*Panax ginseng*)	25 mg	*
Ginkgo Biloba Leaf		
(*Ginkgo biloba*)	25 mg	*
Citrus Bioflavonoids		
Complex	10 mg	*
Lecithin (*Glycine max*)		
(bean)	10 mg	*
Nickel	5 mcg	*
Silicon	2 mcg	*
Boron	60 mcg	*

* Daily Value (%DV) not established

List of Ingredients shows the nutrients and other ingredients used to formulate the supplement, in descending order by weight.

INGREDIENTS: Dicalcium Phosphate, Magnesium Oxide, Ascorbic Acid, Cellulose, Vitamin A Acetate, Beta-Carotene, Vitamin D, dl-Alpha Tocopherol Acetate, Ginseng Root (*Panax ginseng*), Gelatin, Ginkgo Biloba Leaf (*Ginkgo biloba*), Ferrous Fumarate, Niacinamide, Zinc Oxide, Silicon Dioxide, Lecithin, Citrus Bioflavonoids Complex, Pyridoxine Hydrochloride, Riboflavin, Thiamin Mononitrate, Folic Acid, Potassium Iodine, Boron, Cyanocobalamin, Nickelous Sulfate

Contact Information shows the manufacturer's or distributor's name, address, and zip code.

DISTRIBUTED BY COMPANY NAME
P.O. BOX XXX
CITY, STATE 00000-0000

Figure SAN.11 **Supplement Facts panel.** Similar to the Nutrition Facts panel on food labels, the Supplement Facts panel required on dietary supplement labels shows the product composition.

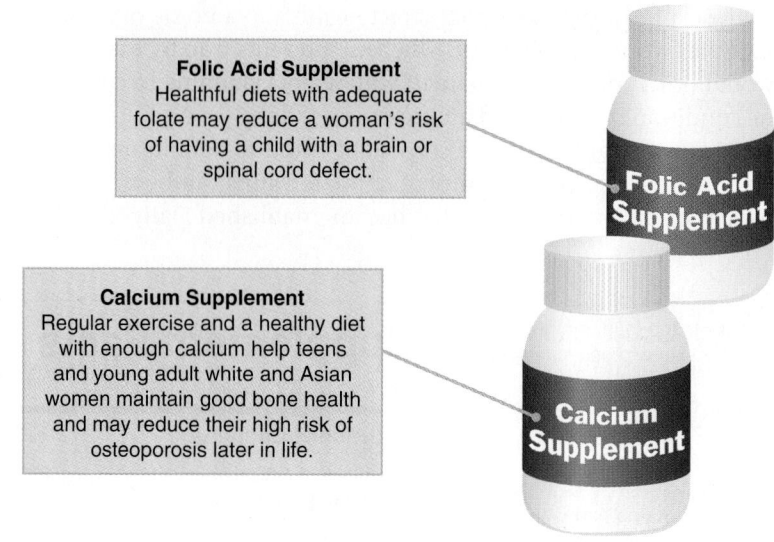

Folic Acid Supplement
Healthful diets with adequate folate may reduce a woman's risk of having a child with a brain or spinal cord defect.

Calcium Supplement
Regular exercise and a healthy diet with enough calcium help teens and young adult white and Asian women maintain good bone health and may reduce their high risk of osteoporosis later in life.

Figure SAN.12 **Health claims for supplements.** Calcium and folic acid supplements may carry health claims similar to these model statements.

For dietary ingredients without a Daily Value, manufacturers may describe the amount of the ingredient. Examples include simple percentage statements, such as "40% omega-3 fatty acids, 10 mg per capsule," and comparative percentage claims, such as "twice the omega-3 fatty acids per capsule (80 mg) as in 100 mg of menhaden oil (40 mg)."[50]

Canadian Regulations

In June 2003, Health Canada's Natural Health Products Directorate published regulations for natural health products.[51] By definition, natural health products include vitamins, minerals, herbal remedies, and homeopathic medicines. Health Canada has developed a product approval system whereby each product acquires a license after it is authorized for sale by the Natural Health Products Directorate. Authorization requires evidence of safety and efficacy. The regulations also include provisions for licensing, good manufacturing practices, labeling and packaging requirements, and adverse reaction reporting. The Canadian regulations took effect January 1, 2004, and go much farther than DSHEA in terms of assuring the safety and efficacy of retail supplements.

Key Concepts: *Dietary supplements are neither foods nor drugs, and the government regulates their manufacture and sale differently than it does for foods, food additives, and drugs. The FTC and FDA monitor advertising and labeling of dietary supplements. A Supplement Facts panel is now required on labels. Canada's regulations for natural health products require premarket approval and product licensing.*

Choosing Dietary Supplements

DSHEA has made many improvements, such as the Supplement Facts panel, to help consumers choose dietary supplements wisely. By loosening previous restrictions, DSHEA also has made many more products available to consumers. However, with the resulting array of supplements, it is a challenge for the FDA to effectively monitor claims, quality, and safety. Because manufacturers can market their products without prior approval, you need to be wary. For tips on choosing supplements, see the FYI "Shopping for

Supplements." Knowledge of nutrition science is your most valuable tool for evaluating a supplement. Read each label and judge each implied claim in light of what you know. Ask the following questions:

- *Is the quantity enough to have an effect or is it trivial?* Consider amino acids, for example. A product contains 25 milligrams of glycine. How does this compare to the amount of glycine you would obtain from a diet with 70 grams of protein? Has glycine been added to the product, or is it a component of the gelatin capsule? Is glycine an essential or a nonessential amino acid? What will happen if you take more than you need?

- *Is the product new to you?* Learn about it from the many reliable resources listed on the Web site for this book. Evaluate the product in light of scientific research. Has it been studied in humans, rodents, or other animals, or only in cell cultures or *in vitro*? If in humans, was the study controlled to eliminate a placebo effect? For case report studies, could the placebo effect influence the results? Consider also the type of preparation and the route of administration. An injected herbal extract may have a very different effect than the same herb in a pill.

- *Consider the dose used in the study. Is it reasonable and an amount found in over-the-counter products?* For example, researchers studied DHEA and found it may help some immune disorders, but at doses 20 to 50 times greater than the dosage of DHEA sold in health-food stores.[52] A consumer who chooses to take 20 of these pills daily to match the dosage used in studies would risk side effects and magnify the effects of potential contaminants. Another example is shark cartilage. In the best-controlled study to date of shark cartilage and cancer, the dose was equivalent to about 75 capsules of shark cartilage daily; even at that high dose, patients with advanced cancer were not helped.[53]

- *Can the supplement cross the intestine and travel to its presumed site of action in the body?* The body digests enzyme preparations, for example, along with other proteins. There is little data on the absorption and **bioavailability** of herbal preparations and other types of non-nutrient supplements.

- *Does the product promise too much?* A product touted to control high blood cholesterol, hangnails, psoriasis, and insomnia is unlikely to do much of anything. Neither will a "low-calorie, high-energy" drink. It's possible that the same results could be achieved more cheaply and more enjoyably by eating regular foods. Why take lycopene capsules when you can eat tomatoes, even ketchup? Why take bilberry extract when blueberries (the American equivalent to European bilberries) are delicious and low in calories?

- *Who is selling the product?* Alternative practitioners, dietitians, and even physicians sometimes sell the supplements they recommend—which is a possible conflict of interest that could compromise their objectivity.[54] In **multilevel marketing**, someone at each level in the system takes a commission on the supplements you buy, so expect to pay extra. When you buy a supplement over the phone, by catalogue, or over the Web, you lose the chance to examine it before you buy it.

A good indicator of quality is the **U.S. Pharmacopeia (USP)** verification mark (see **Figure SAN.13**), which verifies that the product meets the U.S. Pharmacopeia's standards for product purity, accuracy of ingredient labeling, and proper manufacturing practices.[55] Established in 1820, the USP is a

bioavailability A measure of the extent to which a nutrient becomes available to the body tissues after ingestion.

multilevel marketing A system of selling in which each salesperson recruits assistants who then recruit others to help them. The person at each level collects a commission on sales made by the later recruits.

U.S. Pharmacopeia (USP) Established in 1820, the USP is a voluntary, not-for-profit organization that sets quality standards for a range of health care products.

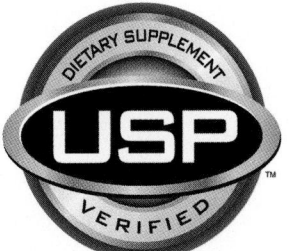

USP has tested and verified ingredients, product, and manufacturing process. USP sets official standards for dietary supplements. See www.usp-dsvp.org.

Figure SAN.13 **U.S. Pharmacopeia verification mark.** Dietary supplements can earn the USP-verified mark through a comprehensive testing and evaluation process.
Source: © 2006 United States Pharmacopeia. All rights reserved. Reprinted with permission.

voluntary, not-for-profit organization that sets quality standards for a range of health care products, including prescription and nonprescription medicines, biotechnology drugs, medical devices, vitamins and minerals, and other dietary supplements. The USP verification mark helps assure consumers, health care professionals, and supplement retailers that a product has passed USP's rigorous program and

- Contains the ingredients declared on the product label
- Contains the amount or strength of ingredients declared on the product label
- Meets requirements for limits on potential contaminants
- Has been manufactured properly by complying with USP and proposed FDA standards for CGMPs

Many nationally known food and drug manufacturers have established their own standards, quality control, and manufacturing practices that they are likely to apply to their dietary supplements as well. Contact the company with your questions; you'll learn a lot, although maybe not what you expected. The "technical representative" may be unable to give you any more information than a brief readout from a computer database. Some companies respond to queries by sending a long printout of journal citations, most of them inappropriate, without text or even abstracts; many references are in a foreign language. On the other hand, some dietary supplement companies have on-site quality control and on-site nutritionists who are knowledgeable and happy to supply helpful information. Once CGMPs are finalized and in place, quality issues will be less of a concern.

Even the best-intentioned, most carefully considered supplement can prove ineffective or even risky. Take the example of beta-carotene supplements. Even though diets rich in beta-carotene are linked with reduced cancer risk, several large, well-controlled studies found that beta-carotene supplements had no protective effect. For some groups of people, such as smokers, these supplements actually increased risk.[56] The results disappointed advocates of beta-carotene, but these studies demonstrate the value of carefully controlled studies and the risk of unproved assumptions about dietary supplements.

Fraudulent Products

Some health advocates consider the burgeoning market of dietary supplements an unwelcome return to the "snake oil" era of the late nineteenth and early twentieth centuries, when "magic" potions and cures were sold door to door and at county fairs and markets. Most manufacturers work hard to assure the quality of their products, yet some supplements on the market are nothing more than a mixture of ineffective ingredients.

In the *FDA Consumer* magazine, the agency had this to say about fraudulent products:

> You often can identify fraudulent products by the types of claims made in their labeling, advertising, and promotional literature. Stephen Barrett, M.D., a board member of the National Council Against Health Fraud, points to the following indicators of possible fraud:
>
> - Claims that the product is a secret cure and use of such terms as *breakthrough, magical, miracle cure,* and *new discovery.* "If the product were a cure for a serious disease, it would be widely reported in the media and used by health-care professionals," he says.

- "Pseudomedical" jargon, such as *detoxify, purify,* and *energize* to describe a product's effects. "These claims are vague and hard to measure," Barrett says. "So, they make it easier for success to be claimed, even though nothing has actually been accomplished," he says.

- Claims that the product can cure a wide range of unrelated diseases. "No product can do that," he says.

- Claims that the supplement has only benefits—and no side effects. "A product potent enough to help people will be potent enough to cause side effects," Barrett says.

- Claims that a product is backed by scientific studies, but with no list of references or references that are inadequate. For instance, if a list of references is provided, the citations cannot be traced, or if they are traceable, the studies are out-of-date, irrelevant, or poorly designed.

- Accusations that the medical profession, drug companies, and the government are suppressing information about a particular treatment. "It would be illogical," Barrett says, "for large numbers of people to withhold information about potential medical therapies when they or their families and friends might one day benefit from them."[57]

Supplement users who suffer a serious harmful effect or illness that they think is related to supplement use should call a doctor or other health care provider. Practitioners can report problems to FDA MedWatch by calling 1-800-FDA-1088 or by going to www.fda.gov/medwatch/report/hcp.htm on the MedWatch Web site. Consumers can call the toll-free MedWatch number or go to www.fda.gov/medwatch/report/consumer/consumer.htm on the MedWatch Web site to report an adverse reaction.

Key Concepts: *When considering a dietary supplement, it is important to consider the product and its claims carefully. Be aware that some products may promise more than they can deliver. A good indicator of quality is the USP verification mark, but even this does not guarantee that a product will fulfill its claims.*

Complementary and Alternative Medicine

Complementary and alternative medicines (CAM) are therapies and treatments outside the medical mainstream. They tend to be based mainly or solely on observation or anecdotal evidence rather than controlled research. One widely used definition is "treatments or health-care practices neither taught widely in U.S. medical schools nor generally available in U.S. hospitals."[58] This definition, however, may need updating; many medical schools and conventional health care providers have begun to teach or use these therapies, sometimes with insurance reimbursement.[59]

The term *alternative* suggests practices that *replace* conventional ones. *Complementary* implies practices that are used *in addition to* conventional ones. For example, using only herbs and megavitamins to treat AIDS would be "alternative," whereas using herbs to combat diarrhea caused by conventional AIDS medications and taking supplements to replace lost vitamins would be "complementary." Many people find the terms *complementary* or *integrative* more acceptable than *alternative,* although all these terms often are used interchangeably. CAM includes a broad range of healing therapies and philosophies. Several among them involve nutrition, including special

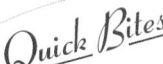
Quick Bites

Mayonnaise Protects Against Strokes

Is this claim science or snake oil? Studies show that foods rich in vitamin E help protect against heart disease and stroke. In one study of stroke reduction in postmenopausal women, mayonnaise was the most concentrated food source of vitamin E. But to claim that mayonnaise prevents strokes is unwarranted and overstates the evidence.

diet therapies, phytotherapy (herbalism), orthomolecular medicine, and other biologic interventions.

In 1990 about 34 percent of the adult U.S. population used CAM;[60] by 1997 that number had grown to 42 percent.[61] In 2002, 62 percent of adults surveyed had used some form of CAM in the previous 12 months.[62] The most commonly used CAM therapies in 2002 were prayer, natural products, deep breathing exercises, meditation, chiropractic care, yoga, massage, and diet-based therapies. People seek out CAM for numerous reasons, including fear of aging, personal beliefs, and distrust of institutional medicine.

Where Does Nutrition Fit In?

A number of alternative therapies involve nutrition, and sometimes the line between standard and alternative nutrition is not clear. A variety of health conditions, such as diabetes, gastrointestinal disorders, and kidney disease, require special diets. Alternative nutrition practices include diets to prevent and treat diseases not shown to be diet-related. (See **Figure SAN.14**.) What often makes these practices "alternative" is the limited nature of the diet, the lack of rigorous scientific evidence showing effectiveness, and the divergence from science-based healthy eating patterns such as the DASH diet or MyPyramid. Other practices outside the nutritional mainstream include reliance on only raw foods and the extensive use of herbal and botanical supplements as well as megadoses of vitamin/mineral supplements, which we have already discussed.

Special Diets, Food Restrictions, and Food Prescriptions

Vegetarian Diets

The specifics of vegetarianism are described in Chapter 6, "Proteins and Amino Acids." Most nutritionists consider vegetarianism a routine variation of a normal diet, particularly if the vegetarian's motivation is religious or philosophical, the result of a concern for animals, or an aversion to animal products. When a meat eater goes vegetarian in an attempt to prevent or cure disease, that's "alternative."

Macrobiotic Diet

Aside from vegetarianism, the **macrobiotic diet** probably is the best-known alternative diet. The original version of this primarily vegetarian diet progressed in ten increasingly restrictive stages, with the "highest level" consisting of little more than brown rice and water. The diet has since evolved to a simpler one-level regimen based on whole-grain cereals and vegetables, a small amount of fish, no other animal products, and no fruit.[63]

Proponents tout the macrobiotic diet as a cure for a variety of illnesses, most notably cancer. To use it as a cancer treatment, the practitioner individualizes the diet according to Eastern philosophy (yin and yang, whose symbol is shown in **Figure SAN.15**) and the location of the cancer. Critics say macrobiotic restrictions interfere with legitimate cancer treatment by causing weight loss in people who are already too thin from their illness. The diet is so limited that it just can't meet the increased nutritional needs of the cancer patient. Advocates of macrobiotics, on the other hand, argue that undernutrition may help fight the cancer by starving it.[64] It looks as if neither opinion is correct: Macrobiotic diets appear to have no clear effect, good or bad, on cancer progression or survival.

macrobiotic diet A highly restrictive dietary approach applied as a therapy for risk factors or chronic disease in general.

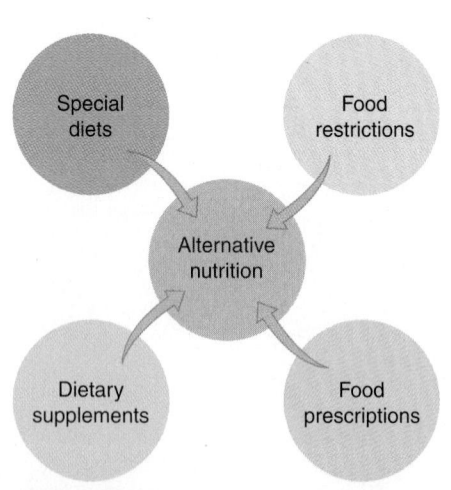

Figure SAN.14 **Alternative nutrition practices.** Although many mainstream medical practices may involve special dietary regimens, alternative nutrition practices often are overly restrictive, depart from established dietary guidelines, and lack rigorous scientific evidence.

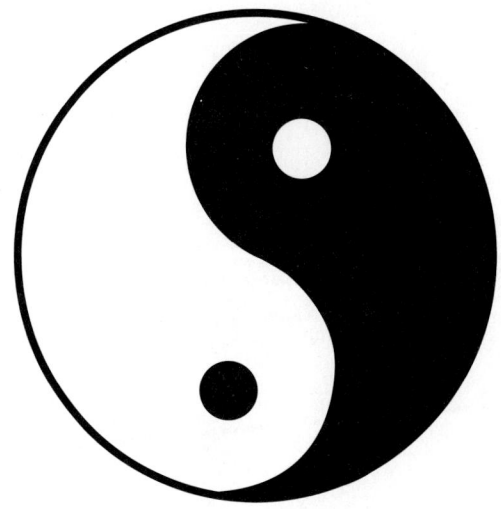

The symbol of yin and yang. In traditional Chinese medicine, practitioners strive to balance opposing life forces of yin and yang through the use of food and herbs.

The Yin and Yang of Food

The early theory of yin and yang had its genesis during the Yin and Zhou dynasties (1766 B.C.E.–256 B.C.E.). The yin force is passive, downward flowing, and cold. Conversely, the yang force is aggressive, upward rising, and hot. The concept of balance and harmony between these life forces is the basis upon which food and herbs are used as medicine. In traditional Chinese healing methods, disease is viewed as the result of an imbalance of these energies in the body. To balance these energies, according to this view, your diet should balance yin foods and yang foods. Yin (cold) foods include milk, honey, fruit, and vegetables; and yang (hot) foods include beef, poultry, seafood, eggs, and cheese. Foods are also classified as sweet (earth), bitter (fire), sour (wood), pungent (metal), and salty (water). Each class supposedly has specific effects on different parts of the body.

Compared to the general public, those who follow a macrobiotic diet tend to have healthier blood lipid levels and higher blood levels of phytochemicals, which reflects vegetable intake.[65] However, the diet is low in calcium and vitamin D, which contributes to the risk for osteoporosis. Pediatricians caution against this diet for children.

Food Restrictions and Food Prescriptions

Societies throughout the world commonly use dietary changes to treat or prevent illness. The specifics vary from place to place, however, which suggests that they are based on cultural factors rather than science.

In recent years we have seen yeast-free diets, dairy-free diets, sugar-free diets, white-flour-free diets, both low-carbohydrate and high-carbohydrate diets, both low-red-meat and high-red-meat diets, caffeine-free diets, salicylate-free diets, and more. We have been advised to load up on molasses, yogurt, honey, vinegar, oysters, mushrooms, and soy nuts. People with subjective symptoms such as headaches, fatigue, or back pain have been instructed to avoid irrational lists of "allergenic foods" based on "blood screening." We've also seen illogical instructions on how to combine foods, such as "don't eat applesauce and asparagus at the same meal." For weight loss, we've had grapefruit diets, hard-boiled-egg diets, cottage-cheese diets, water diets, high-fat diets, low-fat diets, and blue-foods-only diets; the list goes on and on.

Such diets come and go. They are not based on science and eventually fall out of style when they don't work. Those few that prove effective and have a scientific basis become integrated into conventional nutrition and diet therapy. (See **Figure SAN.16**.)

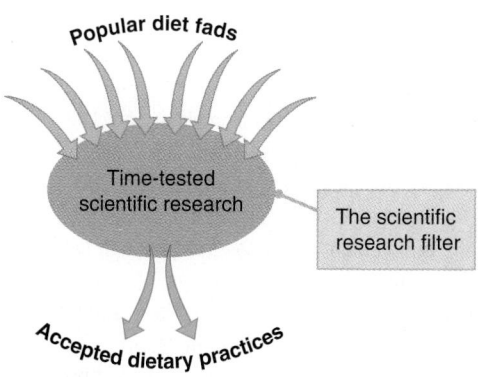

Popular diet fads

Time-tested scientific research

The scientific research filter

Accepted dietary practices

Many apply but few are chosen. Dietary practices with a scientific basis and proven efficacy are incorporated into conventional nutrition and diet therapy.

Key Concepts: *Many types of diet can be described as alternative. Their origins and claims vary, and their proponents often cannot show that they improve health. Some alternative diets can actually be harmful by restricting foods and thereby lowering the body's intake of necessary nutrients.*

Label [to] **Table**

If you picked up a multivitamin/mineral container from your drugstore shelf, would you know how to read the label? Look at this Supplement Facts panel from a basic multivitamin/mineral supplement. Here are some questions that you might have.

1. If you were a 20-year-old woman who knew she wasn't consuming enough calcium, would this supplement allow you to get your recommended intake?
2. If 25 percent of the vitamin A in this supplement comes from beta-carotene, where does the rest come from?
3. What trend do you see in the amounts of B vitamins?
4. What trend do you see in the amounts of bone minerals?
5. What trend do you see in the amounts of antioxidant vitamins?
6. Does the USP statement make this supplement "legitimate"?

Supplement Facts
Daily Multivitamin/Mineral Dietary Supplement

USP Made to U.S. Pharmacopeia (USP) quality, purity, and potency standards. Laboratory tested to dissolve within 60 minutes.

Serving Size 1 tablet

Each Tablet Contains	% DV	Each Tablet Contains	% DV
Vitamin A 10,000 I.U.	200%	Iodine 150 mcg	100%
25% as beta-carotene		Magnesium 100 mg	25%
Vitamin C 120 mg	200%	Zinc 22.5 mg	150%
Vitamin D 400 IU	100%	Selenium 45 mcg	64%
Vitamin E 60 IU	200%	Copper 3 mg	150%
Vitamin K 25 mcg	31%	Manganese 2.5 mg	125%
Thiamin (vit. B$_1$) 1.5 mg	100%	Chromium 100 mcg	83%
Riboflavin (vit. B$_2$) 1.7 mg	100%	Molybdenum 25 mcg	33%
Niacin 20 mg	100%	Chloride 36.3 mg	1%
Vitamin B$_6$ 2 mg	100%	Sodium less than 5 mg	less than 1%
Folate (folic acid) 400 mcg	100%	Potassium 40 mg	1%
Vitamin B$_{12}$ 6 mcg	100%	Nickel 5 mcg	*
Biotin 30 mcg	10%	Tin 10 mcg	*
Pantothenic acid 10 mg	100%	Silicon 2 mg	*
Calcium 162 mg	16%	Vanadium 10 mcg	*
Iron 9 mg	50%	Boron 150 mcg	*
Phosphorus 109 mg	11%		

* Daily Value (%DV) not established

Answers to Questions

1. No. This supplement provides only 162 milligrams, and the Adequate Intake (AI) for a 20-year-old woman is 1,000 milligrams. You may need a calcium supplement if you can't eat enough calcium-rich foods.
2. The other 7,500 IU of vitamin A is most likely retinol in the form of retinyl acetate or retinyl palmitate; check the list of ingredients.
3. With the exception of biotin, this supplement provides 100% Daily Value for the B vitamins. And the 30 micrograms of biotin provides 100 percent of the current AI.
4. This supplement contains very low percentages of the Daily Values for calcium, magnesium, and phosphorus (16%, 11%, and 25%, respectively). Adding more of these minerals would make the pill huge and impossible to swallow! A nutritious diet should provide the rest of these minerals.
5. This supplement contains 200 percent of the Daily Value for each of the antioxidant vitamins C and E, and one-fourth (50% DV) of its vitamin A content comes from the antioxidant beta-carotene.
6. By listing the U.S. Pharmacopeia "stamp of approval," you can be confident that this supplement underwent a test to see how quickly it dissolves. If pills do not dissolve, their contents cannot be absorbed. In this case, the supplement took 60 minutes to dissolve. The USP sets standards for the quality, purity, and potency of supplements.

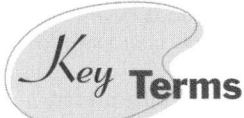

LEARNING *Portfolio*

Key Terms

Study Points

➤ A functional food is considered to be a food that may provide a health benefit beyond basic nutrition.

➤ Phytochemicals are plant chemicals responsible for the health-promoting properties of many functional foods.

➤ Consumption of plant foods containing multiple antioxidants is strongly associated with health benefits. Scientific evidence strongly supports eating at least five or more servings of fruits and vegetables daily and emphasizing whole grains.

➤ The federal government reviews the safety of new food additives before they can be used in foods sold on the market.

➤ The Delaney Clause is a controversial food law that prohibits the approval of a food additive if it has been found to cause cancer in humans or laboratory animals, even if massive doses are required to produce the disease.

➤ Dietary supplements encompass vitamins, minerals, herbal products, amino acids, glandular extracts, enzymes, and many other products.

➤ Vitamin and mineral supplements may be warranted in certain circumstances, although the preferred mode of obtaining adequate nutrition is through foods.

➤ Megadose vitamin or mineral therapy has not been proved effective in the treatment of cancer, colds, or heart disease. Moreover, such megadoses act more like drugs than nutrients in the body and should be approached with caution.

➤ Herbal medicine is a traditional form of healing in many cultures. Some herbal medicines have shown enough promise to warrant large-scale clinical studies involving supplements. However, herbal products can have side effects and can interfere with prescription medications.

➤ Dietary supplements are regulated in the United States according to the provisions of the Dietary Supplement Health and Education Act of 1994. Unlike drugs and food additives, dietary supplements do not need premarket approval.

➤ Claims for dietary supplements can include health claims, structure/function claims, and nutrient content claims.

➤ Dietary supplements must have a Supplement Facts panel on the label.

➤ Consumers should carefully evaluate claims and evidence for dietary supplements and consult their physician before taking a supplement.

➤ Complementary and alternative medicine (CAM) comprises practices outside the medical mainstream that are becoming increasingly popular. CAM includes a broad range of therapies, many of which include nutrition. People seek them for a variety of reasons, including environmental concerns and a fear of aging.

Study Questions

1. **What are phytochemicals, and how do they benefit plants and humans?**
2. **Name three chronic diseases that consuming functional foods may help prevent.**
3. **What purpose(s) do food additives serve?**
4. **What is the purpose of the Delaney Clause? What are the complications surrounding this food law?**
5. **What is a macrobiotic diet?**
6. **How do you know a product is a dietary supplement?**
7. **What things should someone do before purchasing supplements?**
8. **If a dietary supplement product label contains the words "High in vitamin E," what type of claim is it making? What other claims can a supplement make?**
9. **What are some of the possible complications involved in using herbal medicines?**

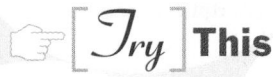

☞ [*Try*] **This**

Finding Functional Beverages

This exercise will familiarize you with the many beverages now available to consumers that contain functional ingredients. Take a trip to your grocery store and spend some time in the beverage aisles. You may want to check out the chilled juice section in addition to the bottled teas and juice beverages. Pick out about 10 different products that have either a nutrient or herbal compound added and try to identify how many have nutrient content claims, health claims, and structure/function claims. Note the prices of these products. How does their nutritional content compare to a 100% fruit juice like orange juice? How does it compare to soda?

Take a Walk on the "Web Side"

This exercise will familiarize you with various Web sites that promote and sell supplements. Log on to the Internet and start doing searches with key words affiliated with supplements. Try *vitamins, minerals, supplements, herbs,* and even some specific terms like *chromium picolinate* and *ginseng*. On the Web sites you visit, how is the nutrition information presented? Do the supplement's benefits sound too good to be true? See if you can spot a fraud. Use the information in the "Fraudulent Products" section of this chapter to identify the accuracy of the product information you find.

References

1 Institute of Food Technologists. *Functional Foods: Opportunities and Challenges.* IFT Expert Report, March 2005. http://www.ift.org/cms/?pid=1001247. Accessed 3/1/06.

2 Heasman M. Addressing the functional food paradox. *Nutraceuticals World.* November 2003. http://www.nutraceuticalsworld.com/Nov031.htm. Accessed 3/1/06.

3 Heber D. Vegetables, fruits and phytoestrogens in the prevention of diseases. *J Postgrad Med.* 2004;50:145–149.

4 Goldwyn S, Lazinsky A, Wei H. Promotion of health by soy isoflavones: efficacy, benefit and safety concerns. *Drug Metabol Drug Interact.* 2000;17:261–289.

5 Shu XO, Jin F, Dai Q, et al. Soyfood intake during adolescence and subsequent risk of breast cancer among Chinese women. *Cancer Epidemiol Biomarkers Prev.* 2001;10:483–488.

6 Maskarinec G. Soy foods for breast cancer surivors and women at high risk for breast cancer? *J Am Diet Assoc.* 2005;105:1524–1528.

7 Stahl W. Macular carotenoids: lutein and zeaxanthin. *Dev Ophthalmol.* 2005;38:70–88.

8 Turner RE, Degnan FH, Archer DL. Label claims for food and supplements: a review of the regulations. *Nutr Clin Pract.* 2005;20(1):21–32.

9 Percival SS, Turner RE. Applications of herbs to functional foods. In: Wildman REC, ed. *Handbook of Nutraceuticals and Functional Foods.* 2nd ed. Boca Raton, FL: CRC Press, 2007.

10 US Food and Drug Administration. Letter to manufacturers regarding botanicals and other novel ingredients in conventional foods. January 30, 2001. http://www.cfsan.fda.gov/~dms/ds-ltr15.html. Accessed 3/1/06.

11 US Food and Drug Administration. Concerns about botanical and other novel ingredients in conventional foods. June 4–5, 2001. http://www.cfsan.fda.gov/~dms/ds-bot5.html. Accessed 3/1/06.

12 Sacks FM, Lichtenstein A, Van Horn L, Harris W, Kris-Etherton P, Winston M. Soy protein, isoflavones, and cardiovascular health: an American Heart Association Science Advisory for professionals from the Nutrition Committee. *Circulation.* 2006;113:1034–1044.

13 Turner RE, Degnan FH, Archer DL. Op. cit.

14 Timbo BB, Ross MP, McCarthy PV, Lin C-TL. Dietary supplements in a national survey: prevalence of use and reports of adverse events. *J Am Diet Assoc.* 2006;106:1966–1974.

15 Multivitamin-mineral supplements: take one—but which one? *Dietary Supplement.* 2002;3(5,6).

16 *Physicians' Desk Reference.* 59th ed. Montvale, NJ: Medical Economics Company, 2005.

17 Lederle FA. Oral cyanocobalamin for pernicious anemia: medicine's best kept secret? *JAMA.* 1991;265:94–95.

18 *Physicians' Desk Reference.* 59th ed. Op. cit.

19 Jacques PF, Taylor A, Hankinson SE, et al. Long-term vitamin C supplement use and prevalence of early age-related lens opacities. *Am J Clin Nutr.* 1997;66:911–916.

20 US Preventive Services Task Force. Routine vitamin supplementation to prevent cancer and cardiovascular disease: recommendations and rationale. *Ann Intern Med.* 2003;139:51–55.

21 *Alternative Medicine, Expanding Medical Horizons. A Report to the National Institutes of Health on Alternative Medical Systems and Practices in the United States.* Washington, DC: US Government Printing Office, 1994:230–232, 237. NIH publication 94-066.

22 Institute of Medicine, Food and Nutrition Board. *Dietary Reference Intakes for Vitamin C, Vitamin E, Selenium, and Carotenoids.* Washington, DC: National Academy Press, 2000.

23 Byers T, Guerrero N. Epidemiologic evidence for vitamin C and vitamin E in cancer prevention. *Am J Clin Nutr.* 1995; 62(suppl):1385S–1392S.

24 Institute of Medicine, Food and Nutrition Board. *Dietary Reference Intakes for Vitamin A, Vitamin K, Arsenic, Boron, Chromium, Copper, Iron, Manganese, Molybdenum, Nickel, Silicon, Vanadium, and Zinc.* Washington, DC: National Academy Press, 2001.

25 Leo MA, Lieber CS. Alcohol, vitamin A, and beta-carotene: adverse interactions, including hepatotoxicity and carcinogenicity. *Am J Clin Nutr.* 1999;69:1071–1085.

26 Timbo BB, Ross MP, McCarthy PV, Lin C-TL. Op. cit.

27 Health Canada. Baseline natural health products survey among consumers, March 2005. http://www.hc-sc.gc.ca/dhp-mps/pubs/natur/eng_cons_survey_e.html. Accessed 3/1/06.

28 Elvin-Lewis M. Should we be concerned about herbal remedies? *J Ethnopharmacol.* May 2001;75:141–164.

29 St. John's wort study launched. NIH news release; October 1, 1997.

30 Hypericum Depression Trial Study Group. Effect of *Hypericum perforatum* (St John's wort) in major depressive disorder: a randomized controlled trial. *JAMA.* 2002;287:1807–1814.

31 *Milk Thistle: Effects on Liver Disease and Cirrhosis and Clinical Adverse Effects.* Rockville, MD: Agency for Healthcare Research and Quality, 2000. Summary, Evidence Report/Technology Assessment, No. 21. http://www.ahrq.gov/clinic/epcsums/milktsum.htm. Accessed 3/1/06.

32 Evans JG, Wilcock G, Birks J. Evidence-based pharmacotherapy of Alzheimer's disease. *Int J Neuropsychopharmacol.* 2004; 7:351–369.

33 Gordon AE, Shaughnessy AF. Saw palmetto for prostate disorders. *Am Fam Physician.* 2003;67:1281–1283.

34 Shinohara K, et al. Saw palmetto for benign prostatic hyperplasia. *N Engl J Med.* 2006;354:557–566.

35 Lowe FC, Fagelman E. Cranberry juice and urinary tract infections: what is the evidence? *Urology.* 2001;57:407–413.

36 Rosenblatt M, Mindel J. Spontaneous hyphema associated with ingestion of ginkgo biloba extract. *N Engl J Med.* 1997; 336:15, 1108.

37 Boullata J. Natural health product interactions with medication. *Nutr Clin Pract.* 2005;20(1):33–51.

38 Edwards C. Lessons from licorice. *N Engl J Med.* 1991;325: 1242–1243.

39 US Food and Drug Administration. Risk of drug interactions with St. John's wort, indinavir and other drugs. FDA public health advisory; February 10, 2000. http://www.fda.gov/cder/drug/advisory/stjwort.htm. Accessed 3/1/06.

40 Gallagher RE. Arsenic: new life for an old potion. *N Engl J Med.* 1998:339:1389–1390; and Centers for Disease Control and Prevention. Lead poisoning associated with use of traditional ethnic remedies—California, 1991–1992. *MMWR.* 1993;42:521–523.

41 Gordon DW, Rosenthal G, Hart J, et al. Chaparral ingestion: the broadening spectrum of liver injury caused by herbal medications. *JAMA.* 1995;273:489–490.

42 DiPaola RS, Zhang H, Lambert GH, et al. Clinical and biologic activity of an estrogenic herbal combination (PC-SPES) in prostate cancer. *N Engl J Med.* 1998;339:785–791.

43 Centers for Disease Control and Prevention. Anticholinergic poisoning associated with herbal tea—New York City, 1994. *MMWR.* 1995;44:193–195; and Plantain adulteration with foxglove. FDA press release; June 12, 1997.

44 Good Housekeeping Consumer Safety Symposium on Dietary Supplements and Herbal Remedies. March 3, 1998; New York, NY.

45 Harkey MR, Henderson GL, Gershwin ME, et al. Variability in commercial ginseng products: an analysis of 25 preparations. *Am J Clin Nutr.* 2001;73(6):1101–1106.

46 US Food and Drug Administration. FDA proposes labeling and manufacturing standards for all dietary supplements. FDA news release; March 7, 2003.

47 Business guide for dietary supplement industry. Federal Trade Commission press release; November 18, 1998.

48 US Food and Drug Administration. *Dietary Supplement Health and Education Act of 1994, Public Law 103-417, 103rd Congress.* http://www.fda.gov/opacom/laws/dshea.html. Accessed 3/1/06.

49 Kurtzweil P. An FDA guide to dietary supplements. *FDA Consumer.* Sept–Oct 1998, revised January 1999. http://www.cfsan.fda.gov/~dms/fdsupp.html. Accessed 3/1/06.

50 US Food and Drug Administration. Claims that can be made for conventional foods and dietary supplements. March 20, 2001. http://www.cfsan.fda.gov/~dms/hclaims.html. Accessed 3/1/06.

51 Health Canada, Natural Health Products Directorate. *Natural Health Products Regulations.* http://www.hc-sc.gc.ca/hpfb-dgpsa/nhpd-dpsn/nhp_regs_e.html. Accessed 3/1/06.

52 Salvato P, Thompson C, Keister R. Viral load response to augmentation of natural dehydroepiandrosterone (DHEA). Presented at: International Conference on AIDS; July 7–12, 1996; Vancouver, BC, Canada.

53 Miller DR, Anderson GT, Stark JJ, et al. Phase I/II trial of the safety and efficacy of shark cartilage in the treatment of advanced cancers. *J Clin Oncol.* 1998;16:3649–3655.

54 Washburn L. Are doctors' side deals prescription for trouble? *Hackensack (NJ) Sunday Record.* August 22, 1999:A1.

55 US Pharmacopeia. USP-verified dietary supplements. http://www.usp.org/USPVerified/dietarySupplements/. Accessed 3/1/06.

56 The Alpha-Tocopherol, Beta-Carotene and Cancer Prevention Study Group. The effect of vitamin E and beta carotene on the incidence of lung cancer and other cancers in male smokers. *N Engl J Med.* 1994;330:1029–1035.

57 Kurtzweil P. Op. cit.

58 Eisenberg DM, Kessler RC, Foster C, et al. Unconventional medicine in the United States: prevalence, costs, and patterns of use. *N Engl J Med.* 1993;328:246–252.

59 Pelletier KR, Marie A, Krasner M, Haskell WL. Current trends in the integration and reimbursement of complementary and alternative medicine by managed care, insurance carriers, and hospital providers. *Am J Health Promotion.* 1997;12:112–123.

60 Eisenberg DM, Kessler RC, Foster C, et al. Op. cit.

61 Eisenberg DM, Davis RB, Ettner SL, et al. Trends in alternative medicine use in the United States 1990–1997: results of a follow-up national survey. *JAMA.* 1998;280:1569–1575.

62 Barnes PM, Powell-Griner E, McFann K, Nahin RL. Op. cit.

63 *Alternative Medicine, Expanding Medical Horizons.* Op. cit.

64 Ibid.

65 Ibid.

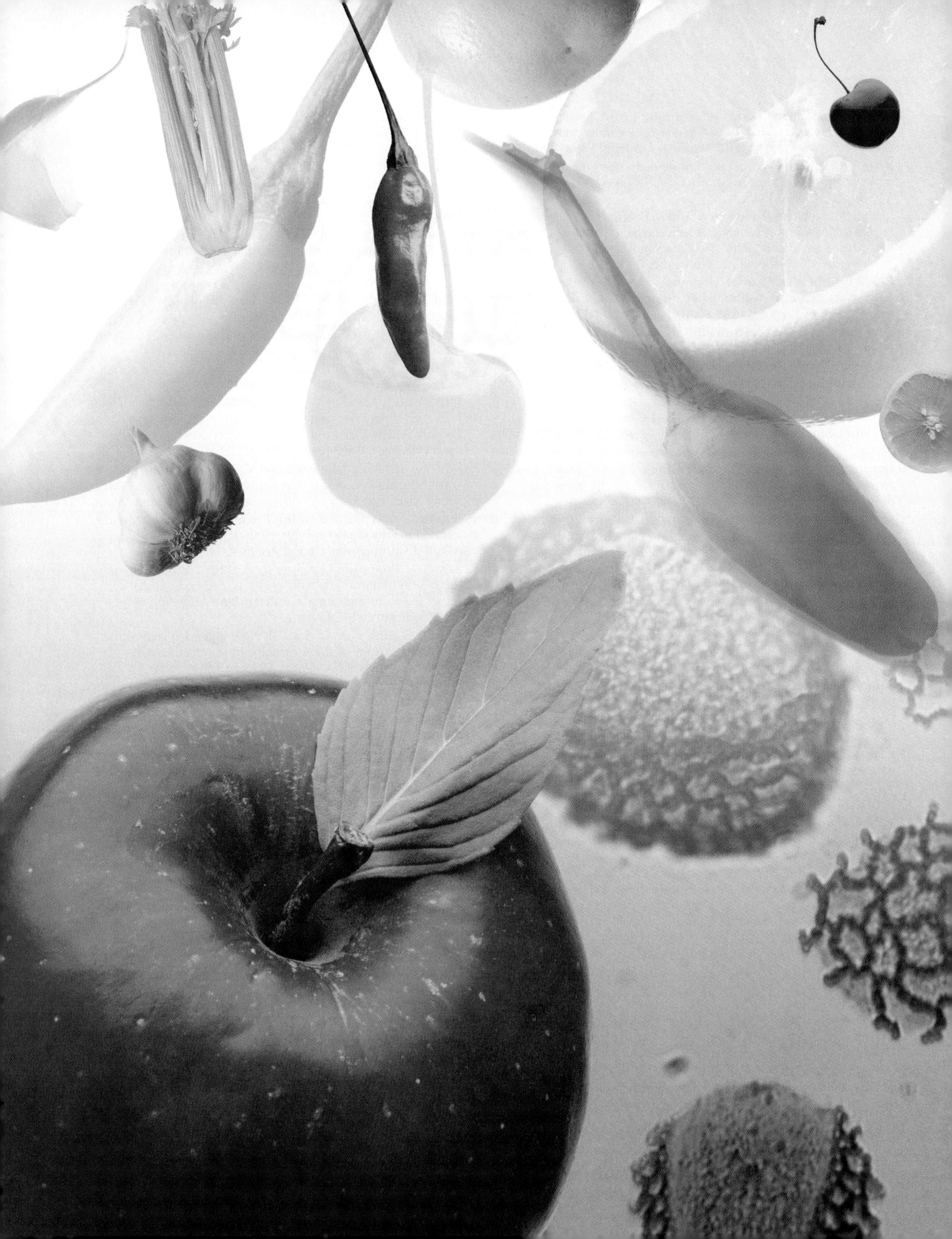

Chapter 3

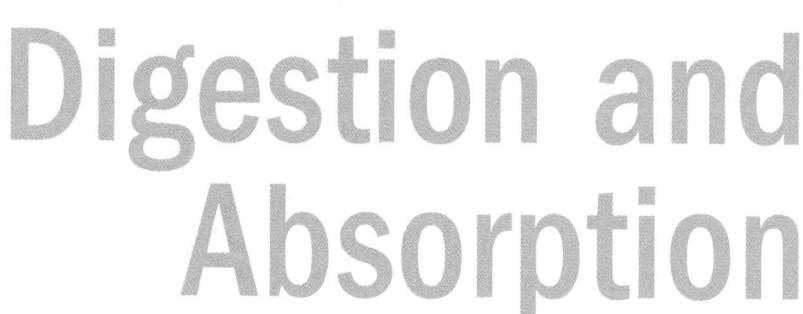

Digestion and Absorption

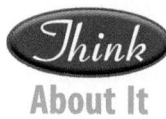
Think About It

1 Your friend warns you that eating some foods together is not healthful. Is this likely to change your eating behavior?

2 How good are you at identifying tastes?

3 Have you ever noticed that food sometimes tastes sweeter after chewing it for awhile?

4 You feel particularly happy and you find that a meal prepared by your friend tastes especially good. Any connection?

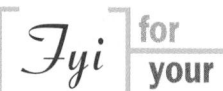
Fyi for your Information

This chapter's FYI boxes include practical information on the following topics:
- Lactose Intolerance
- Bugs in Your Gut? Health Effects of Intestinal Bacteria

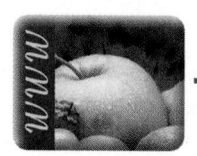

The Web site for this book offers many useful tools and is a great source for additional nutrition information for both students and instructors. Visit the site at **nutrition.jbpub.com** for information on digestion and absorption. You'll find exercises that explore the following topics:
- Gastrointestinal Disorders
- Have You Heard About GERD?
- Gallbladder Health
- Lactose Intolerance

What About 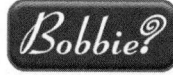 Bobbie?

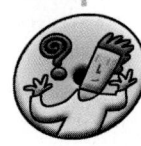

Track the choices Bobbie is making with Nutritionist Pro or EatRight Analysis software.

Key to Illustrations

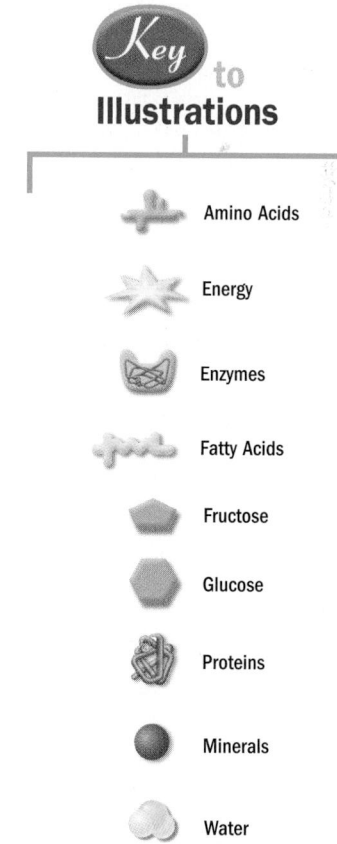

- Amino Acids
- Energy
- Enzymes
- Fatty Acids
- Fructose
- Glucose
- Proteins
- Minerals
- Water

The aroma of a roasting turkey floats past your nose. You haven't eaten for six or seven hours. Anticipating a delicious experience, your mouth waters, and your digestive juices are turned on. Is this virtual reality? Not at all! Before you eat a morsel of food, fleeting thoughts from your brain signal your body to prepare for the feast to come.

The body's machinery to process food and turn it into nutrients is not only efficient but elegant. The action unfolds in the digestive tract in two stages: **digestion**—the breaking apart of foods into smaller and smaller units—and **absorption**—the movement of those small units from the gut into the bloodstream or lymphatic system for circulation. Your digestive system is designed to digest carbohydrates, proteins, and fats simultaneously, while at the same time preparing other substances—vitamins, minerals, and cholesterol, for example—for absorption. Remarkably, your digestive system doesn't need any help! Despite promotions for enzyme supplements and diet books that recommend consuming food or nutrient groups separately, scientific research does not support these claims. Unless you have a specific medical condition, your digestive system is ready, willing, and able to digest and absorb the foods you eat, in whatever combination you eat them.

But go back to the aroma of that roast turkey for a moment. Before we begin digesting and absorbing, our senses of taste and smell first attract us to foods we are likely to consume.

Taste and Smell: The Beginnings of Our Food Experience

You probably wouldn't eat a food if it didn't appeal in some way to your senses. Smell and taste belong to our chemical sensing system, or the **chemosenses**. The complicated processes of smelling and tasting begin when tiny molecules released by the substances around us bind to receptors on special cells in the nose, mouth, or throat. These special sensory cells transmit messages through nerves to the brain, where specific smells or tastes are identified.

The Chemosenses

Olfactory (smell) **cells** are stimulated by the odors around us, such as the fragrance of a gardenia or the smell of bread baking. These nerve cells are found in a small patch of tissue high inside the nose, and they connect directly to the brain.

Gustatory (taste) **cells** react to food and beverages. These surface cells in the mouth send taste information along their nerve fibers. The taste cells are clustered in the taste buds of the mouth and throat. Many of the visible small bumps on the tongue contain taste buds.

A third chemosensory mechanism, the **common chemical sense**, contributes to our senses of smell and taste. In this system, thousands of nerve

digestion The process of transforming the foods we eat into units for absorption.

absorption The movement of substances into or across tissues; in particular, the passage of nutrients and other substances into the walls of the gastrointestinal tract and then into the bloodstream.

chemosenses [key-mo-SEN-sez] The chemical sensing system in the body, including taste and smell. Sensory cells in the nose, mouth, or throat transmit messages through nerves to the brain, where smells and tastes are identified.

olfactory cells Nerve cells in a small patch of tissue high in the nose connected directly to the brain to transmit messages about specific smells. Also called smell cells.

gustatory cells Surface cells in the throat and on the taste buds in the mouth that transmit taste information. Also called taste cells.

common chemical sense A chemosensory mechanism that contributes to our senses of smell and taste. It comprises thousands of nerve endings, especially on the moist surfaces of the eyes, nose, mouth, and throat.

Quick Bites

How Many Taste Buds Do You Have?

We have almost 10,000 taste buds in our mouths, including those on the roofs of our mouths. In general, females have more taste buds than males.

endings—especially on the moist surfaces of the eyes, nose, mouth, and throat—give rise to sensations such as the sting of ammonia, the coolness of menthol, and the irritation of chili peppers.

In the mouth, along with texture, temperature, and the sensations from the common chemical sense, tastes combine with odors to produce a perception of flavor. It is flavor that lets us know whether we are eating a pear or an apple. You recognize flavors mainly through the sense of smell. If you hold your nose while eating chocolate, for example, you will have trouble identifying it—even though you can distinguish the food's sweetness or bitterness. That's because the familiar flavor of chocolate is sensed largely by odor, as is the well-known flavor of coffee.

Many nutritionists have suggested that fat has no taste and that its appeal is due solely to its texture. However, this may not be the case. Animal studies have found a taste receptor for fat, and essential fatty acids (fatty acids that must be obtained from the diet) elicit the strongest taste response.[1]

The sight, smell, thought, taste, and in some cases, even the sound of food can trigger a set of physiologic responses known as the **cephalic phase responses**.[2] These responses (see **Figure 3.1**) involve more than just the digestive tract, and they follow rapidly on the heels of sensory stimulation. In the digestive tract, salivary and gastric secretions flow, preparing for the consumption of food. If no food is consumed, the response diminishes; but eating continues the stimulation of the salivary and gastric cells.

cephalic phase responses The responses of the parasympathetic nervous system to the sight, smell, thought, taste, and sound of food. Also called preabsorptive phase responses.

Figure 3.1 **The cephalic (preabsorptive) phase responses.** In response to sensory stimulation, your body primes its resources to better absorb and use anticipated nutrients.

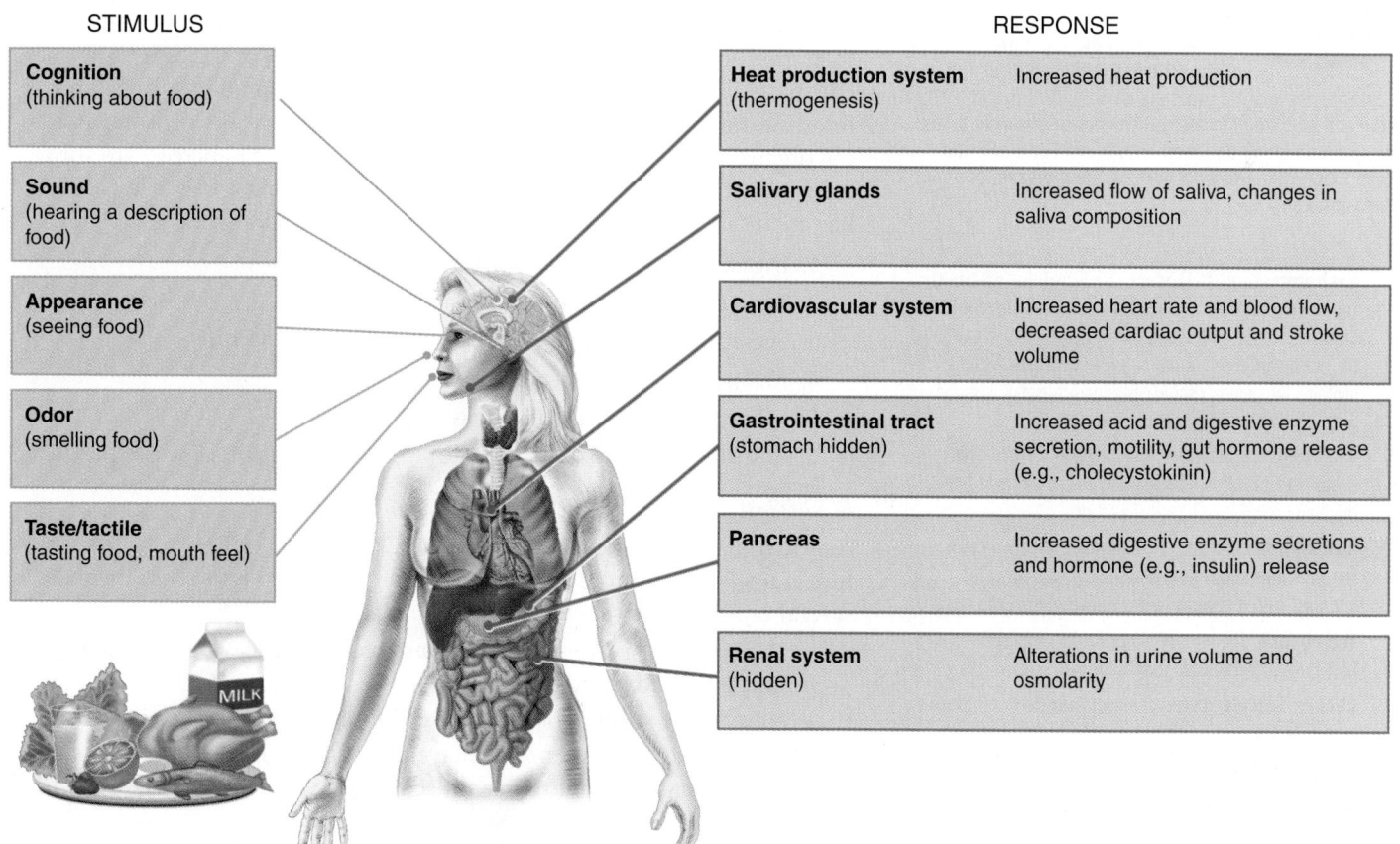

STIMULUS

Cognition
(thinking about food)

Sound
(hearing a description of food)

Appearance
(seeing food)

Odor
(smelling food)

Taste/tactile
(tasting food, mouth feel)

RESPONSE

Heat production system (thermogenesis) — Increased heat production

Salivary glands — Increased flow of saliva, changes in saliva composition

Cardiovascular system — Increased heart rate and blood flow, decreased cardiac output and stroke volume

Gastrointestinal tract (stomach hidden) — Increased acid and digestive enzyme secretion, motility, gut hormone release (e.g., cholecystokinin)

Pancreas — Increased digestive enzyme secretions and hormone (e.g., insulin) release

Renal system (hidden) — Alterations in urine volume and osmolarity

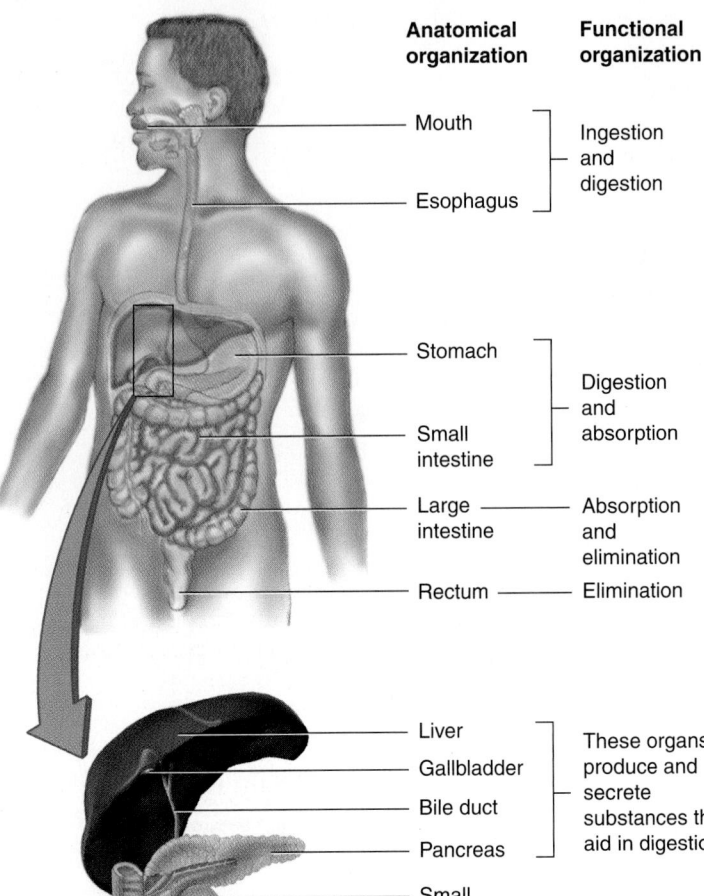

Anatomical organization | **Functional organization**

Mouth ⎱ Ingestion and digestion
Esophagus ⎰

Stomach ⎱ Digestion and absorption
Small intestine ⎰

Large intestine — Absorption and elimination

Rectum — Elimination

Liver ⎱
Gallbladder │ These organs produce and secrete substances that aid in digestion
Bile duct │
Pancreas ⎰
Small intestine

Figure 3.2 **Anatomic and functional organization of the GI tract.** Although digestion begins in the mouth, most digestion occurs in the stomach and small intestine. Absorption primarily takes place in the small and large intestines. For a detailed description of the GI tract and assisting organs, see Appendix E.

gastrointestinal (GI) tract [GAS-troh-in-TES-tin-al] The connected series of organs and structures used for digestion of food and absorption of nutrients; also called the alimentary canal or the digestive tract. The GI tract contains the mouth, esophagus, stomach, small intestine, large intestine (colon), rectum, and anus.

excretion The process of separating and eliminating waste products of metabolism and undigested food from the body.

mucosa [myu-KO-sa] The innermost layer of a cavity. The inner layer of the gastrointestinal tract, also called the intestinal wall. It is composed of epithelial cells and glands.

submucosa The layer of loose, fibrous, connective tissue under the mucous membrane.

circular muscle Layers of smooth muscle that surround organs, including the stomach and the small intestine.

longitudinal muscle Muscle fibers aligned lengthwise.

serosa A smooth membrane composed of a mesothelial layer and connective tissue. The intestines are covered in serosa.

Key Concepts: *Taste and smell are the first interactions we have with food. The flavor of a particular food is really a combination of olfactory, gustatory, and other stimuli. Smell (olfactory) receptors receive stimuli through odor compounds. Taste (gustatory) receptors in the mouth sense flavors. Other nerve cells (the common chemical senses) are stimulated by other chemical factors. If one of these stimuli is missing, our sense of flavor is incomplete.*

The Gastrointestinal Tract

If, instead of teasing the body with mere sights and smells, we actually sit down to a meal and experience the full flavor and texture of foods, the real work of the digestive tract begins. For the food we eat to nourish our bodies, we need to digest it (break it down into smaller units); absorb it (move it from the gut into circulation); and finally transport it to the tissues and cells of the body. The digestive process starts in the mouth and continues as food journeys down the gastrointestinal, or GI, tract. At various points along the GI tract, nutrients are absorbed, meaning they move from the GI tract into circulatory systems so they can be transported throughout the body. If there are problems along the way, with either incomplete digestion or inadequate absorption, the cells will not receive the nutrients they need to grow, perform daily activities, fight infection, and maintain health. A closer look at the gastrointestinal tract will help you see just how amazing this organ system is.

Organization of the GI Tract

The **gastrointestinal (GI) tract**, also known as the alimentary canal, is a long, hollow tube that begins at the mouth and ends at the anus. The specific parts include the mouth, esophagus, stomach, small intestine, large intestine, and rectum. (See **Figure 3.2**.) The GI tract works with the assisting organs—the salivary glands, liver, gallbladder, and pancreas—to turn food into small molecules that the body can absorb and use. The GI tract has an amazing variety of functions, including the following:

1. Ingestion—the receipt and softening of food
2. Transport of ingested food
3. Secretion of digestive enzymes, acid, mucus, and bile
4. Absorption of end products of digestion
5. Movement of undigested material
6. Elimination—the transport, storage, and **excretion** of waste products

A Closer Look at Gastrointestinal Structure

Although it's convenient to describe the GI tract as a hollow tube, its structure is really much more complex. As you can see in **Figure 3.3**, there are several layers to this tube:

- The innermost layer, called the **mucosa**, is a layer of epithelial (lining) cells and glands.
- Next, is the **submucosa**, a layer of loose, fibrous, connective tissue.
- Continuing outward are two layers of muscle fibers:
  - First is a layer of **circular muscle**, where muscle fibers go around the tube.
  - Next is a layer of **longitudinal muscle**, where fibers lie lengthwise along the tube.

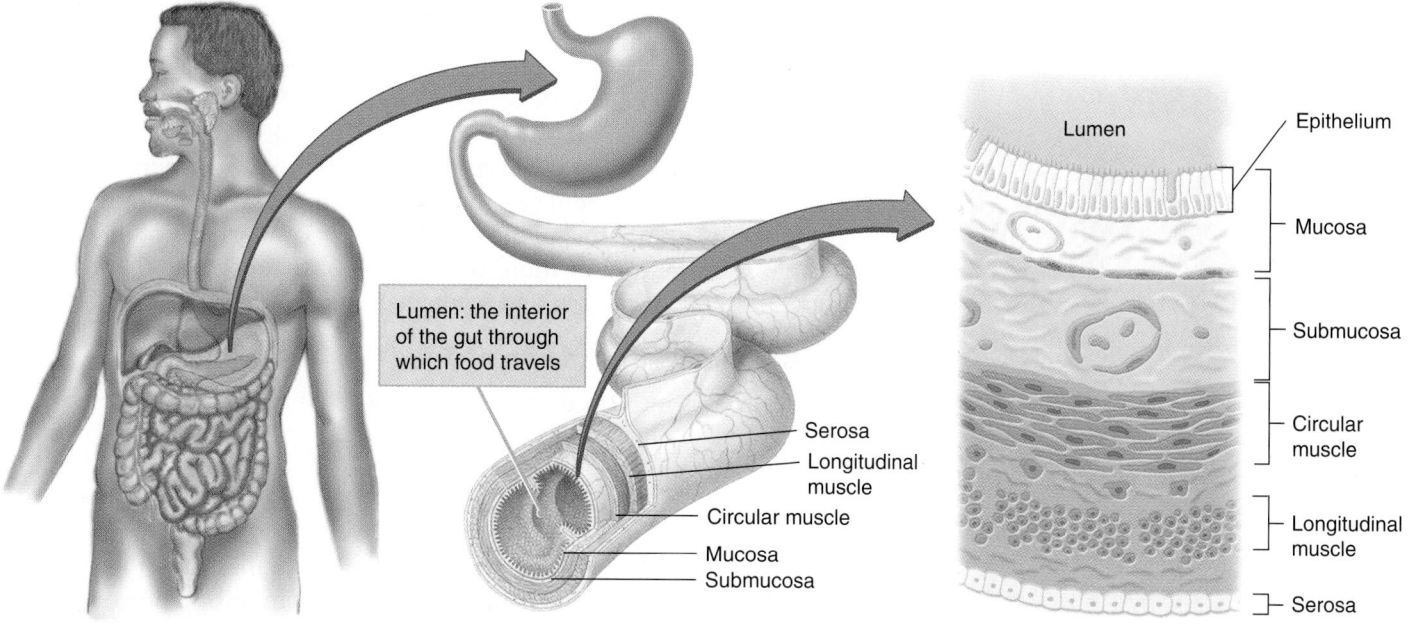

Lumen: the interior of the gut through which food travels

Figure 3.3 **Structural organization of the GI tract wall.** Your intestinal tract is a long, hollow tube lined with mucosal cells and surrounded by layers of muscle cells.

- Finally the outer surface, or **serosa**, provides a covering for the entire GI tract.

At several points along the tract, where one part connects with another (e.g., where the esophagus meets the stomach), the muscles are thicker and form **sphincters**. As you can see in **Figure 3.4**, by alternately contracting and relaxing, a sphincter acts as a valve controlling the movement of food material so that it goes in only one direction.

Key Concepts: *The gastrointestinal tract consists of the mouth, esophagus, stomach, small intestine, large intestine, and rectum. The function of the GI tract is to ingest, digest, and absorb nutrients and eliminate waste. The general structure of the GI tract consists of many layers, including an inner mucosal lining, a layer of connective tissue, layers of muscle fibers, and an outer covering layer. Sphincters are muscular valves along the GI tract that control movement from one part to the next.*

Overview of Digestion: Physical and Chemical Processes

The breakdown of food into smaller units and finally into absorbable nutrients involves both chemical and physical processes. First, there is the physical breaking of food into smaller pieces, such as happens when we chew. In addition, the muscular contractions of the GI tract continue to break food up and mix it with various secretions, while at the same time moving the mixture (called **chyme**) along the tract. Enzymes, along with other chemicals, help complete the breakdown process and promote absorption.

The Physical Movement and Breaking Up of Food

Distinct muscular actions of the GI tract take the food on its long journey. From mouth to anus, wavelike muscular contractions called **peristalsis** transport food and nutrients along the length of the GI tract. Peristaltic waves from the stomach muscles occur about three times per minute. In the small intestine, circular and longitudinal bands of muscle contract approximately every four to five seconds. The large intestine uses slow peristalsis to move the end products of digestion (feces).

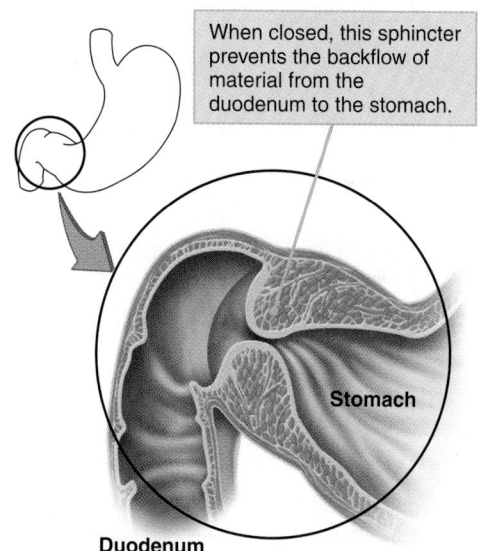

When closed, this sphincter prevents the backflow of material from the duodenum to the stomach.

Stomach

Duodenum

Figure 3.4 **Sphincters in action.** Movement from one section of the GI tract to the next is controlled by muscular valves called sphincters.

sphincters [SFINGK-ters] Circular bands of muscle fibers that surround the entrance or exit of a hollow body structure (e.g., the stomach) and act as valves to control the flow of material.

chyme [KIME] A mass of partially digested food and digestive juices moving from the stomach into the duodenum.

peristalsis [per-ih-STAHL-sis] The wavelike, rhythmic muscular contractions of the GI tract that propel its contents down the tract.

PERISTALSIS

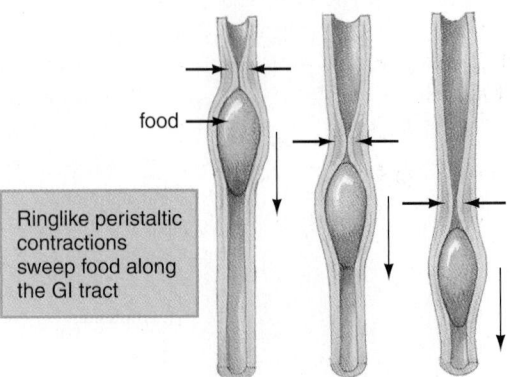

food →

Ringlike peristaltic contractions sweep food along the GI tract

SEGMENTATION

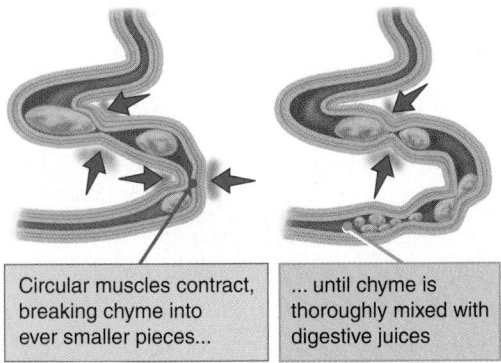

Circular muscles contract, breaking chyme into ever smaller pieces...

... until chyme is thoroughly mixed with digestive juices

Figure 3.5 **Peristalsis and segmentation.** Peristalsis and segmentation help break up, mix, and move food through the GI tract.

segmentation Periodic muscle contractions at intervals along the GI tract that alternate forward and backward movement of the contents, thereby breaking apart chunks of the food mass and mixing in digestive juices.

enzymes [EN-zimes] Large proteins in the body that accelerate the rate of chemical reactions but are not altered in the process.

catalyze To speed up a chemical reaction.

hydrolysis A reaction that breaks apart a compound through the addition of water.

Segmentation, a muscular movement that occurs in the small intestine, divides and mixes the chyme by alternating forward and backward movement of the GI tract contents. Segmentation also enhances absorption by bringing chyme into contact with the intestinal wall. In contrast, peristaltic contractions proceed in one direction for variable distances along the length of the intestine. Some even travel the entire distance from the beginning of the small intestine to the end. Peristaltic contractions of the small intestine often are continuations of contractions that began in the stomach. **Figure 3.5** shows peristalsis and segmentation.

The Chemical Breakdown of Food

Chemically, it is the action of enzymes that divide nutrients into compounds small enough for absorption.

Enzymes are proteins that **catalyze**, or speed up, chemical reactions but are not altered in the process. Most enzymes can catalyze only one or a few related reactions, a property called enzyme specificity. Enzymes act in part by bringing the reacting molecules close together. In digestion, these chemical reactions divide substances into smaller compounds by a process called **hydrolysis** (breaking apart by water), as **Figure 3.6** shows. Most of the digestive enzymes can be identified by name; they commonly end in *–ase* (amylase, lipase, and so on.). For example, the enzyme needed to digest sucr*ose* is sucr*ase*.

In addition to enzymes, other chemicals support the digestive process. These include acid in the stomach, a neutralizing base in the small intestine, bile that prepares fat for digestion, and mucus secreted along the GI tract. This mucus does not break down food but lubricates it and protects the cells that line the GI tract from the strong digestive chemicals. Along the GI tract, fluids containing various enzymes and other substances are

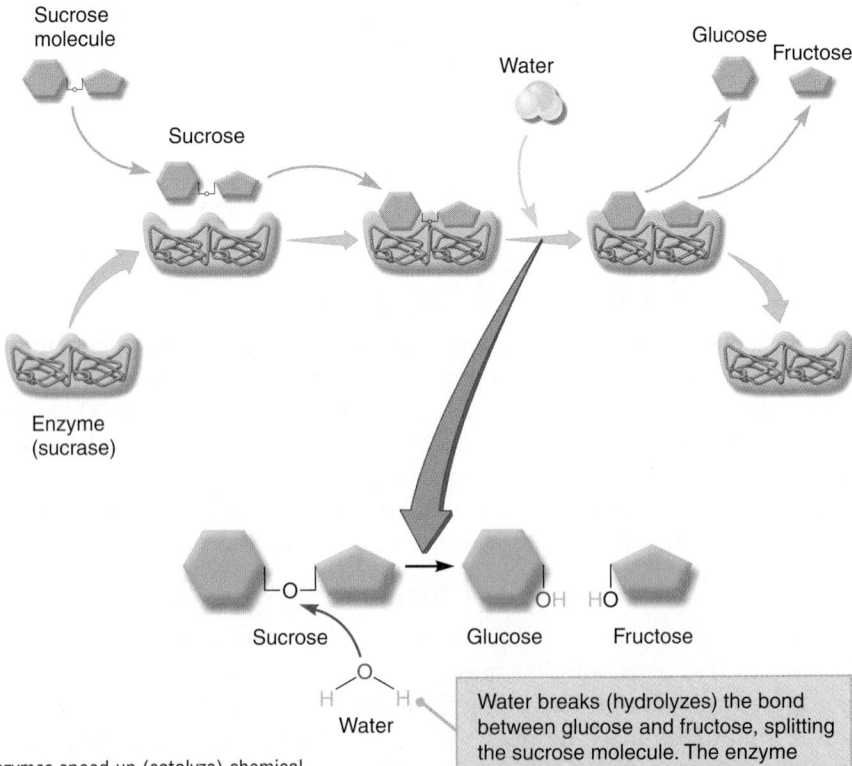

Sucrose molecule

Sucrose

Water

Glucose Fructose

Enzyme (sucrase)

Sucrose

Glucose Fructose

Water

Water breaks (hydrolyzes) the bond between glucose and fructose, splitting the sucrose molecule. The enzyme sucrase speeds up the reaction.

Figure 3.6 **Water and enzymes in chemical reactions.** Enzymes speed up (catalyze) chemical reactions. When water breaks a chemical bond, the action is called hydrolysis.

added to the consumed food. In fact, the volume of fluid secreted into the GI tract is about 7,000 milliliters (about 7¹/₂ quarts) per day.[3] **Table 3.1** shows the average daily fluids in the GI tract.

Key Concepts: Digestion involves both physical and chemical activity. Physical activity includes chewing and the movement of muscles along the GI tract that divide food into smaller pieces and mix it with digestive secretions. Chemical digestion is the breaking of bonds in nutrients, such as carbohydrates or proteins, to produce smaller units. Enzymes—proteins that encourage chemical processes—catalyze these hydrolytic reactions.

Overview of Absorption

Food is broken apart during digestion and moved from the GI tract into circulation and on to the cells. Many of the nutrients—vitamins, minerals, and water—do not need to be digested before they are absorbed. But the energy-yielding nutrients—carbohydrate, fat, and protein—are too large to be absorbed intact and must be digested first. At this point, we need to outline how nutrients are moved from the interior, or **lumen**, of the gut through the lining cells (mucosa) and into circulation.

The Four Roads to Nutrient Absorption

There are four processes by which nutrients are absorbed: passive diffusion, facilitated diffusion, active transport, and endocytosis (see **Figure 3.7**). Let's take a look at each one in turn.

Passive diffusion is the movement of molecules without the expenditure of energy through the cell membrane, through either special watery channels or intermolecular gaps in the cell membrane. Molecules cross permeable cell membranes as a result of random movements that tend to equalize the concentration of substances on both sides of a membrane. **Concentration gradients** (e.g., a high outside concentration and a low inside concentration of molecules) drive passive diffusion. The larger the concentration of molecules on one side of the cell membrane, the faster those molecules move across the membrane to the area of lower concentration.

Since the cell membrane mainly consists of fat-soluble substances, it welcomes fats and other fat-soluble molecules. Oxygen, nitrogen, carbon dioxide, and alcohols are highly soluble in fat and readily dissolve in the cell membrane and diffuse across it. Large amounts of oxygen are delivered this way, passing easily into a cell's interior almost as if it had no membrane barrier at all. Although water crosses cell membranes easily, most water-soluble nutrients (carbohydrates, amino acids, vitamins, and minerals) cannot be absorbed via passive diffusion. They need help to cross into the intestinal cells. This help comes in the form of a carrier, and may also require energy.

In **facilitated diffusion**, special carriers help transport a substance (such as the simple sugar fructose) across the cell membrane. The facilitating carriers are proteins that reside in the cell membrane. The diffusing molecule becomes lightly bound to the carrier protein, which changes its shape to open a pathway for the diffusing molecules to move into the cell. Concentration gradients also help to drive facilitated diffusion, which is passive and can move substances only from a region of higher concentration to one of lower concentration.

Energy is required for **active transport** of substances in an unfavorable direction. Substances cannot diffuse "uphill" against an unfavorable gradient, whether the difference is one of concentration, electrical charge, or

Table 3.1 Average Daily Fluid Input and Output

Source	Amount (mL)
Fluid input	
Food and beverages	2,000
Saliva	1,500
Gastric secretions	2,500
Pancreatic secretions	1,500
Bile	500
Small intestine secretions	1,000
Total input	9,000
Fluid output	
Small intestine absorption	7,500
Large intestine absorption	1,400
Feces	100
Total output	9,000

Source: Klein S, Cohn SM, Alpers DH. Alimentary tract in nutrition. In: Shils ME, Shike M, Ross AC, Cabellero B, Cousins RJ, eds. *Modern Nutrition in Health and Disease.* 10th ed. Philadelphia: Lippincott Williams & Wilkins, 2006:1115–1142.

lumen Cavity or hollow channel in any organ or structure of the body.

passive diffusion The movement of substances into or out of cells without the expenditure of energy or the involvement of transport proteins in the cell membrane. Also called simple diffusion.

concentration gradients Differences between the solute concentrations of two substances.

facilitated diffusion A process by which carrier (transport) proteins in the cell membrane transport substances into or out of cells down a concentration gradient.

active transport The movement of substances into or out of cells against a concentration gradient. Active transport requires energy (ATP) and involves carrier (transport) proteins in the cell membrane.

PASSIVE DIFFUSION

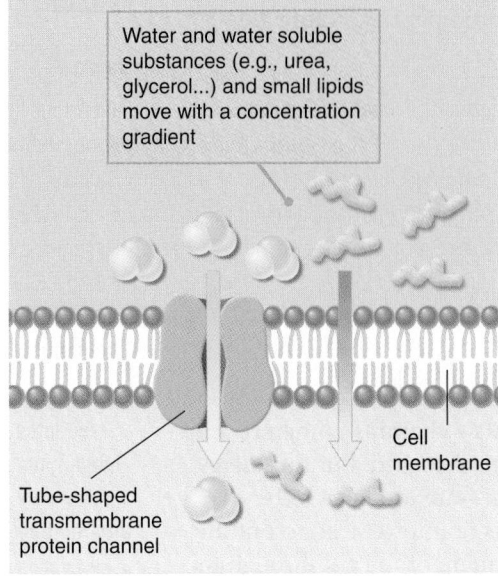

Water and water soluble substances (e.g., urea, glycerol...) and small lipids move with a concentration gradient

Cell membrane

Tube-shaped transmembrane protein channel

(a)

FACILITATED DIFFUSION

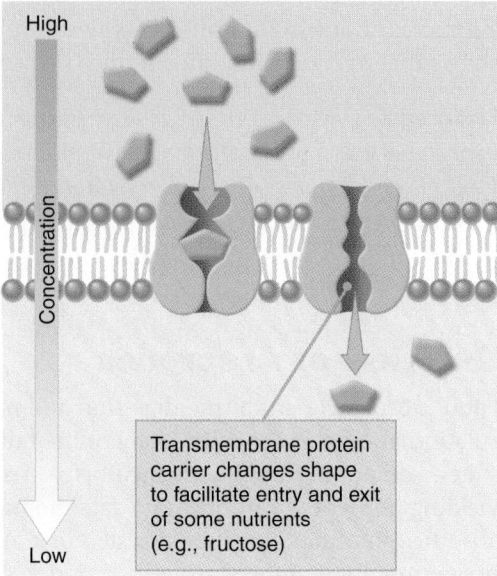

High

Concentration

Low

Transmembrane protein carrier changes shape to facilitate entry and exit of some nutrients (e.g., fructose)

(b)

Figure 3.7 **(a) Passive diffusion.** Using passive diffusion, some substances easily move in and out of cells, either through protein channels or directly through the cell membrane.
(b) Facilitated diffusion. Some substances need a little assistance to enter and exit cells. A transmembrane protein helps out by changing shape.
(c) Active transport. Some substances need a lot of assistance to enter cells. Similar to swimming upstream, energy is needed for the substance to penetrate despite an unfavorable concentration gradient.
(d) Endocytosis. Cells can use their cell membranes to engulf a particle and bring it inside the cell. The engulfing portion of the membrane separates from the cell wall and encases the particle in a vesicle.

ACTIVE TRANSPORT

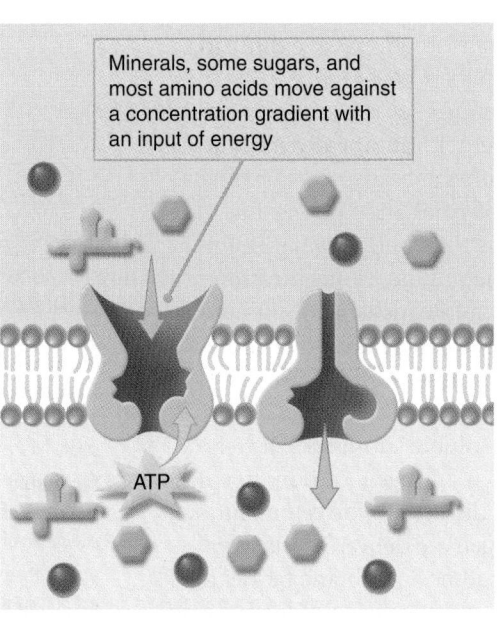

Minerals, some sugars, and most amino acids move against a concentration gradient with an input of energy

ATP

(c)

ENDOCYTOSIS

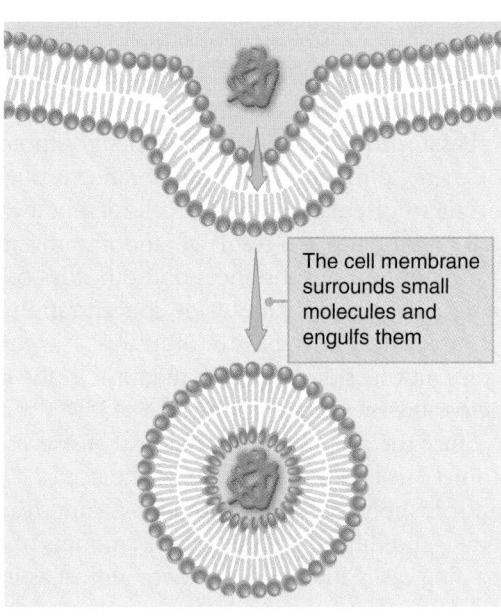

The cell membrane surrounds small molecules and engulfs them

(d)

endocytosis The uptake of material by a cell by the indentation and pinching off of its membrane to form a vesicle that carries material into the cell.

pinocytosis The process by which cells internalize fluids and macromolecules. To do so, the cell membrane invaginates and forms a pocket around the substance. From *pino*, "drinking," and *cyto*, "cell."

phagocytosis The process by which cells engulf large particles and small microorganisms. Receptors on the surface of cells bind these particles and organisms to bring them into large vesicles in the cytoplasm. From *phago*, "eating," and *cyto*, "cell."

pressure. Substances that usually require active transport across some cell membranes include many minerals (sodium, potassium, calcium, iron, chloride, and iodide), several sugars (glucose and galactose), and most amino acids (simple components of protein). These substances can move from the intestine even though their concentration in the intestinal lumen is lower than their concentration in the absorptive cell.

Most substances either diffuse or are actively transported across cell membranes, but some are engulfed and ingested in a process known as **endocytosis**. This occurs, for example, when a newborn infant absorbs antibodies from breast milk.[4] In endocytosis, a portion of the cell membrane forms a sac around the substance to be absorbed, pulling it into the interior of the cell. When cells ingest small molecules and fluids, the process is known as

pinocytosis. A similar ingestion process, **phagocytosis**, is used by specialized cells to absorb large particles.

Key Concepts: *Absorption through the GI cell membranes occurs by one of four basic processes. Passive diffusion occurs when nutrients (e.g., water) permeate the intestinal wall without a carrier or energy expenditure. Facilitated diffusion occurs when a carrier brings substances (e.g., fructose) into the absorptive intestinal cell without expending energy. Active transport requires energy to transport a substance (e.g., glucose or galactose) across a cell membrane in an unfavorable direction. Endocytosis (phagocytosis or pinocytosis) occurs when the absorptive cell's membrane engulfs particles or fluids (e.g., absorption of antibodies from breast milk).*

Assisting Organs

The salivary glands, liver, gall bladder, and pancreas all have critical roles in the digestive process. The GI tract works in concert with these organs, which assist digestion by providing fluid, acid neutralizers, enzymes, and **emulsifiers**.

Salivary Glands

Three pairs of **salivary glands** (parotid, sublingual, and submandibular) located in or near the mouth secrete saliva into the oral cavity (see **Figure 3.8**). Saliva moistens food, lubricating it for easy swallowing. Saliva also contains enzymes that begin the process of chemical digestion. We secrete approximately 1,500 milliliters (about 1.5 quarts) of saliva each day. The mere sight, smell, or thought of food can start the flow of saliva.

Liver

The **liver** produces and secretes 600 to 1,000 milliliters of **bile** daily. Bile is a yellow-green, pasty material that contains water, bile salts and acids, pigments, cholesterol, phospholipids (a type of fat molecule), and electrolytes (electrically charged minerals). Bile tastes bitter, which is why the word "bile" has come to denote bitterness. Bile acts as an emulsifier by reducing large globs of fat to smaller globs. This process breaks no bonds in fat molecules, but rather increases the surface area of fat, allowing more contact between fat molecules and enzymes in the small intestine.

Bile is concentrated in your gallbladder and released to the small intestine on demand. After it has done its work, most bile salts are reabsorbed and returned to the liver for recycling. This recirculation is known as the **enterohepatic** (*entero* meaning "intestines," and *hepatic* referring to the liver) **circulation** of bile salts (see **Figure 3.9**).

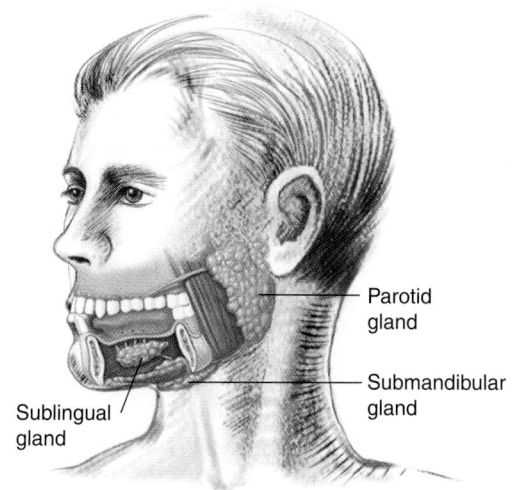

Figure 3.8 **The salivary glands.** The three pairs of salivary glands supply saliva, which moistens and lubricates food. Saliva also contains salivary enzymes that begin the digestion of starch.

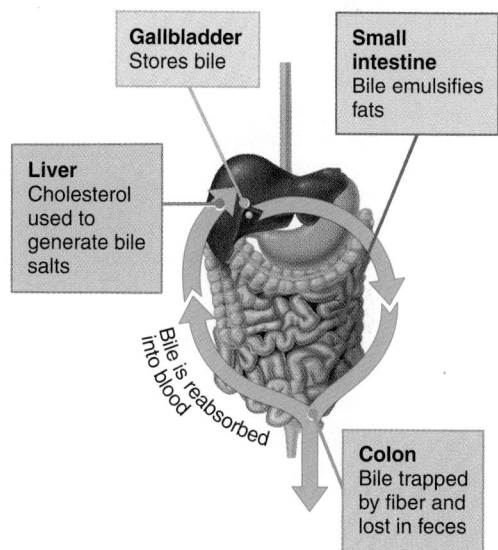

Gallbladder
Stores bile

Small intestine
Bile emulsifies fats

Liver
Cholesterol used to generate bile salts

Bile is reabsorbed into blood

Colon
Bile trapped by fiber and lost in feces

Figure 3.9 **Enterohepatic circulation.** During this recycling process, bile travels from the liver to the gallbladder and then to the small intestine, where it assists digestion. In the small intestine, most of the bile is reabsorbed and sent back to the liver for reuse.

emulsifiers Agents that blend fatty and watery liquids by promoting the breakup of fat into small particles and stabilizing their suspension in aqueous solution.

salivary glands Glands in the mouth that release saliva.

liver The largest glandular organ in the body, it produces and secretes bile, detoxifies harmful substances, and helps metabolize carbohydrates, lipids, proteins, and micronutrients.

bile An alkaline, yellow-green fluid that is produced in the liver and stored in the gallbladder. The primary constituents of bile are bile salts, bile acids, phospholipids, cholesterol, and bicarbonate. Bile emulsifies dietary fats, aiding fat digestion and absorption.

enterohepatic circulation [EN-ter-oh-heh-PAT-ik] Recycling of certain compounds between the small intestine and the liver. For example, bile acids move from the liver to the gallbladder, then into the small intestine, from whence they are absorbed into the portal vein and transported back to the liver.

gallbladder A pear-shaped sac that stores and concentrates bile from the liver.

cholecystokinin (CCK) [ko-la-sis-toe-KY-nin] A hormone produced by cells in the small intestine that stimulates the release of digestive enzymes from the pancreas and bile from the gallbladder.

pancreas An organ that secretes enzymes that affect the digestion and absorption of nutrients and that releases hormones, such as insulin, which regulate metabolism as well as the disposition of the end products of food in the body.

amylase [AM-ih-lace] A salivary enzyme that catalyzes the hydrolysis of amylose, a starch. Also called ptyalin.

lingual lipase A fat-splitting enzyme secreted by cells at the base of the tongue.

bolus [BOH-lus] A chewed, moistened lump of food that is ready to be swallowed.

esophagus [ee-SOFF-uh-gus] The food pipe that extends from the pharynx to the stomach, about 25 centimeters long.

stomach The enlarged, muscular, saclike portion of the digestive tract between the esophagus and the small intestine, with a capacity of about 1 quart.

esophageal sphincter The opening between the esophagus and the stomach that relaxes and opens to allow the bolus to travel into the stomach, and then closes behind it. Also acts as a barrier to prevent the reflux of gastric contents. Commonly called the cardiac sphincter.

hydrochloric acid An acid of chloride and hydrogen atoms made by the gastric glands and secreted into the stomach. Also called gastric acid.

pH A measurement of the hydrogen ion concentration, or acidity, of a solution. It is equal to the negative logarithm of the hydrogen ion (H^+) concentration expressed in moles per liter.

mucus A slippery substance secreted in the GI tract (and other body linings) that protects cells from irritants such as digestive juices.

pepsinogen The inactive form of the enzyme pepsin.

pepsin A protein-digesting enzyme produced by the stomach.

gastric lipase An enzyme in the stomach that hydrolyzes certain triglycerides into fatty acids and glycerol.

gastrin [GAS-trin] A polypeptide hormone released from the walls of the stomach mucosa and duodenum that stimulates gastric secretions and motility.

intrinsic factor A glycoprotein released from parietal cells in the stomach wall that binds to and aids in absorption of vitamin B_{12}.

The liver also is a detoxification center that filters toxic substances from the blood and alters their chemical forms. These altered substances may be sent to the kidney for excretion or carried by bile to the small intestine and removed from the body in feces. The liver is a "chemical factory"—performing over 500 chemical functions that include the production of blood proteins, cholesterol, and sugars. The liver is also a "dynamic warehouse" that stores vitamins, hormones, cholesterol, minerals, and sugars, releasing them to the bloodstream as needed.

Gallbladder

The primary function of the **gallbladder** is to store and concentrate bile from the liver. The gallbladder is a small, muscular, pear-shaped sac nestled in a depression on the right underside of the liver. This organ holds about a quarter of a cup of bile and is the storage stop for bile between the liver and the small intestine. The gallbladder fills with bile and thickens it, until a hormone released after eating signals the gallbladder to squirt out its colorful contents.

The gallbladder is normally relaxed and full between meals. When dietary fats enter the small intestine, they stimulate the production of **cholecystokinin (CCK)**, a hormone, in the intestinal wall. Cholecystokinin causes the gallbladder to contract and the sphincter of Oddi, which is at the end of the common bile duct, to relax. Like a squeeze bulb, the gallbladder squirts bile into the duodenum (the upper part of the small intestine), about 500 milliliters each day. The common bile duct also carries digestive enzymes from the pancreas.

Pancreas

The **pancreas** secretes enzymes that affect the digestion and absorption of nutrients. During the course of a day, the pancreas secretes about 1,500 milliliters of fluid, which contains mostly water, bicarbonate, and digestive enzymes. The pancreas also releases hormones that are involved in other aspects of nutrient use by the body. For example, the pancreatic hormones insulin and glucagon regulate blood glucose levels. The combination of these two functions makes the pancreas one of the most important organs in the digestion and use of food.

Key Concepts: The salivary glands, liver, gallbladder, and pancreas all make important contributions to the digestive process. The salivary glands release saliva, which contains mucus and enzymes, into the mouth. The liver produces bile, which is stored in the gallbladder and released into the small intestine, where bile helps to prepare fats for digestion. The pancreas also secretes liquid that contains bicarbonate and several types of enzymes into the small intestine.

Putting It All Together: Digestion and Absorption

Up to this point, our discussion has centered on structures, mechanisms, and processes to give you a general idea of the workings of the GI tract. Now you're ready for a complete tour, a journey along the GI tract to see what happens and how digestion and absorption are accomplished. Detailed descriptions of specific enzymes and actions on individual nutrients are covered in later chapters.

Mouth

As soon as you put food in your mouth the digestive process begins. As you chew, you break down the food into smaller pieces, increasing the surface area available to enzymes. Saliva contains the enzyme salivary **amylase** (ptyalin), which breaks down starch into small sugar molecules. Food remains in the mouth only for a short time, so only about 5 percent of the starch is completely broken down. The next time you eat a cracker or a piece of bread, chew slowly and notice the change in the way it tastes. It gets sweeter. That's the salivary amylase breaking down the starch into sugar. Salivary amylase continues to work until the strong acid content of the stomach deactivates it. To start the process of fat digestion, the cells at the base of the tongue secrete another enzyme, **lingual lipase**. The overall impact of lingual lipase on fat digestion, though, is small.

Saliva and other fluids, including mucus, blend with the food to form a **bolus**, a chewed, moistened lump of food that is soft and easy to swallow. When you swallow, the bolus slides past the epiglottis, a valvelike flap of tissue that closes off your air passages so you don't choke. The bolus then moves rapidly through the **esophagus** to the stomach, where it will be digested further. **Figure 3.10** shows the process of swallowing.

Stomach

The bolus enters the **stomach** through the **esophageal sphincter**, also called the cardiac sphincter, which immediately closes to keep the bolus from sliding back into the esophagus. Quick and complete closure by the esophageal sphincter is essential to prevent the acidic stomach contents from backing up into the esophagus, causing the pain and tissue damage called heartburn.

Nutrient Digestion in the Stomach

The stomach cells produce secretions that are collectively called gastric juice. Included in this mixture are water, hydrochloric acid, mucus, pepsinogen (the inactive form of the enzyme pepsin), the enzyme gastric lipase, the hormone gastrin, and intrinsic factor.

- **Hydrochloric acid** makes the stomach contents extremely acidic, dropping the **pH** to 2, compared with a neutral pH of 7. (See **Figure 3.11**.) This acidic environment kills many pathogenic (disease-causing) bacteria that may have been ingested, and also aids in the digestion of protein. **Mucus** secreted by the stomach cells coats the stomach lining, protecting these cells from damage by the strong gastric juice.

  Hydrochloric acid works in protein digestion in two ways. First, it demolishes the functional, three-dimensional shape of proteins, unfolding them into linear chains; this increases their vulnerability to attacking enzymes. Second, it promotes the breakdown of proteins by converting the enzyme precursor **pepsinogen** to its active form, **pepsin**.

- Pepsin then begins breaking the links in protein chains, cutting dietary proteins into smaller and smaller pieces.

- Stomach cells also produce an enzyme called **gastric lipase**. It has a minor role in the digestion of lipids, specifically triglycerides with an abundance of short-chain fatty acids.

- **Gastrin**, another component of gastric juice, is a hormone that stimulates gastric secretion and motility.

- **Intrinsic factor** is a substance necessary for the absorption of vitamin B_{12} that occurs farther down the GI tract, near the end of the small intestine. In the absence of intrinsic factor, only about one-fiftieth of ingested vitamin B_{12} is absorbed.

After swallowing, salivary amylase continues to digest carbohydrates. After about an hour, acidic stomach secretions become well mixed with the

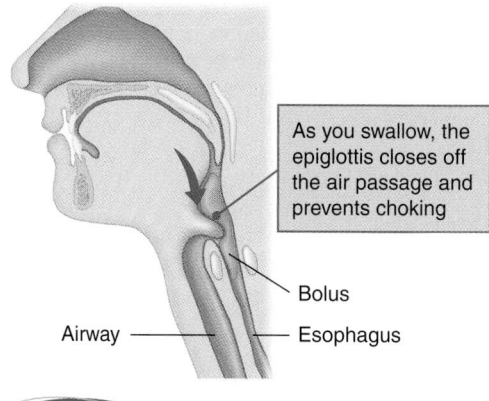

Figure 3.10 **Swallowing.** Your epiglottis didn't completely do its job if you have ever had a drink go "down the wrong pipe" and choked.

As you swallow, the epiglottis closes off the air passage and prevents choking

Bolus

Airway — Esophagus

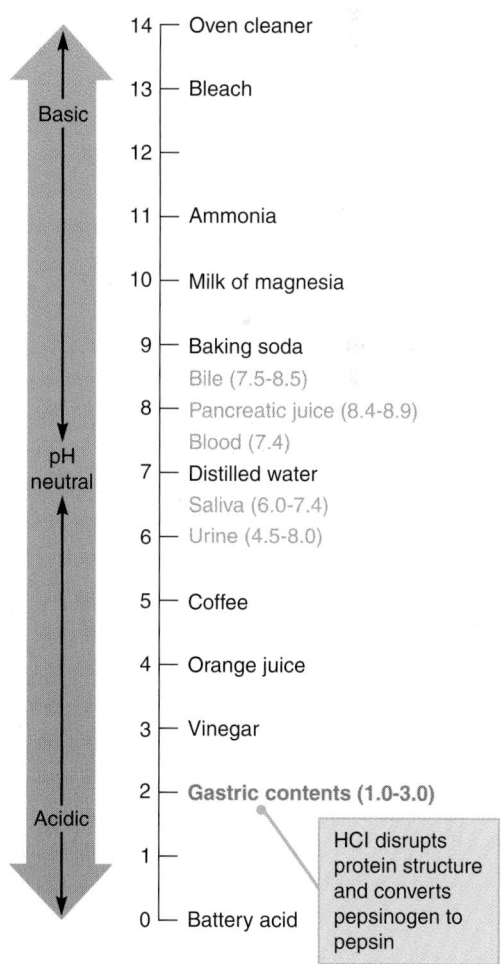

TYPICAL pHs OF COMMON SUBSTANCES

Basic

14 — Oven cleaner

13 — Bleach

12 —

11 — Ammonia

10 — Milk of magnesia

9 — Baking soda
   Bile (7.5-8.5)

8 — Pancreatic juice (8.4-8.9)
   Blood (7.4)

pH neutral

7 — Distilled water
   Saliva (6.0-7.4)

6 — Urine (4.5-8.0)

5 — Coffee

4 — Orange juice

3 — Vinegar

2 — Gastric contents (1.0-3.0)

Acidic

1 —

0 — Battery acid

HCl disrupts protein structure and converts pepsinogen to pepsin

Figure 3.11 **The pH scale.** Because pancreatic juice has a pH around 8, it can neutralize the acidic chyme, which leaves the stomach with a pH around 2.

pyloric sphincter [pie-LORE-ic] A circular muscle that forms the opening between the stomach and the duodenum. It regulates the passage of food into the small intestine.

food. This increases the acidity of the food and effectively blocks further salivary amylase activity.

Do you sometimes feel your stomach churning? An important action of the stomach is to continue mixing food with GI secretions to produce the semiliquid chyme. To accomplish this, the stomach has an extra layer of diagonal muscles. These, along with the circular and longitudinal muscles, contract and relax to mix food completely. When the chyme is ready to leave the stomach, about 30 to 40 percent of carbohydrate, 10 to 20 percent of protein, and less than 10 percent of fat have been digested.[5] The stomach slowly releases the chyme through the **pyloric sphincter** and into the small intestine. The pyloric sphincter then closes to prevent the chyme from returning to the stomach (see **Figure 3.12**).

The stomach normally empties in one to four hours, depending on the types and amounts of food eaten. Carbohydrates speed through the stomach in the shortest time, followed by protein and fat. Thus, the higher the fat content of a meal, the longer it will take to leave the stomach.

Nutrient Absorption in the Stomach

Although a substantial fraction of digestion has been accomplished by the time chyme leaves the stomach, very little absorption has occurred. Only some lipid-soluble compounds and weak acids, such as alcohol and aspirin, are absorbed through the stomach. Chyme moves on to the small intestine, the digestive and absorptive workhorse of the gut.

Figure 3.12 **The stomach.** The stomach churns and mixes food with stomach secretions. Hydrochloric acid unfolds proteins and stops salivary amylase action, while pepsin begins protein digestion. The pyloric sphincter controls movement of chyme from the stomach to the small intestine.

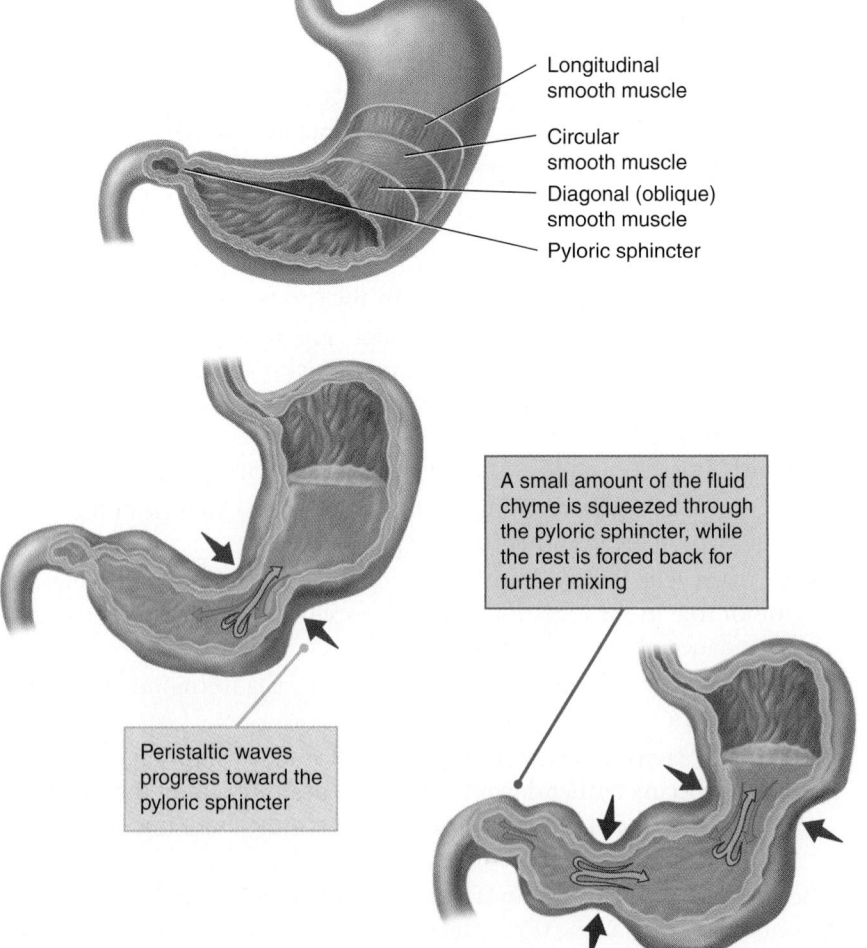

Longitudinal smooth muscle

Circular smooth muscle

Diagonal (oblique) smooth muscle

Pyloric sphincter

A small amount of the fluid chyme is squeezed through the pyloric sphincter, while the rest is forced back for further mixing

Peristaltic waves progress toward the pyloric sphincter

Small Intestine

The **small intestine** is where the digestion of protein, fat, and nearly all carbohydrate is completed and where most nutrients are absorbed. As you can see in **Figure 3.13**, the small intestine is a tube about 3 meters long (about 10 feet), divided into three parts:

- **Duodenum** (the first 25 to 30 centimeters—10 to 12 inches)
- **Jejunum** (about 120 centimeters—about 4 feet)
- **Ileum** (about 150 centimeters—about 5 feet)

Most digestion occurs in the duodenum, where the small intestine receives **digestive secretions** from the pancreas, gallbladder, and its own glands. The remainder of the small intestine primarily absorbs previously digested nutrients.

small intestine The tube (approximately 10 feet long) where the digestion of protein, fat, and carbohydrate is completed, and where the majority of nutrients are absorbed. The small intestine is divided into three parts: the duodenum, the jejunum, and the ileum.

duodenum [doo-oh-DEE-num, or doo-AH-den-um] The portion of the small intestine closest to the stomach. The duodenum is 10 to 12 inches long and wider than the remainder of the small intestine.

jejunum [je-JOON-um] The middle section (about 4 feet) of the small intestine, lying between the duodenum and ileum.

ileum [ILL-ee-um] The terminal segment (about 5 feet) of the small intestine, which opens into the large intestine.

digestive secretions Substances released at different places in the GI tract to speed the breakdown of ingested carbohydrates, fats, and proteins into smaller compounds that can be absorbed by the body.

Figure 3.13 **The small intestine.** The duodenum is mainly responsible for digesting food; the jejunum and ileum primarily deal with the absorption of food. In addition to the digestive juices from assisting organs, the duodenum secretes mucus, enzymes, and hormones to aid digestion. All along the intestinal walls, nutrients are absorbed into blood and lymph. Undigested materials are passed on to the large intestine.

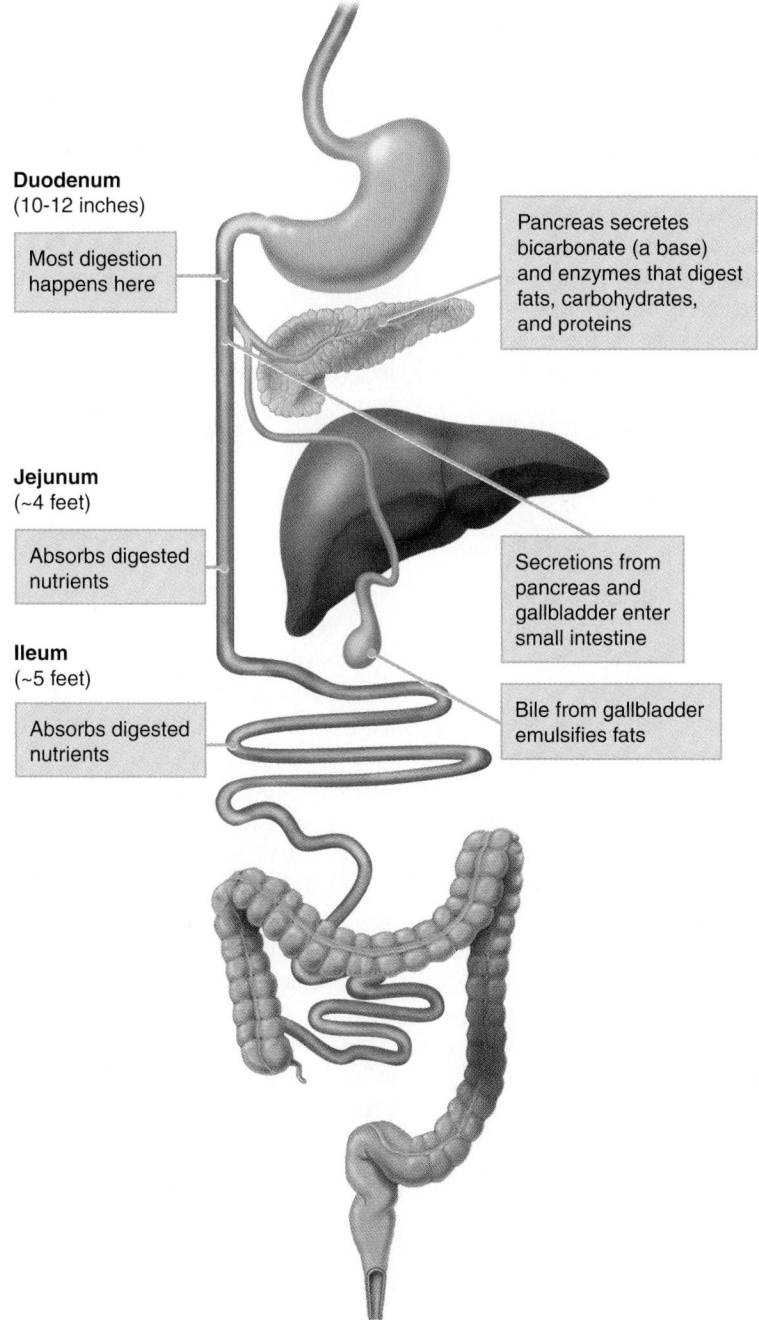

Duodenum (10-12 inches)

Most digestion happens here

Pancreas secretes bicarbonate (a base) and enzymes that digest fats, carbohydrates, and proteins

Jejunum (~4 feet)

Absorbs digested nutrients

Secretions from pancreas and gallbladder enter small intestine

Ileum (~5 feet)

Absorbs digested nutrients

Bile from gallbladder emulsifies fats

secretin [see-CREET-in] An intestinal hormone released during digestion that stimulates the pancreas to release water and bicarbonate.

Nutrient Digestion in the Small Intestine

In the duodenum, the acidic chyme from the stomach is neutralized by a base, bicarbonate, from the pancreas. The slow delivery of chyme through the pyloric sphincter (about 2 milliliters per minute) allows chyme to be adequately neutralized. This is important because the enzymes of the small intestine need a more neutral environment to work effectively. The stimulus for release of bicarbonate from the pancreas is the hormone **secretin**. This hormone is released from intestinal cells in response to the appearance of

Fyi Lactose Intolerance

FOR YOUR INFORMATION

When drinking a milkshake is followed shortly by bloating, gas, abdominal pain, and diarrhea, it could be lactose intolerance—the incomplete digestion of the lactose in milk due to low levels of the intestinal enzyme lactase. Lactose is the primary carbohydrate in milk and other dairy foods. Nondairy foods—such as instant breakfast mixes, cake mixes, mayonnaise, luncheon meats, medications, and vitamin supplements—also contain small amounts of lactose. Lactase is necessary to digest lactose in the small intestine. If lactase is deficient, undigested lactose enters the large intestine, where it is fermented by colonic bacteria, producing short-chain organic acids and gases (hydrogen, methane, carbon dioxide).

With the exception of a rare inherited disorder in which infants are born without lactase, infants have sufficiently high levels of lactase for normal digestion. However, lactase activity declines with weaning in many racial/ethnic groups. This normal, genetically controlled decrease in lactase activity, called lactose maldigestion, is prevalent among Asians, Native Americans, and African Americans. However, among U.S. Caucasians and Northern and Central Europeans, lactose maldigestion is far less common because lactase activity tends to persist. Lactose maldigestion occurs in about 25 percent of the U.S. population and in 75 percent of the worldwide population.

In addition to primary lactose intolerance, lactose intolerance can be secondary to diseases or conditions (e.g., inflammatory bowel disease such as Crohn's disease or celiac disease, gastrointestinal surgery, and certain medications) that injure the intestinal mucosa

where lactase is expressed. Secondary lactose maldigestion is temporary and lactose digestion improves once the underlying causative factor is corrected.

Lactose intolerance is far less prevalent than commonly believed. Many factors unrelated to lactose, including strong beliefs, can contribute to this condition. Studies have demonstrated that among self-described lactose-intolerant individuals, one-third to one-half develop few or no gastrointestinal symptoms following intake of lactose under well-controlled, double-blind conditions.

Self-diagnosis of lactose intolerance is a bad idea because it could lead to unnecessary dietary restrictions, expense, nutritional shortcomings, and failure to detect or treat a more serious gastrointestinal disorder. If lactose maldigestion is suspected, tests are available to diagnose this condition.

People with real or perceived lactose intolerance may limit their consumption of dairy foods unnecessarily and jeopardize their intake of calcium and other essential nutrients. A low intake of calcium is associated with increased risk of osteoporosis (porous bones), hypertension, and colon cancer.

With the exception of the few individuals who are sensitive to even very small amounts of lactose, avoiding all lactose is neither necessary nor recommended because some lactase is still being produced. Lactose maldigesters need to determine the amount of lactose they can comfortably consume at any one time. Here are some strategies for including milk and other dairy foods in your diet without developing symptoms:

1. Initially, consume small servings of lactose-containing foods such as milk (e.g., $\frac{1}{2}$ cup). Gradually increase the serving size until symptoms begin to appear, then back off.
2. Consume lactose with a meal or other foods (e.g., milk with cereal) to improve tolerance.
3. Adjust the type of dairy food. Whole milk may be tolerated better than low-fat milk, and chocolate milk may be tolerated better than unflavored milk. Many cheeses (e.g., Cheddar, Swiss, Parmesan) contain considerably less lactose than does milk. Aged cheeses generally have negligible amounts of lactose. Yogurts with live, active cultures are another option; these bacteria will digest lactose. Sweet acidophilus milk, yogurt milk, and other nonfermented dairy foods may be tolerated better than regular milk by lactose maldigesters. However, factors such as the strain of bacteria used may influence tolerance to these dairy foods.
4. Lactose-hydrolyzed dairy foods and/or commercial enzyme preparations (e.g., lactase capsules, chewable tablets, solutions) are another option. Lactose-reduced (70 percent less lactose) and lactose-free (99.9 percent less lactose) milks are available, although at a higher cost than regular milk.

Lactose maldigestion need not be an impediment to meeting the needs for calcium and other essential nutrients provided by milk and other dairy foods.

chyme. Pancreatic juice contains a variety of digestive enzymes that help to digest fats, carbohydrates, and proteins. Secretions from the intestinal wall cells add enzymes to complete carbohydrate digestion.

The presence of fat in the duodenum stimulates the release of stored bile by the gallbladder. The specific signal comes from the intestinal hormone cholecystokinin. Lipids ordinarily do not mix with water, but bile acts as an emulsifier, keeping lipid molecules mixed with the watery chyme and digestive secretions. Without the action of bile, lipids might not come into contact with pancreatic lipase, and digestion would be incomplete.

Distribution of lactose intolerance worldwide.

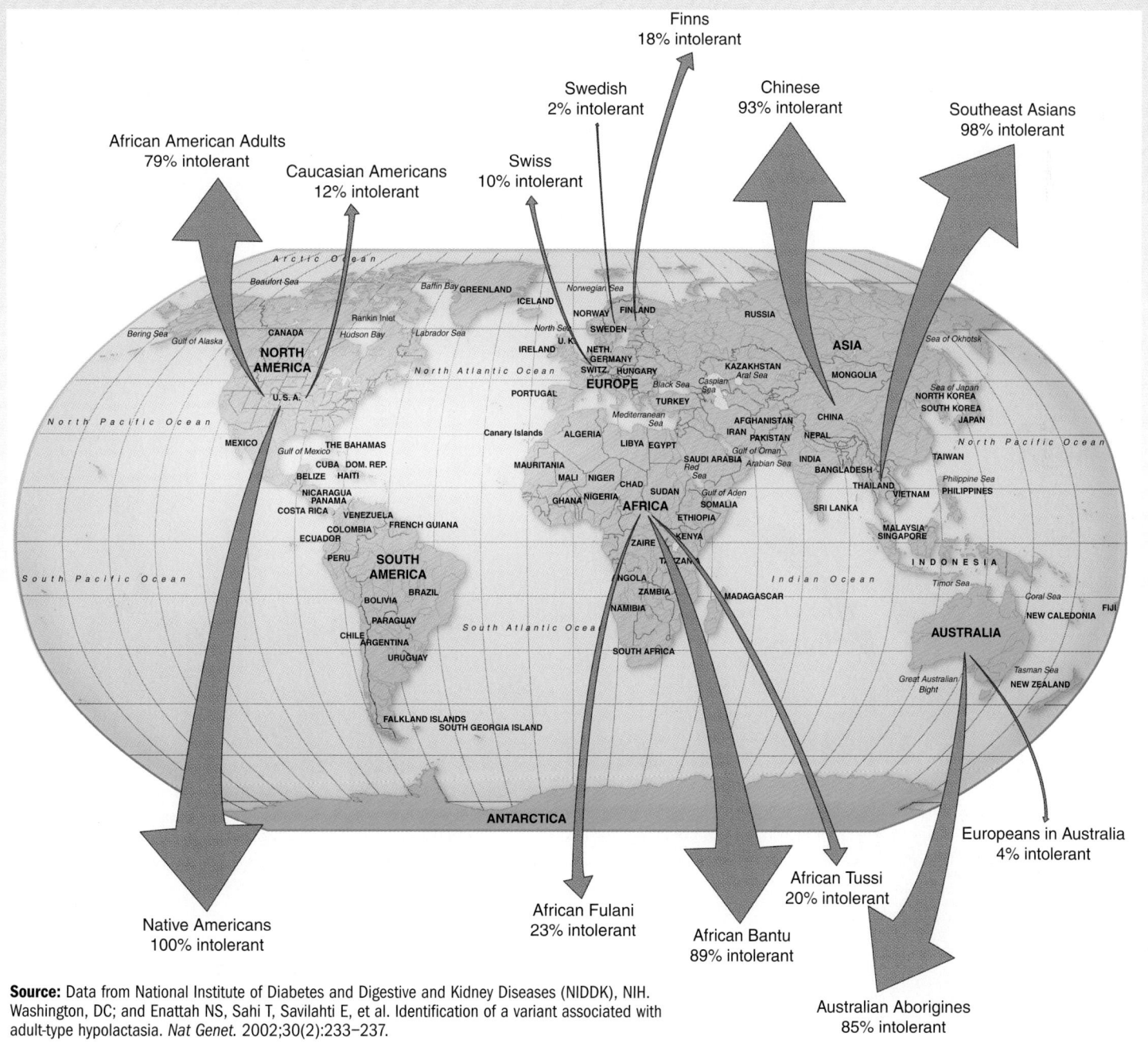

Finns
18% intolerant

Swedish
2% intolerant

Chinese
93% intolerant

Southeast Asians
98% intolerant

African American Adults
79% intolerant

Caucasian Americans
12% intolerant

Swiss
10% intolerant

Native Americans
100% intolerant

African Fulani
23% intolerant

African Bantu
89% intolerant

African Tussi
20% intolerant

Europeans in Australia
4% intolerant

Australian Aborigines
85% intolerant

Source: Data from National Institute of Diabetes and Digestive and Kidney Diseases (NIDDK), NIH. Washington, DC; and Enattah NS, Sahi T, Savilahti E, et al. Identification of a variant associated with adult-type hypolactasia. *Nat Genet.* 2002;30(2):233–237.

With the pancreatic and intestinal enzymes working together, digestion progresses nicely, leaving smaller protein, carbohydrate, and lipid compounds ready for absorption. Other nutrients, such as vitamins, minerals, and cholesterol, are not digested and generally are absorbed unchanged.

Just as the small intestine accomplishes much of the nutrient digestion, it is also responsible for most nutrient absorption. Its structure makes the process of absorption efficient and complete. In most cases, more than 90 percent of ingested carbohydrate, fat, and protein is absorbed. To see how this is possible, we need to examine the structure of the small intestine.

Absorptive Structures of the Small Intestine

The small intestine packs a gigantic surface area into a small space. As you can see in **Figure 3.14**, the interior surface of the small intestine is wrinkled into folds, tripling the absorptive surface area. These folds are carpeted with fingerlike projections called **villi** that expand the absorptive area another tenfold. Each cell lining the surface of each villus is covered with a "brush border" containing as many as 1,000 hairlike projections called **microvilli**. The microvilli increase the surface area another 20 times. Taken together,

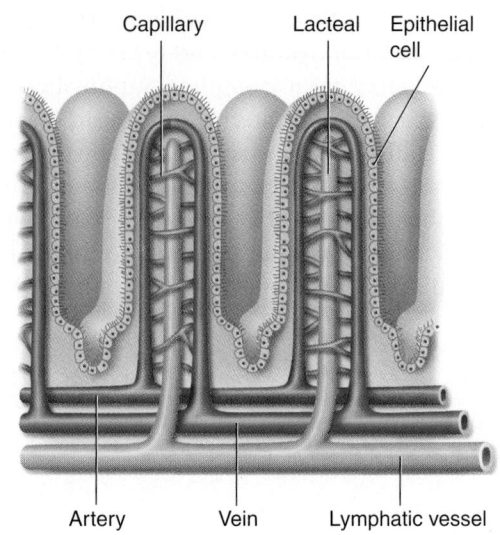

Anatomy of the villi.

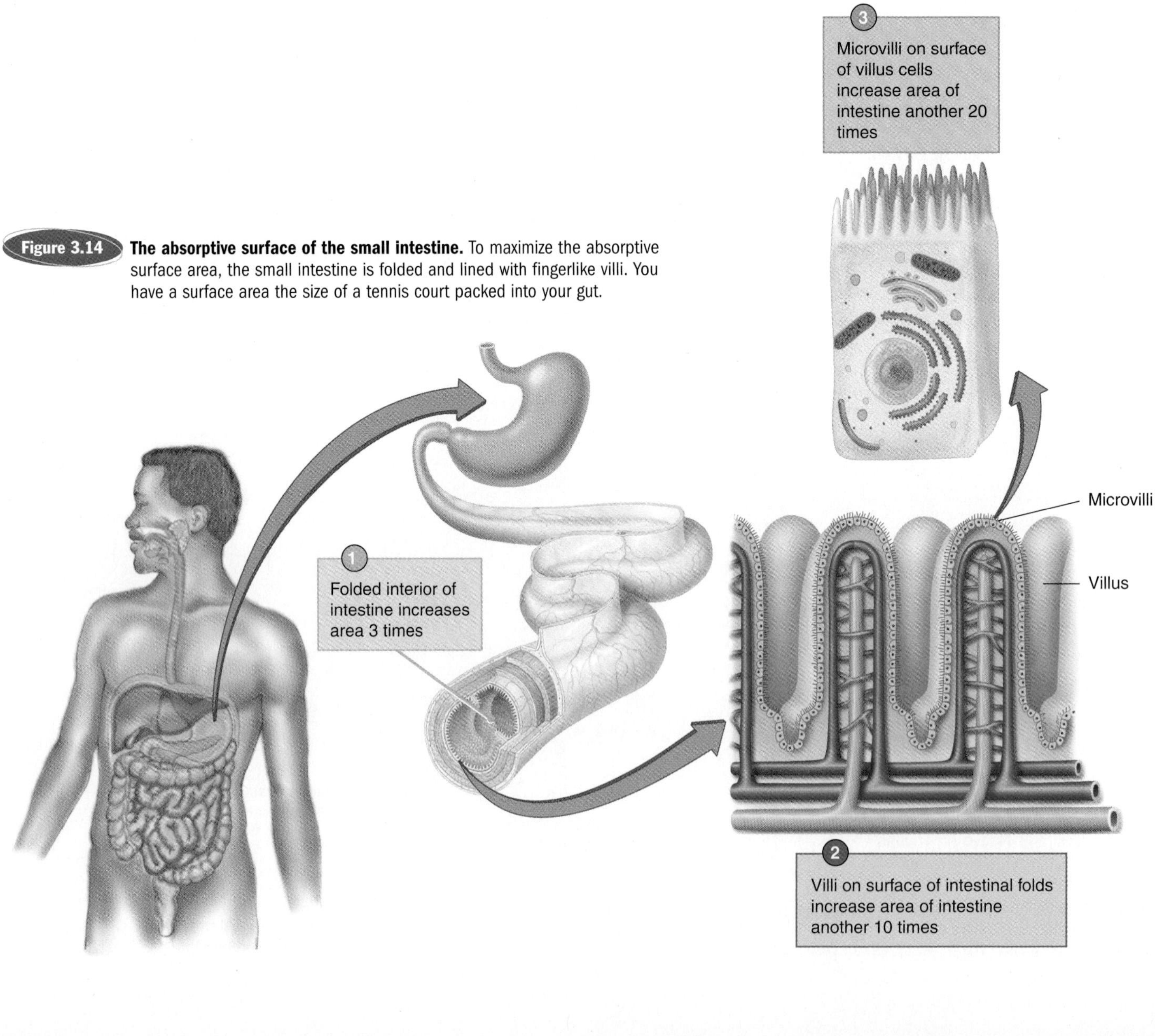

Capillary Lacteal Epithelial cell

Artery Vein Lymphatic vessel

3 Microvilli on surface of villus cells increase area of intestine another 20 times

Microvilli

Villus

Figure 3.14 **The absorptive surface of the small intestine.** To maximize the absorptive surface area, the small intestine is folded and lined with fingerlike villi. You have a surface area the size of a tennis court packed into your gut.

1 Folded interior of intestine increases area 3 times

2 Villi on surface of intestinal folds increase area of intestine another 10 times

the folds plus the villi and microvilli yield a 600-fold increase in surface area. In fact, your 10-foot (3 meters) long intestine has an absorptive surface area of more than 300 square yards (250 or more square meters)—equivalent to the surface of a tennis court!

Nutrient Absorption in the Small Intestine

As nutrients journey through the small intestine, they are trapped in the folds and projections of the intestinal wall and absorbed through the microvilli into the lining cells. Depending on your diet, each day your small intestine absorbs several hundred grams of carbohydrate, 60 or more grams of fat, 50 to 100 grams of amino acids, 3 to 5 grams of vitamins and minerals, and 7 to 8 liters of water. But the total absorptive capacity of the healthy small intestine is far greater. It actually has the capacity to absorb as much as several kilograms of carbohydrate, 500 grams of fat, 500 to 700 grams of amino acids, and 20 or more liters of water per day.[6] Approximately 85 percent of the water absorption by the gut occurs in the jejunum.[7]

Nutrients absorbed through the intestinal lining pass into the interior of the villi. Each villus contains blood vessels (veins, arteries, and capillaries) and a **lymph** vessel (known as a **lacteal**) that transport nutrients to other parts of your body. Water-soluble nutrients are absorbed directly into the bloodstream. Fat-soluble lipid compounds are absorbed into the lymph rather than directly into the blood.

Absorption takes place along the entire length of the small intestine. Most minerals, with the exception of the electrolytes sodium, chloride, and potassium, are absorbed in the duodenum and upper part of the jejunum. Carbohydrates, amino acids, and water-soluble vitamins are absorbed along the jejunum and upper ileum, whereas lipids and fat-soluble vitamins are absorbed primarily in the ileum. At the very end of the small intestine, the terminal ileum is the site of vitamin B_{12} absorption. If there is damage to the lower small intestine, or surgical removal of this section in the treatment of cancer and other diseases, malabsorption of fat-soluble vitamins and vitamin B_{12} is likely.

The small intestine suffers constant wear and tear as it propels and digests the chyme. The intestinal lining is renewed continually as the mucosal cells are replaced every two to five days. When the chyme has completed its 3- to 10-hour journey through the small intestine, it passes through the **ileocecal valve**, the connection to the large intestine.

The Large Intestine

The chyme's next stop is the **large intestine**. As **Figure 3.15** shows, this tube is about 5 feet (1.5 meters) long and includes the **cecum, colon**, rectum, and anal canal. As chyme fills the cecum, a local reflex signals the ileocecal valve to close, preventing material from reentering the ileum of the small intestine.

Digestion in the Large Intestine

The peristaltic movements of the large intestine are sluggish compared with those of the small intestine. Normally 18 to 24 hours are required for material to traverse its length. During that time, the colon's large population of bacteria digests small amounts of fiber, providing a negligible number of calories daily.[8] Of more significance are the other substances formed by this bacterial activity, including vitamin K, vitamin B_{12}, thiamin, riboflavin, biotin, and various gases that contribute to flatulence.[9] Other than bacterial action, no further digestion occurs in the large intestine.

villi Small, fingerlike projections that blanket the folds in the lining of the small intestine. Singular is *villus*.

microvilli Minute, hairlike projections that extend from the surface of absorptive cells facing the intestinal lumen. Singular is *microvillus*.

lymph Fluid that travels through the lymphatic system, made up of fluid drained from between cells and large fat particles.

lacteal A small lymphatic vessel in the interior of each intestinal villus that picks up chylomicrons and fat-soluble vitamins from intestinal cells.

ileocecal valve The sphincter at the junction of the small and large intestines.

large intestine The tube (about 5 feet) extending from the ileum of the small intestine to the anus. The large intestine includes the appendix, cecum, colon, rectum, and anal canal.

cecum The blind pouch at the beginning of the large intestine into which the ileum opens from one side and which is continuous with the colon.

colon The portion of the large intestine extending from the cecum to the rectum. It is made up of four parts—the ascending, transverse, descending, and sigmoid colons. Although often used interchangeably with the term *large intestine*, these terms are not synonymous.

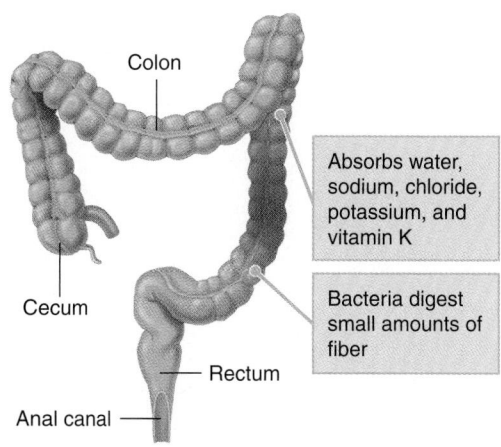

Colon

Absorbs water, sodium, chloride, potassium, and vitamin K

Cecum

Bacteria digest small amounts of fiber

Rectum

Anal canal

Figure 3.15 **The large intestine.** In the large intestine, bacteria break down dietary fiber and other undigested carbohydrates, releasing acids and gas. The large intestine absorbs water and minerals, and forms feces for excretion.

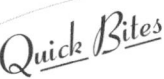

The Clever Colon

Though it has been presumed that the colon has no digestive function, recent research shows that the human colon can be an important digestive site in patients who are missing significant sections of their intestines. These patients can actually absorb energy from starch and nonstarch polysaccharides in the colon.

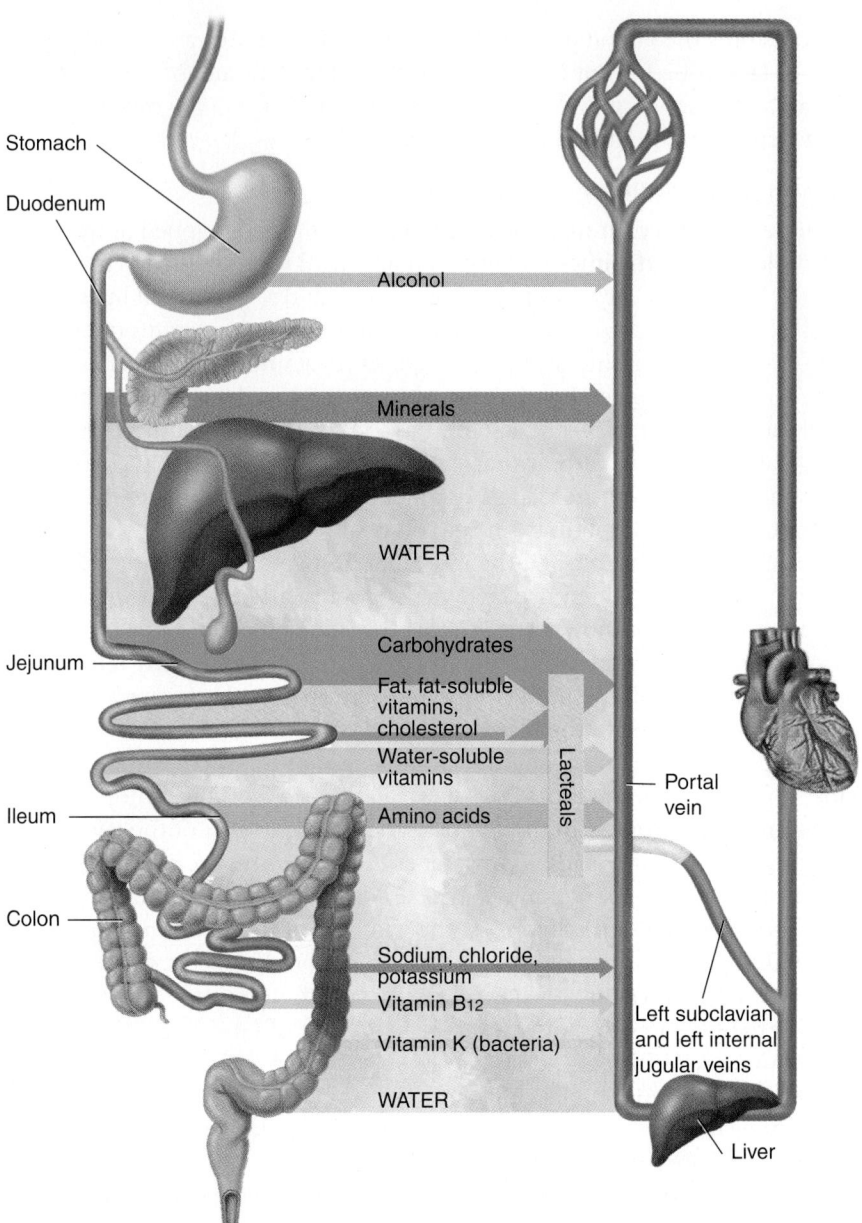

Figure 3.16 **Absorption of nutrients.**

Nutrient Absorption in the Large Intestine

Minimal nutrient absorption takes place in the large intestine, limited to water, sodium, chloride, potassium, and some of the vitamin K produced by bacteria. Although vitamin B_{12} is also produced by colonic bacteria, it is not absorbed. The colon dehydrates the watery chyme, removing and absorbing most of the remaining fluid. Of the approximately 1,000 milliliters of material that enters the large intestine, only about 150 milliliters remains for excretion as feces. The semisolid feces, consisting of roughly 60 percent solid matter (food residues, which include dietary fiber, bacteria, and digestive secretions) and 40 percent water, then passes into the rectum. In the **rectum**, strong muscles hold back the waste until it is time to defecate. The rectal muscles then relax, and the anal sphincter opens to allow passage of the stool out the anal canal.[10] **Figure 3.16** summarizes nutrient absorption along the GI tract.

rectum The muscular final segment of the intestine, extending from the sigmoid colon to the anus.

Key Concepts: *Digestion begins in the mouth with the action of salivary amylase. Food material next moves down the esophagus to the stomach, where it mixes with gastric secretions. Protein digestion is begun through the action of pepsin, while salivary amylase action ceases due to the low pH level of the stomach. Some substances, such as alcohol, are absorbed directly from the stomach. The liquid material (chyme) next moves to the small intestine. Here, secretions from the gallbladder, pancreas, and intestinal lining cells complete the digestion of carbohydrates, proteins, and fats. The end products of digestion, along with vitamins, minerals, water, and other compounds, are absorbed through the intestinal wall and into circulation. Undigested material and some liquid moves on to the large intestine, where water and electrolytes are absorbed, leaving waste material to be excreted as feces.*

Regulation of Gastrointestinal Activity

The processes of digestion and absorption are regulated by interaction of the nervous and hormonal systems. It would be wasteful to use energy for peristalsis or to secrete digestive enzymes when they were not needed. So, a system of signals is necessary to control GI movement and secretions. That's where nerve cells and hormones come in.

Nervous System

Nerves carry information back and forth between tissues and the brain. Chemicals called neurotransmitters send signals to either excite or suppress nerves, thereby stimulating or inhibiting activity in various parts of the body.

The **central nervous system (CNS)** regulates GI activity in two ways. The **enteric nervous system** is a local system of nerves in the gut wall that is stimulated both by the chemical composition of chyme and by the stretching of the GI lumen that results from food in the GI tract. This stimulation leads to nerve impulses that enhance the muscle and secretory activity along the tract. The enteric nervous system plays an essential role in the control of motility, blood flow, water and electrolyte transport, and acid secretion in the GI tract. A branch of the **autonomic nervous system** (the portion of the CNS that controls organ function) responds to the sight, smell, and thought of food. This branch of the CNS carries signals to and from the GI tract via the vagus nerve, and also enhances GI motility and secretion. In the past, treatments for some ulcers and other GI ailments included severing the vagus nerve, a measure that brought temporary, but not long-term, relief.

Hormonal System

Hormones are also involved in GI regulation (see **Figure 3.17**). Hormones are chemical messengers that are produced at one location and travel in the bloodstream to affect another location in the body. Some GI hormones, however, are secreted by and active in the same tissue.

Gastrointestinal hormonal signals increase or decrease GI motility and secretions, and influence your appetite by sending signals to

central nervous system (CNS) The brain and the spinal cord. The central nervous system transmits signals that control muscular actions and glandular secretions along the entire GI tract.

enteric nervous system A network of nerves located in the gastrointestinal wall.

autonomic nervous system The part of the central nervous system that regulates the automatic responses of the body; consists of the sympathetic and parasympathetic systems.

Figure 3.17 **Hormonal regulation of digestion.** In response to food moving through the digestive tract, hormones control the increase and decrease of digestive activities.

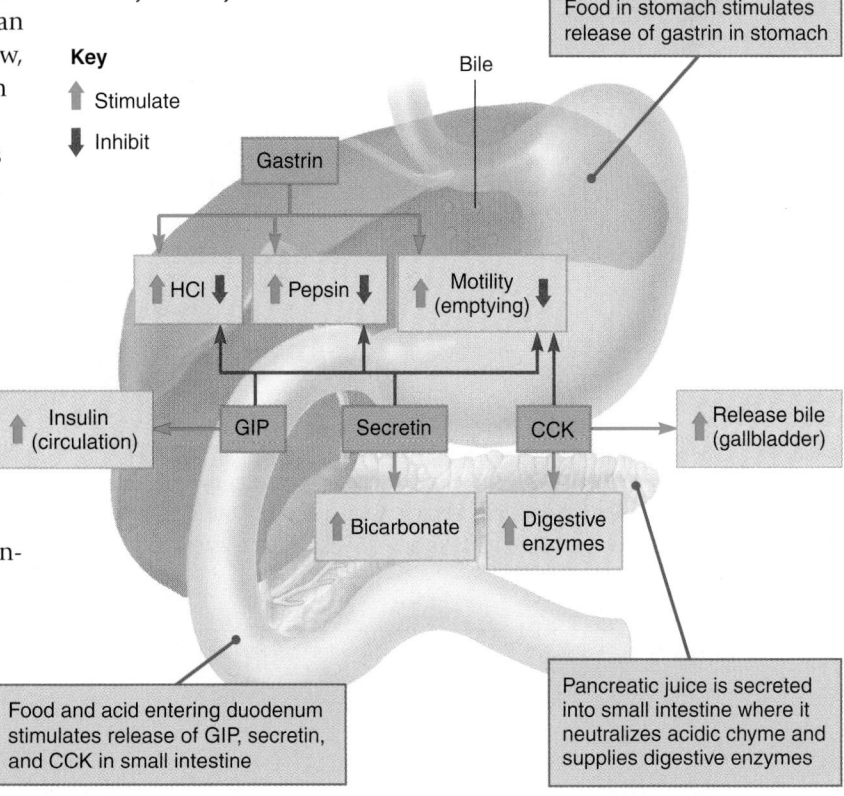

Key
⬆ Stimulate
⬇ Inhibit

Food in stomach stimulates release of gastrin in stomach

Bile

Gastrin

⬆ HCl ⬇   ⬆ Pepsin ⬇   ⬆ Motility (emptying) ⬇

⬆ Insulin (circulation)   GIP   Secretin   CCK   ⬆ Release bile (gallbladder)

⬆ Bicarbonate   ⬆ Digestive enzymes

Food and acid entering duodenum stimulates release of GIP, secretin, and CCK in small intestine

Pancreatic juice is secreted into small intestine where it neutralizes acidic chyme and supplies digestive enzymes

NUTRITION SCIENCE IN ACTION
Gum Chewing After Surgery

Observations: Any abdominal surgery, including colon surgery, can cause a marked decrease or stoppage of intestinal function (ileus). Immediate consequences include pain, vomiting, and bloating. Ileus also can lead to longer hospital stays, increased risk of infection, and breathing difficulties. Chewing gum may stimulate the same nerves in the body as eating, promoting the release of hormones that stimulate muscular contractions and movement along the bowel.

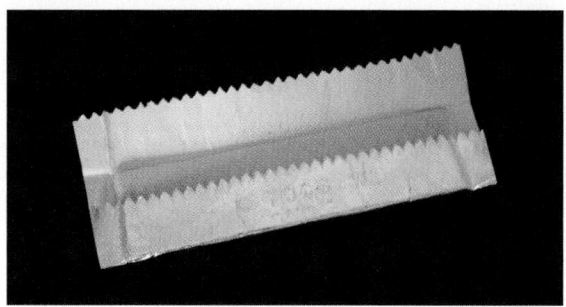

Hypothesis: Chewing gum after colon surgery will shorten hospital stays and the time for appetite and bowel function to return.

Experimental Plan: Recruit 34 patients scheduled for elective colon surgery. Randomly assign study participants to chew gum (experimental group) or not to chew gum (control group) after surgery. Beginning the morning after surgery, the gum-chewing group will chew sugarless gum (one stick) three times daily. For all participants, record the time of first flatus (passing gas), bowel movement, return of appetite, and length of hospital stay.

Results: The hypothesis is confirmed. Compared with control group patients, the gum-chewing patients were quicker to have an appetite, pass gas, have a bowel movement, and leave the hospital.

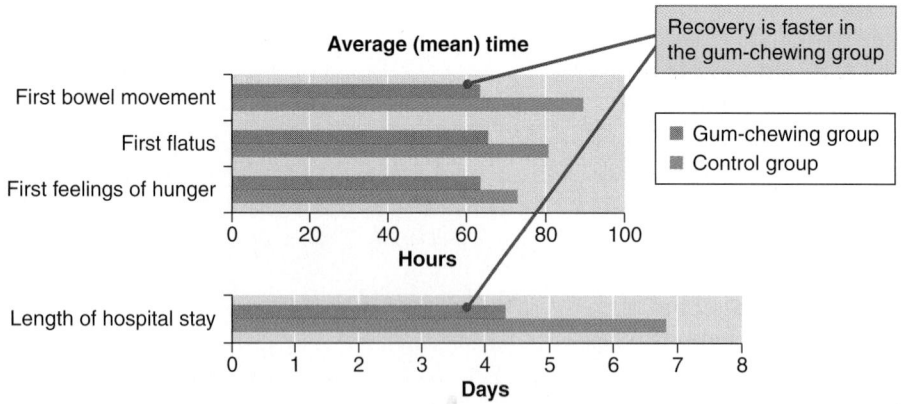

Conclusion and Discussion: Gum chewing early in the postoperative period following colon surgery hastens the time to bowel movement and first feeding. Gum chewing is an inexpensive and effective adjunct to postoperative care. Future studies may reveal the mechanism by which gum chewing activates cephalic response mechanisms and promotes bowel function.

Source: Based on Schuster R, Grewal N, Greaney GC, Waxman K. Gum chewing reduces ileus after elective open sigmoid colectomy. *Arch Surg.* 2006;141:174–176.

the central nervous system. Some GI hormones function as growth factors for the gastrointestinal mucosa and pancreas.

The four major hormones that regulate the GI function are gastrin, secretin, cholecystokinin, and gastric inhibitory peptide.

- Gastrin is released by cells in the stomach in response to distention of the stomach, nerve impulses from the vagus nerve, and the presence of chemicals such as alcohol and caffeine. Gastrin increases muscle movement in the stomach and enhances release of hydrochloric acid and pepsinogen to encourage digestion.

- Secretin is released by cells along the duodenal wall when acidic chyme begins to move into the duodenum. Secretin opposes the action of gastrin; it reduces gastric secretion and motility, and stimulates the pancreas to release bicarbonate so as to neutralize chyme.

- Cholecystokinin (CCK) is released by cells along the small intestine as amino acids and fatty acids from digestion begin to enter the small intestine. CCK stimulates the pancreas to secrete enzymes, stimulates the gallbladder to contract and release bile, and slows gastric emptying.

- **Gastric inhibitory peptide (GIP)** is also released from the intestinal mucosal cells in response to fat and glucose in the small intestine. As its name implies, GIP inhibits gastric secretion, motility, and emptying. In addition, GIP stimulates the release of insulin, which is necessary for glucose utilization.

Taken together, nerve cells and hormones coordinate the movement and secretions of the GI tract so that enzymes are released when and where they are needed and chyme moves at a rate that will optimize digestion and absorption. Side effects from abdominal surgery can slow or halt movement through the GI tract for hours or days. Researchers are investigating strategies for stimulating the release of hormones to improve postoperative GI movement and speed recovery. (See Nutrition Science in Action, "Gum Chewing After Surgery.")

Key Concepts: *Both hormonal and nervous system signals regulate gastrointestinal activity. Nerve cells in both the enteric and autonomic nervous systems control muscle movement and secretory activity. Key hormones involved in regulation are gastrin, secretin, cholecystokinin, and gastric inhibitory peptide. The net effect of these regulators is to coordinate GI movement and secretion for optimal digestion and absorption of nutrients.*

Circulation of Nutrients

After foods are digested and nutrients are absorbed, they are transported via the vascular and lymphatic systems to specific destinations throughout the body. Let's take a closer look at how each of these circulatory systems delivers nutrients to the places they are needed.

Vascular System

The **vascular system** is a network of veins and arteries through which the blood carries nutrients (see **Figure 3.18**). The heart is the pump that keeps the blood circulating through the body. From intestinal cells, water-soluble nutrients are absorbed directly into tiny capillary tributaries of the bloodstream, where they travel to the liver before being dispersed throughout the body. Blood carries oxygen from the lungs and nutrients from the GI system

Quick Bites

Short Bowel Syndrome

Patients who suffer from short bowel syndrome commonly have difficulty absorbing fat-soluble vitamins. To enhance absorption, treatment includes taking a fat-soluble vitamin supplement that easily mingles with water. These patients may also need to take intramuscular shots of B_{12} because they are unable to absorb this water-soluble vitamin.

gastric inhibitory peptide (GIP) [GAS-trik in-HIB-ihtor-ee PEP-tide] A hormone released from the walls of the duodenum that slows the release of the stomach contents into the small intestine and also stimulates release of insulin from the pancreas.

vascular system A network of veins and arteries through which the blood carries nutrients. Also called the circulatory system.

lymphatic system A system of small vessels, ducts, valves, and organized tissue (e.g., lymph nodes) through which lymph moves from its origin in the tissues toward the heart.

to all body tissues. Once the destination cells have used the oxygen and nutrients, carbon dioxide and waste products are picked up by the blood and transported to the lungs and kidneys, respectively, for excretion.

Lymphatic System

The **lymphatic system** is a network of vessels that drain lymph, the clear fluid formed in the spaces between cells. Lymph moves through this system and eventually empties into the bloodstream near the neck. Lymph vessels in the small intestine absorb fat-soluble nutrients and most end products of fat digestion. After a fatty meal, lymph can become as much as 1 to 2 percent fat. Nutrients absorbed into the lymphatic system, unlike those absorbed directly into the vascular system, bypass the liver before entering the bloodstream. We'll discuss the specific process for absorption of lipids into the lymphatic system in Chapter 5, "Lipids."

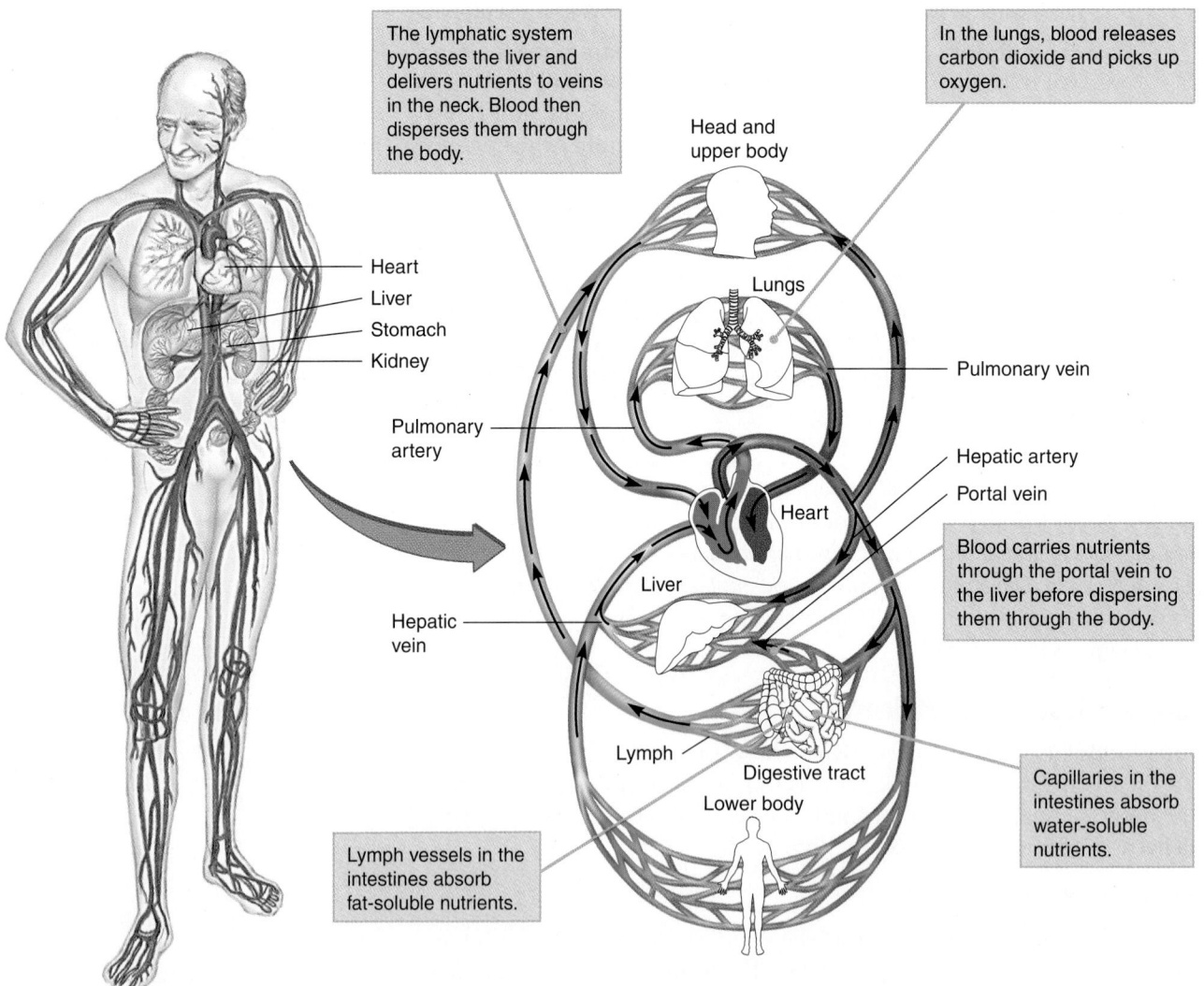

The lymphatic system bypasses the liver and delivers nutrients to veins in the neck. Blood then disperses them through the body.

In the lungs, blood releases carbon dioxide and picks up oxygen.

Head and upper body

Heart
Liver
Stomach
Kidney

Lungs

Pulmonary vein

Pulmonary artery

Hepatic artery
Portal vein

Heart

Blood carries nutrients through the portal vein to the liver before dispersing them through the body.

Liver

Hepatic vein

Lymph

Digestive tract

Lower body

Capillaries in the intestines absorb water-soluble nutrients.

Lymph vessels in the intestines absorb fat-soluble nutrients.

Figure 3.18 **Circulation.** Blood carries oxygen from the lungs and nutrients from the GI system to all body tissues. Intestinal cells absorb water-soluble nutrients and deliver them directly into tiny capillary tributaries of the bloodstream. From there, they travel to the liver before being dispersed throughout the body. Intestinal cells absorb fat-soluble nutrients and deliver most to the lymphatic system, a circulatory system that bypasses the liver before connecting to the bloodstream.

Unlike the vascular system, the lymphatic system has no pumping organ. The major lymph vessels contain one-way valves; when the vessels are filled with lymph, smooth muscles in the vessel walls contract and pump the lymph forward. The succession of valves allows each segment of the vessel to act as an independent pump. Lymph also is moved along by skeletal muscle contractions that squeeze the vessels.

The lymphatic system also performs an important cleanup function. Proteins and large particulate matter in tissue spaces cannot be absorbed directly into the blood capillaries, but they easily enter the lymphatic system, where they are carried away for removal. This removal process is essential—without it a person would die within 24 hours from buildup of fluid and materials around the cells.[11]

Key Concepts: *Absorbed nutrients are carried by either the vascular or lymphatic system. Water-soluble nutrients are absorbed directly into the bloodstream, carried to the liver, and then distributed around the body. Fat-soluble vitamins and large lipid molecules are absorbed into the lymphatic vessels and carried by this system before entering the vascular system.*

Influences on Digestion and Absorption

Psychological Influences

The taste, smell, and presentation of foods can have a positive effect on digestion. Just the thought of food can trigger saliva production and peristalsis. Stressful emotions such as depression and fear can have the reverse effect (see **Figure 3.19**): They stimulate the brain to activate the autonomic nervous system. This results in decreased gastric acid secretion, reduced blood flow to the stomach, inhibition of peristalsis, and reduced propulsion of food.[12] The next time you sit down to a holiday meal, notice how you feel at the sight of your family's traditional foods as well as smells from your childhood. Happiness and positive memories add to the enjoyment of food, whereas sadness can bring on a poor appetite or stomach upset.

Chemical Influences

The type of protein you eat and the way it is prepared affects digestion. Plant proteins tend to be less digestible than animal proteins. Cooking food usually denatures protein (uncoils its three-dimensional structure), which increases digestibility. Cooking meat softens its connective tissue, making chewing easier and increasing the meat's accessibility to digestive enzymes.

Food processing produces chemicals that may influence digestive secretions. For example, frying foods in fat at very high temperatures produces small amounts of **acrolein**,[13] which decreases the flow of digestive secretions; in contrast, meat extracts may stimulate digestion. The physical condition of a food sometimes causes problems with digestion. Cold foods may cause intestinal spasms in people who suffer from irritable bowel syndrome or Crohn's disease. Stomach contents can affect absorption. When food is consumed on an empty stomach, it has more contact with gastric secretions and will be absorbed faster than if it was consumed on a full stomach. Certain medicines may inhibit nutrient absorption, and in turn, certain foods may interact with medicines, making the drugs less effective or toxic. (See Chapter 16, "Life Cycle: From Childhood Through Adulthood.")

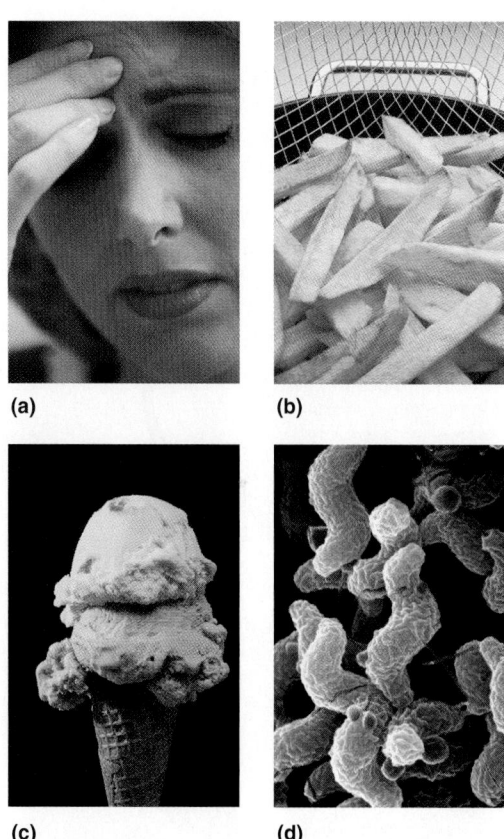

(a)   (b)

(c)   (d)

Figure 3.19 **Negative factors for digestion.** (a) Stress. (b) High-temperature fat frying. (c) Cold foods. (d) Bacteria.

acrolein A pungent decomposition product of fats, generated from dehydrating the glycerol component of fats; responsible for the coughing attacks caused by the fumes released by burning fat. This toxic water-soluble liquid vaporizes easily and is highly flammable.

Quick Bites

Halt! Who Goes There?

*B*e they friend or foe, antibiotics kill micro-organisms in your GI tract, frequently causing diarrhea. About half of pharmaceutical drugs have gastrointestinal side effects.

Bacterial Influences

In the healthy stomach, hydrochloric acid kills most bacteria. In conditions where there is a lower concentration of hydrochloric acid, more bacteria can survive and multiply; harmful bacteria can cause gastritis (an inflammation of the stomach lining) and peptic ulcer (a wound in the mucous membranes lining the stomach or duodenum). Bacteria that cause foodborne illness resist the germicidal effects of hydrochloric acid, so they survive to wreak havoc on the digestive process.

The large intestine maintains a large population of bacteria. These bacteria can form several vitamins and digest small amounts of fiber, producing a small amount of energy. These bacteria also synthesize gases, such as hydrogen, ammonia, and methane, as well as acids and various substances that contribute to the odor of feces. If the digestion and absorption of food in the small intestine are incomplete, the undigested material enters the large intestine, where bacterial action produces excessive gas, and possibly bloating and pain.

Key Concepts: *Psychological, chemical, and bacterial factors can influence the processes of digestion and absorption. Emotions can influence GI motility and secretion. The temperature and form of food can also affect digestive secretions. Although stomach acid kills many types of bacteria, some are resistant to acid and cause foodborne illness. Helpful bacteria in the large intestine can cause bloating and gas if they receive and begin to digest food components that are normally digested in the small intestine.*

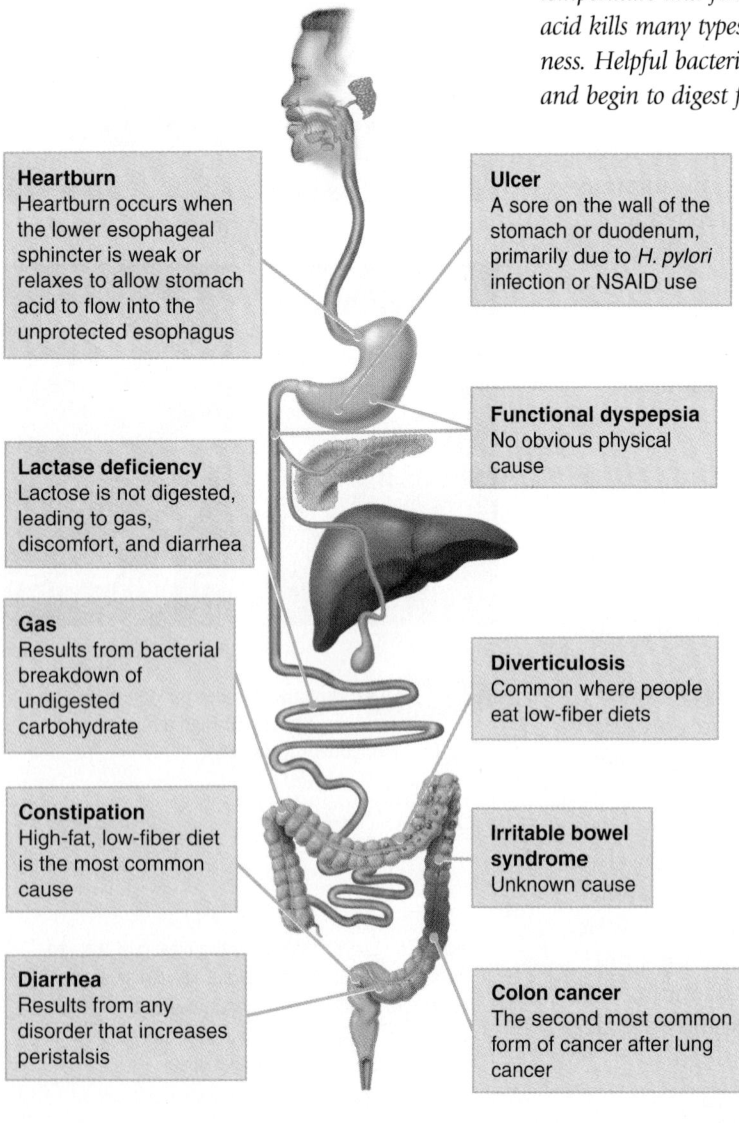

Nutrition and GI Disorders

"I have butterflies in my stomach." "It was a gut-wrenching experience." Our language contains many references to the connection between emotional distress and the GI tract. Most of us have experienced intestinal cramping right before a big date or job interview, or a queasy stomach in response to something very disgusting. The brain, through numerous neurochemical connections with the gut, exerts a profound influence on GI function. Nearly all GI disorders are influenced to some degree by emotional state. On the other hand, a number of illnesses that were once attributed largely to emotional stress, such as peptic ulcer disease, have been shown to be caused primarily by infection and other physical causes. **Figure 3.20** shows some common ailments that affect the GI tract.

Although stress management may help and medical intervention can be required, we can prevent and manage most GI disorders with diet. For instance, adding fiber-rich foods (see **Table 3.2**) and water to the diet reduces intestinal pressure, decreases the time food by-products remain in the colon, and promotes bowel regularity. You can avoid most problems and keep your GI tract operating at peak efficiency if you regularly eat a healthful diet, exercise, and maintain a healthy weight.

Figure 3.20 **Common GI ailments.** Beans are familiar culprits in what is perhaps the most common GI ailment—gas. Rice is the only starch that does not cause gas.

Heartburn
Heartburn occurs when the lower esophageal sphincter is weak or relaxes to allow stomach acid to flow into the unprotected esophagus

Lactase deficiency
Lactose is not digested, leading to gas, discomfort, and diarrhea

Gas
Results from bacterial breakdown of undigested carbohydrate

Constipation
High-fat, low-fiber diet is the most common cause

Diarrhea
Results from any disorder that increases peristalsis

Ulcer
A sore on the wall of the stomach or duodenum, primarily due to *H. pylori* infection or NSAID use

Functional dyspepsia
No obvious physical cause

Diverticulosis
Common where people eat low-fiber diets

Irritable bowel syndrome
Unknown cause

Colon cancer
The second most common form of cancer after lung cancer

Constipation

Constipation is defined as having a bowel movement fewer than three times per week.[14] With constipation, stools are usually hard, dry, small in size, and difficult to eliminate. People who are constipated may find it painful to have a bowel movement and often experience straining, bloating, and the sensation of a full bowel.

Constipation is a symptom, not a disease. Almost everyone experiences constipation at some point, and a poor diet (low in fiber and water and high in fats) typically is the cause. Some fibers, such as the pectins in fruits and gums in beans, dissolve easily in water and take on a soft, gel-like texture in the intestines. Other fibers, such as cellulose in wheat bran, pass almost unchanged through the intestines. The bulk and soft texture of fiber help prevent hard, dry stools that are difficult to pass. People who eat plenty of high-fiber foods are not likely to become constipated.

Liquids such as water and juice add fluid to the colon and bulk to stools, making bowel movements softer and easier to pass. The caffeine in many liquids (e.g., coffee, tea, and many soft drinks) is a mild diuretic (a substance that increases urine production).

Although treatment depends on the cause, severity, and duration, in most cases dietary changes help relieve symptoms and prevent constipation.

constipation Infrequent and difficult bowel movements, followed by a sensation of incomplete evacuation.

Table 3.2 **Fiber Content of Foods**

Food Group	Serving Size	Fiber (g)
Legumes		
Kidney beans	1 cup, cooked	11.3
Lentils	1 cup, cooked	15.6
Split peas	1 cup, cooked	16.3
Fruit		
Dried plums	$\frac{1}{2}$ cup	4.7
Apple with skin	1 small	2.5
Peach with skin	1 large	2.4
Vegetables		
Broccoli	1 cup, raw	2.4
Carrot	2 medium, raw	3.4
Tomato	1 large, raw	2.2
Grains		
Wheat-bran-flake cereal	1 ounce	4.9
Bulgur wheat	$\frac{1}{2}$ cup, cooked	4.1
Whole-wheat bread	1 slice	1.1
Brown rice	$\frac{1}{2}$ cup, cooked	1.8
Spaghetti, enriched white	$\frac{1}{2}$ cup, cooked	1.3
White bread	1 slice	0.6
White rice	$\frac{1}{2}$ cup, cooked	0.3

Source: US Department of Agriculture, Agricultural Research Service. USDA National Nutrient Database for Standard Reference, Release 18. 2005. http://www.nal.usda.gov/fnic/foodcomp. Accessed 3/13/06.

diarrhea Watery stools due to reduced absorption of water.

Diarrhea

Diarrhea—loose, watery stools that occur more than three times in one day—is caused by digestive products moving through the large intestine too rapidly for sufficient water to be reabsorbed.

Diarrhea is a symptom of many disorders that cause increased peristalsis. Culprits include stress, intestinal irritation or damage, and intolerance to gluten, fat, or lactose. Eating food contaminated with bacteria or viruses often causes diarrhea when the digestive tract speeds the offending food along the alimentary canal and out of the body.

Diarrhea can cause dehydration, which means the body lacks enough fluid to function properly. Dehydration is particularly dangerous in children and the elderly, and it must be treated promptly to avoid serious health problems.

Fyi Bugs in Your Gut? Health Effects of Intestinal Bacteria

FOR YOUR INFORMATION

Unseen and unnoticed, millions and millions of bacteria call your GI tract home. Although we often associate bacteria with illness, the right kinds of bacteria in the gut actually protect us from disease. The normal microflora of the gut, specifically strains of *lactobacilli* and *bifidobacteria*, have been linked to improved digestion, intestinal regularity, enhanced GI immune function, improved lactose tolerance, reduced risk of developing allergies, and even reduced risk of colorectal cancer. So how can we be good hosts to our intestinal guests, keeping them well-fed and happy? The answer may be in food products and dietary supplements known as probiotics and prebiotics.

Probiotics are foods (or supplements) that contain live microorganisms such as *Lactobacillus acidophilus*. Such lactic-acid-producing bacteria have been used for centuries to ferment milk into yogurt, cheeses, and other products. The bacteria convert lactose into lactic acid, which causes the milk to gel and imparts a tart flavor to the product. The resulting product has a much longer shelf-life than fresh milk and is associated with good health and longevity in many societies. Other probiotics are *Bifidobacteria* and yeast. When consumed in sufficient quantities, these microorganisms have the potential to improve health.

The term *prebiotic* describes a nondigestible food product that can be fermented by gastrointestinal bacteria and stimulates the growth and/or activity of "good" gut bacteria. For example, it is thought that the composition of breast milk strongly favors the growth of *lactobacilli* and *bifidobacteria* in the newborn gut. Some scientists have found *bifidobacteria* to be the dominant species in breast-fed infants while the microflora of bottle-fed infants is more diverse. The reduced incidence of GI infections in breast-fed infants has been attributed to the dominance of *bifidobacteria*. Substances that may be effective prebiotics include fructooligosaccharides, polydextrose, arabinogalactan, polyols, and inulin.

So how does feeding the bacteria in your gut improve your health? Successful colonization of helpful bacteria allows them to outnumber (and out-eat) disease-causing bacteria, thus reducing the likelihood of food-borne illness and other infections. Studies in young children show that supplementation with *Lactobacillus* reduced the severity and duration of diarrhea due to rotavirus, a common infectious agent in daycare centers. Some probiotics enhance the ability of the gut as a barrier to infectious agents, and may also adjust the activity of the immune system.

"Good" bacteria can digest the lactose that enters the colon of a person with lactose intolerance, reducing symptoms and discomfort. Intestinal bacteria metabolize both indigestible and incompletely digested food material. Probiotics may produce by-products that reduce disease risk. For example, acids produced by probiotic colon bacteria change the pH of the colon, which may interfere with carcinogenesis (development of cancer).

In addition to promoting the growth and function of beneficial bacteria, prebiotics may have other health effects. Some prebiotics have been shown to enhance absorption of calcium and magnesium. Others may inhibit growth of lesions in the gut, which in turn reduces colorectal cancer risk. Although lipid-lowering effects have been attributed to prebiotics, the limited data available show inconsistent effects on cholesterol and triglycerides.

Fermented milk products such as yogurt or kefir are one way to keep your gut happy. Look for a seal adopted by the National Yogurt Association to identify products that contain a minimum of 100 million live lactic acid bacteria per gram of yogurt. Not all brands of yogurt contain live, active cultures. Supplemental probiotics must have sufficient numbers of live bacteria to be useful; currently, identification and standardization procedures are lacking. Prebiotics are found in whole grains, onions, bananas, garlic, artichokes, and a variety of fortified foods, beverages, and dietary supplements. Although results are preliminary, food and supplement sources of probiotics and prebiotics may be another useful way to improve gut microflora and overall health.

A diet of broth, tea, and toast and avoidance of lactose, caffeine, and sorbitol can reduce diarrhea until it subsides. As stools form, you can gradually introduce more foods. Pectin, a form of dietary fiber found in apples and citrus peel, may be helpful. Also, include foods high in potassium, if tolerated, to replace lost electrolytes. Fluid replacement is also important to avoid dehydration.

Diverticulosis

Like an inner tube that pokes through weak places in an old tire, the colon develops small pouches that bulge outward through weak spots as people age. Known as diverticulosis, this condition afflicts about half of all Americans aged 60 to 80, and almost everyone over age 80. Although it usually causes few problems, in 10 to 25 percent of these people, the pouches become infected or inflamed—a condition called diverticulitis.

Diverticulosis and diverticulitis are common in developed or industrialized countries—particularly the United States, England, and Australia—where low-fiber diets are common. Diverticular disease is rare in Asian and African countries, where people eat high-fiber, vegetable-based diets.

A low-fiber diet can make stools hard and difficult to pass. If the stool is too hard, muscles must strain to move it. This is the main cause of increased pressure in the colon, which causes weak spots to bulge outward.

Increasing the amount of fiber in the diet may reduce symptoms of diverticulosis and prevent complications such as diverticulitis. Fiber keeps stools soft and lowers pressure inside the colon so bowel contents can move through easily. Additional benefits of fiber are listed in **Table 3.3**.

Until recently, many doctors suggested avoiding foods with small seeds, such as tomatoes or strawberries, because they believed that particles could lodge in the diverticula and cause inflammation. However, this is now a controversial point and no evidence supports this recommendation.

If cramps, bloating, and constipation are problems, a doctor may prescribe a short course of pain medication. However, many medications cause either diarrhea or constipation, undesirable side effects for people with diverticulosis.

Heartburn and Gastroesophageal Reflux

Heartburn occurs when the lower esophageal sphincter (LES) relaxes inappropriately, allowing the stomach's contents to flow back into the esophagus. Unlike the stomach, the esophagus has no protective mucous lining, so acid can damage it quickly and cause pain. Many people experience occasional heartburn, but for some, heartburn is a chronic, often daily, event and a symptom of a more serious disorder called **gastroesophageal reflux disease (GERD)**. GERD, along with obesity, is a key risk factor for esophageal cancer, a type of cancer that is on the rise in North America.[15] GERD has a variety of causes, and many treatment strategies involve lifestyle and nutrition.

Doctors recommend avoiding foods and beverages that can weaken the LES, including chocolate, peppermint, fatty foods, coffee, and alcoholic beverages. Foods and beverages that can irritate a damaged esophageal lining, such as citrus fruits and juices, tomato products, and pepper, also should be avoided.

Decreasing both the portion size and the fat content of meals may help. High-fat meals remain in the stomach longer than low-fat meals. This creates back pressure on the lower esophageal sphincter. Eating meals at least two to three hours before bedtime may lessen reflux by allowing partial

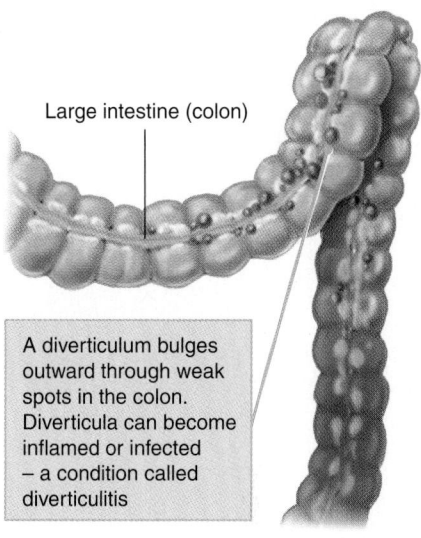

Large intestine (colon)

A diverticulum bulges outward through weak spots in the colon. Diverticula can become inflamed or infected – a condition called diverticulitis

gastroesophageal reflux disease (GERD) A condition in which gastric contents move backwards (reflux) into the esophagus, causing pain and tissue damage.

Table 3.3 Benefits of Fiber

1. Helps control weight by delaying gastric emptying and providing a feeling of fullness.
2. Improves glucose tolerance by delaying the movement of carbohydrate into the small intestine.
3. Reduces risk for heart disease by binding with bile (which contains cholesterol) in the intestine and causing it to be excreted, which in turn helps to lower blood cholesterol levels.
4. Promotes regularity and reduces constipation by increasing stool weight and decreasing transit time.
5. Reduces the risk of diverticulosis by decreasing pressure within the colon, decreasing transit time, and increasing stool weight.

Source: Institute of Medicine, Food and Nutrition Board. *Dietary Reference Intakes for Energy, Carbohydrate, Fiber, Fat, Fatty Acids, Cholesterol, Protein, and Amino Acids.* Washington, DC: National Academy Press, 2005. Reprinted with permission.

emptying and a decrease in stomach acidity. Elevating the head of the bed or sleeping on a specially designed wedge reduces heartburn by allowing gravity to minimize reflux of stomach contents into the esophagus.

In addition, cigarette smoking weakens the LES, and being overweight often worsens symptoms. Stopping smoking is important, and many overweight people find relief when they lose weight.

Irritable Bowel Syndrome

About 20 percent of people in Western countries suffer from **irritable bowel syndrome (IBS)**, a poorly understood condition that causes abdominal pain, altered bowel habits (such as diarrhea or constipation), and cramps.[16] Often IBS is just a mild annoyance, but for some people it can be disabling.

The cause of IBS remains a mystery, but emotional stress and specific foods clearly aggravate the symptoms in most sufferers.[17] Beans, chocolate, milk products, and large amounts of alcohol are frequent offenders. Fat in any form (animal or vegetable) is a strong stimulus of colonic contractions after a meal. Caffeine causes loose stools in many people, but it is more likely to affect those with IBS. Women with IBS may have more symptoms during their menstrual periods, suggesting that reproductive hormones can increase IBS symptoms.

The good news about IBS is that although its symptoms can be uncomfortable, it does not shorten life span or progress to more serious illness. IBS can usually be controlled with diet and lifestyle modifications and judicious use of medication. Stress management is an important part of treatment for IBS and includes stress reduction (relaxation) training and relaxation therapies, such as meditation; counseling and support; regular exercise; changes to stressful situations in your life; and adequate sleep.[18]

irritable bowel syndrome (IBS) A disruptive state of intestinal motility with no known cause. Symptoms include constipation, abdominal pain, and episodic diarrhea.

Label [to] **Table**

As you've learned in this chapter, fiber is one of the few things you do not digest fully. Instead, fiber moves through the GI tract and most of it leaves the body in feces. If it's not digested, then why all the fuss about eating more fiber? You'll learn later in this textbook (in the Carbohydrates chapter) that a healthy intake of fiber may lower your risk of cancer and heart disease and help with bowel regularity. So how do you know which foods have fiber? You have to check out the food label!

This Nutrition Facts panel is from the label on a loaf of whole-wheat bread. The highlighted sections show you that every slice of bread contains 3 grams of fiber. The 12% listed to the right of that refers to the Daily Values below. Look at the Daily Values at the far right of the label, and note that there are two numbers listed for fiber. One (25 g) is for a person who consumes about 2,000 kilocalories per day and the other (30 g) is for a 2,500-kilocalorie level. It should be no surprise that if you are consuming more calories, you should also be consuming more fiber. The 12% Daily Value is calculated using the 2,000-kilocalorie fiber guideline as follows:

$$\frac{3 \text{ grams fiber per slice}}{25 \text{ grams Daily Value}} = .12, \text{ or } 12\%$$

This means if you make a sandwich with 2 slices of whole-wheat bread, you're getting 6 grams of fiber and almost one-quarter (24% Daily Value) of your fiber needs per day. Not bad! Be careful though; many people inadvertently buy wheat bread thinking that it's as high in fiber as *whole-wheat* bread but it's not. Whole-wheat bread contains the whole (complete) grain, but wheat bread often is stripped of its fiber. Check the label before you buy your next loaf.

Many researchers are convinced that IBS sufferers have abnormal patterns of intestinal motility, but studies show no consistent differences in the GI motion patterns of IBS patients compared with normal control subjects. Some researchers have postulated that IBS sufferers may be hypersensitive to GI stimuli, but, again, research results are inconclusive. We are a long way from understanding what causes IBS, but it is likely that a number of physical and psychosocial factors combine to trigger this disorder.

Colorectal Cancer

After lung cancer, colorectal cancer—cancer of the colon or rectum—is the second leading cause of cancer-related deaths in the United States.[19] According to the World Health Organization, "Review of the relationships between diet and colorectal cancer suggests that risk is increased by high intakes of meat and fat, and decreased by high intakes of fruit, vegetables, folate, and calcium. Overweight and obesity increase risk while regular physical activity reduces risk."[20] A study of nearly 149,000 American adults found that those who ate the most red meat and processed meat had a 30 to 40 percent higher risk of developing colorectal cancer.[21]

Observational and case control studies support the idea that fiber-rich diets reduce colorectal cancer risk, and scientists have hypothesized a number of possible ways that fiber might be protective.[22] These include dilution of carcinogens in a bulkier stool, more rapid transit of carcinogens through the GI tract, and lower colon pH due to bacterial fermentation of fiber.

Although there are logical reasons why a high fiber intake may be beneficial, studies in humans and animals fail to support these theories. Fiber has not been shown to reduce risk of colorectal cancer[23] or to prevent recurrence of the colorectal polyps that are precursors to many cancers.[24]

Nutrition Facts

Serving Size: 1 slice (43g)
Servings Per Container: 16

Calories 100
Calories from Fat 15

Amount Per Serving	% Daily Value*
Total Fat 2g	**3%**
Saturated Fat 0g	0%
Trans Fat 0g	
Cholesterol 0mg	**0%**

Amount Per Serving	% Daily Value*
Sodium 230mg	**9%**
Total Carbohydrate 18g	**6%**
Dietary Fibers 3g	**12%**
Sugars 2g	
Protein 5g	

Vitamin A 0%	·	Vitamin C 0%	·	Calcium 6%	·	Iron 6%
Thiamin 10%	·	Riboflavin 4%	·	Niacin 10%	·	Folate 10%

* Percent Daily Values are based on a 2,000 calorie diet. Your daily values may be higher or lower depending on your calorie needs:

	Calories:	2,000	2,500
Total Fat	Less Than	65g	80g
Sat Fat	Less Than	20g	25g
Cholesterol	Less Than	300mg	300mg
Sodium	Less Than	2,400mg	2,400mg
Total Carbohydrate		300g	375g
Dietary Fiber		25g	30g

INGREDIENTS: STONE GROUND WHOLE WHEAT FLOUR, WATER, HIGH FRUCTOSE CORN SYRUP, WHEAT GLUTEN, WHEAT BRAN. CONTAINS 2% OR LESS OF EACH OF THE FOLLOWING: YEAST, SALT, PARTIALLY HYDROGENATED SOYBEAN OIL, HONEY, MOLASSES, RAISIN JUICE CONCENTRATE, DOUGH CONDITIONERS (MAY CONTAIN ONE OR MORE OF EACH OF THE FOLLOWING: MONO- AND DIGLYCERIDES, CALCIUM AND SODIUM STEAROYL LACTYLATES, CALCIUM PEROXIDE), WHEAT GERM, WHEY, CORNSTARCH, YEAST NUTRIENTS (MONOCALCIUM PHOSPHATE, CALCIUM SULFATE, AMMONIUM SULFATE).

flatus Lower intestinal gas that is expelled through the rectum.

ulcer A craterlike lesion that occurs in the lining of the stomach or duodenum; also called a peptic ulcer to distinguish it from a skin ulcer.

Quick Bites

Flatulence Facts

Researchers studying pilots and astronauts during the 1960s made some interesting discoveries. The average person inadvertently swallows air with food and drink, and subsequently expels approximately one pint of gas per day, composed of 50 percent nitrogen. Another 40 percent is composed of carbon dioxide and the products of aerobic bacteria in the intestine.

Gas

Everyone has gas and eliminates it by burping or passing it through the rectum. Gas is made primarily of odorless vapors. The unpleasant odor of flatulence comes from bacteria in the large intestine that release small amounts of gases that contain sulfur. Although having gas is common, it can be uncomfortable and embarrassing.

Gas in the stomach is commonly caused by swallowing air. Everyone swallows small amounts of air when they eat and drink. However, eating or drinking rapidly, chewing gum, smoking, or wearing loose dentures can cause some people to take in more air. Burping, or belching, is the way most swallowed air leaves the stomach. The remaining gas moves into the small intestine, where it is partially absorbed. A small amount travels into the large intestine for release through the rectum. (The stomach also releases carbon dioxide when stomach acid and bicarbonate mix, but most of this gas is absorbed into the bloodstream and does not enter the large intestine.)

Frequent passage of rectal gas may be annoying, but it's seldom a symptom of serious disease. **Flatus** (lower intestinal gas) composition depends largely on dietary carbohydrate intake and the activity of the colon's bacterial population.

Most foods that contain carbohydrates can cause gas. By contrast, fats and proteins cause little gas. In the large intestine, bacteria partially break down undigested carbohydrate, producing hydrogen, carbon dioxide, and, in about one-third of people, methane. Eventually these gases exit through the rectum.

Foods that produce gas in one person may not cause gas in another. Some common bacteria in the large intestine can destroy the hydrogen that other bacteria produce. The balance of the two types of bacteria may explain why some people have more gas than others.

Carbohydrates that commonly cause gas are raffinose and stachyose, found in large quantities in beans; lactose, the natural sugar in milk; fructose, a common sweetener in soft drinks and fruit drinks; and sorbitol, found naturally in fruits and used as an artificial sweetener.

Most starches, including potatoes, corn, noodles, and wheat, produce gas as they are broken down in the large intestine. Rice is the only starch that does not cause gas.

The fiber in oat bran, beans, peas, and most fruits is not broken down until it reaches the large intestine, where digestion causes gas. In contrast, the fiber in wheat bran and some vegetables passes essentially unchanged through the intestines and produces little gas.

Ulcers

A gnawing, burning pain in the upper abdomen is the classic sign of a peptic ulcer, which also can cause nausea, vomiting, loss of appetite, and weight loss. A peptic **ulcer** is a sore that forms in the duodenum (duodenal ulcer) or the lining of the stomach (gastric ulcer).

It was once assumed that stress was a major factor in the development of peptic ulcer disease, particularly in people with "intense" personalities. Diet was also thought to be important, with spicy foods often cast as a major villain. But much to the amazement of most of the medical community, research over the last 10 years has confirmed that the vast majority of ulcers are actually caused by infection with a bacterium, *Helicobacter pylori*.

Excessive use of nonsteroidal anti-inflammatory drugs (NSAIDs), such as aspirin, ibuprofen, and naproxen sodium, is also a common cause of ulcers.

H. pylori causes 80 percent of gastric ulcers and more than 90 percent of duodenal ulcers. These bacteria weaken the protective mucous coating, allowing acid to penetrate to the sensitive lining beneath. Both the acid and the bacteria irritate the lining and cause a sore, or ulcer. *H. pylori* is able to survive in stomach acid because it secretes enzymes that neutralize the acid. This mechanism allows *H. pylori* to make its way to the "safe" area—the protective mucous lining. Once there, the bacterium's spiral shape helps it burrow through the mucous lining.[25]

NSAIDs cause ulcers by interfering with the GI tract's ability to protect itself from acidic stomach juices. Normally the stomach and duodenum employ three defenses against digestive juices: mucus that coats the lining and shields it from stomach acid, the chemical bicarbonate that neutralizes acid, and blood circulation that aids in cell renewal and repair. NSAIDs hinder all these protective mechanisms. With the defenses down, digestive juices can cause ulcers by damaging the sensitive lining of the stomach and duodenum. Fortunately, NSAID-induced ulcers usually heal once the person stops taking the medication.

If you had ulcers in the 1950s, you would have been told to quit your high-stress job and switch to a bland diet. Today, ulcer sufferers are usually treated with an antimicrobial regimen aimed at eradicating *H. pylori*.[26] Although personality and life stress are no longer considered significant factors in the development of most ulcers, relapse after treatment is more common in people who are emotionally stressed or suffering from depression.

Functional Dyspepsia

Chronic pain in the upper abdomen not due to any obvious physical cause (such as inflammation of the esophagus, peptic ulcer, or gallstones) is referred to as **functional dyspepsia**. Like IBS, the cause of functional dyspepsia is unknown. Hypersensitivity to GI stimuli, abnormal GI motility, and psychosocial problems have all been postulated as causes of dyspepsia.[27] *H. pylori* may also be a factor in some cases of functional dyspepsia.

The treatment of functional dyspepsia includes drugs that speed up the transit of food through the upper part of the intestinal tract, agents that decrease stomach acid production, and antibiotics. Just as with IBS, stress reduction techniques such as meditation and biofeedback can often improve the symptoms of functional dyspepsia.

Key Concepts: *GI disorders generally produce uncomfortable symptoms such as abdominal pain, gas, bloating, and change in elimination patterns. Some GI disorders, such as diarrhea, are generally symptoms of some other illness. Although medications are useful in reducing symptoms, many GI disorders are treatable with changes in diet, especially getting adequate fiber and fluids in the diet.*

As you have seen, the gastrointestinal tract is the key to turning food and its nutrients into nourishment for our bodies. **Figure 3.21** shows the sites for digestion and absorption of the macronutrients using a piece of pizza as an example of a food that contains substantial amounts of carbohydrate, fat, and protein. A healthy GI tract is an important factor in our overall health and well-being.

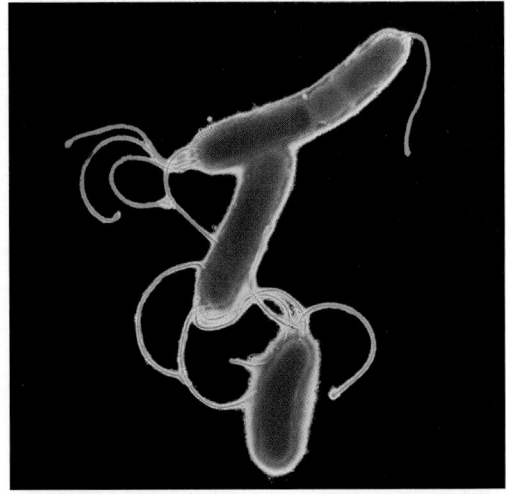

Helicobacter pylori.

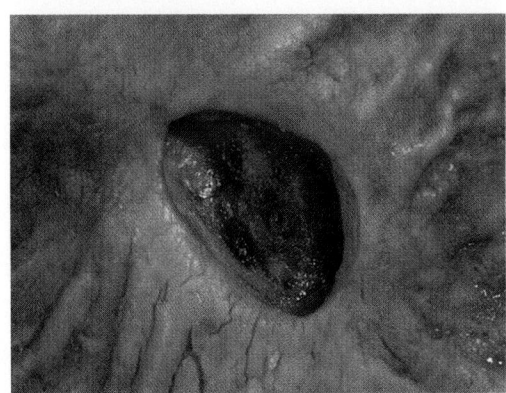

Stomach ulcer.

functional dyspepsia Chronic pain in the upper abdomen not due to any obvious physical cause.

Figure 3.21 **Fate of a piece of pizza.** When you eat a piece of pizza, what happens to the carbohydrate, fat, and protein?

Carbohydrate: Enzymes in the mouth begin the breakdown of starch. Stomach acid halts carbohydrate digestion. In the small intestine, enzymes break down carbohydrate, which is absorbed into the blood. In the large intestine, bacteria digest small amounts of fiber. The remainder is eliminated in feces.

Fat: The stomach absorbs a few short-chain fatty acids into the blood. But most fat is broken down and absorbed in the small intestine, where it enters the lymphatic system.

Protein: Stomach acid unfolds proteins, and enzymes begin protein breakdown. The small intestine completes the breakdown to amino acids, which enter the blood.

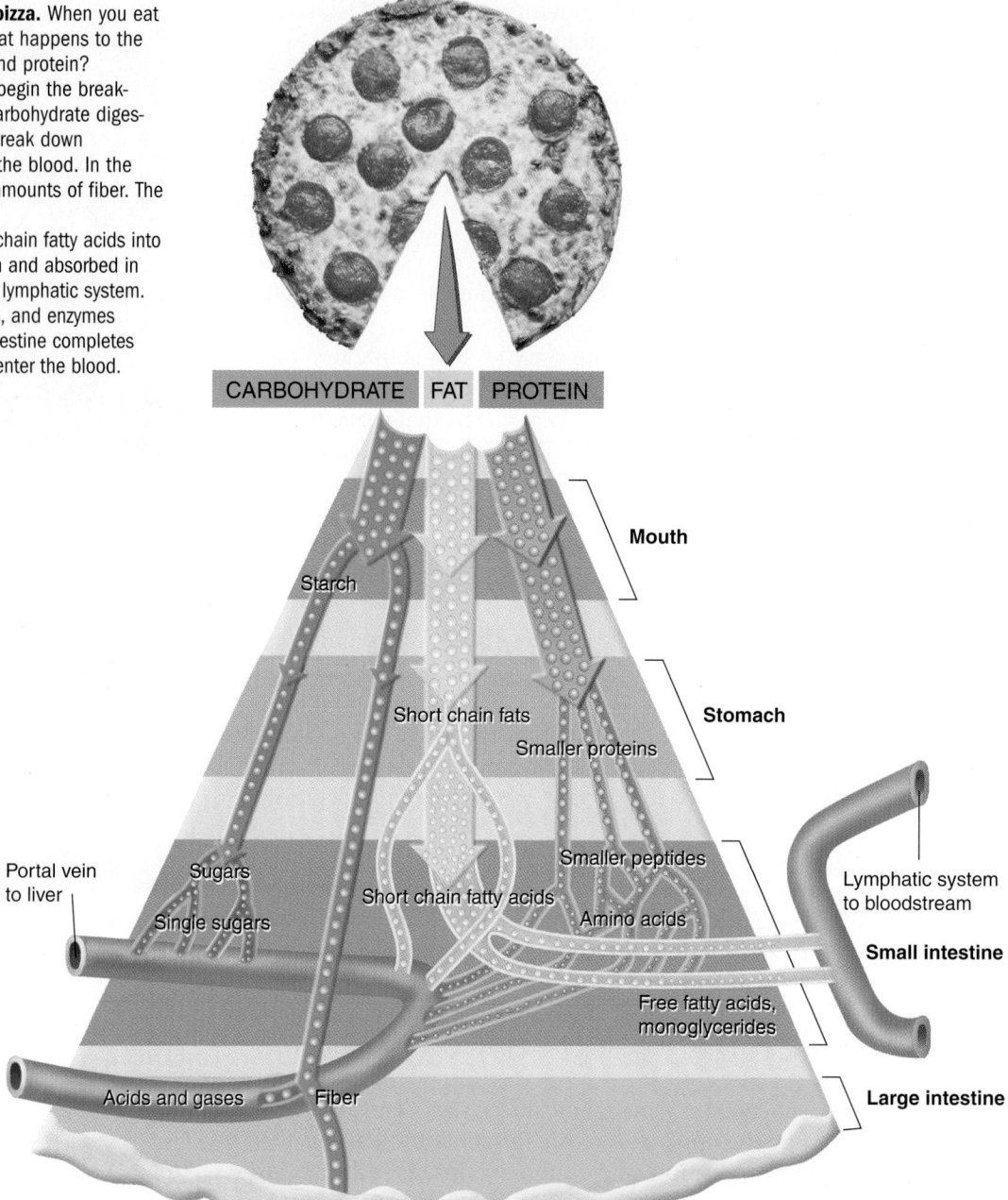

LEARNING *Portfolio* chapter 3

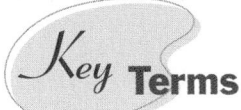

Key Terms

Study Points

- ➤ The GI tract is a tube that can be divided into regions: the mouth, esophagus, stomach, small intestine, large intestine, and rectum.

- ➤ Digestion and absorption of the nutrients in foods occur at various sites along the GI tract.

- ➤ Digestion involves both physical processes (e.g., chewing, peristalsis, and segmentation) and chemical processes (e.g., the hydrolytic action of enzymes).

- ➤ Absorption is the movement of molecules across the lining of the GI tract and into circulation.

- ➤ Four mechanisms are involved in nutrient absorption: passive diffusion, facilitated diffusion, active transport, and endocytosis.

- ➤ In the mouth, food is mixed with saliva for lubrication. Salivary amylase begins the digestion of starch.

- ➤ Secretions from the stomach lower the pH of stomach contents and begin the digestion of proteins.

- ➤ The pancreas and gallbladder secrete material into the small intestine to help with digestion.

- ➤ Most chemical digestion and nutrient absorption occur in the small intestine.

- ➤ Electrolytes and water are absorbed from the large intestine. Remaining material, waste, is excreted as feces.

- ➤ Both the nervous system and the hormonal system regulate GI tract processes.

- ➤ Numerous factors affect GI tract functioning, including psychological, chemical, and bacterial factors.

- ➤ Problems that occur along the GI tract can affect digestion and absorption of nutrients. Dietary changes are important in the treatment of GI disorders.

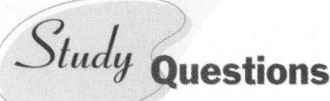
Study Questions

1. The contents of which organ has the lowest pH? Which organ produces an alkaline or basic solution to buffer this low pH?

2. What is the purpose of mucus in the GI tract? What would happen if it didn't line the stomach?

3. Where in the GI tract does the majority of nutrient digestion and absorption take place?

4. List the organs (in order) that make up the GI tract.

5. Name three "assisting" organs that are not part of the GI tract but are needed for proper digestion. What are their roles in digestion?

6. List the four major hormones involved in regulating digestion and absorption. What are their roles?

7. What is gastroesophageal reflux disease?

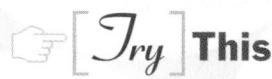
☞ [*Try*] This

The Saltine Cracker Experiment

This experiment will help you understand the effect of salivary amylase. Remember, salivary amylase is the starch-digesting enzyme produced by the salivary glands. Chew two saltine crackers until a watery texture forms in your mouth. You have to fight the urge to swallow so you can pay attention to the taste of the crackers. Do you notice a change in the taste?

The crackers first taste salty and "starchy," but as amylase is secreted it begins to break the chains of starch into sugar. As it does this, the saltines begin to taste sweet like animal crackers!

What About *Bobbie?*

Because both fluid and fiber are important for a healthy gastrointestinal tract, let's check out Bobbie's intake of these. Refresh yourself with her day of eating (see Chapter 1). How do you think Bobbie did in terms of fiber? She did pretty well! At 25 grams of fiber, she's right at the Adequate Intake (AI) for fiber for women for her age—25 grams per day. Here are her best fiber sources:

Food	Fiber Grams
Spaghetti (pasta)	3.5
Tortilla chips	3
Banana	3
Salsa	2
Sourdough bread	2

Are you surprised by the tortilla chips and the amount of fiber they add? Don't misinterpret this to mean that tortilla chips are a great source of fiber. There are two reasons why the chips rank so high. First, the other grain choices were not whole wheat and therefore didn't contribute a lot of fiber. Second, her afternoon snack consisted of just over 200 calories of tortilla chips.

What could Bobbie have done differently if she wanted to keep her fiber intake high, but reduce calories and fat by avoiding the tortilla chips? Here are a few small changes that she could make.

- By choosing a whole-wheat bagel, she'd add 4 grams of fiber.
- By having her sandwich on whole-wheat bread, she'd add at least 3 grams of fiber.
- By substituting the 2 tablespoons of croutons with 2 more tablespoons of kidney beans, she'd add 1.5 grams of fiber.
- If she ate another piece of fruit as a snack sometime in her day, it would add 1 to 3 grams of fiber.

Now let's look at Bobbie's fluid intake. Remember, when you increase your fiber, it is critical to increase your fluid intake so you don't become constipated. Here's a list of Bobbie's drinks:

Breakfast—10 ounces coffee

Snack—none

Lunch—12 ounces diet soda

Snack—16 ounces water

Dinner—12 ounces diet soda

Snack—none

How do you think she did? Her total fluid intake is 50 ounces (1,500 milliliters). Her food also contains fluids and contributes another 1,000 milliliters. The AI for total fluid intake for adult women is 2,700 milliliters per day. If Bobbie's intake is assumed to be about 2,500 milliliters, this is close to the AI. She could add another beverage with one or both of her snacks and be right on target. She also could improve her fluid choices, since most contain caffeine, which is a mild diuretic.

What suggestions do you have that will improve Bobbie's fluid intake? Any of the following would work:

- Carry a water bottle to sip throughout the day.
- Wash down the morning banana snack with a cup or two of water.
- Consider decaffeinated coffee or decaffeinated soda.
- Drink more water with the tortilla chips in the afternoon.
- Add a fluid to dinner.
- Drink water with the piece of pizza at night.

References

1 Gilbertson TA, Fontenot DT, Lui L, et al. Fatty acid modulation of K+ channels in taste receptor cells: gustatory cues for dietary fat. *Am J Physiol.* 1997;272:(4 pt 1):C1203–1210.

2 Mattes RD. Physiologic responses to sensory stimulation by food: nutritional implications. *J Am Diet Assoc.* 1997; 97:406–410.

3 Klein S, Cohn SM, Alpers DH. Alimentary tract in nutrition. In: Shils ME, Shike M, Ross AC, Cabellero B, Cousins RJ, eds. *Modern Nutrition in Health and Disease.* 10th ed. Philadelphia: Lippincott Williams & Wilkins, 2006:1115–1142.

4 Caspary WF. Physiology and pathophysiology of intestinal absorption. *Am J Clin Nutr.* 1992;55:299S–307S; and Yamada T, Alpers DH. *Textbook of Gastroenterology.* New York: JB Lippincott, 1995.

5 Guyton AC, Hall JE. *Textbook of Medical Physiology.* 10th ed. Philadelphia: WB Saunders, 2000.

6 Yamada T, Alper DH. Op. cit.

7 Klein S, Cohn SM, Alpers DH. Op. cit.

8 Scheppach W, Luehrs H, Menzel T. Beneficial health effects of low-digestible carbohydrate consumption. *Br J Nutr.* 2001; 85(suppl 1):S23–S30.

9 Guyton AC, Hall JE. Op. cit.

10 Yamada T, Alper DH. Op. cit.

11 Guyton AC, Hall JE. Op. cit.

12 Mahan LK, Escott-Stump S. *Krause's Food Nutrition and Diet Therapy.* 11th ed. Philadelphia: WB Saunders, 2004.

13 US Department of Health and Human Services, Agency for Toxic Substances and Disease Registry. *Toxicological Profile for Acrolein.* Atlanta, GA: US Public Health Service, 1989.

14 National Digestive Diseases Information Clearinghouse. Constipation. February 2006. NIH publication 06-2754. http://digestive.niddk.nih.gov/ddiseases/pubs/constipation /index.htm. Accessed 3/16/06.

15 Mayne ST, Navarro SA. Diet, obesity, and reflux in the etiology of adenocarcinomas of the esophagus and gastric cardia in humans. *J Nutr.* 2002;132(11):3467S–3470S.

16 Ringel Y, Sperber AD, Drossman DA. Irritable bowel syndrome. *Annu Rev Med.* 2001;52:319–338.

17 National Institute of Diabetes and Digestive and Kidney Diseases. Irritable bowel syndrome. April 2003. NIH publication 03-693. http://digestive.niddk.nih.gov/ddiseases/pubs /ibs/. Accessed 03/13/06.

18 Ibid.

19 Centers for Disease Control and Prevention. Colorectal cancer: the importance of prevention and early detection. 2004/2005 fact sheet. http://www.cdc.gov/cancer/colorctl/about2004.htm. Accessed 03/13/06.

20 World Health Organization. *Diet, Nutrition and the Prevention of Chronic Diseases: A Report of a Joint WHO/FAO Expert Consultation.* Geneva, Switzerland: World Health Organization, 2003. WHO Technical Report Series 916.

21 Chao A, Thun MJ, Connell CJ, et al. Meat consumption and risk of colon cancer. *JAMA.* 2005;293:172–182.

22 Institute of Medicine, Food and Nutrition Board. *Dietary Reference Intakes for Energy, Carbohydrate, Fiber, Fat, Fatty Acids, Cholesterol, Protein, and Amino Acids.* Washington, DC: National Academy Press, 2005.

23 Terry P, Giovannucci E, Michels KB, et al. Fruit, vegetables, dietary fiber, and risk of colorectal cancer. *J Natl Cancer Inst.* 2001;93(7):525–533.

24 Schatzkin A, Lanza E, Corle D, et al. Lack of effect of a low-fat, high-fiber diet on the recurrence of colorectal adenomas. Polyp Prevention Trial Study Group. *N Engl J Med.* 2000; 342(16):1149–1155.

25 National Institute of Diabetes and Digestive and Kidney Diseases. *H. pylori* and peptic ulcer. October 2004. NIH publication 05-4225. http://digestive.niddk.nih.gov/ddiseases/pubs /hpylori/index.htm. Accessed 03/13/06.

26 Ibid.

27 Wiklund J, Butler-Wheelhouse P. Psychosocial factors and their role in symptomatic gastroesophageal reflux disease and functional dyspepsia. *Scand J Gastroenterol.* 1996; 220(suppl):94–100.

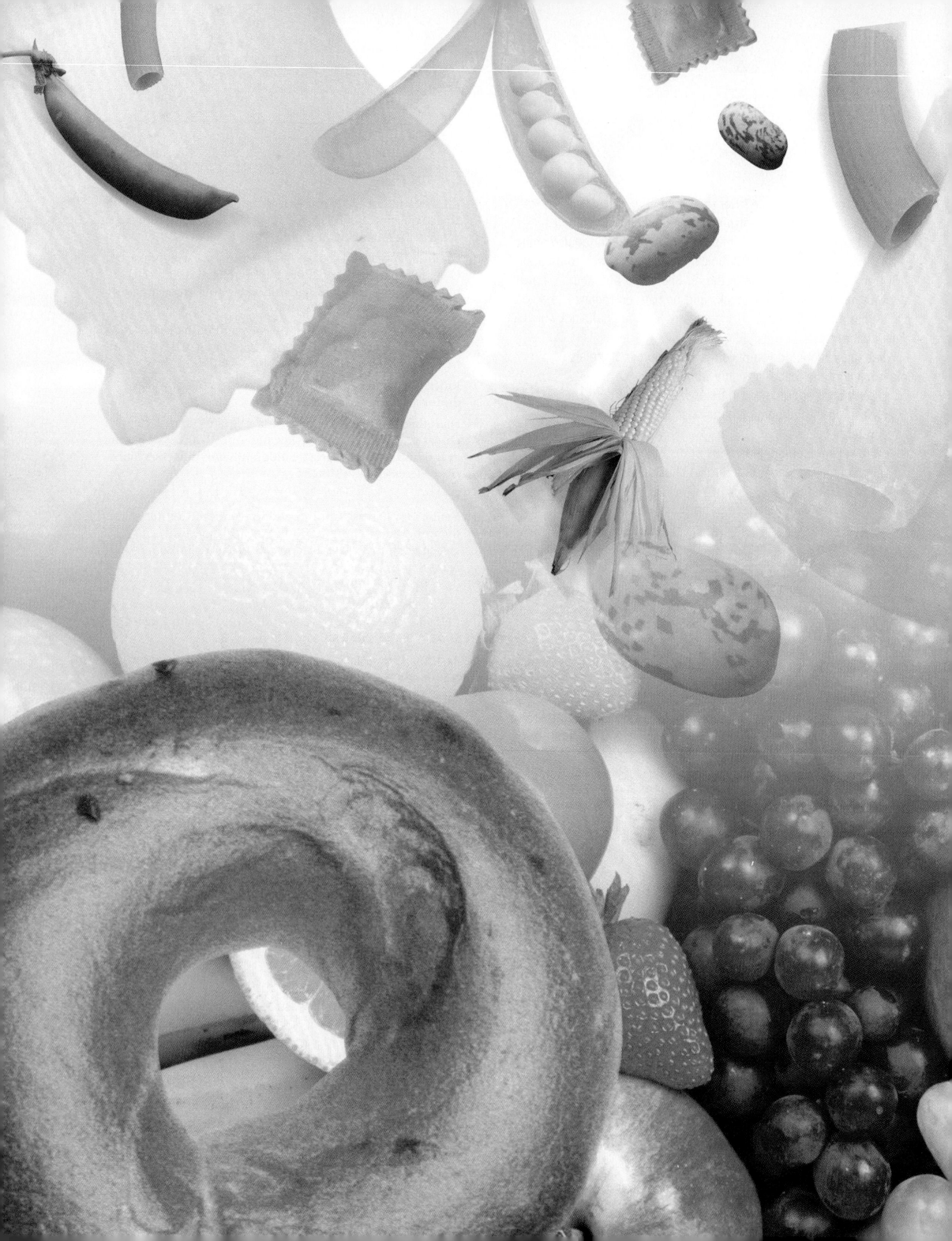

Chapter 4

Carbohydrates

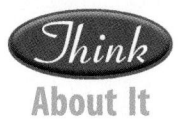 **Think About It**

1 When you think of the word *carbohydrate*, what foods come to mind?

2 How does your dietary fiber intake stack up?

3 Many people choose honey instead of white sugar because they think it's more "natural." What do you think?

4 Do you prefer artificial sweeteners to sugar? Explain your preference.

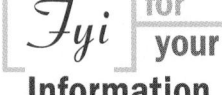 **Fyi for your Information**

This chapter's FYI boxes include practical information on the following topics:
• The Glycemic Index of Foods: Useful or Useless?

• Unfounded Claims Against Sugars

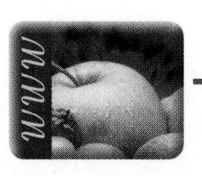

The Web site for this book offers many useful tools and is a great source for additional nutrition information for both students and instructors. Visit the site at **nutrition.jbpub.com** for information on carbohydrates. You'll find exercises that explore the following topics:
• Aspartame: Your Friend or Foe?

• Are You in the Carbohydrate Zone?

• Constant Craving?

Key to Illustrations

Amino Acids		Gas	
ATP/Energy		Glucose	
Carbon Dioxide		Minerals	
Disaccharide		Oxygen	
Enzymes		Short-Chain Fatty Acids	
Fructose		Water	
Galactose			

What About 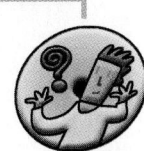 *Bobbie?*

Track the choices Bobbie is making with Nutritionist Pro or EatRight Analysis software.

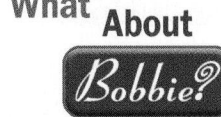

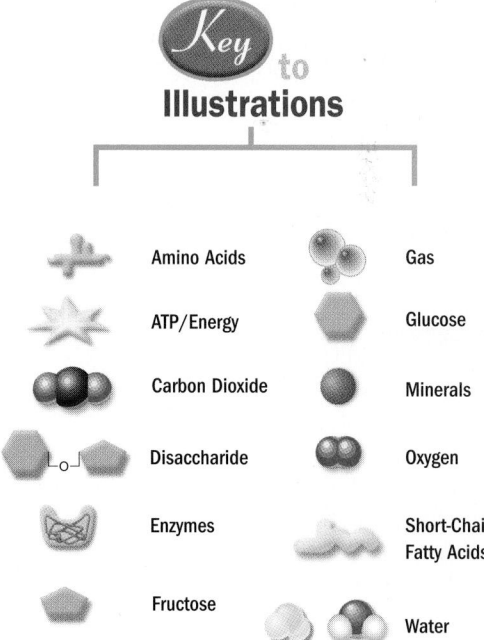

Does sugar causes diabetes? Will too much sugar make a child hyperactive? Does excess sugar contribute to criminal behavior? What about starch? Does it really make you fat? These and other questions have been asked about sugar and starch—dietary carbohydrates—over the years. But where do these ideas come from? What is myth and what is fact? Are carbohydrates important in the diet? Or, as some popular diets suggest, should we eat only small amounts of carbohydrates? What links, if any, are there between carbohydrate in your diet and health?

Most of the world depends on carbohydrate-rich plant foods for daily sustenance. In some countries, 80 percent or more of daily calorie intake is carbohydrate. Rice provides the bulk of the diet in Southeast Asia, as does corn in South America, cassava in certain parts of Africa, and wheat in Europe and North America. (See **Figure 4.1**.) Besides providing energy, foods rich in carbohydrates, such as whole grains, legumes, fruits, and vegetables, are also good sources of vitamins, minerals, dietary fiber, and phytochemicals that can help lower the risk of chronic diseases.

Generous carbohydrate intake should provide the foundation for any healthful diet. Carbohydrates contain only 4 kilocalories per gram, compared with 9 kilocalories per gram for fat. Thus, a diet rich in carbohydrates provides fewer calories and a greater volume of food than the typical fat-laden American diet. As you explore the topic of carbohydrates, think about some claims you have heard for and against a high carbohydrate intake.

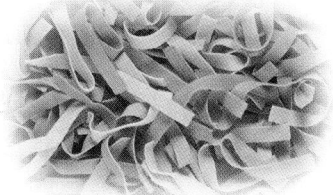

Quick Bites

Is Pasta a Chinese Food?
Noodles were used in China as early as the first century; Marco Polo did not bring them to Italy until the 1300s.

Figure 4.1 **Cassava, rice, wheat, and corn.** These carbohydrate-rich foods are dietary staples in many parts of the world.

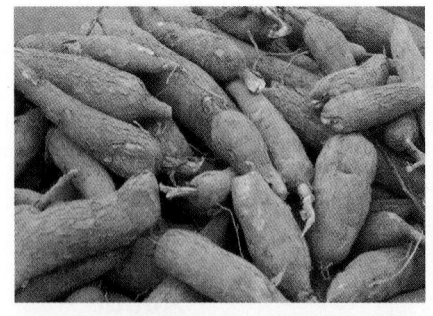
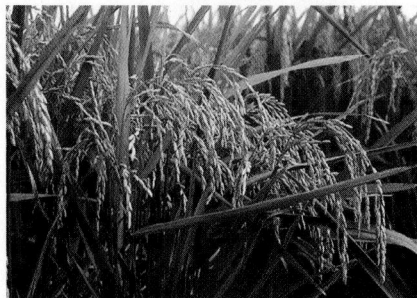
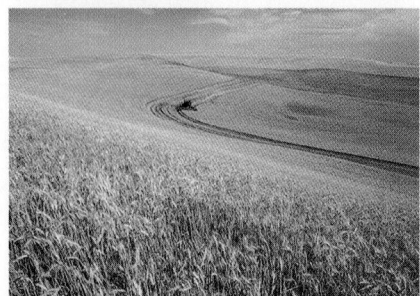
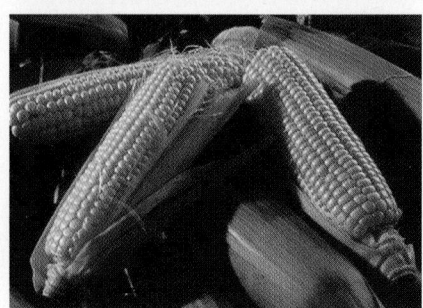

What Are Carbohydrates?

Plants use carbon dioxide from the air, water from the soil, and energy from the sun to produce carbohydrates and oxygen through a process called photosynthesis. (See **Figure 4.2.**) Carbohydrates are organic compounds that contain carbon (C), hydrogen (H), and oxygen (O) in the ratio of two hydrogen atoms and one oxygen atom for every one carbon atom (CH_2O). The sugar glucose, for example, contains 6 carbon atoms, 12 hydrogen atoms, and 6 oxygen atoms, giving this vital carbohydrate the chemical formula $C_6H_{12}O_6$. Two or more sugar molecules can be assembled to form increasingly complex carbohydrates. The two main types of carbohydrates in food are simple carbohydrates (sugars) and complex carbohydrates (starches and fiber).

Simple Sugars: Monosaccharides and Disaccharides

Simple carbohydrates are naturally present as simple sugars in fruits, milk, and other foods. Plant carbohydrates also can be refined to produce sugar products such as table sugar or corn syrup. The two main types of sugars are monosaccharides and disaccharides. **Monosaccharides** consist of a single sugar molecule (*mono* meaning "one" and *saccharide* meaning "sugar"). **Disaccharides** consist of two sugar molecules chemically joined together (*di* meaning "two"). Monosaccharides and disaccharides give various degrees of sweetness to foods.

simple carbohydrates Sugars composed of a single sugar molecule (a monosaccharide) or two joined sugar molecules (a disaccharide).

monosaccharides Any sugars that are not broken down during digestion and have the general formula $C_nH_{2n}O_n$, where $n = 3$ to 7. The common monosaccharides glucose, fructose, and galactose all have six carbon atoms ($n = 6$).

disaccharides [dye-SACK-uh-rides] Carbohydrates composed of two monosaccharide units linked by a glycosidic bond. They include sucrose (common table sugar), lactose (milk sugar), and maltose.

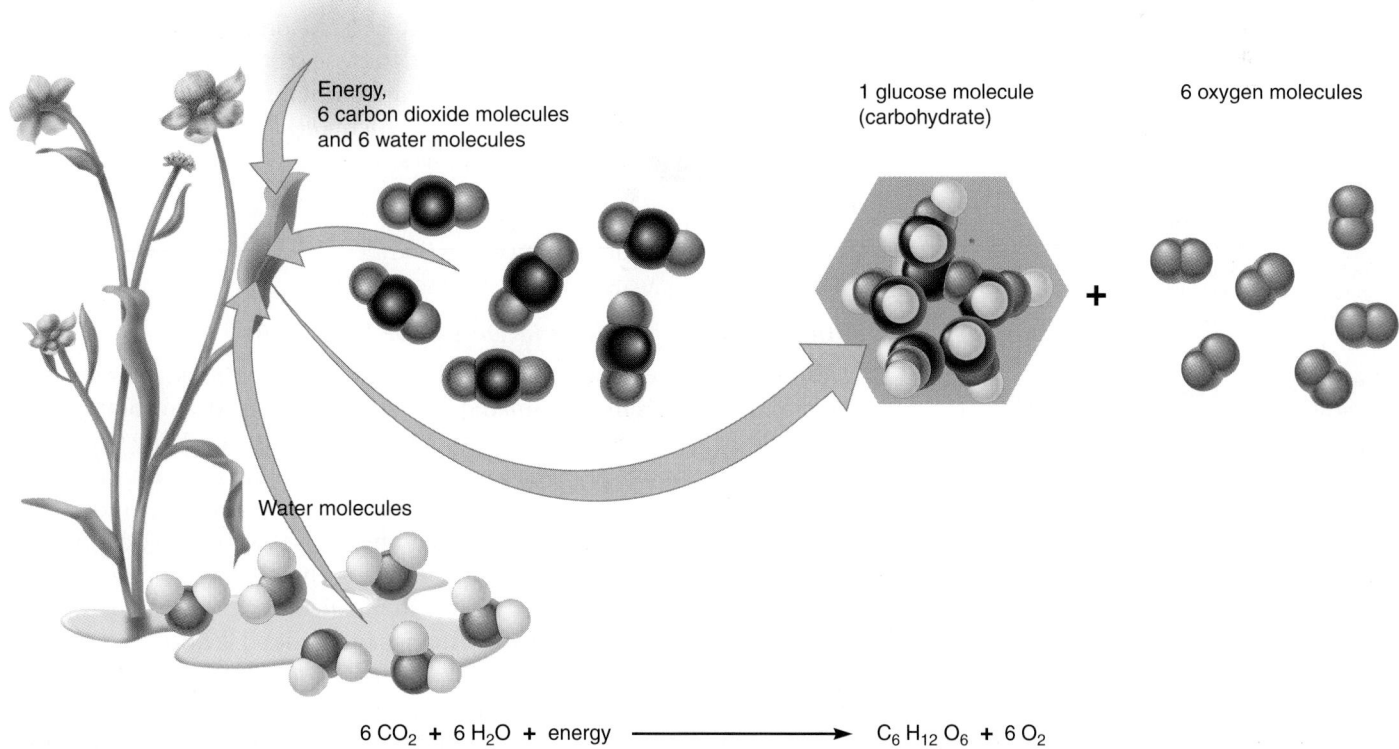

Energy, 6 carbon dioxide molecules and 6 water molecules

1 glucose molecule (carbohydrate)

6 oxygen molecules

Water molecules

$$6\,CO_2 + 6\,H_2O + energy \longrightarrow C_6H_{12}O_6 + 6\,O_2$$

Figure 4.2 **Plants make carbohydrates.** Plants release oxygen as they use water, carbon dioxide, and energy from the sun to make carbohydrate (glucose) molecules.

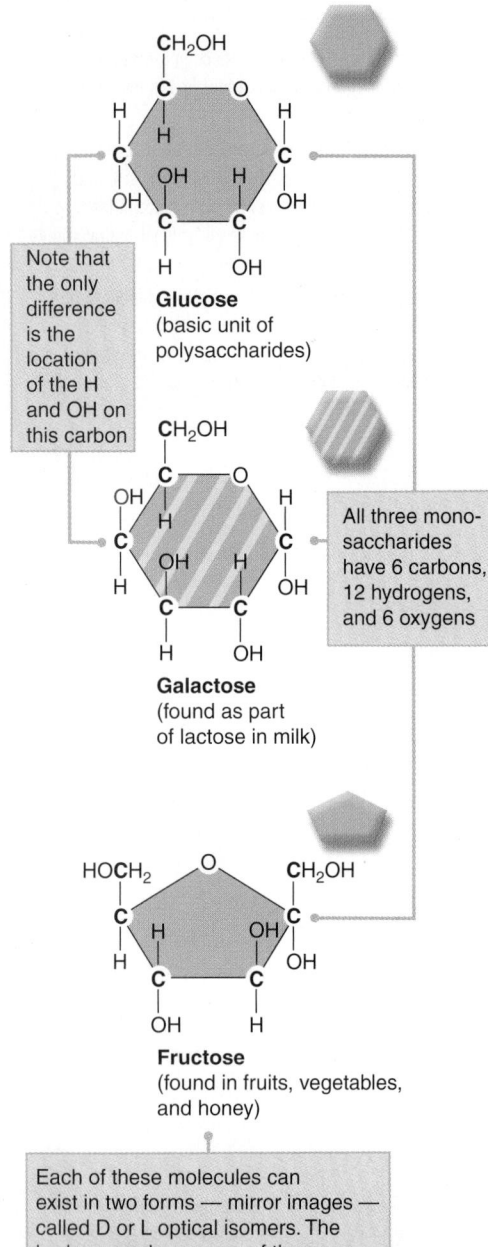

Note that the only difference is the location of the H and OH on this carbon

Glucose
(basic unit of polysaccharides)

All three monosaccharides have 6 carbons, 12 hydrogens, and 6 oxygens

Galactose
(found as part of lactose in milk)

Fructose
(found in fruits, vegetables, and honey)

Each of these molecules can exist in two forms — mirror images — called D or L optical isomers. The body can only use one of these forms, the D isomer

Figure 4.3 **The monosaccharides: glucose, galactose, and fructose.** Since glucose and galactose share similar six-sided hexagonal structures, they can be difficult to tell apart. Fructose's five-sided pentagon stands out.

glucose [GLOO-kose] A common monosaccharide containing six carbons that is present in the blood; also known as dextrose and blood sugar. It is a component of the disaccharides sucrose, lactose, and maltose and various complex carbohydrates.

Monosaccharides: The Single Sugars

The most common monosaccharides in the human diet are the following:

- Glucose
- Fructose
- Galactose

 **Glucose**  **Fructose** 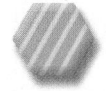 **Galactose**

All three monosaccharides have six carbons, and all have the chemical formula $C_6H_{12}O_6$, but each has a different arrangement of these atoms. The carbon and oxygen atoms of glucose and galactose form a six-sided ring. The structures of glucose and galactose look almost identical except for the reversal of the OH and H groups on one of the carbon atoms. The carbons and oxygen of fructose form a five-sided ring. Look carefully at **Figure 4.3** to find all six carbons.

Glucose

The monosaccharide glucose is the most abundant simple carbohydrate unit in nature. Also referred to as dextrose, **glucose** plays a key role in both foods and the body. Glucose imparts a mildly sweet flavor to food. It seldom exists as a monosaccharide in food but is usually joined to other sugars to form disaccharides, starch, or dietary fiber. Glucose makes up at least one of the two sugar molecules in every disaccharide.

In the body, glucose supplies energy to cells. The body closely regulates blood glucose (blood sugar) levels to assure a constant fuel source for vital body functions. Glucose is virtually the only fuel used by the brain, except during prolonged starvation, when the glucose supply is low.

Fructose

Also called levulose or fruit sugar, **fructose** tastes the sweetest of all the sugars and occurs naturally in fruits and vegetables. Although the sugar in honey is about half fructose and half glucose, fructose is the primary source of the sweet taste. Food manufacturers use high-fructose corn syrup as an additive to sweeten many foods, including soft drinks, fruit beverages such as lemonade, desserts, candies, jellies, and jams. The term *high-fructose* is a little misleading—the fructose content of this sweetener is around 50 percent.

Galactose

Galactose rarely occurs as a monosaccharide in food. It usually is chemically bonded to glucose to form lactose, the primary sugar in milk.

Other Monosaccharides and Derivative Sweeteners

Pentoses are single sugar molecules that contain five carbons. Although they are present in foods in only small quantities, they are essential components of nucleic acids, the genetic material of life. (See **Figure 4.4**.) The five-carbon sugar ribose is part of ribonucleic acid, or RNA. Another five-carbon sugar, deoxyribose, is a part of deoxyribonucleic acid, or DNA. Some pentoses also are components of indigestible gums and mucilages, which are classified as part of the dietary fiber component of foods.[1] Pentoses are synthesized in the body, and therefore are not needed in the diet.

Sugar alcohols are derivatives of monosaccharides. Like other sugars, they taste sweet and supply energy to the body. However, they are absorbed more slowly than sugars and the body processes them differently. Some fruits naturally contain minute amounts of sugar alcohols. Sugar alcohols such as sorbitol, mannitol, lactitol, and xylitol also are used as nutritive sweeteners in foods. For example, sorbitol, which is derived from glucose, sweetens sugarless gum, breath mints, and candy. For more information on sugar alcohols, see the "Nutritive Sweeteners" section later in this chapter.

Disaccharides: The Double Sugars

Disaccharides consist of two monosaccharides chemically joined by a process called condensation. The following disaccharides (see **Figure 4.5**) are important in human nutrition:

- Sucrose (common table sugar)
- Lactose (major sugar in milk)
- Maltose (product of starch digestion)

Joining and Cleaving Sugar Molecules

Sugar molecules are joined or separated (cleaved) by the removal or addition of a molecule of water. A **condensation** reaction chemically joins two monosaccharides while removing an H from one sugar molecule and an OH from the other to form water (H_2O) (see **Figure 4.6**). A hydrolysis reaction separates disaccharides into monosaccharides (see **Figure 4.7**). During hydrolysis, the addition of a molecule of water splits the bond between the two sugar molecules, providing the H and OH groups necessary for the

fructose [FROOK-tose] A common monosaccharide containing six carbons that is naturally present in honey and many fruits; often added to foods in the form of high-fructose corn syrup. Also called levulose or fruit sugar.

galactose [gah-LAK-tose] A monosaccharide containing six carbons that can be converted into glucose in the body. In foods and living systems, galactose usually is joined with other monosaccharides.

pentoses Sugar molecules containing five carbon atoms.

sugar alcohols Compounds formed from monosaccharides by replacing a hydrogen atom with a hydroxyl group (−OH); commonly used as nutritive sweeteners. Also called polyols.

condensation In chemistry, a reaction in which a covalent bond is formed between two molecules by removal of a water molecule.

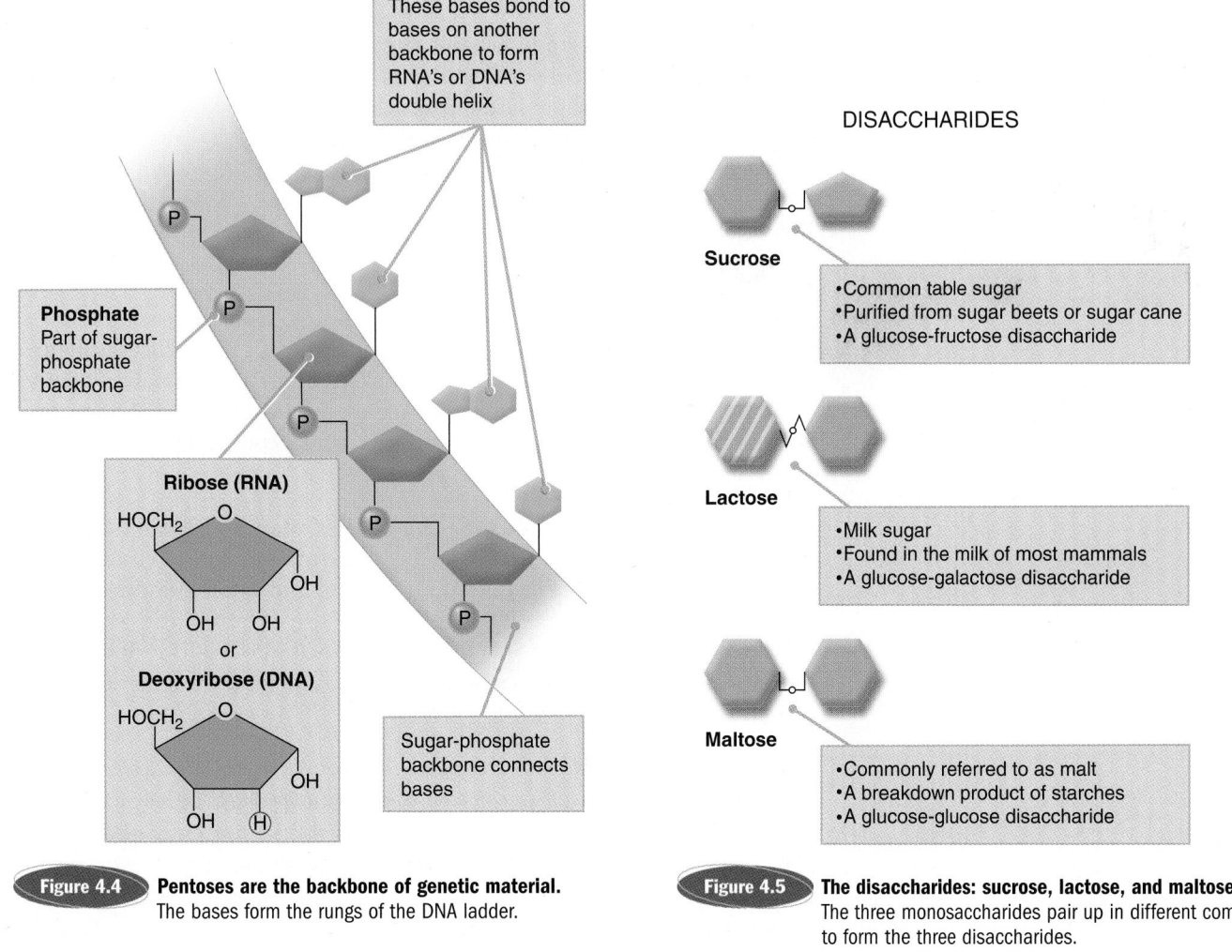

Figure 4.4 **Pentoses are the backbone of genetic material.** The bases form the rungs of the DNA ladder.

Figure 4.5 **The disaccharides: sucrose, lactose, and maltose.** The three monosaccharides pair up in different combinations to form the three disaccharides.

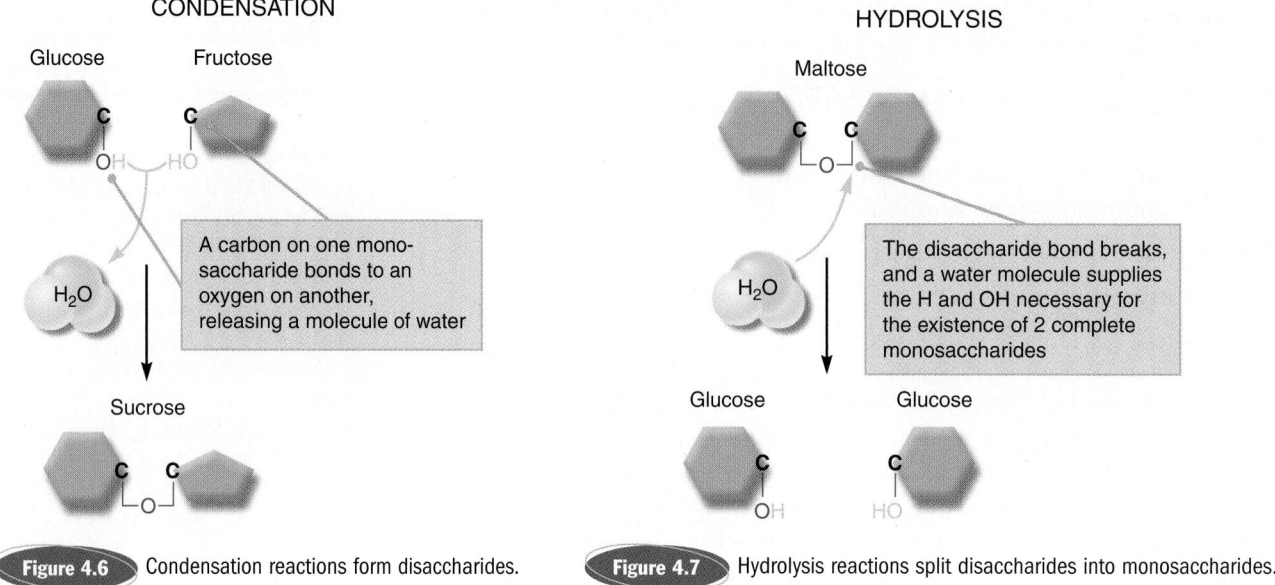

CONDENSATION

Glucose   Fructose

A carbon on one mono-saccharide bonds to an oxygen on another, releasing a molecule of water

H_2O

Sucrose

Figure 4.6 Condensation reactions form disaccharides.

HYDROLYSIS

Maltose

The disaccharide bond breaks, and a water molecule supplies the H and OH necessary for the existence of 2 complete monosaccharides

H_2O

Glucose   Glucose

Figure 4.7 Hydrolysis reactions split disaccharides into monosaccharides.

sugars to exist as monosaccharides. The digestion of carbohydrates involves hydrolysis reactions.

Sucrose

Sucrose, most familiar to us as table sugar, is composed of one molecule of glucose and one molecule of fructose. Sucrose provides some of the natural sweetness of honey, maple syrup, fruits, and vegetables. Manufacturers use a refining process to extract sucrose from the juices of sugar cane or sugar beets. Full refining removes impurities; white sugar and powdered sugar are so highly refined they are virtually 100 percent sucrose. When a food label lists *sugar* as an ingredient, the term refers to sucrose.

Lactose

Lactose, or milk sugar, is composed of one molecule of glucose and one molecule of galactose. Lactose gives milk and other dairy products a slightly sweet taste. Human milk has a higher concentration (approximately 7 grams per 100 milliliters) of lactose than cow's milk (approximately 4.5 grams per 100 milliliters), so human milk tastes sweeter than cow's milk.

Maltose

Maltose is composed of two glucose molecules. Maltose seldom occurs naturally in foods, but is formed whenever long molecules of starch break down. Human digestive enzymes in the mouth and small intestine break down starch into maltose. When you chew a slice of fresh bread, you may detect a slightly sweet taste as starch breaks down into maltose. Starch also breaks down into maltose in germinating seeds. Maltose is fermented in the production of beer.

Key Concepts: *Carbohydrates are composed of carbon, hydrogen, and oxygen and can be categorized as simple or complex. Simple carbohydrates include monosaccharides and disaccharides. The monosaccharides glucose, fructose, and galactose are single sugar molecules. The disaccharides sucrose, lactose, and maltose are double sugar molecules. A condensation reaction joins two monosaccharides to form a disaccharide.*

sucrose [SOO-crose] A disaccharide composed of one molecule of glucose and one molecule of fructose joined together. Also known as table sugar.

lactose [LAK-tose] A disaccharide composed of glucose and galactose; also called milk sugar because it is the major sugar in milk and dairy products.

maltose [MALL-tose] A disaccharide composed of two glucose molecules; sometimes called malt sugar. Maltose seldom occurs naturally in foods but is formed whenever long molecules of starch break down.

Complex Carbohydrates

Complex carbohydrates are chains of more than two sugar molecules. Short carbohydrate chains may have as few as three monosaccharide molecules, but long chains, the polysaccharides, can contain hundreds or even thousands.

Oligosaccharides

Oligosaccharides (*oligo* meaning "scant") are short carbohydrate chains of 3 to 10 sugar molecules. Dried beans, peas, and lentils contain the two most common oligosaccharides—raffinose and stachyose.[2] Raffinose is formed from three monosaccharide molecules—one galactose, one glucose, and one fructose. Stachyose is formed from four monosaccharide molecules—two galactose, one glucose, and one fructose. The body cannot break down raffinose or stachyose, but they are readily broken down by intestinal bacteria and are responsible for the familiar gaseous effects of foods such as beans.

Human milk contains more than one hundred different oligosaccharides, which vary according to the length of a woman's pregnancy, how long she has been nursing, and her genetic makeup.[3] For breastfed infants, oligosaccharides serve a function similar to dietary fiber in adults—making stools easier to pass. Some of these oligosaccharides also protect infants from disease-causing agents by binding to them in the intestine. Oligosaccharides in human milk also provide sialic acid, a compound essential for normal brain development.[4]

Polysaccharides

Polysaccharides (*poly* meaning "many") are long carbohydrate chains of monosaccharides. Some polysaccharides form straight chains, whereas others branch off in all directions. Such structural differences affect how the polysaccharide behaves in water and with heating. The way monosaccharides are linked make them digestible (e.g., starch) or nondigestible (e.g., fiber).

Starch

Plants store energy as **starch** for use during growth and reproduction. Rich sources of starch include (1) grains such as wheat, rice, corn, oats, millet, and barley, (2) legumes such as peas, beans, and lentils, and (3) tubers such

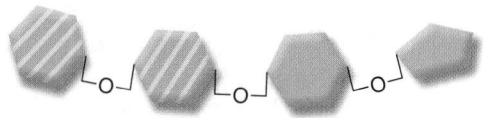

Stachyose

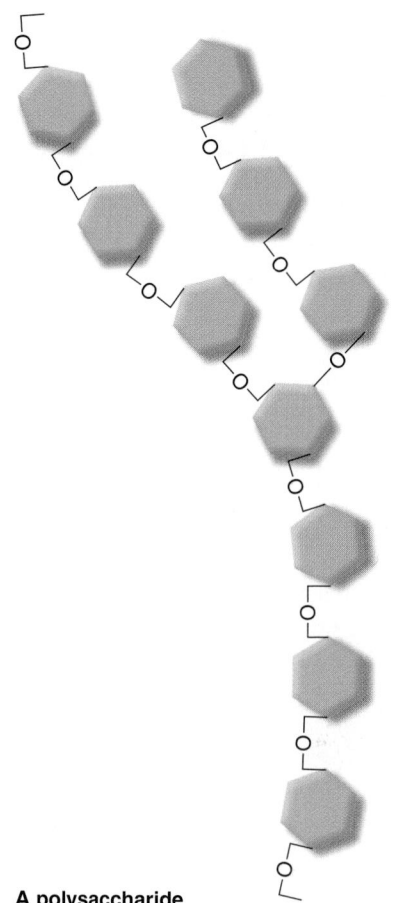

A polysaccharide

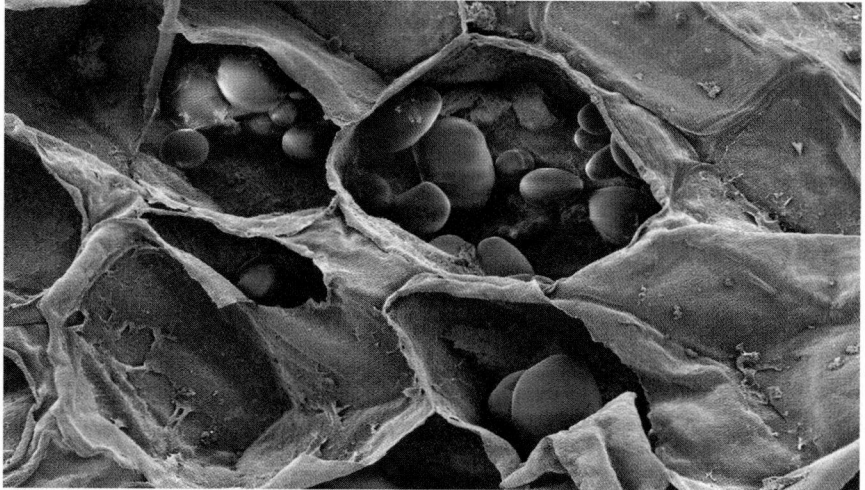

A scanning electron micrograph of a potato tuber cell shows the starch granules where energy is stored.

complex carbohydrates Chains of more than two monosaccharides. May be oligosaccharides or polysaccharides.

oligosaccharides Short carbohydrate chains composed of 3 to 10 sugar molecules.

polysaccharides Long carbohydrate chains composed of more than 10 sugar molecules. Polysaccharides can be straight or branched.

starch The major storage form of carbohydrate in plants; starch is composed of long chains of glucose molecules in a straight (amylose) or branching (amylopectin) arrangement.

amylose [AM-ih-los] A straight-chain polysaccharide composed of glucose units.

amylopectin [am-ih-low-PEK-tin] A branched-chain polysaccharide composed of glucose units.

resistant starch A starch that is not digested.

glycogen [GLY-ko-jen] A very large, highly branched polysaccharide composed of multiple glucose units. Sometimes called animal starch, glycogen is the primary storage form of glucose in animals.

dietary fiber Carbohydrates and lignins that are naturally in plants and are nondigestible; that is, they are not digested and absorbed in the human small intestine.

functional fiber Isolated nondigestible carbohydrates, including some manufactured carbohydrates, that have beneficial effects in humans.

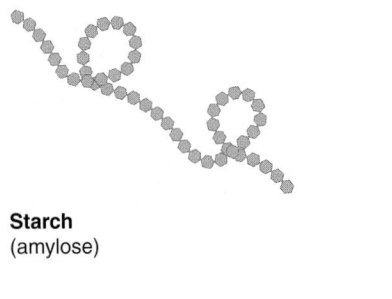

Starch
(amylose)

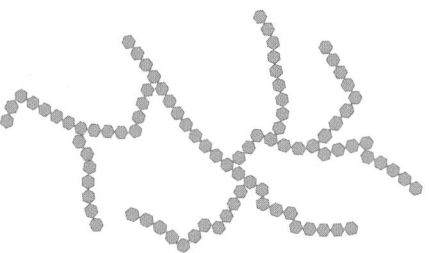

Starch
(amylopectin)

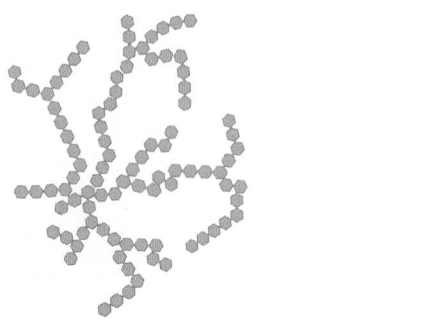

Glycogen

Figure 4.8 **Starch and glycogen.** Plants have two main types of starch—amylose, which has long unbranched chains of glucose, and amylopectin, which has branched chains. Animals store glucose in highly branched chains called glycogen.

as potatoes, yams, and cassava. Starch imparts a moist, gelatinous texture to food. For example, it makes the inside of a baked potato moist, thick, and almost sticky. The starch in flour absorbs moisture and thickens gravy.

Starch takes two main forms in plants: amylose and amylopectin. **Amylose** is made up of long, unbranched chains of glucose molecules, whereas **amylopectin** is made up of branched chains of glucose molecules. (See **Figure 4.8.**) Amylose and amylopectin typically occur in a ratio of about 1:4 in plants, although this proportion can vary.[5] Wheat flour contains a higher proportion of amylose, whereas cornstarch contains a higher proportion of amylopectin.

The proportion of amylose to amylopectin in a food affects its functional properties. For example, food manufacturers often thicken gravies for frozen foods with cornstarch (rich in branched amylopectin) because it forms thicker, more stable gels than gravies thickened with wheat flour (rich in unbranched amylose).

In the body, amylopectin is digested more rapidly than amylose.[6] Although the body easily digests most starches, a small portion of the starch in plants may remain enclosed in cell structures and escape digestion in the small intestine. Starch that is not digested is called **resistant starch**.[7] Some legumes, such as white beans, contain large amounts of resistant starch. Resistant starch also is formed during the processing of starchy foods.

Glycogen

Glycogen, also called animal starch, is the storage form of carbohydrate in living animals. (See Figure 4.8.) After slaughter, tissue enzymes break down most glycogen within 24 hours. Although some organ meats, such as kidney, heart and liver, contain small amounts of carbohydrate, meat from muscle contains none.[8] Since plant foods also contain no glycogen, it is a negligible carbohydrate source in our diets. Glycogen does, however, play an important role in our bodies as a readily mobilizable store of glucose.

Glycogen is composed of long, highly branched chains of glucose molecules. Its structure is similar to amylopectin, but glycogen is much more highly branched. When we need extra glucose, glycogen in our cells can be broken down rapidly into single glucose molecules. Because enzymes can attack only the ends of glycogen chains, the highly branched structure of glycogen multiplies the number of sites available for enzyme activity.

Skeletal muscle and the liver are the two major sites of glycogen storage. In muscle cells, glycogen provides a reservoir of glucose for strenuous muscular activity. Liver cells also use glycogen to regulate blood glucose levels. If necessary, liver glycogen can provide as much as 100 to 150 milligrams of glucose per minute to the blood at a sustained rate for up to 12 hours.[9]

Normally, the body can store only about 200 to 500 grams of glycogen at a time.[10] Some athletes practice a carbohydrate-loading regimen by gradually tapering off rigorous training and emphasizing high-carbohydrate meals a few days to one week before competition. This can increase the amount of stored glycogen by 20 to 40 percent above normal, providing a competitive edge for marathon running and other endurance events.[11] (See Chapter 13, "Sports Nutrition.")

Fiber

The Food and Nutrition Board redefined *fiber* as part of the DRI report on macronutrients.[12] **Dietary fiber** consists of nondigestible carbohydrates and lignins that are intact and intrinsic in plants. **Functional fiber** refers to isolated, nondigestible carbohydrates that have beneficial physiological effects in humans. **Total fiber** is the sum of dietary fiber and functional fiber.

All types of plant foods—including fruits, vegetables, legumes, and whole grains—contain dietary fiber. Many types of dietary fiber resemble starches— they are polysaccharides, but are not digested in the human GI tract. Examples of these nonstarch polysaccharides include cellulose, hemicellulose, pectins, gums, and beta-glucans (β-glucans). Oligosaccharides also are considered to be dietary fiber. Examples of functional fiber include extracted plant pectins, gums, and resistant starches, chitin and chitosan, and commercially produced nondigestible polysaccharides. Fiber is not found in animal foods.

Cellulose **Cellulose** gives plant cell walls their strength and rigidity. It forms the woody fibers that support tall trees. It also forms the brittle shafts of hay and straw and the stringy threads in celery. Cellulose is made up of long, straight chains of glucose molecules. (See **Figure 4.9**.) Grains, fruits, vegetables, and nuts all contain cellulose.

Hemicelluloses The **hemicelluloses** are a diverse group of polysaccharides that vary from plant to plant. They are mixed with cellulose in plant cell walls.[13] Hemicelluloses are composed of a variety of monosaccharides with many branching side chains. The outer bran layer on many cereal grains is rich in hemicelluloses, as are legumes, vegetables, and nuts.

Pectins **Pectins** are gel-forming polysaccharides found in all plants, especially fruits. The pectin in fruits acts like a cement that gives body to fruits and helps them keep their shape. When fruit becomes overripe, pectin breaks down into monosaccharides and the fruit becomes mushy. When

total fiber The sum of dietary fiber and functional fiber.

cellulose [SELL-you-los] A straight-chain polysaccharide composed of hundreds of glucose units linked by beta bonds. It is nondigestible by humans and a component of dietary fiber.

hemicelluloses [hem-ih-SELL-you-los-es] A group of large polysaccharides in dietary fiber that are fermented more easily than cellulose.

pectins A type of dietary fiber found in fruits.

Quick Bites

"An Apple a Day Keeps the Doctor Away"

Most likely this adage persisted over time due to actual health benefits from apples. Apples have a high pectin content, a soluble fiber known to be an effective GI regulator.

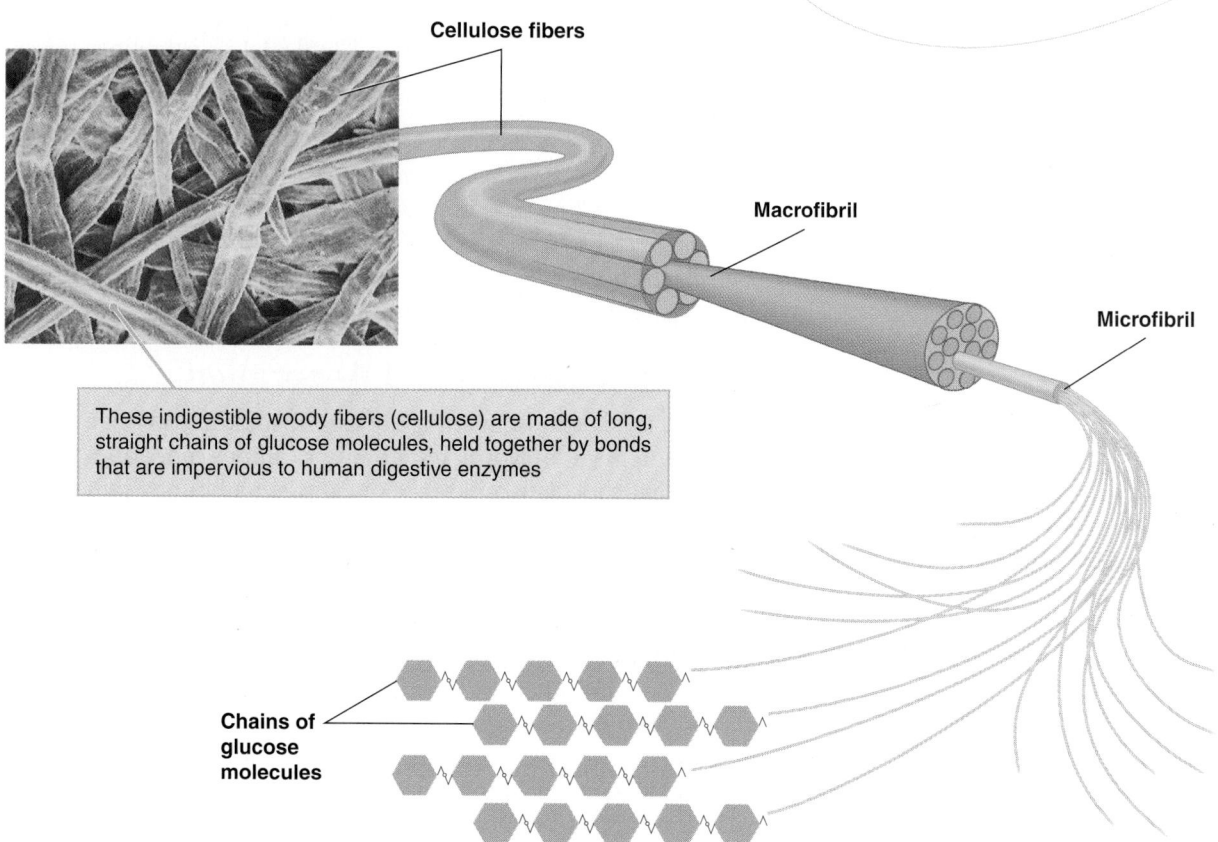

Cellulose fibers

Macrofibril

Microfibril

These indigestible woody fibers (cellulose) are made of long, straight chains of glucose molecules, held together by bonds that are impervious to human digestive enzymes

Chains of glucose molecules

Figure 4.9 **The structure of cellulose.** Cellulose forms the nondigestible, fibrous component of plants and is part of grasses, trees, fruits, and vegetables.

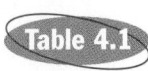

Table 4.1 Foods Rich in Dietary Fiber

Fruits

Apples	Grapefruit
Bananas	Mango
Berries	Oranges
Cherries	Pears
Cranberries	

Vegetables

Asparagus	Green peppers
Broccoli	Red cabbage
Brussels sprouts	Spinach
Carrots	Sprouts

Nuts and Seeds

Almonds	Sesame seeds
Peanuts	Sunflower seeds
Pecans	Walnuts

Legumes

Most legumes

Grains

Brown rice	Wheat-bran cereals
Oat bran	Whole-wheat breads
Oatmeal	

Source: Adapted from Shils ME, Olson JA, Shike M, Ross AC, eds. *Modern Nutrition in Health and Disease.* 10th ed. Philadephia: Lippincott Williams & Wilkins, 2006.

gums Dietary fibers, which contain galactose and other monosaccharides, found between plant cell walls.

mucilages Gelatinous soluble fibers containing galactose, mannose, and other monosaccharides; found in seaweed.

psyllium The dried husk of the psyllium seed.

lignins [LIG-nins] Insoluble fibers composed of multi-ring alcohol units that constitute the only noncarbohydrate component of dietary fiber.

β-glucans Functional fiber, consisting of branched polysaccharide chains of glucose, that helps lower blood cholesterol levels. Found in barley and oats.

chitin A long-chain structural polysaccharide of slightly modified glucose. Found in the hard exterior skeletons of insects, crustaceans, and other invertebrates; also occurs in the cell walls of fungi.

chitosan Polysaccharide derived from chitin.

pancreatic amylase Starch-digesting enzyme secreted by the pancreas.

alpha (α) bonds Chemical bonds linking two mono-saccharides (glycosidic bonds) that can be broken by human intestinal enzymes, releasing the individual mono-saccharides. Maltose and sucrose contain alpha bonds.

beta (β) bonds Chemical bonds linking two monosaccharides (glycosidic bonds) that cannot be broken by human intestinal enzymes. Cellulose contains beta bonds.

mixed with sugar and acid, pectin forms a gel that the food industry uses to add firmness to jellies, jams, sauces, and salad dressings.

Gums and Mucilages Like pectin, **gums** and **mucilages** are thick, gel-forming fibers that help hold plant cells together. The food industry uses plant gums such as gum arabic, guar gum, locust bean gum, and xanthan gum and mucilages such as carrageenan to thicken, stabilize, or add texture to foods such as salad dressings, puddings, pie fillings, candies, sauces, and even drinks. **Psyllium** (the husk of psyllium seeds) is a mucilage that becomes very viscous when mixed with water. It is the main component in the laxative Metamucil, and is being added to some breakfast cereals.

Lignins **Lignins** are not actually carbohydrates. Rather, these nondigestible substances make up the woody parts of vegetables such as carrots and broccoli and the seeds of fruits such as strawberries.

β-Glucans **β-glucans** are polysaccharides of branched glucose units. These fibers are found in large amounts in barley and oats. β-glucan fiber is especially effective in lowering blood cholesterol levels (see the section "Carbohydrates and Health" later in this chapter).

Chitin and Chitosan **Chitin** and **chitosan** are polysaccharides found in the exoskeletons of crabs and lobsters, and in the cell walls of most fungi. Chitin and chitosan are primarily consumed in supplement form. Although they are marketed as being useful for weight control, published research does not support this claim.

Foods rich in dietary fiber include whole-grain foods such as brown rice, rolled oats, and whole-wheat breads and cereals; legumes such as kidney beans, garbanzo beans (chickpeas), peas, and lentils; fruits; and vegetables. **Table 4.1** lists foods rich in dietary fiber, and Table 3.2 lists the fiber content of common foods.

Key Concepts: *Complex carbohydrates include starch, glycogen, and fiber. Starch is composed of straight or branched chains of glucose molecules and is the storage form of energy in plants. Glycogen is composed of highly branched chains of glucose molecules and is the storage form of energy in animals. Fibers include many different substances that cannot be digested by enzymes in the human intestinal tract and are found in plant foods, such as whole grains, legumes, vegetables, and fruits.*

Carbohydrate Digestion and Absorption

Although glucose is a key building block of carbohydrates, you can't exactly find it on the menu at your favorite restaurant or campus hideout. You must first drink that chocolate milkshake or eat that hamburger bun so that your body can convert the food carbohydrate into glucose in the body. Let's see what happens to the carbohydrate foods you eat!

Digestion

Figure 4.10 provides an overview of the digestive process. Carbohydrate digestion begins in the mouth, where the starch-digesting enzyme salivary amylase hydrolyzes starch into shorter polysaccharides and maltose. Chewing stimulates saliva production and mixes salivary amylase with food. Disaccharides, unlike starch, are not digested in the mouth. In fact, only about 5 percent of the starches in food are broken down by the time the food is swallowed.

When carbohydrate enters the stomach, the acidity of stomach juices eventually halts the action of salivary amylase by denaturing it, which

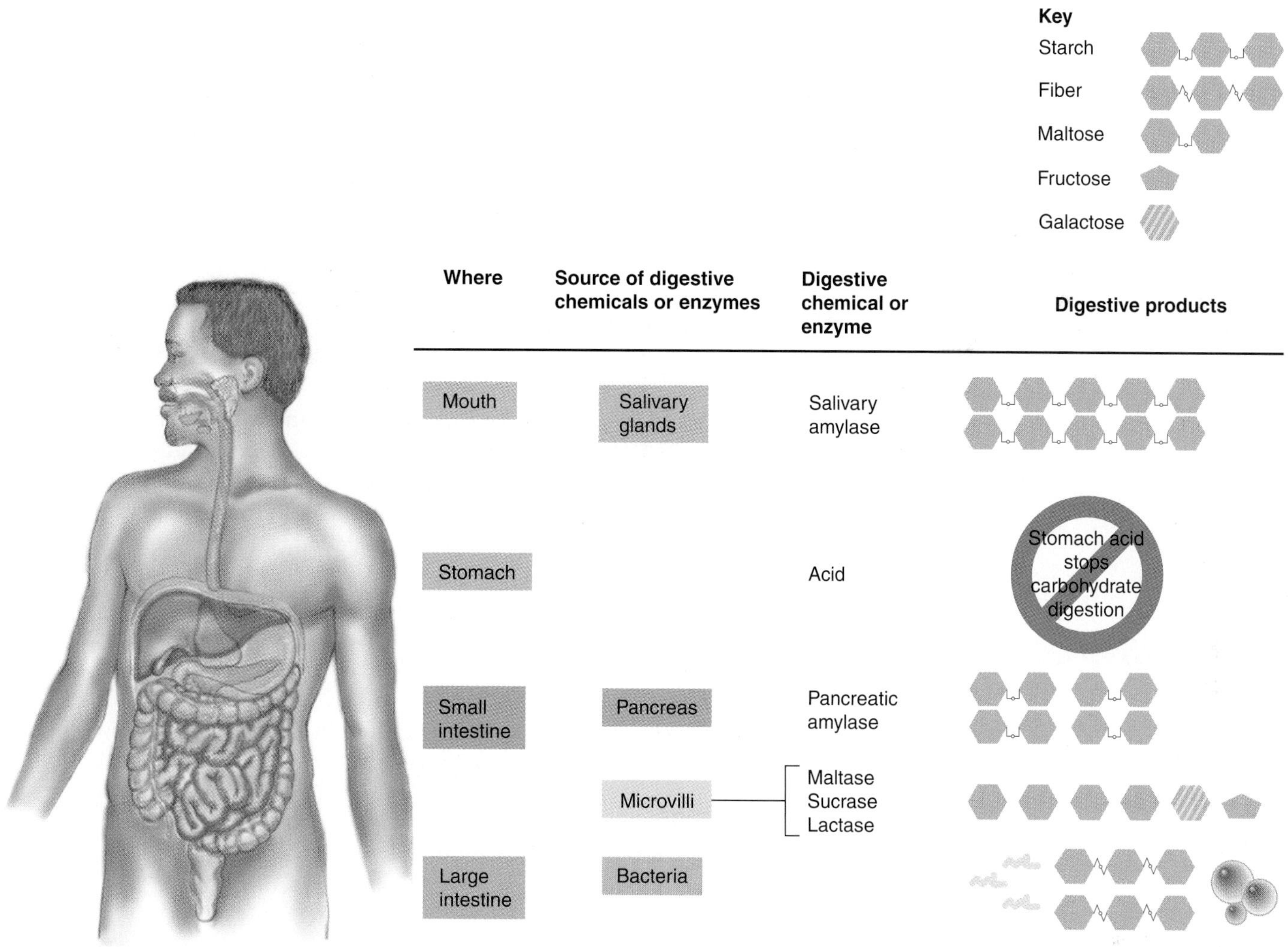

Key

Starch	
Fiber	
Maltose	
Fructose	
Galactose	

Where	Source of digestive chemicals or enzymes	Digestive chemical or enzyme	Digestive products
Mouth	Salivary glands	Salivary amylase	
Stomach		Acid	Stomach acid stops carbohydrate digestion
Small intestine	Pancreas	Pancreatic amylase	
	Microvilli	Maltase Sucrase Lactase	
Large intestine	Bacteria		

Figure 4.10 **Carbohydrate digestion.** Most carbohydrate digestion takes place in the small intestine.

causes the enzyme (a protein) to lose its shape and function. This denaturation stops carbohydrate digestion, which will restart in the small intestine. Certain fibers, such as pectins and gums, provide a feeling of fullness and tend to delay digestive activity by slowing stomach emptying.

Most carbohydrate digestion takes place in the small intestine. As the stomach contents enter the small intestine, the pancreas secretes pancreatic amylase into the small intestine. **Pancreatic amylase** continues the digestion of starch, breaking it into many units of the disaccharide maltose.

Meanwhile, enzymes attached to the brush border (microvilli) of the mucosal cells lining the intestinal tract go to work. (See Chapter 3 for a detailed explanation of the complex structure of the small intestine.) These digestive enzymes, called brush border disaccharidases, break disaccharides into monosaccharides for absorption. The enzyme maltase splits maltose into two glucose molecules. The enzyme sucrase splits sucrose into glucose and fructose. The enzyme lactase splits lactose into glucose and galactose.

The bonds that link glucose molecules in complex carbohydrates are called glycosidic bonds. The two forms of these bonds, **alpha (α) bonds** and **beta (β) bonds**, have important differences. (See **Figure 4.11**.) Human enzymes easily break alpha bonds, making glucose available from the polysaccharides starch and glycogen. Our bodies don't have enzymes to break

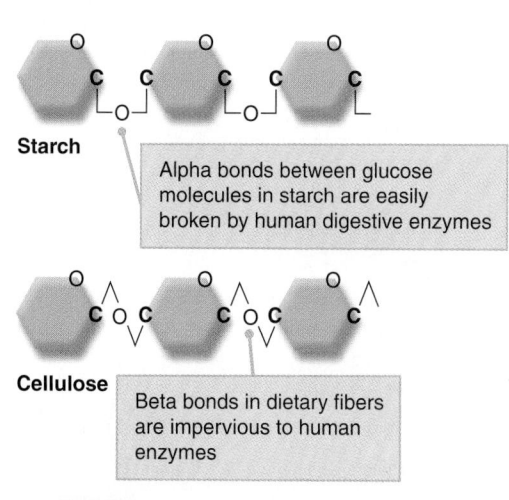

Starch

Alpha bonds between glucose molecules in starch are easily broken by human digestive enzymes

Cellulose

Beta bonds in dietary fibers are impervious to human enzymes

Figure 4.11 **Alpha bonds and beta bonds.** Human digestive enzymes can easily break the alpha bonds in starch, but they cannot break the beta bonds in cellulose.

most beta bonds, such as those that link the glucose molecules in cellulose, a nondigestible polysaccharide. Beta bonds also link the galactose and glucose molecules in the disaccharide lactose, but the enzyme lactase is specifically tailored to attack this small molecule. People with a sufficient supply of the enzyme lactase can break these bonds. When lactase is lacking, however, the beta bonds remain unbroken and lactose remains undigested until bacteria in the colon can attack it. (See Chapter 3 for more on lactose maldigestion.)

Enzymes are highly specific; they speed up only certain reactions and work on only certain molecules. Humans lack the digestive enzymes needed to break down the oligosaccharides raffinose and stachyose, for example. The commercial product Beano is an enzyme preparation. When taken immediately before eating beans or other gas-forming vegetables, Beano helps break oligosaccharides into monosaccharides so that the body can absorb them.

Some carbohydrate remains intact as it enter the large intestine. This carbohydrate may be fiber or resistant starch, or the small intestine may have lacked the necessary enzymes to break it down. In the large intestine, bacteria partially ferment (break down) undigested carbohydrate and produce gas plus a few short-chain fatty acids. These fatty acids are absorbed into the colon and are used for energy by the colon cells. In addition, these fatty acids may reduce the risk of developing gastrointestinal disorders, cancers, and cardiovascular disease.[14]

Some fibers, particularly cellulose and psyllium, pass through the large intestine unchanged and therefore produce little gas. Instead, these fibers add to the stool weight and water content, making it easier to pass.

Absorption

Monosaccharides are absorbed into the mucosal cells lining the small intestine by two different mechanisms that you learned about in Chapter 3. Fructose is absorbed by facilitated diffusion, whereas glucose and galactose depend on an active transport mechanism. A sodium-dependent glucose

Figure 4.12 **Travels with carbohydrate.** (1) Carbo–hydrate digestion begins in the mouth. (2) Stomach acid halts carbohydrate digestion. (3) Carbohydrate digestion resumes in the small intestine, where monosaccharides are absorbed. (4) Monosaccharides enter intestinal cells through a variety of transport proteins and use facilitated diffusion to leave the cells and enter the bloodstream. (5) The liver converts fructose and galactose to glucose, which it can assemble into chains of glycogen, release to the blood, or use for energy.

Key

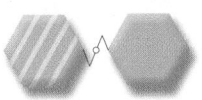
Lactose

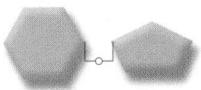
Sucrose

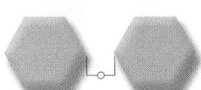
Maltose

Fructose

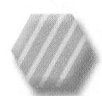
Galactose

Glucose

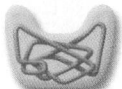
Enzymes

Na⁺

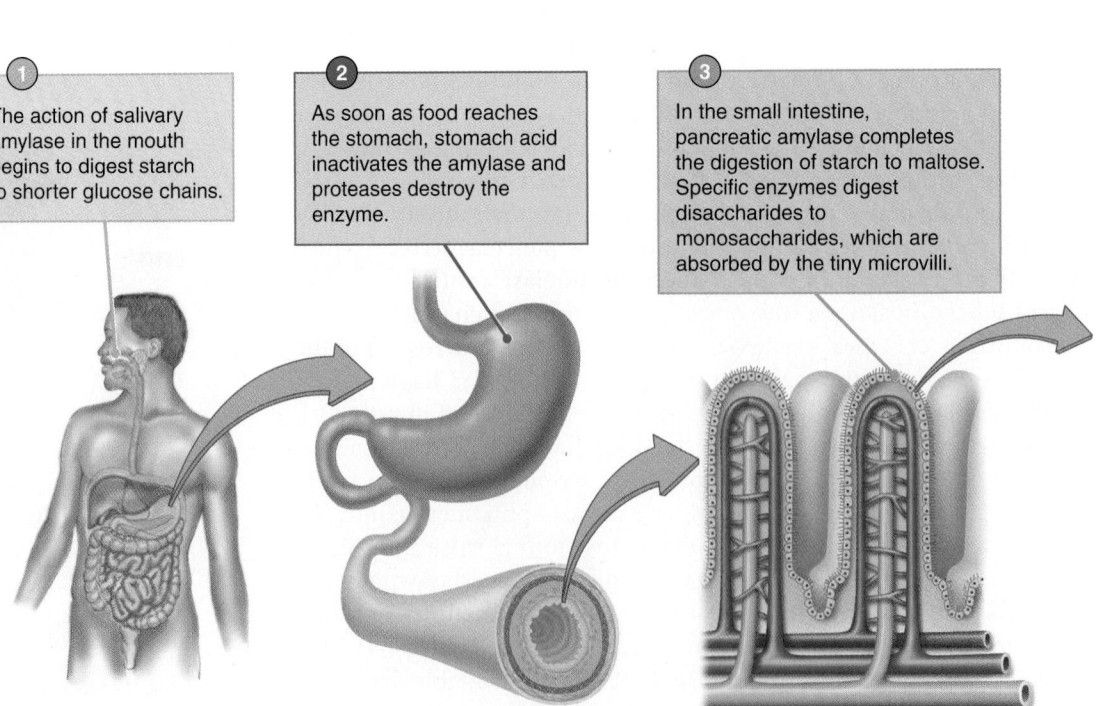

1. The action of salivary amylase in the mouth begins to digest starch to shorter glucose chains.

2. As soon as food reaches the stomach, stomach acid inactivates the amylase and proteases destroy the enzyme.

3. In the small intestine, pancreatic amylase completes the digestion of starch to maltose. Specific enzymes digest disaccharides to monosaccharides, which are absorbed by the tiny microvilli.

transport protein helps move glucose and galactose across the intestinal cell's membrane. The carrier protein in the cell membrane is first loaded with sodium, and then either glucose or galactose can attach to it.[15] Energy for this process is provided by the hydrolysis of adenosine triphosphate (ATP). Fructose absorption is slower than that of glucose or galactose. In the villi, absorbed monosaccharides pass through the intestinal mucosal cells and enter the bloodstream. Glucose, galactose, and fructose molecules travel to the liver via the portal vein, where galactose and fructose are converted into glucose or used for energy. The liver stores and releases glucose as needed to maintain constant blood glucose levels. **Figure** 4.12 illustrates the digestion and absorption of carbohydrates.

Key Concepts: *Carbohydrate digestion takes place primarily in the small intestine, where digestible carbohydrates are broken down and absorbed as monosaccharides.*

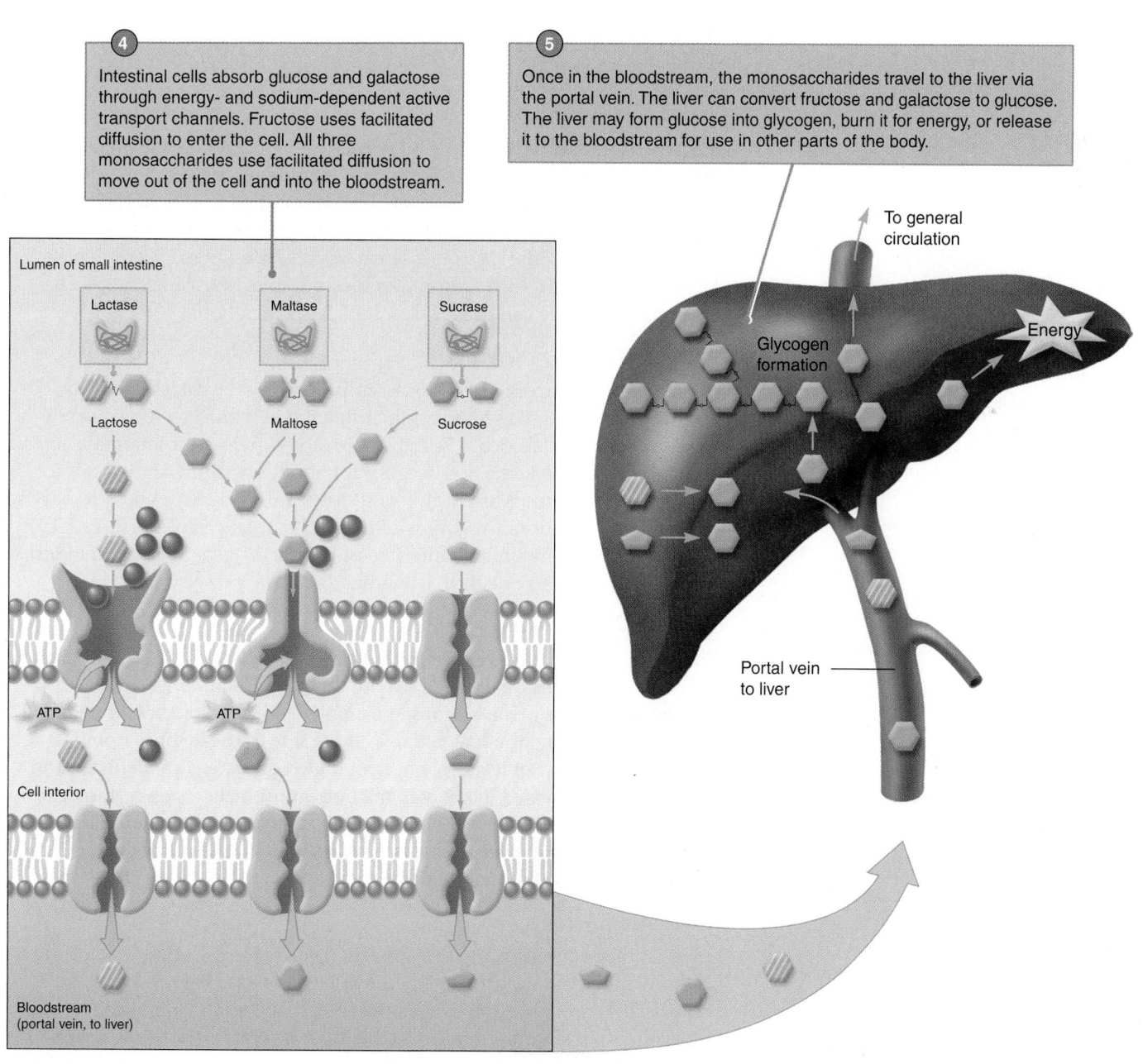

4 Intestinal cells absorb glucose and galactose through energy- and sodium-dependent active transport channels. Fructose uses facilitated diffusion to enter the cell. All three monosaccharides use facilitated diffusion to move out of the cell and into the bloodstream.

5 Once in the bloodstream, the monosaccharides travel to the liver via the portal vein. The liver can convert fructose and galactose to glucose. The liver may form glucose into glycogen, burn it for energy, or release it to the bloodstream for use in other parts of the body.

Lumen of small intestine

Lactase

Maltase

Sucrase

Lactose

Maltose

Sucrose

ATP

ATP

Cell interior

Bloodstream
(portal vein, to liver)

To general circulation

Glycogen formation

Energy

Portal vein to liver

Glucose

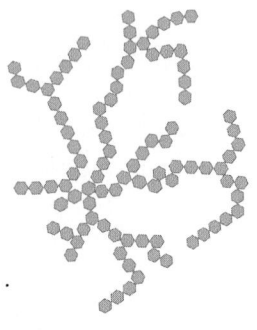

Glycogen

ketone bodies Molecules formed when insufficient carbohydrate is available to completely metabolize fat. Formation of ketone bodies is promoted by a low glucose level and high acetyl CoA level within cells. Acetone, acetoacetate, and beta-hydroxybutyrate are ketone bodies. Beta-hydroxybutyrate is sometimes improperly called a ketone. (See *ketones*.)

ketosis [kee-TOE-sis] Abnormally high concentration of ketone bodies in body tissues and fluids.

blood glucose levels The amount of glucose in the blood at any given time. Also known as blood sugar levels.

insulin [IN-suh-lin] Produced by beta cells in the pancreas, this polypeptide hormone stimulates the uptake of blood glucose into muscle and adipose cells, the synthesis of glycogen in the liver, and various other processes.

glucagon [GLOO-kuh-gon] Produced by alpha cells in the pancreas, this polypeptide hormone promotes the breakdown of liver glycogen to glucose, thereby increasing blood glucose. Glucagon secretion is stimulated by low blood glucose levels and by growth hormone.

epinephrine A hormone released in response to stress or sudden danger, epinephrine raises blood glucose levels to ready the body for "fight or flight." Also called adrenaline.

glycemic index A measure of the effect of food on blood glucose levels. It is the ratio of the blood glucose value after eating a particular food to the value after eating the same amount of white bread or glucose.

Bacteria in the large intestine partially ferment resistant starch and some types of fiber, producing gas and a few short-chain fatty acids that can be absorbed through the large intestine and used for energy. The liver converts absorbed monosaccharides into glucose.

Carbohydrates in the Body

Through the processes of digestion and absorption, our varied diet of carbohydrates from vegetables, fruits, grains, and milk becomes glucose. Glucose has one major role—to supply energy for the body.

Normal Use of Glucose

Cells throughout the body depend on glucose for energy to drive chemical processes. Although most—but not all—cells can also burn fat for energy, the body needs some glucose to burn fat efficiently.

When we eat food, our bodies immediately use some glucose to maintain normal blood glucose levels. We store excess glucose as glycogen in liver and muscle tissue. Insulin and glucagon, two hormones produced by the pancreas, closely regulate blood glucose levels.

Using Glucose for Energy

Glucose is the primary fuel for most cells in the body and the preferred fuel for the brain, red blood cells, nervous system, fetus, and placenta. Even when fat is burned for energy, a small amount of glucose is needed to break down fat completely. To obtain energy from glucose, cells must take up glucose from the blood. Once glucose enters cells, a series of metabolic reactions break it down into carbon dioxide and water, releasing energy in a form that the body can use.[16] (See Chapter 7, "Metabolism.")

Storing Glucose as Glycogen

To store excess glucose, the body assembles it into the long, branched chains of glycogen. Glycogen can be broken down quickly, releasing glucose for energy as needed. Liver glycogen stores are used to maintain normal blood glucose levels and account for about one-third of the body's total glycogen stores. Muscle glycogen stores are used to fuel muscle activity and account for about two-thirds of the body's total glycogen stores.[17] The body can store only limited amounts of glycogen—usually enough to last from a few hours to one day, depending on activity level.[18]

Sparing Body Protein

In the absence of carbohydrate, both proteins and fats can be used for energy. Although most cells can break down fat for energy, brain cells and developing red blood cells require a constant supply of glucose.[19] (After an extended period of starvation, the brain adapts and is able to use ketones from fat breakdown for part of its energy needs.) If glycogen stores are depleted and glucose is not provided in the diet, the body must make its own glucose from protein to maintain blood levels and supply glucose to the brain. Adequate consumption of dietary carbohydrate spares body proteins from being broken down and used to make glucose.

Preventing Ketosis

Even when fat provides the fuel for cells, cells require a small amount of carbohydrate to completely break down fat to release energy. When no carbohydrate is available, the liver cannot break down fat completely. Instead, it produces small compounds called **ketone bodies**.[20] Most cells can use ketone bodies for energy.

When ketone bodies are produced more quickly than the body can use them, ketone levels build up in the blood and can cause a condition known as **ketosis**. People vulnerable to ketosis include those who consume only small amounts of carbohydrate or who cannot metabolize blood glucose normally. Ketosis is most commonly caused by very low carbohydrate diets, starvation, uncontrolled diabetes mellitus, and chronic alcoholism. Ketosis also can develop when fluid intake is too low to allow the kidneys to excrete excess ketone bodies. As the concentration of ketone bodies increases, the blood becomes too acidic. The body loses water as it excretes excess ketones in urine, and dehydration is a common consequence of ketosis. To prevent ketosis, the body needs a minimum of 50 to 100 grams of carbohydrate daily.[21] (See Chapter 7, "Metabolism," for more details on ketosis.)

Key Concepts: *Glucose circulates in the blood to provide immediate energy to cells. The body stores excess glucose in the liver and muscle as glycogen. The body needs adequate carbohydrate intake to prevent the breakdown of body proteins to fulfill glucose or energy needs. The body needs some carbohydrate to completely break down fat and prevent the buildup of ketone bodies in the blood.*

Regulating Blood Glucose Levels

The body closely regulates **blood glucose levels** (also known as blood sugar levels) to maintain an adequate supply of glucose for cells. If blood glucose levels drop too low, a person becomes shaky and weak. If blood glucose levels rise too high, a person becomes sluggish and confused, and may have difficulty breathing.

Two hormones produced by the pancreas tightly control blood glucose levels.[22] When blood glucose levels rise after a meal, special pancreatic cells called beta cells release the hormone insulin into the blood. **Insulin** acts like a key, "unlocking" the cells of the body and allowing glucose to enter and fuel them. Insulin works on receptors on the surface of cells, increasing their affinity for glucose and increasing glucose uptake by cells. It also stimulates liver and muscle cells to store glucose as glycogen. As glucose enters cells to deliver energy or be stored as glycogen, blood glucose levels return to normal. (See **Figure 4.13a**.)

When an individual has not eaten in a while and blood glucose levels begin to fall, alpha cells in the pancreas release another hormone, **glucagon**. Glucagon stimulates the breakdown of glycogen stores to release glucose into the bloodstream. (See **Figure 4.13b**.) It also stimulates gluconeogenesis, or the synthesis of glucose from protein. Another hormone, **epinephrine** (also called adrenaline), exerts effects similar to glucagon to ensure that all body cells have adequate energy for emergencies. Released by the adrenal glands in response to sudden stress or danger, epinephrine is called the fight-or-flight hormone.

Different foods vary in their effect on blood glucose levels. Foods rich in simple carbohydrates or starch but low in fat or fiber tend to be digested and absorbed rapidly. This rapid absorption causes a corresponding large and rapid rise in blood glucose levels.[23] The body reacts to this rise by pumping out extra insulin, which in turn can lower blood sugar levels too far before finally stabilizing. Other foods—especially those rich in dietary fiber, resistant starch, or fat—cause a less dramatic blood glucose response accompanied by smaller swings in blood glucose levels.

The **glycemic index** measures the effect of a food on blood glucose levels. Foods with a high glycemic index cause a faster and higher rise in blood glucose, whereas foods with a low glycemic index cause a slower rise in blood glucose.

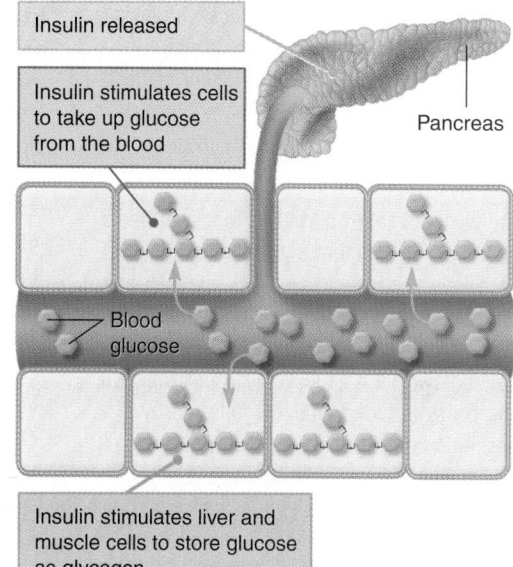

High blood glucose

Insulin released

Insulin stimulates cells to take up glucose from the blood

Pancreas

Blood glucose

Insulin stimulates liver and muscle cells to store glucose as glycogen

(a)

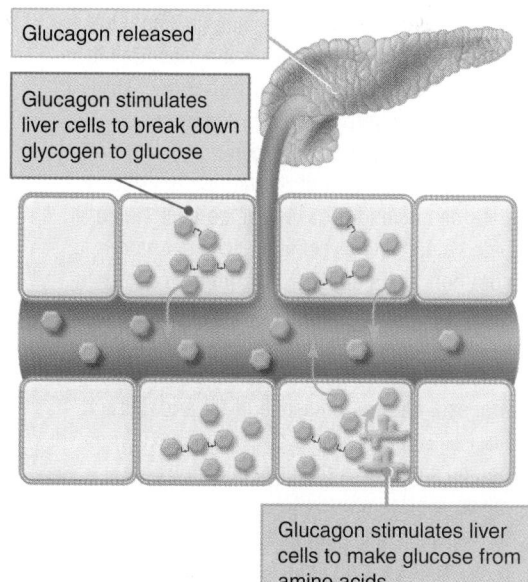

Low blood glucose

Glucagon released

Glucagon stimulates liver cells to break down glycogen to glucose

Glucagon stimulates liver cells to make glucose from amino acids

(b)

Figure 4.13 **Regulating blood glucose levels.** Insulin and glucagon have opposing actions. (a) Insulin acts to lower blood glucose levels, and (b) glucagon acts to raise them.

𝒯𝓎𝒾   The Glycemic Index of Foods: Useful or Useless?

FOR YOUR INFORMATION

The glycemic index is a valuable and easy-to-use concept, claim some researchers.[1] Others contend that although it is promising, more definitive data are needed before this concept should be promoted for widespread public use.[2] Several popular weight-loss diets use the glycemic index to guide food choices.

How Is Glycemic Index Measured?

The glycemic index classifies foods or meals based on their potential to raise blood glucose levels. It is expressed as a percentage of the response to a standard food or carbohydrate, usually white bread or pure glucose.[3]

Foods with a high glycemic index trigger a sharp rise in blood glucose, followed by a dramatic fall, often to levels that are transiently below normal. In contrast, low-glycemic-index foods trigger slower and more modest changes in blood glucose levels.

What Factors Affect the Glycemic Index of a Food or Meal?

The glycemic index of a food is not always easy to predict. Would you expect a high-sugar food such as ice cream to have a high glycemic index? Ice cream actually has a low index because its fat slows sugar absorption. On the other hand, wouldn't you expect complex carbohydrate foods such as bread or potatoes to have a low glycemic index? In fact, the starch in white bread and cooked potatoes is readily absorbed, so each has a high value.[4] The glycemic indices of some common foods are listed in **Table 1**, and lower-glycemic-index substitutions are given in **Table 2**.

The type of carbohydrate, the cooking process, and the presence of fat and dietary fiber all affect a food's glycemic index.[5] In a person's diet, it is the glycemic index of mixed meals, referred to as the *glycemic load* of a meal, rather than the individual foods, that counts.[6]

Why Do Some Researchers Believe the Glycemic Index Is Useful?

Health benefits can be significant. Diets that emphasize low-glycemic-index foods decrease the risk of developing type 2 diabetes and improve blood sugar control in people who are already afflicted.[7] Epidemiological studies suggest that such diets also reduce the risk of colon and other cancers[8] and may help reduce the risk of heart disease as well. Diets with a low glycemic load are associated with higher HDL cholesterol levels,[9] and with reduced incidence of heart attack.[10] Also, studies indicate that the effectiveness of low-fat, high-carbohydrate diets for weight loss can be improved by reducing the glycemic load.[11]

Why Do Some Researchers Believe the Glycemic Index Is Useless?

Some researchers question the usefulness of conclusions drawn primarily from epidemiological studies.[12] Epidemiological studies can show association, but cannot prove causation. Also, researchers worry about the inconsistencies in the use of glucose or white bread as the standard and the wide variations in measured glycemic responses to individual foods.

Many believe the glycemic index is too complex for most people to use effectively. After reviewing current research, the 2005 Dietary Guidelines Advisory Committee concluded that the glycemic index is of little use in providing dietary guidance for Americans.[13] The American Diabetes Association has not yet endorsed widespread adoption of low-glycemic-index diets, stating that "although the use of low-glycemic index food may reduce postprandial hyperglycemia, there is not sufficient evidence of long-term benefit to recommend use of low-glycemic index diets as a primary strategy in food/meal planning for individuals with type 1 diabetes, or for general use by type 2 diabetes patients."[14]

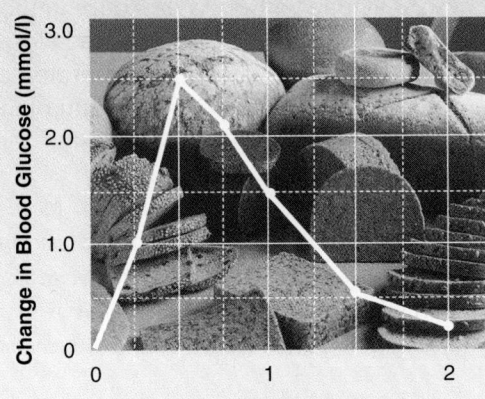

Time (hrs)
HIGH GLYCEMIC INDEX

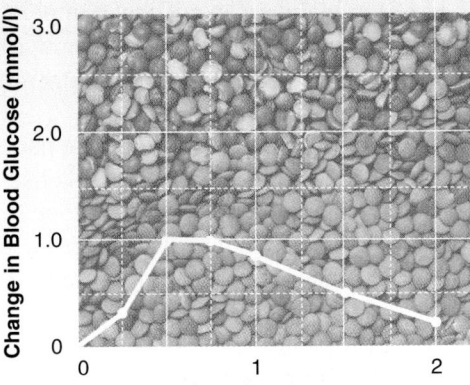

Time (hrs)
LOW GLYCEMIC INDEX

What's the Bottom Line?

Like many other nutrition issues, the glycemic index needs further study. We need to continue to identify the influence of processing techniques on the glycemic index, and agree on methodologies and standards for measuring it. Most researchers also call for prospective, long-term clinical trials to evaluate the effects of low-glycemic-index and low-glycemic-load diets in chronic disease risk reduction and treatment.[15] Until then, encouraging the consumption of whole-grain, minimally refined cereal products and other low-glycemic-index foods won't hurt, and it may help to improve health!

Table 1 Glycemic Index of Some Foods Compared with Pure Glucose*

Food	Glycemic Index	Food	Glycemic Index
BAKERY PRODUCTS		**FRUITS**	
Angel food cake	67	Apples	38
Waffles	76	Bananas	52
		Pineapple	59
BREADS			
White bread	73	**LEGUMES**	
Wheat bread,		Black-eyed peas	42
whole meal flour	71	Lentils	29
BREAKFAST CEREALS		**PASTA**	
All bran	42	Spaghetti	42
Corn flakes	81	Macaroni	47
Oatmeal	58		
		VEGETABLES	
CEREAL GRAINS		Carrots	47
Barley	25	Baked potatoes	85
Sweet corn	53	Green peas	48
White rice, long grain	56		
Bulgur	48	**CANDY**	
		Jelly beans	78
DAIRY FOODS		Life Savers	70
Ice cream	61		
Skim milk	32		

* Glycemic response to pure glucose is 100.

Source: Data compiled from Foster-Powell K, Holt SHA, Brand-Miller JC. International table of glycemic index and glycemic load values: 2002. *Am J Clin Nutr.* 2002;76:5–56.

Table 2 Sample Substitutions for High-Glycemic-Index Foods

High-Glycemic-Index Food	Low-Glycemic-Index Alternative	High-Glycemic-Index Food	Low-Glycemic-Index Alternative
Bread, wheat or white	Oat bran, rye, or pumpernickel bread	Plain cookies and crackers	Cookies made with nuts and whole grains such as oats
Processed breakfast cereal	Unrefined cereal such as oats (either museli or oatmeal); bran cereals	Cakes and muffins	Cakes and muffins made with fruit, oats, or whole grains
		Bananas	Apples
		Potatoes	Pasta or legumes

Low glycemic index = 55 or less, medium = 56–69, high = 70 or more.

1 Miller JB, Colagiuri S, Foster-Powell K. The glycemic index is easy and works in practice. *Diabetes Care.* 1997;20:1628–1629.

2 Pi-Sunyer FX. Glycemic index and disease. *Am J Clin Nutr.* 2002;76(suppl):290S–298S.

3 Jenkins DJA, Kendall CWC, Augustin LSA, et al. Glycemic index: overview of implications in health and disease. *Am J Clin Nutr.* 2002;76(suppl):266S–273S.

4 Foster-Powell K, Holt SH, Brand-Miller JC. International table of glycemic index and glycemic load values: 2002. *Am J Clin Nutr.* 2002;76:5–56.

5 Pi-Sunyer FX. Op. cit.

6 Willett W, Manson J, Liu S. Glycemic index, glycemic load, and risk of type 2 diabetes. *Am J Clin Nutr.* 2002;76(suppl):274S–280S.

7 Ibid.

8 Jenkins DJA, Kendall CWC, Augustin LSA, et al. Op. cit.

9 Leeds AR. Glycemic index and heart disease. *Am J Clin Nutr.* 2002;76(suppl):286S–289S.

10 Jenkins DJA, Kendall CWC, Augustin LSA, et al. Op. cit.

11 Pawlak DB, Ebbeling CB, Ludwig DS. Should obese patients be counseled to follow a low-glycaemic index diet? Yes. *Obes Rev.* 2002;3:235–243.

12 Raben A. Should obese patients be counseled to follow a low-glycaemic index diet? No. *Obes Rev.* 2002;3(4):245–256; and Pi-Sunyer FX. Op. cit.

13 Dietary Guidelines Advisory Committee. *Report of the Dietary Guidelines Advisory Committee on the Dietary Guidelines for Americans, 2005.* January 31, 2005. http://www.health.gov/dietaryguidelines/dga2005/report/. Accessed 4/12/06.

14 Franz MJ, Bantle JP, Beebe CA, et al. Evidence-based nutrition principles and recommendations for the treatment and prevention of diabetes and related complications. *Diabetes Care.* 2002;25(1):148–198.

15 Ludwig DS, Eckel RH. The glycemic index at 20 y. *Am J Clin Nutr.* 2002;76(suppl):264S–265S.

diabetes mellitus A chronic disease in which uptake of blood glucose by body cells is impaired, resulting in high glucose levels in the blood and urine. Type 1 is caused by decreased pancreatic release of insulin. In type 2, target cells (e.g., fat and muscle cells) lose the ability to respond normally to insulin.

hypoglycemia [HIGH-po-gly-SEE-mee-uh] Abnormally low concentration of glucose in the blood; any blood glucose value below 40 to 50 mg/dL of blood.

reactive hypoglycemia A type of hypoglycemia that occurs about one hour after eating carbohydrate-rich food. The body overreacts and produces too much insulin in response to food, rapidly decreasing blood glucose.

fasting hypoglycemia A type of hypoglycemia that occurs because the body produces too much insulin even when no food is eaten.

Although some experts disagree on the usefulness of the glycemic index for humans, diets that emphasize foods with a low glycemic index may offer important health benefits.[24]

High Blood Sugar: Diabetes Mellitus

Diabetes mellitus is a disease in which the body either does not produce enough insulin or does not properly use insulin; as a consequence, blood glucose levels are elevated. Diabetes mellitus is the sixth leading cause of death among Americans.[25] About 1 in 20 people will develop diabetes sometime during their life, and so almost everyone knows someone who has diabetes.[26] In 2005, an estimated 20.8 million Americans—7 percent of the population—had diabetes. Yet, only 14.6 million were aware that they had this disease. The prevalence of diabetes increases with age, and 20.9 percent of adults aged 60 or older have the disease.[27] Although the causes of diabetes are not completely known, both genetics and environmental factors such as obesity and lack of exercise appear to be involved. For more on diabetes, see Chapter 14, "Diet and Health."

Low Blood Sugar: Hypoglycemia

Excess insulin results in low blood sugar, or **hypoglycemia**. Too much glucose enters cells, lowering blood glucose levels too far. When blood glucose levels drop too low, nervousness, irritability, hunger, headache, shakiness, rapid heartbeat, and weakness can develop. A further drop in blood glucose levels can cause coma and death.

A person with diabetes can develop hypoglycemia in response to an overdose of insulin or vigorous exercise. In nondiabetic individuals, two types of hypoglycemia occur. **Reactive hypoglycemia** occurs about one hour after eating carbohydrate-rich food. The body overreacts and produces too much insulin in response to food. Individuals can prevent reactive hypoglycemia by eating frequent, smaller meals to smooth out blood glucose responses to food. **Fasting hypoglycemia** occurs because the body produces too much insulin even when no food is eaten. Pancreatic tumors can cause fasting hypoglycemia.

Key Concepts: *In healthy individuals, two hormones produced by the pancreas closely regulate blood glucose levels. Insulin allows glucose to enter cells and stimulates storage of glucose as glycogen, lowering blood glucose levels. Glucagon stimulates the release of glucose from glycogen and the formation of glucose from protein. Some individuals lack the ability to regulate blood glucose levels properly, resulting in diabetes (characterized by hyperglycemia) or hypoglycemia (low blood sugar).*

Carbohydrates in the Diet

What foods supply our dietary carbohydrates? **Figure 4.14** shows many foods rich in carbohydrates. Plant foods are our main dietary sources of carbohydrates: grains, legumes, and vegetables provide starches and fibers; fruits provide sugars and fibers. Additional sugar (mainly lactose) is found in dairy foods, and various sugars are found in beverages, jams, jellies, and candy.

Recommendations for Carbohydrate Intake

The minimum amount of carbohydrate required by the body is based on the brain's requirement for glucose. This glucose can come either from dietary carbohydrate or from synthesis of glucose from protein in the body. Relying on protein alone is not recommended, however, because adaptation to using protein for glucose and ketone bodies for energy may be incomplete.[28] Therefore,

Quick Bites

Carbohydrate Companions

The word *companion* comes from the Latin word *companio*, meaning "one who shares bread."

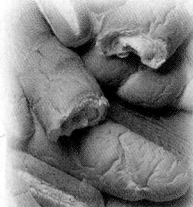

an RDA for carbohydrate of 130 grams per day has been set for individuals aged 1 year and older. The RDA for carbohydrate rises to 175 grams per day for pregnancy and 210 grams per day during lactation.

Most Americans eat more carbohydrate than this amount. In fact, health-promoting diets *should* contain more carbohydrate. In its report on DRIs for macronutrients, the Food and Nutrition Board developed recommended ranges of intake for the energy-yielding nutrients based on evidence of increased risk for heart disease with very high carbohydrate intakes, and increased risk for obesity and heart disease with high fat intake. The Acceptable Macronutrient Distribution Range (AMDR) for carbohydrate is 45 to 65 percent of kilocalories. For an adult who eats about 2,000 kilocalories daily, this represents 225 to 325 grams of carbohydrate. The Daily Value for carbohydrates is 300 grams per day, representing 60 percent of the calories in a 2,000-kilocalorie diet.

The *Dietary Guidelines for Americans* suggests that we "choose carbohydrates wisely."[29] One key recommendation is to choose and prepare foods and beverages with little added sugar. Although the AMDR for added sugars is no more than 25 percent of daily energy intake, a point at which the micronutrient quality of the diet declines, many sources suggest that added sugar intake should be lower. In its 2003 report on diet and chronic disease, the WHO suggested a limit of 10 percent of energy from added sugars.[30] The "discretionary calorie allowance" in the USDA's MyPyramid food guidance system covers calories from added sugars, alcohol, and higher-fat meat or milk choices. For someone consuming 2,000 kilocalories daily, about 250 kilocalories are "discretionary." If no alcohol is consumed, added sugar must then be balanced with extra fat. If fat intake is low (close to 20 percent of energy intake), added sugar could be as much as 18 teaspoons, equivalent to two cans of regular soft drink each day. But if fat intake is higher (35 percent of energy intake), allowable added sugar drops to 0 teaspoons.

The *Dietary Guidelines for Americans* also recommends that we "choose fiber-rich fruits, vegetables, and whole grains often." Fruits, vegetables, and whole grains, along with legumes, are good sources of fiber. The Adequate Intake (AI) value for total fiber is 38 grams per day for men aged 19 to 50 years, and 25 grams per day for women in the same age group. This AI value is based on a level of intake (14 grams per 1,000 kilocalories) that provides the greatest risk reduction for heart disease.[31] The Daily Value for fiber used on food labels is 25 grams.

Current Consumption

Adult Americans currently consume about 49 to 50 percent of their energy intake as carbohydrate. Dietary fiber averages around 18 grams per day for women and 22 grams per day for men.[32] Added sugar intake ranges widely, from 40 to 120 grams per day for adults; on average, sugar intake is about 16 percent of daily energy intake. Although these values for total carbohydrate and added sugar are within the AMDRs, fiber consumption is lower than recommended.

Natural sugars in milk, fruits, and grains make up about half of our sugar intake; refined sugars added to foods make up the other half. About one-third of our added sugar intake comes from nondiet soft drinks. This is of concern because as soft drink intake rises, so does energy intake, while consumption of milk and the vitamin and mineral quality of the diet declines.[33] Many studies suggest that rising soft drink consumption is a factor in overweight and obesity, even among very young children.[34]

Think about It **2**

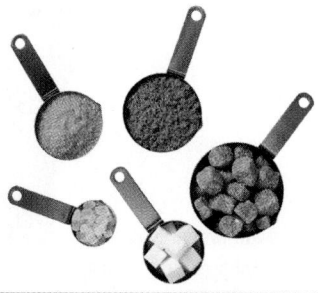

Table sugar, corn syrup, and brown sugar are rich in sucrose, a simple carbohydrate

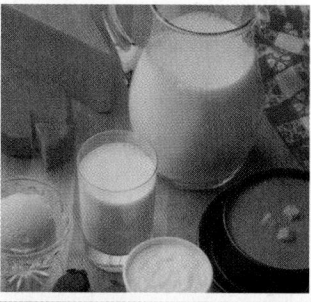

Milk and milk products are rich in lactose, a simple carbohydrate

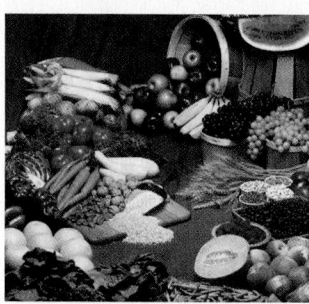

Fruits and vegetables provide simple sugars, starch, and fiber

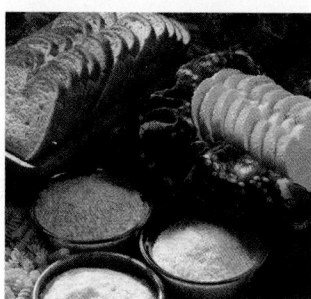

Bread, flour, cornmeal, rice, and pasta are rich in starch and, sometimes, dietary fiber

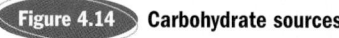

Figure 4.14 Carbohydrate sources.

germ The innermost part of a grain, located at the base of the kernel, that can grow into a new plant. The germ is rich in protein, oils, vitamins, and minerals.

endosperm The largest, middle portion of a grain kernel. The endosperm is high in starch to provide food for the growing plant embryo.

bran The layers of protective coating around the grain kernel that are rich in dietary fiber and nutrients.

husk The inedible covering of a grain kernel. Also known as the chaff.

Choosing Carbohydrates Wisely

The *Dietary Guidelines for Americans* encourages us to increase our intake of fruits, vegetables, whole grains, and fat-free or low-fat milk while keeping calorie intake under control. These foods are all good sources of carbohydrates and many other nutrients. Choosing a variety of fruits and vegetables, and particularly including choices from all five vegetable subgroups (dark-green vegetables, orange vegetables, legumes, starchy vegetables, and other vegetables), provides vitamin A, vitamin C, folate, potassium, and fiber.

Strategies for Increasing Fiber Intake

Along with fruits and vegetables, whole grains are important sources of fiber. Whole kernels of grains consist of four parts: germ, endosperm, bran, and husk. (See **Figure 4.15**.) The **germ**, the innermost part at the base of the kernel, is the portion that grows into a new plant. It is rich in protein, oils, vitamins, and minerals. The **endosperm** is the largest, middle portion of the grain kernel. It is high in starch and provides food for the growing plant embryo. The **bran** is composed of layers of protective coating around the grain kernel and is rich in dietary fiber. The **husk** is an inedible covering.

When grains are refined—making white flour from wheat, for example, or making white rice from brown rice—the process removes the outer husk and bran layers and sometimes the inner germ of the grain kernel. Because the bran and germ portions of the grain contain much of the dietary fiber, vitamins, and minerals, the nutrient content of whole grains is far superior to that of refined grains. Although food manufacturers add iron, thiamin, riboflavin, and niacin back to white flour through enrichment, they usually do not add back dietary fiber and nutrients such as vitamin B_6, calcium, phosphorus, potassium, magnesium, and zinc, which are also lost in processing.

Read labels carefully to choose foods that contain whole grains. Terms such as *whole-wheat*, *whole-grain*, *rolled oats*, and *brown rice* indicate that the entire grain kernel is included in the food. Even better, look for the words *100 percent whole grain* or *100 percent whole wheat*. Several "whole-grain" products on the market may contain some whole grains, but the total amount of whole grains may be very low or refining may have removed most of certain whole-grain components. In early 2006, the FDA proposed that anything labeled as containing whole grains must contain a comparable amount of the fibrous, protein-dense, and nutrient-rich portions of grains—the endosperm, germ and bran—in the same proportion normally present in the intact grain.[35]

To increase your fiber intake:

- Eat more whole-grain breads, cereals, pasta, and rice; and more fruits, vegetables, and legumes.

- Eat fruits and vegetables with the peel, if possible. The peel is high in fiber.

- Add fruits to muffins and pancakes.

- Add legumes, such as lentils and pinto, navy, kidney, and black beans, to casseroles and mixed dishes as a meat substitute.

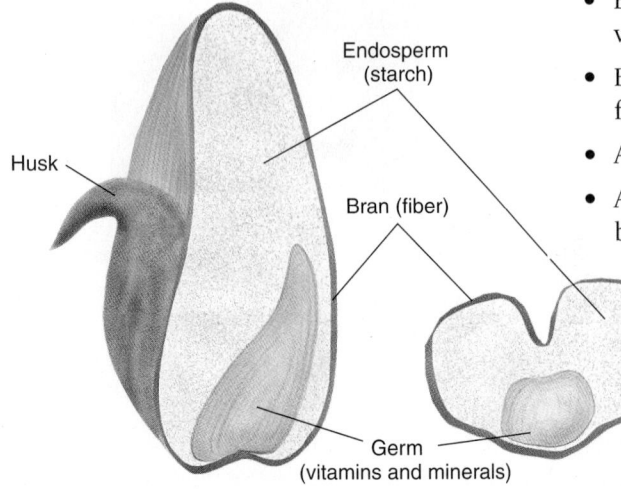

Husk

Endosperm (starch)

Bran (fiber)

Germ (vitamins and minerals)

Figure 4.15 **Anatomy of a kernel of grain.** Whole kernels of grains consist of four parts: germ, endosperm, bran, and husk.

- Substitute whole-grain flour for all-purpose flour in recipes whenever possible.
- Use brown rice instead of white rice.
- Substitute oats for flour in crumb toppings.
- Choose high-fiber cereals.
- Choose whole fruits rather than fruit juices.

When increasing your fiber intake, do so gradually and drink plenty of fluids to allow your body to adjust. Add just a few grams a day; otherwise, abdominal cramps, gas, bloating, and diarrhea or constipation may result. Parents and caregivers should also emphasize foods rich in fiber for children older than 2 years, but must take care that these foods do not fill a child up before energy and nutrient needs are met. **Table 4.2** lists various foods that are high in simple and complex carbohydrates.

Although health food stores, pharmacies, and even grocery stores sell many types of fiber supplements, most experts agree that you should get fiber from food rather than from a supplement. Foods rich in dietary fiber contain a variety of fibers as well as vitamins, minerals, and other phytochemicals that offer important health effects.

Moderating Sugar Intake

Most of us enjoy the taste of sweet foods, and there's no reason why we should not. But for some individuals, habitually high sugar intake crowds out foods that are higher in fiber, vitamins, and minerals.

To reduce added sugars in your diet:

- Use less of all nutritive sugars, including white sugar, brown sugar, honey, and syrups.
- Limit consumption of soft drinks, high-sugar breakfast cereals, candy, ice cream, and sweet desserts.
- Use fresh or frozen fruits and fruits canned in natural juices or light syrup for dessert and to sweeten waffles, pancakes, muffins, and breads.

Read ingredient lists carefully. Food labels list the total grams of sugar in a food, which includes both sugars naturally present in foods and sugars added to foods. Many terms for added sweeteners appear on food labels. Foods likely to be high in sugar list some form of sweetener as the first, second, or third ingredient on labels. **Table 4.3** lists various forms of sugar used in foods.

Sugar substitutes can help many people lower sugar intake, but foods with these substitutes may not provide less energy than similar products containing nutritive sweeteners. Rather than sugar, other energy-yielding nutrients, such as fat, are the primary source of the calories in these foods. Also, as sugar substitute use in the United States has increased, so has sugar consumption—an interesting paradox!

Key Concepts: *Current recommendations suggest that Americans consume at least 130 grams of carbohydrate per day. An intake of total carbohydrates representing between 45 and 65 percent of total energy intake and a fiber intake of 14 grams per 1,000 kilocalories are associated with reduced heart disease risk. Added sugar should account for no more than 25 percent of daily energy and ideally should be much less. Americans generally eat too little fiber. An emphasis on consuming whole grains, legumes, fruits, and vegetables would help to increase fiber intake.*

Table 4.2 High-Carbohydrate Foods

High in Complex Carbohydrates	High in Simple Carbohydrates
Bagels	**Naturally Present**
Tortillas	Fruits
Cereals	Fruit juices
Crackers	Skim milk
Rice cakes	Plain nonfat yogurt
Legumes	
Corn	**Added**
Potatoes	Angel food cake
Peas	Soft drinks
Squash	Sherbet
Popcorn	Syrups
	Sweetened nonfat yogurt
	Candy
	Jellies
	Jams
	Gelatin
	High-sugar breakfast cereals
	Cookies
	Frosting

Table 4.3 Forms of Sugar Used in Foods

Brown rice syrup	Invert sugar
Brown sugar	Lactose
Concentrated fruit juice sweetener	Levulose
Confectioners sugar	Maltose
Corn syrup	Mannitol
Dextrose	Maple sugar
Fructose	Molasses
Galactose	Natural sweeteners
Glucose	Raw sugar
Granulated sugar	Sorbitol
High-fructose corn syrup	Turbinado sugar
	White sugar
	Xylitol

Quick Bites

Sugar Overload

In many affluent countries, sugar consumption is nearly 100 pounds per capita per year. The United States averages 103 pounds of sugar per person per year—roughly half as refined sugar and half as corn sweeteners (especially as high-fructose corn syrup). Boys aged 12 to 19 years consume nearly 160 pounds per year, and girls the same ages consume 114 pounds annually.

nutritive sweeteners Substances that impart sweetness to foods and that can be absorbed and yield energy in the body. Simple sugars, sugar alcohols, and high-fructose corn syrup are the most common nutritive sweeteners used in food products.

refined sweeteners Composed of monosaccharides and disaccharides that have been extracted and processed from other foods.

polyols See *sugar alcohols.*

nonnutritive sweeteners Substances that impart sweetness to foods but supply little or no energy to the body; also called artificial or alternative sweeteners. They include acesulfame, aspartame, saccharin, and sucralose.

saccharin [SAK-ah-ren] An artificial sweetener that tastes about 300 to 700 times sweeter than sucrose.

aspartame [AH-spar-tame] An artificial sweetener composed of two amino acids and methanol. It is 200 times sweeter than sucrose. Its trade name is NutraSweet.

phenylketonuria (PKU) An inherited disorder caused by a lack or deficiency of the enzyme that converts phenylalanine to tyrosine.

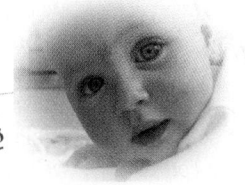

Quick Bites

Why is honey dangerous for babies?

Because honey and Karo syrup (corn syrup) can contain spores of the bacterium *Clostridium botulinum*, they should never be fed to infants younger than one year of age. Infants do not produce as much stomach acid as older children and adults, so these spores can germinate in an infant's GI tract and cause botulism, a deadly foodborne illness.

Nutritive Sweeteners

Nutritive sweeteners are digestible carbohydrates and therefore provide energy. They include monosaccharides, disaccharides, and sugar alcohols from either natural or refined sources. White sugar, brown sugar, honey, maple syrup, glucose, fructose, xylitol, sorbitol, and mannitol are just some of the many nutritive sweeteners used in foods. One slice of angel food cake, for example, contains about 5 teaspoons of sugar. Fruit-flavored yogurt contains about 7 teaspoons of sugar. Even two sticks of chewing gum contain about 1 teaspoon of sugar. Whether sweeteners come from natural sources or are refined, all are broken down in the small intestine and absorbed as monosaccharides and provide energy. Because all these absorbed monosaccharides end up as glucose, the body cannot tell whether the monosaccharides came from honey or table sugar.

The sugar alcohols in sugarless chewing gums and candies are also nutritive sweeteners, but the body does not digest and absorb them fully, so they provide only about 2 kilocalories per gram, compared with the 4 kilocalories per gram that other sugars provide.

Natural Sweeteners Natural sweeteners such as honey and maple syrup contain monosaccharides and disaccharides that make them taste sweet. Honey contains a mix of fructose and glucose—the same two monosaccharides that make up sucrose. Bees make honey from the sucrose-containing nectar of flowering plants. Real maple syrup contains primarily sucrose and is made by boiling and concentrating the sap from sugar maple trees. Most maple-flavored syrups sold in grocery stores, however, are made from corn syrup with maple flavoring added.

Many fruits also contain sugars that impart a sweet taste. Usually the riper the fruit, the higher its sugar content—a ripe pear tastes sweeter than an unripe one.

Refined Sweeteners **Refined sweeteners** are monosaccharides and disaccharides that have been extracted from plant foods. White table sugar is sucrose extracted from either sugar beets or sugar cane. Molasses is a by-product of the sugar-refining process. Most brown sugar is really white table sugar with molasses added for coloring and flavor.

Manufacturers make high-fructose corn syrup by treating cornstarch with acid and enzymes to break down the starch into glucose. Then different enzymes convert about half the glucose to fructose. High-fructose corn syrup has about the same sweetness as table sugar but costs less to produce. An increase in high-fructose corn syrup in soft drinks and other processed foods accounts for much of the increased use of sweeteners in the United States since the 1970s.[36]

Sugar Alcohols The sugar alcohols sorbitol, xylitol, and mannitol occur naturally in a wide variety of fruits and vegetables and are commercially produced from other carbohydrates such as sucrose, glucose, and starch. Also known as **polyols**, these sweeteners are not as sweet as sucrose, but they do have the advantage of being less likely to cause tooth decay. Manufacturers use sugar alcohols to sweeten sugar-free products, such as gum and mints, and to add bulk and texture, provide a cooling sensation in the mouth, and retain moisture in foods. When sugar alcohols are used as the sweetener, the product may be sugar- (sucrose-) free, but it is not calorie-free. Check the label to be sure. An excessive intake of sugar alcohols may cause diarrhea.[37]

Thin About **3**

Nonnutritive Sweeteners

Gram for gram, most **nonnutritive sweeteners** (also called *artificial sweeteners*) are many times sweeter than nutritive sweeteners. As a consequence, food manufacturers can use much less artificial sweetener to sweeten foods. **Figure 4.16** compares the sweetness of sweeteners. Although some nonnutritive sweeteners do provide energy, their energy contribution is minimal given the small amounts used.

The most common nonnutritive sweeteners in the United States are saccharin, aspartame, and acesulfame K. Cyclamates, which were banned in the United States in 1969 because of cancer concerns, are still used in Canada and many other countries. For people who want to decrease their intake of sugar and energy while still enjoying sweet foods, artificial sweeteners offer an alternative. Also, artificial sweeteners do not contribute to tooth decay.

Saccharin Discovered in 1879 and used in foods ever since then, **saccharin** tastes about 300 times sweeter than sucrose. In the 1970s, research indicated that very large doses of saccharin were associated with bladder cancer in laboratory animals. As a result, in 1977 the U.S. Food and Drug Administration (FDA) proposed banning saccharin from use in food. Widespread protests by consumer and industry groups, however, led Congress to impose a moratorium on the saccharin ban. Every few years, the moratorium was extended, and products containing saccharin had to display a warning label about saccharin and cancer risk in animals. In 2000, convincing evidence of safety led to saccharin's removal from the National Toxicology Program's list of potential cancer-causing agents, and the U.S. Congress repealed the warning label requirement.[38] In Canada, although saccharin is banned from food products, it can be purchased in pharmacies and carries a warning label.

Aspartame The artificial sweetener **aspartame** is a combination of two amino acids: phenylalanine and aspartic acid. When digested and absorbed, it provides 4 kilocalories per gram. However, aspartame is so many times sweeter than sucrose that the amount used to sweeten foods contributes virtually zero calories to the diet, and it does not promote tooth decay. The FDA approved aspartame for use in some foods in 1981 and for use in soft drinks in 1983. More than 90 countries allow aspartame in products such as beverages, gelatin desserts, gums, and fruit spreads. Because heating destroys the sweetening power of aspartame, this sweetener cannot be used in products that require cooking.

Several safety concerns have been raised regarding aspartame. Some groups claim that aspartame could cause high blood levels of phenylalanine. In reality, high-protein foods such as meats contain much more phenylalanine than foods sweetened with aspartame. The amounts of phenylalanine in aspartame-sweetened foods are not high enough to cause concern for most people. However, people with a genetic disease called **phenylketonuria (PKU)** cannot properly metabolize the amino acid phenylalanine, so they must carefully monitor their phenylalanine intake from all sources, including aspartame.

Although some people report headaches, dizziness, seizures, nausea, or allergic reactions with aspartame use, scientific studies have failed to confirm these effects, and most experts believe aspartame is safe for healthy people.[39] The FDA sets a maximum allowable daily intake of aspartame of 50 milligrams per kilogram of body weight.[40] This amount of aspartame equals the amount in sixteen 12-ounce diet soft drinks for adults and eight diet soft drinks for children.

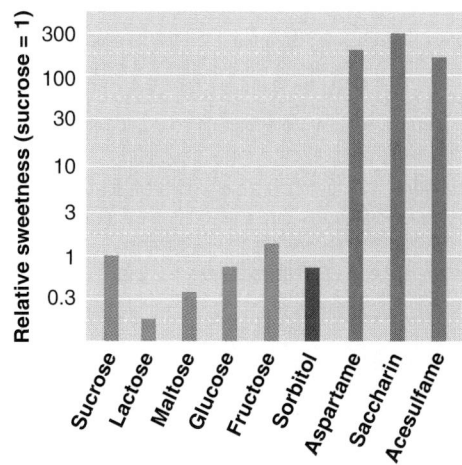

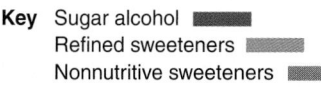

Key Sugar alcohol ▮▮▮
Refined sweeteners ▮▮▮
Nonnutritive sweeteners ▮▮▮

Figure 4.16 **Comparing the sweetness of sweeteners.** Artificial sweeteners are much sweeter than table sugar.

Quick Bites

The Discovery of Saccharin

A German student named Constantine Fahlberg discovered saccharin in 1879, while working with organic chemicals in the lab of Ira Remsen at Johns Hopkins University. One day, while eating some bread, he noticed a strong sweet flavor. He deduced that the flavor came from the compound on his hands, $C_6H_4CONHSO_2$. Fahlberg then patented saccharin by himself, without Remsen.

American Dietetic Association

Use of Nutritive and Nonnutritive Sweeteners

It is the position of the American Dietetic Association that consumers can safely enjoy a range of nutritive and nonnutritive sweeteners when consumed in a diet that is guided by current federal nutrition recommendations, such as the *Dietary Guidelines for Americans* and the Dietary References Intakes, as well as individual health goals.

J Am Diet Assoc. 2004;104:255–275.
Reprinted with permission.

acesulfame K [ay-SUL-fame] An artificial sweetener that is 200 times sweeter than common table sugar (sucrose). Because it is not digested and absorbed by the body, acesulfame contributes no calories to the diet and yields no energy when consumed.

sucralose An artificial sweetener made from sucrose; it was approved for use in the United States in 1998, and has been used in Canada since 1992. Sucralose is non-nutritive and about 600 times sweeter than sugar.

Acesulfame K Marketed under the brand name Sunette, **acesulfame K** is about 200 times sweeter than table sugar. The FDA approved its use in the United States in 1988. Acesulfame K provides no energy, because the body cannot digest it. Food manufacturers use acesulfame K in chewing gum, powdered beverage mixes, nondairy creamers, gelatins, and puddings. Heat does not affect acesulfame K, so it can be used in cooking.

Sucralose Sold under the trade name Splenda, **sucralose** was approved for use in the United States in 1998 and has been used in Canada since 1992. Sucralose is made from sucrose, but the resulting compound is nonnutritive and about 600 times sweeter than sugar. Sucralose has been approved for use in a wide variety of products, including baked goods, beverages, gelatin desserts, and frozen dairy desserts. It also can be used as a "tabletop sweetener," with consumers adding it directly to food.

[*Fyi*] Unfounded Claims Against Sugars

FOR YOUR INFORMATION

Sugar has become the vehicle for diet zealots to create a new crusade. Cut sugar to trim fat! Bust sugar! Break the sugar habit! These battle cries falsely demonize sugar as a dietary villain. But what are the facts?

Sugar and Obesity
Many people believe that sugar is fattening and causes obesity. Sugar is a carbohydrate, and all carbohydrates provide 4 kilocalories per gram. High fat—not sugar—intakes are associated with a greater risk of obesity.[1] Fat is a more concentrated source of energy, and provides 9 kilocalories per gram. However, many foods high in sugar, such as doughnuts and cookies, are also high in fat. Excess energy intake from any source will cause obesity, but sugar by itself is no more likely to cause obesity than starch or protein. The increased availability of low-fat and fat-free foods has not reduced obesity rates in the United States; in fact, the incidence of obesity is still climbing. Some speculate that consumers equate fat-free with calorie-free and eat more of these foods, not realizing that fat-free foods often have a higher sugar content, which makes any calorie savings negligible. Also, foods high in added sugars often have low nutrient value and become "extras" in the diet. High intake of added sugar is associated with increased total energy intake.[2]

Sugar and Heart Disease
Risk factors for heart disease include a genetic predisposition, smoking, high blood pressure, high blood cholesterol levels, diabetes, and obesity. Sugar by itself does not cause heart disease.[3] However, if intake of high-sugar foods contributes to obesity, then risk for heart disease increases. In addition, excessive intake of refined sugar can alter blood lipids in carbohydrate-sensitive people, increasing their risk for heart disease. However, a high fat intake is more likely to promote obesity than a high sugar intake. Thus, total fats, saturated fat, cholesterol, and obesity have a significantly more important relationship to heart disease than sugar.

Sugar and Behavior
Parents continue to talk about kids "bouncing off the walls" at birthday parties because of "all that sugar." So, what's going on? Most likely, the event (a party, trick-or-treating for Halloween, a carnival) is enhancing kids' normal levels of excitement and enthusiasm. From a brain chemistry perspective, carbohydrates actually have a calming effect by increasing production of the sleep-inducing chemical serotonin! Well-controlled research studies have found no link between sugar and hyperactivity, so blame the excitement of the party, but not the sugar, for kids' "wild"

behavior.[4] (See the Nutrition Science in Action feature, "Sugar and Children's Behavior.")

In 1978 Dan White blamed his gunning down the mayor of San Francisco on an emotional state created by eating too many Hostess Twinkies, a legal strategy that became known as the Twinkie defense. Claims that sugar causes criminal behavior in adults are unfounded. Studies show no association between high sugar intake and adult behavior.[5]

1 Lichtenstein AH, Kennedy E, Barrier P, et al. Dietary fat consumption and health. *Nutr Rev.* 1998;56:S3–S19.

2 Dietary Guidelines Advisory Committee. *Report of the Dietary Guidelines Advisory Committee on the Dietary Guidelines for Americans, 2005.* January 31, 2005. http://www.health.gov/dietaryguidelines/dga2005/report/. Accessed 4/12/06.

3 Institute of Medicine, Food and Nutrition Board. *Dietary Reference Intakes for Energy, Carbohydrate, Fiber, Fat, Fatty Acids, Cholesterol, Protein, and Amino Acids.* Washington, DC: National Academy Press, 2005.

4 White JW, Wolraich M. Effect of sugar on behavior and mental performance. *Am J Clin Nutr.* 1995;62:S242–S249; Wolraich ML, Lindgren SD, Stumbo PJ, et al. Effects of diets high in sucrose or aspartame on the behavior and cognitive performance of children. *N Engl J Med.* 1994;330:301–307; and Institute of Medicine, Food and Nutrition Board. Op. cit.

5 White JW, Wolraich M. Op. cit.

NUTRITION SCIENCE IN ACTION

Sugar and Children's Behavior

Observations: Many parents and child-care professionals observe that eating sugary foods "sets some children off." Parents cite cane sugar as the most frequent trigger of hyperactive behavior and provide anecdotal evidence with reports of children who become restless, irritable, and uncontrollable after eating sugar.

Hypothesis: Dietary sucrose adversely affects behavior in children.

Experimental Plan: Conduct a double-blind trial with 23 school-aged children (6 to 10 years) described by parents as sensitive to sugar. For each of three consecutive 3-week periods, provide the children and their families with a different diet (see below). The children, their families, and the research staff are unaware of the sequence of the diets, and all diets are essentially free of additives, artificial food coloring, and preservatives. Use standardized assessments to evaluate each child's behavior at the start and weekly during the experimental diets. The assessments measure 39 variables, such as attention, impulsivity, hyperactivity, aggression, social skills, mood, memory, and learning. Each week, ask the parents to attempt identification of the children's diets.

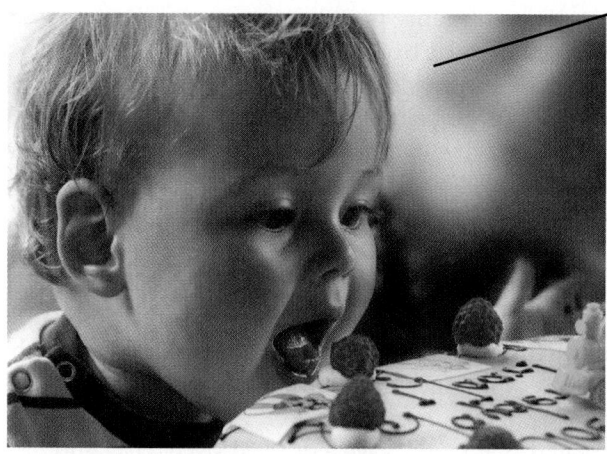

Does eating sugar affect a child's behavior?

Experimental Diets

Diet 1
  High sucrose; no artificial sweeteners

Diet 2
  Low sucrose; sweeten with aspartame

Diet 3
  Low sucrose; sweeten with saccharin

Results: The hypothesis that dietary sugar causes adverse behavior is not confirmed. In this group of school-aged children thought to be sensitive to sugar, none of 39 measured variables differed significantly among the three dietary periods or with the baseline assessment. Only one parent correctly identified the sequence of diets.

Conclusion and Discussion: Overall, comparisons among the three diets and baseline measures are resoundingly negative and do not support opinions and uncontrolled observations that sugar intake affects children's behavior. Additional studies have yielded similar negative results. Sugar-free diets, which can be burdensome and socially inhibiting, should not be endorsed on the basis of unsupported anecdotal evidence.

Source: Based on Wolraich ML, Lindgren SD, Stumbo PJ, et al. Effects of diets high in sucrose or aspartame on the behavior and cognitive performance of children. *New Engl J Med.* 1994;330:301–307.

D-tagatose An artificial sweetener derived from lactose that has the same sweetness as sucrose with only half the calories.

trehalose A disaccharide of two glucose molecules, but with a linkage different from maltose. Used as a food additive and sweetener.

neotame An artificial sweetener similar to aspartame, but one that is sweeter and does not require a warning label for phenylketonurics.

stevioside A dietary supplement, not approved for use as a sweetener, that is extracted and refined from *Stevia rebaudiana* leaves.

stevia See *stevioside*.

glycyrrhizin Nonnutritive sweetener derived from licorice root. Has a licorice flavor and is 50 to 100 times sweeter than sucrose.

dihydrochalcones (DHCs) Nonnutritive sweeteners derived from bioflavonoids of citrus fruits. Approximately 300 to 2,000 times sweeter than sucrose and have a licorice aftertaste.

thaumatin Mixture of sweet-tasting proteins from a West African fruit. Approximately 2,000 times sweeter than sucrose and has licorice aftertaste. Breaks down when heated to cooking temperatures.

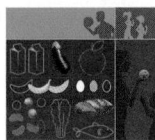

Dietary Guidelines for Americans, 2005
key recommendations

- Choose fiber-rich fruits, vegetables, and whole grains often.
- Choose and prepare foods and beverages with little added sugars or caloric sweeteners, such as amounts suggested by the USDA Food Guide and the DASH Eating Plan.
- Reduce the incidence of dental caries by practicing good oral hygiene and consuming sugar- and starch-containing foods and beverages less frequently.
- Consume a sufficient amount of fruits and vegetables while staying within energy needs. Two cups of fruit and 2½ cups of vegetables per day are recommended for a reference 2,000-calorie intake, with higher or lower amounts depending on the calorie level.
- Choose a variety of fruits and vegetables each day. In particular, select from all five vegetable subgroups (dark green, orange, legumes, starchy vegetables, and other vegetables) several times a week.
- Consume 3 or more ounce-equivalents of whole-grain products per day, with the rest of the recommended grains coming from enriched or whole-grain products. In general, at least half the grains should come from whole grains.
- Consume 3 cups per day of fat-free or low-fat milk or equivalent milk products.

Other Sweeteners

The FDA has accepted the manufacturers' determinations that the sweet substances known as **D-tagatose** and **trehalose** are GRAS (Generally Recognized as Safe) and can be added to foods. Small amounts of tagatose are found naturally in some dairy foods, and tagatose is derived from lactose. Although it has only 75 to 92 percent of the sweetness of sugar, tagatose is incompletely absorbed and provides only 1.5 kilocalories per gram. Trehalose, which is only half as sweet as sucrose, is found naturally in mushrooms, lobster, shrimp, and foods produced using baker's or brewer's yeast. It is made commercially from starch. In foods, trehalose is probably used more often for its textural properties than for sweetness. Trehalose is absorbed completely and provides 4 kilocalories per gram, but produces a lower glycemic response than glucose.[41]

Neotame was approved as a food additive in 2002. It can be used as a tabletop sweetener or added to foods. Neotame is a derivative of a dipeptide containing aspartic acid and phenylalanine—the same two amino acids that make up aspartame. However, chemical modifications to the structure make it 30 to 40 times sweeter than aspartame, or about 7,000 to 13,000 times sweeter than sucrose.

Stevioside (also known as **stevia**) is derived from the stevia plant found in South America. Stevia leaves have been used for centuries to sweeten beverages and make tea. In Japan, stevioside has been used as a sweetener since the 1970s. This substance is 300 times sweeter than sucrose, but its metabolism in the body has been incompletely investigated. Because the FDA has not approved stevioside as a food additive nor accepted it as a GRAS substance, it cannot be used in food in the United States. Although stevia may be sold as a dietary supplement, its labels may not promote its use as a sweetener.

Some sweet food additives are generally recognized as safe (GRAS) flavoring agents but are not approved as sweeteners. **Glycyrrhizin**, an extract of licorice root, is 50 to 100 times sweeter than sucrose, but its pronounced licorice flavor and tendency to increase blood pressure limit widespread use. **Dihydrochalcones (DHCs)**, derived from citrus fruits, can be 300 to 2,000 times sweeter than sucrose. **Thaumatin**, a mixture of sweet-tasting proteins from a West African fruit, is about 2,000 times sweeter than sucrose. DHCs and thaumatin have a delayed sweet taste and licorice aftertaste. Thaumatin cannot be used in products to be baked or boiled.

Key Concepts: *Sweeteners add flavor to foods. Nutritive sweeteners provide energy, whereas nonnutritive sweeteners provide little or no energy. The body cannot tell the difference between sugars derived from natural and refined sources.*

Carbohydrates and Health

Carbohydrates contribute both positively and negatively to health. On the up side, foods rich in fiber help keep the gastrointestinal tract healthy and may reduce the risk of heart disease and cancer. On the down side, excess sugar can contribute to weight gain, poor nutrient intake, and tooth decay.

Sugar and Nutrient Intake

Foods high in sugar are popular in American diets. These empty-calorie foods (e.g., candy, soft drinks, sweetened gelatin, and some desserts) provide most of their energy from sugar but contain little or no dietary fiber, vitamins, or minerals. Studies link the rising prevalence of obesity in children to consumption of sugar-sweetened drinks.[42] On average, Americans drink 53 gallons of soda per year—40 percent more than two decades ago.[43] Consider that one 12-ounce soft drink contains 10 to 12 teaspoons of sugar. Would you add that much sugar to a glass of iced tea?

People with high energy needs, such as active teenagers and young adults, can afford to get a bit more of their calories from high-sugar foods. People with low energy needs, such as some elderly or sedentary people or people trying to lose weight, cannot afford as many calories from high-sugar foods. Most people can include moderate amounts of sugar in their diet and still meet other nutrient needs. But as the amount of added sugar in the diet increases, intake of vitamins and minerals tends to decrease.[44]

Sugar and Dental Caries

High sugar intake contributes to **dental caries**, or cavities. (See **Figure 4.17**.) When bacteria in the mouth feed on sugars, they produce acids that eat away tooth enamel and dental structure, causing dental caries. Although these bacteria quickly metabolize sugars, they feed on any carbohydrate, including starch.

The longer a carbohydrate remains in the mouth or the more frequently it is consumed, the more likely it will promote dental caries. Foods that stick to the teeth, such as caramel, licorice, crackers, sugary cereals, and cookies, are more likely to cause dental caries than foods that are quickly washed out of the mouth. High-sugar beverages such as soft drinks are more likely to cause dental caries when they are sipped slowly over an extended period of time. A baby should never be put to bed with a bottle, because the warm milk or juice may remain in the mouth all night, providing a ready source of carbohydrate for bacteria to break down.

Snacking on high-sugar foods throughout the day provides a continuous intake of carbohydrate that nourishes the bacteria in your mouth, promoting the formation of dental caries. Good dental hygiene, adequate fluoride, and a well-balanced diet for strong tooth formation can help prevent cavities.[45]

Fiber and Obesity

Foods rich in fiber are usually low in fat and energy. They are also more filling, offer a greater volume of food for fewer calories, and take longer to eat. Once eaten, foods high in dietary fiber take longer to leave the stomach and they attract water, giving a feeling of fullness. Consider the following three apple products, which have the same energy content but different fiber content: a large apple containing 5 grams of dietary fiber; $^1/_2$ cup of applesauce containing 2 grams of fiber; and $^3/_4$ cup of apple juice containing 0.2 gram of fiber. For most of us, the whole apple would be more filling and satisfying than the applesauce or apple juice.

Studies show that fiber intakes are higher in lean people than in obese people. Although this suggests that fiber intake has a role in weight control, studies designed to determine how fiber intake might affect overall energy intake have not shown a major effect. Research has not produced conclusive evidence that fiber intake has an effect on satiety or weight maintenance.[46]

Fiber and Type 2 Diabetes

Populations with a high intake of dietary fiber have a low incidence of type 2 diabetes. Epidemiological evidence suggests that intake of certain fibers may delay glucose uptake and smooth out the blood glucose response, thus

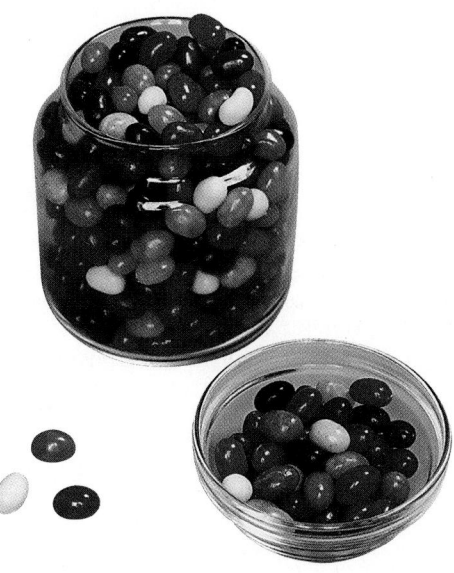

dental caries [KARE-ees] Destruction of the enamel surface of teeth caused by acids resulting from bacterial breakdown of sugars in the mouth.

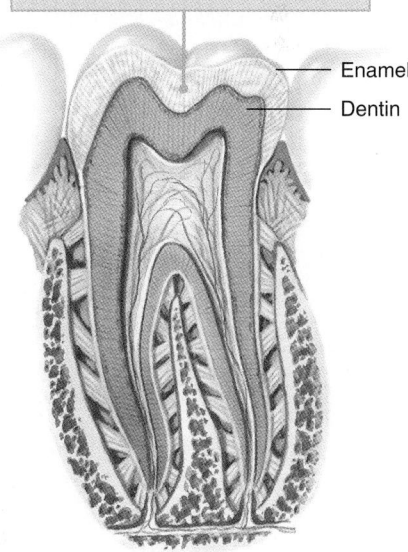

Bacteria feeding on sugar and other carbohydrates produce acids that eat away tooth enamel

Enamel

Dentin

Figure 4.17 **Dental health.** Good dental hygiene, adequate fluoride, and proper nutrition help maintain healthy teeth. A well-balanced diet contains vitamins and minerals crucial for healthy bones and teeth. To help prevent dental caries, avoid continuous snacking on high-sugar foods, especially those that stick to the teeth.

providing a protective effect against diabetes.[47] Current dietary recommendations for people with type 2 diabetes advise a high intake of foods rich in dietary fiber.[48]

Fiber and Cardiovascular Disease

High blood cholesterol levels increase risk for heart disease. Dietary trials using high doses of oat bran, which is high in dietary fiber, show blood cholesterol reductions of 2 percent per gram of intake.[49] Because every 1 percent decrease in blood cholesterol levels decreases the risk of heart disease by 2 percent, high fiber intake can decrease the risk of heart disease substantially. Studies show a 20 to 40 percent difference in heart disease risk between the highest and lowest fiber intake groups.[50]

Fiber from oat bran, legumes, and psyllium may lower serum cholesterol levels by binding bile acids in the gastrointestinal tract and preventing their reabsorption into the body. Bile acids are made from cholesterol in the liver and are secreted into the intestinal tract to aid with fat absorption. (See Chapter 3, "Digestion and Absorption.") When dietary fiber prevents their reabsorption, new bile acids must be made in the liver from cholesterol, reducing blood cholesterol levels. The short-chain fatty acids produced from bacterial fermentation of fiber in the large intestine may also inhibit cholesterol synthesis.[51]

Studies also show an association between high intake of whole grains and low risk of heart disease.[52] Whole grains contain not only fiber but also antioxidants, which may protect against cellular damage that promotes heart disease. It is likely that the combination of compounds found in grains, rather than any one component, explains the protective effects against heart disease.[53] Consuming at least three 1-ounce servings of whole grains each day can reduce heart disease risk.[54]

Fiber and Gastrointestinal Disorders

Fiber, particularly cellulose from cereal grains, helps promote healthy gastrointestinal functioning. High fiber intake also helps in treating certain gastrointestinal disorders.[55]

Diets rich in fiber add bulk and increase water in the stool, softening the stool and making it easier to pass. Fiber also accelerates passage of food through the intestinal tract, promoting regularity. If fluid intake is also ample, high fiber intake helps prevent and treat constipation, hemorrhoids (swelling of rectal veins), and diverticular disease (development of pouches on the intestinal wall).

Negative Health Effects of Excess Fiber

Despite its health advantages, high fiber intake can cause problems, especially for people who drastically increase their fiber intake in a short period of time. If you increase your fiber intake, you also should increase your water intake to prevent the stool from becoming hard and impacted. A sudden increase in fiber intake also can cause increased intestinal gas and bloating. These problems can be prevented both by increasing fiber intake gradually over several weeks and by drinking plenty of fluids.

High fiber intake may also bind small amounts of minerals in the GI tract and prevent them from being absorbed. In particular, fiber binds the minerals zinc, calcium, and iron. For people who get enough of these minerals, the recommended amounts of dietary fiber will not significantly affect mineral status.[56]

American Dietetic Association

Health Implications of Dietary Fiber

It is the position of the American Dietetic Association (ADA) that the public should consume adequate amounts of dietary fiber from a variety of plant foods.

J Am Diet Assoc. 2002;102:993–1000.
Reprinted with permission.

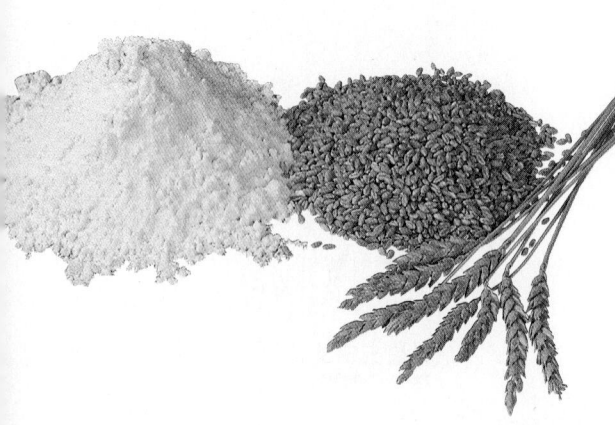

If the diet contains high amounts of fiber, some people, such as young children and the elderly, may become full before meeting their energy and nutrient needs. Because of a limited stomach capacity, they must be careful that their fiber intake does not interfere with their ability to consume adequate energy and nutrients.

Due to the bulky nature of fibers, excess consumption is likely to be self-limiting. Although a high fiber intake may cause occasional adverse gastrointestinal symptoms, serious chronic adverse effects have not been observed. As part of an overall healthy diet, a high intake of fiber will not produce significant deleterious effects in healthy people. Therefore, a Tolerable Upper Intake Level (UL) is not set for fiber.

Key Concepts: *High sugar intake promotes dental caries and can contribute to nutrient deficiencies by replacing more nutritious foods in the diet. High intake of foods rich in dietary fiber offers many health benefits, including reduced risk of obesity, type 2 diabetes, cardiovascular disease, and gastrointestinal disorders. Increase fiber intake gradually while drinking plenty of fluids; children and the elderly with small appetites should take care that their energy needs are still met. The DRIs do not contain a UL for fiber.*

Quick Bites

Fierce Fiber and Flatulence

The Jerusalem artichoke surpasses even dry beans in its capacity for facilitating flatulence. This artichoke contains large amounts of nondigestible carbohydrate. After passing through the small intestine undigested, the fiber is attacked by gas-generating bacteria in the colon.

Label [to] **Table**

This label highlights all the carbohydrate-related information you can find on a food label. Look at the center of the Nutrition Facts label and you'll see the Total Carbohydrates along with two of the carbohydrate "subgroups": Dietary Fiber and Sugars. Recall that carbohydrates are classified into simple carbohydrates and the two complex carbohydrates starch and fiber.

Using this food label you can determine all three of these components. There are 19 total grams of carbohydrate with 14 grams coming from sugars and 0 grams from fiber. This means the remaining 5 grams must be from starch, which is not required to be listed separately on the label. Without even knowing what food this label represents, you can decipher that it contains a high proportion of sugar (14 of the 19 grams) and is probably sweet. If this is a fruit juice, that level of sugar would be expected; but if this is cereal, you'd be getting a lot more sugar than complex carbohydrates, and probably not be making the best choice!

Do you see the 6% listed to the right of "Total Carbohydrates"? This doesn't mean that the food item contains 6% of its calories from carbohydrate. Instead, it refers to the daily allotment (or Daily Value) of carbohydrates listed at the bottom of the label. There you can see that a person consuming 2,000 kcalories per day should consume 300 grams of carbohydrates each day. This product contributes 19 grams per serving, which is just 6% of the Daily Value of 300 grams per day. Note that the % Daily Value for fiber is 0% because this food item lacks fiber.

The last highlighted section on this label, at the bottom of some Nutrition Facts labels, is the number of calories in a gram of carbohydrate. Recall that carbohydrates contain 4 kilocalories per gram. Armed with this information and the product's calorie information, can you calculate the percentage of calories that come from carbohydrate?

Here's how:

19 g carbohydrate × 4 kcal per g = 76 carbohydrate kcal

76 carbohydrate kcal ÷ 154 total kcal = 0.49 or 49% carbohydrate kcal

Nutrition Facts

Serving Size: 1 cup (248g)
Servings Per Container: 4

Amount Per Serving

Calories 154 Calories from fat 35

	% Daily Value*
Total Fat 4g	6%
Saturated Fat 2.5g	12%
Trans Fat 0.5g	
Cholesterol 20mg	7%
Sodium 170mg	7%
Total Carbohydrate 19g	6%
Dietary Fiber 0g	0%
Sugars 14g	
Protein 11g	

Vitamin A 4%	•	Vitamin C 6%
Calcium 40%	•	Iron 0%

* Percent Daily Values are based on a 2,000 calorie diet. Your daily values may be higher or lower depending on your calorie needs:

		Calories:	2,000	2,500
Total Fat	Less Than		65g	80g
Sat Fat	Less Than		20g	25g
Cholesterol	Less Than		300mg	300mg
Sodium	Less Than		2,400mg	2,400mg
Total Carbohydrate			300g	375g
Dietary Fiber			25g	30g

Calories per gram:
Fat 9 · Carbohydrate 4 · Protein 4

LEARNING *Portfolio* chapter 4

Key Terms

	page		page
acesulfame K [ay-SUL-fame]	168	hypoglycemia [HIGH-po-gly-SEE-mee-uh]	162
alpha (α) bonds	154	insulin [IN-suh-lin]	158
amylopectin [am-ih-low-PEK-tin]	152	ketone bodies	158
amylose [AM-ih-lose]	152	ketosis [kee-TOE-sis]	158
aspartame [AH-spar-tame]	166	lactose [LAK-tose]	150
beta (β) bonds	154	lignins [LIG-nins]	154
β-glucans	154	maltose [MALL-tose]	150
blood glucose levels	158	monosaccharides	147
bran	164	mucilages	154
cellulose [SELL-you-los]	153	neotame	170
chitin	154	nonnutritive sweeteners	166
chitosan	154	nutritive sweeteners	166
complex carbohydrates	151	oligosaccharides	151
condensation	149	pancreatic amylase	154
dental caries [KARE-ees]	171	pectins	153
diabetes mellitus	162	pentoses	149
dietary fiber	152	phenylketonuria (PKU)	166
dihydrochalcones (DHCs)	170	polyols	166
disaccharides [dye-SACK-uh-rides]	147	polysaccharides	151
endosperm	164	psyllium	154
epinephrine	158	reactive hypoglycemia	162
fasting hypoglycemia	162	refined sweeteners	166
fructose [FROOK-tose]	149	resistant starch	152
functional fiber	152	saccharin [SAK-ah-ren]	166
galactose [gah-LAK-tose]	149	simple carbohydrates	147
germ	164	starch	151
glucagon [GLOO-kuh-gon]	158	stevia	170
glucose [GLOO-kose]	148	stevioside	170
glycemic index	158	sucralose	168
glycogen [GLY-ko-jen]	152	sucrose [SOO-crose]	150
glycyrrhizin	170	sugar alcohols	149
gums	154	D-tagatose	170
hemicelluloses [hem-ih-SELL-you-loses]	153	thaumatin	170
husk	164	total fiber	153
		trehalose	170

Study Points

➤ Carbohydrates include the simple sugars and complex carbohydrates.

➤ Monosaccharides are the building blocks of carbohydrates.

➤ Three monosaccharides are important in human nutrition: glucose, fructose, and galactose.

➤ The monosaccharides combine to make disaccharides: sucrose, lactose, and maltose.

➤ Starch, glycogen, and fiber are long chains (polysaccharides) of glucose units.

➤ Carbohydrates are digested by enzymes from the mouth, pancreas, and small intestine and absorbed as monosaccharides.

➤ The liver converts the monosaccharides fructose and galactose to glucose.

➤ Blood glucose levels rise after eating and fall between meals. Two pancreatic hormones, insulin and glucagon, regulate blood glucose levels, preventing extremely high or low levels.

➤ Hyperglycemia results from a lack of insulin or ineffective insulin.

➤ Hypoglycemia results when blood glucose falls too low.

➤ The main function of carbohydrates in the body is to supply energy. In this role, carbohydrates spare protein for use in making body proteins, and allow for the complete breakdown of fat as an additional energy source.

➤ Carbohydrates are found mainly in plant foods as starch, fiber, and sugar.

➤ In general, Americans consume more sugar and less starch and fiber than is recommended.

➤ Carbohydrate intake can affect health. Excess sugar can contribute to low nutrient intake, excess energy intake, and dental caries.

➤ Diets high in complex carbohydrates, including fiber, have been linked to reduced risk for GI disorders, heart disease, and cancer.

Study Questions

1. **Describe the difference between starch and fiber.**

2. **How will eating excessive amounts of carbohydrate affect health?**

3. **What are the consequences of eating too little carbohydrate?**

4. **List the benefits of eating more fiber. What are the consequences of eating too much? Too little?**

5. **Which foods contain carbohydrates?**

6. **What advantage does the branched-chain structure of glycogen provide compared to a straight chain of glucose?**

7. **Which blood glucose regulation hormone is secreted in the recently fed state? The fasting state?**

8. **Describe the structure of a monosaccharide, disaccharide, and polysaccharide.**

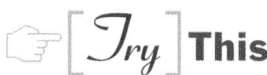

The Fiber Type Experiment

This experiment is to help you understand the difference between sources of dietary fiber. Go to the store and buy a small amount of raw bran. It is usually sold in a bin at a health food store or near the hot cereals in a grocery store. Also purchase some pectin (near the baking items) or some Metamucil (in the pharmacy section). Once you're home, fill two glasses with water and put the raw bran in one glass and the pectin or Metamucil in the other. Stir each glass for a minute or two and watch what happens. Describe the differences. What would happen in your GI tract?

The Sweetness of Soda

This experiment is to help you understand the amount of sugar found in a can of soda. Take a glass and fill it with 12 ounces (1½ cups) of water. Using a measuring spoon, add 10 to 12 teaspoons of sugar to the water. Stir the sugar water until all the sucrose has dissolved. Now sip the water. Does it taste sweet? It shouldn't taste any sweeter than a can of regular soda. This is the amount of sugar found in one 12-ounce can!

What About Bobbie?

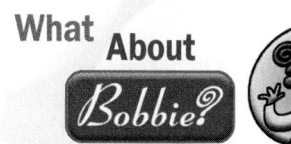

Refer to Chapter 1 to see the complete list of food and drinks from Bobbie's recorded intake. Let's examine her day of eating using the guidelines you've learned in this chapter. How well did Bobbie do? Did she meet her overall carbohydrate goal? Did she consume 45 to 65 percent of her calories from carbohydrates? Was her diet made up mostly of complex carbohydrates or simple sugars? Let's take a look.

Her overall carbohydrate intake was 292 grams or 1,168 kilocalories. Her total energy intake was 2,300 kilocalories, which means 51 percent of her calories were from carbohydrate. This is within the Acceptable Macronutrient Distribution Range (AMDR) for carbohydrate. Here are the biggest contributors, which supply more than 80 percent of Bobbie's carbohydrate intake:

Food	Carbohydrate (g)	Percentage of calorie intake (%)
Spaghetti	60	10
Bread (lunch and dinner)	53	9
Bagel	39	7
Banana	27	5
Tortilla chips	27	5
Pizza	24	4
Spaghetti sauce	10	1.7
Cookie	9	1.5

Review the list of Bobbie's foods again. Do you think her carbohydrate intake comes mostly from complex sources or simple sugars? Very few of her carbohydrate sources are high in sugars: just the banana, the sugar for the coffee, and the chocolate chip cookie.

Let's take a closer look at Bobbie's carbohydrate intake. Which food groups contribute the most to her carbohydrate intake? To answer this question, let's divide her carbohydrate-dense foods into the three carbohydrate-rich food groups:

Food Group	Number of Servings	
	Bobbie's	Recommended*
GRAINS GROUP		
Bagel	2	
Bread (lunch)	2	
Bread (dinner)	1	
Tortilla chips	2	
Pasta	3	
Pizza	1	
Total	11 oz eq	7 oz eq (3.5 as a whole grain)

What About Bobbie?

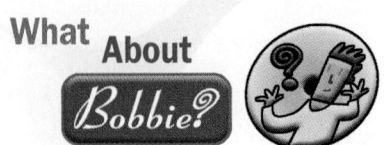

Food Group		Number of Servings	
		Bobbie's	Recommended*
FRUIT GROUP			
Banana		1 cup	
	Total	1 cup	2 cups
VEGETABLE GROUP			
Lettuce		1 cup	
Sandwich and salad toppings		¹/₂ cup	
Salsa		¹/₂ cup	
Green beans		¹/₂ cup	
	Total	2¹/₂ cups	3 cups

*Based on USDA's MyPyramid food intake patterns for 2,200 kilocalories.

So, now that you've reviewed Bobbie's food group totals, what can you conclude about her carbohydrate intake? Her total carbohydrate calories are within the recommended range, but her diet still could use some improvement. Bobbie has plenty of servings for grains, but no whole grains. She is low in fruits, and her vegetable choices could be a little more varied. Adding a half-cup of orange juice for breakfast and another piece of fresh fruit during the day would help. Choosing spinach or romaine lettuce for her salad would broaden her vegetable choices, and a whole-wheat bagel instead of cinnamon raisin would be a good start for adding more whole grains.

References

1 Eastwood M. *Principles of Human Nutrition.* New York: Chapman & Hall, 1997.

2 Institute of Medicine, Food and Nutrition Board. *Dietary Reference Intakes for Energy, Carbohydrate, Fiber, Fat, Fatty Acids, Cholesterol, Protein, and Amino Acids (Macronutrients).* Washington, DC: National Academy Press, 2005.

3 Newburg DS, Ruiz-Palacios GM, Morrow AL. Human milk glycans protect infants against enteric pathogens. *Annu Rev Nutr.* 2005;25:37–58.

4 Wang B, McVeagh P, Petocz P, Brand-Miller J. Brain ganglioside and glycoprotein sialic acid in breastfed compared with formula-fed infants. *Am J Clin Nutr.* 2003;78(5):1024–1029.

5 Eliasson AC. *Carbohydrates in Food.* New York: Marcel Dekker, 1996.

6 Institute of Medicine, Food and Nutrition Board. Op. cit.

7 World Health Organization. *Carbohydrates in Human Nutrition: Report of a Joint FAO/WHO Expert Consultation, Rome, 1997.* Geneva, Switzerland: World Health Organization, 1997. FAO Food and Nutrition Paper 66.

8 Meat processing. *Encyclopaedia Britannica* [online]. http://www.britannica.com/eb/article?eu=120856. Accessed 4/12/06.

9 Robyt JF. *Essentials of Carbohydrate Chemistry.* New York: Springer, 1998.

10 Flatt JP. Use and storage of carbohydrates. *Am J Clin Nutr.* 1995;61(suppl):952S–959S.

11 Miller GD. Carbohydrates in ultra-endurance exercise and athletic performance. In: Wolinski I, ed. *Nutrition in Exercise and Sport.* 3rd ed. Boca Raton, FL: CRC Press, 1998.

12 Institute of Medicine, Food and Nutrition Board. Op cit.

13 Graham LE, Graham JM, Wilcox LW. *Plant Biology.* Upper Saddle River, NJ: Prentice Hall, 2003.

14 Wong JM, de Souza R, Kendall CW, et al. Colonic health: fermentation and short chain fatty acids. *J Clin Gastroenterol.* 2006;40(3):235–243.

15 Martini FH. *Fundamentals of Anatomy and Physiology.* San Francisco, CA: Benjamin Cummings, 2004.

16 Martini FH. Op. cit.; and Berg JM, Tymoczko JL, Stryer L. *Biochemistry.* 5th ed. New York: W.H. Freeman, 2002.

17 Martini FH. Op. cit.

18 Ibid.

19 Ibid.

20 Berg JM, Tymoczko JL, Stryer L. Op. cit.

21 Institute of Medicine, Food and Nutrition Board. Op cit.

22 Martini FH. Op. cit.

23 Institute of Medicine, Food and Nutrition Board. Op. cit.

24 Jenkins DJA, Kendall CWC, Augustin LSA, et al. Glycemic index: overview of implications in health and disease. *Am J Clin Nutr.* 2002;76(suppl):266S–273S.

25 National Digestive Diseases Information Clearinghouse. *National Diabetes Statistics.* November 2005. NIH publication 06-3892. http://diabetes.niddk.nih.gov/dm/pubs/statistics/index.htm. Accessed 4/11/06.

26 Diabetes Prevention Program Research Group. Reduction in the incidence of type 2 diabetes with lifestyle intervention or metformin. *New Engl J Med.* 2002;346:393–403.

27 National Digestive Diseases Information Clearinghouse. Op. cit.

28 Institute of Medicine, Food and Nutrition Board. Op. cit.

29 US Departments of Agriculture and Health and Human Services. *Dietary Guidelines for Americans, 2005.* 6th ed. Washington, DC: US Government Printing Office, 2005.

30 World Health Organization. *Diet, Nutrition and the Prevention of Chronic Diseases: A Report of a Joint WHO/FAO Expert Consultation.* Geneva, Switzerland: World Health Organization, 2003. WHO Technical Report Series 916.

31 Institute of Medicine, Food and Nutrition Board. Op. cit.

32 Ibid.

33 Dietary Guidelines Advisory Committee. *Report of the Dietary Guidelines Advisory Committee on the Dietary Guidelines for Americans, 2005.* http://www.health.gov/dietaryguidelines/dga2005/report/. Accessed 4/12/06.

34 Welsh JA, Cogswell ME, Rogers S, et al. Overweight among low-income preschool children associated with the consumption of sweet drinks: Missouri, 1999–2002. *Pediatrics.* 2005;115:223–229.

35 US Food and Drug Administration. Whole grain label statements—draft guidance. February 17, 2006. http://www.cfsan.fda.gov/~dms/flgragui.html. Accessed 5/7/06.

36 Giboney M, Sigman-Grant M, Stanton JL, Keast DR. Consumption of sugars. *Am J Clin Nutr.* 1995;62(suppl): 178S–194S; and Coulston AM, Johnson RK. Sugar and sugars: myth and realities. *J Am Diet Assoc.* 2002;102:351–353.

37 American Dietetic Association. Position of the American Dietetic Association: use of nutritive and nonnutritive sweeteners. *J Am Diet Assoc.* 2004;104:255–275.

38 US Department of Health and Human Services, National Toxicology Program. *Report on Carcinogens.* 11th ed. January 31, 2005. http://ntp.niehs.nih.gov/index.cfm?objectid= 32BA9724-F1F6-975E-7FCE50709CB4C932. Accessed 4/12/06.

39 Butchko HH, Stargel WW, Comer CP, et al. Aspartame: review of safety. *Regul Toxicol Pharmacol.* 2002;35:S1–S93.

40 American Dietetic Association. Op. cit.

41 Ibid.

42 Murray R, Frankowski B, Taras H. Are soft drinks a scapegoat for childhood obesity? *J Pediatr.* 2005;146(5):586–590.

43 Is sugar bad for you? *Harvard Health Letter.* February 2001; 26:1–2.

44 US Departments of Agriculture and Health and Human Services. Op. cit.

45 American Dental Association. *Fluoridation Facts.* Chicago: American Dental Association, 2005. http://www.ada.org/public/topics/fluoride/facts/index.asp. Accessed 5/8/06.

46 Institute of Medicine, Food and Nutrition Board. Op. cit.

47 Ibid.

48 Anderson JW, Randles KM, Kendall CW, et al. Carbohydrate and fiber recommendations for individuals with diabetes: a quantitative assessment and meta-analysis of the evidence. *J Am Coll Nutr.* 2004;23:5–17.

49 Institute of Medicine, Food and Nutrition Board. Op. cit.

50 Ibid.

51 Pereira DI, Gibson GR. Effects of consumption of probiotics and prebiotics on serum lipid levels in humans. *Crit Rev Biochem Mol Biol.* 2002;37(4):259–281.

52 Jacobs DR, Meyer KA, Kushi LH, Folsom AR. Whole-grain intake may reduce the risk of ischemic heart disease death in postmenopausal women: the Iowa Women's Health Study. *Am J Clin Nutr.* 1998;68:248–257; and Willet WC, Hu FB. Optimal diets for prevention of coronary heart disease. *JAMA.* 2002;288(20):2569–2578.

53 Slavin JL, Jacobs D, Marquart L, Wiemer K. The role of whole grains in disease prevention. *J Am Diet Assoc.* 2001;101: 780–785.

54 US Departments of Agriculture and Health and Human Services. Op. cit.

55 Institute of Medicine, Food and Nutrition Board. Op. cit.

56 Ibid.

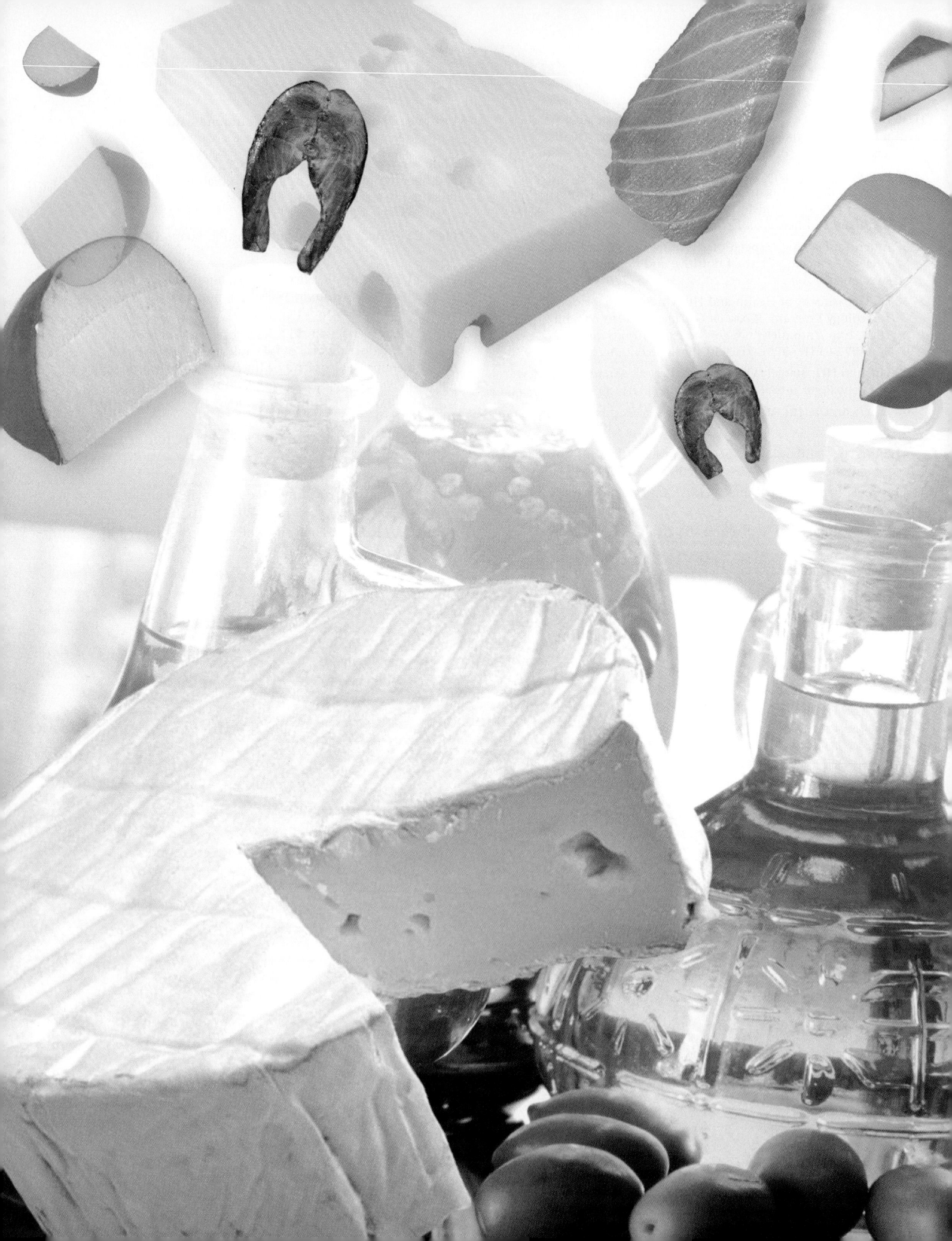

Chapter 5

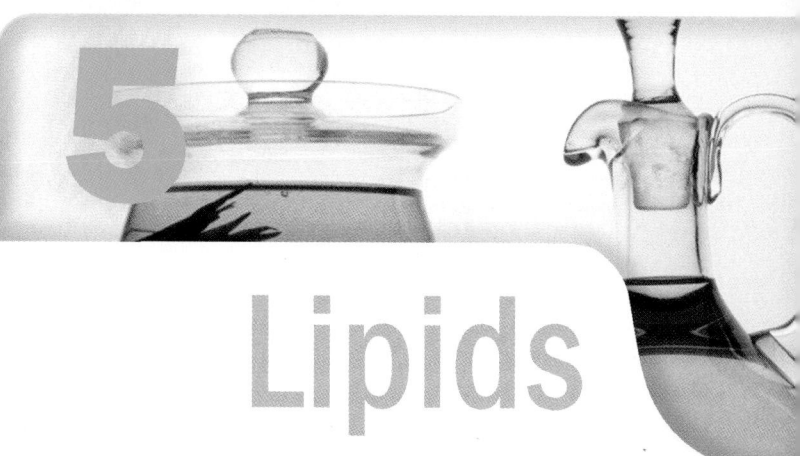

Lipids

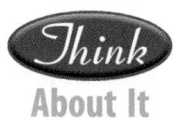

Think About It

1 How important is fat to the foods you think of as tasty?
2 Can one have too little body fat?
3 What's your take on the differences between fat and cholesterol?
4 What's your understanding of "good" versus "bad" cholesterol?

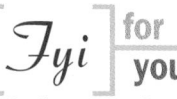

Fyi for your Information

This chapter's FYI boxes include practical information on the following topics:

- Fats on the Health Store Shelf
- Which Spread for Your Bread?
- Does "Reduced Fat" Reduce Calories? That Depends on the Food

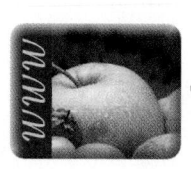

The Web site for this book offers many useful tools and is a great source for additional nutrition information for both students and instructors. Visit the site at nutrition.jbpub.com for information on lipids. You'll find exercises that explore the following topics:

- Olestra: Snack Without the Guilt?
- Fat, Low-Fat, No-Fat?
- Fats and Cholesterol

What About Bobbie?

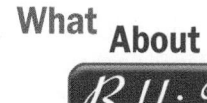

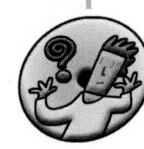

Track the choices Bobbie is making with Nutritionist Pro or EatRight Analysis software.

Key to Illustrations

●	Chylomicron
✦	Energy
⌁	Fatty Acids
⣿	Glycerol
⣿	Phospholipids
⬡⬡	Sterols
⣿	Triglycerides
◌	Water

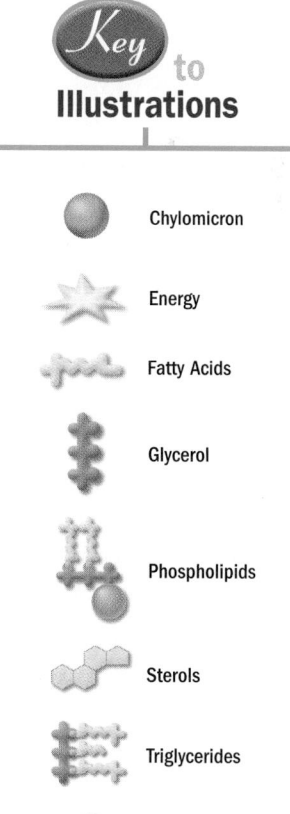

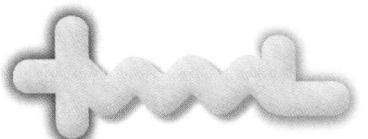

A generic fatty acid

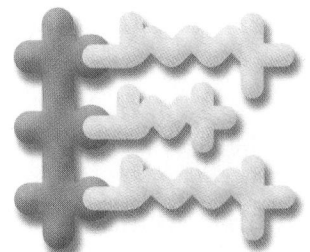

A generic triglyceride

aria and Rachel are trying to lose weight. Maria swears by a new diet program that allows you to eat all the fat you want, but no high-carbohydrate, "starchy" foods. Her diet is working—she's already lost 10 pounds! Then there's Rachel, whose goal in life is to eat zero grams of fat. She's fat-obsessed—always insisting on "fat-free" everything, and driving her friends nuts with information about the number of fat grams in whatever they eat. As you listen to the two of them compare dieting stories, you wonder which one has the right approach to fat consumption, or even whether there *is* a right approach. On the one hand, it seems that you hear a lot about American high-fat diets and high rates of obesity and heart disease. On the other hand, can a "no-fat" diet be healthy? Are all low-fat and no-fat products really more nutritious?

Fat is an essential nutrient. Although our bodies are very good at making and storing fat in the form of triglycerides, they cannot make some types of fatty acids (a component of triglycerides), so these compounds must come from the diet. Triglycerides—the fats we associate with fried foods, cream cheese, vegetable oil, or salad dressing—are one type of a larger group of compounds called lipids. Cholesterol, another lipid, is familiar to most Americans, but you may not realize that your body makes cholesterol and that your dietary cholesterol makes only a small contribution to the total amount in your body. All lipids have important roles, but at the same time, too much triglyceride or too much cholesterol can increase the risk for chronic disease.

Fats contribute greatly to the flavor and texture of foods. When you take out the fat, sometimes you have to boost the flavor with sugar, sodium, or other additives to have a tasty product. This means that fat-free foods sometimes aren't any lower in calories than regular food—so Rachel can't eat the whole box of fat-free cookies and still expect to lose weight!

Once you have an idea of the role of lipids in the body and in foods, you'll be able to apply the principles of moderation, balance, and variety in selecting a healthful, enjoyable diet with neither too much nor too little fat.

What Are Lipids?

The term *lipids* applies to a broad range of organic molecules that dissolve easily in organic solvents such as alcohol, ether, or acetone, but are much less soluble in water. Lipids generally are **hydrophobic** (averse to water; literally "water-fearing") and **lipophilic** (soluble in fat and fat solvents; literally "fat-loving"). In contrast, water-soluble substances are, not surprisingly, **hydrophilic** (attracted to water, "water loving") and

hydrophobic Insoluble in water.

lipophilic Attracted to fat and fat solvents; fat-soluble.

hydrophilic [high-dro-FILL-ik] Readily interacting with water (literally, "water-loving"). Hydrophilic compounds are polar and soluble in water.

lipophobic Adverse to fat solvents; insoluble in fat and fat solvents.

phospholipids Compounds that consist of a glycerol molecule bonded to two fatty acid molecules and to a phosphate group with a nitrogen-containing component. Phospholipids have both hydrophilic and hydrophobic regions that make them good emulsifiers.

sterols A category of lipids that includes cholesterol. Sterols are hydrocarbons with several rings in their structures.

fatty acids Compounds containing a long hydrocarbon chain with a carboxyl group (COOH) at one end and a methyl group (CH_3) at the other end.

chain length The number of carbons that a fatty acid contains. Foods contain fatty acids with chain lengths of 4 to 24 carbons, and most have an even number of carbons.

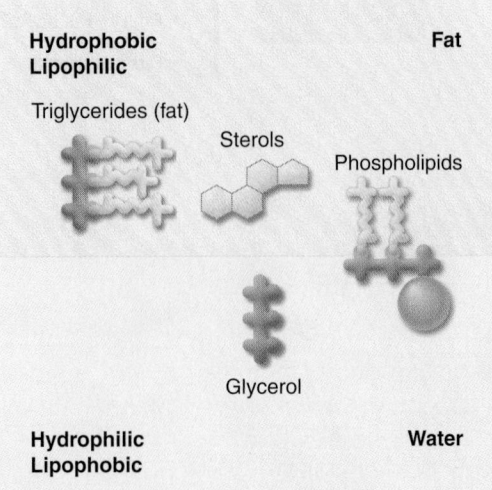

Hydrophobic Lipophilic	**Fat**

Triglycerides (fat)

Sterols

Phospholipids

Glycerol

Hydrophilic Lipophobic	**Water**

Think About It

1

lipophobic (averse to fat solvents, "fat fearing"). Lipids vary in their solubilities, with some being very hydrophobic and others less so. The main classes of lipids found in foods and in the body are triglycerides, phospholipids, and sterols.

Triglycerides are the largest category of lipids. In the body, fat cells store triglycerides in adipose tissue. In foods, we call triglycerides "fats and oils," with fats usually being solid and oils being liquid at room temperature. Overall, however, the choice of terminology—*fat, triglyceride, oil*—is somewhat arbitrary, and the terms are often used interchangeably. In this chapter, when we use the word *fat* or *oil*, we are referring to triglycerides.

About 2 percent of dietary lipids are **phospholipids**. They are found in foods of both plant and animal origin, and the body also makes those that it needs. Unlike other lipids, phospholipids are soluble in both fat and water. These versatile molecules play crucial roles as a major constituent in cell membranes, and in blood and body fluids, where they help keep fats suspended in these watery fluids.

Only a small percentage of our dietary lipids are **sterols**, yet one infamous member, cholesterol, generates much public concern. The body makes cholesterol, which is an important component of cell membranes and a precursor in the synthesis of sex hormones, adrenal hormones (e.g., cortisol), vitamin D, and bile salts.

Lipids share similar functional properties, solubility, and transport mechanisms, although the composition and structure of individual molecules vary. Fatty acids are components of both triglycerides and phospholipids and are often attached to cholesterol.

Fatty Acids Are Key Building Blocks

Fatty acids determine the characteristics of a fat, such as whether it is solid or liquid at room temperature. Fatty acids that are not joined to another compound, such as the glycerol of a triglyceride, are sometimes called "free" fatty acids, to emphasize that they are unattached. Some free fatty acids have their own distinct flavor. Butyric acid, for example, is the fatty acid that gives butter its flavor (see **Figure 5.1**). Caproic, caprylic, and capric acids, all named after the Greek word for "goat," have the undesirable "goaty" flavors and odors that their names suggest. They may be present as free fatty acids in spoiled foods, contributing to a strong unpleasant odor.

Although there are many kinds of fatty acids, they are basically chains of carbon atoms with an organic acid (carboxyl) group (–COOH) at one end and a methyl group (–CH₃) at the other end.

Chain Length

Fatty acids differ in **chain length** (the number of carbons in the chain). Foods contain fatty acids with chain lengths of 4 to 24 carbons, and most have an even number of carbons. They are grouped as short-chain (fewer than 6 carbons), medium-chain (6 to 10 carbons), and long-chain (12 or more carbons) fatty acids. (See **Figure 5.2**.) The shorter the carbon chain, the more liquid the fatty acid (the lower its

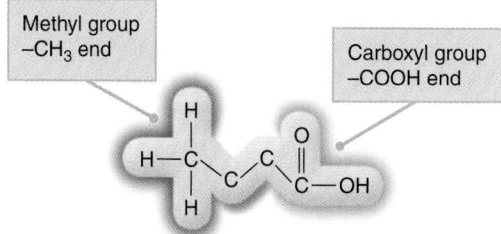

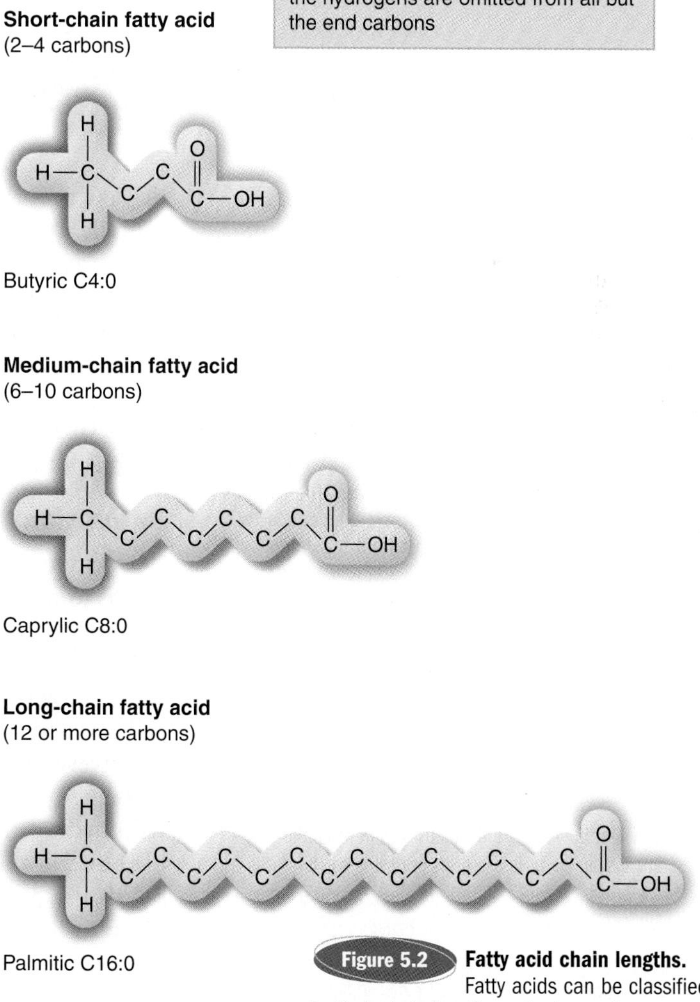

Figure 5.1 **Fatty acid structure.** The basic structure of a fatty acid is a carbon chain with a methyl end (–CH₃) and an acid (carboxyl) end (–COOH). Butyric acid (shown here) is a fatty acid found in butter fat.

Methyl group
–CH₃ end

Carboxyl group
–COOH end

Butyric acid

For simplicity in most of these pictures the hydrogens are omitted from all but the end carbons

Short-chain fatty acid
(2–4 carbons)

Butyric C4:0

Medium-chain fatty acid
(6–10 carbons)

Caprylic C8:0

Long-chain fatty acid
(12 or more carbons)

Palmitic C16:0

Figure 5.2 **Fatty acid chain lengths.** Fatty acids can be classified by their chain length as short-, medium-, or long-chain fatty acids.

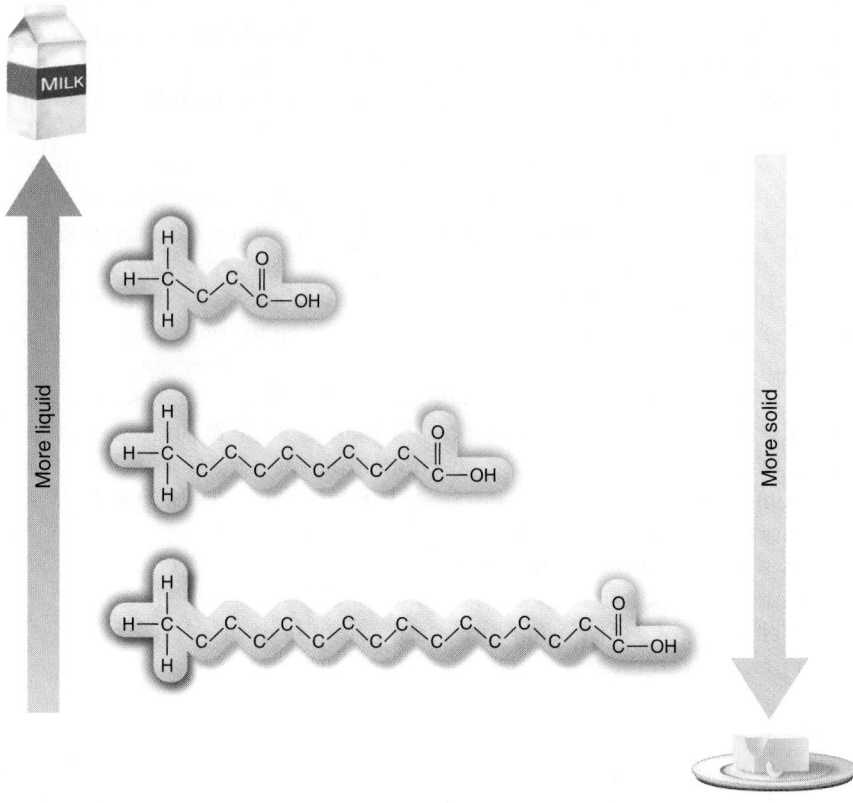

Figure 5.3 **Fatty acid chain lengths and liquidity.** As chain length of saturated fatty acids increases, they become more solid at room temperature.

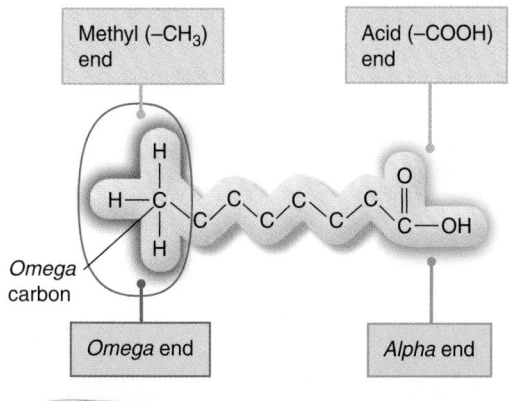

Figure 5.4 **Fatty acid nomenclature.** The carbons are identified by their locations in the chain. While some disciplines count from the *alpha* carbon, nutritionists count from the *omega* carbon.

saturated fatty acid A fatty acid completely filled by hydrogen with all carbons in the chain linked by single bonds.

unsaturated fatty acid A fatty acid in which the carbon chain contains one or more double bonds.

monounsaturated fatty acid A fatty acid in which the carbon chain contains one double bond.

polyunsaturated fatty acid A fatty acid in which the carbon chain contains two or more double bonds.

melting point). (See **Figure 5.3**.) Shorter fatty acids are also more water-soluble, a property that affects their absorption in the digestive tract.

Each carbon in these chains can be numbered for identification, but it's important to know from which end the counting begins. In organic chemistry, the scientific naming of fatty acids counts from the carbon at the acid (–COOH) end. This carbon is the *alpha* carbon, and the carbon at the methyl (–CH₃) end is the *omega* carbon. They are named after the first and last letters of the Greek alphabet, respectively. (See **Figure 5.4**.) Nutritionists identify double bonds by their location relative to the *omega* carbon, as you'll see later.

Saturation

Within a fatty acid chain, each carbon atom has four bonds. When a carbon is joined to adjacent carbons with single bonds (–C–C–C–), it still has two bonds available for other atoms, such as hydrogen atoms. If all the carbons in the chain are joined with single bonds and the remaining bonds are filled with hydrogen, the fatty acid is called a **saturated fatty acid**. It is fully loaded (saturated) with hydrogen.

However, if adjoining carbons are connected by a double bond (C=C), there are two fewer bonds holding hydrogen, so the chain is not saturated with hydrogen. This is an **unsaturated fatty acid**. A fatty acid with one double bond is a **monounsaturated fatty acid**; one with two or more double bonds is a **polyunsaturated fatty acid** (often abbreviated MUFA and PUFA, respectively). **Figure 5.5** illustrates the three types of fatty acids.

Foods never contain only unsaturated or only saturated fatty acids. Instead, food fats are a mixture of fatty acid types, so it is technically wrong to refer to a particular food fat as a "saturated fat." However, food fats with more unsat-

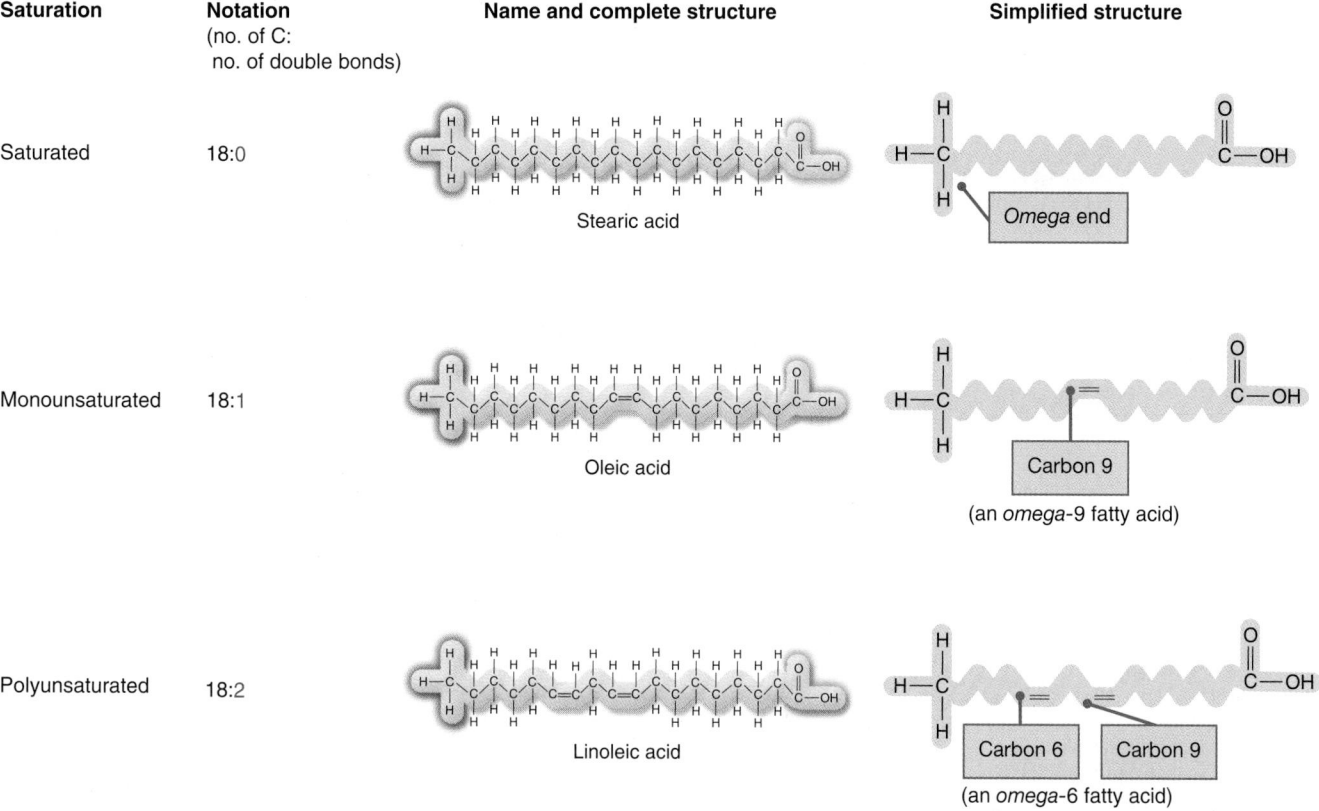

Saturation	Notation (no. of C: no. of double bonds)	Name and complete structure	Simplified structure
Saturated	18:0	Stearic acid	*Omega* end
Monounsaturated	18:1	Oleic acid	Carbon 9 (an *omega*-9 fatty acid)
Polyunsaturated	18:2	Linoleic acid	Carbon 6 Carbon 9 (an *omega*-6 fatty acid)

Figure 5.5 **Saturated, monosaturated, and polyunsaturated fatty acids.** Hydrogens saturate the carbon chain of a saturated fatty acid. Unsaturated fatty acids are missing some hydrogens and have one (mono) or more (poly) carbon–carbon double bonds.

urated fatty acids typically have lower melting points and are more likely to be liquid at room temperature. Foods rich in saturated fatty acids tend to be solid at room temperature and have higher melting points. (See **Figure 5.6**.) For example, stearic acid, an 18-carbon saturated fatty acid, is abundant in chocolate and meat fats, both of which are solid at room temperature. The major fatty acid of olive oil is 18-carbon monounsaturated oleic acid. Olive oil is a thick liquid at room temperature, but may solidify under refrigeration. The major fatty acid of soybean oil is an 18-carbon fatty acid with two double bonds called linoleic acid, and soybean oil is a thin liquid at room temperature. And 18-carbon *alpha*-linolenic acid, a fatty acid with three double bonds, is abundant in flaxseed oil, a very thin liquid at room temperature.

Key Concepts: *The term* lipids *refers to a group of organic molecules that are soluble in organic solvents and less soluble in water, including triglycerides, phospholipids, and sterols. Fatty acids are key structural components of both triglycerides and phospholipids and are sometimes attached to cholesterol. Fatty acids are carbon chains of varying lengths. Those with no double bonds between carbon atoms are called* saturated, *whereas those with at least one double bond are called* unsaturated.

Geometric and Positional Isomers

Otherwise identical unsaturated fatty acids can exist in different geometric forms, or isomers. In most naturally occurring unsaturated fatty acids, the hydrogens next to double bonds are on the same side of the carbon chain. This is called a *cis* formation. The carbon chain of a *cis* **fatty acid** is bent. If

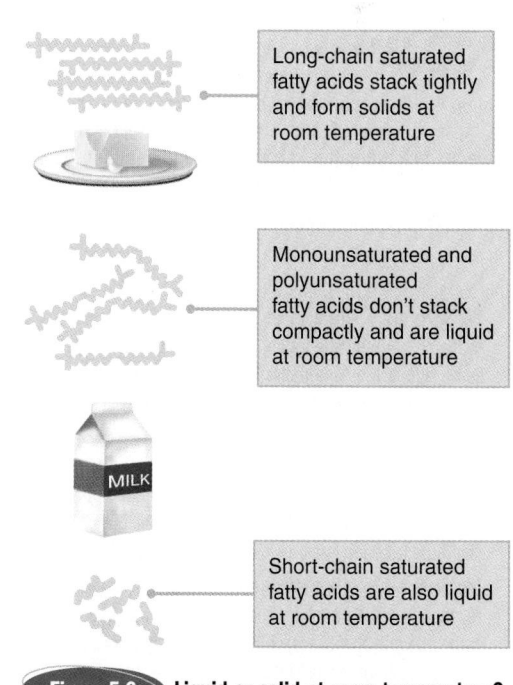

Long-chain saturated fatty acids stack tightly and form solids at room temperature

Monounsaturated and polyunsaturated fatty acids don't stack compactly and are liquid at room temperature

MILK

Short-chain saturated fatty acids are also liquid at room temperature

Figure 5.6 **Liquid or solid at room temperature?** Short-chain and unsaturated fatty acids cannot pack tightly together and tend to be more liquid than long-chain saturated fatty acids.

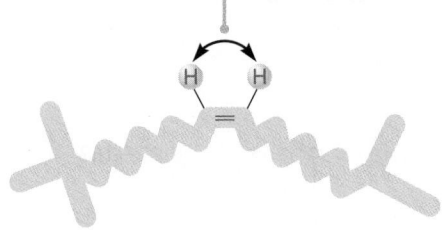

These two neighboring hydrogens repel each other, causing the carbon chain to bend

Cis form (bent)

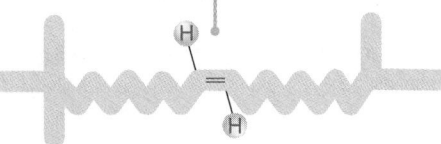

These two hydrogens are already as far apart as they can get

Trans form (straighter)

Figure 5.7 ***Cis* and *trans* fatty acids.** Fatty acids with the bent *cis* form are more common in food than the *trans* form. *Trans* fatty acids are most commonly found in hydrogentated fats, such as those in stick margarine, shortening, and deep-fat fried foods.

the double bond is altered, moving the hydrogens across from each other, the formation is called *trans* and the carbon chain is straighter. (See **Figure 5.7.**) There are small amounts of *trans* **fatty acids** in meats and dairy products from cows and sheep, but the commercial process of **hydrogenation**, or adding hydrogens where some of the double bonds are located in the unsaturated fatty acid, creates most of our dietary *trans* fatty acids.[1] Most *trans* fatty acids are monounsaturated, but a small number are fatty acids with two double bonds. *Trans* fatty acids have become a health concern because they have been shown to raise low-density lipoprotein (LDL) cholesterol levels and therefore increase one's risk for heart disease.

Conjugated linoleic acid (CLA) is a collective term for a group of geometric and positional isomers of linoleic acid in which the double bonds (*trans* or *cis*) are conjugated; that is, the double bonds occur without an intervening carbon atom not part of a double bond. Although present in only trace amounts in cow's milk, conjugated linoleic acid is being studied for potential positive health effects.

Small amounts of *trans* fatty acids and conjugated linoleic acid are present in all diets. They can serve as a source of fuel energy for the body. However, there are no known requirements for *trans* fatty acids and conjugated linoleic acid for specific body functions.[2]

Omega-3, *Omega*-6, and *Omega*-9 Fatty Acids

The location of the double bond closest to the *omega* (methyl) end of the fatty acid chain identifies a fatty acid's family. Oleic acid has one double bond, at carbon 9 (counting from the *omega* end of the chain) and is classified as an ***omega*-9 fatty acid**. Linoleic acid has double bonds both at carbon 6 and carbon 9. Because the first double bond occurs at carbon 6, it is an ***omega*-6 fatty acid**. ***Omega*-3 fatty acids** such as *alpha*-linolenic acid have a double bond at carbon 3, plus two or more additional double bonds. (See **Figure 5.8.**) All of these fatty acids can be burned for energy. When the body uses them to synthesize new compounds, however, the *omega*-3, *omega*-6, and *omega*-9 classes behave quite differently.

Nonessential and Essential Fatty Acids

The body is a good chemist, synthesizing most fatty acids as it needs them. The liver adds carbons in a process called **elongation** to build storage and structural fats, to manufacture the fat in breast milk, or to make fatty acids for use in other compounds. The body also synthesizes oleic acid, an

cis **fatty acid** Unsaturated fatty acid in which the hydrogens surrounding a double bond are both on the same side of the carbon chain, causing a bend in the chain. Most naturally occurring unsaturated fatty acids are *cis* fatty acids.

trans **fatty acids** Unsaturated fatty acids in which the hydrogens surrounding a double bond are on opposite sides of the carbon chain. This straightens the chain, and the fatty acid becomes more solid.

hydrogenation [high-dro-jen-AY-shun] A chemical reaction in which hydrogen atoms are added to carbon–carbon double bonds, converting them to single bonds. Hydrogenation of monounsaturated and polyunsaturated fatty acids reduces the number of double bonds they contain, thereby making them more saturated.

conjugated linoleic acid A polyunsaturated fatty acid in which the position of the double bonds has moved, so that a single bond alternates with two double bonds.

omega-9 fatty acid Any polyunsaturated fatty acid in which the first double bond starting from the methyl (CH_3) end of the molecule lies between the ninth and tenth carbon atoms.

omega-6 fatty acid Any polyunsaturated fatty acid in which the first double bond starting from the methyl (CH_3) end of the molecule lies between the sixth and seventh carbon atoms.

omega-3 fatty acids Any polyunsaturated fatty acid in which the first double bond starting from the methyl (CH_3) end of the molecule lies between the third and fourth carbon atoms.

elongation Addition of carbon atoms to fatty acids to lengthen them into new fatty acids.

desaturation Insertion of double bonds into fatty acids to change them into new fatty acids.

nonessential fatty acids The fatty acids that your body can make when they are needed. It is not necessary to consume them in the diet.

essential fatty acids The fatty acids that the body needs but cannot synthesize, and which must be obtained from diet.

eicosanoids A class of hormonelike substances formed in the body from long-chain fatty acids.

omega-9 fatty acid, by removing hydrogens from carbons 9 and 10 of saturated stearic acid, thus creating a double bond at carbon 9. This process is called **desaturation**. Oleic acid can be elongated further and desaturated to create other necessary fatty acids.

Because your body can make saturated and *omega*-9 fatty acids, it is not essential to get them in your diet. We therefore call them **nonessential fatty acids**. (Do not confuse "nonessential" with "unimportant." Your body ensures an adequate supply of nonessential fatty acids by making them when they are needed.)

Our bodies cannot produce carbon–carbon double bonds before the ninth carbon from the methyl end, so we cannot manufacture certain fatty acids such as *omega*-6 linoleic or *omega*-3 *alpha*-linolenic acids. They must come from food, so they're called **essential fatty acids** (EFA). (See **Figure 5.9**.) Deficiency of essential fatty acids is extremely rare. It typically occurs only with severe fat malabsorption or prolonged intravenous feeding without supplemental fat. A lack of linoleic acid leads to a scaly skin rash and dermatitis, poor growth in children, and a lowered immune response. In the few human cases where *alpha*-linolenic acid was lacking, neuropathy, visual problems, and poor growth were the results.[3]

Building Eicosanoids, *Omega*-3 and *Omega*-6 Fatty Acids

You metabolize most of the fatty acids you eat to supply your energy needs, but a small proportion become crucial chemical regulators. The **eicosanoids** (also called prostanoids) are one such group of regulators. These signaling molecules contain 20 or more carbons (*eikosi* is the Greek word for "twenty"). They have profound localized effects through their influence on inflammatory processes, blood vessel dilation and constriction, blood clotting, and more. Because they don't circulate throughout the body as hormones do, scientists sometimes call eicosanoids "local" hormones.

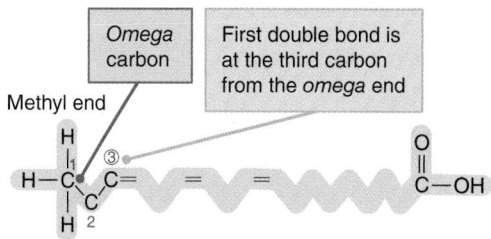

Alpha-linolenic, an *omega*-3 fatty acid

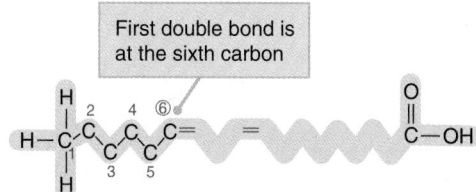

Linoleic, an *omega*-6 fatty acid

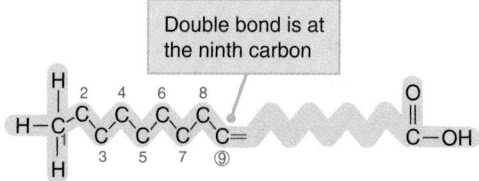

Oleic, an *omega*-9 fatty acid

Figure 5.8 **Omega-3, omega-6, and omega-9 fatty acids.** Unsaturated fatty acids can be classified by counting from the *omega* carbon to the location of the first double bond.

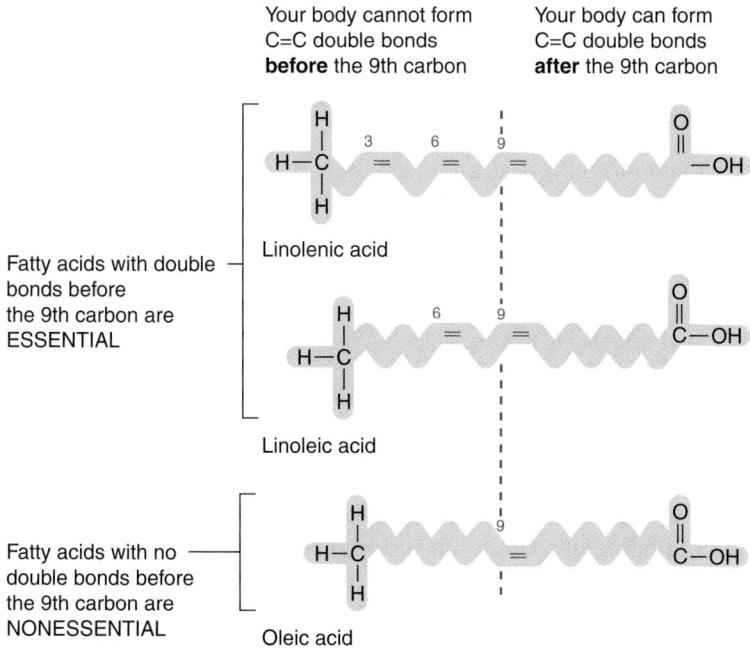

Figure 5.9 **Essential and nonessential fatty acids.** Your body makes some types of fatty acids, but others are essential in your diet.

American Heart Association

Omega-3 Fatty Acids

The American Heart Association recommends eating fish (particularly fatty fish) at least two times a week. Fish is a good source of protein and doesn't have the high saturated fat that fatty meat products do. Fatty fish like mackerel, lake trout, herring, sardines, albacore tuna, and salmon are high in two kinds of *omega*-3 fatty acids, eicosapentaenoic acid (EPA) and docosahexaenoic acid (DHA).

Some people with high triglycerides and patients with cardiovascular disease may benefit from more *omega*-3 fatty acids than they can easily get from diet alone. These people should talk to their doctor about taking supplements to reduce heart disease risk.

Reproduced with permission. www.americanheart.org.
© 2006, American Heart Association, Inc.

Table 5.1 *Omega*-6 to Eicosanoids

Linoleic acid	(18:2)
	desaturation
Gamma-linolenic acid	(18:3)
	elongation
Dihomo-*gamma*-linolenic acid	(20:3)
	desaturation
Arachidonic acid	(20:4)
	elongation
Eicosanoids	(22:4)
• thromboxanes	desaturation
• prostaglandins	(22:5)
• leukotrienes	long-chain fatty acid

Table 5.2 *Omega*-3 to Eicosanoids

Alpha-linolenic acid	(18:3)
	desaturation
	(18:4)
	elongation
	(20:4)
	desaturation
EPA (eicosapentaenoic acid)	(20:5)
	elongation
Eicosanoids	(22:5)
• thromboxanes	
• prostaglandins	
• leukotrienes	
	desaturation
DHA (docosahexaenoic acid)	(22:6)

linoleic acid [lin-oh-LAY-ik] An essential *omega*-6 fatty acid that contains 18 carbon atoms and 2 carbon–carbon double bonds (18:2).

alpha-linolenic acid [al-fah lin-oh-LEN-ik] An essential *omega*-3 fatty acid that contains 18 carbon atoms and 3 carbon–carbon double bonds (18:3).

Eicosanoids are made from unsaturated long-chain fatty acids from membrane phospholipids or circulating free fatty acids. The liver elongates these fatty acids 2 carbons at a time until the carbon chains have 20 or 22 carbons. Elongation alternates with desaturation. Once the fatty acid reaches 20 carbons, the body can convert it to one or more of the eicosanoids, such as thromboxanes, prostaglandins, prostacyclins, lipoxins, and leukotrienes. Eicosanoids can have opposing physiologic effects depending on whether they are derived from *omega*-3, *omega*-6 or *omega*-9 fatty acids. Here, we will concentrate on eicosanoids derived from the essential fatty acids—that is, from the *omega*-3s and *omega*-6s, over which we probably have the most dietary control and where most interest currently lies.

The **Omega-6 Fatty Acids**

Linoleic acid, an 18-carbon essential fatty acid with two double bonds (18:2), is our main dietary *omega*-6 fatty acid. In a sequence of elongation and desaturation steps, our bodies convert linoleic acid to arachidonic acid, a 20-carbon fatty acid with four double bonds (20:4). To simplify a very complex picture, a series of eicosanoids is then formed from arachidonic acid (see **Table 5.1**), and these eicosanoids have the overall effect of constricting blood vessels, promoting blood clotting, and promoting inflammation.

The **Omega-3 Fatty Acids**

Alpha-linolenic acid is an 18-carbon essential fatty acid with three double bonds (18:3). It can ultimately be elongated and desaturated to EPA (eicosapentaenoic acid), with 20 carbons and five double bonds (20:5), and DHA (docosahexaenoic acid), with 22 carbons and six double bonds (22:6). (See **Table 5.2**.) However, for these reactions to take place, it must compete with the *omega*-6s (and even with polyunsaturated *trans* fatty acids) for the same enzymes, so only a portion of *alpha*-linolenic acid is converted to EPA and DHA. The eicosanoids derived from EPA have the overall effect of dilating blood vessels, discouraging blood clotting, and reducing inflammation. Because of these properties, *omega*-3 fatty acids have attracted interest as a potential factor in reducing risk for vascular disease.[4] DHA (along with *omega*-6 arachidonic acid) has been shown to support infant brain and eye development and is now being added to selected infant formulas.

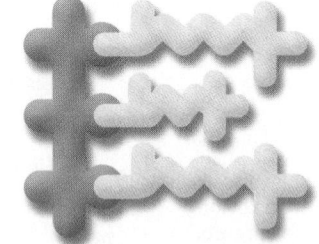

Key Concepts: *Unsaturated fatty acids can have cis or trans double bonds. The body can make many of the fatty acids it needs, but it cannot make linoleic or alpha-linolenic acids, so these are dietary essentials. The body can elongate and desaturate essential fatty acids to form other important compounds, such as eicosanoids.*

A generic triglyceride

Triglycerides

Triglycerides are the major lipids in both the diet and in the body. Triglycerides add flavor and texture (and calories!) to foods and are an important source of the body's energy.

Triglyceride Structure

A triglyceride consists of three fatty acids attached to a molecule of glycerol. Both in food and in the body, most fatty acids exist as part of a triglyceride molecule.

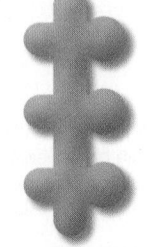

A generic glycerol

Alone, **glycerol** is a thick, smooth liquid often used in the food industry. Chemically it is an alcohol, a simple three-carbon molecule with an alcohol (hydroxyl) group (–OH) at each carbon. Glycerol is the backbone of a triglyceride. It is always the same, whereas the fatty acids attached to it can vary considerably. Chemically speaking, a triglyceride is an **ester**, a combination of an alcohol and a fatty acid. An ester forms when a hydrogen and an oxygen from the fatty acid's carboxyl (acid) group combine with a hydrogen from the alcohol's hydroxyl (alcohol) group. Because the reaction produces a molecule of water, it is called a condensation reaction. An ester linkage now chemically joins the altered fatty acid and alcohol, a process called **esterification**.

Esterification produces triglycerides, **diglycerides**—two fatty acids attached to a glycerol, and **monoglycerides**—one fatty acid attached to a glycerol. **Figure 5.10** illustrates the formation of a triglyceride. Our foods contain relatively small amounts of mono- and diglycerides, mostly as food additives used for their emulsifying or blending qualities.

Triglyceride Functions

Although some of us, like Rachel at the beginning of this chapter, think of fat as something to avoid, fat is a key nutrient with important body functions. **Figure 5.11** shows the functions of triglycerides.

Energy Source

Fat is a rich and efficient source of calories. Under normal circumstances, dietary and stored fat supply about 60 percent of the body's resting energy needs. Like carbohydrate, fat is *protein-sparing*; that is, fat is burned for energy, sparing valuable proteins for their important roles as muscle tissue, enzymes, antibodies, and other functions. Different body tissues preferentially use different sources of calories. Glucose is virtually the sole fuel for the brain except during prolonged starvation, and fat is the preferred fuel of muscle tissue at rest (see **Figure 5.12**). During physical activity, glucose and glycogen join fat in supplying energy.

glycerol [GLISS-er-ol] An alcohol that contains 3 carbon atoms, each of which has an attached hydroxyl group (–OH). It forms the backbone of mono-, di-, and triglycerides.

ester A chemical combination of an organic acid (e.g., fatty acid) and an alcohol. When hydrogen from the alcohol combines with the acid's hydrogen and oxygen, water is released and an ester linkage is formed. A triglyceride is an ester of three fatty acids and glycerol.

esterification [e-ster-ih-fih-KAY-shun] A condensation reaction in which an organic acid (e.g., fatty acid) combines with an alcohol with the loss of water, creating an ester.

diglycerides Molecules composed of glycerol combined with two fatty acids.

monoglycerides Molecules composed of glycerol combined with one fatty acid.

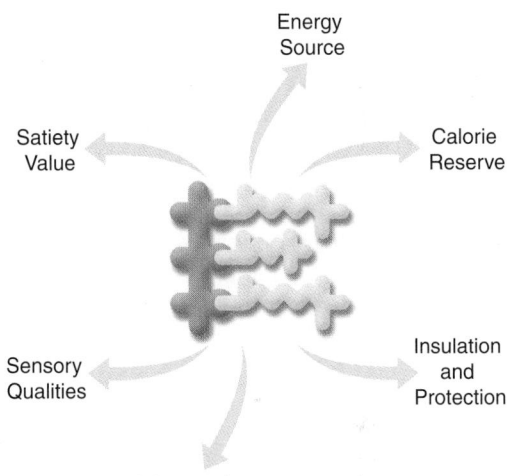

Figure 5.11 **Functions of triglycerides.** Fat performs a number of essential functions in the body.

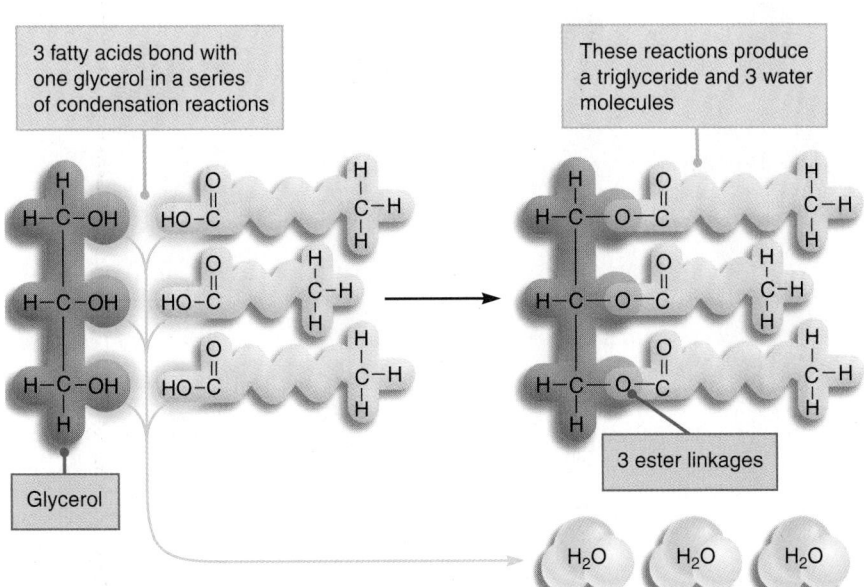

Figure 5.10 **Forming a triglyceride.** Condensation reactions attach three fatty acids to a glycerol backbone to form a triglyceride. These reactions release water.

3 fatty acids bond with one glycerol in a series of condensation reactions

These reactions produce a triglyceride and 3 water molecules

3 ester linkages

Glycerol

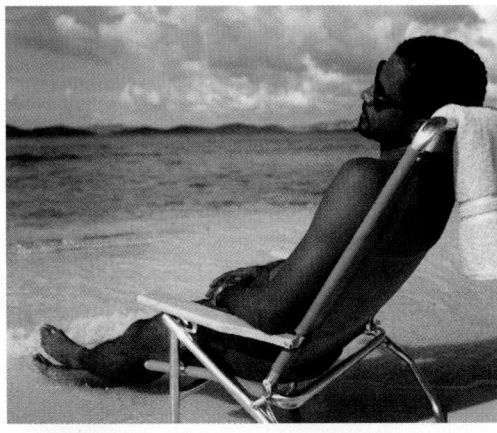

Figure 5.12 **Fat is a major energy source.** When at rest, muscles prefer to use fat for fuel.

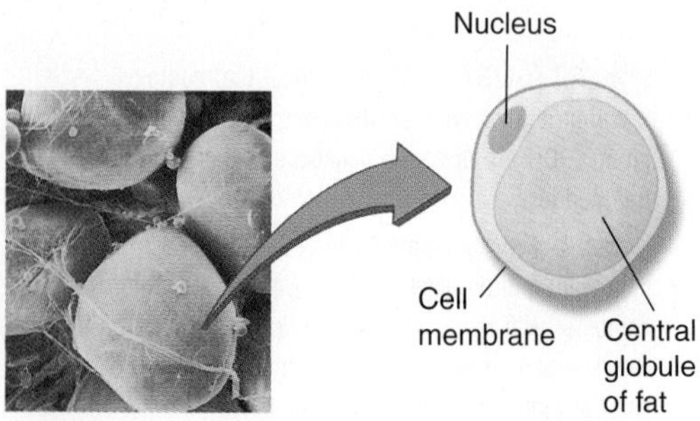

Nucleus

Cell membrane

Central globule of fat

Figure 5.13 **Fat is an efficient storage medium.** Evolution has selected fat, rather than glycogen, as its primary energy storage medium. A gram of fat stores more than six times as much energy as a gram of glycogen. If a 155-pound man (with 20 pounds of fat) could store all his energy reserves as glycogen and none as fat, he would weigh 255 pounds!

adipocytes Fat cells.

adipose tissue Body fat tissue.

visceral fat Fat stores that cushion body organs.

subcutaneous fat Fat stores under the skin.

lanugo [lah-NEW-go] Soft, downy hair that covers a normal fetus from the fifth month but is shed almost entirely by the time of birth. It also appears on semi-starved individuals who have lost much of their body fat, serving as insulation normally provided by body fat.

High-fat foods are higher in calories than either high-protein or high-carbohydrate foods. One gram of fat contains 9 kilocalories, compared with only 4 kilocalories in a gram of carbohydrate or protein, or 7 kilocalories per gram for alcohol. For example, a tablespoon of corn oil (pure fat) has 120 kilocalories, whereas a tablespoon of sugar (pure carbohydrate) has only 50 kilocalories.

Fat's caloric density is especially important when energy needs are high. An infant, for example, who needs ample energy for fast growth but whose stomach can hold only a limited amount of food, needs the high fat content of breast milk or infant formula to get enough calories. When inappropriately put on a low-fat diet, infants and young children do not grow and develop properly. Other people with high-energy needs include athletes, individuals who are physically active in their jobs, and people who are trying to regain weight lost due to illness.

Of course, fat's caloric density has a negative side. In practical terms, 9 kilocalories per gram translates to about 115 to 120 kilocalories per tablespoon of pure fat (e.g., vegetable oil). That makes it very easy to get too many fat calories, and dietary fat in excess of a person's energy needs is a major contributor to obesity.

Energy Reserve

We store excess dietary fat as body fat to tide us over during periods of calorie deficit. Fat's caloric density comes in handy for this task, storing energy away in a small space. The fat is stored inside fat cells called **adipocytes**, which form body fat tissue, technically called **adipose tissue**. (See **Figure 5.13**.) Hibernating animals have perfected this process; the fat stores they build in autumn can see them through a winter's fast.

The body possesses complex mechanisms for freeing triglycerides and fatty acids and delivering them when and where they are needed for energy. Cells then break down these lipids to release energy stored in their chemical bonds.

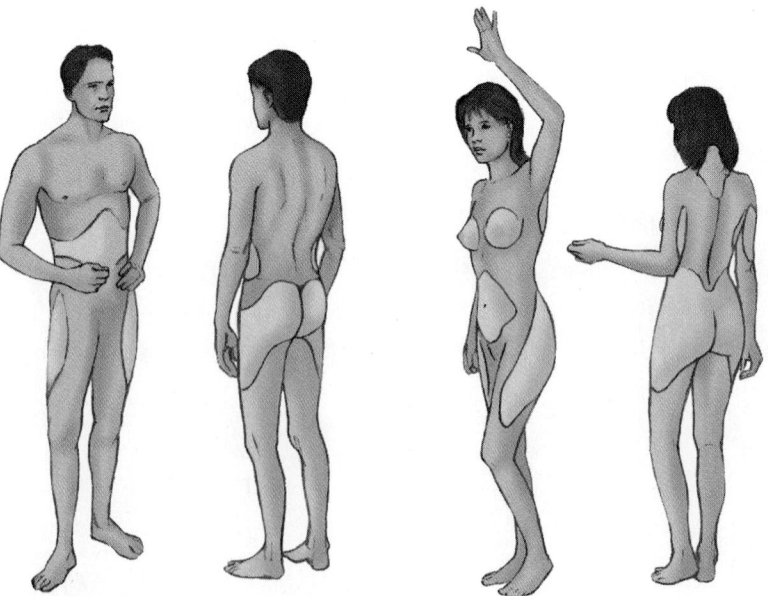

Figure 5.14 **Sites for fat storage differ for men and women.** Whereas men often store excess fat in their abdomens, women tend to store it in their hips.

Insulation and Protection

Fat tissue accounts for about 15 to 30 percent of a person's body weight. Part of this is **visceral fat**, adipose tissue around organs that remains relatively inert until called upon to release stored energy. Meanwhile, it serves an important function by cushioning and shielding delicate organs, especially the kidneys. Women have extra fat, most noticeably in the breasts and hips, to help shield their reproductive organs and to guarantee adequate calories during pregnancy. Other fat tissue is **subcutaneous fat**, lying under the skin, where it protects and insulates the body. Perhaps nowhere is fat's structural role more dramatic than in the brain, which is 60 percent fat.[5] **Figure 5.14** shows the primary areas of fat storage in women and men.

Can a person have too little body fat? Just ask someone whose body fat has been depleted by illness. It hurts to sit and it hurts to lie down. For people without enough body fat, cool temperatures are intolerable and even room temperature may be uncomfortably cool. Women stop menstruating and become infertile. Children stop growing. Skin deteriorates from pressure sores or from fatty acid deficiency and may become covered with fine hair called **lanugo**. Illness, involuntary starvation, and famine can deplete fat to this extent, as can excessive dieting and exercise.

Carrier of Fat-Soluble Compounds

As you can see in **Figure 5.15**, dietary fats dissolve and transport micronutrients such as fat-soluble vitamins and fat-soluble phytochemicals such as carotenoids. Phytochemicals, although not essential (their lack will not cause a deficiency disease), have emerged as contributors to optimal health.

Dietary fats carry other fat-soluble substances through the digestive process, improving intestinal absorption or bioavailability. For example, the body absorbs more lycopene, the healthful red-colored phytochemical in tomatoes, if the tomatoes are served with oil or salad dressing. People who suffer from fat malabsorption disorders risk deficiency of fat-soluble micronutrients, so many must use supplements.

Removing a food's lipid portion—for example, removing butterfat from milk—also removes fat-soluble vitamins. In the case of most dairy products, vitamin A is usually replaced. But the natural vitamin E of whole wheat (vitamin E is in the germ) is not replaced after the lipid-rich germ portion of wheat grain is removed during refinement to white flour. Fat-soluble vitamins may be destroyed in fat processing; for example, some vitamin E is lost in processing vegetable oils. (See "Spotlight on Complementary and Alternative Nutrition.")

Sensory Qualities

As a food component or as an ingredient, fat contributes greatly to the flavor, odor, and texture of food (see **Figure 5.16**). Simply put, it makes food taste good. Flavorful volatile chemicals are dissolved in the fat of a food; heat sends them into the air, producing mouth-watering odors that perk up appetites. Fats have a rich, satisfying feeling in the mouth. Fats make baked goods tender and moist. And fats can be heated to high temperatures for frying, which seals in flavors and cooks food quickly. These are all good qualities—but too good for many people who find high-fat foods irresistible and eat too much of them. Alas, fat's most appealing attributes are also serious drawbacks to maintaining a healthful diet.

Quick Bites

The Marvelous Storage Efficiency of Fat

Why do you think we don't store all our extra energy as readily available glycogen? It would take more than six pounds of glycogen to store the same energy as one pound of fat. Just imagine how much bulkier we would be! How cumbersome it would be to move about! That's why only a very small portion of the body's energy reserve is glycogen.

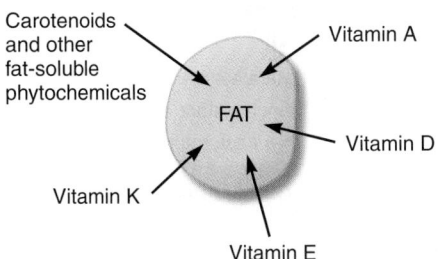

Carotenoids and other fat-soluble phytochemicals

Vitamin A

FAT

Vitamin K

Vitamin D

Vitamin E

Figure 5.15 **Fat is a micronutrient carrier.** Fat holds more than just energy. It also carries important nutrients, such as fat-soluble vitamins and carotenoids.

Figure 5.16 Fat imparts a rich, sensory quality to food.

SATURATED FATS AND OILS

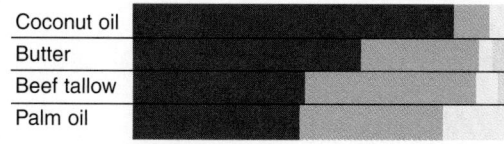

Coconut oil
Butter
Beef tallow
Palm oil

MONOUNSATURATED OILS

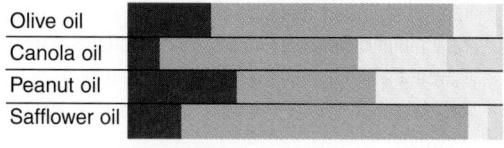

Olive oil
Canola oil
Peanut oil
Safflower oil

POLYUNSATURATED OILS

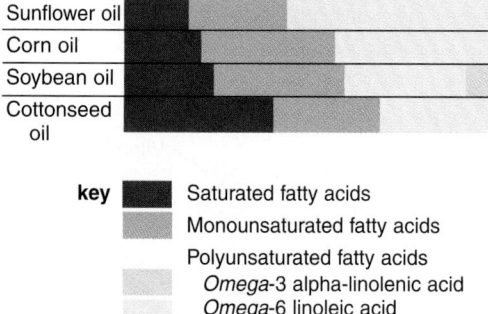

Sunflower oil
Corn oil
Soybean oil
Cottonseed oil

key ■ Saturated fatty acids
■ Monounsaturated fatty acids
Polyunsaturated fatty acids
Omega-3 alpha-linolenic acid
Omega-6 linoleic acid

Figure 5.17 **The diversity of fats.** Fats are mixtures of saturated and unsaturated fatty acids. Depending on which type of fatty acid is most prevalent, the fat is classified as saturated, monounsaturated, or polyunsaturated.
Source: Adapted from *Nutrition Today*, 31(3) May/June 1996.

Key Concepts: *Triglycerides are formed when a glycerol molecule combines with three fatty acids. Dietary triglycerides add texture and flavor to food and are a concentrated source of calories. The body stores excess calories as adipose tissue. While storing energy, adipose tissue also insulates the body and cushions its organs. The fats in food carry valuable fat-soluble nutrients into the body and help with their absorption.*

Triglycerides in Food

Dietary triglycerides are found in a variety of fats and oils and in foods that contain them, such as salad dressing and baked goods. Some food fats are obvious, such as butter, margarine, cooking oil, and fat along a cut of meat or under the skin of chicken. Baked goods, snack foods, nuts, and seeds also provide fat, but it is less noticeable.

Fats and oils are mixtures of many triglycerides, but we often categorize them by their most prevalent type of fatty acid—saturated, monounsaturated, or polyunsaturated. (See **Figure 5.17**.) Canola oil, for example, often is classified as a monounsaturated fat. Its fatty acids are mostly monounsaturated oleic acid; however, 10 percent of its fatty acids are the essential *alpha*-linolenic acid. Although these classifications are useful, they do not always tell the whole story. For example, saturated stearic acid appears to affect blood cholesterol differently than saturated palmitic acid does. As we've seen, *omega*-3 and *omega*-6 fatty acids also behave differently in the body, even though both classes are polyunsaturated. Their food sources often differ as well.

Sources of **Omega-3 Fatty Acid**

Plant foods are generally rich in polyunsaturated fatty acids. Soybean oil, canola oil, and walnuts contain *alpha*-linolenic acid, the essential *omega*-3 fatty acid. However, the most generous source is flaxseed (or linseed) oil, which is more than 50 percent *alpha*-linolenic acid. Longer-chain *omega*-3s, EPA and DHA, are found in fatty fish (e.g., salmon, tuna, and mackerel) and in fish oil supplements. Because fish oil supplements can have potent effects, children, pregnant women, and nursing mothers should not take them without medical supervision.[6] See the FYI feature "Fats on the Health Store Shelf." **Table 5.3** lists the *omega*-3 fatty acids in some foods.

Sources of **Omega-6 Fatty Acid**

Good sources of the 18-carbon *omega*-6 fatty acid linoleic acid include seeds, nuts, and the richest sources, common vegetable oils such as corn oil. Small amounts of arachidonic acid, a 20-carbon *omega*-6 fatty acid, are found in meat, poultry, and eggs, but not in plant foods.

Commercial Processing of Fats

In nature, almost all fats exist in combination with other macronutrients: They generally occur along with starches in plant foods, and with proteins in animal foods. In earlier times, the only concentrated fats and oils available to people were obtained by very simple processing: rendering fats from meats and poultry; skimming or churning the butterfat from milk; skimming the oil from ground nuts; or pressing a few oil-rich plant parts such as coconuts or olives.

Technology that came into use in the 1920s allowed production of pure vegetable oils.[7] By efficiently removing edible oil from its source, processing has increased the availability of calories worldwide. Processing reduces waste and prevents spoilage during normal use and storage. It does so by inhibiting the destructive processes of hydrolysis and oxidation.

Hydrolysis Products containing unrefined fats and oils also contain enzymes that hydrolyze oil by splitting fatty acids from triglycerides. Free fatty acids then perpetuate the damaging hydrolysis. Refining destroys the hydrolytic enzymes and removes most free fatty acids.

Oxidation The more unsaturated an oil (the more double bonds it has), the more vulnerable it is to **oxidation**. Oxidation occurs when an unsaturated fat comes in contact with air and oxygen atoms attach at double-bond sites on the fatty acid chain. Oxidation rapidly turns fats rancid, and oxidized fats damage body tissues, particularly blood vessels.[8] Fortunately, people avoid bad-tasting rancid fats. Exposure to light increases the rate of oxidation and shortens shelf life. The presence of small amounts of metals, which typically are removed by refining, also promotes oxidation. Naturally occurring vitamin E inhibits oxidation, which explains why it and other antioxidants are often added to oils.

Unfortunately, processing also has a negative side. To achieve stability and uniform taste, potentially healthful phospholipids, plant sterols, and other phytochemicals are removed, and a significant portion of the natural vitamin E is lost. Oils have become so familiar that we often forget they are highly processed, highly refined foods. Further processing of oils into solid fats such as margarine or shortening also produces some undesirable changes.

Hydrogenation To get a liquid vegetable oil to act like a solid fat, it must be at least partially hydrogenated. Hydrogenation involves breaking some of the double bonds in unsaturated fatty acids and adding hydrogen. This

oxidation Oxygen attaches to the double bonds of unsaturated fatty acids. Rancid fats are oxidized fats.

Table 5.3 *Omega*-3 Fatty Acids in Selected Foods

	18:3 (mg)	20:5 (EPA) (mg)	22:6 (DHA) (mg)
1 Tbsp canola oil	1,302		
1 Tbsp soybean oil	925		
1 Tbsp walnut oil	1,414		
1 Tbsp flaxseed oil	7,249		
3 oz canned sockeye salmon (fatty fish)		418	564
3 oz cooked mackerel (fatty fish)		555	1,016
3 oz flounder (lean fish)		207	219
3 oz cooked shrimp		145	122
1 Tbsp cod liver oil		938	1,492
1 Tbsp salmon oil		1,771	2,480

Fish and seafood also contain small amounts of 18:3, which are not included on this table.

It sounds like a lot of *omega*-3. But remember, these are milligrams! Dietary fat is usually measured in grams. The 267 milligrams (0.267 g) of EPA and DHA in a serving of shrimp is not much in relation to a diet that has 50+ grams of fat and is a bit less than half the recommendation for daily intake.

Source: Based on data from US Department of Agriculture, Agricultural Research Service. USDA Nutrient Database for Standard Reference, Release 18. 2005. http://www.nal.usda.gov/fnic/foodcompindex.html. Accessed 5/24/06.

process produces a harder, more saturated fat—one that is more effective for making baked goods and snack foods, and one that spreads like butter (most of us recoil at the thought of putting pure corn oil on toast!). Although hydrogenation protects the fat from oxidation and rancidity, it also changes some of the double bonds in the fat's structure to the *trans* configuration. Combined with the increase in saturated fatty acids, this has led many to wonder whether margarine is a better alternative to butter (see the FYI feature "Which Spread for Your Bread?").

Key Concepts: *Triglycerides are found mainly in foods we think of as fats and oils, but also in nuts, seeds, meats, and dairy products. Saturated fatty acids are found mainly in animal foods and tropical oils, whereas polyunsaturated fatty acids are found in vegetable oils and other plant foods. Unsaturated fatty acids are susceptible to spoilage by oxidation. Hydrogenation of oils protects fats from oxidation but creates* trans *fatty acids, which increase risk for heart disease.*

Phospholipids

Phospholipids are similar to triglycerides in that they contain both glycerol and fatty acids. However, important differences in their structure make phospholipids entirely different in terms of function. Phospholipids are synthesized by the body and not needed in the diet.

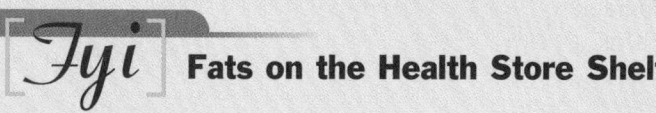

[*Fyi*] Fats on the Health Store Shelf

FOR YOUR INFORMATION

Many claims made for lipid products sold as supplements may not hold up under scientific scrutiny. You may not even recognize these products as lipids, especially because their long, complicated names are often abbreviated. The amount of lipid and calories in most of these products is quite small.

EPA and DHA in Fish Oil Capsules
These *omega*-3 fatty acids are thought to help lower blood pressure, reduce inflammation, reduce blood clotting, and lower high serum triglyceride levels.[1] They were thought to help psoriasis, but studies proved disappointing.[2] Dietary supplementation with *omega*-3 fatty acids is unlikely to reduce the risk of cancer. A large body of scientific literature has failed to find a significant association between *omega*-3 fatty acid consumption and cancer incidence.[3] EPA (eicosapentaenoic acid) and DHA (docosahexaenoic acid) usually make up only about one-third of the fatty acids in fish oil capsules, and research studies often use multiple doses. These should not be taken without close medical supervision, because their blood-thinning properties can cause bleeding.

Because fish oil is highly unsaturated, antioxidant vitamins are included to prevent oxidation. Another problem, though not health related, is that fish oil capsules often leave a fishy aftertaste.

Flaxseed Oil Capsules
Flaxseed oil is an unusually good source of *omega*-3 *alpha*-linolenic acid, which accounts for about 55 percent of its fatty acids. Like fish oil, flaxseed oil is highly unsaturated, and thus very susceptible to rancidity. Capsules protect the oil from oxygen, but limit the dose. A half-tablespoon of canola oil has about as much *omega*-3 as a capsule of flaxseed oil, but adds more calories. DHA and EPA are considered more potent *omega*-3 fatty acids than *alpha*-linolenic.

GLA in Borage, Evening Primrose, or Black Currant Seed Oil Capsules
These oils contain 9 to 24 percent GLA (*gamma*-linolenic acid), the *omega*-6 desaturation product of linoleic acid. Studies of GLA's effects on skin diseases and heart conditions have been disappointing, and research

on potential benefits of GLA supplements in rheumatoid arthritis has been conflicting.[4]

Medium-Chain Triglycerides Oil
Medium-chain triglycerides (MCTs) can be purchased as such, or found as ingredients in "sports" drinks and foods. Because MCTs are absorbed easily, they are marketed to athletes as a noncarbohydrate source of quick, concentrated energy. However, they have no specific performance benefits. A tablespoon of MCT contains about 100 kilocalories.

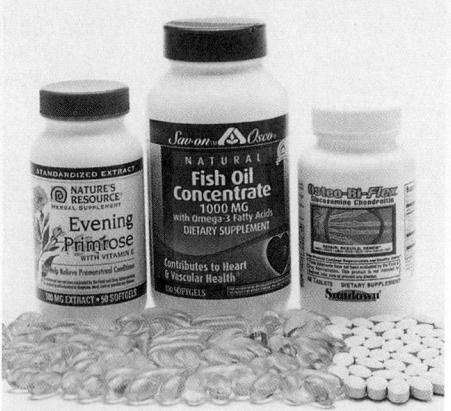

Phospholipid Structure

Phospholipids have a chemical structure similar to that of triglycerides, except that one of the fatty acids is replaced by another compound. Phospholipids are diglycerides—two fatty acids attached to a glycerol backbone. A **phosphate group** with a nitrogen-containing component, such as choline, occupies the third attachment site. **Figure 5.18** shows the structure of a phospholipid.

The phosphate–nitrogen component of phospholipids is hydrophilic, so a phospholipid is compatible with both fat and water: Fatty acids in its diglyceride area attract fats, while its phosphate–nitrogen component attracts water-soluble substances.

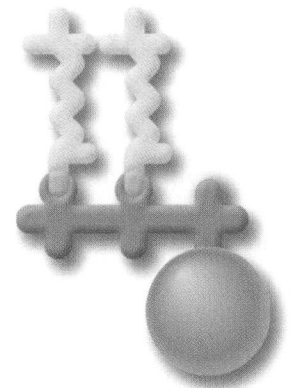

A generic phospholipid

phosphate group A chemical group ($-PO_4$) on a larger molecule, where the phosphorus is single-bonded to each of the four oxygens, and the other bond of one of the oxygens is attached to the rest of the molecule. Often hydrogen atoms are attached to the oxygens. Sometimes there are double bonds between the phosphorus and an oxygen.

Phospholipid Functions

Because phospholipids have both hydrophobic and hydrophilic regions, they are ideal emulsifiers (compounds that help keep fats suspended in a watery environment) and are often used in foods to keep oil and water mixed. This same property makes phospholipids a perfect structural

Lecithin Oil or Granules

Lecithin supplements are derived from soybeans and are a mixture of phospholipids. They are often promoted as emulsifiers that lower cholesterol, but since dietary phospholipids are broken down by the enzyme lecithinase in the intestine, they cannot have this effect. They may be useful as a source of choline. Because choline is the precursor of acetylcholine (a neurotransmitter), lecithin is promoted for treating Parkinson's and Alzheimer's diseases, which are associated with low levels of acetylcholine in the brain. Unfortunately, these claims have little scientific support.[5]

Monolaurin Capsules

Monolaurin is an ester of lauric acid, a 12-carbon fatty acid found in coconut oil. Lauric acid is said to have anti-infective effects, but the amount in these capsules is probably too small to be significant.

CLA

Conjugated linoleic acid (CLA) is linoleic acid with only one saturated bond between its two double bonds. It is promoted as an aid for reducing body fat and has been suggested to have anticancer properties. Studies show promising results,[6] but more work is needed to identify specific functions of CLA and evaluate its long-term safety.[7]

DHEA

Dehydroepiandrosterone (DHEA) is a testosterone precursor formed from cholesterol. It is present in the body in large quantities during adolescence, peaks in the 20s, and gradually declines with age. Many elderly people have low levels, and levels also dip during serious illnesses. With only a few exceptions, attempts to use DHEA for illnesses or to slow aging have been disappointing. Researchers generally use doses many times greater than those in over-the-counter supplements, levels that may cause hairiness in women and, more seriously, a risk of liver problems.[8]

Shark Liver Oil and Squalene Capsules

Squalene, an intermediary compound in the synthesis of cholesterol in the body, and shark liver oil, which contains squalene, are said to help liver, skin, and immune function. The basis for these claims is unclear.

1 Connor SL, Connor WE. Are fish oils beneficial in disease prevention and treatment? *Am J Clin Nutr.* 1997;66:S1020–S1031.

2 Soyland E, Funk J, Rajka G, et al. Effect of dietary supplementation with very-long-chain n-3 fatty acids in patients with psoriasis. *N Engl J Med.* 1993:328:1812–1816.

3 MacLean CH, Newberry SJ, Mojica WA, et al. Effects of omega-3 fatty acids on cancer risk: a systematic review. *JAMA.* 2006;295(4):403–416.

4 Sarubin Fragakis A. *The Health Professional's Guide to Popular Dietary Supplements.* 2nd ed. Chicago: American Dietetics Association, 2003.

5 Higgins JP, Flicker L. Lecithin for dementia and cognitive impairment. *Cochrane Database Syst Rev.* 2000;4:CD001015.

6 Larsson SC, Bergkvist L, Wolk A. High-fat dairy food and conjugated linoleic acid intakes in relation to colorectal cancer incidence in the Swedish mammography cohort. *Am J Clin Nutr.* 2005;82(4):894–900.

7 Belury MA. Dietary conjugated linoleic acid in health: physiological effects and mechanisms of action. *Annu Rev Nutr.* 2002;22:505–531.

8 Khaw KT. Dehydroepiandrosterone, dehydroepiandrosterone sulphate and cardiovascular disease. *J Endocrinol.* 1996;150:S149–S153.

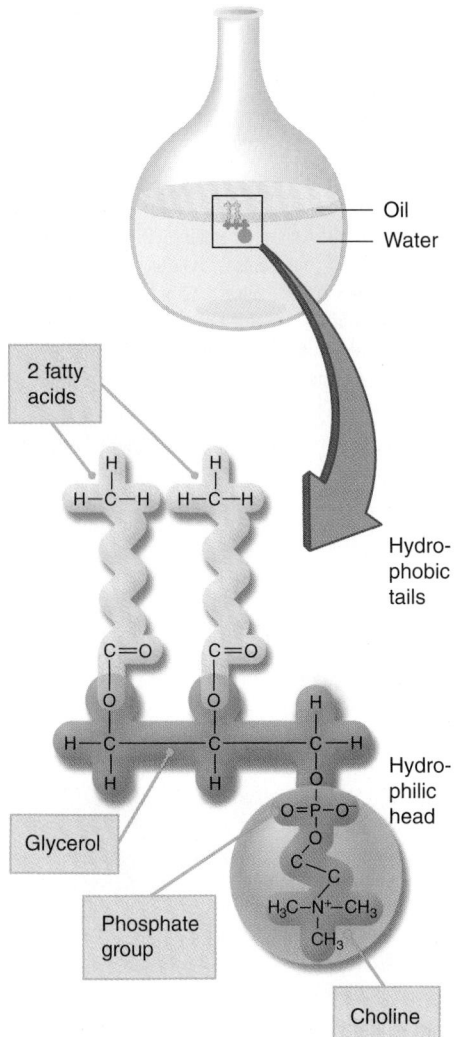

element for cell membranes—able to communicate with the watery environments of blood and cell fluids, yet with a lipid portion that allows other lipids to enter and exit cells.

Cell Membranes

Phospholipids are major components of cell membranes. Cell membranes are a double layer of phospholipids that selectively allow both fatty and water-soluble substances into the cell. (See **Figure 5.19**.) They also provide a temporary store of fatty acids, donating them for short-term energy needs or for synthesis into regulatory chemicals (e.g., eicosanoids). Phosphatidylcholine (a phospholipid), whose **choline** is the precursor to the major neurotransmitter acetylcholine, plays an especially important role in nerve cells. By keeping fatty acids, choline, and other biologically active substances bound in phospholipids and freeing them only as needed, the body is able to regulate them closely.

Lipid Transport

The ability of phospholipids to combine both fatty and watery substances comes in handy throughout the body. In the stomach, dietary phospholipids help break fats into tiny particles for easier digestion. In the intestine, phospholipids from bile continue emulsifying. And in the watery environment of blood, phospholipids coat the surface of the lipoproteins that carry lipid particles to their destinations in the body.

Emulsifiers (Lecithins)

In the body and in foods of animal origin, phosphatidylcholine is also called **lecithin**. However, for food additives or supplements, the term *lecithin* is used for a mix of phospholipids derived from plants (usually soybeans). Understandably, this inconsistent terminology has caused confusion.

Lecithins are used by the food industry as emulsifiers to combine two ingredients that don't ordinarily mix, such as oil and water. (See **Figure 5.20**.) In high-fat powdered products (e.g., dry milk, milk replacers, and coffee creamers), lecithins help to mix hydrophobic compounds with water. Lecithins in salad dressing, chili, and sloppy-joe mixes increase dispersion and reduce fat separation. Lecithin is even added to chewing gum to increase

Figure 5.18 **Phospholipid.** A phospholipid is soluble in both oil and water. This is a useful property for transporting fatty substances in the body's watery fluids.

choline A nitrogen-containing compound that is part of phosphatidylcholine, a phospholipid. Choline is also part of the neurotransmitter acetylcholine. The body synthesizes choline from the amino acid methionine.

lecithin In the body, a phospholipid with the nitrogenous component choline. In foods, lecithin is a blend of phospholipids with different nitrogenous components.

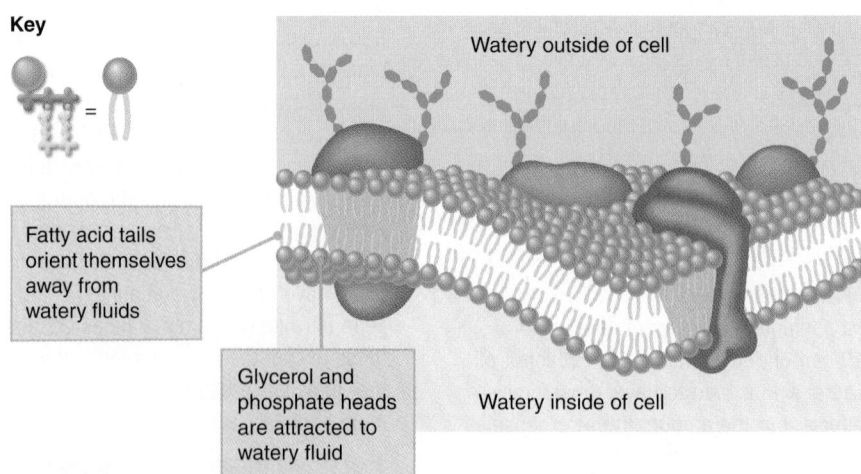

Figure 5.19 **Cell membranes are phospholipid bilayers.** Although proteins and other substances are embedded in cell membranes, these membranes primarily consist of phospholipids.

its shelf life, prolong flavor release, and prevent the gum from sticking to teeth and dental work.

Phospholipids in Food

Phospholipids occur naturally throughout the plant and animal world, albeit in small amounts compared with triglycerides. They are most abundant in egg yolks, liver, soybeans, and peanuts. Naturally occurring phospholipids are often lost when foods are processed, but other phospholipids are frequently used as food additives. Overall, a typical diet contains only about 2 grams per day. However, phospholipids are not a dietary essential because your body can readily synthesize them from available raw materials.

Key Concepts: *Phospholipids are diglycerides (glycerol plus two fatty acids) with a molecule containing a phosphate/nitrogen group attached at the third attachment point of glycerol. This structure gives the phospholipid both hydrophobic and hydrophilic regions, contributing to its functional properties. Phospholipids are major components of cell membranes and act as emulsifiers. They also store fatty acids for release into the cell and serve as a source of choline. Phospholipids are not needed in the diet because the body can synthesize them.*

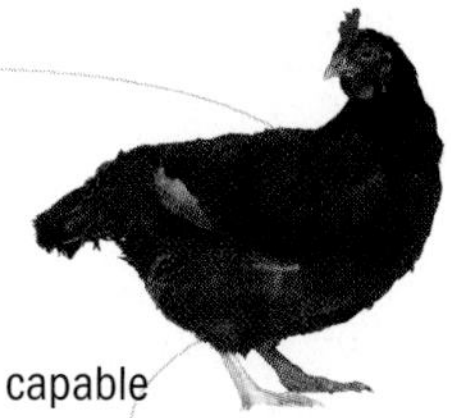

Sterols

Although classified as lipids, sterols are quite different from triglycerides and phospholipids, both in structure and function. The best-known sterol is cholesterol.

Sterol Structure

Whereas triglycerides and phospholipids have fingerlike structures, sterols are hydrocarbons with a multiple-ring structure. (See **Figure 5.21**.) Like triglycerides, sterols are lipophilic and hydrophobic. Unlike triglycerides and phospholipids, most sterols contain no fatty acids.

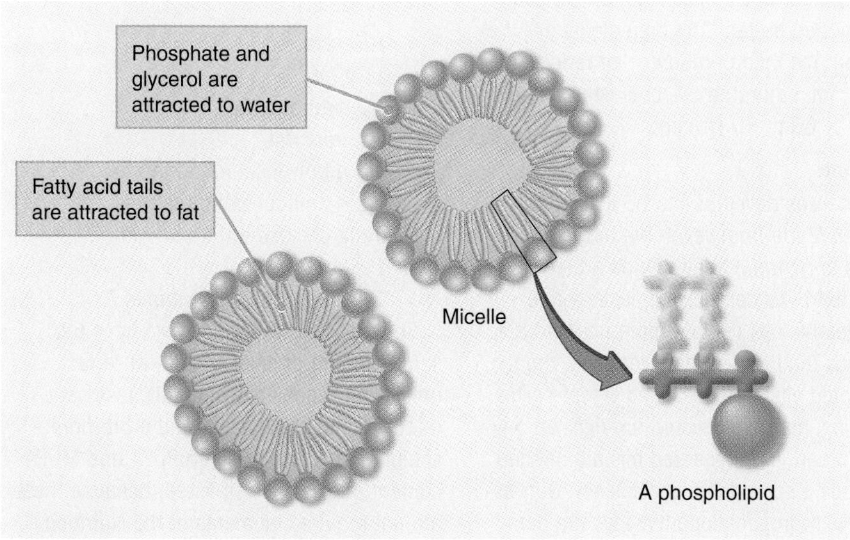

Think About It
3

Figure 5.20 **Phospholipids and emulsification.** Phospholipids form water-soluble packages called *micelles* that suspend fat-soluble compounds in watery media. In a micelle, the phospholipids form into a water-soluble ball with a fatty core. The hydrophilic head of each phospholipid molecule points outward in contact with the watery medium, while the hydrophobic tails point inward in contact with the fatty core.

- Phosphate and glycerol are attracted to water
- Fatty acid tails are attracted to fat
- Micelle
- A phospholipid

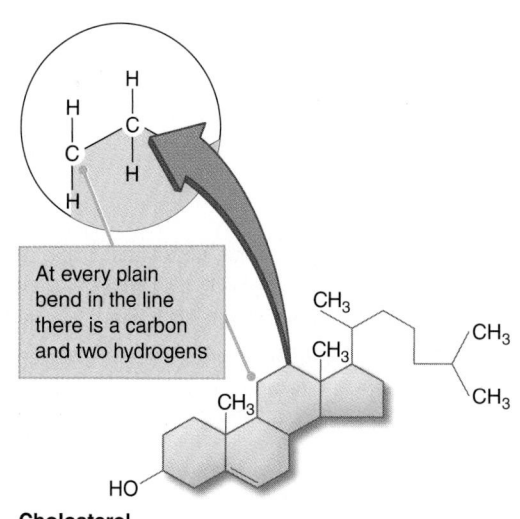

At every plain bend in the line there is a carbon and two hydrogens

Cholesterol

Figure 5.21 **Sterols.** Sterols are multi-ring structures. Because of its role in heart disease, cholesterol has become the best known sterol.

cholesterol [ko-LES-te-rol] A waxy lipid (sterol) whose chemical structure contains multiple hydrocarbon rings.

Cholesterol Functions

Because of the publicity generated by its role in atherosclerosis (heart disease), **cholesterol** is the best-known sterol. But cholesterol is a necessary, important substance in the body; it becomes a problem only when excessive amounts accumulate in the blood. Like phospholipids, it is a major structural component of all cell membranes and is especially abundant in nerve and brain tissue. In fact, most cholesterol resides in body tissue, not in the blood serum or plasma that is routinely tested for cholesterol levels.

High blood cholesterol levels are common, but it is also possible to have undesirably low cholesterol levels. Although less common, very low levels (usually defined as less than 160 mg/dL) are associated with some kinds of stroke; lung, liver, and behavioral illnesses; and reduced immunity.[9] As yet, researchers have not determined whether low cholesterol causes these conditions or results from them. For people with AIDS or cancer, declining cholesterol levels often indicate that their condition is worsening.[10]

Fyi Which Spread for Your Bread?

FOR YOUR INFORMATION

Okay, it's time to see if you can put some of your new knowledge about lipids to work. You're standing in front of the dairy case ready to pick out the best spread. But, wow! So many choices. Of course, there's butter, the traditional spread—wholesome, natural, and creamy; sometimes there's just no substitute for the real thing. Margarine is the choice of many, and has come to be more familiar than butter to some consumers. Then what's this "vegetable oil spread"? Here's one that says it "helps promote healthy cholesterol levels."

Butter

When it comes to heart health, butter has some serious disadvantages: (1) It's high in cholesterol-raising saturated fat, (2) it contains cholesterol, and (3) like other fats, it's high in calories.

Here are the facts: 1 tablespoon of butter provides

  100 kcal
  11 g fat
  7 g saturated fat
  0 g *trans* fat
  30 mg cholesterol
  85 mg sodium
  8% Daily Value for vitamin A

The ingredients are simple: "cream, salt, annatto (added seasonally)." Annatto is a natural coloring (a carotenoid) that is used to keep the color of butter consistent, despite what dairy cows might have been grazing on.

If you like the taste of butter, but want a bit less saturated fat and cholesterol, you can buy "whipped butter." The ingredients are the same, but the incorporation of air reduces calories, fat, saturated fat, cholesterol, and sodium by 60 to 70 percent.

Margarine

Margarine was developed to be a substitute for butter. Made from vegetable oils, it appears to be more healthful; as a plant-derived food, it's certainly cholesterol-free, and vegetable oils contain more unsaturated fatty acids than butter. Inconveniently, though, unsaturated oils are liquid, and without extra processing, margarine would run right off any slice of bread. Hydrogenated oils are needed to produce a spreadable consistency. But, as you know, hydrogenation increases the number of saturated and *trans* fatty acids in a fat, and both of these are associated with higher blood cholesterol levels.

Looking at the label of a standard stick of margarine, you'll find the following per tablespoon:

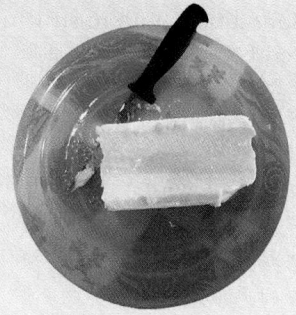

  100 kcal
  11 g fat
  2 g saturated fat
  2 g *trans* fat
  3.5 g polyunsaturated fat
  3.5 g monounsaturated fat
  0 mg cholesterol
  115 mg sodium
  10% Daily Value for vitamin A

So compared with butter, we have the same amount of calories and fat (a fact unknown to many consumers!), less saturated fat and cholesterol, and a bit more sodium and vitamin A. The PUFA and MUFA content of butter is not listed, because these are not required elements of the Nutrition Facts label.

Turning to the list of ingredients, we find "liquid soybean oil, partially hydrogenated soybean oil, water, whey, salt, soy lecithin, and vegetable mono- and diglycerides (emul-

Cholesterol is important not only in cell membranes but also as a precursor molecule. For example, vitamin D is synthesized from cholesterol. Cholesterol is the precursor of five major classes of sterol hormones: progesterones, glucocorticoids, mineralocorticoids, androgens, and estrogens. (See **Figure 5.22**.) Progesterone is essential for maintaining a healthy pregnancy. Glucocorticoids (such as cortisol) increase the formation of liver glycogen and the breakdown of fat and protein. Mineralocorticoids (primarily aldosterone) help control blood pressure. Androgens (such as testosterone) promote the development of male sex characteristics, and estrogens promote the development of female sex characteristics. When testosterone is synthesized from cholesterol, an intermediate called DHEA (dehydroepiandrosterone) is formed. DHEA has become a popular nutritional supplement, marketed with the largely unfulfilled promise that it will boost potency and restore youth.

The liver uses cholesterol to manufacture bile salts, which are secreted in bile. The gallbladder stores and concentrates the bile. On demand, the gallbladder releases the bile into the small intestine, where bile salts emulsify dietary fats.

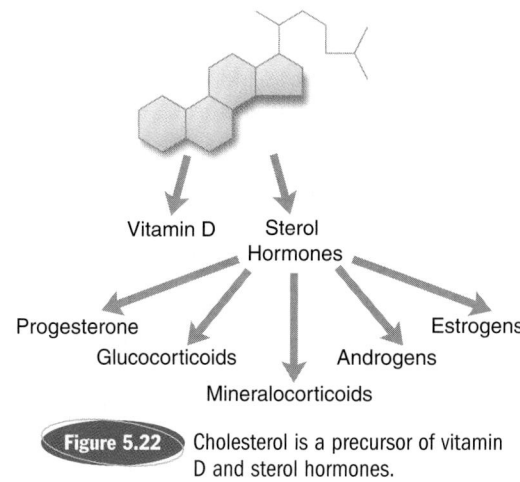

Figure 5.22 Cholesterol is a precursor of vitamin D and sterol hormones.

sifiers), sodium benzoate (a preservative), vitamin A palmitate, beta carotene (color)." Nothing terribly unusual, especially now that you know what lecithin and mono- and diglycerides are.

Spreads and Other Butter Imitators
Beyond the traditional stick margarine, there are numerous "light," "soft," "whipped," "squeeze," and "spread" products. These items do not fit the legal definition of "margarine," and so the term *vegetable oil spread* is generally used. In terms of ingredients, these products have more liquid oil and water and less partially hydrogenated oils than margarine. More emulsifiers may be needed, along with flavors (including salt) and colors. The result typically is fewer calories, saturated fat, and still no cholesterol.

Some products tout the inclusion of canola or olive oil for more healthful MUFA. Others indicate "no *trans* fatty acids" and have no hydrogenated oils on the list. Several spreads contain plant sterols or stanols that reduce intestinal absorption of cholesterol.[1] Another product, still under development, will contain the soluble fiber psyllium, also meant to lower cholesterol absorption.[2]

Cholesterol-Lowering Margarines
Stanols are plant sterols similar in structure to cholesterol. Ingested plant sterols compete with and inhibit cholesterol absorption. Studies show that consumption of stanols reduces total blood cholesterol levels and LDL cholesterol levels.[3] HDL cholesterol levels increased or remained unchanged.[4]

The "cholesterol-lowering" margarines Benecol and Take Control contain plant sterols. Consumption of 3 grams of stanol per day, which is equivalent to three pats of these margarines, can effectively improve lipid profiles and may reduce cardiovascular risk. When consumed as part of a controlled diet, sterol/stanol esters do not change blood levels of fat-soluble vitamins or carotenoids.[5] Unfortunately, these margarines are expensive, about five times the cost of regular margarine.

Making Choices
The spread you choose may depend on your purpose. There are times, and foods, where nothing but real butter will do. If you've ever tried baking cookies with a soft, reduced-fat spread, you know the outcome—and probably will use butter, margarine, or vegetable shortening next time.

Remember, your goal is to limit total fats as well as saturated and *trans* fatty acids. Using less butter or margarine overall will do that. Choosing a margarine or spread with liquid vegetable oil as the first ingredient (meaning that the amount of hydrogenated oil is less) will reduce not only saturated fat but *trans* fat as well. Moderation is the key—making choices that consider your whole diet will help you stay in line with heart-healthy recommendations.

1 Hollingsworth P. Margarine: the over-the-top functional food. *Food Tech.* 2001;55(1):59–62.

2 Ostlund RE. Phytosterols in human nutrition. *Annu Rev Nutr.* 2002;22:533–549.

3 Jones PJ, Ntanios FY, Raeini Sarjaz M, Vanstone CA. Cholesterol-lowering efficacy of a sitostanol-containing phytosterol mixture with a prudent diet in hyperlipidemic men. *Am J Clin Nutr.* 1999; 69(6):1144–1150; Gylling H, Miettinen TA. Cholesterol reduction by different plant stanol mixtures and with variable fat intake. *Metabolism.* 1999;48:(5):575–580; and Jones PJ, MacDougall DE, Ntanios F, Vanstone CA. Dietary phytosterols as cholesterol-lowering agents in humans. *Can J Physiol Pharmacol.* 1997;75:(3):217–227.

4 Gylling H, Miettinen TA. Cholesterol reduction by different plant stanol mixtures and with variable fat intake. *Metabolism.* 1999;48(5):575–580.

5 Raeini-Sarjaz M, Ntanios FY, Vanstone CA, Jones PJ. No changes in serum fat-soluble vitamin and carotenoid concentrations with the intake of plant sterol/stanol esters in the context of a controlled diet. *Metabolism.* 2002;51(5):652–656.

Would You Pay More for Cholesterol-Free Mushrooms?

Several years ago, some plant foods were promoted with labels claiming they were "cholesterol free." As you might expect, the FDA found this misleading because plant foods never contain cholesterol unless an animal product such as butter or egg has been added. Regulations no longer allow the implication that cholesterol has been removed from a naturally cholesterol-free food. Rather than saying "cholesterol-free mushrooms," labels must now say "mushrooms, a cholesterol-free food."

Cholesterol Synthesis

Because the body can synthesize cholesterol, it is not needed in the diet. Although researchers believe all cells synthesize at least some cholesterol, the liver is the primary cholesterol-manufacturing site, and the intestines contribute appreciable amounts. In fact, your body produces approximately 1,000 milligrams of cholesterol per day, far more than is found in the average diet. This production level attests to cholesterol's biological importance. In the lens of the eye, which has a high concentration of cholesterol, on-site cholesterol synthesis may be essential for preventing cataracts.[11] Animal studies suggest that the brain makes almost all the cholesterol incorporated into it during development.[12] Increasing dietary cholesterol reduces synthesis somewhat, but not by an equivalent amount.[13] Less cholesterol is produced when we eat frequent small meals rather than a few large meals. Fasting markedly reduces cholesterol production.[14]

Sterols in Food

Cholesterol occurs only in foods of animal origin. It is distributed based on its biological roles: It is highest in the brain, high in the liver and other organ meats, and moderate in muscle tissue. Because it is fat-

---

Table 5.4 **Cholesterol in Selected Foods**

	Approximate Cholesterol (mg)	
1 oz cheddar cheese	30	
1 cup cottage cheese (1% fat)	9	
1 cup cottage cheese (4% fat)	32	
1 cup skim milk	5	As the fat content of dairy foods drops, so do cholesterol levels.
1 cup whole milk	34	
1 tbsp half & half	6	
1 tbsp whipping cream	21	
1 tbsp butter	31	
1 tbsp lard	12	
1 tbsp margarine or vegetable oil	0	
3 oz lean pork	73	
3 oz lean beef	73	
3 oz ground beef	76	Notice that skeletal muscle from all kinds of animals has similar levels of cholesterol regardless of its differing fat content.
3 oz chicken breast	71	
3 oz flounder	58	
3 oz salmon	60	
3 oz crabmeat	65	
3 oz lobster meat	61	
1 large egg	212	
3 oz beef kidney	609	
3 oz beef liver	337	Cholesterol is especially high in organ meats.
3 oz beef brain	1,696	

The values here give only a general idea of amounts in foods. Cholesterol values are quite variable, differing by time of the year; the animal's origin, species, or breed; processing; and more. One thing is always true, though: Cholesterol is never found in plant foods.

Source: Based on data from US Department of Agriculture, Agricultural Research Service. USDA National Nutrient Database for Standard Reference, Release 18. 2005. http://www.nal.usda.gov/fnic/foodcompindex.html. Accessed 5/24/06.

soluble, cholesterol is found in the butterfat portion of dairy products. Egg yolks are high in cholesterol, with about 212 milligrams per large egg (the egg white contains no cholesterol), and breast milk is moderately high, suggesting the importance of cholesterol during early growth and development.[15] **Table 5.4** lists the amounts of cholesterol in some common foods.

Aside from cholesterol and vitamin D, few dietary sterols have nutritional significance. Whale liver and plants contain the cholesterol precursor **squalene**. Although whale liver is not a common item in U.S. grocery stores, squalene capsules are sold as dietary supplements with the unproved claim that squalene speeds healing. Plants contain a number of other sterols (phytosterols) that are poorly absorbed. **Phytosterols** are of current interest because they reduce intestinal absorption of cholesterol and are used as a cholesterol-lowering food ingredient in certain vegetable oil spreads.

squalene A cholesterol precursor found in whale liver and plants.

phytosterols Sterols found in plants. Phytosterols are poorly absorbed by humans and reduce intestinal absorption of cholesterol. They recently have been introduced as a cholesterol-lowering food ingredient.

Key Concepts: *Sterols are hydrocarbons with a distinctive ring structure. Cholesterol is the best-known sterol; other sterols are hormones or hormone precursors. Cholesterol is an important precursor compound and is a key component of cell membranes. High levels of blood cholesterol increase the risk of heart disease. Cholesterol is found only in foods of animal origin, and because the body can make all it needs, cholesterol is not a dietary essential.*

Lipid Digestion and Absorption

Like the other macronutrients (carbohydrates and proteins), most lipids are broken into smaller compounds for absorption in the gastrointestinal tract. However, because lipids generally are not water-soluble and digestive secretions are all water-based, the body must treat lipids a bit differently to digest them.

Digestion of Triglycerides and Phospholipids

Because triglycerides are not water-soluble and the enzymes needed to digest them are found in a watery environment, preparing triglycerides for digestion is a more elaborate process than for either carbohydrates or proteins. But don't worry! Your digestive system is equal to the task. Physical actions (chewing, peristalsis, and segmentation) combined with various emulsifiers allow digestive enzymes to do their work.

In the mouth, a combination of chewing and the work of lingual lipase gets the digestive process rolling, with the small amount of dietary phospholipid providing emulsification. In the stomach, gastric lipase joins in, and the stomach's churning and contractions keep the fat dispersed. Diglycerides that form in the breakdown process become emulsifiers, too. After two to four hours in the stomach, about 30 percent of dietary triglycerides have been broken down to diglycerides and free fatty acids.[16]

Fat in the small intestine stimulates the release of the hormones cholecystokinin (CCK) and secretin from duodenal cells. CCK signals the gallbladder to contract, sending bile down the bile duct to the duodenum. Secretin signals the pancreas to

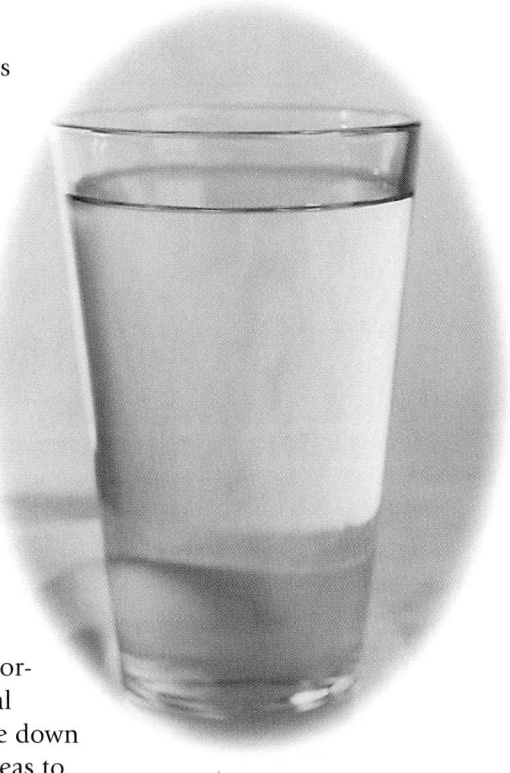

release pancreatic juice rich in pancreatic lipase, which joins bile just before it reaches the duodenum, where the two substances mix with the watery chyme.

Bile contains a large quantity of bile salts and the phospholipid lecithin. These components are the key elements that emulsify fat, breaking globules into smaller pieces so that water-soluble pancreatic lipase can attack the surface. This emulsification process increases the total surface area of fats by as much as 1,000-fold.[17] Many common household detergents remove grease with this same action of emulsification.

As bile breaks up clumps of triglycerides into small pieces and keeps them suspended in solution, pancreatic lipase breaks off one fatty acid at a time. Pancreatic juice contains enormous amounts of pancreatic lipase— enough to digest all accessible triglycerides within minutes. When the lipase has completed its work, most of the dietary triglycerides have been split into monoglycerides and free fatty acids. (See **Figure 5.23**.)

Bile salts surround the products of fat digestion, forming **micelles**— water-soluble globules with a fatty core. The micelles transport the monoglycerides and free fatty acids through the watery intestinal environment to the brush border of the intestinal mucosal cells for absorption.

Phospholipid digestion follows a similar pathway, with phospholipases as well as other lipases participating in the process and with the added release of the phospholipid's phosphate and nitrogen components.

Digestibility

Normally, triglyceride digestion and absorption are very efficient. It is abnormal to find more than 6 or 7 percent of ingested lipids still intact in fecal matter. Production of fatty stools, called **steatorrhea**, indicates fat

micelles Tiny emulsified fat packets that can enter enterocytes. The complexes are composed of emulsifier molecules oriented with their hydrophobic part facing inward and their hydrophilic part facing outward toward the surrounding aqueous environment.

steatorrhea Production of stools with an abnormally high amount of fat.

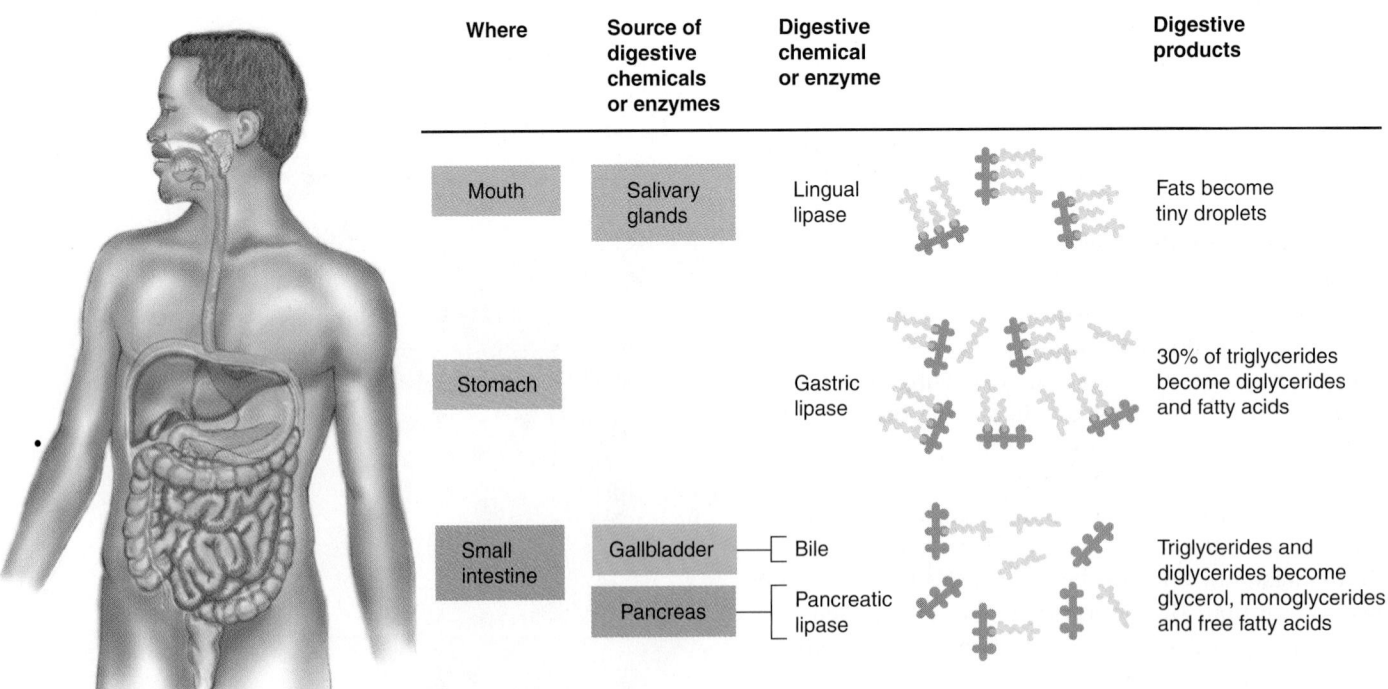

Where	Source of digestive chemicals or enzymes	Digestive chemical or enzyme		Digestive products
Mouth	Salivary glands	Lingual lipase		Fats become tiny droplets
Stomach		Gastric lipase		30% of triglycerides become diglycerides and fatty acids
Small intestine	Gallbladder	Bile		Triglycerides and diglycerides become glycerol, monoglycerides and free fatty acids
	Pancreas	Pancreatic lipase		

Figure 5.23 **Triglyceride digestion.** Most triglyceride digestion takes place in the small intestine.

malabsorption, a condition that may follow radiation therapy or digestive surgery and often accompanies diseases of malabsorption such as cystic fibrosis or Crohn's disease.

Triglycerides of medium-chain fatty acids (medium-chain triglycerides, or MCT) are used in products developed for people with fat malabsorption.[18] Medium-chain fatty acids—those with 6 to 10 carbons—are more water-soluble than longer-chain fatty acids and thus are more readily emulsified, with less need for bile. Because the fatty acid chains are shorter and therefore more water-soluble, MCTs are digested quickly and absorbed efficiently.

Breast milk is easily digestible. It is rich in medium-chain fatty acids and contains its own lipase, which enhances fat digestion despite the immaturity of the baby's digestive system. Some free medium-chain fatty acids released by hydrolysis are even absorbed directly through the baby's stomach lining.

Short-chain fatty acids, with the exception of butyric acid in milk fat, are almost never found in foods. Instead, they are produced by bacteria in the colon from undigested food, especially certain types of fiber. These fatty acids enter the cells of the large intestine (**enterocytes**), where they can be used for energy. A lack of short-chain fatty acids, which can occur when prolonged and exclusive intravenous feeding bypasses bacterial activity, is thought to damage intestinal cells, and nutritionists are studying the use of short-chain fatty acid supplements for these cases. Some research also suggests butyric acid stimulates colon cells to suppress cancer growth, a finding that helps explain how dietary fiber may discourage colon cancer.[19]

Lipid Absorption

Most fat absorption takes place in the duodenum or jejunum of the small intestine. Micelles carry the monoglycerides and long-chain fatty acids to the surfaces of the microvilli in the brush border, even penetrating the recesses between individual microvilli. Here, the monoglycerides and long-chain fatty acids immediately diffuse into the intestinal cells (enterocytes). The unabsorbed bile salts return to the interior of the small intestine to ferry another load of monoglycerides and fatty acids. In the last section of the small intestine (the ileum), bile salts are absorbed. They return via the portal vein to the liver, where they are once again secreted as part of bile. This bile recycling pathway—the liver to the intestine and the intestine to the liver—is called enterohepatic circulation. Figure 3.9 in Chapter 3, "Digestion and Absorption," illustrates enterohepatic circulation.

As monoglycerides and fatty acids pass into the intestinal cells, they reform into triglycerides. Most of the triglycerides, cholesterol, and phospholipids join protein carriers to form a **lipoprotein**. When this assemblage leaves the intestinal cell, it is called a **chylomicron**. The chylomicrons make their way to the central lacteal of the villi, where they enter the lymph system, to be propelled through the thoracic duct and emptied into veins in the neck.

Absorption of glycerol and of short-chain and medium-chain fatty acids is more direct. They are absorbed directly into the bloodstream rather than forming triglycerides and entering the lymph system. These fatty acids can diffuse directly into the capillaries of the villi because they are

enterocytes Intestinal cells.

lipoprotein Complexes that transport lipids in the lymph and blood. They consist of a central core of triglycerides and cholesterol surrounded by a shell composed of proteins and phospholipids. The various types of lipoproteins differ in size, composition, and density.

chylomicron [kye-lo-MY-kron] A large lipoprotein particle formed in intestinal cells following the absorption of dietary fats. A chylomicron has a central core of triglycerides and cholesterol surrounded by phospholipids and proteins.

more water-soluble than longer-chain fatty acids. **Figure 5.24** illustrates the digestion and absorption of triglycerides.

One or two hours after you eat, dietary fat begins to appear in the bloodstream. Fat levels peak after 3 to 5 hours, and fats are generally cleared by 10 hours. That's why health professionals instruct people to fast for 12 hours before having blood drawn for lipid testing.

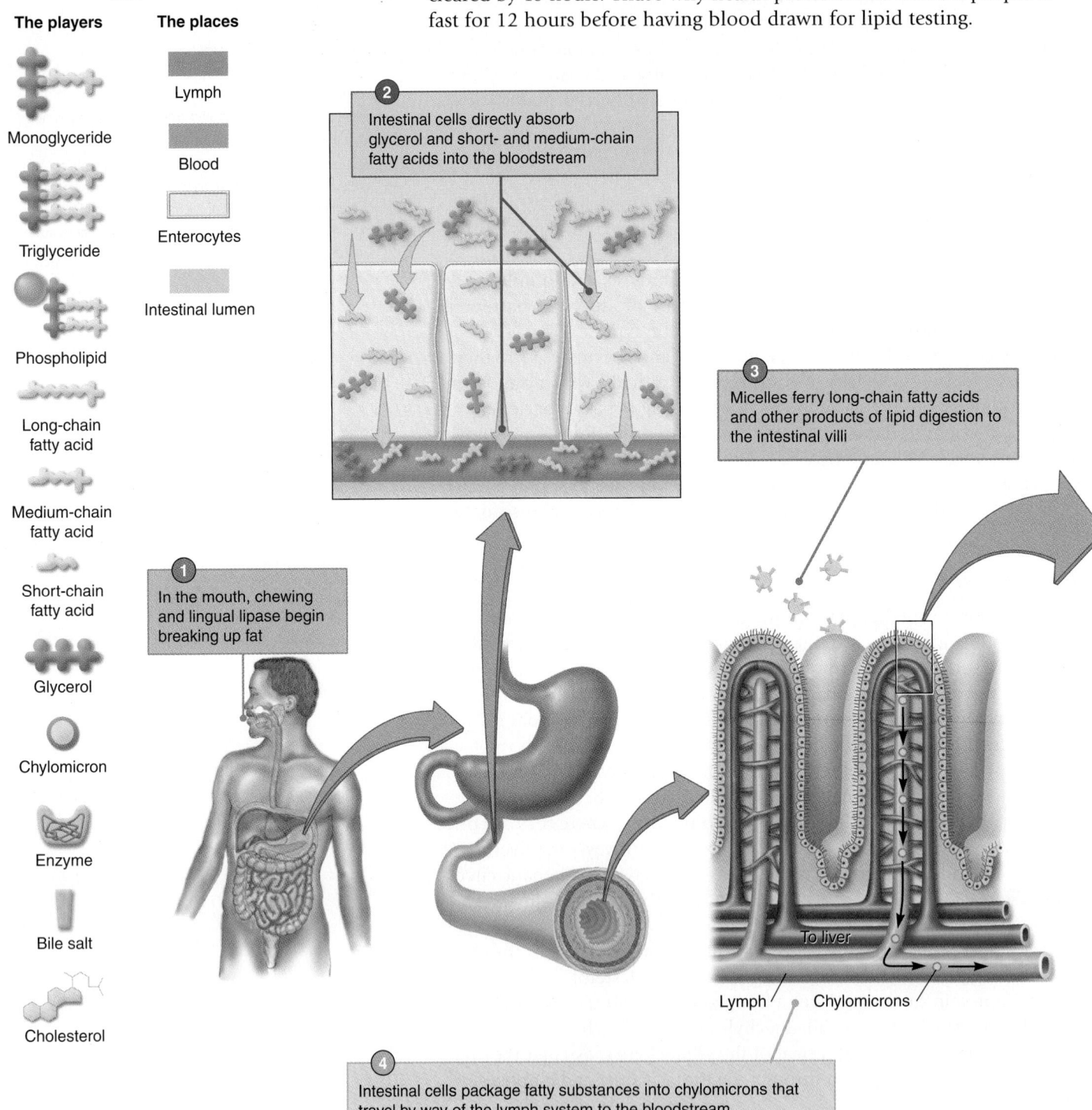

KEY

The players

Monoglyceride

Triglyceride

Phospholipid

Long-chain fatty acid

Medium-chain fatty acid

Short-chain fatty acid

Glycerol

Chylomicron

Enzyme

Bile salt

Cholesterol

The places

Lymph

Blood

Enterocytes

Intestinal lumen

2 Intestinal cells directly absorb glycerol and short- and medium-chain fatty acids into the bloodstream

3 Micelles ferry long-chain fatty acids and other products of lipid digestion to the intestinal villi

1 In the mouth, chewing and lingual lipase begin breaking up fat

To liver

Lymph   Chylomicrons

4 Intestinal cells package fatty substances into chylomicrons that travel by way of the lymph system to the bloodstream

Figure 5.24 **Digestion and absorption of triglycerides.** Minimal fat digestion takes place in the mouth and stomach. In the small intestine, bile salts and lecithin break up and disperse fatty lipids in tiny globules. Enzymes attack these globules, breaking down triglycerides and phospholipids to fatty acids and other component parts. Glycerol and short- and medium-chain fatty acids are absorbed directly into the bloodstream. Bile salts surround the remaining products of fat digestion, forming water-soluble micelles that carry fat to intestinal cells, where it is absorbed and repackaged for transport by the lymphatic system.

Digestion and Absorption of Sterols

Digestion does little to change cholesterol and other sterols, which are poorly absorbed compared with triglycerides. Cholesterol may be esterified (attached to a fatty acid) prior to absorption. When there is dietary fat in the intestine, cholesterol absorption increases. When there are plenty of plant sterols and dietary fiber in the intestine, especially fiber from fruits, vegetables, oats, peas, and beans, cholesterol absorption decreases. Overall, only about 50 percent of dietary cholesterol is absorbed, and that proportion decreases as cholesterol intake increases. Because certain fibers bind bile salts and cholesterol and carry them out of the colon, health professionals often recommend eating foods rich in soluble fiber to lower blood cholesterol.

Key Concepts: *Digestion breaks most lipids down into glycerol, free fatty acids, monoglycerides, and, in the case of phospholipids, a nitrogenous compound. In the small intestine, long-chain fatty acids and monoglycerides are absorbed primarily into the lymphatic system. Glycerol, short-chain fatty acids, and medium-chain fatty acids are absorbed directly into the blood. Sterols are mostly unchanged by digestion, and their absorption is relatively poor.*

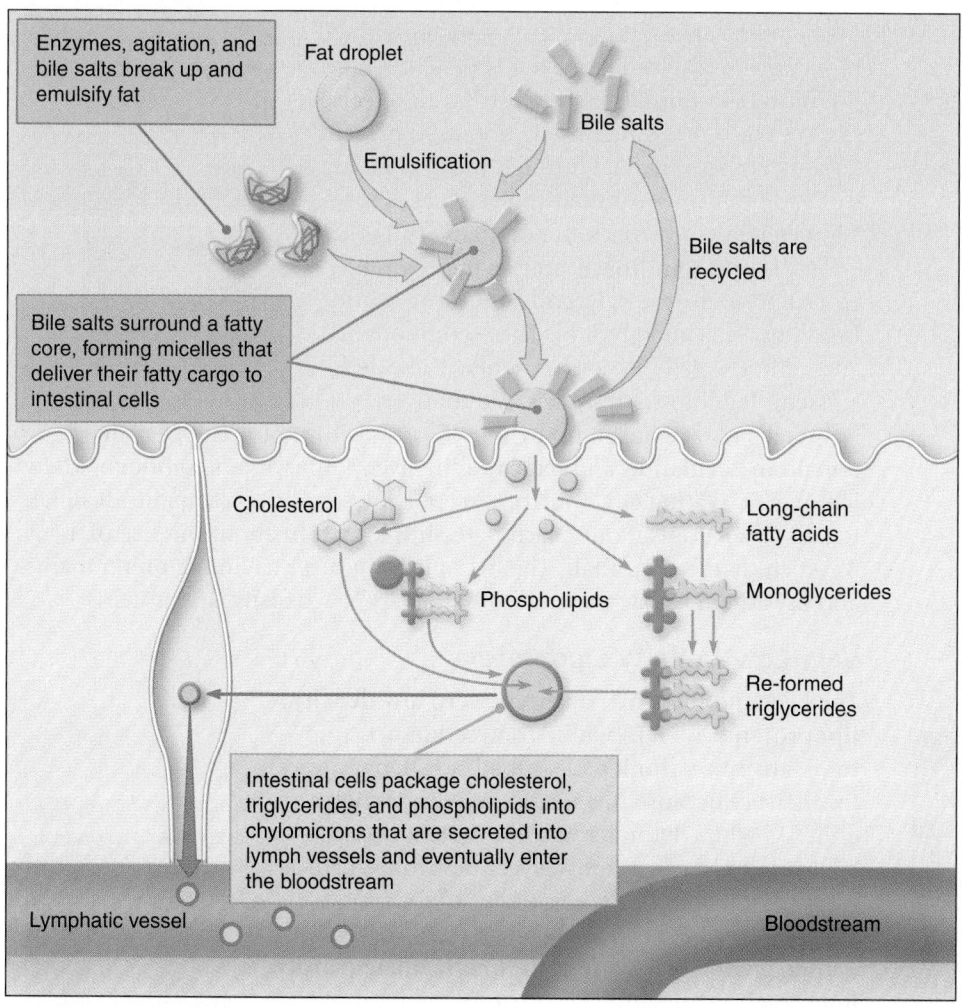

Enzymes, agitation, and bile salts break up and emulsify fat

Fat droplet

Emulsification

Bile salts

Bile salts are recycled

Bile salts surround a fatty core, forming micelles that deliver their fatty cargo to intestinal cells

Cholesterol

Phospholipids

Long-chain fatty acids

Monoglycerides

Re-formed triglycerides

Intestinal cells package cholesterol, triglycerides, and phospholipids into chylomicrons that are secreted into lymph vessels and eventually enter the bloodstream

Lymphatic vessel

Bloodstream

Lipids in the Body

The digestive tract is not the only place where lipids need special handling to move in a water-based environment. To be transported around the body in the bloodstream, lipids must be specially packaged into lipoprotein carriers.

Lipoproteins have a lipid core of triglycerides and cholesterol esters (cholesterol linked to fatty acids) surrounded by a shell of phospholipids with embedded proteins and cholesterol. They can transport water-insoluble (hydrophobic) lipids through the watery environment of the bloodstream. Lipoproteins differ mainly by size, density, and the composition of their lipid cores. In general, as the percentage of triglyceride drops, the density increases. A lipoprotein with a small core that contains little triglyceride is much denser than a lipoprotein with a large core composed mostly of triglycerides. To get a feel for relative sizes, different lipoproteins can be compared to a huge beach ball, softball, baseball, golf ball, and $^3/_4$-inch steel ball bearing. (See **Figure 5.25**.)

Chylomicrons

Chylomicrons formed in the intestinal tract enter the lymphatic system, travel through the thoracic duct, and flow into the bloodstream at the jugular veins of the neck. As they enter the bloodstream, chylomicrons are large, fatty lipoproteins—think of a beach ball 3 to 6 feet in diameter. Chylomicrons are about 90 percent fat, but as they circulate through the capillaries, they gradually give up their triglycerides.

An enzyme located on the capillary walls, called **lipoprotein lipase**, attacks the chylomicrons and removes triglyceride, breaking it into free fatty acids and glycerol. These components enter adipose cells as needed, where they are reassembled into triglycerides. Alternatively, fatty acids may be taken up by muscle and oxidized for energy or may remain in circulation and return to the liver.[20] After about 10 hours, little is left of a circulating chylomicron except cholesterol-rich remnants. It's like the air was let out of our beach ball, shrinking it to about the size of a $4^1/_2$-inch diameter softball. The liver picks up these chylomicron remnants and uses them as raw material to build very low density lipoproteins.

Very Low Density Lipoprotein

The liver and intestines assemble **very low density lipoproteins (VLDL)** with a triglyceride-rich core— for relative size, think of a softball. VLDL has a very low density because it is nearly two-thirds triglyceride. As with chylomicrons, lipoprotein lipase splits off and hydrolyzes triglycerides from VLDL as it circulates through the capillaries of the bloodstream. As VLDL loses triglycerides, it becomes denser, gradually becoming an intermediate-density lipoprotein. Our softball has shrunk to about the size of a $2^3/_4$-inch diameter baseball. When the diet is high in saturated and *trans* fat, more VLDL and triglycerides are released from the liver.[21]

lipoprotein lipase The major enzyme responsible for the hydrolysis of plasma triglycerides.

very low density lipoproteins (VLDL) The triglyceride-rich lipoproteins formed in the liver. VLDL enters the bloodstream and is gradually acted upon by lipoprotein lipase, releasing triglyceride to body cells.

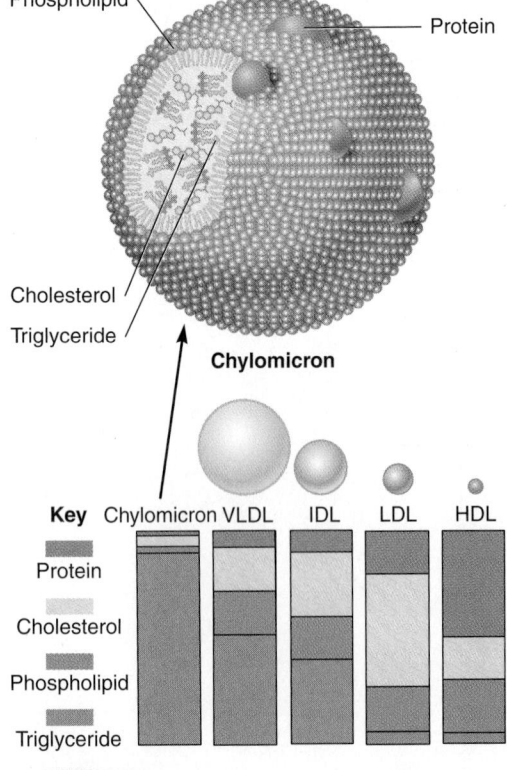

Figure 5.25 **Lipoprotein sizes and composition.** Lipoproteins become less dense as they increase in size. LDL is about double the size of HDL. VLDL is about 60 times larger than HDL. Chylomicrons range from 500–1000 times larger than HDL.

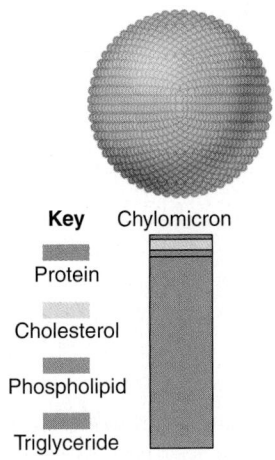

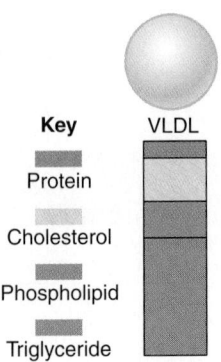

Intermediate-Density Lipoprotein

Intermediate-density lipoproteins (IDL) are about 40 percent triglyceride. As IDL travels through the bloodstream, it acquires cholesterol from another lipoprotein (HDL, see later in this chapter), and circulating enzymes remove some phospholipids. IDL returns to the liver, where liver cells convert it to low-density lipoproteins.

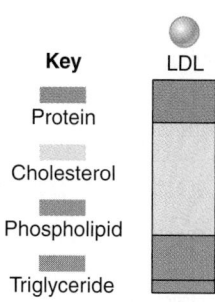

Key IDL

- Protein
- Cholesterol
- Phospholipid
- Triglyceride

Low-Density Lipoprotein

Elevated levels of **low-density lipoproteins (LDL)** in the blood increase the risk of atherosclerosis and heart disease, earning LDL cholesterol the nickname "bad cholesterol." LDL delivers cholesterol to body cells, which use it to synthesize membranes, hormones, and other vital compounds. LDL is more than half cholesterol and cholesterol esters; triglycerides make up only 6 percent. For a relative size, think of a golf ball about $1^5/_8$ inches in diameter.

Key LDL

- Protein
- Cholesterol
- Phospholipid
- Triglyceride

Special receptors on the cell walls bind low-density lipoproteins, which the cell engulfs and ingests via endocytosis. Inside the cell, LDL is broken into its component parts, releasing its load of cholesterol.

When the LDL receptors on liver cells bind LDL, they help control blood cholesterol levels.[22] A lack of LDL receptors reduces the uptake of cholesterol, forcing it to remain in circulation at dangerously high levels. Some research suggests that saturated fats block LDL receptors, limiting their clearance of cholesterol from the blood.[23] However, the main effect of saturated (and also *trans*) fats appears to be on VLDL production, which then leads to elevated LDL levels in the blood.[24]

Low-density lipoprotein also is picked up by scavenger receptors. These are a different type of receptor, one that has a particular affinity for altered (oxidized) LDL. When smoking, diabetes, high blood pressure, or infections injure blood vessel walls, the body's emergency repair team swings into action. It mobilizes white blood cells, which travel to the site of the injury and bury themselves in the blood vessel wall. Certain white blood cells with scavenger receptors bind and ingest LDL. As LDL degrades, it releases its cholesterol. Over several years, this process leads to an accumulation of cholesterol and the development of plaque that thickens and narrows the artery, a condition known as atherosclerosis.

High-Density Lipoprotein

High-density lipoproteins (HDL) appear to protect against atherosclerosis, earning HDL cholesterol the nickname "good cholesterol." The liver and intestines make HDL, which is about 5 percent triglyceride, a fat content similar to LDL. On the other hand, HDL is only about 20 percent cholesterol, much less than LDL, which is more than 50 percent cholesterol. HDL has a higher protein content than any other lipoprotein. For a relative size, think of a steel ball bearing about $3/_4$ inches in diameter.

Key HDL

- Protein
- Cholesterol
- Phospholipid
- Triglyceride

In the bloodstream, HDL picks up cholesterol released by dying cells and from cell membranes as they are renewed. HDL also picks up cholesterol from arterial plaques, reducing their accumulation. HDL hands off cholesterol

intermediate-density lipoproteins (IDL) The lipoproteins formed when lipoprotein lipase strips some of the triglycerides from VLDL. Containing about 40 percent triglycerides, this type of lipoprotein is more dense than VLDL and less dense than LDL. Also called a VLDL remnant.

low-density lipoproteins (LDL) The cholesterol-rich lipoproteins that result from the breakdown and removal of triglycerides from intermediate-density lipoprotein in the blood.

high-density lipoproteins (HDL) The blood lipoproteins that contain high levels of protein and low levels of triglycerides. Synthesized primarily in the liver and small intestine, HDL picks up cholesterol released from dying cells and other sources and transfers it to other lipoproteins.

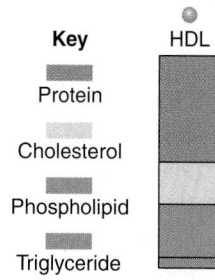

Plaque buildup in a coronary artery.

think
out it

4

to other lipoproteins, especially IDL, which return the cholesterol to the liver for recycling. Low HDL levels increase risk for atherosclerotic heart disease, whereas high HDL levels have a protective effect. About 1 percent of the population who have extremely high HDL levels have extremely low rates of heart disease and stroke.[25]

Key Concepts: *Lipoprotein carriers transport lipids in the blood. Chylomicrons, formed in the intestinal mucosal cells, transport lipids from the digestive tract into circulation. VLDL carries lipids from the liver to the other body tissues, delivering triglycerides and gradually becoming IDL. The liver takes up IDL and assembles LDL, the main carrier of cholesterol. High blood levels of LDL cholesterol, the "bad cholesterol," have been shown to be a risk factor for heart disease. Circulating HDL picks up cholesterol and sends it back to the liver for recycling or excretion. A relatively high level of HDL cholesterol, the "good cholesterol," reduces risk for heart disease.*

Lipids in the Diet

Now that you know something about lipids and their importance in the body, you can see that Rachel's no-fat approach to life has serious flaws. However, consumption of too much dietary fat can contribute unwanted calories, and high intake of saturated and *trans* fat has been linked to heart disease. Read on for a discussion of the recommended amounts and balance of lipids in a healthful diet.

Recommended Intakes

As interest in the relationship between fat intake and health grew in the 1970s and 1980s, the American Heart Association (AHA), the National Cholesterol Education Program (NCEP) of the National Institutes of Health, and the *Dietary Guidelines for Americans* set specific target levels for intake of lipids. These guidelines set limits on total fat and saturated fat intake as a percentage of calories and on the total amount of cholesterol in the diet.

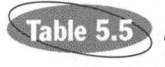 **American Heart Association Diet and Lifestyle Recommendations**

Improving diet and lifestyle is a critical component of the AHA's strategy for cardiovascular disease risk reduction.
- Balance calorie intake and physical activity to achieve or maintain a healthy body weight.
- Consume a diet rich in vegetables and fruit.
- Choose whole-grain, high-fiber foods.
- Consume fish, especially oily fish, at least twice a week.
- Limit your intake of saturated fat to <7% of energy, *trans* fat to <1% of energy, and cholesterol to <300 mg per day.
- Minimize your intake of beverages and foods with added sugars.
- Choose and prepare foods with little or no salt.
- If you consume alcohol, do so in moderation.
- When you eat food that is prepared outside of the home, follow the ADA Diet and Lifestyle Recommendations.

Source: *Circulation.* 2006;114:82–96.

In 2006, the AHA released revised diet and lifestyle recommendations. (See **Table 5.5**.) One of the most significant changes from prior guidelines was a recommendation to consume at least two weekly servings of oily fish, such as tuna or salmon. These recommendations support the AHA's Diet and Lifestyle Goals for Cardiovascular Disease Risk Reduction.[26] Consuming an overall healthy diet and aiming for a healthy body weight are two of the AHA's goals.

Recently, researchers also have focused on the balance of calories from fat and carbohydrate rather than just targeting a reduction in fat. A high-fat, low-carbohydrate diet tends to contribute extra calories that lead to weight gain. When high-fat diets are high in saturated and *trans* fat, increased LDL cholesterol levels and higher heart disease risk result.[26] On the other hand, low-fat, high-carbohydrate diets are associated with lower HDL cholesterol and higher blood triglyceride levels—also increasing heart disease risk. Very low fat intake can make it difficult to get adequate amounts of vitamin E and essential fatty acids.[27]

In 2002, the National Academy of Sciences published its report on Dietary Reference Intakes (DRIs) for the macronutrients.[28] This report recommends an Acceptable Macronutrient Distribution Range (AMDR) for fat of 20 to 35 percent of calories for adults. This is balanced with 45 to 65 percent of calories from carbohydrates and 10 to 35 percent of calories from protein. Because children have higher energy needs, the AMDR for younger ages is more liberal: 30 to 40 percent of calories for children aged 1 to 3 years, and 25 to 35 percent of calories for those aged 4 to 18 years. For infants, the Adequate Intake (AI) for fat is 31 grams per day for birth to 6 months of age, and 30 grams per day for ages 7 to 12 months. AIs or RDAs were not set for older children and adults because there is no defined fat intake level that promotes optimal growth, maintains fat balance, or reduces chronic disease risk. In short, humans can adapt to a wide range of fat intakes.

Many nutritionists were surprised to find that the DRI committee did not set UL levels for fat or cholesterol. The committee concluded that there were no defined levels of intake that separated "healthful" from "harmful" and that any increase in saturated fat, *trans* fat, or cholesterol in the diet increased LDL cholesterol levels and heart disease risk. Because it would be virtually impossible to completely exclude these lipids from the diet, the committee recommended that saturated fat, *trans* fat, and cholesterol intake be minimized. Substituting monounsaturated and polyunsaturated sources improves blood lipid values, with the most favorable results produced by replacing saturated fat with monounsaturated fat.[29]

The 2005 *Dietary Guidelines* merge recommendations from the DRI committee with those of the American Heart Association. (See **Figure 5.26**.) The recommendation for total fat intake is the AMDR: 20 to 35 percent of calories for adults. Saturated fat should be limited to no more than 10 percent of calories, and cholesterol intake limited to less than 300 milligrams per day. The *Dietary Guidelines* also suggest that we keep *trans* fat intake as low as possible. The Daily Values on food labels are 65 grams of total fat (29 percent of the calories in a 2,000-kilocalorie diet), 20 grams of saturated fat (9 percent of calories), and 300 milligrams of cholesterol. Although *trans* fat information is now required on food labels, no Daily Value has been set; consumers should choose foods to minimize *trans* fat intake along with saturated fat and cholesterol.[30] Complete or near-complete avoidance of industrially produced *trans* fats—consumption of less than 0.5 percent of

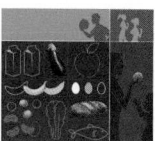

Dietary Guidelines for Americans, 2005
key recommendations

- Consume less than 10 percent of calories from saturated fatty acids and less than 300 mg/day of cholesterol, and keep *trans* fatty acid consumption as low as possible.
- Keep total fat intake between 20 to 35 percent of calories, with most fats coming from sources of polyunsaturated and monounsaturated fatty acids, such as fish, nuts, and vegetable oils.
- When selecting and preparing meat, poultry, dry beans, and milk or milk products, make choices that are lean, low-fat, or fat-free.
- Limit intake of fats and oils high in saturated and/or *trans* fatty acids, and choose products low in such fats and oils.

Key Recommendations for Specific Population Groups

- *Children and adolescents.* Keep total fat intake between 30 to 35 percent of calories for children 2 to 3 years of age and between 25 to 35 percent of calories for children and adolescents 4 to 18 years of age, with most fats coming from sources of polyunsaturated and monounsaturated fatty acids, such as fish, nuts, and vegetable oils.

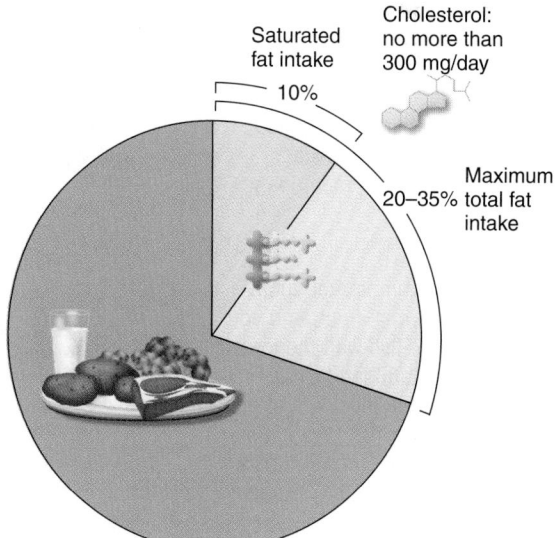

Figure 5.26 **Recommended fat intake.** The *Dietary Guidelines for Americans* recommends a maximum fat intake of 20 to 35 percent of total calories. Saturated fat should supply no more than 10 percent of our total calories, or about one-third of our fat calories.

total energy intake—may be necessary to avoid adverse effects and would be prudent to minimize health risks.[31]

Essential Fatty Acid Requirements

Although too much fat in the diet is not healthful, we still need to get enough fat to meet our need for essential fatty acids. Because essential fatty acid deficiency is virtually nonexistent in the United States and Canada, the DRI committee relied on median intake levels of essential fatty acids to set AI levels. For adults aged 19 to 50, the AI for linoleic acid is 17 grams per day for men and 12 grams per day for women. The AI for *alpha*-linolenic acid is 1.6 grams per day for men and 1.1 grams per day for women. To fulfill our need for *omega*-6 fatty acids, linoleic acid should provide about 2 percent of our calories. Average U.S. consumption is much more than that. Two teaspoons of corn oil, which is a little more than half linoleic acid, would supply more than 2 percent of the calories in a 2,000-kilocalorie diet.

Because science has recognized the importance of *omega*-3 fatty acids only recently, we know less about our requirements.

Omega-6 and *Omega*-3 Balance

The AIs for essential fatty acids reflect the balance of *omega*-6 linoleic acid and *omega*-3 *alpha*-linolenic acid in our modern food supply. Before commercial processing made large quantities of vegetable oils widely available, *omega*-6 linoleic acid was hard to come by. In contrast, availability of *omega*-3s in the food supply has increased very little over time. In fact, some were even removed from foods to discourage rancidity. As a result, the ratio of *omega*-3 to *omega*-6 in the American diet has fallen. The low intake of *omega*-3 fatty acids in relation to the high intake of *omega*-6 fatty acids has caused concerns about an unhealthy imbalance.

Some researchers suggest that to reduce cardiovascular disease risk we should get about 0.75 percent of our calories as *alpha*-linolenic acid (about 1.7 grams per day for a 2,000-kilocalorie diet) and increase EPA and DHA intake to 0.25 to 0.5 percent of calories, or about 500 to 1,000 milligrams per day for a 2,000-kilocalorie diet.[32] A ratio of 6:1 for *omega*-6 fatty acids to *omega*-3 fatty acids is also recommended.[33] To meet these recommendations for *omega*-3 fatty acids, we would need about 1½ to 2 tablespoons of canola or soybean oil per day along with four meals containing fatty fish each week—a threefold increase in current U.S. fish consumption! **Figure 5.27** gives an overview of the dietary sources of fatty acids. Because shark, swordfish, king mackerel, and tilefish contain high levels of mercury, the FDA and EPA recommend that women who may become pregnant, pregnant women, nursing mothers, and young children avoid eating these fish.[34]

It is important to remember that consuming too much of the *omega*-3 fatty acids can suppress immune function and prolong bleeding time, so we should be cautious about the high levels of these fatty acids found in some supplements. The DRI committee set an AMDR for *omega*-6 fatty acids of 5 to 10 percent of energy and an AMDR for *alpha*-linolenic acid of 0.6 to 1.2 percent of energy.

Current Dietary Intakes

Dietary surveys report that mean fat intake is just under 33 percent of calories.[35] Although this value is within the recommended AMDR, about 25 percent of the population has a fat intake greater than 35 percent of calories.

BASIC FATTY ACIDS

Saturated
Animal products (including dairy products), palm and coconut oils, and cocoa butter.

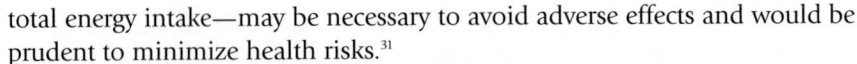

Polyunsaturated
Sunflower, corn, soybean, and cottonseed oils.

Monounsaturated
Most nuts and olive, canola, peanut, and safflower oils.

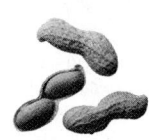

TRANS FATTY ACIDS
Stick margarine (not soft or liquid margarine) and many fast foods and baked goods.

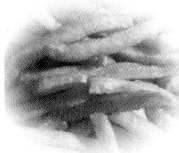

ESSENTIAL FATTY ACIDS

Omega-3 fatty acids

Alpha-*linolenic acid*
Canola oil, soybeans, olive oil, many nuts (e.g., walnuts, peanuts, filberts, pistachios, pecans, almonds), seeds, and purslane (a green, leafy vegetable).

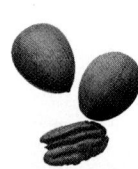

DHA and EPA
Fish such as mackerel, tuna, salmon, herring, trout, and cod liver oil. The fish with the lowest amount of total fat include Atlantic cod, haddock, and pink salmon. Other fish high in *omega*-3 but also high in total fat are sardines and bluefish. Human milk.

Omega-6 fatty acids

Linoleic acid
Plants (flax) and some vegetable oils (soybean and canola oil).

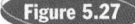 **Figure 5.27** **Overview of dietary sources of fatty acids. Source:** Cancer smart. *Scientific American.* July, 1998;4(3):9.

Fat intake as a percentage of calories is down from 36 percent in the early 1970s, and down markedly from 45 percent in 1965. See "What About Bobbie?" at the end of this chapter to see how to calculate the percentage of calorie intake from fat.

Although the percentage of calories from fat dropped, average calorie intake increased, which means Americans actually are consuming more total grams of fat. Desserts, hamburgers, and french-fried potatoes are the largest contributors to fat intake, according to the NCEP.[36] Although fat intake from meats has fallen markedly since 1970, fat intake from salad and cooking oils and shortenings has risen dramatically.[37]

Current intake of saturated fat is about 11 percent of calories, a little higher than recommended. Cholesterol intake averages 341 milligrams per day for adult men, and 242 milligrams per day for adult women.[38] Intake of linoleic acid is estimated to be 6 percent of calories, with *alpha*-linolenic acid providing 0.75 of calories and EPA plus DHA another 0.1 percent of calories. By keeping total fat intake within the AMDR and getting most of our fat from vegetable oils, fish, and nuts, we can move closer to meeting recommendations.

Role of Fat Replacers

The food industry responded to the public health challenge of the 1990s to lower fat intake by making low-fat, low-calorie goodies that still taste good. More than 15 different types of **fat replacers** have been developed, and over the years, thousands of fat-free, low-fat, and reduced-fat foods have hit grocery shelves.[39]

Fat Replacers: What Are They Made Of?

Some fat replacers are carbohydrates: generally starches and fibers such as vegetable gums, cellulose, maltodextrins, and Oatrim (a fat replacer made from oats). Some are more digestible than others, but all provide far fewer than the 9 kilocalories per gram of fat. They also incorporate extra water into food by binding with it, which further dilutes calories. With their moist, thick textures, they mimic fat's richness and smooth "mouth feel."

Proteins are the raw ingredients of other fat replacers. Food manufacturers can modify egg whites and whey from milk so that they are thick and smooth and hold water. Because this protein and water combination has fewer calories per gram than fat, it cuts calories. However, high heat denatures the protein structure, which changes the properties of these replacers and limits their usefulness. Manufacturers used the protein-based product Simplesse in frozen desserts, but it was not well accepted by consumers.

The most high-tech fat replacers—and the most controversial—are the "fat-based" replacers. This group includes Olean and the poorly digested Caprenin and Salatrim (or Benefat). Caprenin is a blend of medium-chain fatty acids and a 22-carbon fatty acid. Salatrim is primarily a blend of 18-carbon stearic acid and short-chain fatty acids. The fatty acids are arranged on glycerol in a way that inhibits digestion. They provide about half the calories of fat, although this is only an estimate because people differ in their ability to digest them. Manufacturers use these fat replacers in reduced-fat candies and baked goods.

One advantage of fat-based fat replacers is their ability to withstand heat. That's fortunate for **olestra** (Olean), because few food ingredients have had to take as much "heat." Technically, olestra is a sucrose polyester: Sucrose (instead of glycerol) is the "backbone" molecule, with six to eight fatty acids attached (instead of triglyceride's three). (See **Figure 5.28.**)

fat replacers Compounds that imitate the functional and sensory properties of fats, but contain less available energy than fats.

olestra A fat replacer that can withstand heat and is stable at frying temperatures. Olestra, whose trade name is Olean, is a sucrose polyester: Sucrose (instead of glycerol) is the "backbone" molecule, with six to eight fatty acids attached (instead of triglyceride's three). The fatty acid arrangement prevents hydrolysis by digestive lipases, so the fatty acids are not absorbed.

American Dietetic Association

Fat Replacers

It is the position of the American Dietetic Association that the majority of fat replacers, when used in moderation by adults, can be safe and useful adjuncts to lowering the fat content of foods and may play a role in decreasing total dietary energy and fat intake. Moderate use of low-calorie, reduced-fat foods, combined with low total energy intake, could potentially promote dietary intake consistent with the objectives of *Healthy People 2010* and the 2005 *Dietary Guidelines for Americans.*

J Am Diet Assoc. 2005;105:266–275.
Reprinted with permission.

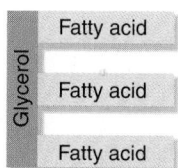

A triglyceride has three fatty acids attached to a glycerol backbone

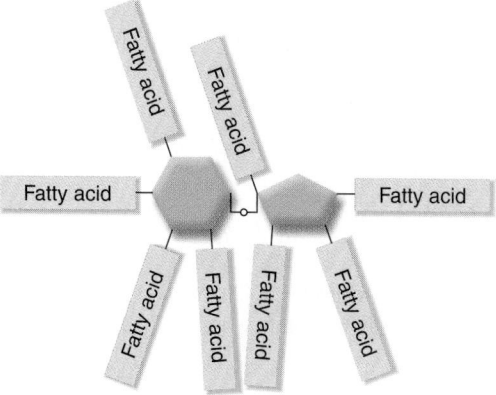

Olestra has six to eight fatty acids attached to a sucrose backbone

Figure 5.28 **The structure of olestra is unlike the structure of a triglyceride.** Although olestra imparts triglyceride-like qualities to food, your digestive enzymes cannot break it down.

Fyi Does "Reduced Fat" Reduce Calories? That Depends on the Food

Reducing fat intake is a common dietary recommendation, one that can help reduce risk for heart disease, cancer, and obesity. Given that fat is our most concentrated source of calories, we expect that a reduced-fat or low-fat food would have fewer calories than its unmodified counterpart. But is this always true?

Sometimes low-fat and fat-free foods make a big difference in calories.

Food	Kilocalories
1 oz American cheese	105
1 oz low-fat cheese product	50
2 oz bologna	180
2 oz fat-free bologna	45
1 tbsp mayonnaise	100
1 tbsp fat-free mayonnaise/dressing	12

But sometimes they make almost no difference at all.

Food	Kilocalories
1 cup canned chicken vegetable soup	75
1 cup reduced-fat chicken vegetable soup	95
3 chocolate cookies (30 g)	145
3 reduced-fat chocolate chip cookies (30 g)	135
2 tbsp peanut butter	190
2 tbsp reduced-fat peanut butter	170
1 oz potato chips	150
1 oz reduced-fat potato chips	135

Many reduced-fat products contain added sugar. Although sugar has fewer calories per gram than fat, the amount added may negate any difference in calories. If fat is your concern, low-fat or fat-free makes sense. But if you're trying to reduce fat *and* calories, modified products may not be a big help. So, be a smart shopper—check the label before you check out with a cartload of reduced-fat foods.

Source: US Department of Agriculture, Agricultural Research Service. USDA National Nutrient Database for Standard Reference, Release 18. 2005. http://www.nal.usda.gov/fnic/foodcomp. Accessed 6/8/06.

Regular mayonnaise

Nutrition Facts

Serving Size: 1 Tbsp (14g)
Servings: 32

Calories 100
  Fat Cal 100

Amount/serving

	%DV
Total Fat 11g	17%
Saturated Fat 1.5g	8%
Trans Fat 0g	
Cholesterol 5mg	2%
Sodium 80mg	3%
Total Carbohydrate 0g	0%
Protein 0g	

* Percent Daily Values (DV) are based on a 2,000 calorie diet.

INGREDIENTS: SOYBEAN OIL, WHOLE EGGS AND EGG YOLKS, WATER, VINEGAR, SALT, SUGAR, LEMON JUICE, NATURAL FLAVORS, CALCIUM DISODIUM SULFATE EDTA USED TO PROTECT QUALITY.

Light mayonnaise

Nutrition Facts

Serving Size: 1 Tbsp (14g)
Servings: 32

Calories 50
  Fat Cal 45

Amount/serving

	%DV
Total Fat 5g	8%
Saturated Fat 1g	4%
Trans Fat 0g	
Cholesterol 5mg	2%
Sodium 115mg	5%
Total Carbohydrate 0g	0%
Protein 0g	

* Percent Daily Values (DV) are based on a 2,000 calorie diet. Not a significant source of dietary fiber, vitamin A, vitamin C, calcium, and iron.

INGREDIENTS: WATER, SOYBEAN OIL, VINEGAR, FOOD STARCH-MODIFIED*, EGG YOLKS, SUGAR, SALT, LEMON JUICE, MUSTARD FLOUR, XANTHAN GUM*, BETA-CAROTENE (COLOR)*, AND NATURAL FLAVORS, POTASSIUM SORBATE, AND CALCIUM DISODIUM SULFATE EDTA USED TO PROTECT QUALITY.

*INGREDIENTS NOT FOUND IN MAYONNAISE.

The number and arrangement of fatty acids and the length and saturation of each fatty acid determine the characteristics of the sucrose polyester. This allows manufacturers to vary properties such as melting point and consistency, to make olestra appropriate for each intended use. The fatty acid arrangement prevents hydrolysis by digestive lipase, so the fatty acids are not absorbed. This makes olestra calorie-free, even though its fatty acids give it the flavor and cooking performance of fat. It is stable even at frying temperatures.

The Olestra Controversy: Are Fat Replacers Safe?

Consumers have expressed few safety concerns about carbohydrate- and protein-based fat replacers. Most safety issues center on olestra, which aroused controversy long before it received FDA approval as a food additive in January 1996. The approval process itself was controversial,[40] and even after FDA approval, olestra continued to evoke strong, conflicting opinions.[41]

Because the GI tract does not absorb olestra, some people suffer fat malabsorption symptoms—diarrhea, gas, and cramps. Olestra also acts as a solvent for fat-soluble nutrients. Thus, when it leaves the body unabsorbed, it carries these nutrients with it. Manufacturers are required to replace fat-soluble vitamins, but critics counter that healthful phytochemicals such as the carotenoids are lost and not replaced.

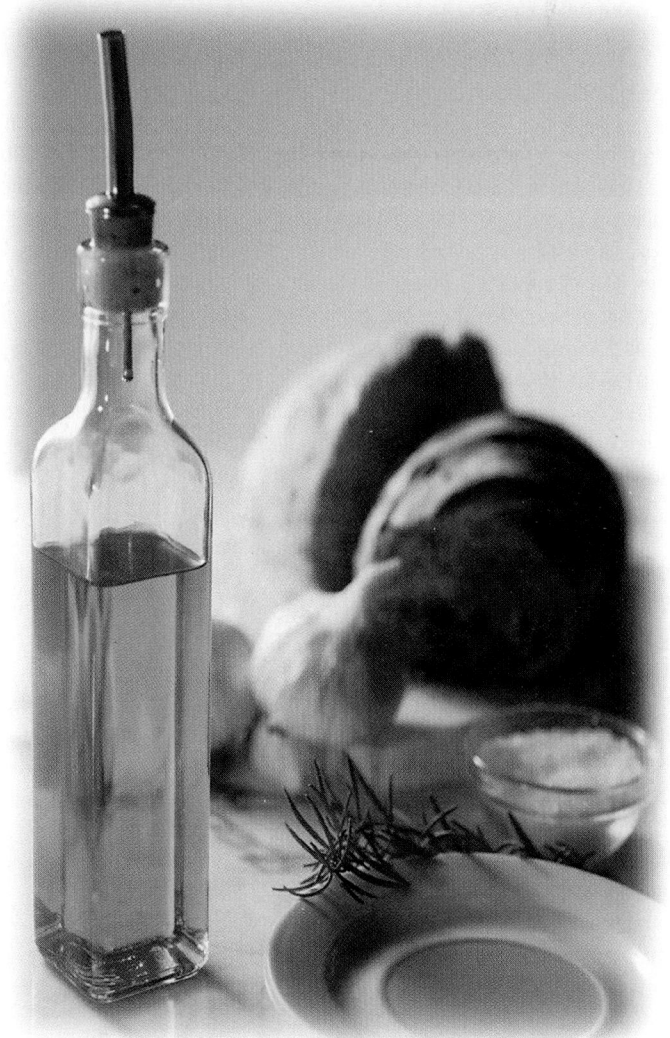

The FDA, concerned about malabsorption and nutrient loss, has limited olestra's use to just a few snack foods. Critics would like to see olestra eliminated altogether, whereas the food industry wants to expand its usage. Postmarketing surveillance (mandated by the FDA) shows that only a small percentage (5 percent) of those surveyed were "heavy consumers" with an average intake of more than 2.0 grams per day.[42] The calorie savings from even a small amount (1 to 2 grams per day) of fat replacement with olestra may be enough to prevent gradual weight gain in adulthood.[43] Surveillance has also not found evidence of reduced blood levels of carotenoids and fat-soluble vitamins.[44]

The power of suggestion, brought on by adverse publicity, may be responsible for some consumers' digestive discomfort after eating olestra-containing chips. In fact, in a large double-blind study of volunteers that pitted olestra-containing chips against regular chips, more people had indigestion after eating the regular chips. Will using olestra subtly encourage people to eat more? In another study, when subjects ate unlabeled olestra-containing potato chips, they ate fewer total calories and less fat than when they ate unlabeled regular potato chips. But when they knew the chips they were eating were fat-free, the subjects ate more.[45] If consumers eat too many olestra-containing snacks, they may be more likely to suffer side effects.

When used in moderation, fat replacers pose no specific risks to adult consumers. There is still a need for research to determine whether long-term consumption increases health risks or if there are specific risks to children.[46]

Do Fat Replacers Save Calories? Do They Reduce Total Fat Intake?

Considering the American population as a whole, the answer to these questions seems to be "no." American fat and calorie intake has not declined with the growth in the fat-replacer market. It is clear that fat replacers won't help if people treat them simply as an excuse to eat more. Nor should "low-fat foods" be confused with "low-calorie foods"; the calories saved by eating low-fat foods are often negligible.[47]

Label [to] Table

The Nutrition Facts panel shown here highlights all of the lipid-related information you can find on a food label. Look at the top of the label, where it states that this product contains 35 calories from fat. Do you know how you can estimate this number from another part of the label? Recall (or look at the bottom of the label) that each gram of fat contains 9 kilocalories. If this food item has 4 grams of fat, then it should make sense that there are approximately 36 kilocalories provided by fat.

Total fat is the second thing you'll see, along with saturated and *trans* fat. Manufacturers are required to list only saturated and *trans* fat content on the label, but they can voluntarily list monounsaturated and polyunsaturated fat. Using this food label, you can estimate the amount of unsaturated fat by simply looking at the highlighted sections. There are 4 total grams of fat—2.5 of them are saturated and 0.5 are *trans*. That means the remaining 1.0 gram is either polyunsaturated, monounsaturated, or a mix of both. Without even knowing what food item this label represents, you can see that it contains more saturated and *trans* fat than unsaturated fat (3.0 grams versus 1.0 gram).

Do you see the "6 percent" to the right of "Total Fat"? It does not mean that the food item contains 6 percent of its calories from

fat. In fact, this food item contains 23 percent of its calories from fat (35 fat kilocalories ÷ 154 total kilocalories = 0.23, or 23% fat kilocalories). The 6 percent refers to the Daily Values found below. You can see that a person who consumes 2,000 kilocalories per day could consume up to 65 grams of fat per day. This product contributes just 4 grams per serving, which is 6 percent of that amount (4 ÷ 65 = 0.06, or 6%). Note that the % Daily Value for saturated fat is 12 percent, which means that just a few servings of this food can contribute quite a bit of saturated fat to your diet. There is no DV for *trans* fat, but intake should be kept as low as possible. Cholesterol is also highlighted on this label (20 mg) along with its Daily Value contribution (7%).

Nutrition Facts

Serving Size: 1 cup (248g)
Servings Per Container: 4

Amount Per Serving

Calories 154   Calories from fat 35

	% Daily Value*
Total Fat 4g	6%
Saturated Fat 2.5g	12%
Trans Fat 0.5g	
Cholesterol 20mg	7%
Sodium 170mg	7%
Total Carbohydrate 19g	6%
Dietary Fiber 0g	0%
Sugars 14g	

Protein 11g

Vitamin A 4%	•	Vitamin C 6%
Calcium 40%	•	Iron 0%

* Percent Daily Values are based on a 2,000 calorie diet. Your daily values may be higher or lower depending on your calorie needs:

		Calories:	2,000	2,500
Total Fat	Less Than		65g	80g
Sat Fat	Less Than		20g	25g
Cholesterol	Less Than		300mg	300mg
Sodium	Less Than		2,400mg	2,400mg
Total Carbohydrate			300g	375g
Dietary Fiber			25g	30g

Calories per gram:
Fat 9 · Carbohydrate 4 · Protein 4

Lipids and Health

Moderation and balance are the keys to a healthful diet. When diets are consistently high in fat, several problems emerge. High-fat diets are typically high in calories, and contribute to weight gain and obesity. High intakes of saturated fat and *trans* fat increase risk for heart disease, and high-fat diets have been weakly linked to several types of cancer.[48] The dietary recommendations discussed earlier suggest levels of fat intake that should reduce risk for these conditions.

Obesity

Obesity is defined as the excessive accumulation of body fat leading to a body weight in relation to height that is substantially greater than some accepted standard (see Chapter 8, "Energy Balance, Body Composition, and Weight Management"). Approximately 65 percent of American adults are overweight or obese, and the rates are climbing, especially among children and teens.[49]

Eating large amounts of dietary fat contributes to this obesity epidemic.[50] Fat is a dense source of calories, it makes food taste good, and it's often unnoticed or "hidden" in restaurant and convenience foods. **Table 5.6** shows how fat increases the calorie content of foods. Standard advice to Americans trying to attain or maintain normal weight usually includes cutting back on fats and fatty foods, along with increasing physical activity and eating fewer calories. For more on obesity and weight management, see Chapter 8.

Quick Bites

What Does the Color of Beef Fat Reveal?

Yellow-tinged fat indicates that a steer was grass fed, while white fat suggests that the animal was fed corn or cereal grain, at least during its final months. Thus, steak surrounded by pearly white fat should be more tender and, consequently, more expensive.

Table 5.6 Fat Can Markedly Increase Calories in Food

	Approximate Kcalories	Approximate Fat (g)
4 oz fried potatoes	188	5.8
4 oz boiled potatoes	98	0.1
$\frac{1}{2}$ cup creamed cottage cheese	108	4.7
$\frac{1}{2}$ cup 1% low-fat cottage cheese	82	1.2
$\frac{1}{2}$ cup green beans + 1 tsp butter	56	4.0
$\frac{1}{2}$ cup green beans without butter	22	0.2
3 oz T-bone steak, untrimmed	260	19.4
3 oz T-bone steak, trimmed	161	7.4
$\frac{1}{2}$ cup vanilla ice cream	145	7.92
$\frac{1}{2}$ cup fat-free vanilla ice cream	105	0.0

Source: Based on data from US Department of Agriculture, Agricultural Research Service. USDA National Nutrient Database for Standard Reference, Release 18. 2005. http://www.nal.usda.gov/fnic/foodcompindex.html. Accessed 5/24/06.

NUTRITION SCIENCE IN ACTION

A Matter of Fat

Observations: Cardiovascular disease (CVD) is the leading cause of death in women in the United States, Canada, and throughout most of the world. Clinical trials and observational studies have identified strong associations between diet and CVD risk factors. To confirm that reducing fat intake reduces risk of CVD, long-term intervention data are needed.

Hypothesis: A dietary intervention that reduces intake of total fat and increases intakes of fruits, vegetables, and grains will reduce the risk of cardiovascular disease.

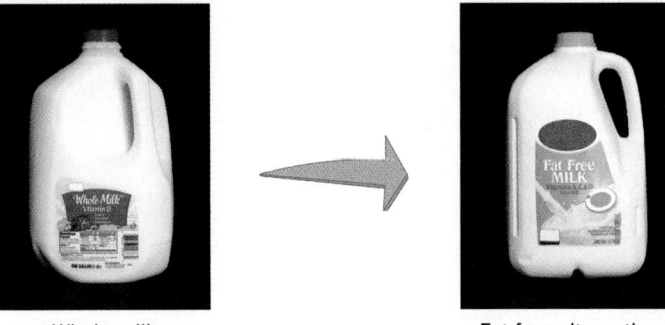

Whole milk   Fat-free alternative

Experimental Plan: The Women's Health Initiative (WHI) enrolled 48,835 women (mean age 62.3 years; 20 percent nonwhite). Investigators randomly assigned 19,541 women to an intervention group that participated in a behavioral modification program aimed at reducing intake of total fat and increasing intakes of grains and fruits and vegetables; the remainder were the control group. For both groups, dietary adherence and health outcomes were recorded for eight years.

Results: The hypothesis was not confirmed. The main CVD findings were that the intervention had no effect on risk of coronary heart disease, stroke, or overall cardiovascular disease. Compared with the control group, the intervention group reported significant changes in all dietary components, resulting in an 8.2 percent reduction in total fat intake and increased intakes of fiber, vegetables and fruits, grains, and soy.

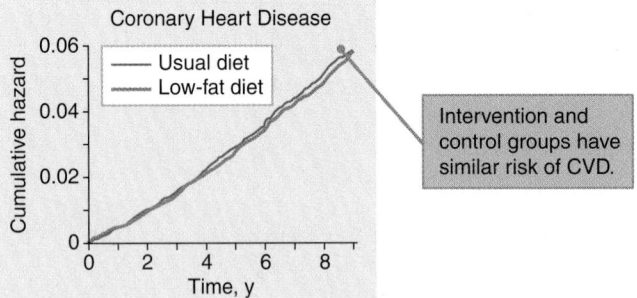

Conclusion and Discussion: The intervention focused on total fat, thus reducing intakes of fats that increase CVD risk (saturated and *trans* fat) *and* those that may reduce risk (unsaturated fats). Since this study was initiated, scientific thinking has evolved to focus on modifying intakes of specific types of fat. Future dietary intervention studies of dietary fat and CVD risk could examine changes in the intakes of different types of dietary fat or other dietary factors, such as fish and fish oil, for which a compelling body of evidence suggests protective effects.

Source: Based on Howard BV, Van Horn L, Hsia J, et al. Low-fat dietary pattern and risk of cardiovascular disease—the Women's Health Initiative randomized controlled dietary modification trial. *JAMA.* 2006;295:655–666.

Heart Disease

Heart disease is the leading cause of death in the United States and Canada, and fat intake is a key factor in its development. High saturated and *trans* fat intake raises blood cholesterol levels, particularly LDL cholesterol.[51] High blood cholesterol is one of the major risk factors for atherosclerosis, a type of heart disease in which arteries become progressively clogged with deposits of fatty material. To reduce the risk of heart disease, reducing intakes of saturated and *trans* fats appears more important than modifying total fat intake.[52] See Nutrition Science in Action, "A Matter of Fat." For more on diet and heart disease, see Chapter 14, "Diet and Health."

Cancer

The evidence linking dietary fat to cancer is inconclusive. The case looks strong when we compare cancer rates between countries: Overall cancer rates are generally higher in countries with high fat intake, and lower in countries where people eat less fat. But in population studies within those countries, the evidence linking fat to cancer is weaker. For more on diet and cancer, see Chapter 14, "Diet and Health."

Key Concepts: *Current recommendations suggest eating 20 to 35 percent of calories from fat, while keeping saturated fat,* trans *fat, and cholesterol intake as low as possible. Over the years, Americans have reduced their percentage of calories from fat but are eating more total calories and, as a result, more grams of fat. This is in spite of the increased availability of a wide variety of fat substitutes and lower-fat foods. Excessive fat intake has been linked to obesity, heart disease, and cancer.*

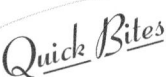

NCEP Tips for Healthful Eating Out

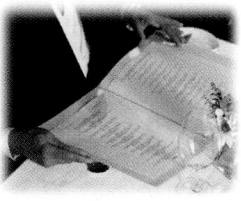

- Choose restaurants that have low-fat, low-cholesterol menu items.

- Don't be afraid to ask for foods that follow your eating pattern.

- Select poultry, fish, or meat that is broiled, grilled, baked, steamed, or poached rather than fried.

- Choose lean deli meats like fresh turkey or lean roast beef instead of higher-fat cuts like salami or bologna.

- Look for vegetables seasoned with herbs or spices rather than butter, sour cream, or cheese. Ask for sauces on the side.

- Order a low-fat dessert like sherbet, fruit ice, sorbet, or low-fat frozen yogurt.

- Control serving sizes by asking for a small serving, sharing a dish, or taking some home.

- At fast-food restaurants, go for grilled chicken and lean roast beef sandwiches or lean plain hamburgers (but remember to hold the fatty sauces), salads with low-fat salad dressing, low-fat milk, and low-fat frozen yogurt. Pizza topped with vegetables and minimum cheese is another good choice.

LEARNING *Portfolio* chapter 5

Key Terms

Study Points

- Lipids are a group of compounds that are soluble in organic solvents but not in water. Fats and oils are part of the lipids group.
- There are three main classes of lipids: triglycerides, phospholipids, and sterols.
- Fatty acids—long carbon chains with methyl and carboxyl groups on the ends—are components of both triglycerides and phospholipids and are often attached to cholesterol.
- Saturated fatty acids have no double bonds between carbons in the chain, monounsaturated fatty acids have one double bond, and polyunsaturated fatty acids have more than one double bond.
- Two polyunsaturated fatty acids, linoleic acid and *alpha*-linolenic acid, are essential; they must be supplied in the diet. Phospholipids and sterols are made in the body and do not have to be supplied in the diet.
- Essential fatty acids are elongated and desaturated in the process of making "local hormones" called eicosanoids. These compounds regulate many body functions.
- Triglycerides are food fats and storage fats. They are composed of glycerol and three fatty acids.
- In the body, triglycerides are an important source of energy. Stored fat provides an energy reserve.
- Phospholipids are made of glycerol, two fatty acids, and a phosphate group with a nitrogen-containing component.
- Phospholipids are components of cell membranes and lipoproteins. Their unique affinity for both fat and water allows them to be effective emulsifiers in foods and in the body.
- Cholesterol is found in cell membranes and is used to synthesize vitamin D, bile salts, and steroid hormones. High levels of blood cholesterol are associated with heart disease risk.
- For adults, the Acceptable Macronutrient Distribution Range (AMDR) for fat is 20 to 35 percent of calories.
- Diets high in fat and saturated fat tend to increase blood levels of LDL cholesterol and increase risk for heart disease.
- Excess fat in the diet is linked to obesity, heart disease, and some types of cancer.

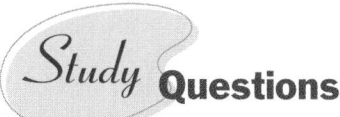

Study Questions

1. **How can different oils contain a mixture of polyunsaturated, monounsaturated, and saturated fats?**

2. **What does the hardness or softness of a triglyceride typically signify?**

3. **What is the most common form of lipid found in food?**

4. **What are the positive and negative consequences of hydrogenating a fat?**

5. **List the many functions of triglycerides.**

6. **Describe the difference between LDL and HDL in terms of cholesterol and protein composition.**

7. **What foods contain cholesterol?**

8. **Name the two essential fatty acids.**

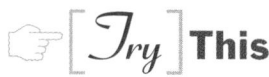 **This**

The Fat = Fullness Challenge

The goal of this experiment is to see whether fat affects your desire to eat between meals. Do this experiment for two consecutive breakfasts. Each meal is to include *only* the foods listed here. Try to eat normally for the other meals of the day and to eat around the same time of day. Each of these breakfasts has approximately the same calories, but one has a high percentage of them from fat, the other from carbohydrate. After each breakfast, take note of how many hours pass before you feel hungry again.

Day 1 ($\sim$ 420 kilocalories; 1.5 grams fat)

One 3-oz bagel with 3 Tbsp of jelly

Day 2 ($\sim$ 430 kilocalories; 28 grams fat)

2 eggs fried

1 biscuit (2½ inch diameter) with 1 tsp butter or margarine

What About Bobbie?

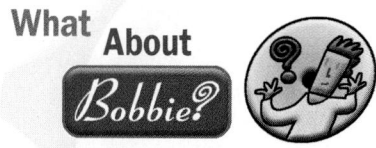

Let's take a look at Bobbie's fat intake. Review her day of eating (see Chapter 1) and pay special attention to the foods you know contain fat. What percentage of her calories do you think came from fat? Did she eat more saturated or unsaturated fat? How about her cholesterol intake? Do you think she came in below the guideline?

Bobbie's total fat intake was 86 grams. Here are the foods that contributed the most fat:

Food	Fat (g)
Salad dressing	13
Meatballs	11
Tortilla chips	11
Garlic bread	10
Cream cheese	8
Mayonnaise	7
Pizza	6

Bobbie's diet has 34 percent of its calories from fat, which is within the AMDR for fat. Here's how to calculate this:

86 grams fat $\times$ 9 kcal/g = 774 kcal fat

774 kcal fat $\div$ 2,300 total kcal = 0.34, or 34% kcal from fat

Are you surprised her fat intake is on the high end of the recommended range? Her intake doesn't look too unusual, but you can see how the "extras" along the way add up. Look at the list of fat-containing foods again. Do you think her diet is higher in saturated or unsaturated fat? Well, three of the foods listed are animal products (meatballs, pizza, and cream cheese), so you know they contribute to the amount of saturated fat. Both the tortilla chips and garlic bread contain a mixture of saturated and unsaturated fats, and the Italian dressing contains mostly unsaturated fat. Her overall saturated fat intake is 27 grams. That's about 11 percent of her caloric intake, which is more than recommended by the *Dietary Guidelines for Americans* (no more than 10 percent of energy as saturated fat). If Bobbie wanted to lower her saturated fat and total fat intake, what changes could she make ? Here are some suggestions.

Bobbie can lower her saturated fat intake by
- Topping her bagel with peanut butter instead of cream cheese
- Decreasing the number of meatballs on her pasta
- Snacking on pizza less often

What About Bobbie?

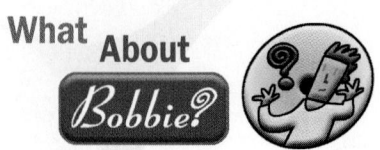

Bobbie can lower her overall fat intake by

- Using cream cheese on only half her bagel and using jelly on the other half
- Using only mustard on her sandwich, not mustard *and* mayonnaise
- Reducing the amount of tortilla chips she eats by half and having a piece of fruit in their place
- Reducing the amount of Italian dressing she puts on her salad (2 tablespoons contain 11 grams of fat and more than 100 kilocalories!)
- Having a plain piece of bread with dinner, not the garlic bread made with butter or margarine

In terms of cholesterol, how do you think Bobbie did? She consumed 261 milligrams in this day. If she follows the tips to lower her saturated fat intake, she'll find that her overall cholesterol intake will be cut in half!

References

1 Mozaffarian D, Katan MB, Ascherio A, et al. Trans fatty acids and cardiovascular disease. *New Engl J Med.* 2006;354(15): 1601–1613.

2 Institute of Medicine, Food and Nutrition Board. *Dietary Reference Intakes for Energy, Carbohydrate, Fiber, Fat, Fatty Acids, Cholesterol, Protein, and Amino Acids.* Washington, DC: National Academy Press, 2005.

3 Ibid.

4 Connor WE. Importance of n-3 fatty acids in health and disease. *Am J Clin Nutr.* 2000;71(suppl):171S–175S; Djoussé L, Arnett DK, Carr AJ, et al. Dietary linolenic acid is inversely associated with calcified atherosclerotic plaque in the coronary arteries: the National Heart, Lung, and Blood Institute Family Heart Study. *Circulation.* 2005;111:2921–2926.

5 Crawford MA. The role of essential fatty acids in neural development: implications for perinatal nutrition. *Am J Clin Nutr.* 1993;57:S703–S710.

6 Hendler SS, Rorvik D, eds. *PDR for Nutritional Supplements.* Montvale, NJ: Medical Economics/Thompson Healthcare, 2001.

7 Wan PJ, Hron RJ. Extraction solvents for oilseeds. *Inform.* July 1998;9:707–709.

8 Seidner DL. Clinical uses for omega-3 polyunsaturated fatty acids and structured triglycerides. *Support Line.* June 1994; 16:7–11.

9 Neaton JD, Blackburn H, Jacobs D, et al. Serum cholesterol level and mortality findings for men screened in the Multiple Risk Factor Intervention Trial. Multiple Risk Factor Intervention Trial Research Group. *Arch Intern Med.* 1992;152: 1490–1500; and El-Sadr WM, Mullin CM, Carr A, et al. Effects of HIV disease on lipid, glucose and insulin levels: results from a large antiretroviral-naïve cohort. *HIV Med.* 2005; 6:114–121.

10 Cheblowski RT, Grosvenor M, Lillington L. Dietary intake and counseling, weight management, and the course of HIV infection. *J Am Diet Assoc.* 1995;95:428–432.

11 Cendella RJ. Cholesterol and cataracts. *Surv Opthalmol.* 1996; 40(4):320–337.

12 Morell P, Jurevics H. Origin of cholesterol in myelin. *Neurochem Res.* 1996;21(4):463–470.

13 Jones PJH. Regulation of cholesterol biosynthesis by diet in humans. *Am J Clin Nutr.* 1997;66:438–446.

14 Ibid.

15 Strauss E. One-eyed animals implicate cholesterol in development. *Science.* 1998;280:1528–1529.

16 Jones PJH, Kubow S. Lipids, sterols, and their metabolites. In: Shils ME, Shike M, Ross CA, Cabellero B, Cousins RJ, eds. *Modern Nutrition in Health and Disease.* 10th ed. Philadephia: Lippincott Williams & Wilkins. 2006;92–122.

17 Guyton AC, Hall JE. *Textbook of Medical Physiology.* 10th ed. Philadelphia: WB Saunders, 2000.

18 Craig GB, Darnell DE, Weinsier RL, et al. Decreased fat and nitrogen losses in patients with AIDS receiving medium-chain-triglyceride-enriched formula vs those receiving long-chain-triglyceride-containing formula. *J Am Diet Assoc.* 1997;97(6):605–611.

19 Nkondjock A, Shatenstein B, Maisonneuve P, Ghadirian P. Specific fatty acids and human colorectal cancer: an overview. *Cancer Detect Prev.* 2003;27:55–66.

20 Institute of Medicine, Food and Nutrition Board. Op. cit.

21 Lin J, Yang R, Tarr PT. Hyperlipidemic effects of dietary saturated fats mediated through PGC-1β coactivation of SREBP. *Cell.* 2005;120:261–273.

22 Brown MS, Goldstein JL. A receptor-mediated pathway for cholesterol homeostasis. *Science.* 1986;232:34–47.

23 Dietschy JM, Turley SD, Spady DK. Role of liver in the maintenance of cholesterol and low density lipoprotein homeostasis in different animal species, including humans. *J Lipid Res.* 1993;34:1637–1659.

24 Wijendran V, Hayes KC. Dietary n-6 and n-3 fatty acid balance and cardiovascular health. *Ann Rev Nutr.* 2004;24:597–615.

25 National Cholesterol Education Program. *Detection, Evaluation, and Treatment of High Blood Cholesterol in Adults (Adult Treatment Panel III) Final Report.* Washington, DC: National Institutes of Health, 2002.

26 Lichtenstein AH, Appel LJ, Brands M, et al. Diet and lifestyle recommendations revision 2006: a scientific statement from the American Heart Association Nutrition Committee. *Circulation.* 2006;114:82–96.

27 Mozafarrian D, Katan MB, Ascherio A, et al. Op cit.

28 Institute of Medicine, Food and Nutrition Board. Op. cit.

29 Ibid.

30 US Departments of Agriculture and Health and Human Services. Op. cit.

31 Mozaffarian D, Katan MB, Ascherio A, et al. Op. cit.

32 Wijendran V, Hayes KC. Op. cit.

33 Ibid.

34 US Department of Health and Human Services and Environmental Protection Agency. *What You Need to Know About Mercury in Fish and Shellfish.* March 2004. http://www.cfsan.fda.gov/~dms/admehg3.html. Accessed 12/3/06.

35 Briefel RR, Johnson CL. Secular trends in dietary intake in the United States. *Ann Rev Nutr.* 2004;24:401–431.

36 High blood cholesterol: what's known, what's new, what's ahead. *Heart Memo.* Summer 1998:5–17.

37 Borrud L, Enns LW, Mickle S. What we eat in America: USDA surveys food consumption changes. *Food Review.* September–December 1996;19(3):14–19.

38 Briefel RR, Johnson CL. Op. cit.

39 Akoh CC. Fat replacers. *Food Tech.* 1998;52:47–53.

40 Blackburn H. Olestra and the FDA. *N Engl J Med.* 1996;334:984–986.

41 Jacobsen M, Corcoran L. Olestra. *Nutrition Action Healthletter.* March 1998:9–11; and Callaway CW. Role of fat-modified foods in the American diet. *Nutrition Today.* July/Aug 1998;33:156–163.

42 Patterson RE, Kristal AR, Peters JC, et al. Changes in diet, weight, and serum lipid levels associated with olestra consumption. *Arch Intern Med.* 2000;160:2600–2604.

43 Thornquist MD, Kristal AR, Patterson RE, et al. Olestra consumption does not predict serum concentrations of carotenoids and fat-soluble vitamins in free-living humans: early results from the sentinel site of the Olestra Post-Marketing Surveillance Study. *J Nutr.* 2000;130:1711–1718.

44 Eldridge AL, Cooper DA, Peters JC. A role for olestra in body weight management. *Obesity Reviews.* 2002;3:17–25.

45 Miller DL, Casteollanos VH, Shide DJ, et al. Effect of fat-free potato chips with and without nutrition labels on fat and energy intakes. *Am J Clin Nutr.* 1998;68:282–290.

46 The American Dietetic Association. Position of the American Dietetic Association: fat replacers. *J Am Diet Assoc.* 2005;105:266–275.

47 Are reduced-fat foods keeping Americans healthier? *Tufts University Health & Nutrition Letter.* March 1998;16:4–5.

48 Zock PL. Dietary fats and cancer. *Curr Opin Lipidol.* 2001;12:5–10; and Smith-Warner SA, Spiegelman D, Adami HO, et al. Types of dietary fat and breast cancer: a pooled analysis of cohort studies. *Int J Cancer.* 2001;92:767–774.

49 National Center for Health Statistics. *Prevalence of Overweight and Obesity Among Adults: United States, 2003–2004.* Available at http://www.cdc.gov/nchs/products/pubs/pubd/hestats/obese03_04/overwght_adult_03.htm. Accessed 12/4/06.

50 Satia-About a J, Patterson RE, Schiller RN, Kristal AR. Energy from fat is associated with obesity in U.S. men: results from the Prostate Cancer Prevention Trial. *Prev Med.* 2002;34:493–501.

51 Mozaffarian D, Katan MB, Ascherio A, et al. Op. cit.

52 Anderson CA, Appel LJ. Dietary modification and CVD prevention. *JAMA.* 2006;295(6):693–695.

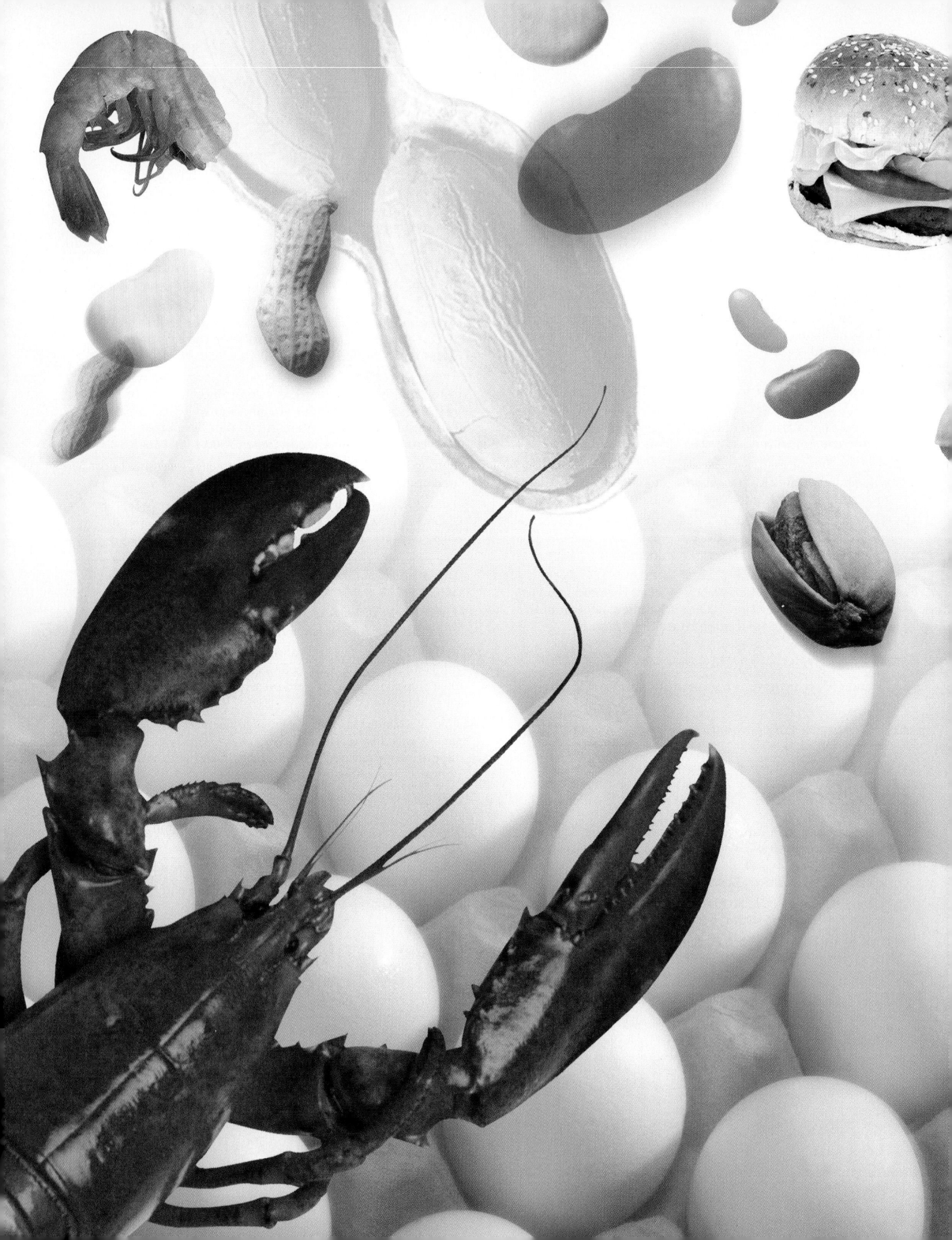

Chapter 6

Proteins and Amino Acids

Think About It

1 What's your understanding of the term *protein-sparing*?

2 Do you take amino acid supplements? If so, do you know how well they are absorbed?

3 What's your estimate of the percentage of your energy intake that comes from protein?

4 Have you ever considered a vegetarian diet?

Fyi for your Information

This chapter's FYI boxes include practical information on the following topics:
- Scrabble Anyone?
- Do Athletes Need More Protein?
- High-Protein Plant Foods

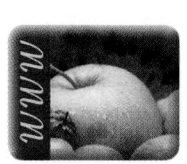

The Web site for this book offers many useful tools and is a great source for additional nutrition information for both students and instructors. Visit the site at **nutrition.jbpub.com** for information on proteins and amino acids. You'll find exercises that explore the following topics:
- Protein Supplements
- Different Proteins, Different Benefits
- Around the World with Proteins
- Chemical Structures

What About Bobbie?

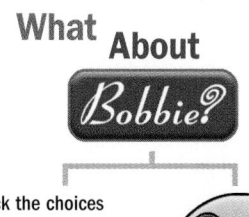
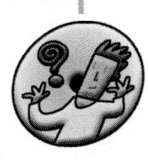

Track the choices Bobbie is making with Nutritionist Pro or EatRight Analysis software.

Key to Illustrations

	Amino Acids
	Dipeptide
	Energy
	Enzymes
	Fatty Acids
	Fructose
	Glucose
	Minerals
	Proteins
	Water

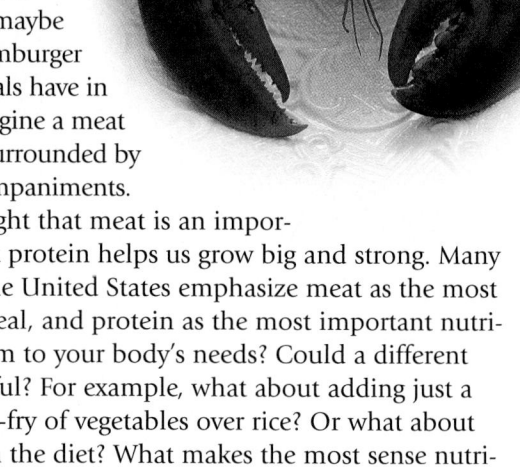

Think of your favorite meal—perhaps a holiday feast, the foods you always ask for on your birthday, or something from a special restaurant. If you are like most Americans, you have probably conjured up something along the lines of steak and baked potato; a lobster feast with corn on the cob; turkey with dressing, mashed potatoes, and all the trimmings; or maybe something simpler—a juicy hamburger and fries. What do all these meals have in common? In each case you imagine a meat item as the focus of the plate, surrounded by various grain or vegetable accompaniments.

From a young age, we're taught that meat is an important source of protein and that protein helps us grow big and strong. Many traditional ways of eating in the United States emphasize meat as the most important ingredient of the meal, and protein as the most important nutrient. But do such meals conform to your body's needs? Could a different style of eating be more healthful? For example, what about adding just a small amount of meat to a stir-fry of vegetables over rice? Or what about eliminating meat entirely from the diet? What makes the most sense nutritionally?

From the body's perspective, protein is critically important. Protein is part of every cell, it is needed in thousands of chemical reactions, and it keeps us "together" structurally. But, as you are about to learn, the human body is so good at using the protein we feed it that our actual needs for dietary protein are relatively small—meat doesn't need to be at the center of the plate to keep you healthy!

Why Is Protein Important?

The word *protein* was coined by the Dutch chemist Gerardus Mulder in 1838, and comes from the Greek word *protos*, meaning "of prime importance." Mulder discovered that proteins are a major component of all plant and animal tissues, second only to water. Today we know that these intricately constructed molecules are vital to many aspects of health and play an integral role in every living cell. Our bodies constantly assemble, break down, and use proteins, so we count on our diet to provide enough protein each day to replace what is being used. When we eat more protein than we need, the excess is either used to make energy or is stored as fat.

Most people associate protein with animal foods such as beef, chicken, fish, or milk. However, plant foods such as dried beans and peas, grains, nuts, seeds, and vegetables also provide protein. Many protein-rich plant foods are also rich in vitamins and minerals. These plant foods usually are low in fat and calories.

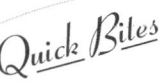

People living in poverty may suffer from a shortage of both protein and energy in the diet. When the diet lacks protein, the body breaks down tissue such as muscle and uses it as a protein source. This causes loss, or **wasting**, of muscles, organs, and other tissues. Protein deficiency also increases susceptibility to infection, and impairs digestion and absorption of nutrients. In the United States and other industrialized countries, most people are able to get more than enough protein to meet their physiological needs. In fact, a more common problem in these areas is excess intake of protein.

Amino Acids Are the Building Blocks of Proteins

Just as glucose is the basic building block of carbohydrates, amino acids are the basic building blocks of proteins. Proteins are sequences of amino acids. When building these sequences, your body has 20 different amino acids from which to choose. Nine of these amino acids are called **indispensable amino acids** because your body cannot make them and must get them in the diet. Your body can manufacture the remaining 11, called **dispensable amino acids**, when enough nitrogen, carbon, hydrogen, and oxygen are available. Dispensable amino acids do not need to be supplied in your diet.

Sometimes, certain dispensable amino acids can become indispensable. This is true of dispensable amino acids that are synthesized from other amino acids or when synthesis is limited due to special physiological conditions.[1] Tyrosine and cysteine are both considered **conditionally indispensable amino acids**. Under normal circumstances, your body makes tyrosine from the indispensable amino acid phenylalanine, and cysteine from either methionine or serine. If a disease or condition interferes with your ability to synthesize tyrosine or cysteine from their amino acid precursors, then your body will need tyrosine or cysteine from the diet. **Table 6.1** lists the indispensable, dispensable, and conditionally indispensable amino acids.

Tyrosine becomes an indispensable amino acid for people with phenylketonuria (PKU), a rare genetic disorder that impairs phenylalanine metabolism (see Chapter 4, "Carbohydrates"). Because people with PKU lack sufficient amounts of an enzyme needed to convert phenylalanine to

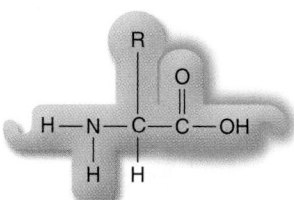

Table 6.1 Indispensable, Dispensable, and Conditionally Indispensable Amino Acids

Indispensable	Dispensable	Conditionally Indispensable
Histidine	Alanine	
Isoleucine	Arginine	Arginine
Leucine	Asparagine	
Lysine	Aspartic acid	
Methionine	Cysteine	Cysteine
Phenylalanine	Glutamic acid	
Threonine	Glutamine	Glutamine
Tryptophan	Glycine	Glycine
Valine	Proline	Proline
	Serine	
	Tyrosine	Tyrosine

wasting The breakdown of body tissue such as muscle and organ for use as a protein source when the diet lacks protein.

indispensable amino acids Amino acids that the body cannot make at all or cannot make enough of to meet physiological needs. Indispensable amino acids must be supplied in the diet.

dispensable amino acids Amino acids that the body can make if supplied with adequate nitrogen. Dispensable amino acids do not need to be supplied in the diet.

conditionally indispensable amino acids Amino acids that are normally made in the body (dispensable) but become indispensable under certain circumstances, such as during critical illness.

Figure 6.1 **Structure of an amino acid.** All amino acids have a similar structure. Attached to a carbon atom is a hydrogen (H), shown here but not in later illustrations of amino acids, an amino group (−NH₂), an acid group (−COOH), and a side group (R). The side group gives each amino acid its unique identity.

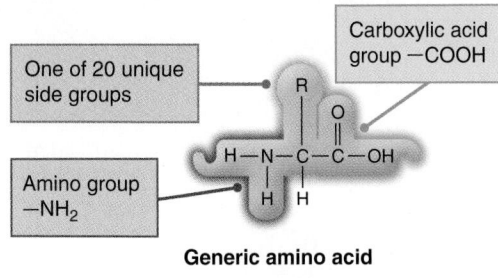

Generic amino acid

Glycine

Phenylalanine

Figure 6.2 **Forming a peptide bond.** Imagine a row of people facing forward with their hands joined—the right hand joined to the left hand. Similarly, when two amino acids join together, the carboxyl group of one amino acid is matched with the amino group of another. A condensation reaction forms a peptide bond and releases water.

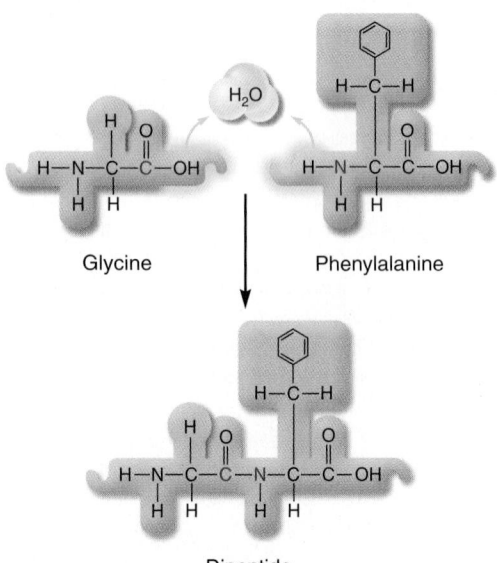

Dipeptide

tyrosine, tyrosine must be supplied in the diet. Phenylalanine intake must be carefully controlled because excess phenylalanine and its metabolic by-products (phenylketones) can build up and contribute to irreversible brain damage.[2] Because foods that have aspartame contain phenylalanine, they can be dangerous for people with PKU. When babies with PKU receive treatment starting at birth, their IQ development is unaffected. Without treatment, they suffer severe mental retardation.

Other amino acids also can become indispensable under certain circumstances. The amino acid glutamine is the main fuel for rapidly dividing cells and plays a key role in transporting nitrogen between organs.[3] Although normally considered dispensable, glutamine can become indispensable after trauma or during periods of critical illness that increase the body's need for it.[4] The amino acid arginine can also become indispensable in conditions of intestinal metabolic dysfunction or severe physiological stress.[5]

Amino Acids Are Identified by Their Side Groups

Amino acids (with the exception of proline) uniformly consist of a central carbon atom chemically bonded to one hydrogen atom (H), one carboxylic acid group (−COOH), one amino (nitrogen-containing) group (−NH₂), and one side group unique to each amino acid (R). The side group gives each amino acid its identity. It can vary from a simple hydrogen atom, as in glycine, to a complex ring of carbon and hydrogen atoms, as in phenylalanine. The side groups mean that amino acids differ in shape, size, composition, electrical charge, and pH. When amino acids are linked to form a protein, these characteristics work together to determine that protein's specific function. **Figure 6.1** shows the structure of an amino acid.

Key Concepts: *Amino acids, which consist of a central carbon atom bonded to a hydrogen, a carboxyl group, an amino group, and a side group, are the building blocks of proteins. Indispensable amino acids cannot be made by the body and must be supplied in the diet. Dispensable amino acids can be made in the body, given an adequate supply of nitrogen, carbon, hydrogen, and oxygen.*

Protein Structure: Unique Three-Dimensional Shapes and Functions

Proteins are very large molecules. Their chains of linked amino acids twist, fold, or coil into unique shapes. Just as we combine letters of the alphabet in different sequences to form an infinite variety of words, the body combines amino acids in different sequences to form a nearly infinite variety of proteins. For this reason, protein molecules are more diverse than either carbohydrates or lipids.

Amino Acid Sequence

Amino acids link in specific sequences to form strands of protein (often called peptides) up to hundreds of amino acids long. One amino acid is joined to the next by a **peptide bond**. To form a peptide bond, the carboxyl (−COOH) group of one amino acid bonds to the amino (−NH₂) group of another amino acid, releasing water (H₂O) in the process. (See **Figure 6.2**.) A **dipeptide** is two amino acids joined by a peptide bond, and a **tripeptide** is three amino acids joined by peptide bonds. The term **oligopeptide** refers to a chain of 4 to 10 amino acids, whereas a **polypeptide** contains more than 10 amino acids.[6] Proteins in the body and in the diet are long polypeptides, most with hundreds of linked amino acids.

Protein Shape

As its amino acids are assembled in the cell's cytoplasm, each protein chain assumes a unique three-dimensional shape that derives from the sequence and properties of its amino acids. The three-dimensional shape of a protein determines its function and its interaction with other molecules. As an example, **Figure 6.3** illustrates the unique folded and twisted shape of **hemoglobin**, the iron-carrying protein in red blood cells. In the lungs, hemoglobin binds oxygen and releases carbon dioxide. It then travels throughout the body, delivering oxygen to other tissues and picking up carbon dioxide for the return trip to the lungs.

Some amino acids carry electrical charges and therefore are attracted to the charged ends of water molecules (**hydrophilic amino acids**). In a watery environment, hydrophilic amino acids orient themselves on the outside of the folded protein chain in close contact with water molecules. Other amino acids are electrically neutral and do not interact with water (**hydrophobic amino acids**). In a watery environment, hydrophobic amino acids fold to the inside of the protein molecule. The amino acid cysteine, which has sulfur atoms in its side group, sometimes will chemically bond to another cysteine in the chain, creating a **disulfide bridge**, which helps stabilize the protein's structure.

peptide bond The bond between two amino acids formed when a carboxyl (–COOH) group of one amino acid joins an amino (–NH₂) group of another amino acid, releasing water in the process.
dipeptide Two amino acids joined by a peptide bond.
tripeptide Three amino acids joined by peptide bonds.
oligopeptide Four to 10 amino acids joined by peptide bonds.
polypeptide More than 10 amino acids joined by peptide bonds.
hemoglobin [HEEM-oh-glow-bin] The oxygen-carrying protein in red blood cells that consists of four heme groups and four globin polypeptide chains. The presence of hemoglobin gives blood its red color.
hydrophilic amino acids Amino acids that are attracted to water (water-loving).
hydrophobic amino acids Amino acids that are repelled by water (water-fearing).
disulfide bridge A bond between the sulfur components of two sulfur-containing amino acids that helps stabilize the structure of protein.

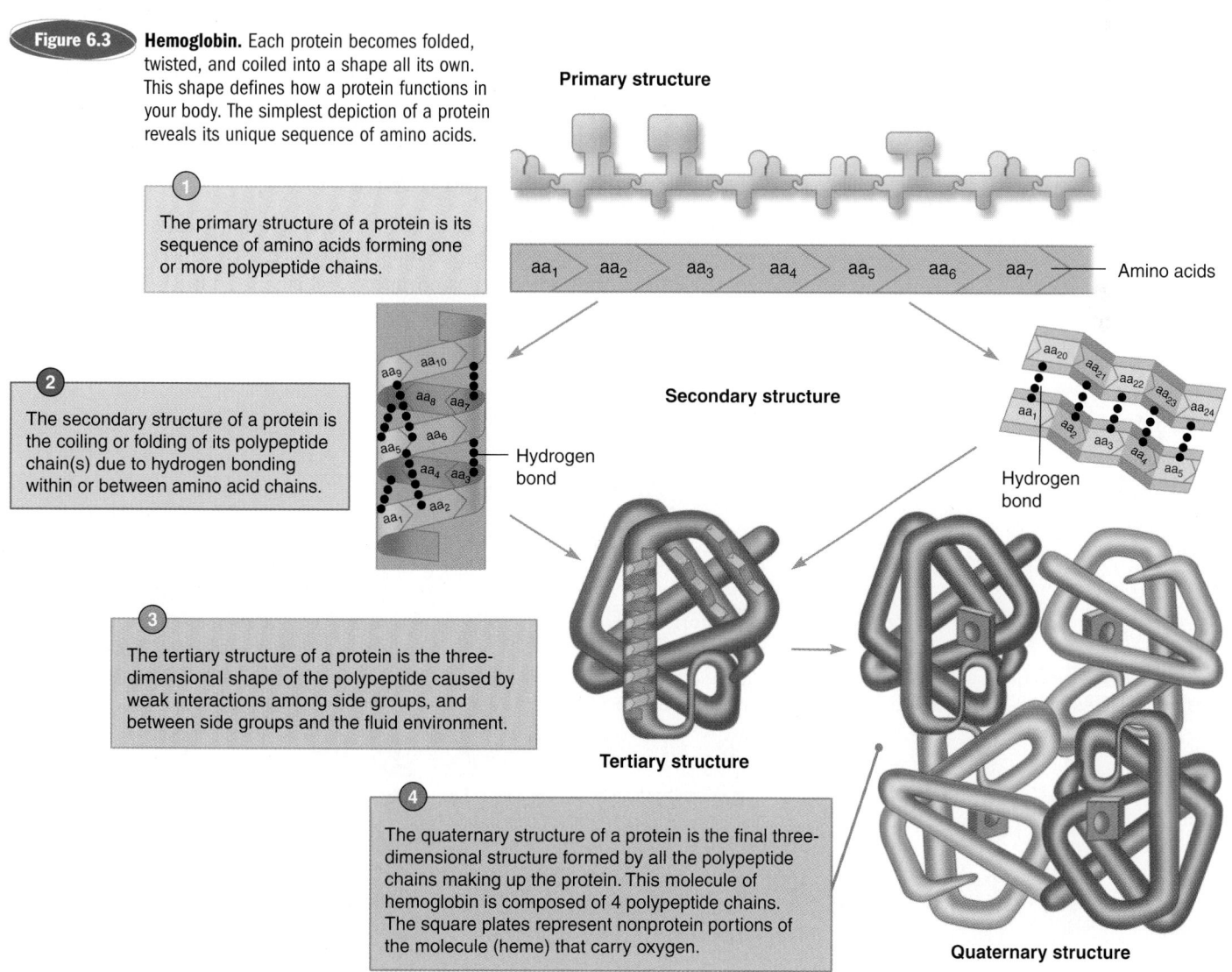

Figure 6.3 **Hemoglobin.** Each protein becomes folded, twisted, and coiled into a shape all its own. This shape defines how a protein functions in your body. The simplest depiction of a protein reveals its unique sequence of amino acids.

Primary structure

1. The primary structure of a protein is its sequence of amino acids forming one or more polypeptide chains.

aa₁ aa₂ aa₃ aa₄ aa₅ aa₆ aa₇ — Amino acids

2. The secondary structure of a protein is the coiling or folding of its polypeptide chain(s) due to hydrogen bonding within or between amino acid chains.

Secondary structure

Hydrogen bond

Hydrogen bond

3. The tertiary structure of a protein is the three-dimensional shape of the polypeptide caused by weak interactions among side groups, and between side groups and the fluid environment.

Tertiary structure

4. The quaternary structure of a protein is the final three-dimensional structure formed by all the polypeptide chains making up the protein. This molecule of hemoglobin is composed of 4 polypeptide chains. The square plates represent nonprotein portions of the molecule (heme) that carry oxygen.

Quaternary structure

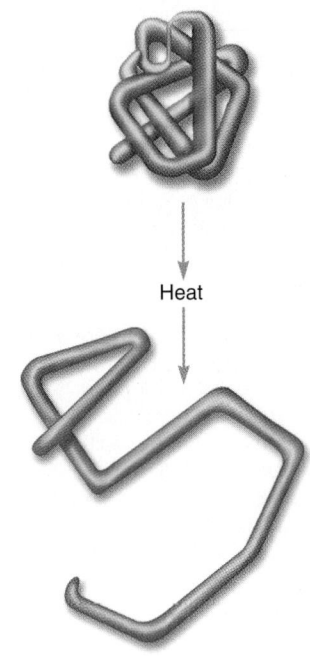

Heat

Figure 6.4 **Denaturation.** Heat, pH, oxidation and mechanical agitation are some of the forces that can denature a protein, causing it to unfold and lose its functional shape.

denaturation An alteration in the three-dimensional structure of a protein resulting in an unfolded polypeptide chain that usually lacks biological activity.

Protein Denaturation: Destabilizing a Protein's Shape

Acidity, alkalinity, heat, alcohol, oxidation, and agitation can all disrupt the chemical forces that stabilize a protein's three-dimensional shape, causing it to unfold and lose its shape (denature), as shown in **Figure 6.4**. Because a protein's shape determines its function, denatured proteins lose their ability to function properly.

If you've ever cooked an egg, you've witnessed protein **denaturation**. As the egg cooks, some of its protein bonds break. As these proteins unfold, they bump into and bind to each other. Eventually, as these interconnections increase, the liquid egg coagulates to form a solid. Raw egg white proteins denature and stiffen as they are whipped, and milk proteins denature and curdle when acid is added.

If an egg is eaten raw, its avidin protein can bind to the B vitamin biotin in the digestive tract, making the vitamin unavailable for absorption. Cooking the egg denatures the avidin and destroys its ability to bind biotin. Denaturation is the first step in breaking down protein for digestion. Stomach acids denature protein, uncoiling the structure into a simple amino acid chain that digestive enzymes can start breaking apart.

Key Concepts: Proteins are large molecules made up of amino acids joined in various sequences. Amino acids are joined by peptide bonds. Each protein assumes a unique three-dimensional shape depending on the sequence of its amino acids and the properties of their side groups. Acid, alkaline, heat, alcohol, and agitation can disrupt chemical forces that stabilize proteins, causing the proteins to denature, or lose their shape.

Functions of Body Proteins

The human body contains thousands of different proteins, each with a specific function determined by its unique shape. Some act as enzymes, speeding up chemical reactions. Others act as hormones, which are a kind of chemical

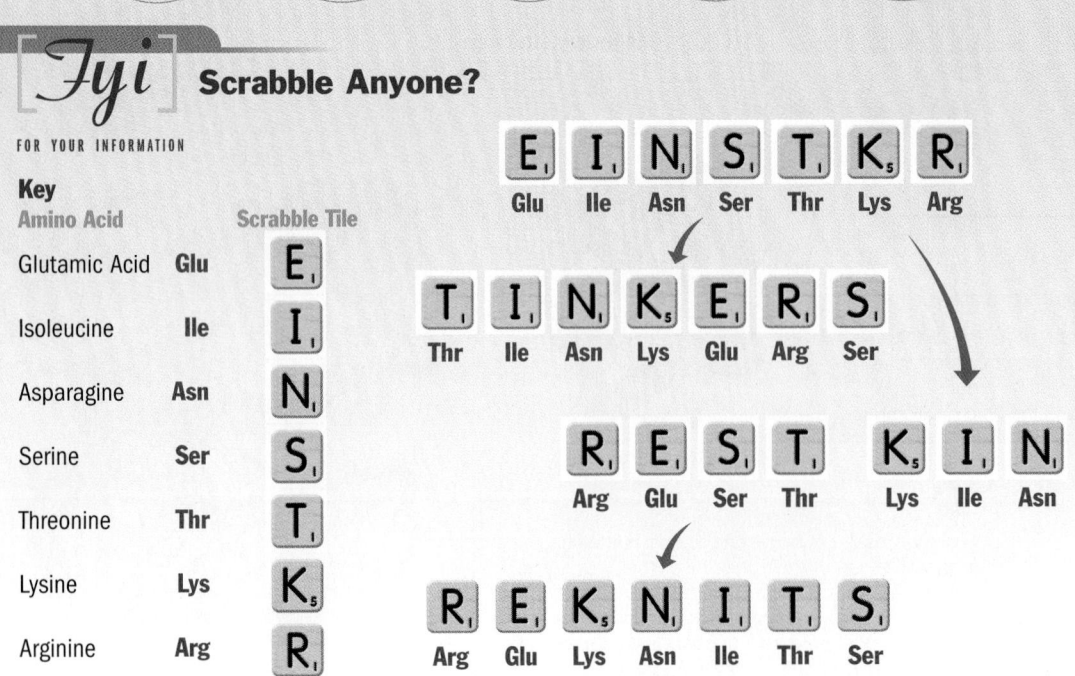

[*Fyi*] **Scrabble Anyone?**

FOR YOUR INFORMATION

Key

Amino Acid		Scrabble Tile
Glutamic Acid	**Glu**	E
Isoleucine	**Ile**	I
Asparagine	**Asn**	N
Serine	**Ser**	S
Threonine	**Thr**	T
Lysine	**Lys**	K
Arginine	**Arg**	R

E I N S T K R
Glu Ile Asn Ser Thr Lys Arg

T I N K E R S
Thr Ile Asn Lys Glu Arg Ser

R E S T K I N
Arg Glu Ser Thr Lys Ile Asn

R E K N I T S
Arg Glu Lys Asn Ile Thr Ser

Scrabble tile = amino acid
word = protein chain

Making a meaningful word from available Scrabble tiles is a good analogy for the making of a functional protein chain from available amino acids. Just as we can make many different words from the same tiles, cells can make many different proteins from the same amino acids.

If your cells have all 20 amino acids at their disposal, these can be arranged in a bewildering number of combinations to create tens of thousands of different protein chains, just as all the letters of the alphabet can be used to make an almost unlimited number of words.

messenger. Antibodies made of protein protect us from foreign substances. Proteins maintain fluid balance by pumping molecules across cell membranes and attracting water. They maintain the acid and base balance of body fluids by taking up or giving off hydrogen ions as needed. Finally, proteins transport many key substances such as oxygen, vitamins, and minerals to target cells throughout the body. **Figure 6.5** illustrates the functions of proteins in the human body.

Structural and Mechanical Functions

Structures such as bone, skin, and hair owe their physical properties to unique proteins. **Collagen**, which appears microscopically as a densely packed long rod, is the most abundant protein in mammals and gives skin and bone their elastic strength. Hair and nails are made of **keratin**, which is another dense protein made of coiled helices. Protein is essential for building these anatomical structures; therefore, protein deficiencies during a child's development can be disastrous. **Figure 6.6** shows structural proteins.

Motor proteins are exactly what their name implies: proteins that turn energy into mechanical work. In fact, these proteins are the final step in converting our food into physical work. When you bike down a road or up a mountain, you are using your stored food energy to power minuscule molecular motors in your muscles. These molecular motors slide muscle proteins past each other, causing muscles to contract. As you pump the pedals, proteins turn that energy bar you ate into work! Similarly, specialized motor proteins are involved in a variety of processes, including cell division, muscle contraction, and sperm swimming.

Quick Bites

How to Beat the Stiffest Egg Whites

Whenever you want the greatest possible lightness or fluffiness, beat egg whites alone. A single drop of yolk or fat may reduce the foam's maximum volume by as much as two-thirds. Also avoid plastic bowls because plastics tend to retain fatty material on their surfaces.

collagen The most abundant fibrous protein in the body. Collagen is the major constituent of connective tissue, forms the foundation for bones and teeth, and helps maintain the structure of blood vessels and other tissues.

keratin A water-insoluble fibrous protein that is the primary constituent of hair, nails, and the outer layer of the skin.

motor proteins Proteins that use energy and convert it into some form of mechanical work. Motor proteins are active in processes such as dividing cells, contracting muscle, and swimming sperm.

Figure 6.5 **Functions of proteins.** There are many different types of proteins, each with its particular role in the body.

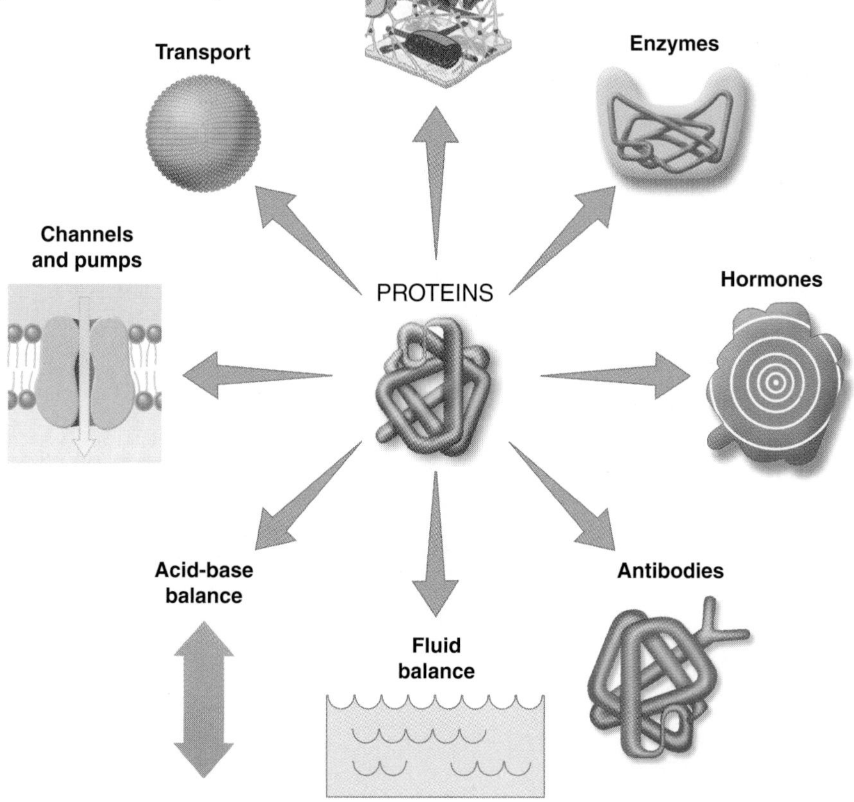

Structure
Transport
Enzymes
Channels and pumps
PROTEINS
Hormones
Acid-base balance
Fluid balance
Antibodies

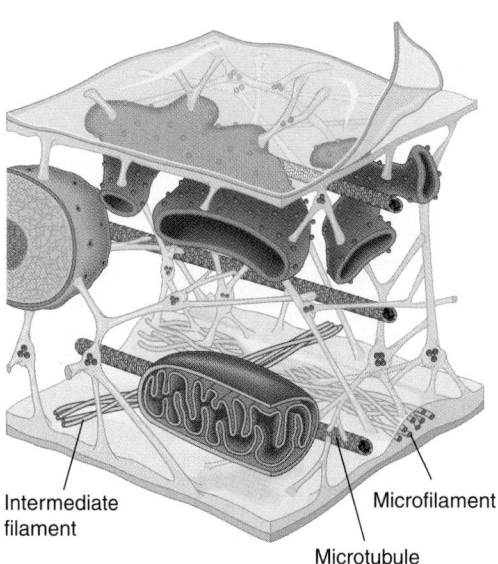

Intermediate filament
Microfilament
Microtubule

Figure 6.6 **Structural proteins.** Proteins provide structure to all cells, including hair, skin, nails, and bone. As part of muscle, they transform energy into mechanical movement.

antibodies [AN-tih-bod-ees] Large blood proteins produced by B lymphocytes in response to exposure to particular antigens (e.g., a protein on the surface of a virus or bacterium). Each type of antibody specifically binds to and helps eliminate its matching antigen from the body. Once formed, antibodies circulate in the blood and help protect the body against subsequent infection.

immune response A coordinated set of steps, including production of antibodies, that the immune system takes in response to an antigen.

intracellular fluid The fluid in the body's cells. It usually is high in potassium and phosphate and low in sodium and chloride. It constitutes about two-thirds of total body water.

extracellular fluid The fluid located outside of cells. It is composed largely of the liquid portion of the blood (plasma) and the fluid between cells in tissues (interstitial fluid), with fluid in the GI tract, eyes, joints, and spinal cord contributing a small amount. It constitutes about one-third of body water.

interstitial fluid [in-ter-STISH-ul] The fluid between cells in tissues. Also called intercellular fluid.

Enzymes

Enzymes are proteins that catalyze chemical reactions without being destroyed in the process. (See **Figures 6.7A** and **B.**) Every cell contains thousands of types of enzymes, each with its own purpose. During digestion, for example, enzymes help break down carbohydrates, proteins, and fats into monosaccharides, amino acids, and fatty acids for absorption into the body. Cellular enzymes release energy from these nutrients to fuel thousands of body processes. Enzymes also trigger the reactions that build muscle and tissue.

Our foods also contain enzymes, but these are inactivated (denatured) by cooking. Stomach acid denatures the enzymes in raw foods. You may notice special purified enzymes being sold as supplements to enhance digestion. Most of the time, stomach acid denatures these enzymes so that they are unable to function in the intestinal tract. However, some enzyme supplements are coated with a special substance to protect them from stomach acid. For example, a specially coated tablet form of the enzyme lactase can help people with lactose intolerance. Coated enzymes temporarily help break down foods in the small intestine but eventually are digested themselves.

Hormones

Hormones are chemical messengers that are made in one part of the body but act on cells in other parts of the body. (See **Figure 6.8.**) Many are proteins with important regulatory functions. Insulin, for example, is a protein hormone that plays a key role in regulating the amount of glucose in the blood. It is released from the pancreas in response to a rise in blood glucose levels, and functions to lower those levels (see Chapter 4, "Carbohydrates"). People with type 1 diabetes must take insulin injections to control blood glucose. Insulin cannot be taken as a pill—if it were, it would be denatured and digested just like any other protein.

Thyroid-stimulating hormone (TSH) and leptin are two other protein hormones. The pituitary gland produces TSH, which stimulates the thyroid gland to produce the hormone thyroxine. Thyroxine, a modified form of

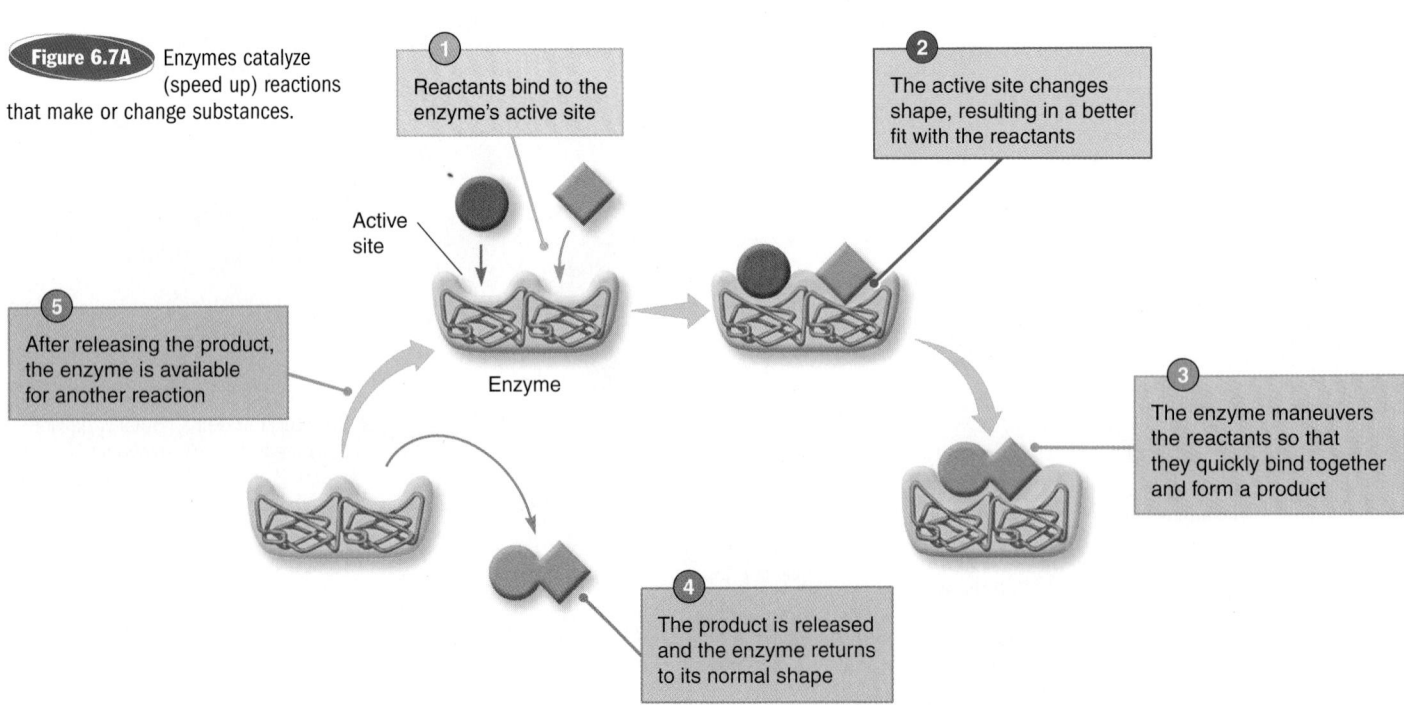

Figure 6.7A Enzymes catalyze (speed up) reactions that make or change substances.

1 Reactants bind to the enzyme's active site

2 The active site changes shape, resulting in a better fit with the reactants

3 The enzyme maneuvers the reactants so that they quickly bind together and form a product

4 The product is released and the enzyme returns to its normal shape

5 After releasing the product, the enzyme is available for another reaction

Active site

Enzyme

the amino acid tyrosine, increases the body's metabolic rate. Leptin is produced by fat cells and plays an important role in body weight regulation.[7] For more information on leptin, see Chapter 8, "Energy Balance, Body Composition, and Weight Management."

Immune Function

Proteins play an important role in the immune system, which is responsible for fighting invasion and infection by foreign substances. (See **Figure 6.9**.) **Antibodies** are blood proteins that attack and inactivate bacteria and viruses that cause infection. When your diet does not contain enough protein, your body cannot make as many antibodies as it needs. Your immune response is weakened and your risk of infection and illness increases. Each protein antibody has a specific shape that allows it to attack and destroy a specific foreign invader. Once your immune system learns how to make a certain kind of antibody, your body can protect itself by quickly making that antibody the next time the same germ invades.

Viruses, such as those that cause the common cold, take over cells to replicate. In a series of steps known as the **immune response**, your body mobilizes its defenses against the viral invaders. As part of the defense strategy, you produce protein antibodies that bind to the viruses, marking them for destruction. Even when the viruses are gone, special cells retain a memory of the particular virus so that a faster immune response can be mounted against future invasions. When people are immunized for a disease such as measles or mumps, they are actually getting a small amount of dead or inactivated virus in the injection. The dead virus cannot cause infection, but it does cue the body to make antibodies to the disease.

Fluid Balance

Fluids in the body are found inside cells (**intracellular fluid**) or outside cells (**extracellular fluid**). There are two types of extracellular fluid: fluid between cells (called intercellular fluid, or **interstitial fluid**) and fluid in

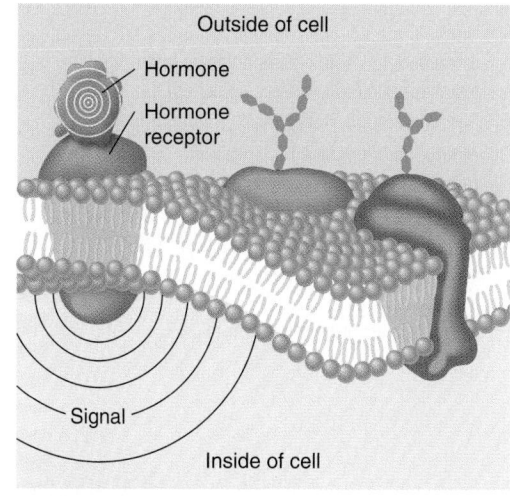

Figure 6.8 **Hormones.** Hormones are formed in one part of the body and carried in the blood to a different location where they signal cells to alter activities.

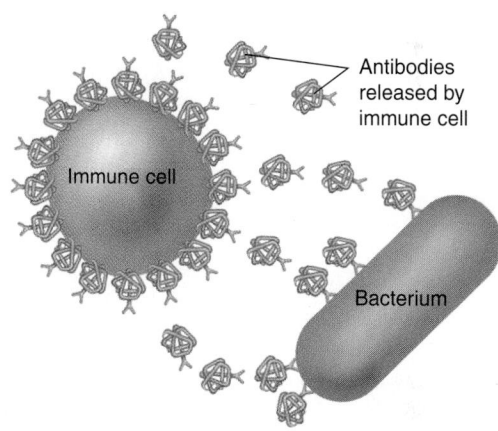

Figure 6.9 **Proteins and the immune system.** Protein antibodies are a crucial line of defense against invading bacteria and viruses.

Figure 6.7B Enzymes catalyze reactions that break down molecules.

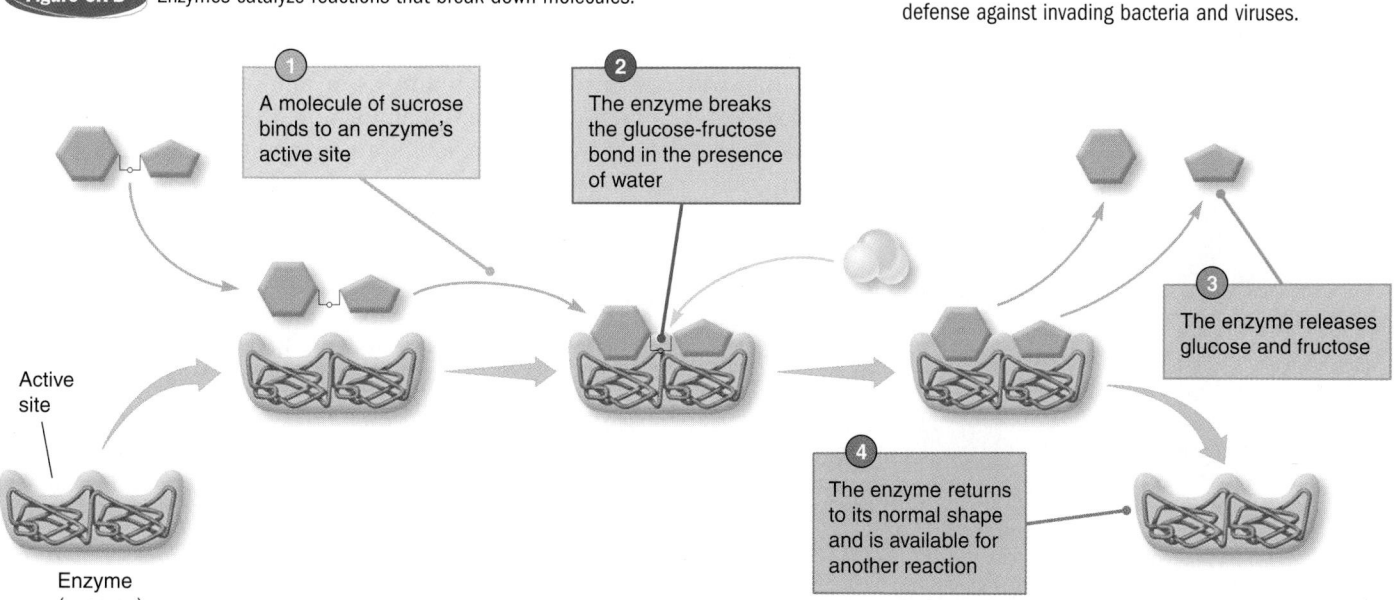

1 A molecule of sucrose binds to an enzyme's active site

2 The enzyme breaks the glucose-fructose bond in the presence of water

3 The enzyme releases glucose and fructose

4 The enzyme returns to its normal shape and is available for another reaction

Active site

Enzyme (sucrase)

intravascular fluid The fluid portion of the blood (plasma) contained in arteries, veins, and capillaries. It accounts for about 15 percent of the extracellular fluid.

edema Swelling caused by the buildup of fluid between cells.

buffers Compounds or mixtures of compounds that can take up and release hydrogen ions to keep the pH of a solution constant. The buffering action of proteins and bicarbonate in the bloodstream plays a major role in maintaining the blood pH at 7.35 to 7.45.

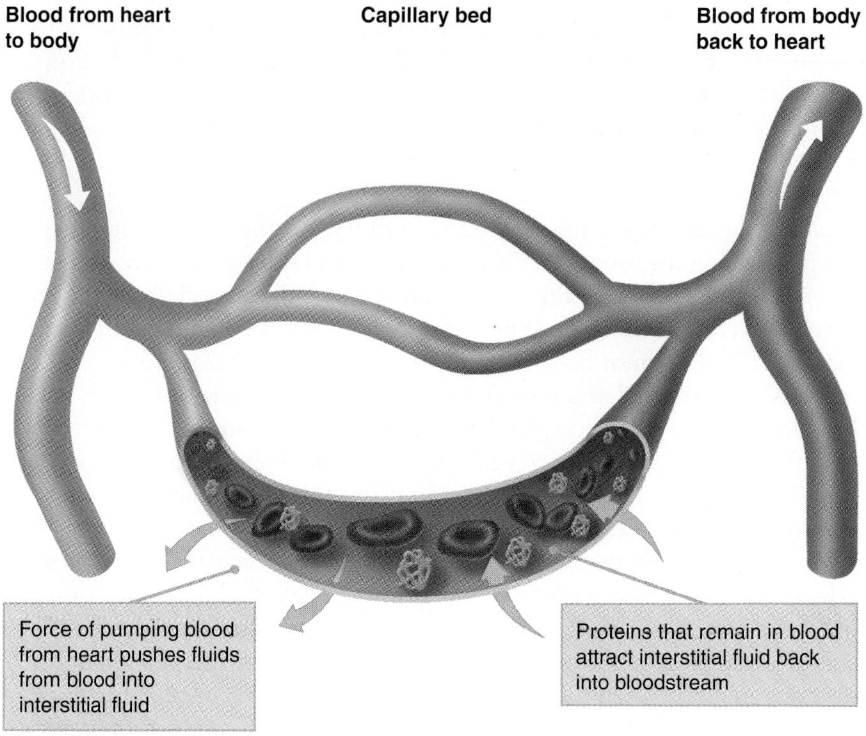

Blood from heart to body   Capillary bed   Blood from body back to heart

Force of pumping blood from heart pushes fluids from blood into interstitial fluid

Proteins that remain in blood attract interstitial fluid back into bloodstream

Figure 6.10   **Proteins in the blood.** Blood proteins attract fluid into capillaries. This counteracts the force of the heart beating, which pushes fluid out of capillaries.

the blood (**intravascular fluid**). These interior and exterior fluid levels must stay in balance for body processes to work properly.

Proteins in the blood help to maintain appropriate fluid levels in the vascular system. (See **Figure 6.10**.) The force of the heart's beating pushes fluid and nutrients from the capillaries out into the fluid surrounding the cells. But blood proteins such as albumin and globulin are too large to leave the capillary beds. These proteins remain in the capillaries, where they attract fluid. This provides a balancing and partially counteracting force that keeps fluid in the circulatory system.

If the diet lacks enough protein to maintain normal levels of blood proteins, fluid will leak into the surrounding tissue and cause swelling, also called **edema**. Children with protein malnutrition often suffer from severe edema. Reestablishing a diet adequate in protein and energy will allow the edema to subside.

Acid–Base Balance

Using a scale of 0 to 14, pH is a measure of the concentration of hydrogen ions in a substance. The higher the concentration of hydrogen ions, the lower the pH. Acids, with a high concentration of hydrogen ions, have a pH lower than 7; bases, with a low concentration of hydrogen ions, have a pH higher than 7. The lower the pH, the stronger the acid. The higher the pH, the stronger the base. The body works hard to keep the pH of the blood near 7.4, or nearly neutral. We can tolerate only small blood pH fluctuations without disastrous physiological consequences. Only a few hours with a blood pH above 8.0 or below 6.8 will cause death.

Proteins help maintain stable pH levels in body fluids by serving as **buffers**; they pick up extra hydrogen ions when conditions are acidic, and they donate hydrogen ions when conditions are alkaline. (See **Figure 6.11**.)

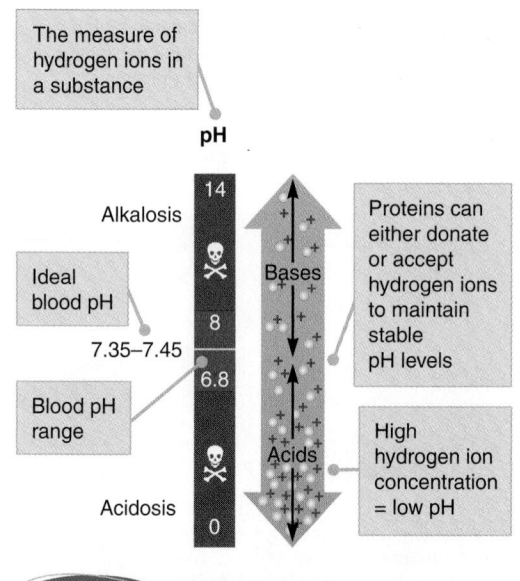

The measure of hydrogen ions in a substance

pH

Alkalosis

Ideal blood pH

7.35–7.45

Blood pH range

Acidosis

14

8

6.8

0

Bases

Acids

Proteins can either donate or accept hydrogen ions to maintain stable pH levels

High hydrogen ion concentration = low pH

Figure 6.11   **Proteins help maintain stable pH levels.** Proteins act as buffers. When conditions are acidic, they pick up extra hydrogen ions. When conditions are alkaline, they donate hydrogen ions.

If proteins are not available to buffer acidic or alkaline substances, the blood can become too acidic or too alkaline, resulting in either **acidosis** or **alkalosis**. Both conditions can be serious; either can cause proteins to denature, which can lead to coma or death.

Transport Functions

Many substances pass in and out of cells via proteins that cross cell membranes and act as channels and pumps. Channels allow substances to flow rapidly through the membranes by passive diffusion and require no input of energy. Pumps (active transporters), in contrast, must use energy to drive the transport of substances across membranes. In fact, sodium-potassium pumps—proteins that control cell volume and nerve impulses and drive the active transport of monosaccharides and amino acids—use more than one-third of the energy your body consumes at rest.[8] **Figure 6.12** shows a transmembrane protein.

Proteins also act as carriers, transporting many important substances in the bloodstream for delivery throughout the body. Lipoproteins, for example, package proteins with lipids so that lipid particles can be carried in the blood. (See **Figure 6.13**.) Other proteins carry fat-soluble vitamins, such as vitamin A, and certain other vitamins and minerals. Because protein carries vitamin A in the blood, protein deficiency contributes to vitamin A deficiency. The protein transferrin carries iron in the blood. In the liver, iron is stored as part of ferritin, a different protein.

Source of Energy and Glucose

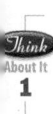

Although your body preferentially burns carbohydrate and fat for energy, if necessary it can use protein for energy or to make glucose. Thus, carbohydrate and fat are protein-sparing: They spare amino acids from being burned for energy and allow them to be used for protein synthesis.

If the diet does not provide enough energy to sustain vital functions, the body will sacrifice its own protein from enzymes, muscle, and other tissues to make energy and glucose for use by the brain, lungs, and heart. This is what happens in cases of starvation. (See Chapter 7, "Metabolism.")

When the body uses protein for energy, it first breaks the protein into individual amino acids. To release energy from an amino acid, the body removes the nitrogen group—a process called **deamination**. It can use the remaining carbon skeleton for energy. The carbon skeleton from most amino acids can be used to make glucose.

If the diet contains more protein than is needed for protein synthesis, most of the excess is converted to glucose or stored as fat. Thus, people who take protein supplements or eat high-protein diets in hopes of increasing muscle mass may instead be expensively adding to their body fat.

This review of protein functions illustrates that protein is of "prime importance," just as the Greeks believed. For proteins to perform all these functions, the diet must provide adequate amounts of protein components. In addition, the body needs adequate energy from carbohydrates and fats, and adequate digestibility of protein foods.

Key Concepts: In the body, proteins perform numerous vital functions that are determined by each protein's shape. As enzymes, they speed up chemical reactions; as hormones, they are chemical messengers. Protein antibodies protect the body from infection and illness; proteins also maintain fluid balance and acid–base balance, and transport substances throughout the body. If needed, protein can also be used as a source of energy or glucose.

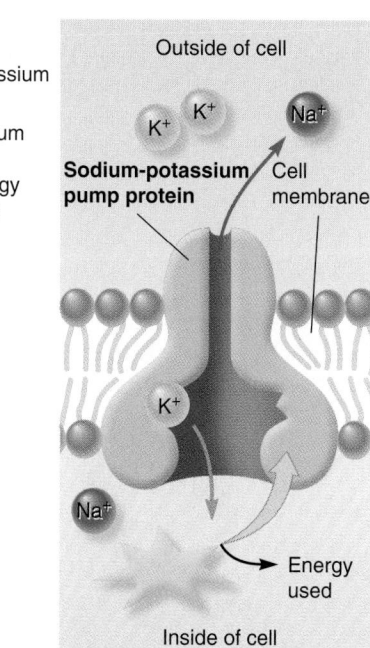

Key

K+ Potassium

Na+ Sodium

Energy input

Outside of cell

Sodium-potassium pump protein

Cell membrane

Inside of cell

Energy used

Figure 6.12 **A transmembrane protein.** Proteins form channels and pumps that help move substances in and out of cells.

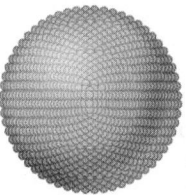

A lipoprotein is a transport protein

Figure 6.13 **Proteins act as carriers.** Lipoproteins have embedded proteins that help them transport fat and cholesterol in the blood.

acidosis An abnormally low blood pH (below about 7.35) due to increased acidity.

alkalosis An abnormally high blood pH (above about 7.45) due to increased alkalinity.

deamination The removal of the amino group (–NH$_2$) from an amino acid.

Protein Digestion and Absorption

Before your body can make a body protein from food protein, it must digest and absorb the protein you eat. **Figure 6.14** shows the process of protein digestion and absorption.

Protein Digestion

The first step in using dietary protein is digesting its long polypeptide chains into amino acids. As with the other energy-yielding nutrients, digestion requires enzymes from a number of sources. Digestion of protein begins in the stomach.

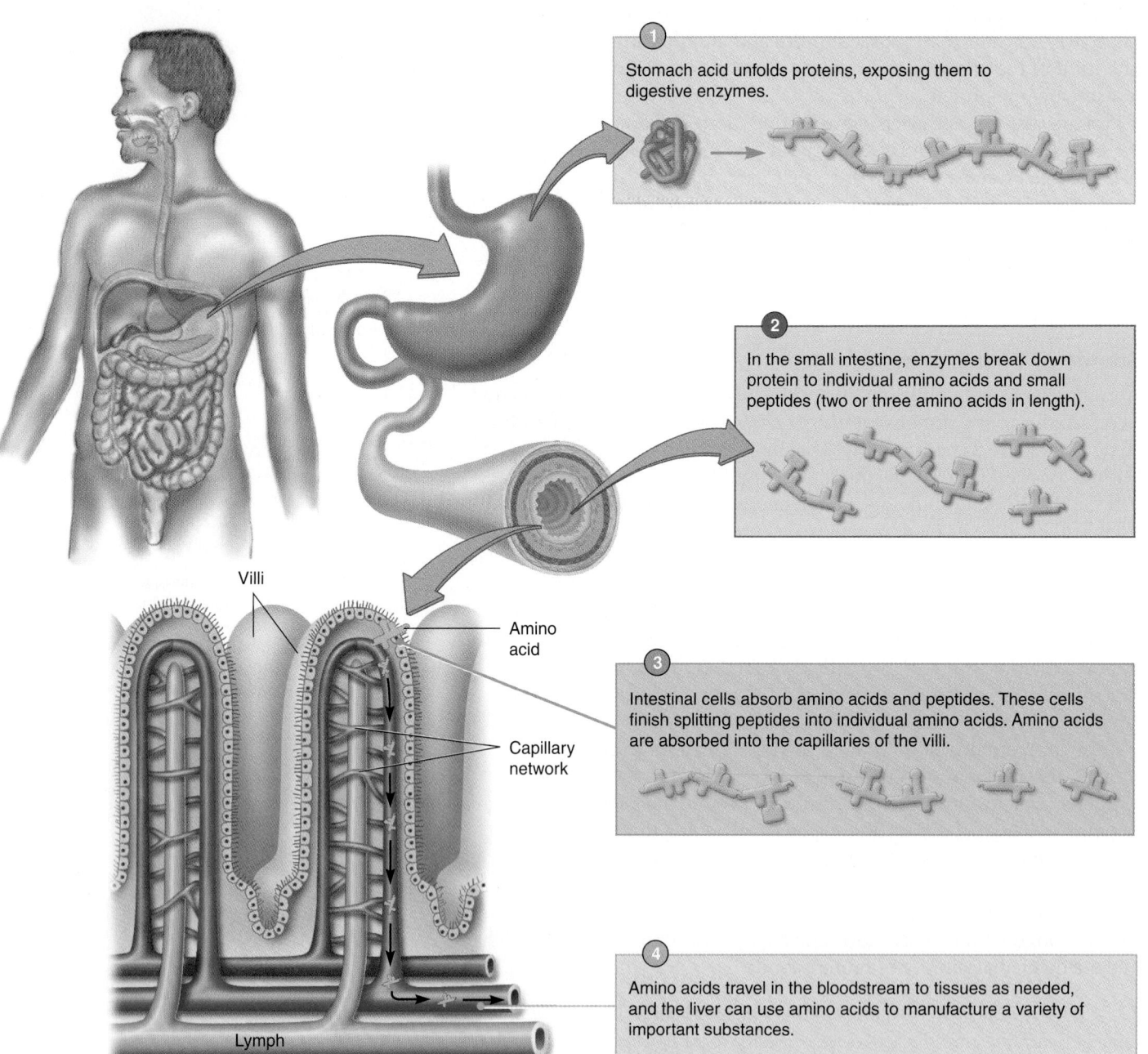

1 Stomach acid unfolds proteins, exposing them to digestive enzymes.

2 In the small intestine, enzymes break down protein to individual amino acids and small peptides (two or three amino acids in length).

Villi

Amino acid

Capillary network

3 Intestinal cells absorb amino acids and peptides. These cells finish splitting peptides into individual amino acids. Amino acids are absorbed into the capillaries of the villi.

4 Amino acids travel in the bloodstream to tissues as needed, and the liver can use amino acids to manufacture a variety of important substances.

Lymph

Figure 6.14 **The breakdown of protein in the body.** Digestion breaks down protein to amino acids that can be absorbed into the bloodstream.

In the Stomach

In the stomach, hydrochloric acid (HCl) denatures a protein, unfolding it and making the amino acid chain more accessible to the action of enzymes. Glands in the stomach lining produce the proenzyme pepsinogen, an inactive **precursor** of the enzyme pepsin. When pepsinogen comes in contact with hydrochloric acid, it is converted to the active enzyme pepsin. Gastric juices must be acidic for this enzyme to be active; it is most active at a (very acidic) pH of 2.5 and is inactive at a pH above 5.0. Gastric glands secrete hydrochloric acid at a pH of approximately 0.8. Once the acid is mixed with the gastric contents, the pH of the gastric juices falls to 2.5—the ideal medium for pepsin activity. By the time dietary protein leaves the stomach, pepsin has broken it down into individual amino acids and peptides of various lengths. Pepsin is responsible for about 10 to 20 percent of protein digestion.[9]

In the Small Intestine

From the stomach, amino acids and polypeptides pass into the small intestine, where most protein digestion takes place. In the small intestine, **proteases** (protein-digesting enzymes) break down large peptides into smaller peptides. If a cell produces active forms of proteases, it will digest itself and break down its own cellular protein. However, cells employ a protective strategy. They produce and secrete most proteases as **proenzymes**, inactive forms of the enzymes, for later activation. This delayed activation protects the integrity of the cell.

Both the pancreas and the small intestine make digestive proenzymes. The pancreas makes **trypsinogen** and **chymotrypsinogen**, which are secreted into the small intestine in response to the presence of protein. Here, these proenzymes are cleaved into their active forms, **trypsin** and **chymotrypsin**, respectively. These activated proteases then break polypeptides into smaller peptides. Pancreatic enzymes completely digest only a small percentage of proteins into individual amino acids; most of the proteins at this point are dipeptides, tripeptides, and still larger polypeptides.

The final stages of protein digestion take place on the surface of the intestine's lining and require enzymes secreted by the intestinal lining cells. Brush border (microvilli) **peptidases** react with intestinal fluids that come in contact with the cell surface and split the remaining larger polypeptides into tripeptides, dipeptides, and individual amino acids. These smaller units are transported across the microvilli membranes into the cell. Inside the cell, many other peptidases specifically attack the linkages between the amino acids. Within minutes, these peptidases digest virtually all the remaining dipeptides and tripeptides into individual amino acids for absorption into the bloodstream.

Undigested Protein

Any parts of proteins not digested and absorbed in the small intestine continue through the large intestine and pass out of the body in the feces. Normally the body efficiently digests and absorbs protein. Diseases of the intestinal tract, however, decrease the efficiency of absorption and increase nitrogen losses in the feces.[10] People with **celiac disease**, for example, cannot properly digest gluten—a protein found in wheat, rye, and oats. Unless treated with a gluten-free diet, people with celiac disease show poor growth, weight loss, and other symptoms resulting from poor absorption of protein and other nutrients. When people have **cystic fibrosis**, thick, sticky mucus prevents digestive enzymes, including proteases, from reaching the small intestine and results in poor digestion and absorption of protein and

precursor A substance that is converted into another active substance. Enzyme precursors are also called proenzymes.

proteases [PRO-tea-ace-ez] Enzymes that break down protein into peptides and amino acids.

proenzymes Inactive precursors of enzymes.

trypsin/trypsinogen A protease produced by the pancreas that is converted from the inactive proenzyme form (trypsinogen) to the active form (trypsin) in the small intestine.

chymotrypsin/chymotrypsinogen A protease produced by the pancreas that is converted from the inactive proenzyme form (chymotrypsinogen) to the active form (chymotrypsin) in the small intestine.

peptidases Enzymes that act on small peptide units by breaking peptide bonds.

celiac disease [SEA-lee-ak] A disease that involves an inability to digest gluten, a protein found in wheat, rye, oats, and barley. If untreated, it causes flattening of the villi in the intestine, leading to severe malabsorption of nutrients. Symptoms include diarrhea, fatty stools, swollen belly, and extreme fatigue.

cystic fibrosis An inherited disorder that causes widespread dysfunction of the exocrine glands, resulting in chronic lung disease, abnormally high levels of electrolytes (e.g., sodium, potassium, chloride) in sweat, and deficiency of pancreatic enzymes needed for digestion.

Quick Bites

Softening Tough Meat

Cooking tough meat in liquid for hours helps dissolve the source of its toughness, fibrous protein called connective tissue.

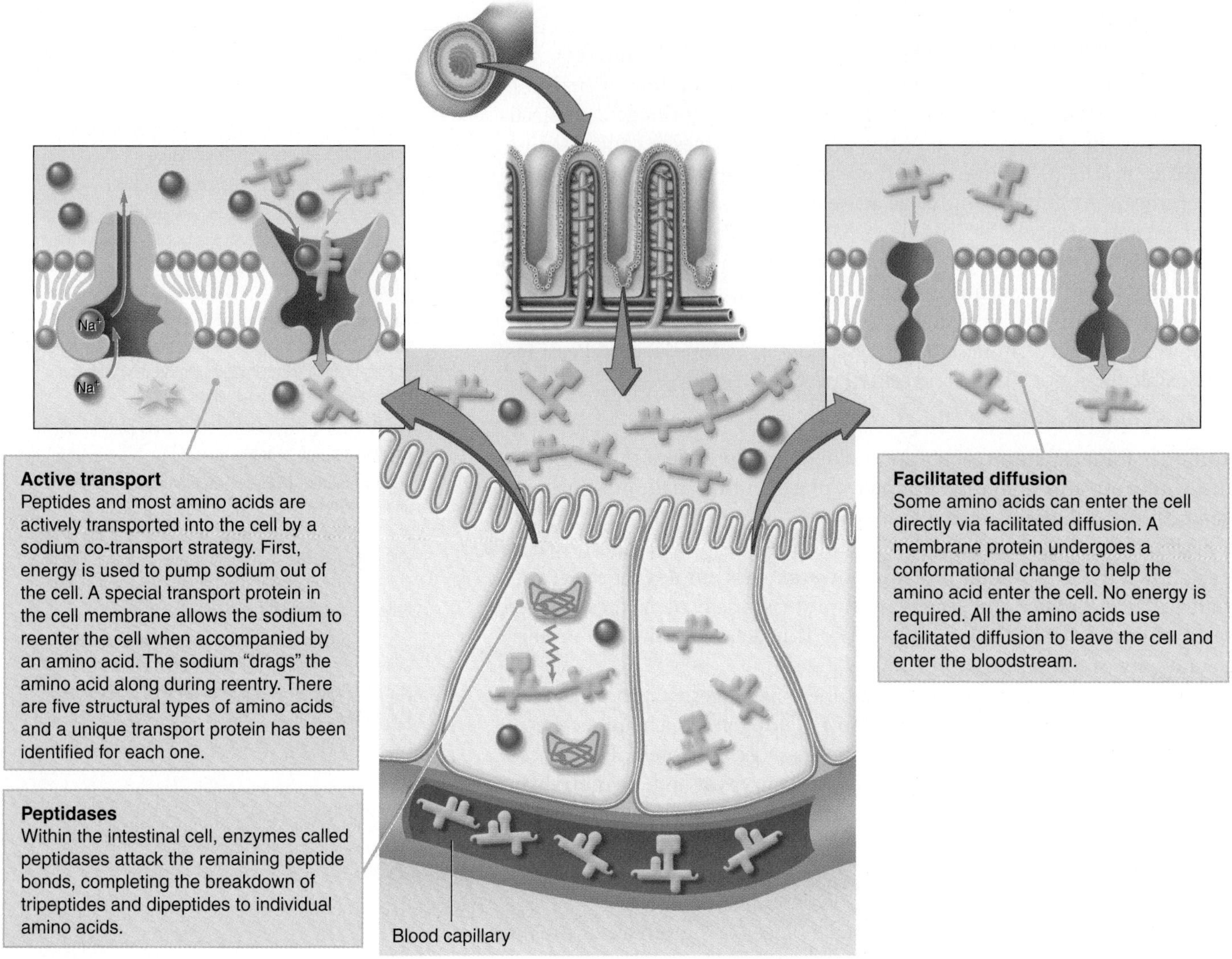

Active transport
Peptides and most amino acids are actively transported into the cell by a sodium co-transport strategy. First, energy is used to pump sodium out of the cell. A special transport protein in the cell membrane allows the sodium to reenter the cell when accompanied by an amino acid. The sodium "drags" the amino acid along during reentry. There are five structural types of amino acids and a unique transport protein has been identified for each one.

Peptidases
Within the intestinal cell, enzymes called peptidases attack the remaining peptide bonds, completing the breakdown of tripeptides and dipeptides to individual amino acids.

Blood capillary

Facilitated diffusion
Some amino acids can enter the cell directly via facilitated diffusion. A membrane protein undergoes a conformational change to help the amino acid enter the cell. No energy is required. All the amino acids use facilitated diffusion to leave the cell and enter the bloodstream.

Figure 6.15 **Protein absorption into an intestinal cell.** Intestinal cells use active transport and facilitated diffusion to absorb amino acids.

other nutrients.[11] Special enzyme preparations that contain protease, lipase, and amylase are needed to prevent malnutrition.

Amino Acid and Peptide Absorption

Absorption of some amino acids requires active transport, whereas other amino acids are absorbed via facilitated diffusion. (See **Figure 6.15.**) Although the active transport process is the same for amino acids as it is for glucose and galactose, amino acids and monosaccharides use different transport proteins.

Although there are several active transport mechanisms, similar amino acids share the same active transport system. The amino acids leucine, isoleucine, and valine, for example, all depend on the same carrier molecule for absorption. Normally proteins in foods supply a mix of many amino acids, so amino acids that share the same transport system are absorbed fairly equally. If a person consumes a large amount of one particular amino acid, however, absorption of other amino acids that share the same transport system will be deficient. Thus, if you take a supplement of one amino acid, you may be interfering with the absorption of another amino acid from your diet.

Most protein absorption takes place in the cells that line the duodenum and jejunum. After they are absorbed, most amino acids and the few

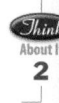

Think About It

2

absorbed peptides are transported via the portal vein to the liver and then released into general circulation. Some amino acids remain in the intestinal cells and are used to synthesize intestinal enzymes and new cells. More than 99 percent of protein enters the bloodstream as individual amino acids. Peptides are rarely absorbed, and whole proteins that escape digestion hardly ever are. The absorption of only a few molecules of whole protein can cause a severe allergic reaction or immune dysfunction.[12]

Key Concepts: *Protein digestion begins in the stomach, where the enzyme pepsin breaks proteins into smaller peptides. Digestion continues in the small intestine, where proteases break polypeptides into smaller peptide units, which are then absorbed into cells, where additional enzymes complete digestion to amino acids. Key enzymes are pepsin in the stomach, and trypsin and chymotrypsin from the pancreas. Proteases (protein-digesting enzymes) are synthesized and secreted as inactive proenzymes, so that cells do not digest themselves.*

Proteins in the Body

Once in the bloodstream, amino acids are transported throughout the body and are available for synthesizing cellular proteins. To build proteins, cells use peptide bonds to link amino acids.

Protein Synthesis

Genetic material in the nucleus of every cell is the blueprint for the thousands of proteins needed to perform life functions. Cells store this genetic material in the form of long, coiled molecules of **DNA (deoxyribonucleic acid)** in each cell's nucleus.

To synthesize a protein, the cell uses a specific length of the DNA in the cell nucleus, called a gene, as a pattern to make a special type of ribonucleic acid (RNA) called **messenger RNA (mRNA)**. This mRNA carries the code for the sequence of amino acids needed in the protein. The mRNA leaves the nucleus of the cell and attaches itself to one of the **ribosomes**, or protein-making machines, in the cell's cytoplasm.

Another type of RNA, **transfer RNA (tRNA)**, then gathers the necessary amino acids from cell fluid and carries them to the mRNA, where enzymes bind each amino acid to the growing protein chain. During protein synthesis, thousands of tRNAs each carry their own specific amino acid to the site of protein synthesis, but only one mRNA controls the sequencing of amino acids for a given protein.

A third type of RNA, **ribosomal RNA (rRNA)**, is the major component of ribosomes. For many years, scientists assumed that rRNA primarily served as a structural framework for protein synthesis and had little catalytic function. With the discovery that RNA in general can play many catalytic roles, scientists now believe that rRNA has a major role in directing protein synthesis. **Figure 6.16** illustrates protein synthesis.

Just as one missing part of a car can stop an entire auto assembly line, one missing amino acid can stop synthesis of an entire protein in the cell. If a dispensable amino acid is missing during protein synthesis, the cell will either make that amino acid or obtain it from the liver via the

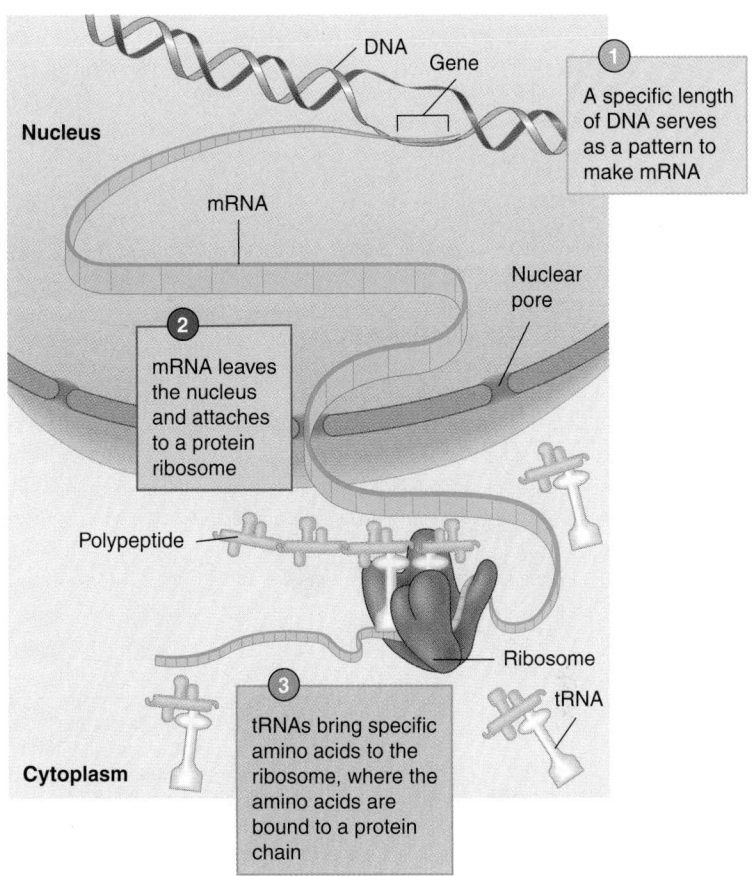

Figure 6.16 **Protein synthesis.** Ribosomes are our protein synthesis factories. mRNA carries manufacturing instructions from DNA in the cell nucleus to the ribosomes. tRNA collects amino acids in the correct sequence, and rRNA in the ribosome directs protein synthesis.

DNA (deoxyribonucleic acid) The carrier of genetic information. Specific regions of each DNA molecule, called genes, act as blueprints for the synthesis of proteins.

messenger RNA (mRNA) Long, linear, single-stranded molecules of ribonucleic acids formed from DNA templates that carry the amino acid sequence of one or more proteins from the cell nucleus to the cytoplasm, where the ribosomes translate mRNA into proteins.

ribosomes Cell components composed of protein located in the cytoplasm that translate messenger RNA into protein sequences.

transfer RNA (tRNA) A type of ribonucleic acid that is composed of a complementary RNA sequence and an amino acid specific to that sequence. It inserts the appropriate amino acid when the messenger RNA sequence and the ribosome call for it.

ribosomal RNA (rRNA) A type of ribonucleic acid that is a major component of ribosomes. It provides a structural framework for protein synthesis and orchestrates the process.

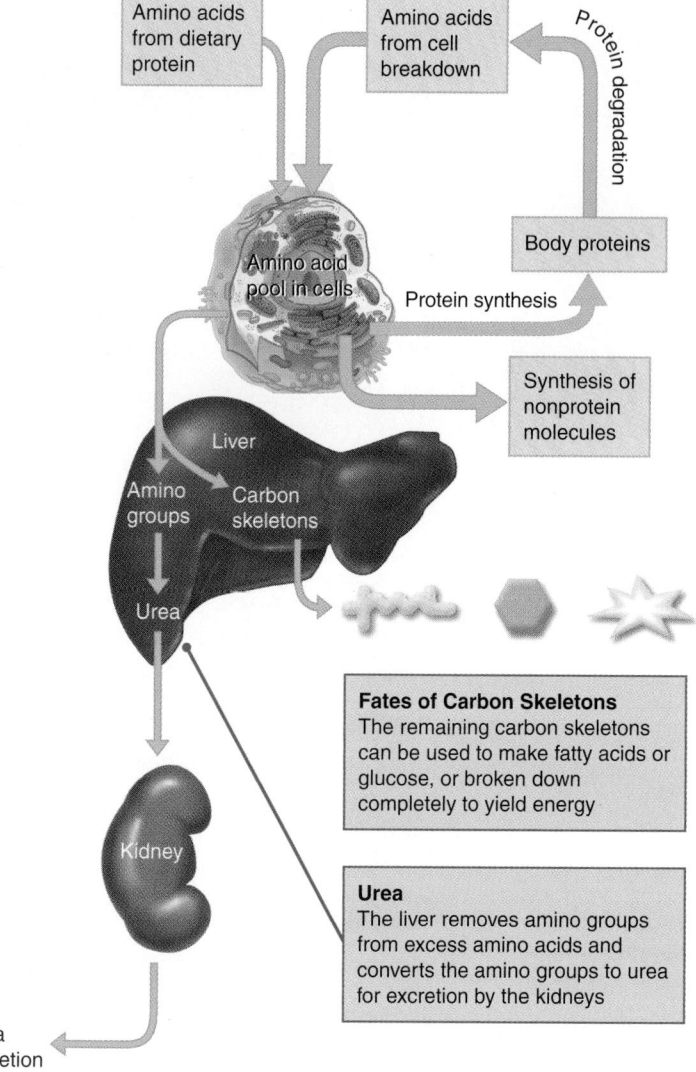

Amino acids from dietary protein

Amino acids from cell breakdown

Protein degradation

Amino acid pool in cells

Body proteins

Protein synthesis

Synthesis of nonprotein molecules

Liver

Amino groups

Carbon skeletons

Urea

Kidney

Fates of Carbon Skeletons
The remaining carbon skeletons can be used to make fatty acids or glucose, or broken down completely to yield energy

Urea
The liver removes amino groups from excess amino acids and converts the amino groups to urea for excretion by the kidneys

Urea excretion

Figure 6.17 **Protein turnover.** Cells draw upon their amino acid pools to synthesize new proteins. These small pools turn over quickly, and must be replenished by amino acids from dietary protein and degradation of body protein. Dietary protein supplies about one-third and the breakdown of body protein supplies about two-thirds of the amino acids needed to synthesize roughly 300 grams of body protein daily.

amino acid pool The amino acids in body tissues and fluids that are available for new protein synthesis.

protein turnover The constant synthesis and breakdown of proteins in the body.

neurotransmitters Substances released at the end of a stimulated nerve cell that diffuse across a small gap and bind to another nerve cell or muscle cell, stimulating or inhibiting it.

bloodstream, and protein synthesis will continue. If an indispensable amino acid is missing, the body may break its own protein down to supply the missing amino acid. If a missing indispensable amino acid is unavailable, protein synthesis halts, and the partially completed protein is broken down into individual amino acids for use elsewhere in the body.

Genetic defects in DNA can also cause problems in protein synthesis. People who have sickle cell anemia have a defect in the amino acid sequencing of their hemoglobin. A genetic error causes the substitution of the amino acid valine for glutamic acid in two locations in the protein chain. This simple error causes the shape of hemoglobin to change so much that the red blood cell becomes stiff and sickle-shaped instead of soft and disk-shaped. Because this faulty protein cannot carry oxygen efficiently, it causes serious medical problems.

The Amino Acid Pool and Protein Turnover

Cells throughout the body constantly and simultaneously synthesize and break down protein. When cells break down protein, the protein's amino acids return to circulation. (See **Figure 6.17**.) These available amino acids, found throughout body tissues and fluids, are collectively referred to as the **amino acid pool**.[13] Some of these amino acids may be used for protein synthesis; others may have their amino group removed and be used to produce energy or nonprotein substances such as glucose.

The constant recycling of proteins in the body is known as **protein turnover**.[14] Each day, more amino acids in your body are recycled than are supplied in your diet. Of the approximately 300 grams of protein synthesized by the body each day, 200 grams are made from recycled amino acids. This remarkable recycling capacity is the reason we need so little protein in our diet. Although our requirements are small, dietary protein is extremely important. When dietary protein is inadequate, increased breakdown of body protein replenishes the amino acid pool. This can lead to the breakdown of essential body tissue.

Synthesis of Nonprotein Molecules

Amino acids have roles other than as components of peptides and proteins; they are precursors of many molecules with important biological roles. Your body makes nonprotein molecules from amino acids and the nitrogen they contain. The vitamin niacin, for example, is made from the amino acid tryptophan. Precursors of DNA, RNA, and many coenzymes derive in part from amino acids. Your body also uses amino acids to make **neurotransmitters**, chemicals that send signals from nerve cells to other parts of the body. The neurotransmitter serotonin, which helps regulate mood, is made from tryptophan. Norepinephrine and epinephrine (also called noradrenaline and adrenaline, respectively), which ready the body for action, are neurotransmitters made from tyrosine. Your body also uses tyrosine to make the skin pigment melanin and a hormone called thyroxine. The simple amino acid glycine combines with many toxic substances to make less harmful substances that the body can excrete. Your body uses the amino acid histidine to make histamine, a potent vasodilator (dilator of blood vessels) and a culprit in allergic reactions.

Protein and Nitrogen Excretion

Cells break down and recycle amino acids. Breakdown of an amino acid yields an amino group ($-NH_2$). This NH_2 molecule is unstable and is quickly converted to ammonia (NH_3). However, ammonia is toxic to cells, so it is expelled into the bloodstream as a waste product and carried to the liver. In the liver, an amino group and an ammonia group react with carbon dioxide through a series of reactions (known collectively as the urea cycle) to generate **urea** and water. The nitrogen-rich urea is transported from the liver by way of the bloodstream to the kidneys, where it is filtered from the blood and sent to the bladder for excretion in the urine. Small amounts of other nitrogen-containing compounds, such as ammonia, uric acid, and creatinine, are excreted in the urine as well. Some nitrogen is also lost through skin, sloughed-off GI cells, mucus, hair and nail cuttings, and body fluids.

Nitrogen Balance

Because nitrogen is excreted as proteins are recycled or used, we can use the balance of nitrogen in the body to evaluate whether the body is getting enough protein. (See **Figure 6.18**.) We can estimate the balance of nitrogen, and therefore protein, in the body by comparing nitrogen intake to the sum of all sources of nitrogen excretion (urine, feces, skin, hair, and body fluids).[15]

urea The main nitrogen-containing waste product in mammals. Formed in liver cells from ammonia and carbon dioxide, urea is carried via the bloodstream to the kidneys, where it is excreted in the urine.

$$\text{nitrogen balance} = \text{grams of nitrogen intake} - \text{grams of nitrogen output}$$

Figure 6.18 **Protein (nitrogen) balance.** Nitrogen balance reflects whether a person is gaining or losing protein.

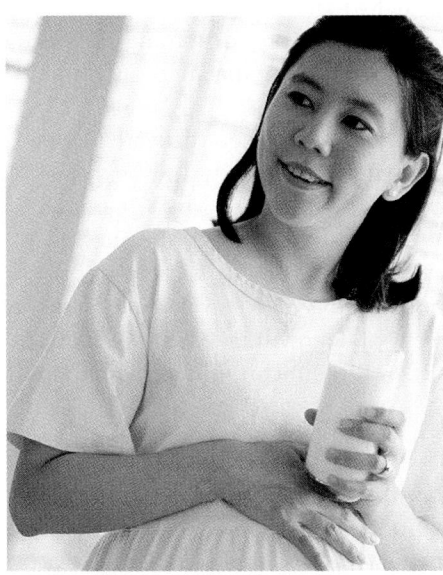

A pregnant woman is adding protein so she has a positive nitrogen balance.

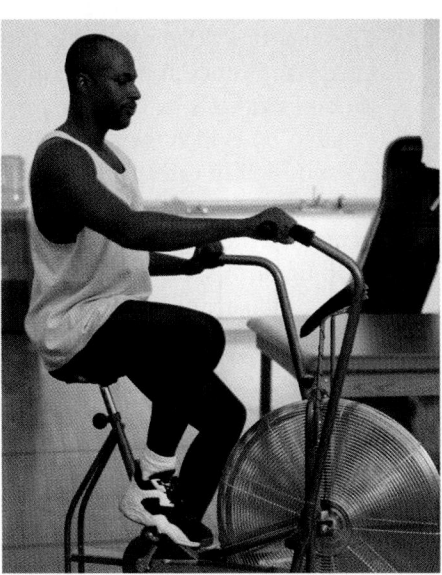

A healthy person who is neither gaining nor losing protein is in nitrogen equilibrium.

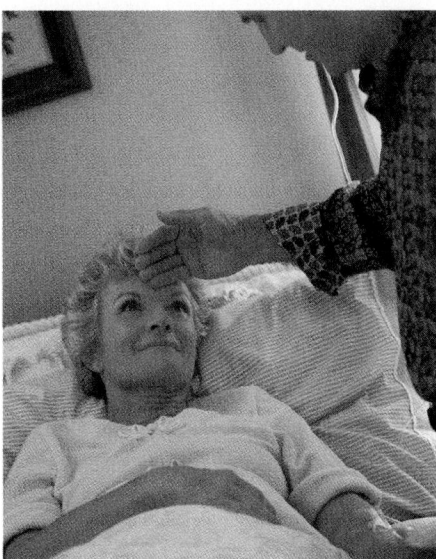

A person who is severely ill and losing protein has a negative nitrogen balance.

positive nitrogen balance Nitrogen intake exceeds the sum of all sources of nitrogen excretion.

negative nitrogen balance Nitrogen intake is less than the sum of all sources of nitrogen excretion.

nitrogen balance Nitrogen intake minus the sum of all sources of nitrogen excretion.

nitrogen equilibrium Nitrogen intake equals the sum of all sources of nitrogen excretion; nitrogen balance equals zero.

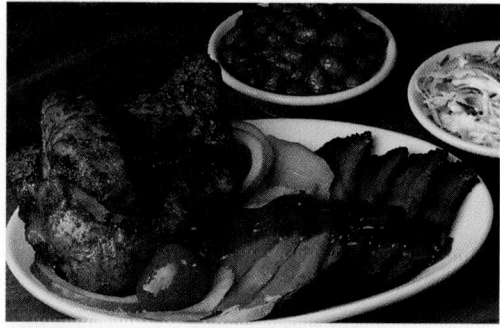

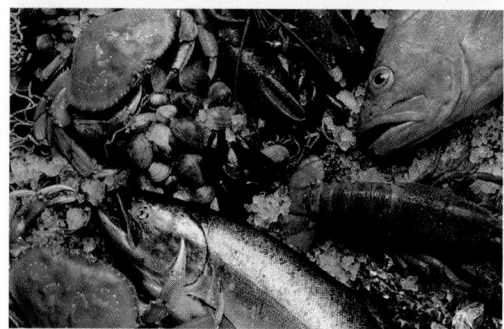

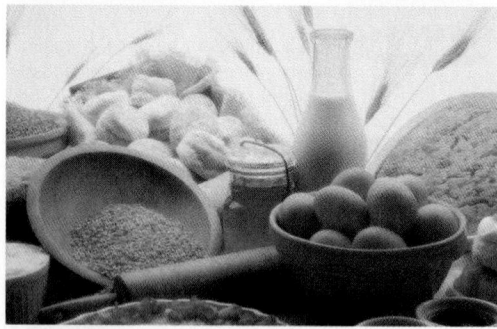

Figure 6.19 Protein sources.

Convert weight to kg
(pounds ÷ 2.2)
Multiply kg by 0.8 = Protein RDA in g

Male, 19–24 years old, 70 kg (154 lb)

70 kg × 0.8 g/kg = 56 g protein

Female, 19–24 years old, 57 kg (125 lb)

57 kg × 0.8 g/kg = 46 g protein

If nitrogen intake exceeds nitrogen excretion, the body is said to be in **positive nitrogen balance**. Positive nitrogen balance means that the body is adding protein, as is the case for growing children, pregnant women, or people recovering from protein deficiency or illnesses. If nitrogen excretion exceeds nitrogen intake, the body is in **negative nitrogen balance**. This means that the body is losing protein. People who are starving or on extreme weight-loss diets or who suffer from fever, severe illnesses, or infections are in a state of negative nitrogen balance. If nitrogen intake equals nitrogen excretion, **nitrogen balance** is zero and the body is in **nitrogen equilibrium**. Healthy adults are in nitrogen equilibrium, which means that their dietary protein intake is adequate to maintain and repair tissue. They have no net gain or loss of body protein, and they simply excrete excess dietary nitrogen.

Key Concepts: *The information that allows a cell to make a particular protein is stored in cellular DNA. Three forms of RNA—mRNA, tRNA, and rRNA—are needed to build body proteins. Cells throughout the body constantly synthesize and break down protein simultaneously, a process known as protein turnover. Nitrogen-containing end products of protein metabolism are excreted in urine via the kidneys. Comparison of nitrogen intake (from dietary protein) to nitrogen excretion gives a measure of nitrogen balance and indicates protein status in the body.*

Proteins in the Diet

Many government and health organizations have made recommendations about the amount of protein in a healthful diet, just as they have for other nutrients. Meat, eggs, milk, legumes, grains, and vegetables are all sources of protein. Fruits contain minimal amounts and, along with fats, are not considered protein sources. **Figure 6.19** shows some good sources of protein.

Recommended Intakes of Protein

In the United States and Canada, the Recommended Dietary Allowance (RDA; see Chapter 2, "Nutrition Guidelines and Assessment") is the accepted dietary standard for protein. RDAs are set to meet the nutritional needs of most healthy people, so most people actually require somewhat less protein than the RDA. RDA values also assume that people are consuming adequate energy and other nutrients to allow their bodies to use dietary protein for protein synthesis, rather than for energy.

Based on evidence of increased heart disease risk when diets are low in fat and high in carbohydrate, and increased risk of obesity and heart disease when diets are high in fat, the Food and Nutrition Board developed Acceptable Macronutrient Distribution Ranges (AMDRs) for the energy-yielding nutrients.[16] For adults, the AMDR for fat is 20 to 35 percent of energy intake, and the AMDR for carbohydrate is 45 to 65 percent of energy intake. This leaves about 10 to 35 percent of energy intake from protein, a level that is typically higher than the RDA. Protein currently provides about 14 to 15 percent of the energy for adults in the United States.[17]

Adults

For adults, the RDA for protein intake is 0.8 gram per kilogram of body weight.[18] In clinical situations that require precise assessments, ideal body weight (rather than actual body weight) is typically used to determine protein needs. The RDA for adults translates into a daily protein recommendation of 56 grams for the average adult male and 46 grams for the average adult female aged 19 to 24. When calculated as a percentage of average energy intake, the protein RDA for adults provides about 8 to 11 percent of energy intake.

Other Life Stages

Infants have the highest protein needs relative to body weight of any time of life (see **Table 6.2**). Protein is needed to support rapid growth during infancy. The Adequate Intake (AI) value for infants 0 to 6 months of age is based on the protein content of human milk and the average milk consumption of breastfed babies. Protein requirements per kilogram body weight gradually fall throughout childhood and adolescence until a person reaches adulthood. (See **Figure 6.20**.)

Both pregnancy and lactation (production of breast milk) increase a woman's need for protein. The RDA for pregnant and lactating women is 1.1 grams per kilogram. This is an increase of about 25 grams per day over the female RDA for protein. Most American women already consume more than enough protein to support pregnancy and lactation.

Some nutritionists suggest that people older than 50 should consume up to 1.2 grams of protein per kilogram body weight. Although elderly people on average have less lean body mass to maintain than younger people, the body becomes less efficient at digesting, absorbing, and using protein as it ages.[19] However, because a statistical analysis of nitrogen balance studies found no significant effect of age on protein requirements, the RDA for this age group is the same as for younger adults—0.8 grams per kilogram.[20] But, since energy needs decline with age, protein should provide a larger percentage of energy intake.

Physical Stress

Severe physical stress can increase the body's need for protein. Infections, burns, fevers, and surgery all increase protein losses, and the diet must replace that lost protein. A severe infection can increase protein requirements by one-third. Severe burns can increase requirements two to four times. Less severe physical stressors, such as a viral illness with a mild fever lasting only a few days, rarely increase protein requirements. Muscle-building activities, such as intense weight training, increase protein need much less than most people think. In fact, the typical American diet supplies an ample amount of protein for most people, even for bodybuilders. (See the FYI feature "Do Athletes Need More Protein?")

Protein Consumption

According to national survey data, the median daily intake of protein for adult males ranges from 71 to 101 grams. This is approximately 1.0 to 1.4 grams per kilogram using a reference body weight of 70 kilograms. For females, the median protein intake is 55 to 62 grams per day, or 0.96 to 1.1 grams per kilogram using a reference body weight of 57 kilograms.[21] Generally speaking, Americans eat more protein than the adult RDA and more than the Daily Value, which is 50 grams per day.

Key Concepts: *Infants, who are growing rapidly, have the highest protein needs relative to body weight. The recommended intakes (AIs or RDAs) decline from 1.52 grams per kilogram for infants 0 to 6 months old to 0.8 gram per kilogram for adults. Pregnancy, lactation, and severe physical stress all can alter protein requirements. Adults currently consume about 15 percent of their energy as protein, a level that provides ample protein for most people.*

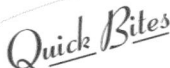

Quick Bites

Mother's Milk

*B*ecause it contains less protein, and in particular less casein protein, infants digest human milk more readily than cow's milk. Milks high in casein protein tend to form curds (clumps) in the stomach upon exposure to stomach acid. These tough curds are hard for digestive enzymes to break apart.

Table 6.2 **Protein AI or RDA for Infants, Children, and Teens**

Age	Protein AI or RDA (g/kg body weight)
0–6 months	1.52
7–12 months	1.2
1 to 3 years	1.05
4 to 8 years	0.95
9 to 13 years	0.95
14 to 18 years	0.85

Source: Institute of Medicine, Food and Nutrition Board. *Dietary Reference Intakes for Energy, Carbohydrate, Fiber, Fat, Fatty Acids, Cholesterol, Protein, and Amino Acids.* Washington, DC: National Academy Press, 2005. Reprinted with permission.

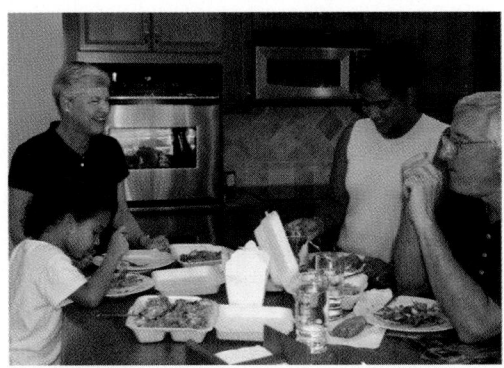

Figure 6.20 **Protein needs change as we age.** Growing children have higher protein needs (as grams per kilogram body weight) than older adults.

complete (high-quality) proteins Proteins that supply all of the indispensable amino acids in the proportions the body needs.

incomplete (low-quality) proteins Proteins that lack one or more amino acids.

complementary protein An incomplete food protein whose assortment of amino acids makes up for, or complements, another food protein's lack of specific indispensable amino acids so that the combination of the two proteins provides sufficient amounts of all the indispensable amino acids.

Protein Quality

Although both animal and plant foods contain protein, the quality of protein in these foods differs. Foods that supply all the indispensable amino acids in the proportions needed by the body are called **complete**, or **high-quality**, **proteins**. Foods that lack adequate amounts of one or more indispensable amino acids are called **incomplete**, or **low-quality**, **proteins**.

When a variety of foods provides ample dietary protein, the protein quality of foods is not a primary dietary concern. But whenever protein or energy intake is marginal, or when only one or a few plant foods are the main protein sources in the diet, protein quality is a critical issue.

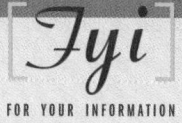

[Fyi] Do Athletes Need More Protein?

FOR YOUR INFORMATION

Athletes are not just pumping iron these days; they're also pumping protein supplements in hopes of building muscle and improving performance. Look inside many sports magazines and you'll see ads for protein or amino acid supplements targeted to athletes. You cannot force your body to build muscle by pumping in more protein than you need, any more than you can make your car run faster by adding more gas to a full tank. Extra protein does not build muscles; only regular workouts fueled by a mix of nutrients can achieve this goal.

Protein Requirements for Athletes

Many people assume that because muscle fibers are protein, building muscle must require protein. This is only partially true. The heavy resistance-type exercise that is needed to stimulate muscle growth must first be fueled by glucose and fatty acids (glucose will be the predominant fuel). Little protein is used as a fuel source in resistance-type exercise. Some studies have shown that men who consume the RDA for protein (0.8 gram per kilogram of body weight) and engage in heavy resistance exercise go into negative nitrogen balance. However, another study in older adults showed positive nitrogen balance during resistance training with intake at the RDA.[1] For endurance athletes, less protein is used for muscle building, but more protein is used as a fuel source. Unfortunately, a study of protein requirements of endurance-trained men did not include non-exercising

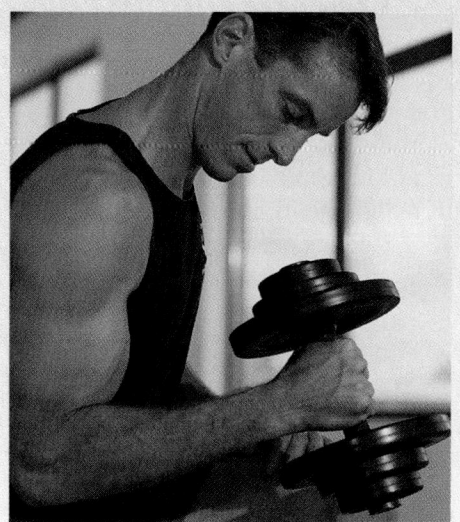

controls, making it difficult to draw specific conclusions.[2] The DRI committee reviewing evidence on macronutrients concluded that a higher RDA was not warranted for healthy adults doing resistance or endurance exercise.[3]

Because Americans, on average, consume much more protein than they actually need, any increased need for athletes is most likely already being met. An athlete in training (let's make his weight 70 kilograms) might consume as many as 5,000 kilocalories per day. Even if his diet contained only 10 percent of calories as protein (the low side of the AMDR for protein, and lower than average), he would be getting about 126 grams of protein daily, about 1.8 grams per kilogram. It is unlikely that an athlete would not be able to meet his or her protein needs from a normal, mixed diet—especially one that follows the MyPyramid food guidance system recommendations.

Risks of Supplements

Maybe there's no benefit to taking protein or amino acid supplements, but there's no harm either, right? Not necessarily. If excess protein means excess calories, it adds weight as fat, not muscle, which can slow down your performance. Purified protein supplements can contribute to calcium losses, thereby harming bone health. Excess protein means excess nitrogen that must be excreted, which poses a risk for dehydration if fluid intake is inadequate. Supplements of single amino acids can interfere with absorption of other amino acids and can alter neurotransmitter activity.

If you are a weekend athlete, there's no need to increase the protein in your diet, and no reason to expect that doing so will help your performance. If you are a competitive athlete, choosing adequate calories from a wide variety of foods will ensure an adequate protein intake. Supplements are unnecessary and expensive, and they may disrupt normal protein balance in the body. Play it safe; choose a healthful diet to fuel your exercise.

1 Campbell WW, Crim MC, Young VR, et al. Effects of resistance training and dietary protein intake on protein metabolism in older adults. *Am J Physiol.* 1995;268:E1143–E1153.

2 Meredith CN, Zackin MJ, Frontera WR, Evans WJ. Dietary protein requirements and body protein metabolism in endurance-trained men. *J Appl Physiol.* 1989;66:2850–2856.

3 Institute of Medicine, Food and Nutrition Board. *Dietary Reference Intakes for Energy, Carbohydrate, Fiber, Fat, Fatty Acids, Cholesterol, Protein, and Amino Acids.* Washington, DC: National Academy Press; 2005.

Complete Proteins

Animal foods generally provide complete protein; that is, they provide all the indispensable amino acids in approximately the right proportions. One exception is gelatin, a protein derived from animal collagen that lacks the indispensable amino acid tryptophan.

Red meats, poultry, fish, eggs, milk, and milk products (all animal foods) contain complete protein. More than 20 percent of these foods' energy content is protein. Protein provides about 80 percent of the energy in water-packed tuna. The protein isolated from soybeans also provides a complete, high-quality protein equal to that of animal protein.[22] Although soy protein contains a lower proportion of the amino acid cysteine than animal protein, the amount of soy typically consumed provides all the amino acids in sufficient amounts to meet the body's needs. Moreover, soybeans contain no cholesterol or saturated fat.

Americans, on the average, obtain about 63 percent of their protein intake from animal foods.[23] (See **Table 6.3**.) In other parts of the world, animal proteins play a smaller role. In Africa and East Asia, for example, animal foods provide only 20 percent of protein intake.[24]

Incomplete and Complementary Proteins

With the exception of soy protein, the protein in plant foods is incomplete; that is, it lacks one or more indispensable amino acids and does not match the body's amino acid needs as closely as animal foods do. Although the protein in one plant food may lack certain amino acids, the protein in another plant food may be a **complementary protein** that completes the amino acid pattern. So the protein of one plant food can provide the indispensable amino acid(s) that the other plant food is missing. **Table 6.4** lists some examples of complementary food combinations.

For example, grain products such as pasta are low in the indispensable amino acid lysine but high in the indispensable amino acids methionine and cysteine. Legumes such as kidney beans are low in methionine and cysteine but high in lysine. In a dish that combines these foods, such as a pasta–kidney bean salad, the protein from pasta complements the protein from kidney beans, so together they provide a complete protein. Generally, when you combine grains with legumes, or legumes with nuts or seeds, you will get complete, high-quality protein.

Small amounts of animal foods can also complement the protein in plant foods. For example, Asians often flavor rice with small amounts of beef, chicken, or fish, complementing the protein in the rice. Americans eat breakfast cereal with milk, which complements the protein in the cereal.

Protein complementation is important only for people who consume little to no animal proteins. For these people, eating a wide variety of plant protein sources is the key to obtaining adequate amounts of all the indispensable amino acids. When protein and energy intake are adequate, there is no need to plan complementary proteins at each meal.[25] Complementary proteins may still need to be combined in the same meal for very young children.[26]

Boosting your intake of plant protein foods can provide benefits. High-protein plant foods are usually rich in vitamins, minerals, and dietary fiber. Plant foods contain no cholesterol and little fat, and they usually cost less than animal foods high in protein. Lentil loaf, for example, is substantially cheaper to make than meat loaf.

Table 6.3 Top Ten Sources of Protein in the United States

Rank	Food	% of Protein Contributed
1	Beef	18
2	Poultry	14
3	Milk	9
4	Yeast bread	7
5	Cheese	6
6	Fish/shellfish*	4
7	Eggs	3
8	Pork, fresh	3
9	Ham	3
10	Pasta	2

* Does not include tuna.
Source: 1989–1991 Continuing Survey of Food Intake by Individuals.

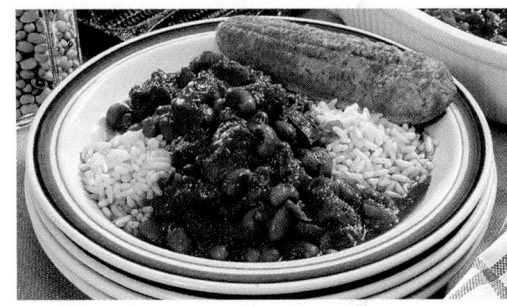

Table 6.4 Examples of Complementary Food Combinations

Beans and rice

Beans and corn or wheat tortillas

Rice and lentils

Rice and black-eyed peas

Pea soup with bread or crackers

Garbanzo beans (chickpeas) with sesame paste

Pasta with beans

Peanut butter on bread

Quick Bites

Paleolithic Protein

*D*idn't our ancestors eat a lot of meat, too? Researchers estimate that hunter/gatherer populations' diets were about one-third meat and two-thirds vegetable. The meat from wild game, however, averages only one-seventh the fat of domesticated beef (about 4 g of fat per 100 g of wild meat, compared to 29 g of fat per 100 g of domestic meat). In addition, compared to the meat at your local supermarket, the fat contained in game animals that graze on the free range has five times as much polyunsaturated fat.

$$\text{chemical score*} = \frac{\text{mg of the essential amino acid in 1 g of test protein}}{\text{mg of the essential amino acid in 1 g of reference protein}}$$

*For a percent value, multiply this result by 100.

$$\text{protein efficiency ratio (PER)} = \frac{\text{weight gain in grams}}{\text{protein intake in grams}}$$

$$\text{net protein utilization (NPU)} = \frac{\text{nitrogen retained}}{\text{nitrogen intake}} \times 100$$

Evaluating Protein Quality

A high-quality protein (1) provides all the indispensable amino acids in the amounts the body needs, (2) provides enough other amino acids to serve as nitrogen sources for synthesis of dispensable amino acids, and (3) is easy to digest. If a food protein contains the right proportion of amino acids but cannot be digested and absorbed, it is useless to the body. We can measure protein quality in many ways, but any assessment of protein quality requires, at the least, information about the amino acid composition of the food protein. Protein quality might be assessed to plan a special diet or develop a new product such as infant formula.

Chemical, or Amino Acid, Scoring

A simple way to determine a food's protein quality is to compare its amino acid composition to that of a reference pattern of amino acids. This method is referred to as **chemical scoring**, or **amino acid scoring**. The amino acid composition of the reference pattern closely reflects the amounts and proportions of amino acids that humans need. The Food and Nutrition Board has proposed an amino acid scoring pattern that uses the pattern of amino acids required by children aged 1 to 3 years.[27] If a protein meets the amino acid needs of growing preschool-aged children, then it should also meet the needs of almost all other segments of the population.

For each of the nine indispensable amino acids, researchers take the number of milligrams of the amino acid in one gram of food and divide it by the number of milligrams of that amino acid in the reference pattern. The result is multiplied by 100 to convert the figure to a percentage. For example, if a food contains only 65 percent of the lysine in the reference, the chemical score for the amino acid lysine is 65. The amino acid with the lowest score is the **limiting amino acid** (the amino acid present in the smallest amount relative to biological need). The chemical score of the food protein is the score of its limiting amino acid.

Protein Efficiency Ratio

The **protein efficiency ratio (PER)** measures amino acid composition *and* accounts for digestibility. Researchers compare the weight gain of growing animals fed a test protein with the weight gain of growing animals fed a high-quality reference protein (e.g., casein, the main protein in cow's milk). Thus, this method measures how well the body can use the test protein, which reflects amino acid composition, digestibility, and availability. The PER is used to determine the protein quality of infant formulas.

Net Protein Utilization

Net protein utilization (NPU) measures how much dietary protein the body actually uses. Scientists carefully measure the nitrogen content of a test food, and then give the food to laboratory animals as their sole protein source. They then measure the animals' nitrogen excretion to determine how much of the food's nitrogen content was retained. The more nitrogen the animal retains from a food, the higher the protein quality of that food—that is, the more efficiently the animal was able to use the food protein to make body proteins.

Biological Value

The **biological value (BV)** method determines how much of the nitrogen absorbed from a particular food protein is retained by the body for growth and/or maintenance. Because nitrogen retention is a function of absorption (if it's not absorbed, it can't be retained), measuring nitrogen absorption is a key element of this method. In general, if a protein has an indispensable amino acid composition similar to our needs, it will be more efficiently retained by the body.

Determining biological value is a tedious process because the key measures of urinary and fecal nitrogen output must be measured while subjects (human or animal) are consuming the test protein and again while they are on a nitrogen-free diet. The final value expresses nitrogen retention as a percentage of nitrogen absorption. Egg protein has a biological value of 100. This means that all the absorbed egg protein is retained by growing laboratory animals (100 percent). The biological value of the protein in corn is 60, meaning only 60 percent of the absorbed corn protein (and not all of it is absorbed) is retained for use by the body.

$$\text{biological value (BV)} = \frac{\text{nitrogen retained}}{\text{nitrogen absorbed}} \times 100$$

Protein Digestibility Corrected Amino Acid Score

The **protein digestibility corrected amino acid score (PDCAAS)** accounts for both the amino acid composition of a food and the digestibility of the protein. The first step in determining the PDCAAS is the same as that used to determine the chemical score—divide the amount of the limiting amino acid by the amount of the same amino acid in the reference pattern. Then, instead of multiplying by 100 to get a percentage, multiply by the percentage of digestible food protein. This will produce a score between 0 and 1. Egg protein provides all the amino acids that preschool children need (the reference standard) and is fully digested, so it has a PDCAAS of 1.0.

Thus, if a protein food has a chemical score of 0.70 based on its limiting amino acid, and 80 percent of the protein in that food is digestible, the PDCAAS score would be 80 percent of 0.70, or 0.56. The PDCAAS value of isolated soybean protein is 0.99. The scores for beef, canned garbanzo beans (chickpeas), and whole wheat are 0.92, 0.66, and 0.40, respectively.

The U.S. Food and Drug Administration (FDA) recognizes the PDCAAS as the official method for determining the protein quality of most food.[28] If the %DV for protein is listed on a food label, it must be based on the food's PDCAAS. It would be misleading to say that, for example, 8 grams of protein from tuna and 8 grams of protein from kidney beans would contribute equally to amino acid needs. Consequently, even though the number of grams of protein per serving might be the same, the %DV would be different for these two foods. For baby foods and infant formulas, the PER method is used to determine protein quality.

$$\text{PDCAAS} = \text{chemical score} \times \frac{\% \text{ digestibility of}}{\text{the protein}}$$

chemical scoring A method to determine the protein quality of a food by comparing its amino acid composition to that of a reference protein. Also called amino acid scoring.

amino acid scoring A method to determine the protein quality of a food by comparing its amino acid composition to that of a reference protein. Also called chemical scoring.

limiting amino acid The amino acid in shortest supply during protein synthesis. Also the amino acid in the lowest quantity when evaluating protein quality.

protein efficiency ratio (PER) Protein quality calculated by comparing the weight gain of growing animals fed a test protein with growing animals fed a high-quality reference protein. It depends on both the digestibility and the amino acid composition of a protein.

net protein utilization (NPU) Percentage of ingested protein nitrogen retained by the body. It measures the amount of dietary protein the body uses.

biological value (BV) The extent to which protein in a food can be incorporated into body proteins. BV is expressed as the percentage of the absorbed dietary nitrogen retained by the body.

protein digestibility corrected amino acid score (PDCAAS) A measure of protein quality that takes into account the amino acid composition of the food and the digestibility of the protein. It is calculated by multiplying the amino acid score by the percentage of the digestible food protein.

Key Concepts: *In general, animal foods provide complete protein that contains the right mix of all the indispensable amino acids. With the exception of soybean protein, plant foods contain incomplete protein—that is, proteins lacking in one or more amino acids. Plant foods can be combined to complement each other's amino acid patterns. Researchers use many methods to determine protein quality, including chemical analysis of amino acid content and biological measures of the protein's digestibility, its retention in the body, or its ability to support growth.*

Estimating Your Protein Intake

By this time, you may be wondering how much protein you consume in a typical day. To be accurate, you would need an inconvenient and expensive chemical analysis of your food intake. Instead, you can estimate your protein intake using more readily available information. First, food labels list the quantity of protein (in grams) in a serving of food. If you have a label for every food you consume, just add up the grams.

Another way to estimate your protein intake is to use the Exchange Lists found in Figure 2.8 and Appendix B. In the Exchange Lists, one starch exchange provides an average of 3 grams of protein, one milk exchange provides 8 grams, one vegetable exchange provides 2 grams, and one meat exchange provides 7 grams. Fruit and fat exchanges contribute 0 protein. You can also use food composition tables or computer software to calculate your protein intake.

As a reference point, if you consume the minimum number of servings recommended in MyPyramid (see Chapter 2), you will get an ample amount of protein—more than enough to meet most people's protein needs.

Proteins and Amino Acids as Additives and Supplements

Proteins contribute to the structure, texture, and taste of food. They are often added to foods to enhance these properties. The milk protein casein is added to frozen dessert toppings. Gelatin is added to yogurt and fillings. **Protein hydrolysates**—protein that has been broken down into amino acids and polypeptides—are added to many foods as thickeners, stabilizers, or flavor enhancers.

Amino acids are also used as additives. Monosodium glutamate (sodium bound to the amino acid glutamic acid) is a flavor enhancer added to many foods. The artificial sweetener aspartame is a dipeptide composed of aspartic acid and phenylalanine.

Protein and amino acid supplements are sold to dieters, athletes, and people who suffer from certain diseases. Despite a lack of scientific evidence, some people buy the amino acid lysine for cold sores and the amino acid tryptophan in the hope that it will relieve pain, depression, and sleep disorders. A number of protein powders and amino acid cocktails are marketed with the claims that they enhance muscle building and exercise performance. Although the anecdotal evidence (stories from friends and health food store clerks) for these products may be convincing, few scientific studies back up these claims. Remember, muscle work builds muscle strength and size, and muscles prefer carbohydrate to fuel this type of work.

There are no documented health benefits from consuming large amounts of individual amino acids, and the risks are unknown. An excess of a single amino acid in the digestive tract can impair absorption of other amino acids that use the same carrier for absorption, which could cause a deficiency of one or more amino acids and an unhealthy excess of the supplemented amino acid.

Key Concepts: *You can use food labels or Exchange List values to estimate your protein intake. Eating a diet that follows MyPyramid will supply adequate amounts of protein. Supplements of protein or amino acids are rarely necessary and might be harmful.*

protein hydrolysates Proteins that have been treated with acid or enzymes to break them down into amino acids and polypeptides.

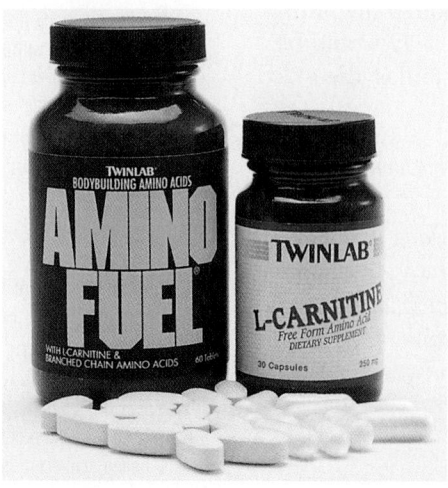

Vegetarian Diets

What did Socrates, Plato, Albert Einstein, Leonardo da Vinci, William Shakespeare, Charles Darwin, and Mahatma Gandhi have in common? They all advocated a vegetarian lifestyle.[29] George Bernard Shaw, vegetarian, famous writer, and political analyst of the early 1900s, wrote, "A man fed on whiskey and dead bodies cannot do the finest work of which he is capable."[30]

Meat-eaters often contend that vegetarian diets do not provide enough protein and other essential nutrients, but this is not necessarily the case. With careful planning, a diet that contains no animal products can be nutritionally complete and offer many health benefits. Poorly planned vegetarian diets, however, can pose health risks.

Why People Become Vegetarians

In parts of the world where food is scarce, vegetarianism is not a choice but a necessity. Where food is abundant, people choose vegetarianism for many reasons. People may choose a vegetarian diet because of religious beliefs, concern for the environment, a desire to reduce world hunger and make better use of scarce resources, an aversion to eating another living creature, or concerns about cruelty to animals. Still others become vegetarians because they believe it is healthier for them. **Table 6.5** shows three religious groups and their vegetarian practices. Today, more than 12 million Americans consider themselves vegetarians.[31]

Types of Vegetarians

Although all vegetarians share the common practice of not eating meat and meat products, they differ greatly in specific dietary practices. Lacto-ovo-vegetarians use animal products such as milk, cheese, and eggs, but abstain from eating the flesh of animals. Vegans eat no animal-based foods and usually avoid products such as cosmetics made with animal-based ingredients. Fruitarians eat only raw fruit, nuts, and green foliage.

Some people eat a semi-vegetarian diet, avoiding red meats but eating small amounts of chicken or fish. The Mediterranean diet, known for reducing the risk of heart disease, is a semi-vegetarian diet rich in grains, pasta, vegetables, cheeses, and olive oil supplemented with small amounts of chicken and fish. **Table 6.6** lists the types of vegetarian diets and the foods typically included and excluded.

Zen macrobiotic diets are mostly vegan and stress whole grains, locally grown vegetables, beans, sea vegetables, and soups. Extreme Zen macrobiotic diets can be very limited, such as a diet of primarily brown rice.

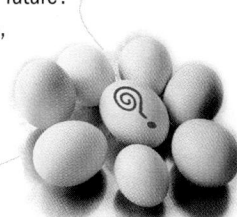

Quick Bites

Prophetic Eggs

Can an egg predict the future? In Trinidad and Tobago, people say you can tell the future by the shape an egg white makes when added to warm water on Good Friday.

Table 6.5 **Religious Groups with Vegetarian Dietary Practices**

Religious Group	Dietary Practices
Buddhism	Some sects lacto-vegetarian, other sects vegan
Hinduism	Generally lacto-vegetarian, but mutton or pork eaten occasionally
Seventh-Day Adventists	Lacto-ovo vegetarian emphasizing whole-grain foods. Also avoid alcohol, tobacco, and caffeine.

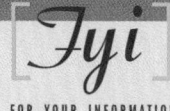

[Fyi] High-Protein Plant Foods

FOR YOUR INFORMATION

Of the top 10 sources of protein in the American diet, only two sources—yeast breads and pasta—are plant-based (see Table 6.3). Lentils, a dense source of plant protein, don't even make the list. Yet look at the comparison between the nutritional profile of lentils and the profile of beef in **Table 1**.

Table 1: How Do Lentils Stack Up Against Beef?

	Cooked Lentils	Lean, Broiled Sirloin
Amount	1 cup	5 ounces
Energy	230 kcal	260 kcal
Protein	18 grams	43 grams
Fat	<1 gram	8 grams
Cholesterol	0	82 milligrams
Carbohydrate	40 grams	0
Dietary fiber	16 grams	0
Percent calories from fat	3%	28%

Source: US Department of Agriculture, Agricultural Research Service. USDA National Nutrient Database for Standard Reference, Release 18. 2005. http://www.nal.usda.gov/fnic/foodcompindex.html. Accessed 6/1/06.

When we consider these two foods in light of the *Dietary Guidelines for Americans* (see Chapter 2), it's no contest. To reduce fat, saturated fat, and cholesterol while increasing fiber, the lentils win hands down! With all that lentils have going for them, you'd think more Americans would be eating them. Yet dried beans, peas, and lentils combined contribute less than 1 percent of the daily protein intake of Americans, while beef contributes 17.7 percent.

High-protein plant foods also contribute complex carbohydrates, dietary fiber, and vitamins and minerals to the diet. Since these plant foods contain little fat, they are nutrient dense; that is, they provide a high amount of protein and nutrients relative to their energy contribution.

Sources of Plant Protein

Grains and grain products, legumes (lentils and dried beans and peas such as kidney beans or chickpeas), starchy vegetables, and nuts and seeds all provide protein (**Table 2**). A serving of a grain product or starchy vegetable provides an average of about 5 grams of protein, a serving of legumes provides 10 to 20 grams of protein,

and a serving of vegetables provides about 3 grams of protein. Although a serving of these foods contains less protein than a serving of meat, you can eat more plant protein foods for fewer calories.

Complementing Plant Proteins

It's important to remember that plant proteins lack one or more of the indispensable amino acids needed to build body proteins, so individual plant proteins need to complement each other. A simple rule to remember in complementing plant proteins is that combining grains and legumes or combining legumes and nuts or seeds provides complete, high-quality protein.

Table 2: Plant Sources of Protein

Plant Protein Source	Grams of Protein	Kilocalories
GRAIN PRODUCTS		
1 oat bran bagel (3 in.)	6	145
1 whole English muffin, mixed grain	6	155
1 large flour tortilla (10 in.)	6	218
1 cup cooked spaghetti	8	221
1 cup cooked brown rice	5	216
1 cup cooked oatmeal	6	147
2 slices whole-wheat bread	5	138
1/2 cup low-fat granola	5	209
STARCHY VEGETABLES		
1 cup cooked corn	5	177
1 cup baked winter squash	5	102
1 medium baked potato with skin	3	145
LEGUMES		
1/2 cup tofu	10	94
1 cup cooked lentils	18	230
1 cup cooked kidney beans	16	219
VEGETABLES		
1 cup cooked broccoli	4	55
1 cup cooked cauliflower	2	29
1 cup cooked Brussels sprouts	4	56
NUTS AND SEEDS		
2 tablespoons peanut butter	8	188
1/4 cup peanuts	10	216
1/4 cup sunflower seeds	7	200

Source: US Department of Agriculture, Agricultural Research Service. USDA National Nutrient Database for Standard Reference, Release 18. 2005. http://www.nal.usda.gov/fnic/foodcompindex.html. Accessed 6/1/06.

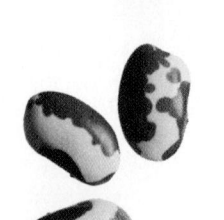
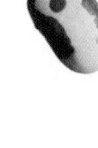
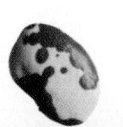

Soy Protein

The protein in soybeans is a notable exception to the rule that most plant proteins are incomplete. Soy provides complete, high-quality protein comparable to that in animal foods. In addition, soybeans provide no saturated fat or cholesterol, and are rich in isoflavonoids— phytochemicals that help reduce risk of heart disease and cancer and improve bone health.

Isoflavonoids act as antioxidants, protecting cells and tissues from damage. One specific isoflavonoid, genistein, inhibits growth of both breast and prostate cancer cells in the laboratory. Isoflavonoids protect LDL cholesterol (the kind of cholesterol associated with greater risk of heart disease) from oxidation. Oxidized LDL cholesterol contributes to the plaque buildup in arteries. The isoflavones in soybeans also act as phytoestrogens, helping to protect older women from cardiovascular disease and osteoporosis. Soy foods that contain most or all of the bean, such as soy milk, sprouts, flour, and tofu, are the best sources of these phytochemicals.

It is easy to incorporate a variety of soy foods into your diet. Tofu, tempeh, ground soy, soy milk, soy flour, and textured soy protein are soy-based products that can be included in many meals and snacks (**Table 3**).

The nutritional benefits of plant protein sources such as soy foods and other legumes, grains, and vegetables deserve a closer look. Most Americans would benefit from emphasizing plant protein foods in their diet. The next time you plan to make meat loaf, make lentil loaf instead.

Table 3: **Soy Food Products and Uses**

Tofu A solid cake of curdled soy milk similar to soft cheese. Tofu comes in hard and soft varieties. It absorbs the flavors of the foods it is mixed with. Soft tofu can be substituted for cheese in pasta dishes, stuffed in large shell pasta, blended with fruit, or used to make pie filling. Hard tofu can be used in salads, shish-ka-bobs, and in place of meat in stir-fry or mixed dishes.

Tempeh Tempeh is a flat cake made from fermented soybeans. It has a mild flavor and chewy texture. Tempeh can be grilled, included in sandwiches, or combined in casseroles.

Meat Analogues Meat analogues are meat alternatives made primarily of soy protein. Flavored and textured to resemble chicken, beef, and pork, they can be substituted for meat in mixed dishes, pizza, tacos, or sloppy joes.

Soy Milk Soy milk is the liquid of the soybean. It comes in regular and low-fat versions and in different flavors. Soy milk can be used plain or substituted for regular milk on cereals, in hot cocoa, puddings, or desserts.

Soy Flour Soy flour is made from roasted soybeans ground into flour. Soy flour can replace up to one-quarter of the regular flour in a recipe.

Textured Soy Protein Textured soy protein resembles ground beef. It can be rehydrated and substituted for ground beef in any recipe.

Table 6.6 Types of Vegetarian Diets

Type	Animal Foods Included	Foods Excluded
Semi-vegetarian	Dairy products, eggs, chicken, fish	Red meats (beef, pork)
Pesco-vegetarian	Dairy products, eggs, and fish	Beef, pork, poultry
Lacto-ovo-vegetarian	Dairy products, eggs	Any animal flesh
Lacto-vegetarian	Dairy products	Eggs, all animal flesh
Ovo-vegetarian	Eggs	Dairy products and animal flesh
Vegan	None	All animal products
Fruitarian	None	All foods except raw fruits, nuts, and green foliage

Health Benefits of Vegetarian Diets

Vegetarian diets usually contain less fat, saturated fat, and cholesterol and more magnesium and folate than nonvegetarian diets.[32] Vegetarian diets that emphasize fresh fruits and vegetables contain higher amounts of antioxidants such as beta-carotene and vitamins C and E, which protect the body from cell and tissue damage. Fruits and vegetables also contain dietary fiber and phytochemicals—substances that are not essential in the diet but that can have important health effects.

On average, vegetarians have lower blood cholesterol levels and are less likely to develop heart disease than nonvegetarians. Vegetarian diets low in fat and saturated fat combined with other healthy lifestyle habits can reverse the clogging of arteries that eventually can lead to heart attack or stroke.[33]

Vegetarians usually weigh less for their height than nonvegetarians, partly because their diets provide less energy and partly because of other healthful lifestyle factors such as regular exercise. High blood pressure occurs less frequently among vegetarians than among nonvegetarians, regardless of body weight or sodium intake.

Vegetarians, especially vegans, have lower rates of cancer than nonvegetarians, particularly prostate and colorectal cancer.[34] Vegetarian diets generally include more fruits, vegetables, phytochemicals, and fiber, and less fat. Intake of red meat has been linked to a higher risk of colorectal cancer.

Health Risks of Vegetarian Diets

Although vegetarian diets offer many health benefits, certain types of vegetarian diets pose some unique nutritional risks. The more limited the vegetarian diet, the more likely are nutritional problems. Lacto-ovo-vegetarian diets that contain a variety of foods generally are nutritionally adequate but can be high in fat and cholesterol. Iron content may be low if the diet contains large amounts of milk products.

Vegan diets tend to be low in zinc, calcium, vitamin D, riboflavin, and vitamin B_{12}. The best sources of these nutrients are animal foods—red meat for zinc; milk for calcium, vitamin D, and riboflavin; and any animal foods for B$_{12}$. Because plant foods contain a form of iron called non-heme iron that is not as well absorbed as the heme iron in animal foods, vegetarians need to include more iron in their diets. Vitamin C and other compounds in fruits and vegetables aid iron absorption in the body.

Vegans tend to have higher intakes of phytates (found in whole grains, bran, and soy products), oxalates (found in spinach, rhubarb, and chocolate), and tannins (found in tea). These compounds can bind minerals, making them less available to the body for absorption. Very limited vegan diets, such as fruitarian diets or extreme Zen macrobiotic diets, pose the greatest nutritional risks. These diets are likely to be deficient in many essential nutrients.

Although vegetarian diets may be adequate for most people, vegetarian diets must be planned carefully for periods of rapid growth, such as for infants and young children and for women who are pregnant or breastfeeding.

Dietary Recommendations for Vegetarians

Dietitians from the United States and Canada have developed a food guide for use in planning vegetarian diets.[35] This food guide includes the following food groups: grains, vegetables and fruits, legumes, nuts and other protein-rich foods, fats, and calcium-rich foods. Vegetarians who include milk, milk products, and eggs in their diet can easily meet their nutritional needs for protein and other essential nutrients but must take care to choose low-fat milk products and limit eggs to avoid excess saturated fat and cholesterol.

Since grains, vegetables, and legumes (dried beans and peas) all provide protein, vegans who eat a variety of foods also can meet their protein needs easily. Although most plant foods do not contain complete protein, eating complementary plant protein sources during the same day adequately meets the body's needs for protein production.

Vegans who avoid all animal products must supplement their diets with a reliable source of vitamin B$_{12}$, such as fortified soy milk. Although bacteria in some fermented foods and in the knobby growths of some seaweeds produce vitamin B$_{12}$, most vegans do not eat enough seaweeds and fermented foods to meet their vitamin B$_{12}$ needs. Vegans also need a dietary source of vitamin D when sun exposure is limited.

The American Dietetic Association and Dietitians of Canada give the following nutritional guidelines for vegetarians:[36]

1. Choose a variety of foods, including whole grains, vegetables, fruits, legumes, nuts, seeds, and, if desired, dairy products and eggs.

2. Choose whole, unrefined foods often and minimize intake of highly sweetened, fatty, and heavily refined foods.

3. Choose a variety of fruits and vegetables.

4. If animal foods such as dairy products and eggs are used, choose lower-fat dairy products and use both eggs and dairy products in moderation.

5. Use a regular source of vitamin B$_{12}$ and, if sun exposure is limited, of vitamin D.

Key Concepts: *Vegetarian diets eliminate animal products to various degrees. Lacto-ovo-vegetarians include milk and eggs in their diets, whereas vegans eat no animal foods. Vegetarian diets tend to be low in fat and high in fiber and phytochemicals, which may help reduce chronic disease risks. Careful diet planning is necessary for vegans and growing children to ensure that all nutrient needs are met.*

American Dietetic Association

Vegetarian Diets

It is the position of the American Dietetic Association and Dietitians of Canada that appropriately planned vegetarian diets are healthful, nutritionally adequate, and provide health benefits in the prevention and treatment of certain diseases.

J Am Diet Assoc. 2003;103:748–765.
ADA and Dietitians of Canada Joint Position.
Reprinted with permission.

The Health Effects of Too Little or Too Much Protein

Because protein plays such a vital role in so many body processes, protein deficiency can wreak havoc in numerous body systems. A lack of available protein means insufficient amounts of indispensable amino acids, which stops the synthesis of body proteins.

Protein deficiency occurs when energy and/or protein intake is inadequate. Adequate energy intake spares dietary and body proteins so they can be used for protein synthesis. Without adequate energy intake, the body burns dietary protein for energy rather than using it to make body proteins. Protein deficiency can occur even in people who eat seemingly adequate amounts of protein if the protein they eat is of poor quality or cannot be absorbed.

Although protein deficiency is widespread in poverty-stricken communities and in some nonindustrialized countries, most people in industrialized countries face the opposite problem—protein excess. Although the RDA for a 70-kilogram (154-pound) person is 56 grams, the average American man consumes approximately 100 grams of protein daily, and the average woman about 70 grams. Many meat-loving Americans eat far more protein.

Some research suggests that high protein intake contributes to risk for heart disease, cancer, and osteoporosis. However, because high protein intake often goes hand-in-hand with high intakes of saturated fat and cholesterol, the independent effects of high protein intake are difficult to determine.

Protein-Energy Malnutrition

A deficiency of protein, energy, or both in the diet is called **protein-energy malnutrition (PEM)**. Protein and energy intake are difficult to separate because diets adequate in energy usually are adequate in protein, and diets inadequate in energy inhibit the body's use of dietary protein for protein synthesis.

Although it can occur at all stages of life, PEM is most common during childhood, when protein is needed to support rapid growth. PEM affects every fourth child worldwide and is a factor in more than half of the 104 million annual deaths of children younger than age 5.[37] PEM symptoms can be mild or severe and exist in either acute or chronic forms.

Protein-energy malnutrition occurs in all parts of the world but is most common in Africa, South and Central America, East and Southeast Asia, and the Middle East. In industrialized countries, PEM occurs most often in populations living in poverty, in the elderly, and in hospitalized patients with other conditions such as anorexia nervosa, AIDS, cancer, or malabsorption syndromes.[38]

There are two forms of severe PEM: **kwashiorkor** and **marasmus**. Sometimes people have symptoms of both. Researchers do not understand fully why PEM causes symptoms of kwashiorkor in some people and symptoms of marasmus in others.[39] Historically, kwashiorkor was thought to result from inadequate intake of protein but adequate intake of energy. Marasmus was thought to result from inadequate intake of both protein and energy. Now researchers know that the lines between these two diseases are not so clear and that protein deficiency rarely develops with adequate energy intake.

Researchers believe that kwashiorkor develops from acute PEM, whereas marasmus develops from chronic PEM. Some researchers also believe that kwashiorkor is an abnormal adaptation to PEM, whereas marasmus is a normal adaptation. Other factors, such as infections or toxins in the diet, may trigger the development of kwashiorkor rather than marasmus.[40] See **Figure 6.21** for the signs and symptoms of kwashiorkor and marasmus.

protein-energy malnutrition (PEM) A condition resulting from long-term inadequate intakes of energy and protein that can lead to wasting of body tissues and increased susceptibility to infection.

kwashiorkor A type of malnutrition that occurs primarily in young children who have an infectious disease and whose diets supply marginal amounts of energy and very little protein. Common symptoms include poor growth, edema, apathy, weakness, and susceptibility to infections.

marasmus A type of malnutrition resulting from chronic inadequate consumption of protein and energy that is characterized by wasting of muscle, fat, and other body tissue.

Kwashiorkor

The term *kwashiorkor* is a Ghanian word that describes the "evil spirit that infects the first child when the second child is born." In many cultures, babies are breastfed until the next baby comes along. When the new baby arrives, the first baby is weaned from nutritious breast milk and placed on a watered-down version of the family's diet. In areas of poverty, this diet is often low in protein, or the consumed protein is not digested and absorbed easily.

One symptom of kwashiorkor that sets it apart from marasmus is edema, or swelling of body tissue, usually in the feet and legs. Lack of blood proteins reduces the force that keeps fluid in the bloodstream, allowing fluid to leak out into the tissues. Because proteins are unavailable to transport fat, it accumulates in the liver. Combined with edema, this accumulation produces a bloated belly. Other features of kwashiorkor include stunted weight and height; increased susceptibility to infection; dry, flaky skin, and sometimes skin sores; dry, brittle, and unnaturally blond hair; and changes in skin color. Because the energy deficit is usually not as severe (or as long-standing) in kwashiorkor as in marasmus, people with kwashiorkor may still have some body fat stores left.

Kwashiorkor usually develops in children between 18 and 24 months of age, about the time weaning occurs. Its onset can be rapid and is often triggered by an infection or illness that increases the child's protein needs. In hospital settings, kwashiorkor can develop in situations where protein needs are extremely high (trauma, infection, burns) but dietary intake is poor.

Marasmus

Marasmus is derived from the Greek word *marasmos*, which means "withering" or "to waste away." It develops more slowly than kwashiorkor and results from chronic PEM. Protein, energy, and nutrient intake are all grossly inadequate, depleting body fat reserves and severely wasting muscle tissue, including vital organs such as the heart. Growth slows or stops, and children are both short and very thin for their age. Metabolism slows and body temperature drops as the body tries to conserve energy. Children with marasmus are apathetic, often not even crying in an effort to conserve energy. Their hair is sparse and falls out easily. Because muscle and fat are used up, a child with marasmus often looks like a frail, wrinkled, elderly person.

Marasmus occurs most often in infants and children aged 6 to 18 months who are fed diluted or improperly mixed formulas. Because this is a time of rapid brain growth, marasmus can permanently stunt brain development and lead to learning disabilities. Marasmus also occurs in adults during cancer and starvation, including the self-imposed starvation of the eating disorder known as anorexia nervosa.

Nutritional Rehabilitation

To recover, people with PEM need gradual and careful refeeding to correct protein, energy, fluid, and vitamin and mineral imbalances.[41] People with PEM are often dehydrated and have low body potassium stores as a result of diarrhea. These imbalances in fluids and electrolytes are corrected first to raise blood pressure and strengthen the heart. Once these imbalances have been corrected, the patient receives protein and other nutrients in small amounts that are gradually increased as tolerated.

Excess Dietary Protein

In industrialized countries, an excess of protein and energy is more common than a deficiency. Generally, self-selected diets do not contain more than 40 percent of calories from protein.[42] Although high protein intake has been

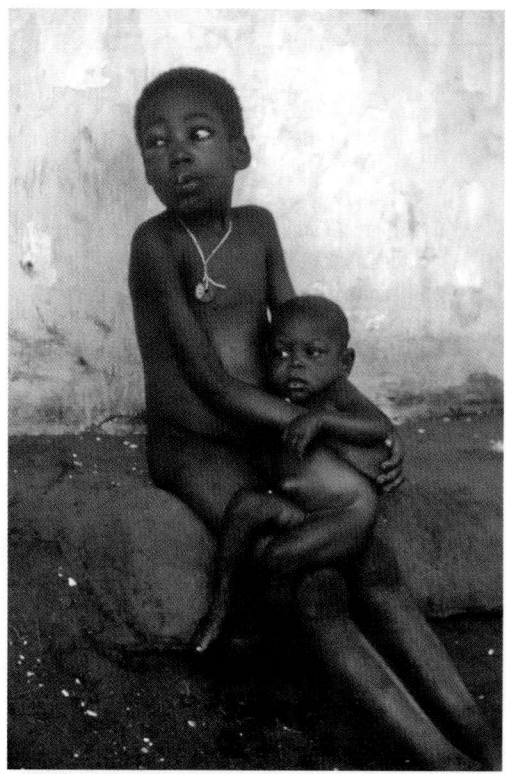

(a)

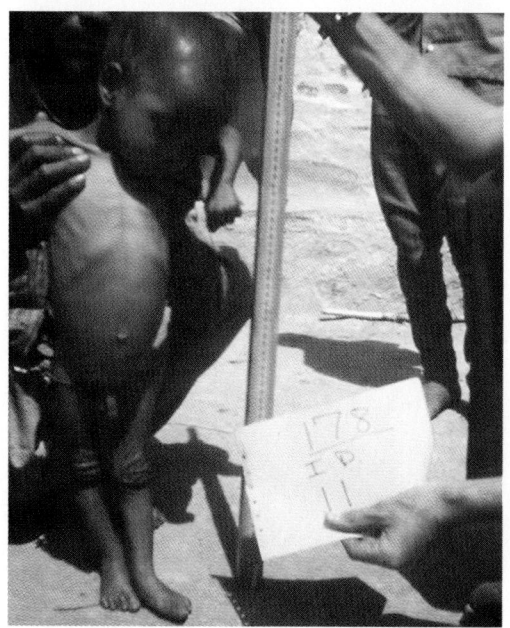

(b)

Figure 6.21 **Kwashiorkor and marasmus.** (a) Edema in the feet and legs and a bloated belly are symptoms of kwashiorkor. (b) Children with marasmus are short and thin for their age and can appear frail and wrinkled.

The Source of Salisbury Steak

r. James Salisbury, a London physician who lived in the late 1800s, believed man to be two-thirds carnivorous and one-third herbivorous. He recommended a diet low in starch and high in lean meat, with lots of hot water to rinse out the products of fermentation. His diet regimen included broiled, lean, minced beef three times a day. Although we call it Salisbury steak as a courtesy to Dr. Salisbury's heritage, minced beef patties are really more like hamburgers.

suggested to contribute to kidney problems, osteoporosis, heart disease, and cancer (see **Figure 6.22**), the Food and Nutrition Board did not find the evidence supporting these links to be strong enough to set a UL for protein.[43]

Kidney Function

Since the kidneys must excrete the products of protein breakdown, high protein intake can strain kidney function and is especially harmful for people with kidney disease or diabetes.

To prevent dehydration, it is important to drink plenty of fluids to dilute the by-products of protein breakdown for excretion. Human infants should not be fed unmodified cow's milk until they are at least 1 year old because the high protein concentration in cow's milk combined with an immature kidney system can cause excessive fluid losses and dehydration.

Mineral Losses

The link between high-protein diets and osteoporosis is based on studies showing that a high protein intake increases calcium excretion, which could then contribute to bone mineral losses. However, these studies generally used purified proteins rather than food proteins. Studies of postmenopausal women have shown that a high meat intake combined with a calcium intake of 600 milligrams per day did not result in increased calcium loss[44] and that substitution of soy protein for meat protein had no effect on calcium balance.[45] Other studies of older men and women have found favorable effects on bone mineral density from increasing both protein and calcium intake.[46]

Obesity

Some epidemiological studies have shown a correlation between high protein intake and body fatness.[47] High-protein foods often are high in fat. A diet high in fat and protein may provide too much energy, contributing to

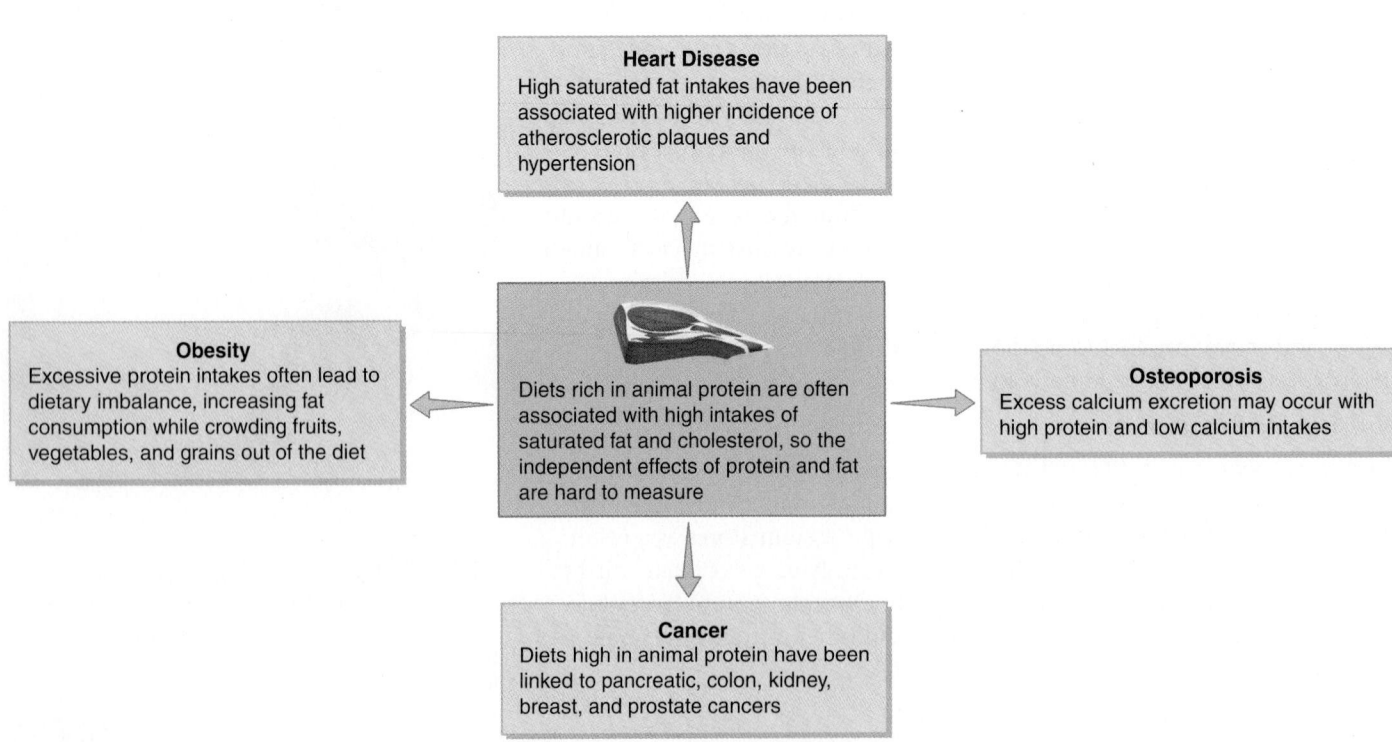

Heart Disease
High saturated fat intakes have been associated with higher incidence of atherosclerotic plaques and hypertension

Obesity
Excessive protein intakes often lead to dietary imbalance, increasing fat consumption while crowding fruits, vegetables, and grains out of the diet

Diets rich in animal protein are often associated with high intakes of saturated fat and cholesterol, so the independent effects of protein and fat are hard to measure

Osteoporosis
Excess calcium excretion may occur with high protein and low calcium intakes

Cancer
Diets high in animal protein have been linked to pancreatic, colon, kidney, breast, and prostate cancers

Figure 6.22 **Excess animal protein.** In developed countries, excess protein and energy are a greater problem than protein deficiency.

obesity. Large amounts of high-protein foods will displace fruits, vegetables, and grains—foods that contain fewer calories. Researchers have suggested that high dietary protein intake alters hormones and the body's response to hormones, including leptin, which regulates feeding centers in the brain to reduce food intake.[48] Some studies suggest that because of this effect on hormones, a high protein intake early in life increases the risk of obesity later in life.[49]

Heart Disease

Research has linked high intake of animal protein to high blood cholesterol levels and increased risk of heart disease. Foods high in animal protein are also high in saturated fat and cholesterol. Whether protein alone—independent of fat—plays a role in the development of heart disease is less clear. Based on studies that showed beneficial effects from consumption of soy protein,[50] the FDA approved a health claim saying that soy protein is beneficial in reducing the risk of heart disease. A recent review by the American Heart Association, however, found that consuming soy protein has little or no effect on the risk factors for heart disease.[51] The researchers also concluded that consuming soy protein products, such as tofu, soy butter, soy nuts, and some soy burgers, could be beneficial. Soy protein foods, with their high content of polyunsaturated fats, fiber, vitamins, and minerals and low content of saturated fat, could replace other protein foods that are high in fat.[52]

Cancer

Some studies suggest a link between a diet high in animal protein foods and an increased risk for certain types of cancers.[53] The evidence is strongest for a relationship between animal protein and colon cancer.[54] Prolonged high intake of both red meat (beef, pork) and processed meat (ham, smoked meats, sausage, bacon) has been associated with increased colon cancer risk.[55]

Gout

Gout is an immensely painful inflammatory arthritis caused by the accumulation of uric acid crystals in joints. Uric acid forms from the breakdown of nitrogen-containing compounds called purines. Uric acid normally dissolves in the blood and passes through the kidneys into the urine. In people with gout, uric acid builds up and forms sharp crystals that can collect around the joints, causing swelling and intense pain. Diets high in meats (especially red meats) and seafood and low in dairy products significantly increase the risk of gout—the most common form of inflammatory arthritis in men.[56] Total protein intake, however, was not correlated with an increased risk of gout. (See the Nutrition Science in Action feature "Protein and Gout.")

Key Concepts: *Protein-energy malnutrition (PEM) is a common form of malnutrition in the developing world, with potentially devastating effects for children. PEM can manifest in two forms: kwashiorkor and marasmus. Among other symptoms, kwashiorkor is distinguished by edema, or swelling of the tissues. Marasmus results from chronic PEM and is distinguished by severe wasting of body fat and muscles. Excess dietary protein may contribute to obesity, heart disease, and certain forms of cancer. These links, however, may be attributable to the high fat intake that often accompanies high protein intake.*

Quick Bites

Protein Makes for Springy Bugs

Resilin is an elastic rubberlike protein in insects, scorpions, and crustaceans. The springiness in the wing hinges of some insects, like locusts and dragonflies, comes from the unique mechanical properties of resilin. The protein also is found in the stingers of bees and ants, the eardrums and sound organs of cicadas, and the little rubber balls in the hips of jumping fleas. The structural properties of resilin are similar to true rubber, which makes it very unusual among structural proteins.

gout An intensely painful form of inflammatory arthritis that results from deposits of needlelike crystals of uric acid in connective tissue and/or the joint space between bones.

NUTRITION SCIENCE IN ACTION
Protein and Gout

Observations: High protein intake and intake of various foods rich in purines have long been thought to increase the risk of gout, but this has not been confirmed by prospective studies. Purine-rich foods include meats, seafood, and certain vegetables. Although protein-rich diets tend to be high in purines, protein also stimulates excretion of uric acid in urine.

Hypothesis: The risk of gout is independently increased by consumption of (1) a protein-rich diet, (2) a diet high in meat, and (3) a diet high in seafood.

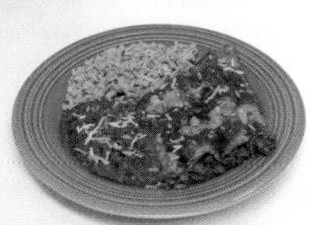

1. High-protein diet

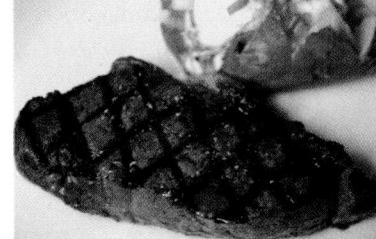

2. High-meat diet

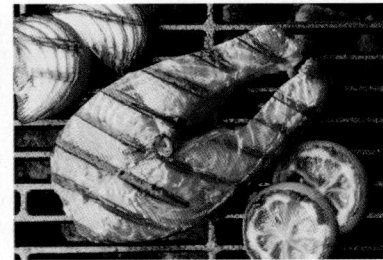

3. High-seafood diet

Experimental Plan: The Health Professionals Follow-up Study is an ongoing study of 51,529 males. Exclude men with a history of gout and follow the remaining 47,150 men for 12 years. Annually assess dietary intake with food frequency questionnaires. Record all newly diagnosed cases of gout.

Results: Hypothesis 1 is not confirmed. A higher total intake of protein was not associated with an increased risk of gout. Hypotheses 2 and 3 are confirmed. The risk of gout increased 21 percent per additional portion of meat per day, and 7 percent per additional portion of seafood per week. The study also found that consumption of dairy protein (especially in low-fat dairy products) reduced the risk of gout.

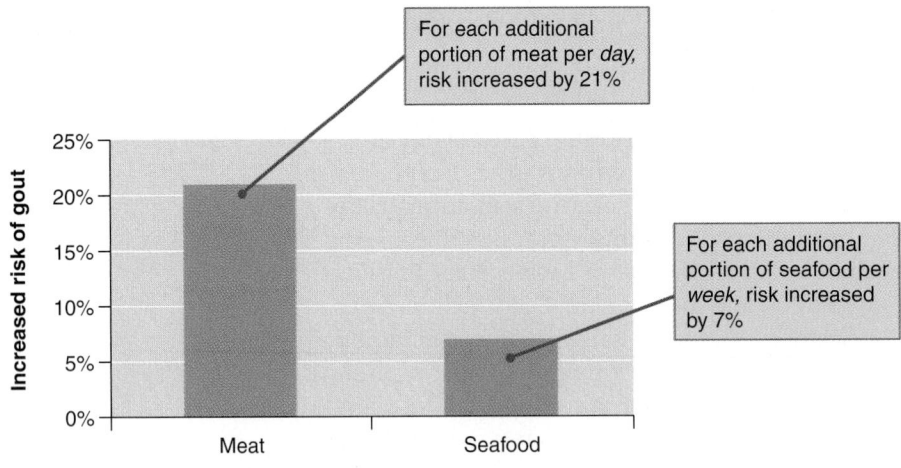

For each additional portion of meat per *day*, risk increased by 21%

For each additional portion of seafood per *week*, risk increased by 7%

Conclusion and Discussion: This large prospective study provides scientific verification of the long-standing view that gout is most common among people whose diet is rich in meats (especially red meats) and low in dairy products. Total protein intake is not associated with the development of gout, and vegetable protein intake may have a protective effect. Because high-protein diets lead to increased urinary uric acid excretion, this may reduce blood uric acid levels. Also, the protein content of foods may not be a good indicator of their purine content. Given the role of increased fish intake in the prevention of heart disease, findings by future studies may lead to more refined fish intake recommendations that account for both gout and heart disease.

Source: Based on Choi HK, Atkinson K, Karlson EW, et al. Purine-rich foods, dairy and protein intake, and the risk of gout in men. *New Engl J Med*. 2004;350(11):1093–1103.

Label [to] **Table**

Have you ever visited a health food store and noticed all the protein powders, amino acid supplements, and high-protein bars? Do you believe claims like "protein boosts your energy level" or "amino acid X helps you build muscle" or "protein shakes are the best pre-workout fuel"? You know from this chapter that protein is an important nutrient and it's used to build and repair tissue. But do you need one of these supplements? Before reaching into your wallet, check out the Nutrition Facts of this protein powder and determine whether it's a good buy.

Take a look at this label and note how far down protein is on the list of nutrients. This de-emphasized placement of protein was intentional to try to get consumers to de-emphasize protein in their diets. You may recall that most Americans eat more protein than they need, and because much of that protein comes from animal foods, they are often getting excess saturated fat. Although there is a DV for protein (50 grams), manufacturers must first determine a food protein's quality by the PDCAAS method before they can determine %DV. Manufacturers are not required to give the %DV for protein on food labels.

Do protein and amino acid supplements do what they claim to do? In terms of building muscle, exercise physiologists agree that it takes consistent muscle work (i.e., weight lifting) and a healthy diet that meets the body's calorie needs. Muscle building does not depend on extra protein. In fact, muscles use carbohydrate and fat for fuel, not protein, so these other nutrients are more important for effective workouts.

In terms of protein's ability to boost your energy level, recall that anything with calories (carbohydrates, proteins, and fats) provides the body with "energy." In fact, unlike carbohydrates and fats, only a small amount of protein is used for energy expenditure. Research shows that the best thing to eat prior to a workout is carbohydrate, not protein, because carbohydrate provides glucose for the muscle cells. Review this label again. What percentage of this protein powder's calories is from protein?

kcal	154
Protein	11 grams × 4 kcal per gram
	= 44 protein kcal

44 ÷ 154 = 0.28 or 28% protein kcal

Surprise! Surprise! Only one-quarter of the powder's calories are protein anyway, so it's okay as a pre-workout fuel not because of its protein content but because of its ample carbohydrate!

Nutrition Facts

Serving Size: 2 scoops
Servings Per Container: 18

Amount Per Serving

Calories 154 Calories from fat 35

	% Daily Value*
Total Fat 4g	6%
Saturated Fat 2.5g	12%
Trans Fat 0g	
Cholesterol 20mg	7%
Sodium 170mg	7%
Total Carbohydrate 17g	6%
Dietary Fiber 0g	0%
Sugars 14g	
Protein 11g	

Vitamin A 4%	.	Vitamin C 6%
Calcium 40%	.	Iron 0%

* Percent Daily Values are based on a 2,000 calorie diet. Your daily values may be higher or lower depending on your calorie needs:

		Calories:	2,000	2,500
Total Fat	Less Than		65g	80g
Sat Fat	Less Than		20g	25g
Cholesterol	Less Than		300mg	300mg
Sodium	Less Than		2,400mg	2,400mg
Total Carbohydrate			300g	375g
Dietary Fiber			25g	30g

Calories per gram:

Fat 9 . Carbohydrate 4 . Protein 4

LEARNING *Portfolio* c h a p t e r 6

Key Terms

Study Points

- Many vital compounds are proteins, including enzymes, hormones, transport proteins, and regulators of both acid–base and fluid balance.

- Proteins are long chains of amino acids.

- Amino acids are composed of a central carbon atom bonded to hydrogen, carboxyl, amino, and side groups.

- At least 20 amino acids are important in human nutrition; 9 of these amino acids are considered indispensable (must come from the diet), while the body can make the other 11 (dispensable) amino acids.

- The amino acid sequence of a protein determines its shape and function.

- Denaturing of proteins changes their shape and therefore their functional properties.

- Protein digestion begins in the stomach through the action of hydrochloric acid and the enzyme pepsin.

- Proteins are digested completely in the small intestine and absorbed by facilitated diffusion and active transport.

- Dietary protein is found in meats, dairy products, legumes, nuts, seeds, grains, and vegetables.

- In general, animal foods contain higher-quality protein than is found in plant foods.

- Protein needs are highest when growth is rapid, such as during infancy, childhood, and adolescence.

- The protein intake of most Americans exceeds their RDA.

- Protein deficiency is most common in developing countries and results in the conditions known as marasmus and kwashiorkor.

- Protein excess is also harmful and may affect risk for osteoporosis, heart disease, cancer, and gout.

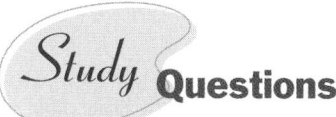

Study Questions

1. **List the functions of body proteins.**

2. **Describe the differences among indispensable, dispensable, and conditionally indispensable amino acids.**

3. **Among the nutrient molecules, which element is unique to protein and how does it fit into the basic structure of an amino acid?**

4. **Why are most plant proteins considered incomplete?**

5. **What are complementary proteins? List three examples of food combinations that contain complementary proteins.**

6. **What health effects occur if you are protein deficient?**

7. **How is protein related to immune function?**

8. **Describe a vegan diet.**

9. **List the potential health benefits of a vegetarian diet.**

☞ [*Try*] **This**

The Sweetness of NutraSweet

The purpose of this experiment is to see the effect of high temperatures on the dipeptide known as NutraSweet (aspartame). Make a cup of hot tea (or coffee) and add one packet of Equal (one brand of aspartame). Stir and taste the tea; note its sweetness. Reheat the tea (via a microwave or stovetop) so that it boils for 30 to 60 seconds. After the tea cools, taste it. Does it still taste sweet? Why or why not?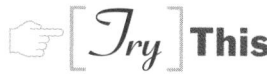

The Vegetarian Challenge

The purpose of this activity is to eat a completely vegan diet for one day. Begin by making a list of your typical meals and snacks. Once the list is complete, review each food item and determine whether it contains animal products. Cross off items that contain animal products and circle the remaining vegan-friendly options. Double-check the circled list with a friend or roommate. You may have missed something! Create a full day's worth of meals and snacks using your circled foods as well as additional vegan options. Make sure your menu looks complete and nutritionally balanced. Try to stick to this menu for at least one day. Pay attention to deviations you make and whether these are vegan food choices.

What About *Bobbie?*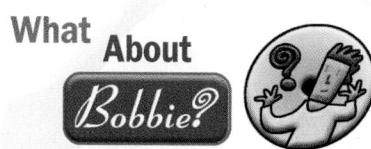

Take a minute to review Bobbie's food intake with a special eye on protein. How do you think she did? Do you think she's lower or higher than her RDA? Let's first calculate her protein RDA. Since Bobbie weighs 155 pounds, her protein RDA is as follows:

155 pounds ÷ 2.2 pounds = 70.5 kilograms
70.5 kilograms X 0.8 gram protein = 56.40 grams

Her protein intake is 96 grams. This is quite high compared to her RDA! Are you surprised to learn she eats twice as much protein as she needs? Her diet doesn't look *that* high in protein, does it? Here are the foods that contribute the most protein to her diet:

Food	Protein (grams)
Meatballs	24
Turkey breast	17
Spaghetti	10
Pizza	9
Bagel	7

Another way to evaluate Bobbie's protein intake is in terms of calories. If her total protein intake is 96 grams, then 384 kilocalories come from protein. Remember, her total kilocalorie intake is 2,300, which means protein accounts for 17 percent of her energy intake. General guidelines recommend that 10 to 35 percent of energy come from protein.

So, what's the deal? Is Bobbie eating way too much protein or just the right amount? She's certainly high compared to her RDA of 56 grams, but using the AMDR, she could consume as much as 200 grams at her current energy intake level! We've already seen that her diet could use more servings of fruits and vegetables, and in future chapters we'll see whether her balance of energy sources is appropriate for obtaining all the needed vitamins and minerals.

References

1 Institute of Medicine, Food and Nutrition Board. *Dietary Reference Intakes for Energy, Carbohydrate, Fiber, Fat, Fatty Acids, Cholesterol, Protein, and Amino Acids.* Washington, DC: National Academy Press, 2005.

2 National Institutes of Health. *Phenylketonuria: Screening and Management.* NIH Consensus Statement. 2000;17(3):1–27.

3 Institute of Medicine, Food and Nutrition Board. Op. cit.

4 Ibid.

5 Ibid.

6 Voet D, Voet JG. *Biochemistry.* 2nd ed. New York: Wiley, 1995.

7 Greenberg AS, Obin MS. Obesity and the role of adipose tissue in inflammation and metabolism. *Am J Clin Nutr.* 2006; 83(2):461S–465S.

8 Berg JM, Tymoczko JL, Stryer L. *Biochemistry.* 5th ed. New York: W.H. Freeman, 2002.

9 Guyton A, Hall J. *Textbook of Medical Physiology.* 10th ed. Philadelphia: WB Saunders, 2000.

10 Kelly DG. Assessment of malnutrition. In Shils ME, Shike M, Ross AC, Cabellero B, Cousins RJ, eds. *Modern Nutrition in Health and Disease.* 10th ed. Philadephia: Lippincott Williams & Wilkens, 2006;1143–1151.

11 Ibid.

12 Guyton A, Hall J. Op. cit.

13 Mathews DE. Proteins and amino acids. In: Shils ME, Shike M, Ross AC, Cabellero B, Cousins RJ, eds. *Modern Nutrition in Health and Disease.* 10th ed. Philadelphia: Lippincott Williams & Wilkins, 2006;23–61.

14 Ibid.

15 Mathews DE. Op. cit.

16 Institute of Medicine, Food and Nutrition Board. Op. cit.

17 Briefel RR, Johnson CL. Secular trends in dietary intake in the United States. *Ann Rev Nutr.* 2004;24:401–431.

18 Institute of Medicine, Food and Nutrition Board. Op. cit.

19 Millward DJ, Roberts SB. Protein requirements of older individuals. *Nutr Res Rev.* 1996;9:67–87.

20 Rand WM, Pellett PL, Young VR. Meta-analysis of nitrogen balance studies for estimating protein requirements in healthy adults. *Am J Clin Nutr.* 2003;77:109–127.

21 Institute of Medicine, Food and Nutrition Board. Op. cit.

22 Young VR. Soy protein in relation to human protein and amino acid nutrition. *J Am Diet Assoc.* 1991;91:828–835; and Institute of Medicine, Food and Nutrition Board. Op. cit.

23 US Department of Agriculture. Nutrient content of the U.S. food supply. http://209.48.219.50/NFSDatabase/QueAV.asp. Accessed 6/8/06.

24 Young VR, Pellett PL. Plant proteins in relation to human protein and amino acid nutrition. *Am J Clin Nutr.* 1994; 59:1203S–1212S.

25 Young VR, Pellett PL. Op. cit.; and American Dietetic Association. Position of the American Dietetic Association and the Dietitians of Canada: vegetarian diets. *J Am Diet Assoc.* 2003;103:748–765.

26 Dwyer JT. Nutritional consequences of vegetarianism. *Ann Rev Nutr.* 1991;11:61–91.

27 Institute of Medicine, Food and Nutrition Board. Op. cit.

28 Food and Agriculture Organization. *Protein Quality Evaluation: Report of the Joint FAO/WHO Expert Consultation.* Rome: Food and Agriculture Organization of the United Nations, 1991. FAO Food and Nutrition Paper 51; and Sarwar G, McDonough RE. Evaluation of protein digestibility-corrected amino acid score method for assessing protein quality of foods. *J Assoc Official Analytic Chem.* 1990;73:347–356.

29 Ballenntine R. *Transition to Vegetarianism: An Evolutionary Step.* Honesdale, PA: Himalayan International Institute of Yoga Science and Philosophy, 1987; and Null G. *The Vegetarian Handbook: Eating Right for Total Health.* New York: St. Martin's Press, 1987.

30 Null G. Op. cit.

31 The Vegetarian Resource Group. How many vegetarians are there? *Vegetarian Journal.* May 21, 2003. http://www.vrg.org /journal/vj2003issue3/vj2003issue3poll.htm. Accessed 12/21/06.

32 American Dietetic Association. Op. cit.

33 Gould KL, Ornish D, Scherwitz L, et al. Changes in myocardial perfusion abnormalities by positron emission tomography after long-term intense risk factor modification. *JAMA.* 1995;274:894–901; and Leitzman C. Vegetarian diets: what are the advantages? *Forum Nutr.* 2005;57:147–156.

34 American Dietetic Association. Op. cit.

35 Messina V, Melina V, Mangels AR. A new food guide for North American vegetarians. *J Am Diet Assoc.* 2003;103:771–775.

36 American Dietetic Association. Op. cit.

37 World Health Organization. *Turning the Tide of Malnutrition: Responding to the Challenge of the 21st Century.* Geneva: World Health Organization, 2000. Document WHO/NHD/00.7.

38 Muller O, Krawinkel M. Malnutrition and health in developing countries. *Can Med Assoc J.* 2005;173(3):279–286; and Swail WS, Samour PQ, Babineau TJ, Bistrian BR. A proposed revision of current ICD-9-CM malnutrition code definitions. *J Am Diet Assoc.* 1996;96:370–373.

39 Manary MJ, Broadhead RL, Yarasheski KE. Whole-body protein kinetics in marasmus and kwashiorkor during acute infection. *Am J Clin Nutr.* 1998;67:1205–1209.

40 Fuhrman MP, Charney P, Mueller CM. Hepatic proteins and nutrition assessment. *J Am Diet Assoc.* 2004;104:1258–1264; and Krawinkel M. Kwashiorkor is still not fully understood. *Bull World Health Organ.* 2003;81:910–911.

41 Hoffer JJ. Metabolic consequences of starvation. In: Shils ME, Shike M, Ross AC, Cabellero B, Cousins RJ, eds. *Modern Nutrition in Health and Disease.* 10th ed. Philadelphia: Lippincott Williams & Wilkins, 2006;730–748.

42 Institute of Medicine, Food and Nutrition Board. Op. cit.

43 Ibid.

44 Roughead ZK, Johnson LK, Lykken GI, Hunt JR. Controlled high meat diets do not affect calcium retention or indices of bone status in healthy postmenopausal women. *J Nutr.* 2003;133:1020–1026.

45 Roughead ZK, Hunt JR, Johnson LK, et al. Controlled substitution of soy protein for meat protein: effects on calcium retention, bone, and cardiovascular health indices in post-menopausal women. *J Clin Endocrinol Metab.* 2005;90:181–189.

46 Dawson-Hughes B, Harris SS. Calcium intake influences the association of protein intake with rates of bone loss in elderly men and women. *Am J Clin Nutr.* 2002;75:773–779; and Promislow JH, Goodman-Gruen D, Slymen DJ, Barrett-Connor E. Protein consumption and bone mineral density in the elderly: the Rancho Bernardo Study. *Am J Epidemiol.* 2002;155:636–644.

47 Institute of Medicine, Food and Nutrition Board. Op. cit.

48 Schwartz M, Seeley RJ. The new biology of body weight regulation. *J Am Diet Assoc.* 1997;97:54–58; and Weigle DS, Breen PA, Matthys CC, et al. A high-protein diet induces sustained reductions in appetite, ad libitum caloric intake, and body weight despite compensatory changes in diurnal plasma leptin and ghrelin concentrations. *Am J Clin Nutr.* 2005;82(1):41–48.

49 Parizkova J, Rolland-Cachera MF. High proteins early in life as a predisposition for later obesity and further health risks. *Nutrition.* 1997;13:818–819; and Koletzko B, Broekaert I, Demmelmair H, et al. Protein intake in the first year of life: a risk factor for later obesity? The E.U. childhood obesity project. *Adv Exp Med Biol.* 2005;569:69–79.

50 Anderson JW, Johnstone RM, Cook-Newell ME. Meta-analysis of the effects of soy protein intake on serum lipids. *N Engl J Med.* 1995;333:276–282.

51 Sacks FM, Lichtenstein A, Van Horn L, et al. Soy protein, isoflavones, and cardiovascular health: an American Heart Association science advisory for professionals from the nutrition committee. *Circulation.* 2006;113:1034–1044.

52 Ibid.

53 Giovannuci E. Intake of fat, meat, and fiber in relation to colon cancer in men. *Cancer Res.* 1994;54:2390.

54 Willett WC. Diet and cancer: an evolving picture. *JAMA.* 2005;293:233–234.

55 Chao A, Thun MJ, Connell CJ. Meat consumption and risk of colorectal cancer. *JAMA.* 2005;293:172–182.

56 Choi HK, Atkinson K, Karlson EW, et al. Purine-rich foods, dairy and protein intake, and the risk of gout in men. *New Engl J Med.* 2004;350(11):1093–1103.

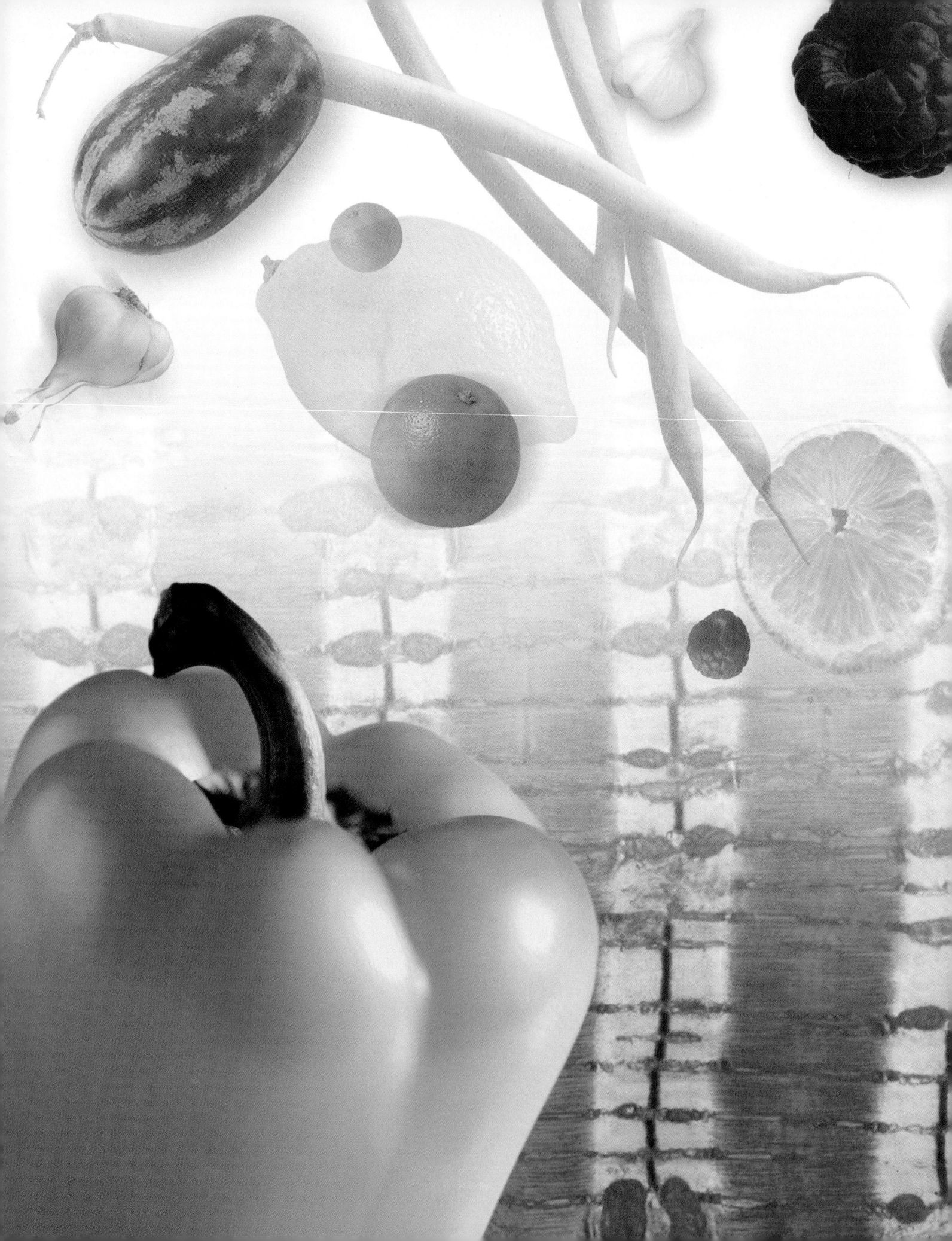

Chapter

Metabolism

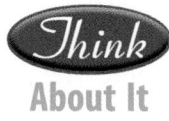

Think About It

1　You are driving on "the energy highway." You stop at the tollbooth. What kind of currency do you need to pay the toll?

2　When you think of "cell power," what comes to mind?

3　What do you think is meant by the saying "Fat burns in a flame of carbohydrate"?

4　When it comes to fasting, what's your body's first priority?

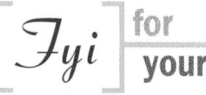

Fyi for your Information

This chapter's FYI boxes include practical information on the following topics:

- Do Carbohydrates Turn into Fat?

- Key Intersections Direct Metabolic Traffic

- Metabolic Profiles of Important Sites

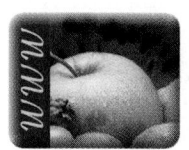

The Web site for this book offers many useful tools and is a great source for additional nutrition information for both students and instructors. Visit the site at nutrition.jbpub.com for information on metabolism. You'll find exercises that explore the following topics:

- Mitochondria Malfunctions

- Deadly Dinitrophenol

- The Ketosis Diet

- The Citric Acid Cycle (Krebs Cycle)

Key to Illustrations

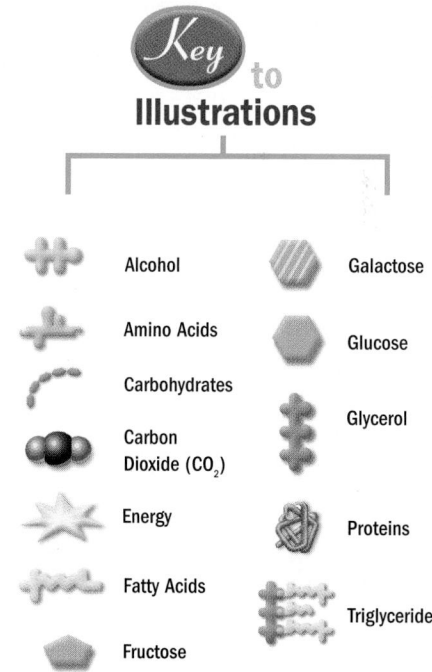

Alcohol

Amino Acids

Carbohydrates

Carbon Dioxide (CO_2)

Energy

Fatty Acids

Fructose

Galactose

Glucose

Glycerol

Proteins

Triglycerides

EXTRACTION OF ENERGY

| Proteins (amino acids) | Carbohydrates (sugars) | Fats (fatty acids) |

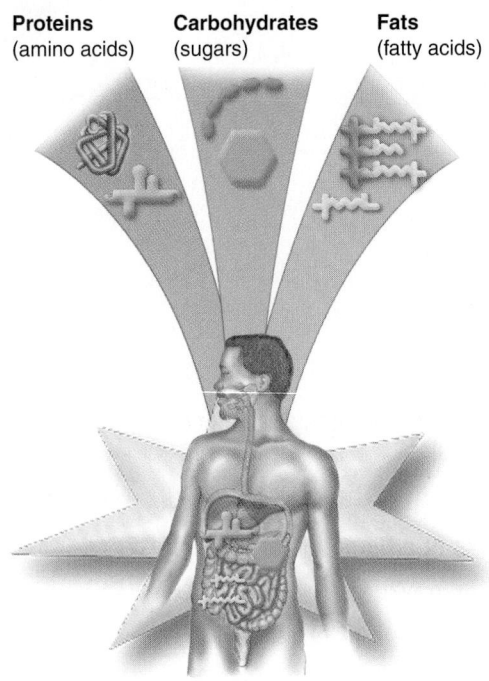

Molecular building blocks

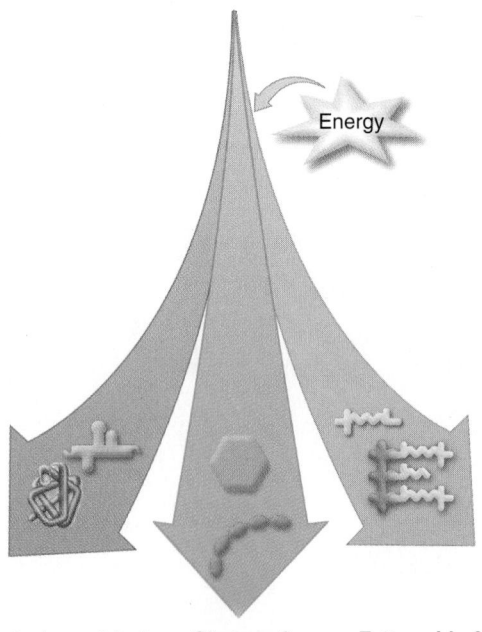

Energy

| Amino acids & body proteins | Glucose & glycogen | Fatty acids & lipids |

BIOSYNTHESIS

Figure 7.1 **Metabolism.** Cells use metabolic reactions to extract energy from food and to form building blocks for biosynthesis.

$\mathcal{Y}$our body is a wonderfully efficient factory. It accepts raw materials (food), burns some to generate power, uses some to produce finished goods, routes the rest to storage, and discards waste and by-products. Constant turnover of your stored inventory keeps it fresh. Your body draws on these stored raw materials to produce compounds, and nutrient intake replenishes the supply.

Do you ever wonder how your biological factory responds to changing supply and demand? Under normal circumstances, it hums along nicely with all processes in balance. When supply exceeds demand, your body stores the excess raw materials in inventory. When supply fails to meet demand, your body draws on these stored materials to meet its needs. Your biological factory never stops; even though a storage or energy-production process may dominate, all your factory operations are active at all times.

Collectively, these processes are known as **metabolism**. (See **Figure 7.1**.) While some metabolic reactions break down molecules to extract energy, others synthesize building blocks to produce new molecules. To carry out metabolic processes, thousands of chemical reactions occur every moment in cells throughout your body. The most active metabolic sites include your liver, muscle, and brain cells.

Energy: Fuel for Work

To operate, machines need energy. Cars use gasoline for fuel, factory machinery uses electricity, and windmills rely on wind power. So what about you? All cells require energy to sustain life. Even during sleep your body uses energy for breathing, pumping blood, maintaining body temperature, delivering oxygen to tissues, removing waste products, synthesizing new tissue for growth, and repairing damaged or worn-out tissues. When awake, you need additional energy for physical movement (such as standing, walking, and talking) and for the digestion and absorption of foods.

Where does the energy come from to power your body's "machinery"? Biological systems use heat, mechanical, electrical, and chemical forms of energy. Our cells get their energy from **chemical energy** held in the molecular bonds of carbohydrates, fats, and protein—the energy macronutrients—as well as alcohol. The chemical energy in foods and beverages originates as light energy from the sun. Green plants use light energy to make carbohydrate in a process called **photosynthesis**. In photosynthesis, carbon dioxide (CO_2) from the air combines with water (H_2O) from the earth to form a carbohydrate, usually glucose ($C_6H_{12}O_6$), and oxygen (O_2). Plants store glucose as starch and release oxygen into the atmosphere. Plants such as corn, peas, squash, turnips, potatoes, and rice store especially high amounts of starch in their edible parts. In the glucose molecule, the chemical bonds between the carbon (C) and hydrogen (H) atoms hold energy from the sun.[1]

Within any system (including the universe), the total amount of energy is constant. Although energy can change from one form to another and can move from one location to another, the system never gains or loses energy. This principle, called the first law of thermodynamics, is known as conservation of energy.

Transferring Food Energy to Cellular Energy

Although burning food releases energy as heat, we cannot use heat to power the many cellular functions that maintain life. Rather than using combustion, we transfer energy from food to a form that our cells can use. (See **Figure 7.2**.) This transfer is not completely efficient; we lose roughly half of the total food energy as heat as our bodies extract energy from food in three stages:[2]

Stage 1: Digestion, absorption, and transportation. Digestion breaks food down into small subunits—simple sugars, fatty acids, monoglycerides, glycerol, and amino acids—that the small intestine can absorb. The circulatory system then transports these nutrients to tissues throughout the body.

Stage 2: Breakdown of many small molecules to a few key metabolites. Inside individual cells, chemical reactions convert simple sugars, fatty acids,

metabolism All chemical reactions within organisms that enable them to maintain life. The two main categories of metabolism are catabolism and anabolism.

chemical energy Energy contained in the bonds between atoms of a molecule.

photosynthesis The process by which green plants use radiant energy from the sun to produce carbohydrates (hexoses) from carbon dioxide and water.

STAGES IN THE EXTRACTION OF ENERGY FROM FOOD

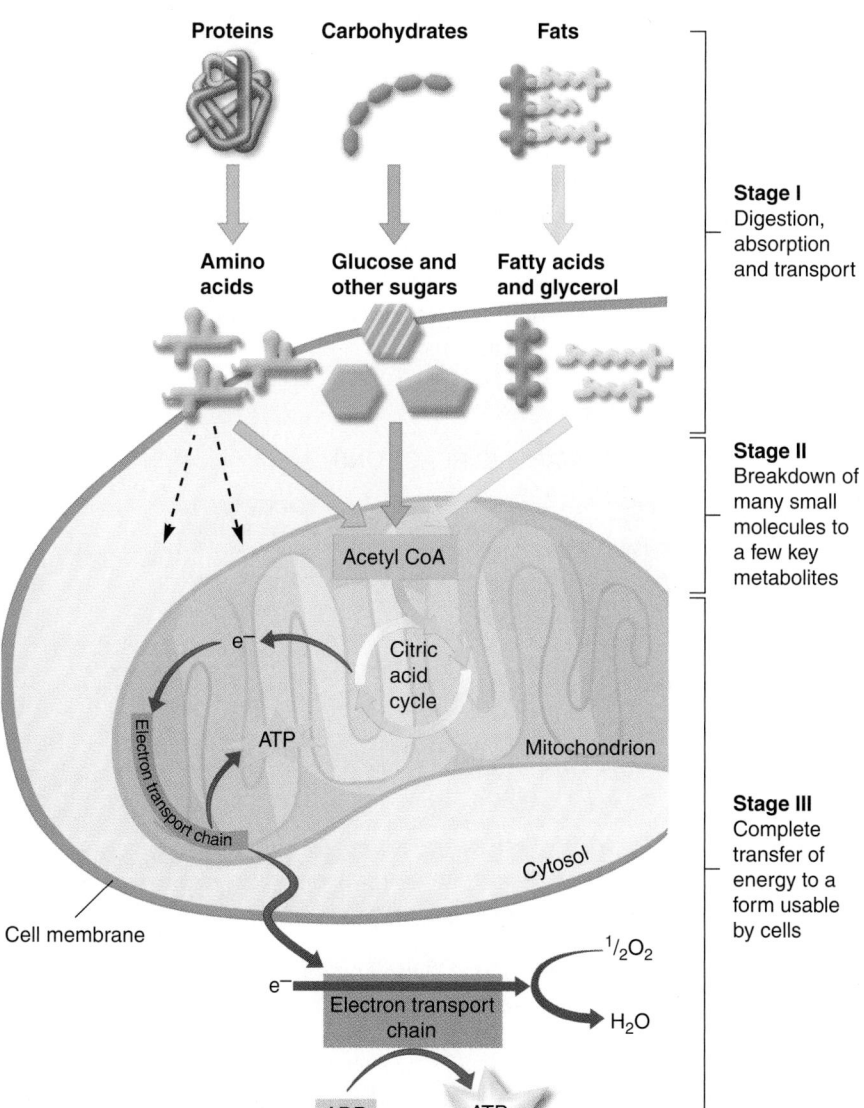

Figure 7.2 **Energy extraction from food.** In the first stage, the body breaks down food into amino acids, monosaccharides, and fatty acids. In the second stage, cells degrade these molecules to a few simple units, such as acetyl CoA, that are pervasive in metabolism. In the third stage, the oxygen-dependent reactions of the citric acid cycle and electron transport chain liberate large amounts of energy in the form of ATP.

metabolites Any substances produced during metabolism.

metabolic pathway A series of chemical reactions that either break down a large compound into smaller units (catabolism) or synthesize more complex molecules from smaller ones (anabolism).

catabolism [ca-TA-bol-iz-um] Any metabolic process whereby cells break down complex substances into simpler, smaller ones.

anabolism [an-A-bol-iz-um] Any metabolic process whereby cells convert simple substances into more complex ones.

cells The basic structural units of all living tissues, which have two major parts—the nucleus and the cytoplasm.

nucleus The primary site of genetic information in the cell, enclosed in a double-layered membrane. The nucleus contains the chromosomes and is the site of messenger RNA (mRNA) and ribosomal RNA (rRNA) synthesis, the "machinery" for protein synthesis in the cytosol.

cytoplasm The material of the cell, excluding the cell nucleus and cell membranes. The cytoplasm includes the semifluid cytosol, the organelles, and other particles.

cytosol The semifluid inside the cell membrane, excluding organelles. The cytosol is the site of glycolysis and fatty acid synthesis.

organelles Various membrane-bound structures that form part of the cytoplasm. Organelles, including mitochondria and lysosomes, perform specialized metabolic functions.

mitochondria (mitochondrion) The sites of aerobic production of ATP, where most of the energy from carbohydrate, protein, and fat is captured. Called the "power plants" of the cell, the mitochondria contain two highly specialized membranes, an outer membrane and a highly folded inner membrane, that separate two compartments, the internal matrix space and the narrow intermembrane space. A human cell contains about 2,000 mitochondria.

glycerol, and amino acids into a few key **metabolites** (products of metabolic reactions). This process liberates a small amount of usable energy.

Stage 3: Transfer of energy to a form that cells can use. The complete breakdown of metabolites to carbon dioxide and water liberates large amounts of energy. The reactions during this stage are responsible for converting more than 90 percent of the available food energy to a form that our bodies can use.

What Is Metabolism?

Metabolism is a general term that encompasses all chemical changes occurring in living organisms. The term **metabolic pathway** describes a series of chemical reactions that either break down a large compound into smaller units (**catabolism**) or build more complex molecules from smaller ones (**anabolism**).[3] For example, when you eat bread or rice, the GI tract breaks down the starch into glucose units. Cells can further catabolize these glucose units to release energy for activities such as muscle contractions. Conversely, anabolic reactions take available glucose molecules and assemble them into glycogen for storage. **Figure 7.3** illustrates catabolism and anabolism.

Metabolic pathways are never completely inactive. Their activity continually ebbs and flows in response to internal and external events. Imagine, for example, that your instructor keeps you late and you have only five minutes to get to your next class. As you hustle across campus, your body ramps up energy production to fuel the demand created by your rapidly contracting muscles. As you sit in your next class, your body continues to break down and extract glucose from the banana you recently ate. Your body assembles the glucose into branched chains to replenish the glycogen stores you depleted while running across campus.

CATABOLIC REACTIONS

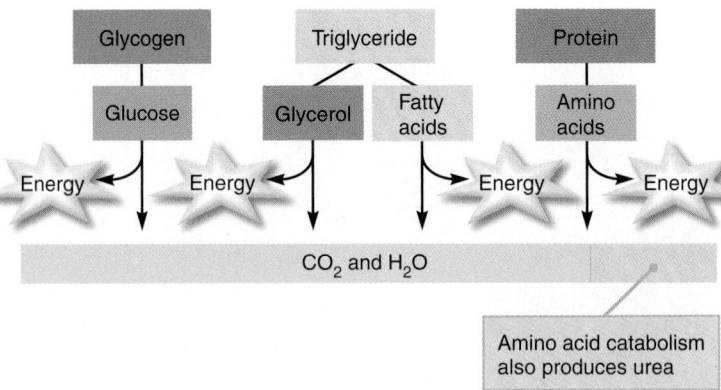

ANABOLIC REACTIONS

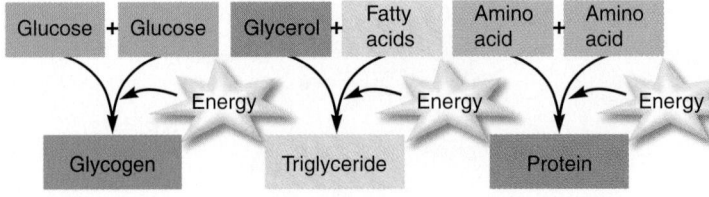

Figure 7.3 **Catabolism and anabolism.** Catabolic reactions break down molecules and release energy and other products. Anabolic reactions consume energy as they assemble complex molecules.

The Cell Is the Metabolic Processing Center

Cells are the "work centers" of metabolism. (See **Figure 7.4**.) Although our bodies are made up of different types of cells (e.g., liver cells, brain cells, kidney cells, muscle cells), most have a similar structure. The basic animal cell has two major parts: the cell **nucleus** and a membrane-enclosed space called the **cytoplasm**. As we zoom in for a closer look, we see that the semi-fluid **cytosol** fills the cytoplasm. Floating in the cytosol are many **organelles**, small units that perform specialized metabolic functions. A large number of these organelles—the capsule-like **mitochondria**—are power generators that contain many important energy-producing pathways.

Figure 7.4 **Cell structure.** Liver cells, brain cells, kidney cells, muscle cells, and so forth, all have a similar structure.

Organelles

Endoplasmic reticulum (ER)
- An extensive membrane system extending from the nuclear membrane.
- Rough ER: The outer membrane surface contains ribosomes, the site of protein synthesis.
- Smooth ER: Devoid of ribosomes, the site of lipid synthesis.

Golgi apparatus
- A system of stacked membrane-encased discs.
- The site of extensive modification, sorting and packaging of compounds for transport.

Lysosome
- Vesicle containing enzymes that digest intracellular materials and recycle the components.

Mitochondrion
- Contains two highly specialized membranes, an outer membrane and a highly folded inner membrane. Membranes separated by narrow intermembrane space. Inner membrane encloses space called mitochondrial matrix.
- Often called the power plant of the cell. Site where most of the energy from carbohydrate, protein, and fat is captured in ATP (adenosine triphosphate).
- About 2,000 mitochondria in a cell.

Ribosome
- Site of protein synthesis.

Nucleus
- Contains genetic information in the base sequences of the DNA strands of the chromosomes.
- Site of RNA synthesis – RNA needed for protein synthesis.
- Enclosed in a double-layered membrane.

Cytoplasm
- Enclosed in the cell membrane and separated from the nucleus by the nuclear membrane.
- Filled with particles and organelles, which are dispersed in a clear semifluid called cytosol.

Cytosol
- The semifluid inside the cell membrane.
- Site of glycolysis and fatty acid synthesis.

Cell membrane
- A double-layered sheet, made up of lipid and protein, that encases the cell.
- Controls the passage of substances in and out of the cell.
- Contains receptors for hormones and other regulatory compounds.

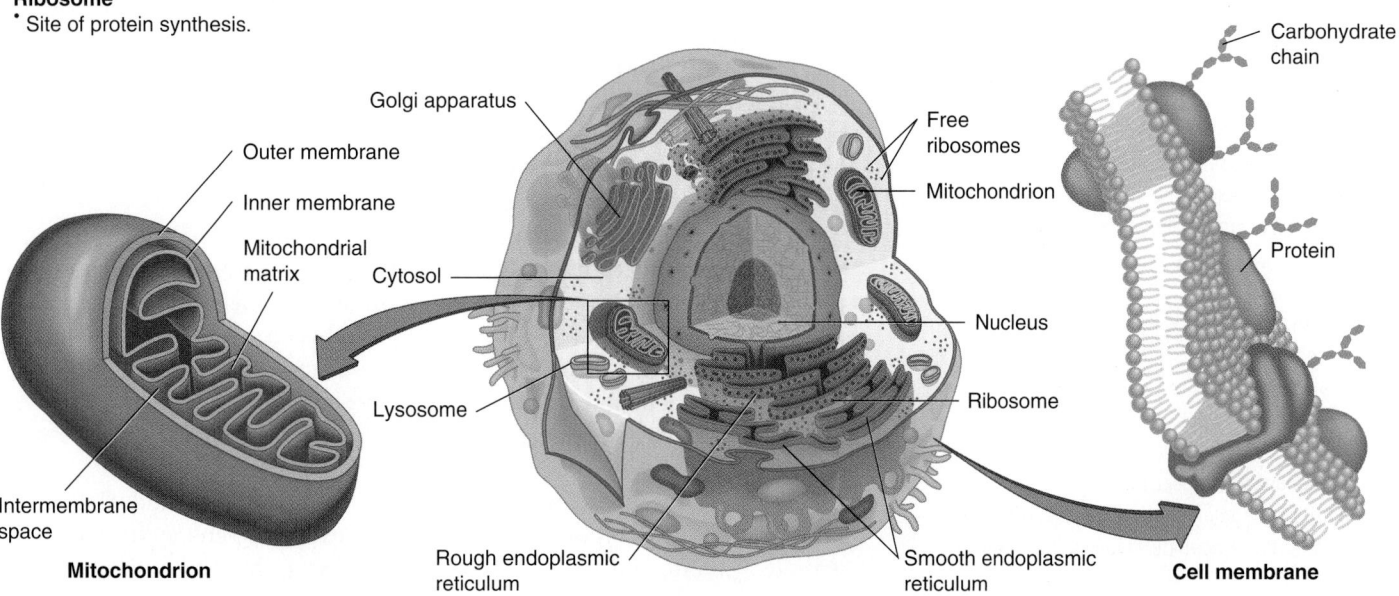

Golgi apparatus

Outer membrane

Inner membrane

Mitochondrial matrix

Cytosol

Lysosome

Free ribosomes

Mitochondrion

Nucleus

Ribosome

Carbohydrate chain

Protein

Intermembrane space

Mitochondrion

Rough endoplasmic reticulum

Smooth endoplasmic reticulum

Cell membrane

cofactors Compounds required for an enzyme to be active. Cofactors include coenzymes and metal ions such as iron (Fe^{2+}), copper (Cu^{2+}), and magnesium (Mg^{2+}).

coenzymes Organic compounds, often B vitamin derivatives, that combine with an inactive enzyme to form an active enzyme. Coenzymes associate closely with these enzymes, allowing them to catalyze certain metabolic reactions in a cell.

adenosine triphosphate (ATP) [ah-DEN-oh-seen try-FOS-fate] A high-energy compound that is the main direct fuel that cells use to synthesize molecules, contract muscles, transport substances, and perform other tasks.

NADH The reduced form of nicotinamide adenine dinucleotide (NAD^+), this coenzyme, derived from the B vitamin niacin, acts as an electron carrier in cells, and undergoes reversible oxidation and reduction.

$FADH_2$ The reduced form of flavin adenine dinucleotide (FAD). This coenzyme, which is derived from the B vitamin riboflavin, acts as an electron carrier in cells and undergoes reversible oxidation and reduction.

NADPH The reduced form of nicotinamide adenine dinucleotide phosphate. This coenzyme, which is derived from the B vitamin niacin, acts as an electron carrier in cells, undergoing reversible oxidation and reduction. The oxidized form is $NADP^+$.

biosynthesis Chemical reactions that form simple molecules into complex biomolecules, especially carbohydrate, lipids, protein, nucleotides, and nucleic acids.

adenosine diphosphate (ADP) The compound produced upon hydrolysis of ATP, and used to synthesize ATP. Composed of adenosine and two phosphate groups.

pyrophosphate Inorganic phosphate. This high-energy phosphate group is an important component of ATP, ADP, and AMP.

Quick Bites

Key Players in the Energy Game

Each of these "key players" in the energy game has a common acronym by which it is usually called:
ATP: adenosine triphosphate
NAD^+: nicotinamide adenine dinucleotide (oxidized)
NADH: nicotinamide adenine dinucleotide (reduced)
$NADP^+$: nicotinamide adenine dinucleotide phosphate (oxidized)
NADPH: nicotinamide adenine dinucleotide phosphate (reduced)
FAD^+: flavin adenine dinucleotide (oxidized)
$FADH_2$: flavin adenine dinucleotide (reduced)

To remember the major parts of a cell, think about a bowl of thick vegetable soup with a single meatball floating in it. For our example, think of the broth as having a runny, jellylike consistency and the bowl as a thin flexible structure with the consistency of a wet paper bag. The bowl surrounds and holds the mixture, similar to the way a cell membrane encloses a cell. The meatball represents the cell nucleus, and the remaining mixture is the cytoplasm. This cytoplasmic soup is made up of a thick, semiliquid fluid (cytosol) and vegetables (organelles). Among the vegetables, think of those kidney beans as mitochondria.

Enzymes, which are catalytic proteins, speed up chemical reactions in metabolic pathways. Many enzymes are inactive unless they are combined with certain smaller molecules called **cofactors**, which usually are derived from a vitamin or mineral. Vitamin-derived cofactors are also called **coenzymes**. All the B vitamins form coenzymes used in metabolic reactions. (For more on coenzymes, see Chapter 10, "Water-Soluble Vitamins.")

Key Concepts: *Metabolism encompasses the many reactions that take place in cells to build tissue, produce energy, break down compounds, and do other cellular work. Anabolism refers to reactions that build compounds, such as protein or glycogen. Catabolism is the breakdown of compounds to yield energy. Mitochondria, the power plants within cells, contain many of the breakdown pathways that produce energy.*

Who Are the Key Energy Players?

Certain compounds have recurring roles in metabolic activities. **Adenosine triphosphate (ATP)** is the fundamental energy molecule used to power cellular functions, so it is known as the universal energy currency. Two other molecules, **NADH** and **$FADH_2$**, are important couriers that carry energy for the synthesis of ATP. A similar energy carrier, **NADPH**, delivers energy for **biosynthesis**.

ATP: The Body's Energy Currency

To power its needs, your body must convert the energy in food to a readily usable form—ATP. This universal energy currency kick-starts many energy-releasing processes, such as the breakdown of glucose and fatty acids, and powers energy-consuming processes, such as building glucose from other compounds. Remember that making large molecules from smaller ones, like constructing a building from bricks, requires energy.

Production of ATP is the fundamental goal of metabolism's energy-producing pathways. Just as the ancient Romans could claim that all roads lead to Rome, you can say that, with a few exceptions, your body's energy-producing pathways lead to ATP production.

The ATP molecule has three phosphate groups attached to adenosine, which is an organic compound. Because breaking the bonds between the phosphate groups releases a tremendous amount of energy, ATP is an energy-rich molecule. (See **Figure 7.5**.) Cells can use this energy to power biological work. When a metabolic reaction breaks the first phosphate bond, it breaks down ATP to **adenosine diphosphate (ADP)** and **pyrophosphate** (P_i). Breaking the remaining phosphate bond releases an equal amount of energy and breaks down ADP to **adenosine monophosphate (AMP)** and P_i.

Because the reaction can proceed in either direction, ATP and ADP are interconvertible, as **Figure 7.6** shows. When extracting energy from carbohydrate, protein, and fat, ADP binds P_i, forming a phosphate bond and capturing energy in a new ATP molecule. When the reaction flows in the opposite direction, ATP releases P_i, breaking a phosphate bond and liberating energy while re-forming ADP. This liberated energy can power biological activities such as motion, active transport across cell membranes, biosynthesis, and signal amplification.

The body's pool of ATP is a small, immediately accessible energy reservoir rather than a long-term energy reserve. The typical lifetime of an ATP molecule is less than one minute, and ATP production increases or decreases in direct relation to energy needs. At rest, you use about 40 kilograms of ATP in 24 hours (an average rate of about 28 grams per minute). In contrast, if you are exercising strenuously, you can use as much as 500 grams per minute! On average, you turn over your body weight in ATP every day.[4]

The molecule **guanosine triphosphate (GTP)** is similar to ATP and holds the same amount of available energy. Like ATP, GTP has high-energy phosphate bonds and three phosphate groups, but they are linked to guanosine rather than to adenosine. Energy-rich GTP molecules are crucial for vision and supply part of the power needed to synthesize protein and glucose. GTP readily converts to ATP.

NADH and FADH$_2$: The Body's Energy Shuttles

When breaking down nutrients, metabolic reactions release high-energy electrons. Further reactions transfer energy from these electrons to ATP. (See **Figure 7.7.**) To reach the site of ATP production, high-energy electrons

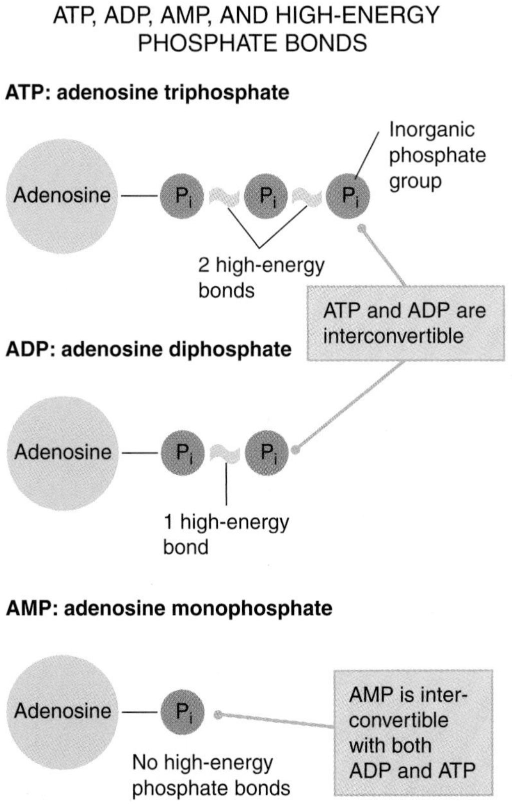

adenosine monophosphate (AMP) Hydrolysis product of ADP and of nucleic acids. Composed of adenosine and one phosphate group.

guanosine triphosphate (GTP) A high-energy compound, similar to ATP, but with three phosphate groups linked to guanosine.

ATP   Adenosine–P~P~P

GTP   Guanosine–P~P~P

ATP, ADP, AMP, AND HIGH-ENERGY PHOSPHATE BONDS

ATP: adenosine triphosphate

Adenosine — P_i ~ P_i ~ P_i

Inorganic phosphate group

2 high-energy bonds

ATP and ADP are interconvertible

ADP: adenosine diphosphate

Adenosine — P_i ~ P_i

1 high-energy bond

AMP: adenosine monophosphate

Adenosine — P_i

No high-energy phosphate bonds

AMP is interconvertible with both ADP and ATP

Figure 7.5 **ATP, ADP, and AMP.** Your body can readily use the energy in high-energy phosphate bonds. During metabolic reactions, phosphate bonds form or break to capture or release energy.

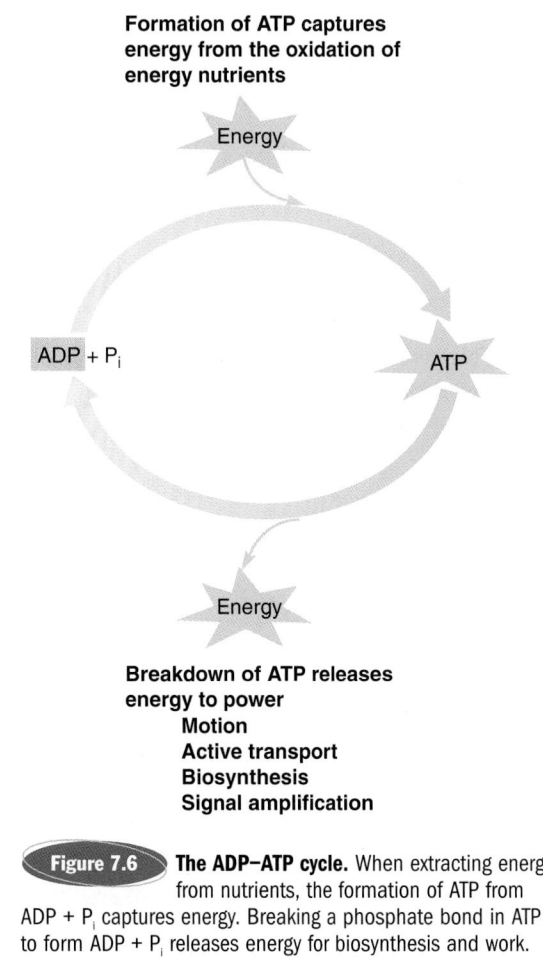

Formation of ATP captures energy from the oxidation of energy nutrients

Energy

ADP + P_i

ATP

Energy

Breakdown of ATP releases energy to power
Motion
Active transport
Biosynthesis
Signal amplification

Figure 7.6 **The ADP–ATP cycle.** When extracting energy from nutrients, the formation of ATP from ADP + P_i captures energy. Breaking a phosphate bond in ATP to form ADP + P_i releases energy for biosynthesis and work.

$$NAD^+ + 2H^+ \leftrightarrow NADH + H^+$$
NADH carries two high-energy electrons

$$FAD + 2H^+ \leftrightarrow FADH_2$$
$FADH_2$ carries two high-energy electrons

$$NADPH + H^+ \leftrightarrow NADP^+ + 2H^+$$
**NADPH releases energy for biosynthesis
when converted to $NADP^+$**

hitch a ride on special molecular carriers. One major electron acceptor is **nicotinamide adenine dinucleotide (NAD^+)**, a derivative of the B vitamin niacin. The metabolic pathways have several energy-transfer points where an NAD^+ accepts two high-energy electrons and two **hydrogen ions** (two protons [$2H^+$]) to form $NADH + H^+$. For simplicity, the "$+ H^+$" is often dropped when talking about NADH.

The other major electron acceptor is **flavin adenine dinucleotide (FAD)**, a derivative of the B vitamin riboflavin. When FAD accepts two high-energy electrons, it picks up two protons ($2H^+$) and forms $FADH_2$.

NADPH: An Energy Shuttle for Biosynthesis

Energy powers the assembly of building blocks into complex molecules of carbohydrate, fat, and protein. NADPH, an energy-carrying molecule similar to NADH, delivers much of the energy these biosynthetic reactions require. The only structural difference between NADPH and NADH is the presence or absence of a phosphate group. Although both molecules are energy carriers, their metabolic roles are vastly different. Whereas the energy carried by NADH primarily produces ATP, nearly all the energy carried by NADPH drives biosynthesis. When a reaction transforms NADPH into $NADP^+$ (nicotinamide adenine dinucleotide phosphate), NADPH releases its cargo of two energetic electrons.

Key Concepts: *ATP is the energy currency of the body. Your body extracts energy from food to produce ATP. NADH and $FADH_2$ are hydrogen and electron carriers that shuttle energy to ATP production sites. NADPH is also a hydrogen and electron carrier, but it shuttles energy for anabolic processes.*

nicotinamide adenine dinucleotide (NAD^+) The oxidized form of nicotinamide adenine dinucleotide. This coenzyme, which is derived from the B vitamin niacin, acts as an electron carrier in cells, undergoing reversible oxidation and reduction. The reduced form is NADH.

hydrogen ions Also called a proton. This lone hydrogen has a positive charge (H^+). It does not have its own electron, but it can share one with another atom.

flavin adenine dinucleotide (FAD) A coenzyme synthesized in the body from riboflavin. It undergoes reversible oxidation and reduction and thus acts as an electron carrier in cells. FAD is the oxidized form; $FADH_2$ is the reduced form.

ENERGY TRANSFER

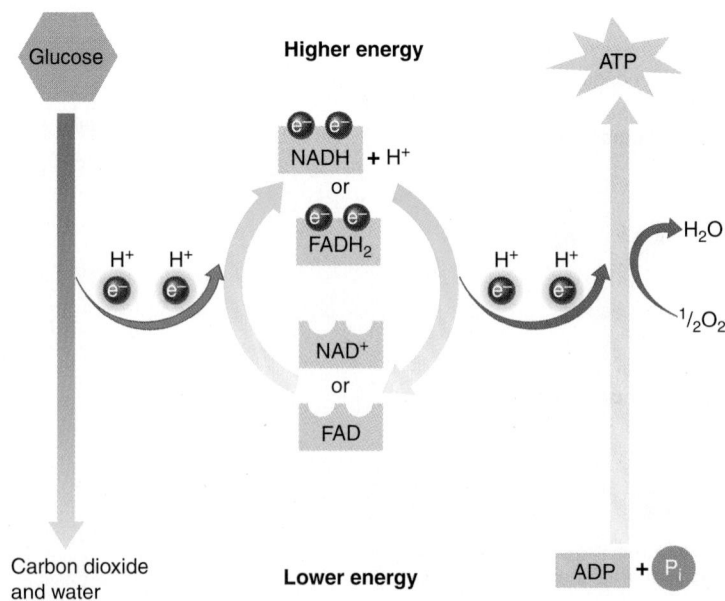

Figure 7.7 **Energy transfer.** As energy moves from glucose to ATP, molecules become high-energy or low-energy as they collect and transfer high-energy electrons and hydrogen ions (protons).

Breakdown and Release of Energy

The complete catabolism of carbohydrate, protein, and fat for energy occurs via several pathways. Although different pathways initiate the breakdown of these nutrients, complete breakdown eventually proceeds along two shared catabolic pathways—the citric acid cycle and the electron transport chain. This section first describes the pathways that catabolize glucose. It then discusses the steps that start the breakdown of fat and protein.

Extracting Energy from Carbohydrate

Cells extract usable energy from carbohydrate via four main pathways: glycolysis, conversion of pyruvate to acetyl CoA, the citric acid cycle, and the electron transport chain. (See **Figure 7.8.**) Although glycolysis and the citric acid cycle produce small amounts of energy, the electron transport chain is the major ATP production site.

Glycolysis

Glycolysis ("glucose splitting") is an **anaerobic** process; that is, it does not require oxygen. In the cytosol, this sequence of reactions splits each six-carbon glucose molecule into *two* three-carbon **pyruvate** molecules while producing a relatively small amount of energy.

Just as a pump requires priming, glycolysis requires the input of two ATP molecules to get started. In the later stages, various reactions produce energy-rich molecules of NADH and release four ATP molecules. Although glycolysis both consumes and releases energy, it produces more than it uses. Glycolysis is rapid, but it produces a comparatively small amount of ATP. The glycolysis of one glucose molecule yields a net of two NADH and two ATP, along with the two pyruvates. (See **Figure 7.9.**)

Although most glycolytic reactions can flow in either direction, some are irreversible, one-way reactions. These one-way reactions prevent glycolysis from running backward.

What about the other simple sugars, fructose and galactose? In liver cells, glycolysis usually breaks them down, and normally they are not available to other tissues.[5] Although fructose and galactose enter glycolysis at intermediate points, the end result is the same as for glucose. One molecule of glucose, fructose, or galactose produces two NADH, a net of two ATP, and two pyruvates. Once glycolysis is complete, the pyruvate molecules easily pass from the cytosol to the interior of mitochondria, the cell's power generators, for further processing.

Conversion of Pyruvate to Acetyl CoA

When a cell requires energy, and oxygen is readily available, **aerobic** reactions in the mitochondria convert each pyruvate molecule to an **acetyl CoA** molecule. These reactions produce CO_2 and transfer a pair of high-energy electrons to form NADH. (See **Figure 7.10.**) The NADH shuttle carries the electrons to the electron transport chain.

Although many metabolic pathways can proceed either forward or backward, the formation of acetyl CoA is a one-way (irreversible) process. To form acetyl CoA, reactions remove one carbon from the three-carbon pyruvate and add **coenzyme A**, a molecule derived from the B vitamin pantothenic acid. After combining with oxygen, the carbon is released as part

glycolysis [gligh-COLL-ih-sis] The anaerobic metabolic pathway that breaks a glucose molecule into two molecules of pyruvate and yields two molecules of ATP and two molecules of NADH. Glycolysis occurs in the cytosol of a cell.

anaerobic [AN-ah-ROW-bic] Referring to the absence of oxygen or the ability of a process to occur in the absence of oxygen.

pyruvate The three-carbon compound that results from glycolytic breakdown of glucose. Pyruvate, the salt form of pyruvic acid, also can be derived from glycerol and some amino acids.

aerobic [air-ROW-bic] Referring to the presence of or need for oxygen. The complete breakdown of glucose, fatty acids, and amino acids to carbon dioxide and water occurs only via aerobic metabolism. The citric acid cycle and electron transport chain are aerobic pathways.

acetyl CoA A key intermediate in the metabolic breakdown of carbohydrates, fatty acids, and amino acids. It consists of a two-carbon acetate group linked to coenzyme A, which is derived from pantothenic acid.

coenzyme A Coenzyme A is a cofactor derived from the vitamin pantothenic acid.

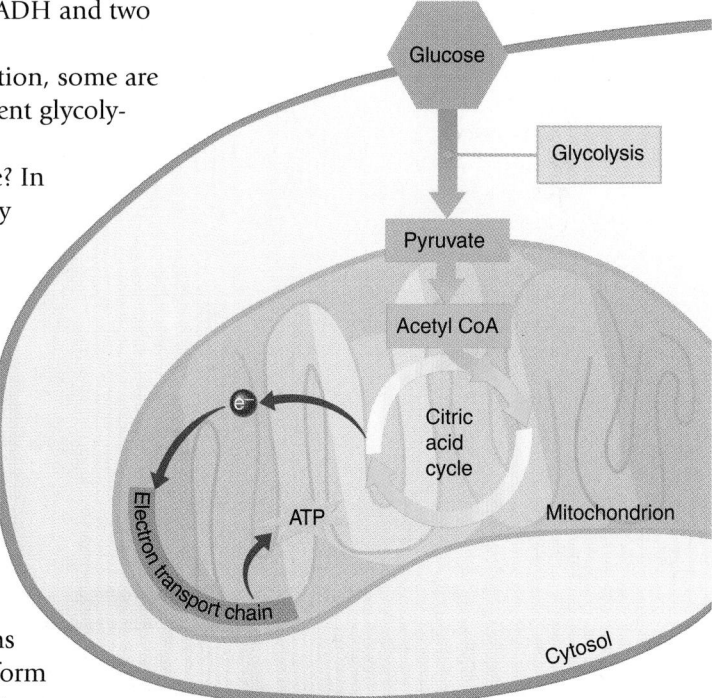

Figure 7.8 **Obtaining energy from carbohydrate.** The complete oxidation of glucose uses four major metabolic pathways: glycolysis, conversion of pyruvate to acetyl CoA, the citric acid cycle, and the electron transport chain. Glycolysis takes place in the cytosol. The remaining reactions take place in the mitochondria.

Quick Bites

When Glycolysis Goes Awry

Red blood cells do not have mitochondria, so they rely on glycolysis as their only source of ATP. They use ATP to maintain the integrity and shape of their cell membranes. A defect in red blood cell glycolysis can cause a shortage of ATP, which leads to deformed red blood cells. Destruction of these cells by the spleen leads to a type of anemia called hemolytic anemia.

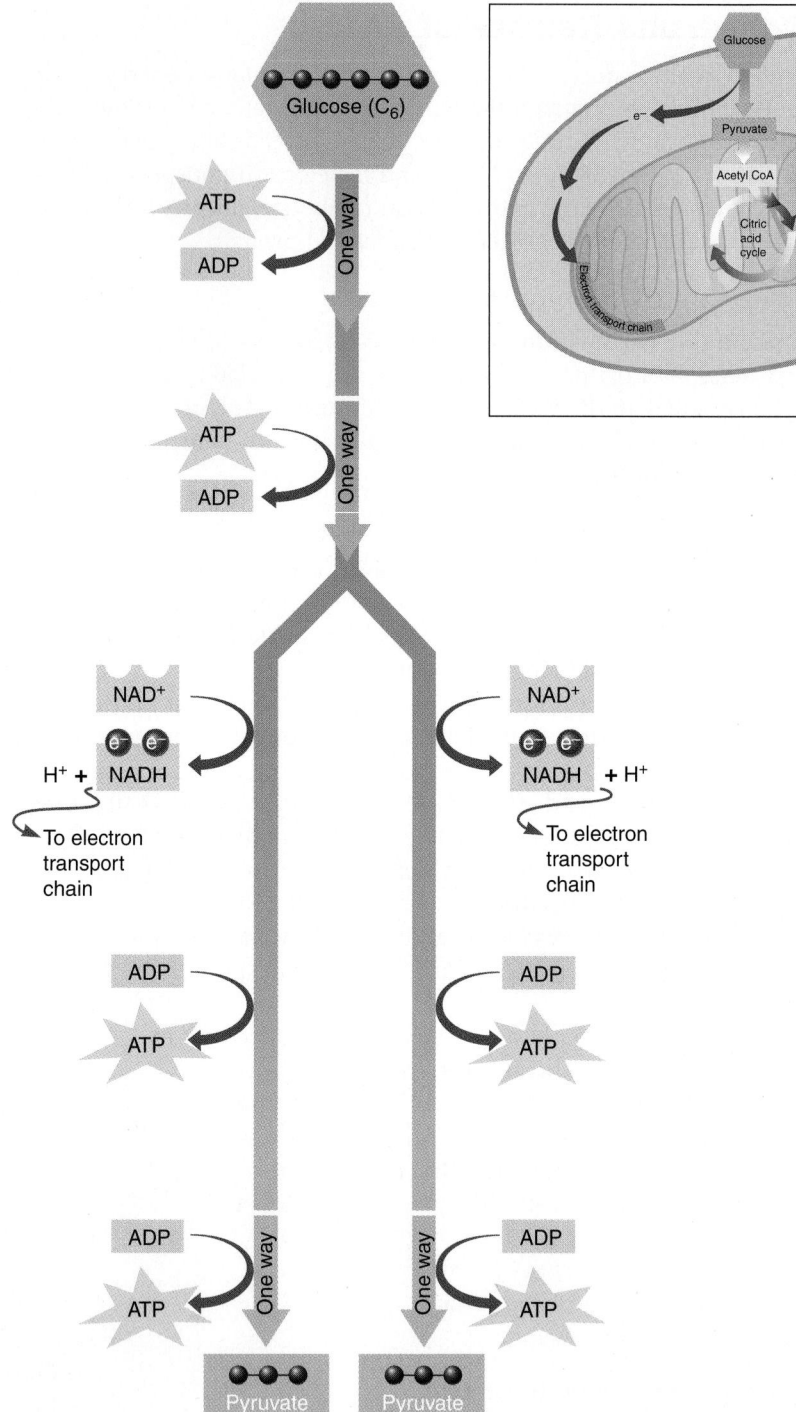

Figure 7.9 **Glycolysis.** The breakdown of one glucose molecule yields two pyruvate molecules, a net of two ATP and two NADH molecules. The two NADH molecules shuttle pairs of high-energy electrons to the electron transport chain for ATP production. Glycolytic reactions do not require oxygen, and some steps are irreversible.

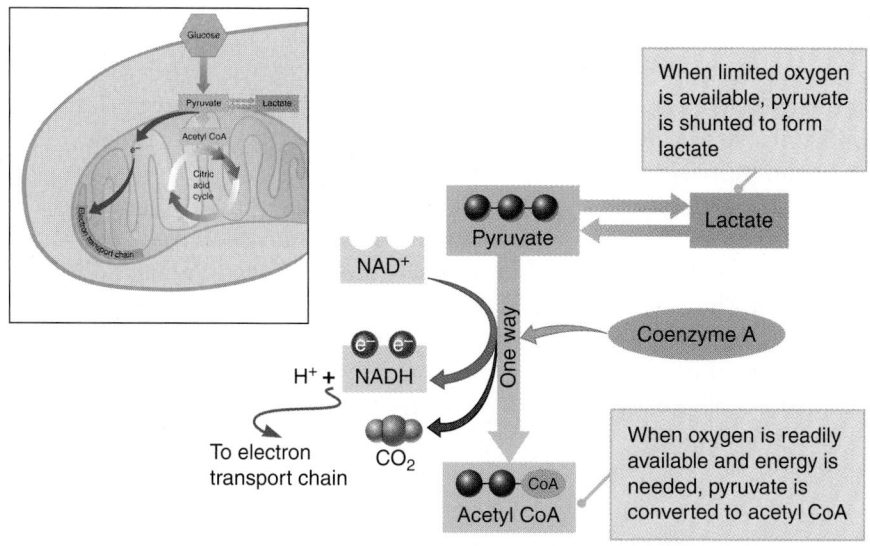

lactate The ionized form of lactic acid, a three-carbon acid. It is produced when insufficient oxygen is present in cells to oxidize pyruvate.

citric acid cycle The metabolic pathway occurring in mitochondria in which the acetyl portion (CH_3COO-) of acetyl CoA is oxidized to yield two molecules of carbon dioxide and one molecule each of NADH, $FADH_2$, and GTP. Also known as the Krebs cycle and the tricarboxylic acid cycle.

oxaloacetate A four-carbon intermediate compound in the citric acid cycle. Acetyl CoA combines with free oxaloacetate in the mitochondria, forming citrate and beginning the cycle.

> **Figure 7.10** **Conversion of pyruvate to acetyl CoA.** When oxygen is readily available, each pyruvate formed from glucose yields one acetyl CoA, one CO_2, and one NADH. The NADH shuttles high-energy electrons to the electron transport chain for ATP production.

of carbon dioxide. Recall that glycolysis splits glucose into two pyruvate molecules, so we now have two NADH and two acetyl CoA molecules.

In rapidly contracting muscle, oxygen is in short supply, and pyruvate cannot form acetyl CoA. Instead, pyruvate is rerouted to form **lactate**, another three-carbon compound. Lactate is an alternative fuel that muscle cells can use or that liver cells can convert to glucose. When oxygen again becomes readily available, lactate is converted back to pyruvate, which irreversibly forms acetyl CoA. You will learn more about lactate production, cycling, and use in Chapter 13, "Sports Nutrition."

Although pyruvate passes easily between the cytosol and the mitochondria, the mitochondrial membrane is impervious to acetyl CoA. The acetyl CoA produced from pyruvate is trapped inside the mitochondria, ready to enter the citric acid cycle.

Citric Acid Cycle

The **citric acid cycle** is an elegant set of reactions that proceed along a circular pathway in the mitochondria. To begin the cycle, acetyl CoA combines with **oxaloacetate**, freeing coenzyme A and yielding a six-carbon compound called citrate (citric acid). The coenzyme A leaves the cycle, becoming available to react with another pyruvate and form a new acetyl CoA. Subsequent reactions in the citric acid cycle transform citrate into a sequence of intermediate compounds as they remove two carbons and release them in two molecules of CO_2. Because acetyl CoA adds two carbons to the cycle and the cycle releases two carbons as CO_2, there is no net gain or loss of carbon atoms. The final step in the citric acid cycle regenerates oxaloacetate.

The citric acid cycle extracts most of the energy that ultimately powers the generation of ATP. For each acetyl CoA entering the cycle, one complete "turn" produces one GTP and transfers pairs of high-energy electrons to three NADH and one $FADH_2$. Because the breakdown of one glucose molecule yields two molecules of acetyl CoA, the citric acid cycle "turns" twice for each glucose molecule and produces twice these amounts (i.e., six NADH, two $FADH_2$, and two GTP).

The citric acid cycle goes by many names. It often is called the **Krebs cycle** after Sir Hans Krebs, the first scientist to explain its operation, who was awarded the Nobel Prize in 1953 for his work. It also is called the **tricarboxylic acid (TCA) cycle** because a tricarboxylic acid (citrate) is formed in the first step. Most nutritionists use the term *citric acid cycle.* **Figure 7.11** shows an overview of the citric acid cycle.

The citric acid cycle is also an important source of building blocks for the biosynthesis of amino acids and fatty acids. Rather than using the cycle's intermediate molecules to complete the cycle, the cell may siphon them off for biosynthesis. Cells may use oxaloacetate, for example, to make glucose or certain amino acids. If alternate uses deplete the supply of oxaloacetate, the citric acid cycle can slow or even stop. Fortunately, cells can make oxaloacetate directly from pyruvate, easily replenishing the citric acid cycle's supply.

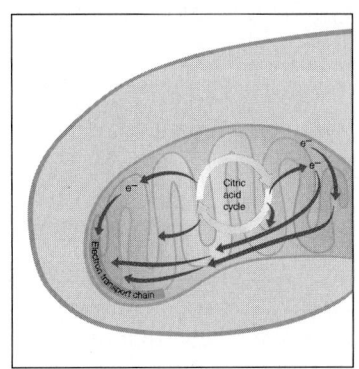

Figure 7.11 **The citric acid cycle.** This circular pathway accepts one acetyl CoA and yields two CO_2, three NADH, one $FADH_2$ and one GTP (readily converted to ATP). The electron shuttles NADH and $FADH_2$ carry high-energy electrons to the electron transport chain for ATP production.

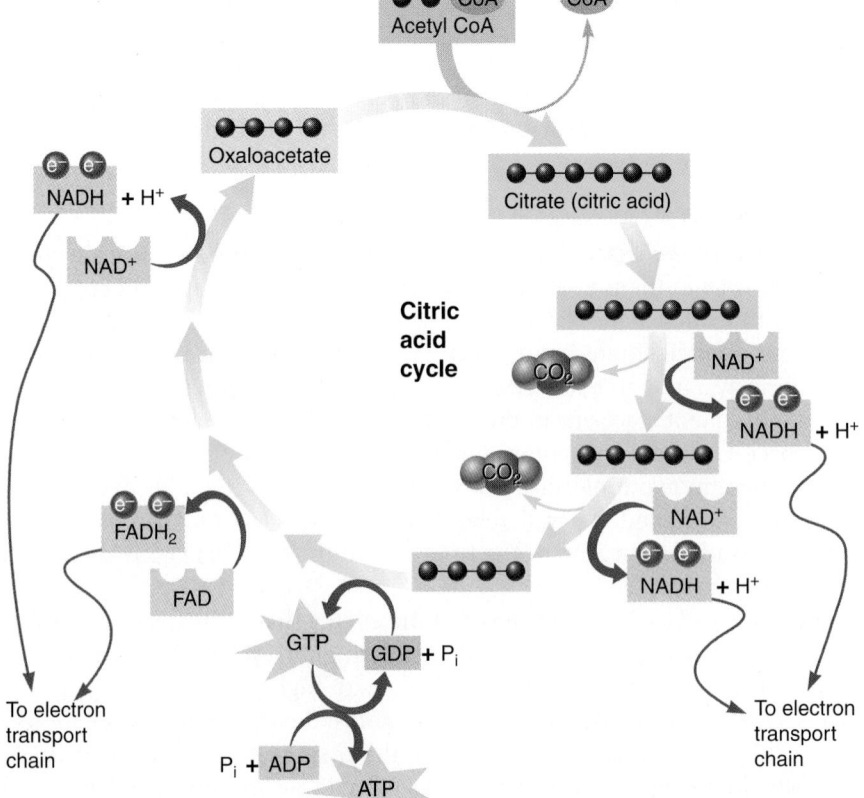

Electron Transport Chain

The final step in glucose breakdown is a sequence of linked reactions that take place in the **electron transport chain**, which is located in the inner **mitochondrial membrane**. Most ATP is produced here, and as long as oxygen is available, it can dispense ATP and maintain exercise for hours. Because the mitochondrion is the site of both the citric acid cycle and the electron transport chain, it truly is the energy power plant of the cell.

NADH and $FADH_2$ now deliver their cargo of high-energy electrons. NADH produced in the mitochondria by the citric acid cycle delivers its pair of high-energy electrons to the beginning of the chain. In the inner mitochondrial membrane, these electrons are passed along a chain of linked reactions, giving up energy along the way to power the final production of ATP. At the end of the electron transport chain, oxygen accepts the energy-depleted electrons and reacts with hydrogen to form water. This formation of ATP coupled to the flow of electrons along the electron transport chain is called **oxidative phosphorylation** because it requires oxygen, and it phosphorylates ADP (joins it to P_i) to form ATP. (See **Figure 7.12**.)

Without an oxygen "basket" at the end to accept the energy-depleted electrons, the transport of electrons down the chain would halt, stopping ATP production. Without ATP, there would be no power for our body's essential functions. If our oxygen supply was not rapidly restored, we would die.

What about $FADH_2$? The high-energy electrons from $FADH_2$ enter the electron transport chain at a later point than the electrons from NADH. Because they travel through fewer reactions, the electrons from $FADH_2$ generate fewer ATP molecules.

Biochemists have revised their estimates of the amount of ATP produced by the electron transport chain. Scientists had estimated that electron pairs from NADH produced 3 ATP and those from $FADH_2$ produced 2 ATP. Experiments have shown, however, that the actual amounts are slightly smaller—2.5 ATP from NADH and 1.5 ATP from $FADH_2$. Because each pair of electrons that traverses the electron transport chain produces slightly fewer ATP molecules than once thought, biochemists have revised their estimates for the total amount of ATP produced from one glucose molecule. Historically, they believed that the complete breakdown of glucose produced 36 to 38 ATP, but the current estimate is 30 to 32 ATP.[6]

electron transport chain An organized series of carrier molecules—including flavin mononucleotide (FMN), coenzyme Q, and several cytochromes—that are located in mitochondrial membranes and shuttle electrons from NADH and $FADH_2$ to oxygen, yielding water and ATP.

mitochondrial membrane The mitochondria are enclosed by a double shell separated by an intermembrane space. The outer membrane acts as a barrier and gatekeeper, selectively allowing some molecules to pass through while blocking others. The inner membrane is where the electron transport chains are located.

oxidative phosphorylation Formation of ATP from ADP and P_i coupled to the flow of electrons along the electron transport chain.

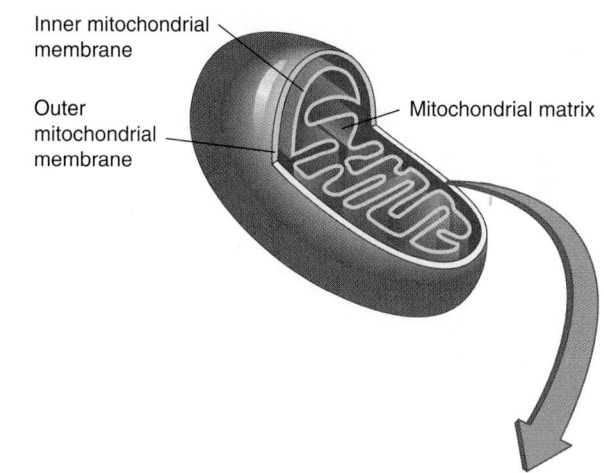

Figure 7.12 **Electron transport chain.** This pathway produces most of the ATP available from glucose. NADH molecules deliver pairs of high-energy electrons to the beginning of the chain. The pairs of high-energy electrons carried by $FADH_2$ enter this pathway farther along and produce fewer ATP than electron pairs carried by NADH. Water is the final product of the electron transport chain.

What about the electron pairs carried by NADH from glycolysis? Recall that glycolysis takes place in the cytosol, whereas the citric acid cycle and electron transport chain are located in the mitochondria. NADH in the cytosol cannot penetrate the outer mitochondrial membrane. Instead, cytosolic NADH transfers its high-energy electrons to special molecules that shuttle them across the outer mitochondrial membrane. Once inside the mitochondrion, the electron pair may be picked up by the formation of either NADH or $FADH_2$. Depending on which shuttle is formed, an electron pair from glycolytic NADH generates either 2.5 or 1.5 ATP. Because of this difference, the complete oxidation of a glucose molecule does not always produce the same amount of ATP. (See **Figure 7.13**.)

End Products of Glucose Catabolism

Now you've seen all the steps in glucose breakdown. What has the cell produced from glucose? The end products of complete catabolism are carbon dioxide (CO_2), water (H_2O), and ATP. Both the conversion of pyruvate to acetyl CoA and the citric acid cycle produce CO_2. The electron transport chain produces water. While glycolysis makes small amounts of ATP and the citric acid cycle makes a little ATP as GTP, the electron transport chain generates the vast majority of this universal energy currency. **Table 7.1** summarizes the pathways of glucose metabolism.

Key Concepts: *The metabolism of glucose to yield energy occurs in several steps. Glycolysis breaks the six-carbon glucose molecule into two pyruvate molecules. Each pyruvate loses a carbon and combines with coenzyme A to form acetyl CoA, which then enters the citric acid cycle. Two carbons enter the cycle as part of acetyl*

Quick Bites

The Latest ATP Count

The number of ATP (or GTP) molecules formed directly in glycolysis and the citric acid cycle is unequivocally known, but the number of ATP molecules formed from NADH and $FADH_2$ in the electron transport chain is less certain. Old estimates credited NADH from the citric acid cycle with 3 ATP and $FADH_2$ with 2 ATP. The best current estimates are 2.5 and 1.5, respectively. "Hence, about 30 ATP are formed when glucose is completely oxidized to CO_2; this value supersedes the traditional estimate of 36 ATP." *—Lubert Stryer, Professor of Biochemistry, Stanford University*

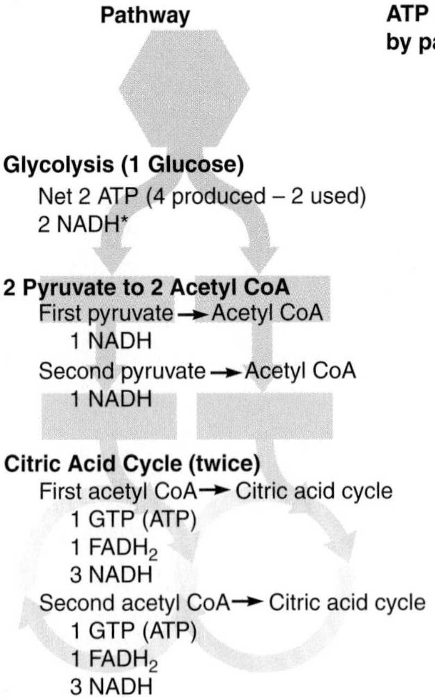

COMPLETE OXIDATION OF GLUCOSE

Pathway	ATP formed by pathway	ATP formed in electron transport chain
Glycolysis (1 Glucose)		
Net 2 ATP (4 produced – 2 used)	2	
2 NADH*		3 to 5
2 Pyruvate to 2 Acetyl CoA		
First pyruvate → Acetyl CoA		
1 NADH		2.5
Second pyruvate → Acetyl CoA		
1 NADH		2.5
Citric Acid Cycle (twice)		
First acetyl CoA → Citric acid cycle		
1 GTP (ATP)	1	
1 $FADH_2$		1.5
3 NADH		7.5
Second acetyl CoA → Citric acid cycle		
1 GTP (ATP)	1	
1 $FADH_2$		1.5
3 NADH		7.5
Subtotal	4	26 to 28
	Total = 30 to 32	

*Each NADH formed in the cytosol by glycolysis will produce either 2.5 or 1.5 ATP in the electron transport chain.

Figure 7.13 **Complete oxidation of glucose.** These metabolic pathways and molecules move energy from glucose to ATP. Complete oxidation of one glucose molecule yields 30 to 32 ATP.

CoA, and two carbons leave as part of two carbon dioxide molecules. Because two acetyl CoA molecules are formed from a single glucose molecule, the citric acid cycle operates twice. Finally, the NADH and FADH₂ formed in these pathways carry pairs of high-energy electrons to the electron transport chain, where ATP and water are produced. When completely oxidized, each glucose molecule yields carbon dioxide, water, and ATP.

Extracting Energy from Fat

To extract energy from fat, the body first breaks down triglycerides into their component parts, glycerol and fatty acids. Glycerol, a small three-carbon molecule, carries a relatively small amount of energy and can be converted by the liver to pyruvate or glucose. Fatty acids store nearly all the energy found in triglycerides.

The breakdown of fatty acids takes place inside the mitochondria. Before a fatty acid can cross into a mitochondrion, it must be linked to coenzyme A, which activates the fatty acid. Just as the input of ATP launched glycolysis, the input of ATP powers fatty acid activation. The breakdown of one ATP molecule to one AMP and two P_i provides the energy to drive this reaction. Although this activation reaction requires only one molecule of ATP, it breaks both of ATP's high-energy phosphate bonds and consumes the energetic equivalent of two ATP molecules (double the amount of energy released from the reaction ATP → ADP + P_i).

Carnitine Shuttle

Without assistance, the activated fatty acid cannot get inside the mitochondria where fatty acid oxidation and the citric acid cycle operate. This entry problem is solved by **carnitine**, a compound formed from the amino acid lysine. Carnitine has the unique task of ferrying activated fatty acids across the mitochondrial membrane, from the cytosol to the interior of the mitochondrion. When carnitine is in short supply, the production of ATP slows. Moderate carnitine deficiency in heart or skeletal muscle reduces muscle endurance; more extreme deficiency causes muscular strength to fail more quickly.[7] Based on its role in fatty acid oxidation, some people claim that

carnitine [CAR-nih-teen] A compound that transports fatty acids from the cytosol into the mitochondria, where they undergo beta-oxidation.

Table 7.1 **Summary of the Major Metabolic Pathways in Glucose Metabolism**

Pathways	Location	Type	Summary	Starting Materials	End Products
Glycolysis	Cytosol	Anaerobic	A series of reactions that convert one glucose molecule to two pyruvate molecules.	Glucose, ATP	Pyruvate, ATP, NADH
Pyruvate to acetyl CoA	Mitochondria	Aerobic	Pyruvate from glycolysis combines with coenzyme A to form acetyl CoA while releasing carbon dioxide.	Pyruvate, coenzyme A	Acetyl CoA, carbon dioxide, NADH
Citric acid cycle	Mitochondria	Aerobic	This cycle of reactions degrades the acetyl portion of acetyl CoA and releases the coenzyme A portion. This cycle releases carbon dioxide and produces most of the energy-rich molecules, NADH and FADH₂, generated by the breakdown of glucose.	Acetyl CoA	Carbon dioxide, NADH, FADH₂, GTP
Electron transport chain	Mitochondria (membrane)	Aerobic	As the electrons from NADH and FADH₂ pass along this chain of transport proteins, they release energy to power the generation of ATP. Oxygen is the final electron acceptor and combines with hydrogen to form water.	NADH, FADH₂	ATP, water

beta-oxidation The breakdown of a fatty acid into numerous molecules of the two-carbon compound acetyl coenzyme A (acetyl CoA).

carnitine supplements act as "fat burners." Research data show that carnitine supplementation in healthy people has little or no effect on fatty acid oxidation rates or athletic performance.[8]

Beta-Oxidation

Once in the mitochondria, a process called **beta-oxidation** disassembles the fatty acid and converts it into several molecules of acetyl CoA. (See **Figure 7.14**.) Starting at the beta carbon of the fatty acid (the second carbon from the acid end), enzymes clip a two-carbon "link" off the end of the chain. Reactions convert this two-carbon link to one acetyl CoA, while also transferring one pair of electrons to $FADH_2$ and another pair to NADH. This process repeats, in stepwise fashion, shortening the chain by two carbons at a time until only one two-carbon segment remains. This final two-carbon link simply becomes one acetyl CoA without producing $FADH_2$ and NADH.

In nature, almost all fatty acids have an even number of carbons. Although they can vary in length from 4 to 26 carbons, they often are 16 or 18 carbons long. If your body encounters an odd-numbered fatty acid, it breaks down this chain in the same way until it reaches a final three-carbon link. Rather than try to clip this link into smaller segments, a reaction joins it with coenzyme A. This three-carbon compound enters the citric acid cycle at a point farther along than acetyl CoA's entry point. Because it skips some of the early citric acid cycle reactions, it has a shorter journey than acetyl CoA and produces two fewer NADH molecules.

The Citric Acid Cycle and Electron Transport Chain Complete Fatty Acid Breakdown

Beta-oxidation of a fatty acid produces a flood of acetyl CoA that can enter the citric acid cycle. The citric acid cycle and electron transport chain complete the extraction of energy from fatty acids. Just as they processed acetyl CoA, NADH, and $FADH_2$ from glucose, these same pathways use acetyl CoA, NADH, and $FADH_2$ from fatty acids to produce ATP.

The end products of fatty acid breakdown are the same as those of glucose breakdown: carbon dioxide, water, and ATP. The exact amount of ATP depends on the length of the fatty acid chain. Because longer chains have more carbon bonds, beta-oxidation of longer chains produces more acetyl CoA and thus more ATP. The complete breakdown of an 18-carbon fatty acid, for example, produces 120 ATP (see **Figure 7.15**), whereas a 10-carbon fatty acid produces only 66 ATP. Because a fatty acid chain typically contains many more carbon atoms than a molecule of glucose, a single fatty acid produces substantially more ATP. For a single triglyceride with three 18-carbon fatty acids, complete breakdown of the fatty acids produces 360 ATP, more than 10 times the 30 to 32 ATP produced from the complete oxidation of glucose.

Fat Burns in a Flame of Carbohydrate

Acetyl CoA from beta-oxidation can enter the citric acid cycle only when fat and carbohydrate breakdown are synchronized. Without available oxaloacetate, acetyl CoA cannot start the citric acid cycle. Conditions such as starvation and consumption of high-fat, low-carbohydrate diets can deplete oxaloacetate, blocking acetyl CoA from entry. This reroutes the acetyl CoA to form a family of compounds called ketone bodies. (See the section "Making Ketone Bodies" later in this chapter.) Production of ketone bodies can occur with popular high-protein diets that are low in carbohydrate but also high in fat.

Pathway	ATP yield
Beta-oxidation – stearic acid (C18:0)	
8 NADH	20
8 FADH$_2$	12
Citric acid cycle – 9 acetyl CoA	
1 GTP x 9 = 9 GTP	9
3 NADH x 9 = 27 NADH	67.5
1 FADH$_2$ x 9 = 9 FADH$_2$	13.5
Subtotal	122
ATP needed to start beta-oxidation	−2
Net yield	**120**

The grand total:
120 ATP from one molecule of stearic acid

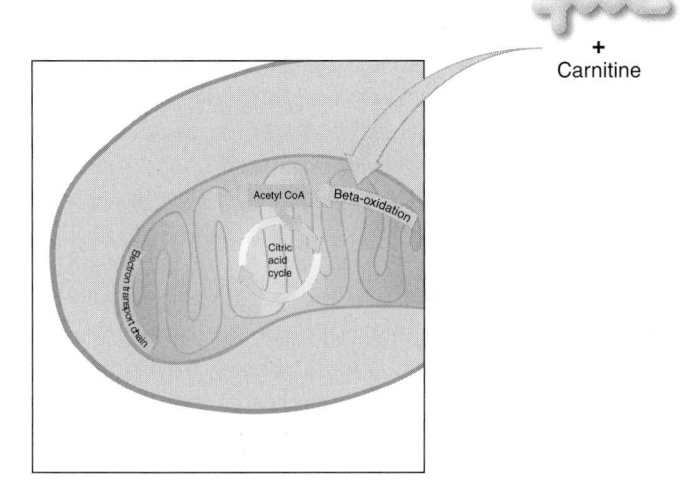

Figure 7.15 **The complete breakdown of stearic acid.** The complete oxidation of one 18-carbon fatty acid yields about four times as much ATP as the complete oxidation of one glucose molecule.

BETA-OXIDATION

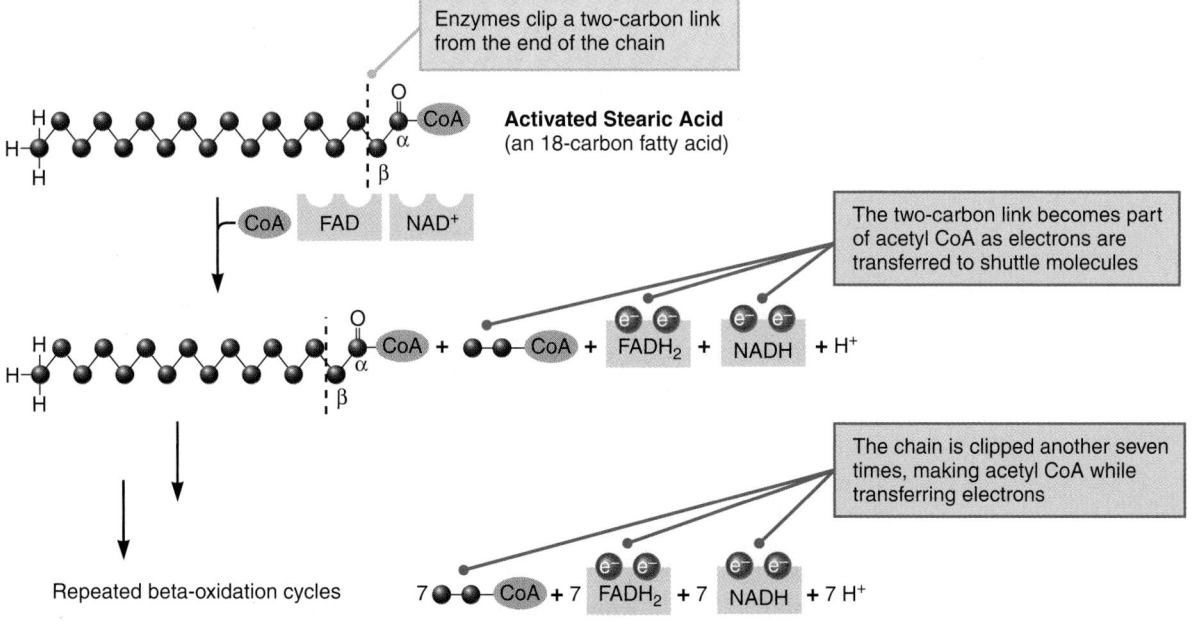

Enzymes clip a two-carbon link from the end of the chain

Activated Stearic Acid
(an 18-carbon fatty acid)

The two-carbon link becomes part of acetyl CoA as electrons are transferred to shuttle molecules

The chain is clipped another seven times, making acetyl CoA while transferring electrons

Repeated beta-oxidation cycles

The final two-carbon link becomes part of acetyl CoA without a transfer of electrons

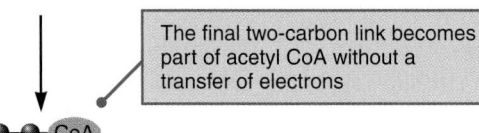

Figure 7.14 **Beta-oxidation.** Beta-oxidation reactions repeatedly clip the two-carbon end off a fatty acid until it is degraded entirely. Beta-oxidation of 18-carbon stearic acid produces 9 acetyl CoA, 8 FADH$_2$, and 8 NADH.

For fatty acid oxidation to continue efficiently and unchecked, reactions in the mitochondria must ensure a reliable supply of oxaloacetate. These reactions convert some pyruvate directly to oxaloacetate rather than to acetyl CoA. Since carbohydrate (glucose) is the original source of the pyruvate, and hence this oxaloacetate, scientists coined the adage "Fat burns in a flame of carbohydrate."

Key Concepts: *Extracting energy from fat involves several steps. First, triglycerides are separated into glycerol and three fatty acids. Glycerol forms pyruvate and can be broken down to yield a small amount of energy. Beta-oxidation breaks down fatty acid chains to two-carbon links that form acetyl CoA, which enters the citric acid cycle. Beta-oxidation and the citric acid cycle form NADH and FADH$_2$, which carry pairs of high-energy electrons to the electron transport chain, where ATP and water are made. The complete breakdown of one triglyceride molecule yields water, carbon dioxide, and substantially more ATP than the complete breakdown of one glucose molecule.*

Extracting Energy from Protein

Because protein has vital structural and functional roles, proteins and amino acids are not considered primary sources of energy. The primary and unique role of amino acids is to serve as building blocks for the synthesis of body protein and nitrogen-containing compounds. However, if energy production falters due to a lack of available carbohydrate and fat, protein comes to the rescue. During starvation, for example, energy needs take priority, so the body breaks down protein and extracts energy from the amino acid building blocks.

To use amino acids as an energy source, a process called deamination first strips off the amino group (–NH2), leaving a "carbon skeleton." (See **Figure 7.16.**) The liver quickly converts the amino group first to ammonia and then to urea, which the kidneys excrete in urine. When you eat more protein than you need, your kidneys excrete the excess nitrogen and your liver uses the carbon skeletons to produce energy, glucose, or fat. Much to the dismay of bodybuilders, when they attempt to build muscle by drinking pricey protein drinks, they can end up gaining fat instead!

Carbon Skeletons Enter Pathways at Different Points

Like a crowd of people streaming into a concert through five different doors rather than one main entrance, carbon skeletons—unlike glucose—can enter the breakdown pathways at several different points. The carbon skeleton from each type of amino acid has a unique structure and number of carbon atoms. These characteristics determine the carbon skeleton's fate, be it pyruvate, acetyl CoA, ketone bodies, or one of the intermediates of the citric acid cycle.

End Products of Amino Acid Catabolism

The complete breakdown of an amino acid yields urea, carbon dioxide, water, and ATP. The carbon skeleton's point of entry into the breakdown pathways determines the amount of ATP it produces. Whereas the complete breakdown of alanine, for example, produces 12.5 ATP, methionine produces only 5 ATP. Compared with glucose and fatty acids, no amino acid produces much ATP. (See **Figure 7.17.**)

Key Concepts: *To extract energy from amino acids, first deamination removes the amino groups, leaving behind carbon skeletons. The liver quickly converts these amino groups to urea and sends them to the kidneys for excretion. The carbon*

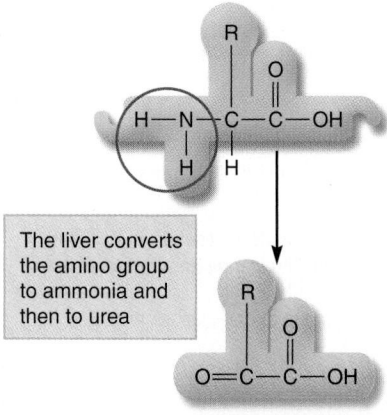

The liver converts the amino group to ammonia and then to urea

The structure of the carbon skeleton determines where it can enter the energy-producing pathways

Figure 7.16 **Deamination.** A deamination reaction strips the amino group from an amino acid.

skeleton structure determines where it enters the catabolic pathways. Some carbon skeletons become pyruvate, others become acetyl CoA, and still others become intermediate compounds of the citric acid cycle. Complete breakdown of amino acids yields water, carbon dioxide, urea, and ATP.

Biosynthesis and Storage

Uh oh! Surveying the results of those holiday dinners and treats, you cringe with regret. Your clothes no longer fit, and you hate the idea of stepping on the scale. Your biosynthetic pathways have been hard at work, building fat stores from your excess intake of energy.

You head for the gym. After sweating through many workouts, your body begins to firm. You drop fat and add muscle. Now any problem with clothes fitting is due to muscle gain, not fat gain. To build muscle protein, different biosynthetic pathways have been busy making amino acids and assembling proteins.

Perhaps you've heard of "carb loading." (See Chapter 13, "Sports Nutrition.") This strategy uses high-carbohydrate meals to pack carbohydrate into your muscle glycogen stores before a race. Biosynthetic pathways assemble glucose into glycogen chains for storage. When needed, your body also can make glucose from certain amino acids and other precursors.

Both the breakdown and biosynthetic pathways are active at all times. While some cells are breaking down carbohydrate, fat, and protein to

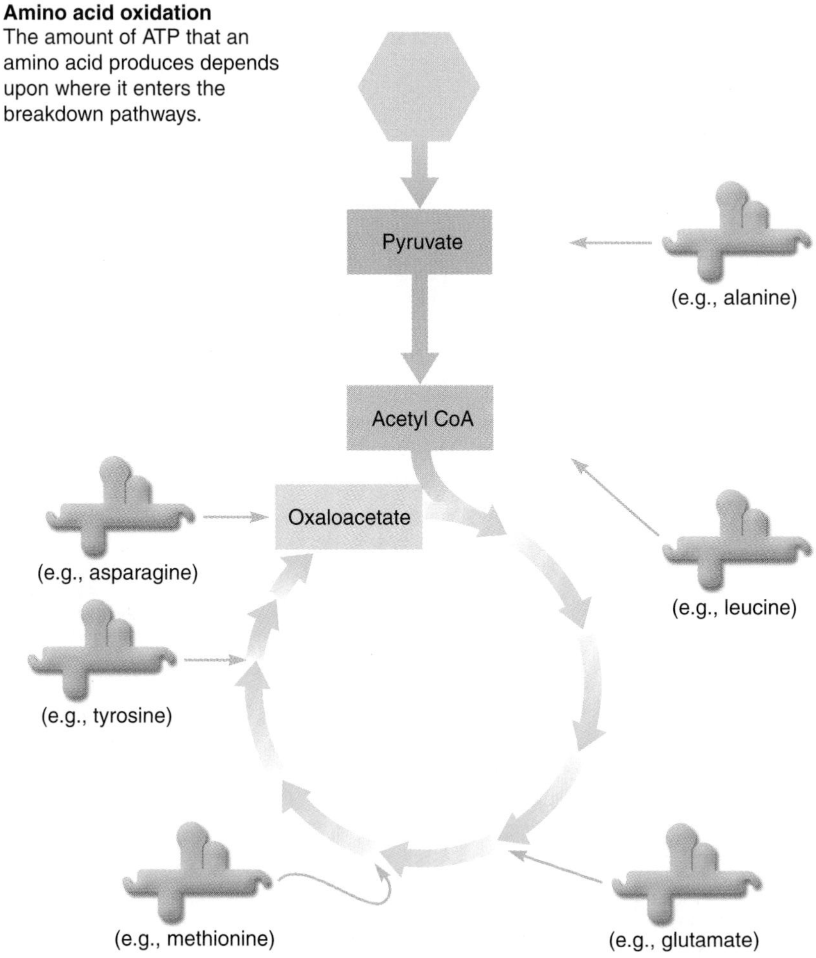

Amino acid oxidation
The amount of ATP that an amino acid produces depends upon where it enters the breakdown pathways.

Figure 7.17 Extracting energy from amino acids. The carbon skeletons of amino acids have several different entrances to the breakdown pathways. Compared with glucose and fatty acids, amino acids yield much smaller amounts of energy (ATP).

gluconeogenesis [gloo-ko-nee-oh-JEN-uh-sis]
Synthesis of glucose within the body from noncarbohydrate precursors such as amino acids, lactate, and glycerol. Fatty acids cannot be converted to glucose.

Quick Bites

Sweet Origins

The word *gluconeogenesis* is derived from the Greek words *glyks*, meaning "sweet," *neo*, meaning "new," and *genesis*, meaning "origin" or "generation."

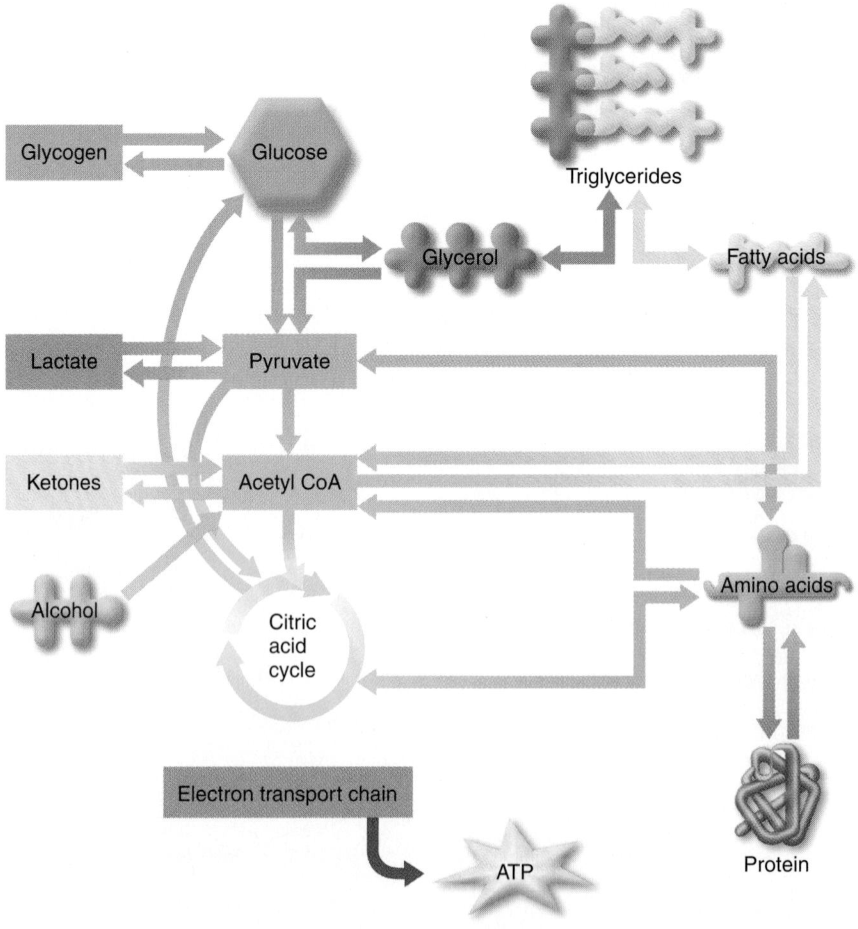

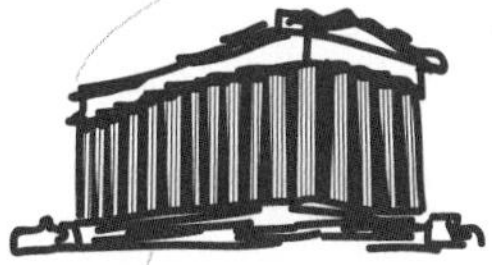

extract energy, other cells are busy building glucose, fatty acids, and amino acids. When your body needs energy, the breakdown pathways prevail. When it has an excess of nutrients, the biosynthetic pathways dominate. The activities in these pathways ebb and flow so that they proceed at just the right rate, not too rapidly and not too slowly. **Figure 7.18** illustrates the interconnections among the metabolic pathways.

Making Carbohydrate (Glucose)

Your body sets a high priority on maintaining an adequate amount of glucose circulating in the bloodstream. **Table 7.2** shows the amount of energy, in kilocalories, that a typical 70-kilogram man has available. Blood glucose is the primary source of energy for your brain, central nervous system, and red blood cells. In fact, while you're at rest, your brain consumes about 60 percent of the energy consumed by your entire body.

The brain stores little glucose—only about 8 kilocalories. About 140 kilocalories of glucose circulate in the blood or are stored in adipose tissue. Your primary carbohydrate stores are in the form of glycogen. Muscle tissue holds about 1,200 kilocalories of glycogen, and the liver stores another 400 kilocalories.

Gluconeogenesis: Pathways to Glucose

When you are exercising intensely or when you aren't taking in enough carbohydrate, your body can remake glucose from pyruvate by using a clever strategy called **gluconeogenesis**. (See **Figure 7.19**.) Your liver is the major site of gluconeogenesis, accounting for about 90 percent of glucose production. Your kidneys make the rest.

Figure 7.18 **Overview of metabolic pathways.** As if they were traveling through a maze of city streets, molecules move through a network of breakdown and biosynthetic pathways. Not all pathways are available to a molecule. Just as traffic lights and one-way streets regulate traffic flow, cellular mechanisms control the flow of molecules in metabolic pathways. These mechanisms include hormones, irreversible reactions, and the location of the reactions in the cell.

Key

■ Major noncarbohydrate precursors to glucose

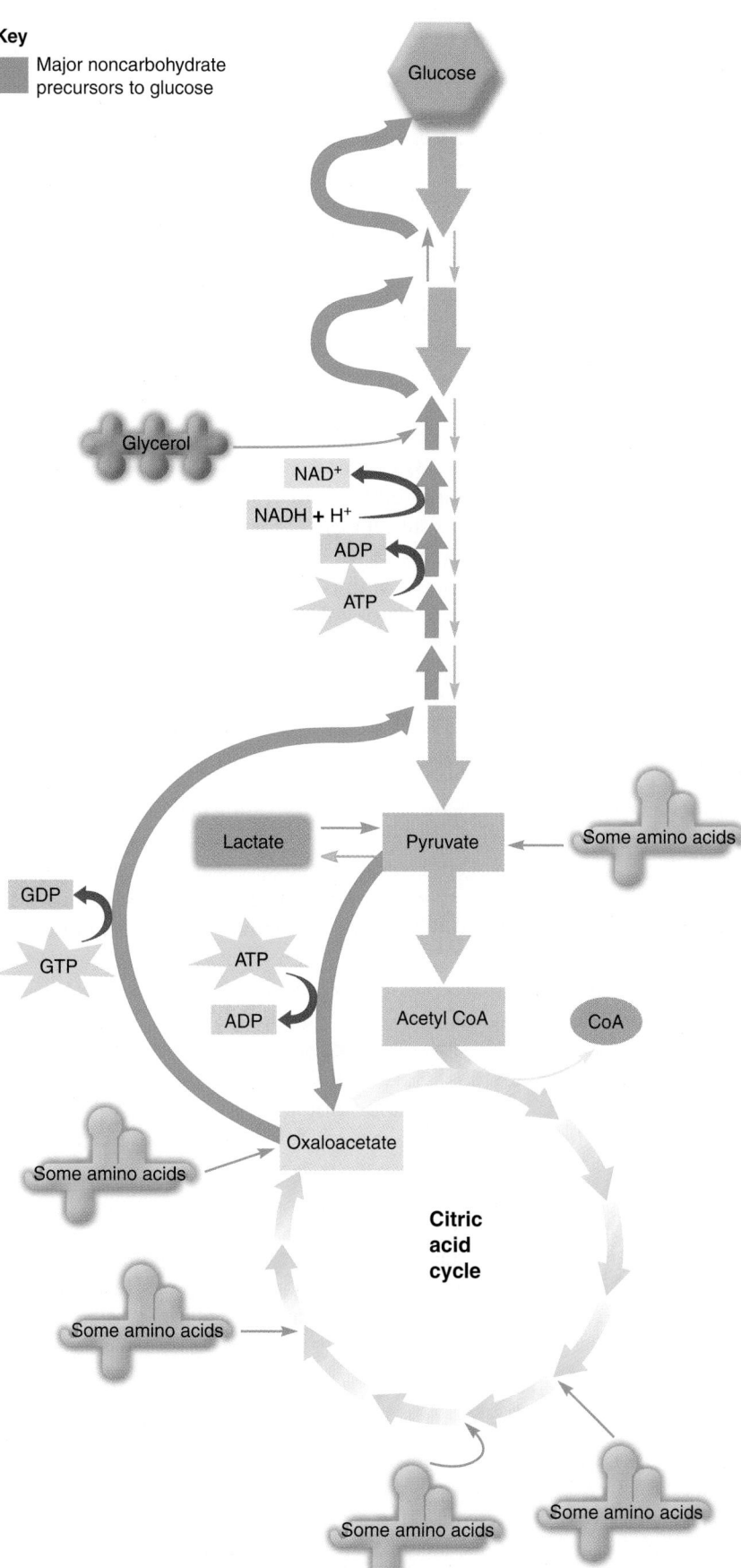

Table 7.2 **Available Energy (kcal) in a Typical 70-kg Man**

Organ	Glucose or Glycogen	Triglycerides	Mobilizable Proteins
Blood	60	45	0
Liver	400	450	400
Brain	8	0	0
Muscle	1,200	450	24,000
Adipose tissue	80	135,000	40

Source: Adapted from Berg JM, Tymoczko JL, Stryer L. *Biochemistry.* 5th ed. New York: WH Freeman, 2002.

Figure 7.19 **Gluconeogenesis.** Liver and kidney cells make glucose from pyruvate by way of oxaloacetate. Gluconeogenesis is NOT the reverse of glycolysis. Although these pathways share many reactions, albeit in the reverse direction, gluconeogenesis must detour around the irreversible steps in glycolysis.

Cori cycle The circular path that regenerates NAD⁺ and glucose when oxygen is low and lactate and NADH build up in excess in muscle tissue.

glucogenic In the metabolism of amino acids, a term describing an amino acid broken down into pyruvate or an intermediate of the citric acid cycle; that is, any compound that can be used in gluconeogenesis to form glucose.

ketogenic In the metabolism of amino acids, a term describing an amino acid broken down into acetyl CoA (which can be converted into ketone bodies).

glycogenesis The formation of glycogen from glucose.

glycogenolysis The breakdown of glycogen to glucose.

lipogenesis [lye-poh-JEN-eh-sis] Synthesis of fatty acids, primarily in liver cells, from acetyl CoA derived from the metabolism of alcohol and some amino acids.

Gluconeogenesis and glycolysis share many—but not all—reactions. During gluconeogenesis, reactions flow in the opposite direction as they do during glycolysis. Because some reactions of glycolysis flow only one way, however, gluconeogenesis must use energy-consuming detours to bypass them. Thus gluconeogenesis is *not* simply a reversal of glycolysis.

Your body can make glucose from pyruvate, lactate, and some noncarbohydrate sources—glycerol and most amino acids. Although gluconeogenesis can use the glycerol portion of fat, it cannot make glucose from fatty acids.

Although some lactate is continually formed and degraded, lactate production increases substantially in exercising muscle. Low oxygen levels in actively contracting muscle cells inhibit the conversion of pyruvate to acetyl CoA. In the liver, gluconeogenesis converts some of the lactate back to glucose via the **Cori cycle**. For more on the Cori cycle, see Chapter 13, "Sports Nutrition."

If the carbon skeleton of an amino acid can be made into glucose, the amino acid is called **glucogenic**. Glucogenic amino acids provide carbon skeletons that become pyruvate or directly enter the citric acid cycle at intermediate points without forming acetyl CoA. If the carbon skeleton of an amino acid directly forms acetyl CoA (which your body can convert to ketone bodies but not glucose), the amino acid is called **ketogenic** (see the section "Ketogenesis: Pathways to Ketone Bodies" later in this chapter).

Key Concepts: *Your body can make glucose from pyruvate, lactate, glucogenic amino acids, and glycerol, but not from fatty acids. Although most gluconeogenesis takes place in the liver, the kidneys are responsible for about 10 percent of glucose synthesis.*

Storage: Glucose to Glycogen

Our main storage form of glucose is glycogen, a branched-chain polysaccharide made of glucose units (see Chapter 4, "Carbohydrates"). Both the liver and muscle store glycogen. Liver glycogen serves as a glucose reserve for the blood, and muscle glycogen supplies glucose to exercising muscle tissue. Glycogen stores are limited; fasting or strenuous exercise can deplete them rapidly.

A pathway called **glycogenesis** assembles glucose molecules into branched chains for storage as glycogen. When the body needs glucose, a different series of reactions known as **glycogenolysis** breaks down the glycogen chains into individual glucose molecules. In muscle, these glucose molecules enter glycolysis and continue along the metabolic pathways to produce ATP. In the liver, glycogenolysis yields glucose that moves into the bloodstream to maintain blood glucose levels.

Making Fat (Fatty Acids)

Acetyl CoA is the most important ingredient in fatty acid synthesis. Compounds that can be metabolized to form acetyl CoA can feed fatty acid synthesis. Such precursors include ketogenic amino acids, alcohol, and fatty acids themselves.

Lipogenesis: Pathways to Fatty Acids

When your body has a plentiful supply of energy (ATP) and abundant building blocks, it can make long-chain fatty acids using a process called **lipogenesis**. To do this, your body assembles two-carbon acetyl CoA "links" into fatty acid chains. Where do these acetyl CoA building blocks come from? Ketogenic amino acids, alcohol, and fatty acids themselves supply acetyl CoA for lipogenesis.

Although you can think of fatty acid synthesis as reassembling the links broken apart by beta-oxidation, lipogenesis is *not* the reversal of beta-oxidation. These pathways use different reactions and take place in different locations—fatty acid synthesis occurs in the cytosol, whereas beta-oxidation operates inside the mitochondria. Another important distinction is that beta-oxidation releases energy, and fatty acid synthesis requires energy. In beta-oxidation, reactions deliver high-energy electrons to NADH for ultimate ATP synthesis. In lipogenesis, NADPH supplies energy to power the synthesis of fatty acids. Your endoplasmic reticulum, a type of organelle in cells, assembles surplus fatty acids and glycerol into triglycerides for storage as body fat.

Storage: Dietary Energy to Stored Triglyceride

When you overeat, your body uses body fat as a long-term energy storage depot. When you eat an excess of fat, most extra dietary fatty acids head straight to your fat stores. If you eat more protein than your tissues can use, your body converts most of the excess protein to body fat. Interestingly, excess carbohydrate does not readily become fat. In research studies, massive overfeeding of carbohydrate in normal men caused only minimal amounts of fat synthesis. (See the FYI feature, "Do Carbohydrates Turn Into Fat?") So are carbohydrate calories "free"? Unfortunately, no. The first law of thermodynamics—the law of conservation of energy—still holds. Although excess carbohydrate does not dramatically increase fat synthesis, it shifts your body's fuel preferences toward burning more carbohydrate and fewer fatty acids.[9] Thus, eating excess carbohydrates still can make you fat by allowing your fat intake to go directly to storage rather than to make ATP. (See **Table 7.3**.)

Key Concepts: *When ATP is plentiful and the diet supplies an excess of energy, your cells make fatty acids and triglycerides. Energy carried by NADPH powers the synthesis of fatty acids from acetyl CoA building blocks. Glycerol and fatty acids are assembled into triglycerides on the endoplasmic reticulum. Although excess dietary carbohydrate is not readily converted to fat, it does shift the body's selection of fuel and encourages the accumulation of dietary fat in body fat stores.*

Making Ketone Bodies

Ketone bodies (sometimes incorrectly called **ketones**) include three compounds: acetoacetate, beta-hydroxybutyrate, and acetone. Acetoacetate and beta-hydroxybutyrate are acids, so they are sometimes referred to as keto

ketones [KEE-tones] Organic compounds that contain a chemical group consisting of C=O (a carbon–oxygen double bond) bound to two hydrocarbons. Pyruvate and fructose are examples of ketones. Acetone and acetoacetate are both ketones and ketone bodies. While beta-hydroxybutyrate is not a ketone, it is a ketone body.

Table 7.3 **Summary of Energy Yield and Interconversions**

Dietary Nutrient	Yields Energy?	Convertible to Glucose?	Convertible to Amino Acids and Body Proteins?	Convertible to Fat?
Carbohydrate (glucose, fructose, galactose)	Yes	Yes	Yes, can yield certain amino acids when amino groups are available	Insignificant
Fat (triglycerides)				
Fatty acids	Yes, large amounts	No	No	Yes
Glycerol	Yes, small amounts	Yes, small amounts	Yes (see carbohydrate)	Insignificant
Protein (amino acids)	Yes, generally not much (see starvation in text)	Yes, if insufficient carbohydrate is available	Yes	Yes, from some amino acids
Alcohol (ethanol)	Yes	No	No	Yes

ketogenesis The process in which excess acetyl CoA from fatty acid oxidation is converted into the ketone bodies acetoacetate, beta-hydroxybutyrate, and acetone.

ketoacidosis Acidification of the blood caused by a buildup of ketone bodies. It is primarily a consequence of uncontrolled type 1 diabetes mellitus and can be life threatening.

Quick Bites

Why Didn't My Cholesterol Levels Drop?

Your body can make cholesterol from acetyl CoA by way of ketones. In fact, all 27 carbons in synthesized cholesterol come from acetyl CoA. The rate of cholesterol formation is highly responsive to cholesterol levels in cells. If levels are low, the liver makes more. If levels are high, synthesis decreases. This is why dietary cholesterol in the absence of dietary fat often has little effect on blood cholesterol levels.

acids. You may recognize the term *acetone*, since this chemical is a common solvent. In fact, you can smell the strong odor of acetone on the breath of people with high levels of ketone bodies in their blood: Their breath smells like some nail polish removers!

Your body makes and uses small amounts of ketone bodies at all times. Although long considered to be just an emergency energy source or the result of an abnormal condition such as starvation or uncontrolled diabetes, ketone bodies are normal, everyday fuels. In fact, your heart and kidneys prefer to use the ketone body acetoacetate rather than glucose as a fuel source.[10]

Ketogenesis: Pathways to Ketone Bodies

During the breakdown of fatty acids, not all acetyl CoA enters the citric acid cycle. Your liver converts some acetyl CoA to ketone bodies, a process called **ketogenesis**. (See **Figure 7.20**.)

Ketogenesis is highly active when fatty acid oxidation in the liver produces such an abundance of acetyl CoA that it overwhelms the available supply of oxaloacetate. Unable to enter the citric acid cycle, the excess acetyl CoA is shunted to ketone body production. When a person has uncontrolled diabetes or is actually starving, ketone bodies help provide emergency energy to all body tissues, especially the brain and the rest of the CNS. Other than glucose, ketone bodies are your central nervous system's only other effective fuel.[11] (See the section "Special States" for more details on starvation and diabetes mellitus.) After the liver makes ketone bodies from acetyl CoA molecules, the ketone bodies travel to other tissues via the bloodstream. Tissue cells can convert the ketone bodies back to acetyl CoA for ATP production via the citric acid cycle and electron transport chain.[12]

To dispose of excess ketone bodies, your kidneys excrete them in urine and your lungs exhale them. If this removal process cannot keep up with the production process, ketone bodies accumulate in the blood—a condition called ketosis. (See Chapter 4, "Carbohydrates.") During even a brief fast, the catabolism of fat and protein increases the production of ketone bodies and results in ketosis.[13] Ketosis is likely to occur in uncontrolled type 1 diabetes mellitus, and in this situation, blood acidity rises quickly. This **ketoacidosis** can lead to a coma and eventually death if untreated.[14] During a short fast, ketoacidosis rarely occurs.

Figure 7.20 **Ketogenesis.** For acetyl CoA from fatty acid oxidation to enter the citric acid cycle, fat and carbohydrate metabolism must be synchronized. When acetyl CoA cannot enter the citric acid cycle, it is shunted to form ketone bodies, a process called ketogenesis.

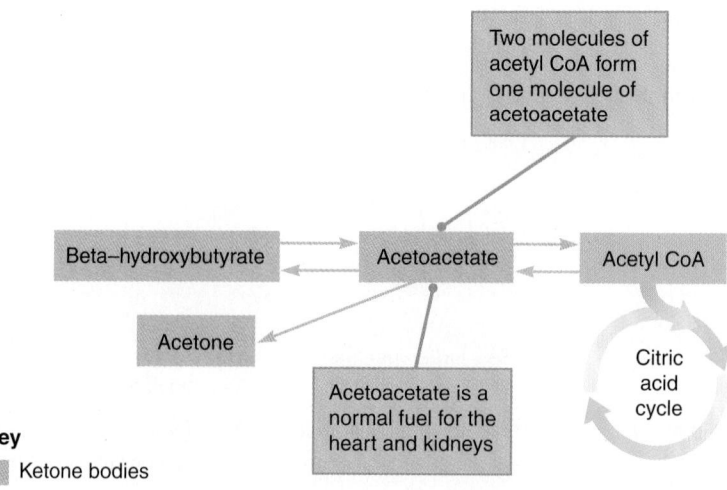

KETONE BODY FORMATION

Two molecules of acetyl CoA form one molecule of acetoacetate

Beta–hydroxybutyrate ⟷ Acetoacetate ⟷ Acetyl CoA

Acetone

Acetoacetate is a normal fuel for the heart and kidneys

Citric acid cycle

Key
Ketone bodies

Because "fat burns in a flame of carbohydrate," a very high-fat, low-carbohydrate diet promotes ketosis. The lack of carbohydrate inhibits formation of oxaloacetate, slowing entry of acetyl CoA into the citric acid cycle and rerouting acetyl CoA to form ketone bodies. Given time, however, the body can adapt to a very high-fat, low-carbohydrate diet and avoid ketosis. Eskimos, for example, sometimes live almost entirely on fat but do not develop ketosis. Even brain cells can adapt to derive 50 to 75 percent of their fuel from ketone bodies (principally beta-hydroxybutyrate) after a few weeks of a low supply of glucose, their preferred fuel.[15]

Key Concepts: *Although some ketone bodies are made and used for energy all the time, a lack of available carbohydrate accelerates ketone body production. Three types of ketone bodies—acetoacetate, beta-hydroxybutyrate, and acetone—can be made from any precursor of acetyl CoA: pyruvate, fatty acids, glycerol, and certain amino acids. Ketone bodies become an important fuel source during*

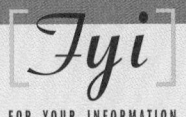

FOR YOUR INFORMATION

Do Carbohydrates Turn into Fat? Marc Hellerstein, M.D., Ph.D.

Thirty years ago, Jules Hirsch and his colleagues addressed this question indirectly. They found that the composition of fatty acids in adipose tissue closely resembled the subjects' dietary fat intake. Moreover, when they put these subjects on controlled diets of different fatty acid composition for six months, adipose fatty acids slowly changed to reflect the new dietary fatty acid composition. These studies concluded that "we are what we eat" with regard to body fat and that fatty acid synthesis is minimal at best.

The body's ability to make fat from carbohydrate is called *de novo lipogenesis* (DNL). Numerous studies using a technique called indirect calorimetry have shown that net DNL is absent or very low in humans under most dietary conditions, even after a large carbohydrate meal. But could there be concurrent synthesis *and* use of fat that results in no net change?

Concurrent DNL and burning of fatty acids is called *futile cycling.* About 25 to 28 percent of the carbohydrate energy is lost during the inefficient conversion to fatty acids. Does this costly conversion really happen? New stable isotopic methods have helped answer this question.

Direct Evidence

Direct evidence from stable isotopic methods shows that DNL is minimal in normal (nonobese, nondiabetic, nonoverfed) men. DNL represents less than 1 gram of saturated fat per day, whether the subjects are given large meals, intravenous glucose, or a liquid diet.

Do any circumstances stimulate DNL? Jean-Marc Schwarz gave fructose and glucose orally to lean and obese subjects. The dietary fructose increased DNL up to twentyfold compared with equal calorie loads of glucose. Nevertheless, fat synthesis still represented only a small percentage of the fructose load given (< 5 percent). Scott Siler has shown that drinking alcohol stimulates DNL. Again, however, only a small percentage (< 5 percent) of the alcohol was converted to fat; the great majority was released from the liver as acetate.

My laboratory studied the effect of five to seven days of carbohydrate overfeeding or underfeeding in normal men. Fat synthesis by the liver was highly sensitive to the degree of dietary carbohydrate excess. In fact, we could determine exactly which diet a person was eating by measuring DNL. Even so, the absolute amount of fat synthesis remained low, even on massively excessive carbohydrate intakes. DNL may be a sensitive *signal* of excess carbohydrate in the diet, but it is not a quantitatively important route for excess carbohydrate disposal.

Other conditions yield similar findings. Very low-fat diets (10 percent of energy as fat; 70 percent as carbohydrate) stimulate lipogenesis, but, again, not a large amount. In young women, lipogenesis increases during the follicular phase of the menstrual cycle, but the amount is small, representing only one to two pounds of extra fat per year. A high rate of DNL has been documented in humans only under conditions of massive carbohydrate overfeeding—for example, 5,000 to 6,000 carbohydrate calories per day for more than a week.

Are Carbohydrate Calories "Free"?

Alas, we still become fatter if we overeat carbohydrate. At rest, our bodies normally burn fat as our primary fuel source. An excess of dietary carbohydrate energy causes a fat-sparing shift in fuel selection as it markedly reduces the use of fat to fuel the body. Dietary fat makes a beeline for body fat storage rather than being burned to release energy. Thus, excess dietary carbohydrate is not "free" when the diet also contains fat, because the carbohydrate spares fat use.

Dr. Hellerstein is Professor of Medicine at the University of California, San Francisco, and Professor of Nutritional Sciences at the University of California at Berkeley.

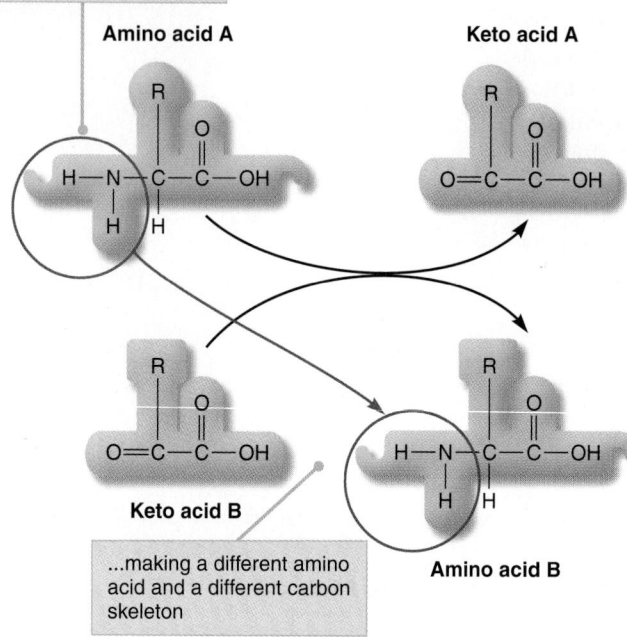

The amino group from one amino acid is transferred to a new carbon skeleton...

Amino acid A

Keto acid A

Keto acid B

...making a different amino acid and a different carbon skeleton

Amino acid B

Figure 7.21 **Transamination.** A transamination reaction transfers the amino group from one amino acid to form a different amino acid.

starvation, uncontrolled diabetes mellitus, and very high-fat, low-carbohydrate diets. In type 1 diabetes mellitus, an accumulation of ketone bodies can acidify the blood, a dangerous condition known as ketoacidosis.

Making Protein (Amino Acids)

Your body rebuilds proteins from a pool of amino acids in your cells. But how is that amino acid pool replenished? Your diet supplies some amino acids, the breakdown of body proteins supplies some, and cells make some. During protein synthesis, your cells can make dispensable amino acids and retrieve indispensable amino acids from the bloodstream. Your cells cannot make indispensable amino acids, however. If a cell lacks an indispensable amino acid and your diet doesn't supply it, protein synthesis stops. The cell breaks down this incomplete protein into its constituent amino acids, which are returned to the bloodstream. (See Chapter 6, "Proteins and Amino Acids," for more details of protein synthesis.)

Biosynthesis: Making Amino Acids

Your body uses many different pathways to synthesize dispensable amino acids. Each pathway is short, involving just a few steps, and builds amino acids from carbon

---

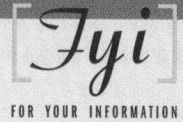

FOR YOUR INFORMATION

Key Intersections Direct Metabolic Traffic

PYRUVATE IS PIVOTAL

Pyruvate is a pivotal point in the metabolic pathways. How does it select a path? What determines its destination? When ATP levels are low, cellular energy is in short supply, so the metabolic pathways flow toward the production of ATP. Depending on oxygen availability, low ATP routes pyruvate to acetyl CoA or lactate. When ATP is abundant, cells have ample energy, so the biosynthetic pathways prevail as pyruvate is converted to oxaloacetate or the amino acid alanine; oxaloacetate is converted to glucose and stored as glycogen.

To Acetyl CoA

When cells need ATP and have readily available oxygen, they rapidly convert pyruvate to acetyl CoA. This irreversible reaction commits the carbons of carbohydrates to oxidation by the citric acid cycle or to the biosynthesis of lipids. Acetyl CoA cannot be converted to glucose.

To and from Lactate

When cells need ATP but lack readily available oxygen, they reroute most pyruvate to form lactate. Although this route is always at least minimally active, it prevails when oxygen levels are low. Reversible reactions convert pyruvate to lactate, so these substances are interconvertible. For more about lactate and its various fates, see the feature "Lactate Is Not a Metabolic Dead End" in Chapter 13. The reaction that converts pyruvate to lactate uses energy carried by NADH, so it also produces NAD⁺. This regeneration of NAD⁺ is critical to continued glycolysis. Anaerobic conditions cut off the supply of NAD⁺ from other sources, so without the NAD⁺ generated in the production of lactate, glycolysis would stop.

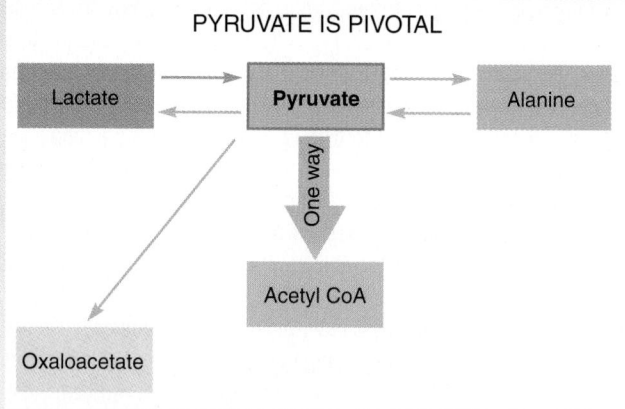

The demand for ATP and the availability of oxygen determine pyruvate's destination.

To Oxaloacetate

Cells also can convert pyruvate to oxaloacetate, another pivotal molecule. Oxaloacetate can react with acetyl CoA to start the citric acid cycle when ATP is needed, or it can provide the building blocks to make glucose.

Oxaloacetate is essential for acetyl CoA's entry into the citric acid cycle. A steady supply of oxaloacetate is critical to the citric acid

skeletons. Pyruvate, along with intermediates of glycolysis and the citric acid cycle supply the carbon skeletons.

To make dispensable amino acids, the body transfers the amino group from one amino acid to a new carbon skeleton, a process called **transamination** (see **Figure 7.21**). To make the amino acid alanine, for example, pyruvate swipes an amino group from the amino acid glutamic acid to yield alanine and alpha-ketoglutaric acid. Transamination requires several enzymes. One group of enzymes, known as the aminotransferases, is derived from the B vitamin pyridoxine (B_6). Although vitamin B_6 deficiency is rare, a lack of B_6 will inhibit amino acid synthesis and impair protein formation.

Key Concepts: *Proteins are made from combinations of indispensable and dispensable amino acids. The body synthesizes dispensable amino acids from pyruvate, other glycolytic intermediates, and compounds from the citric acid cycle. To form amino acids, transamination reactions transfer amino groups to carbon skeletons.*

> **transamination [TRANS-am-ih-NAY-shun]**
> The transfer of an amino group from an amino acid to a carbon skeleton to form a different amino acid.

Regulation of Metabolism

Just as the cruise control on your car regulates the vehicle's speed within a narrow range, your body tightly controls the reactions of your metabolic pathways. Whether highly or minimally active, each pathway proceeds at just the right speed, not too fast and not too slow. How does your body achieve this remarkable control? Although a number of strategies operate simultaneously, certain hormones are the master regulators.

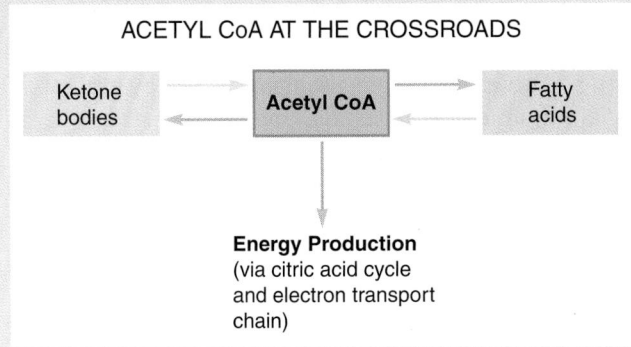

ACETYL CoA AT THE CROSSROADS

Acetyl CoA sits at a key intersection of the carbohydrate and fatty acid breakdown pathways.

cycle's efficient extraction of energy from fatty acids. Carbohydrate feeds the pool of oxaloacetate as reactions break down carbohydrate to pyruvate and irreversibly convert the pyruvate to oxaloacetate. Cells can also make glucose from this oxaloacetate and store energy in the branched glucose chains of glycogen.

When cells have abundant ATP, they restrict the activities of certain enzymes, thus slowing the entry of acetyl CoA into the citric acid cycle. This reroutes the acetyl CoA into energy-storage pathways to form fatty acids so as to store energy as fat.

To and from Alanine
Since a reversible process converts pyruvate to the amino acid alanine, pyruvate and alanine are interconvertible. Although alanine is the only amino acid made from pyruvate, many other amino acids can be converted to pyruvate. Thus, pyruvate is located at a major junction of amino acid and carbohydrate metabolism.

ACETYL CoA AT THE CROSSROADS
Acetyl CoA, like pyruvate, stands at a pivotal point in metabolism. The breakdown pathways for glucose, fatty acids, and some amino acids converge at acetyl CoA. Once formed, what are acetyl CoA's options? It cannot return to pyruvate or make glucose, but acetyl CoA can enter major energy-producing and biosynthetic pathways. The body's energy status determines the predominant route.

To Energy Production
When cells need ATP and have oxaloacetate available, acetyl CoA enters the citric acid cycle for the ultimate production of ATP by the electron transport chain.

To and from Ketone Bodies
When the production of oxaloacetate does not match acetyl CoA production, acetyl CoA cannot enter the citric acid cycle, so the metabolic pathways shunt acetyl CoA to form ketone bodies.

To and from Fatty Acids
When energy is abundant, acetyl CoA molecules become building blocks for fatty acid chains. The body assembles these fatty acid chains into triglycerides and stores them in adipose tissue.

Hormones of Metabolism

Hormones are chemical messengers that help determine whether metabolic processing favors catabolic (breakdown) or anabolic (building) pathways. The major regulatory hormones are insulin, glucagon, cortisol, and epinephrine.

The pancreas secretes insulin, the leader of the storage (anabolic) team. Its mission is to decrease the amount of glucose in the blood, so it promotes carbohydrate use and storage (as glycogen). Because insulin stimulates the use of glucose over fat, its actions are said to be *fat-sparing*. In addition, insulin promotes fat storage in adipose tissue, cellular uptake of amino acids, and assembly of these amino acids into proteins. It also inhibits the breakdown of body proteins.

The pancreas also secretes glucagon, the leader of the breakdown (catabolic) team. Glucagon's mission is to increase the amount of glucose in circulation; it stimulates the breakdown of liver glycogen. The adrenal glands secrete two other members of the breakdown team—the hormones cortisol and epinephrine. Cortisol promotes the breakdown of amino acids for gluconeogenesis and helps increase the activity of the enzymes that drive gluconeogenic reactions.[16] Epinephrine stimulates the conversion of glycogen to glucose in muscle, increasing the amount of glucose available.

The actions of each team ebb and flow in response to the levels of available nutrients.[17] Although both the storage and the breakdown teams are always active, storage dominates in times of plenty, and breakdown dominates in times of need.

Key Concepts: *Hormones and other factors regulate the balance of anabolic and catabolic pathways in energy metabolism. The hormone insulin stimulates glycogen, protein, and triglyceride synthesis. The hormones glucagon, cortisol, and epinephrine stimulate breakdown of glycogen and triglycerides.*

Special States

Now you can put your new knowledge of metabolism to work by evaluating case studies of special physiological states: feasting, fasting, stress, diabetes mellitus, and exercising. What happens to your metabolism under each situation? Read on to find out which states stimulate breakdown and which stimulate biosynthesis.

Feasting

You're stuffed. You just ate a huge holiday dinner: two servings of turkey with a big ladle of gravy and ample servings of dressing, mashed potatoes, caramelized sweet potatoes, green peas, and two bread rolls. To top it off, you ate a piece of pumpkin pie with whipped cream. You meant to stop there; you loudly proclaimed, "I'm so full, I can't eat another bite!" But eventually your grandmother convinced you to taste her special pecan pie. Gosh, that was good! But now you are lying prostrate on the couch, uncomfortable and bloated, with your belt loosened. Your feasting may be finished for now, but your body's work has just begun.

Your meal led to a huge influx of carbohydrate, fat, and protein—a plentiful supply for your tissues and far more energy than you need for life as a couch potato. The influx of food triggers the rapid secretion of the storage hormone insulin and inhibits the release of the breakdown hormones glucagon, cortisol, and epinephrine. Insulin is sometimes called the "hormone of plenty" because when energy is abundant, it promotes the replenishment of energy stores (glycogen and fat), the synthesis of protein, and the maintenance and repair of tissues. Its suppression of glucagon and cortisol reduces the rate of breakdown.

The storage hormone insulin signals your cells to "store, store, store!" Consequently, much of your holiday dinner will wind up stored as fat. The surplus carbohydrate first enters glycogen stores, filling their limited capacity. In the short term, excess carbohydrate primarily readjusts your body's fuel preferences.[18] In a fat-sparing shift, your body maximizes its use of carbohydrate and minimizes its use of fat, thus promoting fat storage.[19] Although your body does not directly make appreciable amounts of fat from carbohydrate, the shift in fuel use triggered by excess carbohydrate still leads to increased fat stores and weight gain.

What happens to the surplus fat and protein? Fat tissue is the perfect energy storage package for both. Although some ATP is produced from dietary fat, nearly all excess dietary fat becomes body fat. Excess protein, beyond what's needed to replenish the overall body pool of amino acids, also heads to fat storage. (See **Figure 7.22**.)

The Return to Normal

After this frenzied bout of storage, the amount of glucose and triglyceride circulating in the bloodstream drops to the fasting level. The level of amino acids in the blood also returns to baseline, and the secretion of insulin slows.

Hours later, after a nap and perhaps a game of touch football, a further decline in blood glucose levels signals the pancreas to secrete the breakdown hormone glucagon. Glucagon broadcasts the order "Release the glucose!" and your body swings into action to counteract falling blood glucose levels. The body breaks down liver glycogen to glucose, which is released into the bloodstream. Glucagon also stimulates the production of glucose from amino acids and slows the synthesis of glycogen and fatty acids. If blood glucose levels continue to fall, the adrenal glands secrete epinephrine, which signals the liver to further increase its release of glucose into the bloodstream. Epinephrine also stimulates the breakdown of muscle glycogen to form glucose that muscles can use. This glucose does not enter the bloodstream and is immediately available for muscle tissue to mount a fight-or-flight response to danger.

If low blood glucose levels persist for hours or days, the pituitary and adrenal glands join the battle by secreting growth hormone and cortisol, respectively. These hormones cause most cells to shift their fuel usage from glucose to fatty acids. Cortisol also promotes the breakdown of amino acids, and gluconeogenesis begins to ramp up and make glucose from circulating amino acids.[20] All breakdown hormones work in concert to maintain blood glucose levels and assure a constant supply of glucose for the central nervous system and red blood cells[21]—until it is time to attack the leftovers!

Key Concepts: *Feasting, or taking in too many calories, stimulates anabolic processes such as glycogen and triglyceride synthesis. Insulin is the key hormone that promotes synthesis and storage of glycogen and fat. Your body resists making fat from excess carbohydrate, but shifts its fuel preferences. This shift still leads to the accumulation of fat stores.*

FEASTING

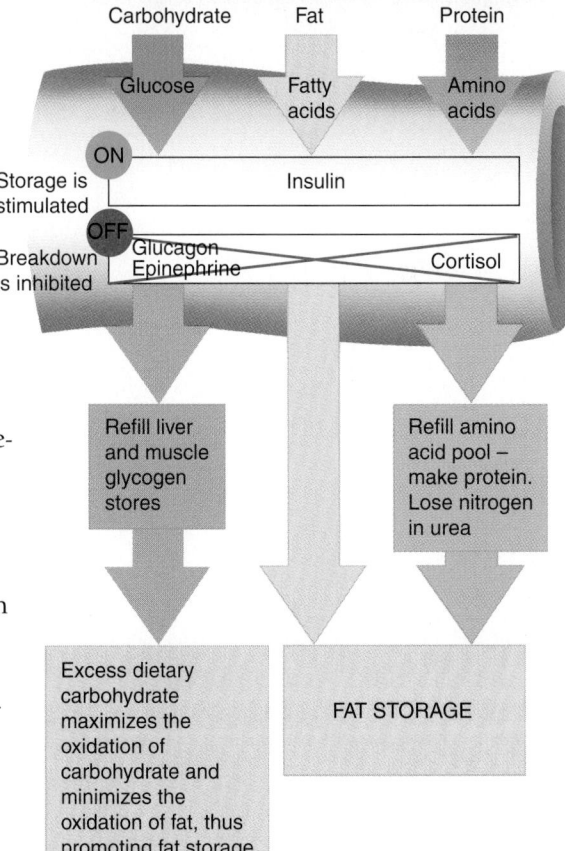

Figure 7.22 **Feasting.** Your body deals with a large influx of energy-yielding nutrients by increasing cellular uptake of glucose and promoting fat storage.

SHORT-TERM FASTING

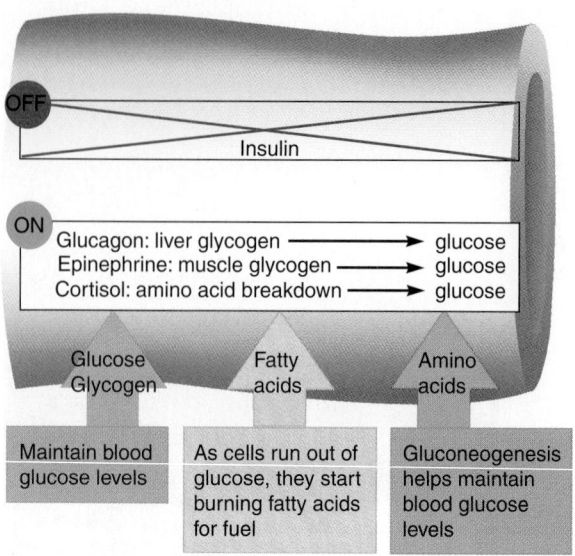

Figure 7.23 **Fasting.** During a short fast, cells first break down liver glycogen to maintain blood glucose levels. They also burn fatty acids and ramp up the production of glucose from amino acids.

Fasting

Feasting on a holiday dinner floods your body with excess energy that is stored for future use. In contrast, fasting and starvation deprive you of energy, so your body must employ an opposing strategy—the mobilization of fuel. (See **Figure 7.23.**) Whether starvation occurs in a child during a famine, a young woman with anorexia nervosa, a patient with AIDS wasting syndrome, or a person who is intentionally fasting, the body responds in the same way.

Some people deprive themselves of food for a particular purpose—to lose weight, to stage a political protest, to participate in a religious fast, or to "cleanse" their bodies. The cleansing motivation is ironic, because fasting actually unleashes potentially damaging toxins to circulate throughout the body. Over time, fat stores accumulate environmental toxins, such as DDT, PCBs, and benzene.[22] In the case of PCBs, despite the fact that Congress banned their use decades ago, more than 9 of 10 Americans still have traces of these compounds in their body fat.[23] When bound in adipose tissue, toxins are relatively harmless. Fasting, however, breaks down adipose tissue and releases these toxins, giving them a second chance to damage cells. Although the liver—the body's detoxification center—and the intestines remove a small portion of these liberated toxins, the balance remain in circulation, where they can wreak havoc.

Survival Priorities and Potential Energy Sources

Starvation confronts your body with several dilemmas. Where will it get energy to fuel survival needs? Which should it burn first—fat, protein, or carbohydrate? Can it conserve its energy reserves? Which tissues should it sacrifice to ensure survival?

Your body's first priority is to preserve glucose-dependent tissue: red blood cells, brain cells, and the rest of the central nervous system. Your brain will not tolerate even a short interruption in the supply of adequate energy. Once your body depletes its carbohydrate reserves, it begins sacrificing readily available circulating amino acids to make glucose and ATP.

Your body's second priority is to maintain muscle mass. In the face of danger, we rely upon our ability to mount a fight-or-flight response. This survival mechanism requires a large muscle mass, allowing us to move quickly and effectively. Your body grudgingly uses muscle protein for energy and breaks it down rapidly only in the final stages of starvation.

Although your body stores most of its energy reserve in adipose tissue, triglycerides are a poor source of glucose. Although your body can make a small amount of glucose from the glycerol backbone, it cannot make any glucose from fatty acids. As a consequence, your body's primary energy stores—fat—are incompatible with your body's paramount energy priority—glucose for your brain. To meet this metabolic challenge, your body's anti-starvation strategies include a glucose-sparing mechanism. It shifts to fatty acids and ketone bodies to fuel its needs. In time, even your brain adapts as most, but not all, brain cells come to rely on ketone bodies for fuel.

The Prolonged Fast: In the Beginning

What happens during the fasting state? Let's take a metabolic look at Fasting Frank, a political activist determined to make a dramatic statement.

Frank begins fasting at sundown, planning to drink only water and consume no other foods or liquids.

The first few hours are no different from your nightly fast between dinner and breakfast. As blood glucose drops to fasting baseline levels, the liver breaks down glycogen to glucose. Gluconeogenesis becomes highly active and begins churning out glucose from circulating amino acids. The liver pours glucose into the bloodstream to supply other organs and shifts to fatty acids for its own energy needs. Muscle cells also start burning fatty acids. After about 12 hours, the battle to maintain a constant supply of blood glucose exhausts nearly all carbohydrate stores.[24]

The First Few Days

During the next few days, fat and protein are the primary fuels. To preserve structural proteins, especially muscle mass, Frank's body first turns to easily metabolized amino acids. It uses some to produce ATP and others to make glucose. Glucogenic amino acids, especially alanine, furnish about 90 percent of the brain's glucose supply. Glycerol from triglyceride breakdown supplies the remaining 10 percent. After a couple of days, production of ketone bodies ramps up, augmenting the fuel supply. (See **Figure 7.24**.)

The Early Weeks

As starvation continues, Frank's body initiates several energy-conservation strategies. It ratchets down its energy use by lowering body temperature, pulse rate, blood pressure, and resting metabolism. Frank becomes lethargic, reducing the amount of energy expended in activity. He also begins to have detectable signs of mild vitamin deficiencies as his body depletes its small reserves of vitamin C and most B vitamins.

If Frank's body continued to rapidly break down protein, he would survive less than three weeks. To avoid such a quick demise, protein breakdown slows drastically and gluconeogenesis drops by two-thirds or more.[25] To pick up the slack, Frank's body doubles the rate of fat catabolism to supply fatty acids for fuel and glycerol for glucose. Ketone bodies pour into the bloodstream and provide an important glucose-sparing energy source for the brain and red blood cells. After about 10 days of fasting, ketone bodies meet most of the nervous system's energy needs. Some brain cells, however, can use only glucose. To maintain a small, but essential, supply of blood glucose, protein breakdown crawls along, supplying small amounts of amino acids for gluconeogenesis.

Several Weeks of Fasting

After several weeks of fasting, Frank is increasingly susceptible to disease and infection. His severe micronutrient deficiencies add to his overall poor health.

The average person has about three weeks of fat stores, and the rate of fat depletion is fairly constant. As the later stages of starvation exhaust the final fat stores, the body turns again to protein, its sole remaining fuel source. Normally, Frank's body breaks down about 30 to 55 grams of protein each day, but now it accelerates the rate to several hundred grams daily. (See **Figure 7.25**.) You can see some of the effects of accelerated protein breakdown in starving children suffering from kwashiorkor. The loss of blood proteins causes the swollen limbs and bulging

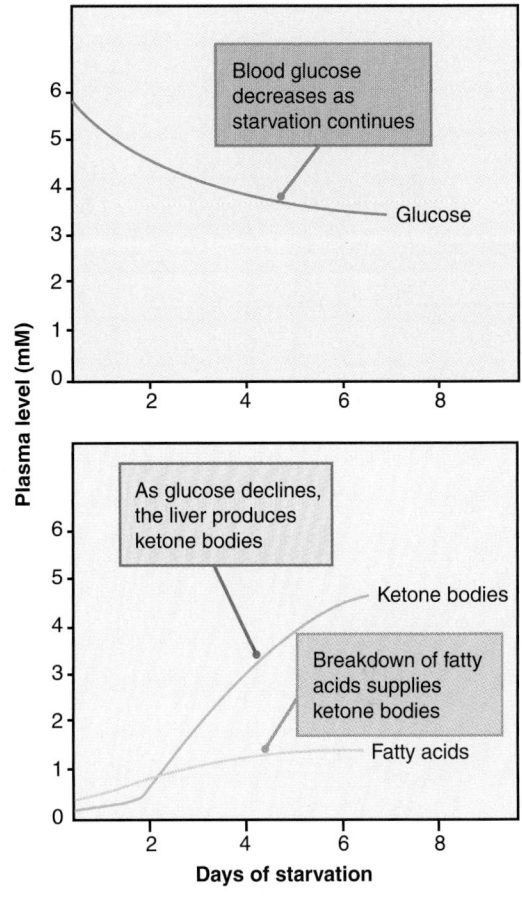

Figure 7.24 **Shifting fuel selection during starvation.** To fuel its needs as blood glucose levels decline, the body shifts from glucose to fatty acids and ketone bodies.

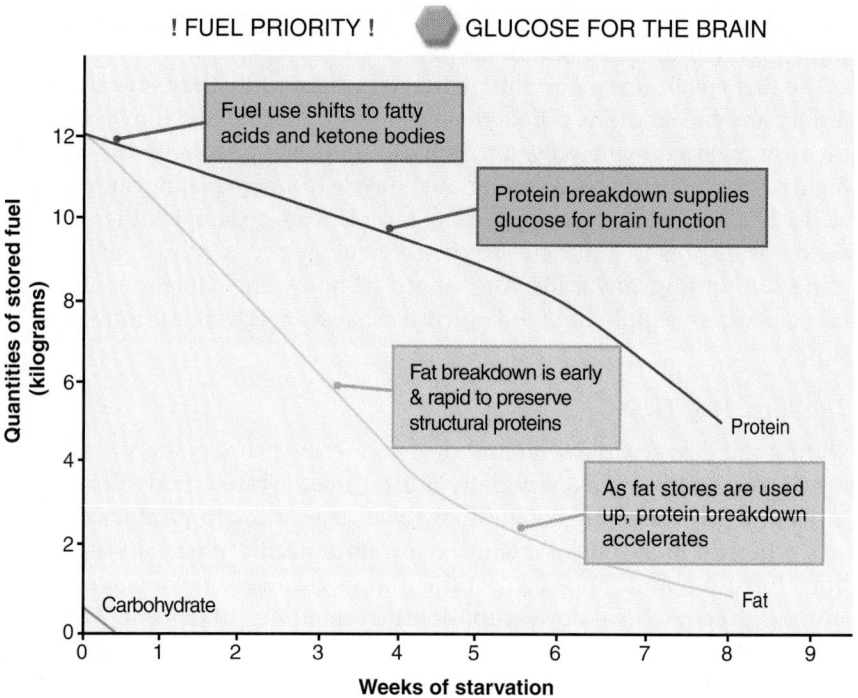

! FUEL PRIORITY ! GLUCOSE FOR THE BRAIN

Fuel use shifts to fatty acids and ketone bodies

Protein breakdown supplies glucose for brain function

Fat breakdown is early & rapid to preserve structural proteins

Protein

As fat stores are used up, protein breakdown accelerates

Carbohydrate

Fat

Figure 7.25 **Starvation and fuel sources.** During starvation, carbohydrate is exhausted quickly, and fat becomes the primary fuel. Burning fat without available carbohydrate produces ketone bodies, a by-product that the body can use as fuel. Glucose produced from amino acids and the glycerol portion of fatty acids help fuel the brain. The body conserves protein and breaks it down rapidly only after most fat stores are depleted.

stomachs that typify this type of protein-energy malnutrition (PEM). (For more detail on PEM, see Chapter 6, "Proteins and Amino Acids.").

The End Is Near

In the final stage of protein depletion, the body deteriorates rapidly. You can see the severe muscle atrophy and emaciation in photos of Holocaust victims. Their bodies sacrificed muscle tissue in attempts to preserve brain tissue. Even organ tissues were not spared. The final stage of starvation attacks the liver and intestines, greatly depleting them. It moderately depletes the heart and kidneys, and even mounts a small attack on the nervous system. Amazingly, starving people can cling to life until they lose about half their body proteins, after which death generally occurs.

How long can a person survive total starvation? Several years ago, some Irish prisoners starved themselves to death—the average time was 60 days.[26] Most people survive total starvation for one to three months. Starvation survival factors include the following:

- *Starting percentage of body fat:* Ample adipose tissue prolongs survival.

- *Age:* Middle-aged people survive longer than children and the elderly.

- *Sex:* Women fare better due to their higher proportion of body fat.

- *Energy expenditure levels:* Increased activity leads to an earlier demise.

Key Concepts: *Fasting, or underconsumption of energy (calories), favors catabolic pathways. The body first obtains fuel from stored glycogen, and then from stored fat and functional proteins, such as muscle. Over time, the body adapts to using increasing amounts of ketone bodies as fuel because limited carbohydrate is available. Larger stores of fat in adipose tissue extend survival time during starvation. In prolonged starvation, the body catabolizes muscle tissue to continue minimal production of glucose from amino acids.*

Psychological Stress

Our bodies respond to stress in the same way that they respond to danger—we mobilize for "fight or flight." In primitive times, this response would culminate in intense physical activity; we actually did fight or flee. In modern times, there often is no such physical outlet. Also, the specific short-term triggering event, such as an attack by a lion, has been largely replaced by a never-ending assault from noise, overcrowding, competition, and economic pressures. Today, many people suffer from chronic stress—a condition that scientists have linked to diseases such as hypertension and heart disease that are common in the modern world.

Chronic psychological stress can increase glucose production while impairing glucose uptake, so that a person needs more insulin for glucose to enter cells. When stressed, our bodies increase the availability of biological building blocks and ramp up energy production, especially in muscle tissues that are related to movement. Stress hormones, including epinephrine, cortisol, growth hormone, and glucagon, stimulate the breakdown of glycogen and the production of glucose. The elevated levels of blood glucose and increased metabolic rate provide energy to help us respond to threats, whether real or perceived.

Cells prepare for action by taking up glucose at a near maximal rate.[27] This uptake slows the assimilation of new glucose. When the danger passes, cells need higher than normal amounts of insulin to return blood glucose to baseline levels. This condition, called glucose intolerance, is a known complication of chronic stress.[28]

Diabetes and Obesity

In type 1 diabetes mellitus, a lack of insulin limits the cellular uptake of glucose. The starving, glucose-deprived cells signal the liver to make more glucose. This combination of limited uptake and increased production causes abnormally high blood glucose levels. The starving cells turn to fatty acids for energy. Inside the cells, the increased rate of fatty acid oxidation, along with a lack of glucose, leads to the production of ketone bodies. In untreated type 1 diabetes mellitus, ketone bodies accumulate rapidly, causing ketosis and producing the characteristic smell of acetone on the breath. The blood becomes acidic, and the condition of a person with untreated type 1 diabetes mellitus can progress quickly to coma and death.

Obese people and individuals with type 2 diabetes mellitus often have only mildly elevated blood glucose levels, elevated fasting insulin levels, and glucose intolerance. Although insulin levels are adequate, their cells have difficulty taking up glucose, possibly due to a problem with insulin receptors. Because some glucose enters the cells, ketosis is less common among people with type 2 diabetes. (For more details on diabetes, see Chapter 14, "Diet and Health.")

Exercise

Exercise increases not only muscle fitness, but also "cell fitness" by enhancing the ability of cells to take up glucose. In fact, regular exercise often can reduce the need for insulin in a person with diabetes.

Carbohydrate and fat are the primary fuels for physical activity, providing more than 90 percent of the energy used by contracting skeletal muscle. During low-intensity aerobic activities, such as walking, fat is a good fuel source. Carbohydrate is better suited to fuel high-intensity anaerobic efforts, such as fast running, that can be maintained for only a few minutes. As exercise intensity moves from low to high, the mix of fuels burned moves gradually from mostly fat to mostly carbohydrate. Which fuel pre-

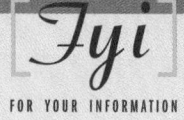

Metabolic Profiles of Important Sites

Brain

What powers your brain? Glucose! But brain cells cannot store glucose, so they need a constant supply. Your brain uses about 120 grams of glucose daily, which corresponds to a dietary energy intake of about 420 kilocalories. When your body's at rest, your brain accounts for about 60 percent of your glucose use.[1]

What happens during starvation? When glucose is in short supply, the liver comes to the rescue by converting fatty acids to ketone bodies. Ketone bodies are a critical source of replacement fuel that augments the supply of glucose to the brain.

Still, some brain cells can use only glucose. These cells survive by breaking down amino acids to make glucose via gluconeogenesis.[2]

Muscle

Muscle can use a variety of fuels—lactate, fatty acids, ketone bodies, glucose, and pyruvate. Unlike your brain, muscle stores large amounts of carbohydrate fuel—about 1,200 kilocalories—in the form of glycogen. This represents about three-fourths of the glycogen in your body. To fuel bursts of activity, muscle cells readily obtain glucose from glycogen.[3]

When your muscles actively contract, they rapidly deplete available oxygen, thus inhibiting the production of ATP via the aerobic breakdown pathways. ATP formed during glycolysis becomes the primary fuel. Muscle cells use the pyruvate from glycolysis to form lactate. The lactate travels to the liver, which converts it to glucose. The glucose returns to your muscle cells and undergoes anaerobic glycolysis. Known as the Cori cycle, this pathway rapidly produces ATP while shifting part of the metabolic burden from your muscles to your liver.

While fatty acids are the primary fuel for muscles at rest, glycogen and glucose fuel short, intense activity, such as when you are sprinting to arrive at class on time. During prolonged exercise, such as running a marathon, fatty acid oxidation kicks in to help out. Fatty

acids can directly supply energy or form ketone bodies to augment the fuel supply.

Your muscle cells are major sites for glycolysis, beta-oxidation, and the common aerobic breakdown pathways—the citric acid cycle and the electron transport chain.

Adipose Tissue

Adipose tissue is your body's primary energy storage depot. A 55-kilogram (121-pound) woman with 25 percent body fat (a healthy body composition) stores about 105,000 kilocalories in adipose tissue, enough energy to

dominates has important implications for how long an activity can be maintained. (See the Science in Action feature "Fuel for Distance Walking.")

Key Concepts: *Chronic psychological stress can cause glucose intolerance, so that a person needs more insulin for glucose to enter cells. In uncontrolled diabetes mellitus, cells react much as they do in starvation. Untreated type 1 diabetes mellitus can cause a dangerous accumulation of ketone bodies and acidification of the blood. Exercise enhances glucose uptake. Depending on the duration and intensity of exercise, your body chooses different mixes of metabolic fuels.*

Quick Bites

Sweet Urine

The word *diabetes* is Greek for "siphon," from *dia*, meaning "through," and *bainein*, meaning "to go." The word *mellitus* is Latin for "sweetened with honey." *Diabetes mellitus* means the flow of sweetened water. The disease causes a rise in blood sugar that spills into the urine. As early as the 1600s, some doctors would taste a patient's urine to confirm a diagnosis of diabetes mellitus.

run 40 marathons! Your liver assembles fatty acids into triglycerides and sends them to adipose tissue for storage. Eighty to 90 percent of the volume of an adipose cell is pure triglyceride.[4]

To supply fatty acids for energy production, adipose cells break down triglycerides to glycerol and free fatty acids.

Liver

Most substances absorbed by your intestines eventually pass through the liver, the body's main metabolic factory. This versatile organ performs glycolysis, gluconeogenesis, beta-oxidation, lipogenesis, ketogenesis, and cholesterol synthesis.

Your liver can store up to 400 kilocalories of glucose as glycogen. When blood glucose levels are low, the liver breaks down stored glycogen to glucose or makes glucose from noncarbohydrate precursors. Several sources pitch in to provide glucose building blocks: muscle supplies lactate and the amino acid alanine; adipose tissue supplies glycerol; and your diet supplies glucogenic amino acids.

The liver is the traffic cop for lipid metabolism. When energy is abundant, the liver directs fatty acids to storage. When energy is scarce, the liver breaks down fatty acids to form ATP. If an inadequate amount of carbohydrate blocks the entry of acetyl CoA into the citric acid cycle, the liver redirects fatty acids to ketone bodies.

Kidney

Your kidneys are important disposal systems of metabolic wastes. Without rapid elimination, these wastes can build up to toxic levels. When your liver deaminates amino acids (removes amino groups), a cooperative effort eliminates the released nitrogen. Your liver captures the nitrogen in urea, which it releases into the bloodstream. The kidneys filter out the urea and excrete it in urine.

The kidneys can make glucose (gluconeogenesis) from amino acids and other precursors. During prolonged starvation, the kidneys produce glucose in amounts that rival production by the liver![5]

Heart

Your heart relies on an interesting mix of fuels. Rather than glucose, which it uses in only small amounts, your heart relies on free fatty acids, lactate, and ketone bodies. During normal conditions, free fatty acids supply the bulk of its energy.[6] When glucose is in short supply, your heart makes a special effort to spare its use. It uses ketone bodies, then free fatty acids, and finally glucose as its fuel source.[7] During heavy exercise, your body releases large amounts of lactate into the bloodstream. Compared to other types of tissue, your heart is particularly capable of using lactate to supply the energy it needs.[8]

Red Blood Cells

Just like the brain, red blood cells rely primarily on glucose for fuel. In these cells, glycolysis and the pentose phosphate pathway (an alternative energy-producing pathway), extract energy from glucose. Since red blood cells have no mitochondria, they do not contain the pathways for beta-oxidation, the citric acid cycle, or the electron transport chain.

The pentose phosphate pathway generates the NADPH that is critical for a red blood cell's health. Energy carried by NADPH helps maintain cell membrane pliability and ion transport capabilities. NADPH also helps preserve iron in the cell's hemoglobin and prevent premature breakdown of the cell's proteins.[9]

1 Berg JM, Tymoczko JL, Stryer L. *Biochemistry*. 5th ed. New York: WH Freeman, 2002.

2 Guyton AC, Hall JE. *Textbook of Medical Physiology*. 10th ed. Philadelphia: WB Saunders, 2000.

3 Berg JM, Tymoczko JL, Stryer L. Op. cit.

4 Guyton AC, Hall JE. Op. cit.

5 Ibid.

6 Schaap FG, van der Vusse GJ, Glatz JF. Fatty acid-binding proteins in the heart. *Mol Cell Biochem*. 1998;180:1–2, 43–51.

7 Murray RK, et al. *Harper's Biochemistry*. 25th ed. Stamford, CT: Appleton & Lange, 1999.

8 Guyton AC, Hall, JE. Op. cit.

9 Ibid.

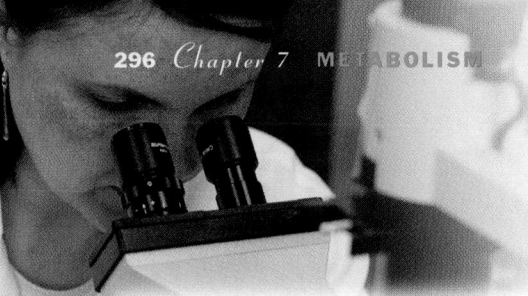
NUTRITION SCIENCE IN ACTION
Fuel for Distance Walking

Observations: Humans naturally select a preferred walking speed (PWS), and the body's fuel selection can be critical to the total distance traveled. The body primarily uses carbohydrate (CHO) to fuel short, intense bursts of activity and uses fat to fuel endurance exercise. Lean humans store far more energy as fat than as CHO, and the choice of fuel may produce a 30-fold difference in the distance traveled.

Hypothesis: Humans select a preferred walking speed that primarily uses fat as fuel and does not deplete carbohydrate stores.

Experimental Plan: Recruit 12 healthy adults. Time the subjects as they walk four laps at their natural rate around a 53-meter track. After resting 10 minutes, subjects walk on a level treadmill for 10-minute increments at 3.2, 4.0, 4.8, 5.6, 6.4, and 7.2 kilometers per hour (kph). Using indirect calorimetry, estimate fat and CHO oxidation during each increment.

Treadmill data collection

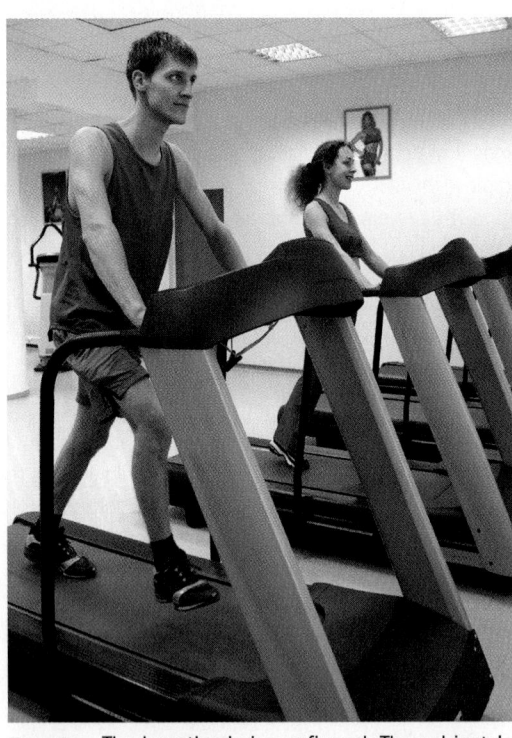

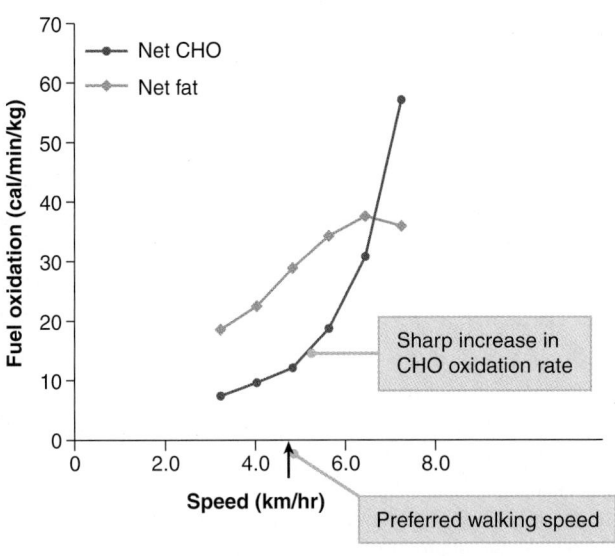

Results: The hypothesis is confirmed. The subjects' natural PWS was 4.7 kph. At speeds less than 4.8 kph, CHO oxidation rates remain low and fat oxidation is the primary fuel. At about 4.8 kph and beyond, CHO oxidation increases abruptly and rises rapidly.

Conclusion and Discussion: The major finding of this study was that able-bodied subjects naturally selected a walking speed just below the speed preceding an abrupt rise in CHO oxidation that would deplete the body's small stores of CHO quickly.

In a historical context, people able to naturally select the walking speed resulting in the greatest range would have a survival advantage when challenged with walking away from a region of food scarcity. Moreover, minimizing CHO depletion would defend the person's ability to engage in burst activity to escape predators or capture prey during the trek.

Source: Based on Willis WT, Ganley KJ, Herman RM. Fuel oxidation during human walking. *Metabolism.* 2005;54(6):793–799.

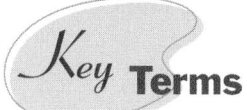

LEARNING *Portfolio* chapter 7

Key Terms

Study Points

➤ Energy is necessary to do any kind of work. The body converts chemical energy from food sources—carbohydrates, proteins, and fats—into a form usable by cells.

➤ Anabolic reactions (anabolism) build compounds. These reactions require energy.

➤ Catabolic reactions (catabolism) break compounds into smaller units. These reactions produce energy.

➤ Adenosine triphosphate, ATP, is the energy currency of the body.

➤ NADH, FADH₂, and NADPH are important carriers of hydrogen and high-energy electrons. NADH and FADH₂ are used in making ATP, while NADPH is used in biosynthetic reactions.

➤ Cells extract energy from carbohydrate via four main pathways: glycolysis, conversion of pyruvate to acetyl CoA, the citric acid cycle, and the electron transport chain.

➤ The citric acid cycle and electron transport chain require oxygen. Glycolysis does not.

➤ The electron transport chain produces more ATP than other catabolic pathways.

➤ To extract energy from fat, first triglycerides are separated into glycerol and fatty acids. Next, beta-oxidation breaks down the fatty acids to yield acetyl CoA, NADH, and FADH₂. The acetyl CoA enters the citric acid cycle, producing more NADH and FADH₂. The NADH and FADH₂ molecules deliver their high-energy electrons to the electron transport chain to make ATP.

➤ To extract energy from an amino acid, first it is deaminated (the amino group is removed). Depending on the structure of the remaining carbon skeleton, it enters the catabolic pathways as pyruvate, acetyl CoA, or a citric acid cycle intermediate. The citric acid cycle and the electron transport chain complete the production of ATP.

➤ The liver converts the nitrogen portion of amino acids to urea, which the kidneys excrete.

➤ Tissues differ in their preferred source of fuel. The brain, nervous system, and red blood cells rely primarily on glucose, while other tissues use a mix of glucose, fatty acids, and ketone bodies as fuel sources.

➤ When carbohydrate is available, glucose can be stored as glycogen in liver and muscle tissue.

➤ Glucose can be produced from the noncarbohydrate precursors glycerol and some (glucogenic) amino acids, but not from fatty acids.

➤ The hormone insulin regulates metabolism by favoring anabolic pathways. It promotes the uptake of glucose by cells, thus removing it from the bloodstream.

➤ Glucagon, cortisol, and epinephrine stimulate catabolic pathways. These hormones promote the breakdown of glycogen to glucose and of amino acids to make glucose via gluconeogenesis. The breakdown of liver glycogen increases the amount of glucose in the blood.

➤ Feasting, or overconsumption of energy, leads to glycogen and triglyceride storage.

➤ Fasting, or underconsumption of energy, leads to the mobilization of liver glycogen and stored triglycerides. Starvation, the state of prolonged fasting, leads to protein breakdown as well and can be fatal.

Study Questions

1. What is the "universal energy currency"? Where is most of it produced?

2. Name the two energy-equivalent molecules that contain three phosphates as part of their structure. What makes these two molecules different? How many high-energy phosphate bonds do they contain?

3. In the catabolic pathways, which two molecules are major electron acceptors? After they accept electrons, which electron carriers do they become? What is the primary function of the electron carriers?

4. How many pyruvate molecules does glycolysis produce from one glucose molecule? What does the oxidative step after glycolysis produce? What does the citric acid cycle produce from a single glucose molecule?

5. Which two-carbon molecules does beta-oxidation form as it "clips" the links of a fatty acid chain? Which other molecules important to the production of ATP does beta-oxidation produce?

6. What dictates whether an amino acid is considered ketogenic or glucogenic?

7. What are ketone bodies and when are they produced?

8. Name the three tissues where energy is stored. Which contains the largest store of energy?

9. Define gluconeogenesis and lipogenesis. Under what conditions do they predominantly occur? What are their primary inputs and outputs?

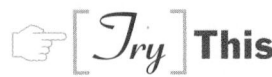 ☞ [*Try*] **This**

Comparing Fad Diets

The purpose of this exercise is to have you evaluate two fad diets in regard to their metabolic consequences. The two diets, Cabbage Soup and Super Protein, are described below. Once you've reviewed them, answer the following questions: Will these diets result in weight loss? Why or why not? On the seventh day of each diet, which of the following metabolic pathways will be highly active?

- Glycogen breakdown
- Fat breakdown
- Gluconeogenesis
- Ketogenesis

Diet 1: The Cabbage Soup Diet

A person following the Cabbage Soup diet eats only a water-based soup made out of cabbage and a few other vegetables. Three to four meals per day of this restricted diet supply approximately 500 kilocalories per day. The diet is devoid of protein and fat and gets its calories from the small amount of carbohydrate in the vegetables. Think about what happens during starvation.

Diet 2: The Super Protein Diet

In the Super Protein diet, a person can eat an unlimited amount of protein-rich foods such as meat, poultry, eggs, and seafood, but no added fats or carbohydrates are allowed. The average person can consume about 1,400 kilocalories if he or she eats three or four small meals each day. Think about what happens when little carbohydrate is available as a person metabolizes fat and protein.

Fasting for Ketones

The purpose of this experiment is to see whether a day without eating will cause your body to produce measurable ketones in your urine. Before starting your fast, check with your physician to be sure this won't pose any health risks. Go to your local pharmacy and ask the pharmacist for urine ketone strips (often called Ketostix). Bring them home and read the directions. Before you start your one-day fast, test your urine to see whether it has a detectable amount of ketones. Start a 24-hour fast (or fast for as long as you can go without food or calorie-containing fluids, but no longer than 24 hours) and test your urine at 6-hour intervals. Do you detect a color change on the strips as the day goes on? Why? What has happened metabolically as the day progresses?

Remember to drink lots of water!

References

1 Alberts B, Johnson A, Lewis J, et al. *Molecular Biology of the Cell.* 4th ed. New York: Garland, 2002.

2 Stipanuk MH. *Biochemical and Physiological Aspects of Human Nutrition.* Philadelphia: WB Saunders, 2000.

3 Murray RK, Granner DK, Mayes PA, Rodwell VW. *Harper's Biochemistry.* 25th ed. Stamford, CT: Appleton & Lange, 1999.

4 Berg JM, Tymoczko JL, Stryer L. *Biochemistry.* 5th ed. New York: W.H. Freeman, 2002.

5 Stipanuk MH. Op. cit.

6 Campbell MK. *Biochemistry.* 3rd ed. Philadelphia: Saunders College Publishing, 1999; and Berg JM, Tymoczko JL, Stryer L. Op. cit.

7 Burge B. Carnitine in energy production. *Healthline.* July 1999.

8 Hawley JA, Brouns F, Jeukendrup A. Strategies to enhance fat utilization during exercise. *Sports Med.* 1998;25(4):241–257; and Brass EP, Hiatt WR. The role of carnitine and carnitine supplementation during exercise in man and individuals with special needs. *J Am Coll Nutr.* 1998;17(3):207–215.

9 Hellerstein MK, Schwartz JM, Neese RA. Regulation of hepatic de novo lipogenesis in humans. *Ann Rev Nutr.* 1996;16: 527–557; and Hellerstein MK. No common energy currency: de novo lipogenesis as the road less traveled. *Am J Clin Nutr.* 2001;74:707–708.

10 Berg JM, Tymoczko JL, Stryer L. Op. cit.

11 Stein JH. *Internal Medicine.* 4th ed. St. Louis, MO: Mosby-Yearbook, 1994.

12 Murray RK, et al. Op. cit.

13 Martini FH. *Fundamentals of Anatomy and Physiology.* 6th ed. San Francisco: Benjamin Cummings, 2004.

14 Anderson JW. Prevention and management of diabetes mellitus. In: Shils ME, Shike M, Ross CA, Cabellero B, Cousins RJ, eds. *Modern Nutrition in Health and Disease.* 10th ed. Philadelphia: Lippincott Williams & Wilkins, 2006; 1043–1066.

15 Guyton AC, Hall JE. *Textbook of Medical Physiology.* 10th ed. Philadelphia: WB Saunders, 2000.

16 Murray RK, et al. Op. cit.

17 Griffin JE, Ojeda SR. *Textbook of Endocrine Physiology.* 4th ed. New York: Oxford University Press, 2000.

18 Shah M, Garg A. High-fat and high-carbohydrate diets and energy balance. *Diabetes Care.* 1996;19(10):1142–1152.

19 Stubbs RJ, Prentice AM, James WP. Carbohydrates and energy balance. *Ann NY Acad Sci.* 1997;819:44–69.

20 Murray RK, et al. Op. cit.

21 Martini FH. Op. cit.

22 Scheele JS. A comparison of the concentrations of certain pesticides and polychlorinated hydrocarbons in bone marrow and fat tissue. *J Environ Pathol Toxicol Oncol.* 1998:17(1): 65–68.

23 Gower T. The fasting cure. *Health.* April 1999:61–63.

24 Guyton AC, Hall JE. Op. cit.

25 Ibid.

26 Ganong WF. *Review of Medical Physiology.* 24th ed. Stamford, CT: McGraw-Hill, 2003.

27 Battilana P, Seematter G, Schneiter P, et al. Effects of free fatty acids on insulin sensitivity and hemodynamics during mental stress. *J Clin Endocrinol Metab.* 2001;86:124–128.

28 Summers RL, Woodward LH, Sanders DY, Hall JE. Graphic analysis for the study of metabolic states. *Adv Physiol Ed.* 1996;15(1):S81–S87.

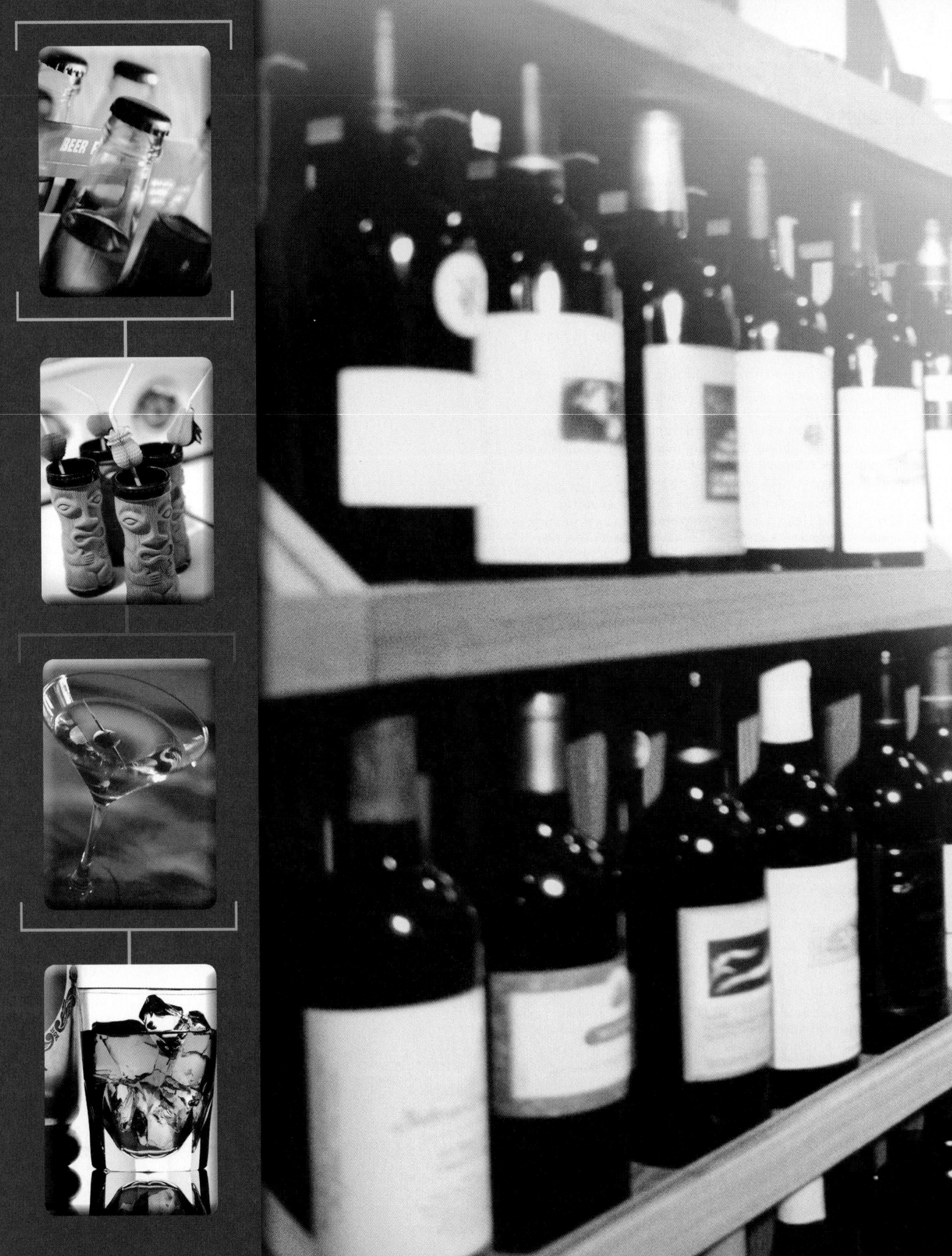

Spotlight on

Alcohol

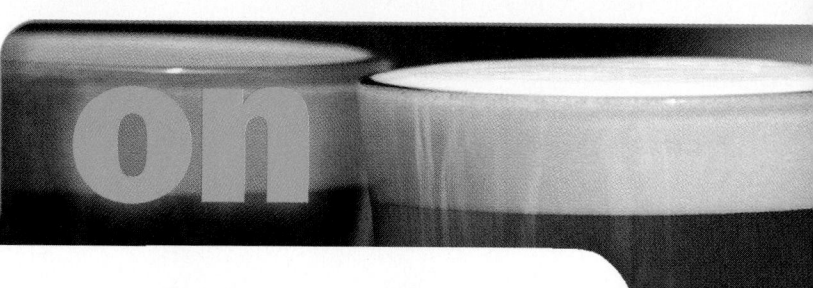

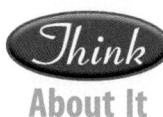
Think About It

1 Have you ever thought of alcohol as a poison?

2 In a word or two, how would you describe alcohol? Is it a nutrient?

3 What's your impression of the alcohol content of wine compared to that of beer? How about compared to vodka?

4 After a night of drinking and carousing, your friend awakens with a splitting headache and asks you for a pain reliever. What would you recommend?

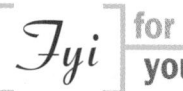
Fyi for your Information

This chapter's FYI boxes include practical information on the following topics:

• Changing the Culture of Campus Drinking

• Myths About Alcohol

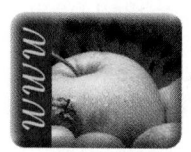

The Web site for this book offers many useful tools and is a great source for additional nutrition information for both students and instructors. Visit the site at **nutrition.jbpub.com** for information on alcohol. You'll find exercises that explore the following topics:

• Time to Hand over the Car Keys?

• Diabetics and Alcohol

• The Culture of Alcohol

Key to Illustrations

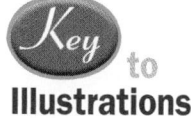 Alcohol

 Enzymes

 Fatty Acids

 Glycerol

 Triglycerides

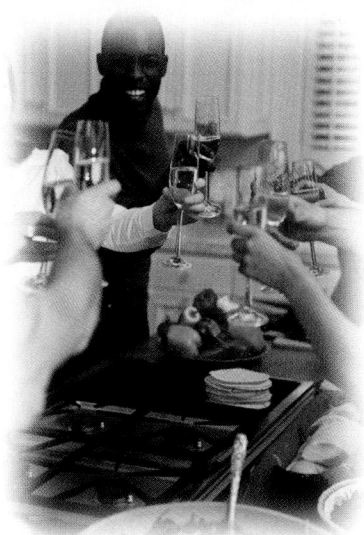

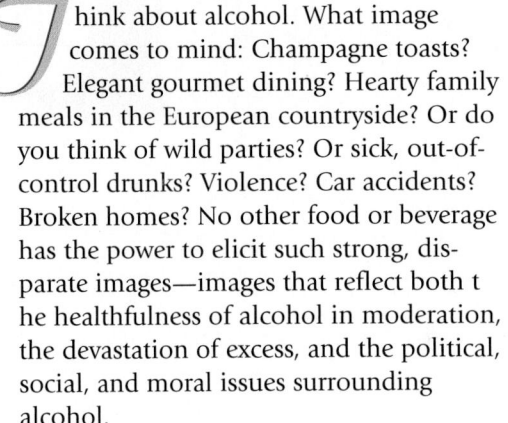

*T*hink about alcohol. What image comes to mind: Champagne toasts? Elegant gourmet dining? Hearty family meals in the European countryside? Or do you think of wild parties? Or sick, out-of-control drunks? Violence? Car accidents? Broken homes? No other food or beverage has the power to elicit such strong, disparate images—images that reflect both the healthfulness of alcohol in moderation, the devastation of excess, and the political, social, and moral issues surrounding alcohol.

Alcohol has a long and checkered history. More drug than food, alcoholic beverages produce druglike effects in the body while providing little, if any, nutrient value other than energy. Yet it still is important to consider alcohol in the study of nutrition. Alcohol is common to the diets of many people. In moderation, it may impart significant health benefits, yet even small quantities can raise risks for birth defects and breast cancer. In large amounts, it interferes with our intake of nutrients as well as the body's ability to use them, and it causes significant damage to every organ system in the body. The *Dietary Guidelines for Americans* advises us, "Those who choose to drink alcohol should do so sensibly and in moderation—defined as the consumption of up to one drink per day for women and up to two drinks per day for men."[1]

For most people, alcohol consumption is a pleasant social activity. Moderate alcohol use does not harm most adults. Nonetheless, many people have serious trouble with drinking. Episodes of heavy drinking are common among adult populations and are on the rise.[2] Adult excessive drinkers and underage drinkers currently account for half of all alcohol consumption and half of consumer spending on alcohol.[3] Heavy drinking can increase the risk for certain cancers. It can also cause liver cirrhosis, brain damage, and harm to the fetus during pregnancy. In addition, drinking increases the number of deaths from automobile crashes, recreational accidents, on-the-job accidents, homicide, and suicide. Underage alcohol use is more likely to kill young people than all illegal drugs combined.[4] A recent analysis found that alcohol use is the third leading actual cause of death in the United States, after tobacco use and poor diet and/or inactivity.[5]

History of Alcohol Use

Alcohol has had a prominent role throughout history. Old religious and medical writings frequently recommend its use, although with warnings for moderation. Thanks to alcohol's antiseptic properties, fermented drinks were safer than water during the centuries before modern sanitation, especially as people moved to towns and villages where water supplies were contaminated. Even mixing alcohol with dirty water afforded some protection from bacteria.[6]

At a time when life was filled with physical and emotional hardships, people valued alcohol for its analgesic and euphoric qualities. People relied on it to lift spirits, ease boredom, numb hunger, and dull the discomfort, even pain, of daily routine. Before the twentieth century, it was one of the few painkillers available in the Western world.

In sharp contrast to what is allowed today, drinking was often encouraged at the worksite. Workers might be given alcohol as an inducement to do boring, painful, or dangerous jobs. Distilled spirits, beers, and wines accompanied sailors and passengers on all long voyages, supplying relatively pathogen-free fluid and calories. Legend has it that even the Puritans, a group known for rigid morality, disembarked at Plymouth Rock because their beer supply was depleted.[7]

The Chemistry and Character of Alcohol

An **alcohol** is an organic compound that has one or more hydroxyl (–OH) groups (also called alcohol groups) in its structure. A compound name that ends in *ol* usually indicates an alcohol structure. For example, tocopherol is the alcohol form of vitamin E, retinol is the alcohol form of vitamin A, and glycerol is the alcohol that forms the backbone of triglycerides and phospholipids.

Forms of Alcohol

Outside of chemistry class, the term *alcohol* usually refers to the specific alcohol compound in beer, wine, and spirits. Its technical name is **ethanol**, or **ethyl alcohol**, a two-carbon compound with one hydroxyl group (see **Figure SA.1**). Ethanol is commonly abbreviated to "EtOH," shorthand often preferred by health professionals. In this chapter, when we use the term *alcohol*, we are referring to ethanol.

Not all alcohols are safe to drink. The simplest alcohol is **methanol**, also called **methyl alcohol** or **wood alcohol**, a solvent used in paints and for woodworking. Some years ago, down-on-their-luck alcoholics thought they had discovered a way to save money—wood alcohol used at that time to heat chafing dishes was intoxicating but considerably cheaper than beer or wine. Unfortunately, methanol caused blindness and death. Methanol is no longer used in these products, but methanol poisoning from other sources still occurs.[8] Today, methanol is used in a number of consumer products, including paint strippers, model airplane fuel, and dry gas. Most windshield washer fluids are 50 percent methanol.

Alcohol (ethanol) is a small molecule. Consequently, unlike starch, protein, and fat, it requires no digestive breakdown to be absorbed, and gastrointestinal absorption is quick and easy. Because of alcohol's unusual ability to cross the **blood–brain barrier**, it affects the brain directly. The blood–brain barrier prevents the passage of many compounds from the blood into the brain, and vice versa.

Organic Solvent

Fats and other lipophilic substances dissolve in alcohol. Thus, alcohol is used as an extract for fat-soluble flavors (in vanilla extract, for example) and as a carrier of medications. Ethanol can also dissolve microbial cell membranes and, until it was replaced by inedible isopropyl alcohol, was used as a topical disinfectant. Unfortunately, alcohol can irritate and damage human cells, making it a potent toxin.

Boiling Point

Alcohol boils at 172°F (78°C), a much lower temperature than water, which allows the distillation of pure alcohol. Many cooks use alcoholic beverages as an ingredient. During cooking, alcohol evaporates. When heated long enough, it dissipates almost entirely, leaving behind the flavors that were in the original alcohol product.

Think About It 1

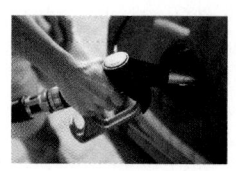

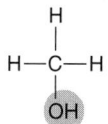
Methanol
(wood alcohol)

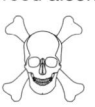

Methanol is an alcohol used as an alternative car fuel and in paint strippers, duplicator fluid, and model airplane fuels.

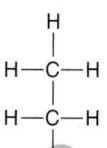
Ethanol
(EtOH)

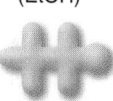

Ethanol is the alcohol in beer, wine, and liquor.

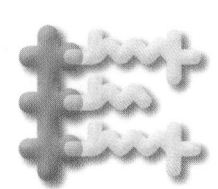
Glycerol

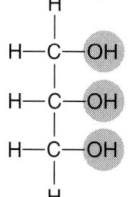

Glycerol is the alcohol that forms the backbone of triglyceride molecules.

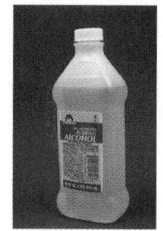
Isopropanol
(rubbing alcohol)

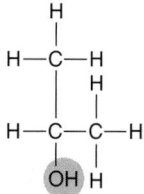

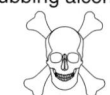

Isopropanol is an alcohol that is used as a disinfectant or solvent, and in making many commercial products.

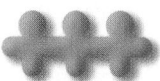

Figure SA.1 **Alcohols.** Ethanol is not the only alcohol people consume. When people eat fat, they consume the alcohol glycerol. Consuming the alcohol methanol or isopropanol can be deadly.

Quick Bites

Nutrients in Beer?

Most of the carbohydrate used in the production of alcohol is converted to ethanol. In beer, however, some carbohydrate remains, along with a little protein and some vitamins. So while it is technically correct to say there are nutrients in beer, the amounts are small when beer is consumed at recommended low levels.

fermentation The anaerobic conversion of various carbohydrates to carbon dioxide and an alcohol or organic acid accompanied by production of ATP.

congeners Biologically active compounds that include nonalcoholic ingredients as well as other alcohols such as methanol. Congeners contribute to the distinctive taste and smell of the beverage and may increase intoxicating effects and subsequent hangover.

Figure SA.2 **A moral and physical thermometer of temperance and intemperance.**
Created by physician and political figure Benjamin Rush (1745–1813).
Source: Reprinted with permission from *Quarterly Journal of Studies on Alcohol*, vol 4, pp. 321–341, 1943 (presently *Journal of Studies on Alcohol*), Copyright Journal of Studies on Alcohol, Inc., Rutgers Center of Alcohol Studies, Piscataway, NJ 08854.

Alcohol: Is It a Nutrient?

Alcohol eludes easy classification. Like fat, protein, and carbohydrate, it provides energy when metabolized. Laboratory experiments in the nineteenth century demonstrated that upon oxidation pure alcohol releases 7 kilocalories per gram, but many people doubted that it actually produced energy in the body. These doubts were the basis of the controversial conclusion that alcohol was not food—a conclusion used by early Prohibitionists as a weapon in their fight against alcohol. (See **Figure SA.2**.) However, a classic series of experiments by energy researchers Francis Atwater and Wilbur Benedict showed that alcohol did indeed produce 7 kilocalories per gram in the body—findings that were a great disappointment to the temperance movement, because the researchers showed that alcohol *was* a food.[9]

But alcohol's status as a *nutrient* is more questionable. It is certainly different from any other substance in the diet. It provides energy but is not essential, performing no necessary function in the body. Unlike the nutrients, alcohol is not stored in the body. And for no nutrient are the dangers of overconsumption so dramatic and the window of safety so narrow. In the small amounts most people usually consume, alcohol acts as a drug, producing a pleasant euphoria. For some people, it is addictive, with the characteristics of tolerance, dependence, and withdrawal symptoms. Certainly, alcohol is a substance available in the diet, but it does *not* meet the technical definition of a nutrient. (See Chapter 1, "Nutrients and Nourishment," for the definition of a nutrient.)

Think About
2

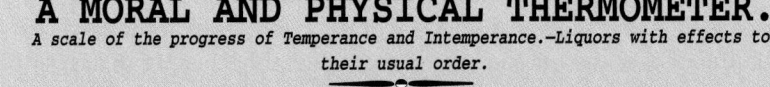

A MORAL AND PHYSICAL THERMOMETER.
A scale of the progress of Temperance and Intemperance.–Liquors with effects to their usual order.

TEMPERANCE.
Health and Wealth.

70	Water,	
60	Milk and Water,	
50	Small Beer,	} Serenity of Mind, Reputation, Long Life, & Happiness.
40	Cider and Perry	
30	Wine,	} Cheerfulness, Strength, and Nourishment, where taken
20	Porter,	only in small quantities, and at meals.
10	Strong Beer,	
0		

INTEMPERANCE.

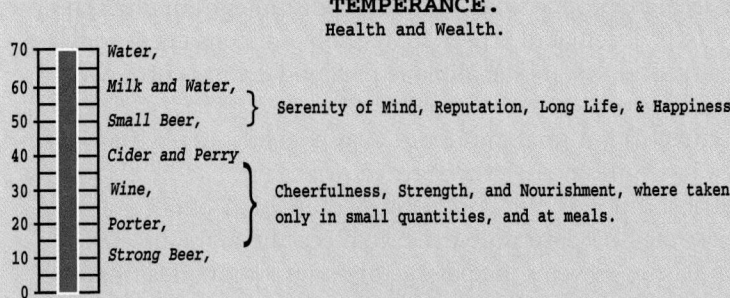

		VICES.	DISEASES.	PUNISHMENTS.
0		Idleness,	Sickness,	Debt.
10	Punch	Gaming,	Tremors of the hands in	Jail.
		peevishness,	the morning, puking,	
20	Toddy and Egg Rum,	quarreling	bloatedness,	Black eyes,
30	Grog–Brandy and Water,	Fighting	Inflamed eyes, red nose	and Rags,
		Horse–	and face,	Hospital or
40	Flip and Shrub,	Racing,	Sore and swelled legs,	Poor house.
	Bitters infused in	Lying and	jaundice,	
50	Spirits and Cordials.	Swearing,	Pains in the hands, burn–	Bridewell.
	Drams of Gin, Brandy,	Stealing &	ing in the hands, and feet	
60	and Rum, in the morning,	Swindling,	Dropsy, Epilepsy,	State prison
70	The same morning and	Perjury,	Melancholy, Palsy, Appe–	do for Life.
	evening, The same during	Burglary,	plexy, Madness, Despair	
	day & night,	Murder,		Gallows.

Key Concepts: *Alcohol, or more specifically, the compound ethyl alcohol, is a small organic molecule that has been part of people's diets for thousands of years. Although it provides calories, alcohol performs no essential function in the body and therefore is not a nutrient.*

Alcohol and Its Sources

When yeast cells metabolize sugar, they produce alcohol and carbon dioxide by a process called **fermentation**. If little oxygen is present, these cells produce more alcohol and less carbon dioxide. **Figure SA.3** shows living yeast cells.

Fermentation can occur spontaneously in nature—all that's needed is sugar, water, a warm environment, and yeast (whose spores are present in air and soil). Human experience with alcohol probably began at least 10,000 years ago with spontaneously fermented fruits or honey. Because all humans possess the enzymes to metabolize at least minimal amounts of alcohol, it's reasonable to assume that humans have always had small quantities of alcohol in their diets.[10] Very small amounts of alcohol are even produced by the microorganisms in our intestines.

Humans learned to make wine from fruits, mead from honey, and beer from grain, probably about 5,000 years ago. In some areas, people made alcohol-containing dairy products. Using simple yeast fermentation, they could not produce beverages with alcohol levels exceeding 16 percent—the point at which alcohol kills off the yeast, halting alcohol production. Later, seventh-century Egyptian chemists discovered how to use distillation to capture concentrated alcohol, which could be added to drinks to boost alcohol content. Distilled alcoholic beverages (such as rum, gin, and whiskey) are called spirits, liquor, or hard liquor.

Beer, wine, and liquor have different alcohol levels: Most beer is up to 5 percent alcohol, although some beers exceed 6 percent; wine is 8 to 14 percent alcohol; and hard liquor is typically 35 to 45 percent alcohol. Beer and wine are labeled with the percentage of alcohol, but hard liquor is labeled by "proof," which is twice the alcohol percentage (an 80-proof whiskey is 40 percent alcohol).

Pure alcohol—a clear, colorless liquid used in chemistry labs—is 95 percent alcohol. (Even "pure" alcohol contains some water.) The beverage closest to pure alcohol is vodka, which is alcohol, water, and almost nothing else; gin is similar but is flavored with juniper berries. Scotch, rum, rye, whiskeys, and other liquors have residual flavor traces of the grain from which they were fermented or flavors introduced during storage. All liquors, however, offer little nutritional value besides energy. Beer and wine do contain unfermented carbohydrates and a trace of protein but, like liquor, have negligible minerals. With the exception of niacin in beer (a 12-ounce beer contains 1.8 milligrams of niacin, nearly 10 percent of the Daily Value), alcoholic beverages have negligible vitamins as well. **Table SA.1** shows the amounts of calories in various alcoholic beverages.

Distillation can yield more than just ethanol. Traces of other volatile compounds, such as methanol, evaporate and then condense in the distilled product. Called **congeners**, these biologically active compounds help to create the distinctive taste, smell, and appearance of alcoholic beverages such as whiskey,

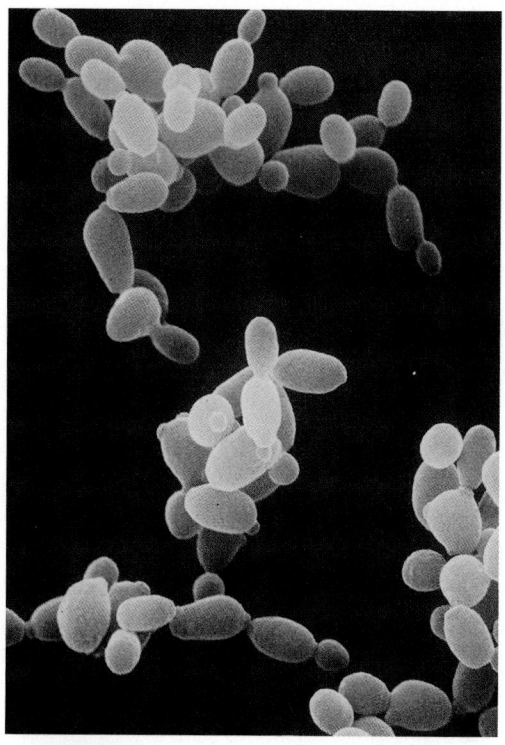

Figure SA.3 A yeast plant micrograph.

Table SA.1 Calories in Selected Alcoholic Beverages

Beverage	Serving Size (fl oz)	Approximate Kcalories
Beer (regular)	12	153
Beer (light)	12	103
White wine	5	122
Red wine	5	125
Sweet dessert wine	3.5	165
80-proof distilled spirits (gin, rum, vodka, whiskey)	1.5	97

This table is a guide to estimate the caloric intake from various alcoholic beverages. Higher alcohol content and mixing alcohol with other beverages, such as calorically sweetened soft drinks, tonic water, fruit juice, or cream, increases the amount of calories in the beverage. Alcoholic beverages supply calories but provide few essential nutrients.

Source: US Department of Agriculture, Agricultural Research Service, USDA National Nutrient Database for Standard Reference, Release 18. 2005. http://www.nal.usda.gov/fnic/foodcomp/search/. Accessed 7/9/06; and US Department of Health and Human Services and US Department of Agriculture, *Dietary Guidelines for Americans, 2005.* 6th ed. Washington, DC: US Government Printing Office, January 2005.

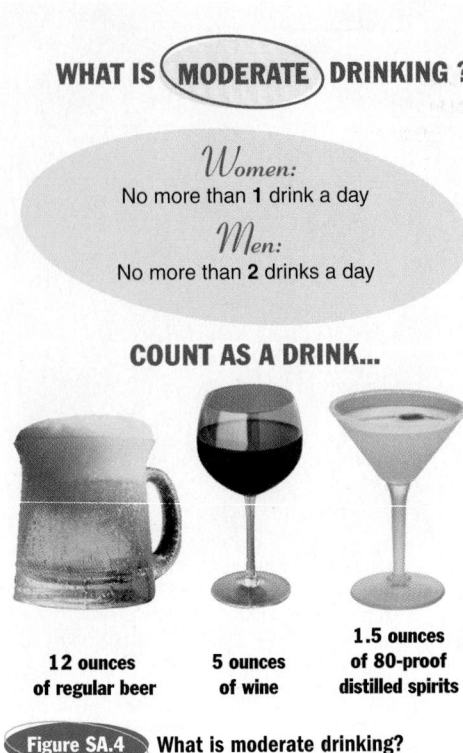

WHAT IS MODERATE DRINKING ?

Women:
No more than **1** drink a day

Men:
No more than **2** drinks a day

COUNT AS A DRINK...

12 ounces of regular beer

5 ounces of wine

1.5 ounces of 80-proof distilled spirits

Figure SA.4 **What is moderate drinking?** **Source:** USDA Center for Nutrition Policy and Promotion.

ALCOHOL ABSORPTION

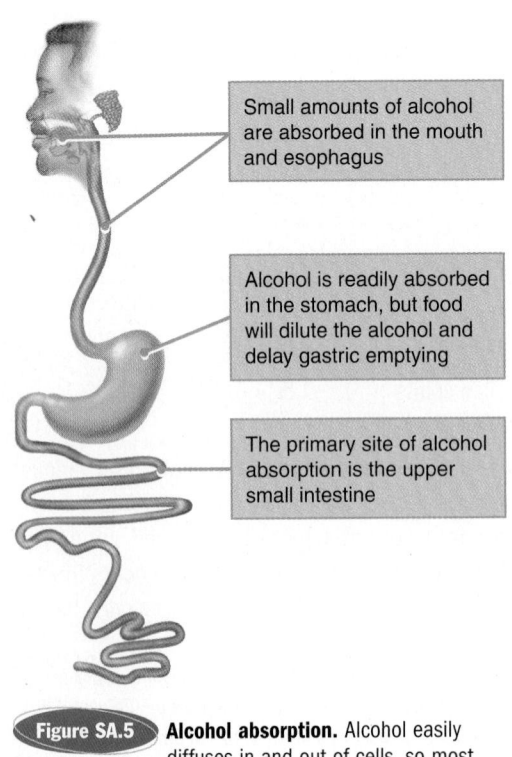

Small amounts of alcohol are absorbed in the mouth and esophagus

Alcohol is readily absorbed in the stomach, but food will dilute the alcohol and delay gastric emptying

The primary site of alcohol absorption is the upper small intestine

Figure SA.5 **Alcohol absorption.** Alcohol easily diffuses in and out of cells, so most alcohol is absorbed unchanged.

brandy, and red wine. But congeners are also suspected of causing or contributing to hangovers, and they may play a role in alcohol's relationship to cancer.[11]

One serving of alcohol, or a **standard drink**, is defined as 12 ounces of regular beer, 5 ounces of wine (12 percent alcohol), or 1.5 ounces (a "jigger") of 80-proof liquor.[12] All contain roughly 15 grams (one measuring tablespoon) of pure alcohol. (See **Figure SA.4**.) Most health professionals who speak of "moderate alcohol intake" usually mean no more than one (for women) or two (for men) servings in a day.[13] Moderate intake is *not* an average of seven drinks per week, when there are six days of abstinence followed by seven drinks in one night! That's **binge drinking** and it's dangerous.

Key Concepts: *Alcohol is formed when yeast ferments sugars to yield energy. Distillation methods produce concentrated solutions containing up to 95 percent alcohol. A typical serving of beer, wine, or distilled spirits contains about 15 grams of alcohol.*

Alcohol Absorption

Alcohol absorption begins immediately in the mouth and esophagus, where small quantities enter the bloodstream. Although alcohol absorption continues in the stomach, the small intestine efficiently absorbs most of the alcohol a person consumes.[14] (See **Figure SA.5**.)

You've heard it before: "Don't drink on an empty stomach." Eating before or with a drink slows down the rush of alcohol into the bloodstream in several ways. Food, especially if it contains fat, delays gastric emptying into the small intestine. The delay also provides a longer opportunity for oxidizing stomach enzymes to work. And food dilutes the stomach contents, lowering the concentration of alcohol and its rate of absorption.

About 80 to 95 percent of alcohol is absorbed unchanged. However, some oxidation does take place in the digestive tract, mainly in the stomach, and products of this metabolism join alcohol as it diffuses into the gut cells.[15] These products travel via the portal vein directly to the liver, where most alcohol metabolism takes place. When all goes well, metabolism achieves two goals: energy production and protection from the damaging effects of alcohol and its even more toxic metabolite **acetaldehyde**.

standard drink One serving of alcohol (about 15 grams), defined as 12 ounces of beer, 4 to 5 ounces of wine, or 1.5 ounces of liquor.

binge drinking Consuming excessive amounts of alcohol in short periods of time.

acetaldehyde A toxic intermediate compound (CH_3CHO) formed by the action of enzyme systems during the metabolism of alcohol.

alcohol dehydrogenase (ADH) The enzyme that catalyzes the oxidation of ethanol and other alcohols.

aldehyde dehydrogenase (ALDH) The enzyme that catalyzes the conversion of acetaldehyde to acetate, which forms acetyl CoA.

fatty liver Accumulation of fat in the liver, a sign of increased fatty acid synthesis.

microsomal ethanol-oxidizing system (MEOS) An energy-requiring enzyme system in the liver that normally metabolizes drugs and other foreign substances. When the blood alcohol level is high, alcohol dehydrogenase cannot metabolize it fast enough, and the excess alcohol is metabolized by MEOS.

Alcohol Metabolism

The body cannot store potentially harmful alcohol and so works extra hard to get rid of it. To prevent alcohol from accumulating and destroying cells and organs, the body quickly metabolizes it and removes it from the blood. The liver selectively metabolizes alcohol before other compounds and has alternative pathways to handle excess consumption. Alcohol is metabolized in three stages:

1. Alcohol is converted to acetaldehyde, a toxic and highly reactive substance.
2. Acetaldehyde is rapidly converted to acetate and then acetyl CoA.
3. Acetyl CoA either enters the citric acid cycle or is made into fatty acids.

Metabolizing Small Amounts of Alcohol

Alcohol dehydrogenase (ADH) is a zinc-containing enzyme that catalyzes the conversion of small to moderate amounts of alcohol to acetaldehyde, a toxic substance. (See **Figure SA.6**.) To avoid toxic buildup, another enzyme, **aldehyde dehydrogenase (ALDH)**, quickly and effectively converts acetaldehyde to acetate. People differ in their ability to eliminate toxic acetaldehyde, and small amounts of it are found in the blood of intoxicated people.[16]

Dehydrogenases in the gastrointestinal tract and the liver are responsible for almost all alcohol metabolism. Probably about 4 to 9 percent, but possibly as much as 20 percent, of alcohol is changed to acetaldehyde in the digestive tract.[17] Gastrointestinal aldehyde dehydrogenase does not completely convert acetaldehyde to acetate, however. The remaining acetaldehyde is more destructive than alcohol itself and can damage the mucous membranes lining the gut.[18]

The metabolic reactions that convert alcohol to acetaldehyde and acetaldehyde to acetate consume NAD+ while forming NADH. Acetate combines with coenzyme A to form acetyl CoA. The conversion of NAD+ to NADH and the resulting buildup of NADH dramatically slow the citric acid cycle, blocking the entry of acetyl CoA into this pathway. In the competition for the limited supply of NAD+, the detoxification of alcohol always takes priority over the operation of the citric acid cycle. This slowed citric acid cycle can process little acetyl CoA, be it from alcohol, carbohydrate, or fat. As a result, cells route most of the acetyl CoA to the synthesis of fatty acids, which are assembled into fat.

Fat accumulation in the liver can be seen after a single bout of heavy drinking, and fatty acid synthesis accelerates with chronic alcohol consumption. **Fatty liver** is the first stage of liver destruction in alcoholics.

Metabolizing Large Amounts of Alcohol

Large amounts of alcohol can overwhelm the alcohol dehydrogenase system, the usual metabolic path. As alcohol builds up, the body identifies it as a foreign substance and routes it into the primary overflow pathway, the **microsomal ethanol-oxidizing system (MEOS)**. The liver ordinarily uses the MEOS bypass pathway to metabolize drugs and detoxify "foreign" substances. Chronic heavy drinking appears to activate MEOS enzymes, which may be responsible for transforming the pain reliever acetaminophen into chemicals that can damage the liver. (See **Figure SA.7**.)

Quick Bites

Alcohol Aversion Therapy

*I*n alcohol aversion therapy, the medication disulfiram (Antabuse) deliberately blocks the conversion of toxic acetaldehyde to acetate (acetic acid). Even small amounts of alcohol trigger the highly unpleasant Antabuse–alcohol reaction, which includes a throbbing headache, breathing difficulties, nausea, copious vomiting, flushing, vertigo, confusion, and a drop in blood pressure.

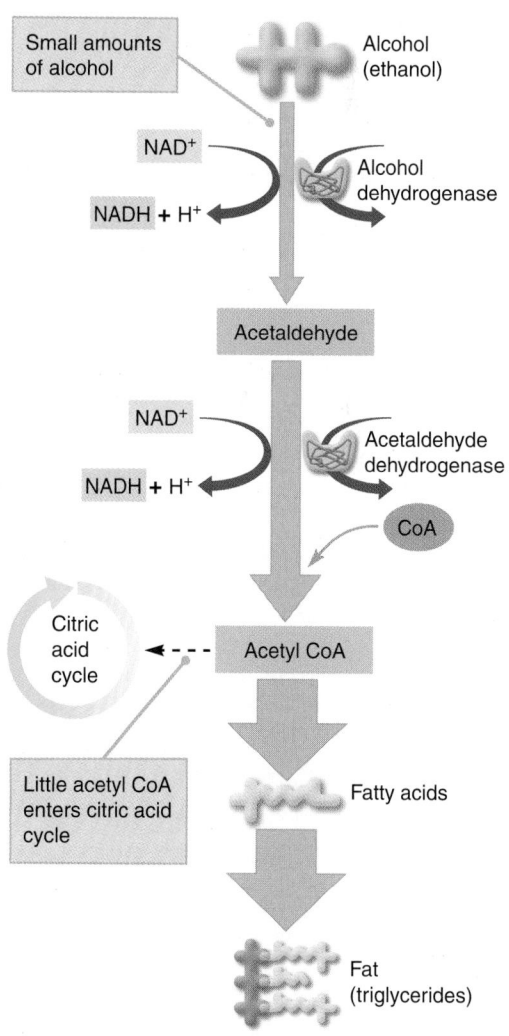

METABOLIZING SMALL TO MODERATE AMOUNTS OF ALCOHOL

Small amounts of alcohol — Alcohol (ethanol)

NAD+ → NADH + H+ — Alcohol dehydrogenase

Acetaldehyde

NAD+ → NADH + H+ — Acetaldehyde dehydrogenase — CoA

Citric acid cycle ◄--- Acetyl CoA

Little acetyl CoA enters citric acid cycle

Fatty acids

Fat (triglycerides)

Figure SA.6 Metabolizing alcohol. The metabolism of alcohol inhibits the citric acid cycle and primarily forms fat.

Quick Bites

How to Shock Your Surgeon

*I*f a former alcoholic neglects to disclose past alcohol use before undergoing surgery, the surgeon could be in for a big surprise. Even if the patient is now a teetotaler, his MEOS could still act like that of an alcoholic—operating at the faster speed it once needed to process alcohol quickly. The overactive MEOS would deplete anesthesia much quicker than expected. Theoretically, the patient could wake up in the middle of surgery, much to the shock of the surgeon. That's why anesthesiologists and surgeons ask their patients about alcohol use, past and present.

The MEOS pathway uses different enzymes than the alcohol dehydrogenase system. When transforming alcohol into acetaldehyde, it oxidizes NADPH to NADP (rather than reducing NAD⁺ to NADH). If this pathway is repeatedly exposed to large doses of alcohol, the MEOS pathway increases its capacity and processing speed. Whether alcoholics metabolize alcohol differently from nonalcoholics is unknown. Clearly, chronic ingestion of alcohol leads to changes in the liver, and the alcohol abuser acquires an increased tolerance to alcohol and to drugs such as sedatives, tranquilizers, and antibiotics.

Removing Alcohol from Circulation

Despite its multiple alcohol-processing pathways, the liver can metabolize only a certain amount of alcohol per hour, regardless of the amount in the bloodstream. The rate of alcohol metabolism depends on several factors, including the amount of metabolizing enzymes in the liver, and varies greatly between individuals. In general, after one standard drink, the amount of alcohol in the drinker's blood (blood alcohol concentration, or

THE MEOS OVERFLOW PATHWAY

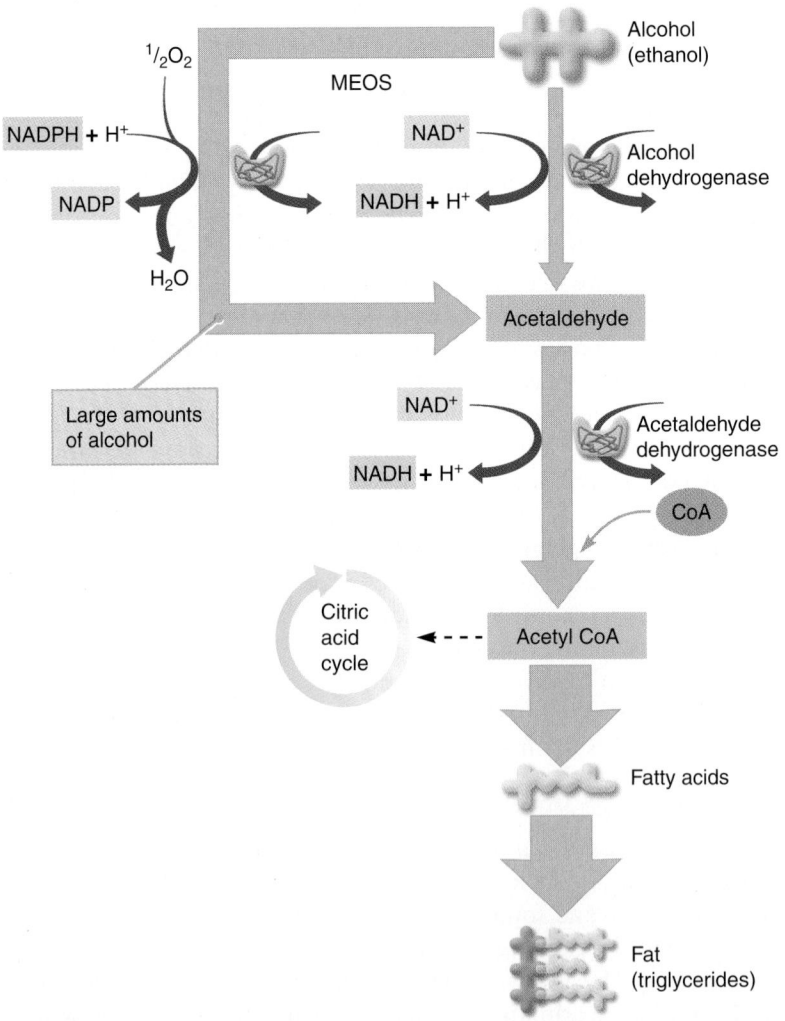

Figure SA.7 **The MEOS overflow pathway.** Large amounts of alcohol can overwhelm its typical metabolic route, so excess alcohol enters an overflow pathway called the microsomal ethanol-oxidizing system (MEOS).

BAC) peaks in 30 to 45 minutes. (See **Figure SA.8**.) When absorption exceeds the liver's capacity, a bottleneck develops and alcohol enters the general circulation. Alcohol diffuses rapidly, dispersing equally into all body fluids, including cerebrospinal fluid and the brain and, during pregnancy, into the placenta and fetus. About 10 percent of circulating alcohol is lost in urine, through the lungs, and through skin. Consequently, urine tests and breathalyzer tests both reflect concentrations of blood alcohol as well as alcohol levels in the brain, and can indicate how much a person's mental and motor functions may be impaired.

Excessive alcohol consumption deprives the brain of oxygen. The struggle to deal with an overdose of alcohol and lack of oxygen eventually causes the brain to shut down functions that regulate breathing and heart rate. This shutdown leads to a loss of consciousness and in some cases coma and death. When a drinker passes out, the body is actually protecting itself: When you lose consciousness, you can't add more alcohol to your system. When you hear of an **alcohol poisoning** death, it usually is the result of consuming such a large quantity of alcohol in such a short period of time that the brain of the victim is overwhelmed. Heart and lung functions shut down, and the person dies.

Even after a person stops drinking, alcohol in the stomach and intestine continues to enter the bloodstream and circulate throughout the body. Blood alcohol concentration continues to rise, and it is dangerous to assume that the person will be fine by sleeping it off. Rapid binge drinking (which often happens on a bet or a dare) is especially dangerous because the victim can ingest a fatal dose before becoming unconscious. Even if the victim lives, an alcohol overdose can lead to irreversible brain damage.

alcohol poisoning An overdose of alcohol. The body is overwhelmed by the amount of alcohol in the system and cannot metabolize it fast enough.

— One drink	0.10% - - -	
— Two drinks	0.05% - - -	
— Three drinks		
— Four drinks		

Figure SA.8 **Blood alcohol concentration over time.** Because the body metabolizes alcohol at a relatively constant rate, it clears small amounts faster than large amounts.
Source: National Institute on Alcohol Abuse and Alcoholism. Alcohol Alert No. 35. PH371; January 1997. http://pubs.niaaa.nih.gov/publications/aa35.htm. Accessed 7/9/06.

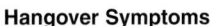

hangover The collection of symptoms experienced by someone who has consumed a large quantity of alcohol. Symptoms can include pounding headache, fatigue, muscle aches, nausea, stomach pain, heightened sensitivity to light and sound, dizziness, and possibly depression, anxiety, and irritability.

Hangover Symptoms

Constitutional—fatigue, weakness, and thirst

Pain—headache and muscle aches

Gastrointestinal—nausea, vomiting, and stomach pains

Sleep and biological rhythms—decreased sleep, decreased dreaming when asleep

Sensory—vertigo and sensitivity to light and sound

Cognitive—decreased attention and concentration

Mood—depression, anxiety, and irritability

Sympathetic hyperactivity—tremor, sweating, increased pulse, and blood pressure

Possible Contributing Factors

Direct effects of alcohol
- Dehydration
- Electrolyte imbalance
- Gastrointestinal disturbances
- Low blood sugar
- Sleep and biological rhythm disturbances

Alcohol withdrawal

Alcohol metabolism (i.e., acetaldehyde toxicity)

Nonalcohol factors
- Compounds other than alcohol in beverages, especially the congener methanol
- Use of other drugs, especially nicotine
- Personality traits such as neuroticism, anger, and defensiveness
- Negative life events and feelings of guilt about drinking
- Family history for alcoholism

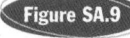 **Figure SA.9** **Hangover causes and symptoms.** Factors other than just alcohol contribute to the misery of a hangover.

The Morning After

After a night of heavy alcohol consumption, the drinker may suffer from a pounding headache, fatigue, muscle aches, nausea, and stomach pain as well as a heightened sensitivity to light and noise—a **hangover** in full force. The sufferer may be dizzy, have a sense that the room is spinning, and be depressed, anxious, and irritable. Usually a hangover begins within several hours after the last drink, when the blood alcohol level is dropping. Symptoms normally peak about the time the alcohol level reaches zero, and they may continue for an entire day.[19]

What causes a hangover? Scientists have identified several causes of the painful symptoms of a hangover. (See **Figure SA.9**.) Alcohol causes dehydration, which leads to headache and dry mouth. Alcohol directly irritates the stomach and intestines, contributing to stomach pain and vomiting. The sweating, vomiting, and diarrhea that can accompany a hangover cause additional fluid loss and electrolyte imbalance. Alcohol's hijack of the metabolic process diverts liver activity away from glucose production and can lead to low blood sugar (hypoglycemia), causing light-headedness and lack of energy. Alcohol also disrupts sleep patterns, interfering with the dream state and contributing to fatigue. The symptoms of a hangover are largely due to inflammation. During a hangover, blood levels of C-reactive protein are elevated and strongly associated with hangover severity.[20] In general, the greater the amount of alcohol consumed, the more likely a hangover will strike. However, some people experience a hangover after only one drink, whereas some heavy drinkers do not have hangovers.[21]

In addition, factors other than alcohol may contribute to the hangover. A person with a family history of alcoholism has increased vulnerability to hangover. Mixing alcohol and drugs is also suspected of increasing the likelihood of a hangover. The congeners in most alcoholic beverages can contribute to more vicious hangovers. Research shows that gin and vodka—beverages that contain less of these biologically active compounds—cause fewer headaches.[22]

Treating a Hangover

So what can you do about a hangover? Few treatments have undergone rigorous, scientific investigation. Time is the most effective treatment—symptoms usually disappear in 8 to 24 hours. Eating bland foods that contain complex carbohydrates, such as toast or crackers, can combat low blood sugar and possibly nausea. Sleep can ease fatigue, and drinking nonalcoholic, noncaffeinated beverages can alleviate dehydration (caffeine is a diuretic and increases urine production). Taking vitamin B_6 or an extract from *Optunia ficus indica* (a type of prickly pear cactus) before drinking may reduce the severity of hangover symptoms.[23] The prickly pear cactus extract may reduce three symptoms of hangover—nausea, dry mouth, and loss of appetite.[24] The best way to prevent a hangover, of course, is to abstain from alcohol.

Certain medications can also relieve some symptoms. Antacids, for example, may relieve nausea and stomach pains. Aspirin may reduce headache and muscle aches but could increase stomach irritation. Avoid acetaminophen because alcohol metabolism enhances its toxicity to the liver.[25] In fact, people who drink three or more alcoholic beverages per day should avoid all over-the-counter pain relievers and fever reducers. These heavy drinkers may have an increased risk of liver damage and stomach bleeding from medicines that contain aspirin, acetaminophen (Tylenol), ibuprofen (Advil), naproxen sodium (Aleve), or ketoprofen (Orudis KT and Actron).[26]

Think About

4

People with hangovers should avoid "the hair of the dog that bit you," a remedy that calls for drinking more alcohol. Additional drinking only enhances the toxicity of the alcohol previously consumed and extends the recovery time.

Individual Differences in Alcohol Metabolism

Individuals vary in their ability to metabolize alcohol and acetaldehyde. As a consequence, they differ in their susceptibility to intoxication, hangover, and, in the long term, addiction and organ damage.

The result of individual differences is easiest to see in acute responses to alcohol. For example, when people of Asian descent drink alcohol, about half experience flushing around the face and neck, probably as a result of high blood acetaldehyde levels.[27] These individuals lack gastric alcohol dehydrogenase, and their livers have an inefficient form of aldehyde dehydrogenase. This may explain why their ancestors depended on boiled water (for teas) as a source of safe fluid. In contrast, Europeans are able to metabolize larger quantities of alcohol and historically have relied on fermentation to produce fluids that were safer to drink.[28]

Elderly people often find that their tolerance for alcohol is less than it used to be. Due to decreased tolerance, the effects of alcohol, such as impaired coordination, occur at lower intakes in the elderly than in younger people, whose tolerance *increases* with increased consumption. This reduced tolerance is compounded by an age-related decrease in body water, so that blood alcohol concentrations in older people are likely to rise higher after drinking.[29]

Women and Alcohol

Men and women respond differently to alcohol. (See **Figure SA.10**.) Blood alcohol rises faster in women, so they become more intoxicated than men at an equivalent dose of alcohol.[30] Accordingly, moderate drinking is usually defined as two standard drinks for men and one for women.[31] Women also metabolize alcohol more slowly than men. Several factors are responsible for alcohol's greater effect on women:

- *Body size and composition.* Women on average are smaller than men and have smaller livers; thus, they have less capacity for metabolizing alcohol. Women also have lower total body water and higher body fat than men of comparable size. After alcohol is consumed, it diffuses uniformly into all body water, both inside and outside cells. Because of their smaller quantity of body water, women have higher concentrations of alcohol in their blood than men do after drinking equivalent amounts of alcohol.[32]

- *Less enzyme activity.* Women also have less alcohol dehydrogenase (the primary enzyme involved in the metabolism of alcohol) activity than men—about 40 percent less.[33] This contributes to higher blood alcohol concentrations and lengthens the time needed to metabolize and eliminate alcohol. The gender difference in blood alcohol levels is due mainly to the significantly lower activity of gastric enzymes in women.[34]

- *Chronic alcohol abuse.* Alcoholism and other alcohol abuse exact a greater physical toll on women than men. Female alcoholics have death rates 50 to 100 percent higher than those of male alcoholics. Furthermore, a higher percentage of female alcoholics die from suicides, alcohol-related accidents, circulatory disorders, and cirrhosis of the liver.

Body composition

Women have a higher percentage of fat than men (size for size women have less water than men to dilute alcohol).

Less enzyme activity

Alcohol dehydrogenase, the primary enzyme involved in the metabolism of alcohol, is up to 40% less active in women than in men.

Body size

Women are smaller on average than men (smaller livers and less total water).

Hormonal fluctuations

Women typically have a heightened response to alcohol which is increased when they are about to have their periods, or when taking birth control pills.

Figure SA.10 **Women and men respond differently to alcohol.** Women tend to have a lower capacity for alcohol than men.

Key Concepts: *Alcohol does not need to be digested prior to absorption and moves easily across the lining of the GI tract into the bloodstream. Once alcohol is absorbed, the liver metabolizes it. The primary metabolic enzymes are alcohol dehydrogenase and aldehyde dehydrogenase. When large amounts of alcohol are consumed, some is metabolized by the MEOS pathway. Genetic and gender differences in the amount and activity levels of alcohol-metabolizing enzymes influence a person's response to consuming alcohol.*

When Alcohol Becomes a Problem

Alcohol affects every organ system in the body. In the short term, small amounts of alcohol change the levels of neurotransmitters in the brain, reducing inhibitions and physical coordination. In the long term, chronic intake of large amounts of alcohol damages the heart, liver, GI tract, and brain. When a pregnant woman drinks, alcohol can have a devastating effect on the development of her baby.

Alcohol in the Brain and the Nervous System

Alcohol diffuses readily into the brain. Because a small amount is absorbed from the mouth directly into circulating blood, its effects can be almost immediate, reaching the brain in as little as one minute after consumption. Alcohol can produce detectable impairments in memory after only a few drinks, and as the amount of alcohol increases, so does the degree of impairment. Large quantities of alcohol, especially when consumed quickly and on an empty stomach, can produce a blackout, that is, an interval of time for which the intoxicated person cannot recall key details of events, or even entire events. **Figure SA.11** shows the effects alcohol has on the brain.

Because alcohol is soluble in fat, it easily can cross the protective fatty membrane of nerve cells. There, it disrupts the brain's complex system for communicating between nerve cells. Neurotransmitters that excite nerve cells and those that inhibit nerve cells are thrown out of balance. Excess of some neurotransmitters produces sleepiness; high levels of others cause a loss of coordination; an imbalance of others impairs judgment and mental ability; and still other neurotransmitters perpetuate the desire to keep drinking, even when it's clearly time to stop. Changes in these messengers are suspected of leading to addiction and symptoms of alcohol withdrawal.[35] In the short run, they probably contribute to a hangover.

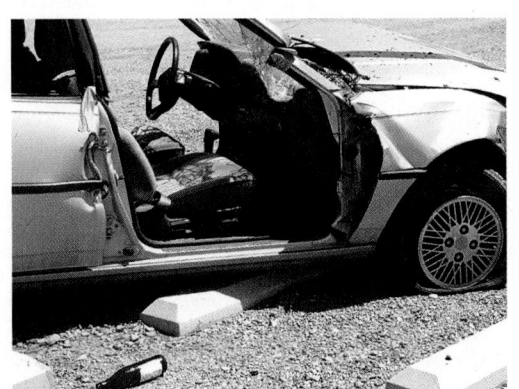

Figure SA.11 **Effects of alcohol on the brain.** As blood alcohol concentration rises, different parts of the brain are affected.

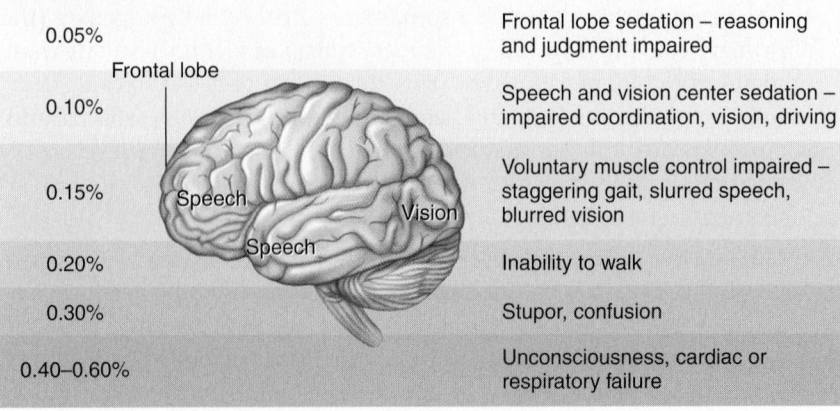

Blood alcohol concentration

0.05%	Frontal lobe sedation – reasoning and judgment impaired
0.10%	Speech and vision center sedation – impaired coordination, vision, driving
0.15%	Voluntary muscle control impaired – staggering gait, slurred speech, blurred vision
0.20%	Inability to walk
0.30%	Stupor, confusion
0.40–0.60%	Unconsciousness, cardiac or respiratory failure

Alcohol's short-term effects are related to how much a person drinks. One or two drinks typically bring alcohol blood levels to 0.04 percent and usually cause only mild, pleasant changes in mood and release of inhibitions. With more drinks and rising blood alcohol levels, coordination, judgment, reaction time, and vision become increasingly impaired. In the United States and Canada, it is illegal for a person whose blood level of alcohol has reached or exceeds 0.08 percent to drive a motor vehicle. A review of 112 studies concluded that certain skills required to drive a motor vehicle can become significantly impaired at a blood alcohol concentration as low as 0.05 percent.[36] For commercial drivers, a BAC of 0.04 percent is illegal nationwide. **Table SA.2** shows the effects that various amounts of alcohol have on mood and behavior.

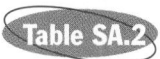 **Table SA.2** **Alcohol Impairment Chart**

Men
BODY WEIGHT IN POUNDS

DRINKS	100	120	140	160	180	200	220	240	
	APPROXIMATE BLOOD ALCOHOL PERCENTAGE								
0	.00	.00	.00	.00	.00	.00	.00	.00	ONLY SAFE DRIVING LIMIT
1	.04	.03	.03	.02	.02	.02	.02	.02	IMPAIRMENT BEGINS
2	.08	.06	.05	.05	.04	.04	.03	.03	DRIVING SKILLS AFFECTED
3	.11	.09	.08	.07	.06	.06	.05	.05	
4	.15	.12	.11	.09	.08	.08	.07	.06	POSSIBLE CRIMINAL PENALTIES
5	.19	.16	.13	.12	.11	.09	.09	.08	
6	.23	.19	.16	.14	.13	.11	.10	.09	
7	.26	.22	.19	.16	.15	.13	.12	.11	LEGALLY INTOXICATED
8	.30	.25	.21	.19	.17	.15	.14	.13	
9	.34	.28	.24	.21	.19	.17	.15	.14	CRIMINAL PENALTIES
10	.38	.31	.27	.23	.21	.19	.17	.16	

Women
BODY WEIGHT IN POUNDS

DRINKS	90	100	120	140	160	180	200	220	240	
	APPROXIMATE BLOOD ALCOHOL PERCENTAGE									
0	.00	.00	.00	.00	.00	.00	.00	.00		ONLY SAFE DRIVING LIMIT
1	.05	.05	.04	.03	.03	.03	.02	.02	.02	IMPAIRMENT BEGINS
2	.10	.09	.08	.07	.06	.05	.05	.04	.04	DRIVING SKILLS AFFECTED
3	.15	.14	.11	.10	.09	.08	.07	.06	.06	
4	.20	.18	.15	.13	.11	.10	.09	.08	.08	POSSIBLE CRIMINAL PENALTIES
5	.25	.23	.19	.16	.14	.13	.11	.10	.09	
6	.30	.27	.23	.19	.17	.15	.14	.12	.11	
7	.35	.32	.27	.23	.20	.18	.16	.14	.13	LEGALLY INTOXICATED
8	.40	.36	.30	.26	.23	.20	.18	.17	.15	
9	.45	.41	.34	.29	.26	.23	.20	.19	.17	CRIMINAL PENALTIES
10	.51	.45	.38	.32	.28	.25	.23	.21	.19	

Note: Subtract .01% for each 40 minutes of drinking. Your body can get rid of one drink per hour. One drink is 1.25 oz of 80-proof liquor, 12 oz of beer, or 5 oz of table wine. Data supplied by the Pennsylvania Liquor Control Board.

Source: Pennsylvania Liquor Control Board. Alcohol impairment chart. http://www.lcb.state .pa.us/edu/cwp/view.asp?a=1346&Q=555292. Accessed 7/9/06. Reprinted with permission.

Fyi Changing the Culture of Campus Drinking

From car crashes to alcohol poisonings, the culture of drinking on many college campuses puts students at grave risk. Alcohol use is pervasive among college students, many of whom are younger than the legal drinking age.

Annually, at least 1,700 student deaths and nearly 600,000 unintentional injuries involve alcohol.[1] College students who drink are more likely to drink and drive, have failing grades, and have medical and legal problems. Increased rates of crime, traffic crashes, rapes and assaults, property damage, and other alcohol-related consequences affect both drinking and nondrinking students, as well as members of the surrounding community. Each year, for example, students who have been drinking assault more than 696,000 of their classmates.[2]

The Culture of College Drinking

On many campuses, alcohol consumption is a rite of passage, and the influence of peers is an especially powerful force driving college problem drinking.[3] Traditions and beliefs handed down through generations of college drinkers reinforce the perception that alcohol is a necessary component of social success.[4] Many students arrive at college with a history of alcohol consumption and positive expectations about alcohol's effects. Thirty percent of twelfth-graders, for example, report heavy episodic drinking in high school, slightly more report having "been drunk," and almost three-fourths report drinking in the past year.[5]

Rates of excessive alcohol use are highest at colleges and universities where fraternities and sororities are popular, where sports teams have a prominent role, and at schools located in the Northeast.[6] In the local community, tolerance of student drinking may permit alcoholic beverage outlets and advertising to be located near campus. Due to lax enforcement, selling alcohol to students below the legal drinking age often has few consequences. Also, underage students who

are caught using fake IDs to obtain alcohol are seldom penalized.[7] Just look at the advertising and sale of alcoholic beverages on or near campuses, and the role of alcohol in college life is evident.

Alcohol Use and Abuse by College Students

Approximately 70 percent of college students consumed some alcohol within 30 days of being surveyed.[8] Although some of these students are problem drinkers (e.g., frequent heavy episodic drinkers or those who display symptoms of dependence), others may drink moderately or may misuse alcohol only occasionally (e.g., drink and drive infrequently). Surveys of drinking patterns show that college students are more likely than nonstudents of similar age to consume any alcohol, to drink heavily, and to engage in heavy episodic drinking. Young people who are not in college, however, are more likely to consume alcohol every day.[9] Even though college students tend to drink more, they are not at greater risk of alcohol-related problems.[10]

A survey questioned students about patterns and consequences of their alcohol use during the past year.[11] Thirty-one percent reported symptoms associated with alcohol abuse (e.g., drinking in hazardous situations and alcohol-related school problems), and 6 percent reported three or more symptoms of alcohol dependence (e.g., drinking more or longer than initially planned and experiencing increased tolerance to alcohol's effects). What happens when these student imbibers leave college? Surprisingly, most high-risk student drinkers reduce their consumption of alcohol. Nevertheless, some continue frequent, excessive drinking, leading to alcoholism or medical problems associated with chronic alcohol abuse.[12]

Binge Drinking

Binge drinking is especially worrisome, and it is widespread on college campuses. What is binge drinking? Binge drinking is defined as the consumption of at least five drinks in a

row for men or four drinks in a row for women. Just over two in five students (44 percent) report binge drinking behaviors, and about one in four (23 percent) report bingeing frequently, defined as three or more times in a two-week period. Frequent binge drinkers average more than 14 drinks per week and account for more than two-thirds of the alcohol consumed by college students.[13] Most college binge drinkers drink not for sociability, but solely and purposefully to get drunk.

Binge drinkers often do something they later regret—argue with friends, make fools of themselves, get sick, engage in unplanned (and often unprotected) sexual activity, or drive drunk. Afterward they may forget where they were or what they did, but the consequences of the binge remain. These consequences may include alienated friends, a hangover, and embarrassment. Or the consequences could be much more serious—sexually transmitted disease, hospitalization, permanent injury, rape, pregnancy, or death.

Abstaining

There is a polarizing trend in college drinking, with binge drinkers at one extreme and abstainers at the other. The number of college students who drink no alcohol is rising and now nearly equals the number who binge frequently. About one in five students (19 percent) report consuming no alcohol within the past year.[14] In a survey of colleges, one in three reported banning the use of alcohol on campus by all students regardless of age.[15]

Prevention Strategies *and* Changing the Culture of Drinking

Changing the culture of college drinking represents the first step toward an effective prevention strategy, according to a task force of college presidents, alcohol researchers, and students established by the National Institute on Alcohol Abuse and Alcoholism. Their report emphasizes the need for collaboration between academic institutions, researchers, and the community to effect lasting change.[16]

The task force strongly supports the use of a "3-in-1 Framework" to target three primary audiences simultaneously: (1) individual students, including high-risk drinkers; (2) the student body as a whole; and (3) the surrounding community.[17] The task force reviewed potentially useful preventive interventions, grouping them into "tiers" according to evidence for their effectiveness.

Tier 1: Strategies Effective Among College Students

Strong evidence supports the following strategies:

1. Simultaneously address alcohol-related attitudes and behaviors (e.g., refuting false beliefs about alcohol's effects while teaching students how to cope with stress without resorting to alcohol).
2. Use survey data to counter students' misperceptions about their fellow students' drinking practices and attitudes toward excessive drinking.
3. Increase student motivation to change drinking habits by providing nonjudgmental advice and progress evaluations.

Programs that combine these three strategies have proved effective in reducing alcohol consumption.[18]

Tier 2: Strategies Effective Among the General Population That Could Be Applied to College Environments

These strategies have proved successful in populations similar to those found on college campuses. Measures include the following:

1. Increase enforcement of minimum legal drinking age laws.[19]
2. Implement, enforce, and publicize other laws to reduce alcohol-impaired driving, such as zero-tolerance laws that reduce the legal blood alcohol concentration for underage drivers to near zero.[20]
3. Increase the prices or taxes on alcoholic beverages.[21]

4. Institute policies and training for servers of alcoholic beverages to prevent sales to underage or intoxicated patrons.[22]

Tier 3: Promising Strategies That Require Research

These strategies make sense intuitively or show theoretical promise, but their usefulness requires further testing. They include more consistent enforcement of campus alcohol regulations and increasing the severity of penalties for violating them, regulating happy hours, enhancing awareness of personal liability for alcohol-related harm to others, establishing alcohol-free dormitories, restricting or eliminating alcohol-industry sponsorship of student events while promoting alcohol-free student activities, and conducting social norms campaigns to correct exaggerated estimates of the overall level of drinking among the student body.

1 Hingson RW, Heeren T, Winter M, et al. Magnitude of alcohol-related mortality and morbidity among U.S. college students ages 18–24: changes from 1998 to 2001. *Ann Rev Pub Health.* 2005;26:259–279.

2 Ibid.

3 Ham LS, Hope DA. Incorporating social anxiety into a model of college student problematic drinking. *Addict Behav.* 2005;30(1):127–150.

4 National Institute on Alcohol Abuse and Alcoholism (NIAAA). *A Call to Action: Changing the Culture of Drinking at U.S. Colleges.* Bethesda, MD: NIAAA, 2002. NIH publication 02–5010; and NIAAA. *Young Adult Drinking.* Bethesda, MD: NIAAA, 2006. Alcohol Alert, No. 68.

5 Johnston LD, O'Malley PM, Bachman JG. *Monitoring the Future: National Survey Results on Drug Use, 1975–2000. Volume I: Secondary School Students.* Bethesda, MD: National Institute on Drug Abuse, 2001. NIH publication 01–4924.

6 Presley CA, Meilman PW, Leichliter JS. College factors that influence drinking. *J Stud Alcohol.* 2002(suppl 14):82–90.

7 Toomey TL, Wagenaar AC. Environmental policies to reduce college drinking: options and research findings. *J Stud Alcohol.* 2002(suppl 14):193–205.

8 O'Malley PM, Johnston LD. Epidemiology of alcohol and other drug use among American college students. *J Stud Alcohol.* 2002(suppl 14):23–39.

9 Slutske WS. Alcohol use disorders among US college students and their non-college-attending peers. *Arch Gen Psychiatry.* 2005;62:321–327.

10 Ibid.

11 Knight JR, Wechsler H, Kuo M, et al. Alcohol abuse and dependence among U.S. college students. *J Stud Alcohol.* 2002;63(3):263–270.

12 Schulenberg J, O'Malley PM, Bachman JG, et al. Getting drunk and growing up: trajectories of frequent binge drinking during the transition to young adulthood. *J Stud Alcohol.* 1996;57(3):289–304.

13 Wechsler H, Lee JE, Kuo M, et al. Trends in college binge drinking during a period of increased prevention efforts: findings from 4 Harvard School of Public Health College Alcohol Study Surveys: 1993–2001. *J Am Coll Health.* 2002;50(5):203–217.

14 Ibid.

15 Wechsler H, Seibring M, Liu IC, Ahl M. Colleges respond to student binge drinking: reducing student demand or limiting access. *J Am Coll Health.* 2004;52(4):159–168.

16 NIAAA, 2002. Op cit.

17 Hingson RW, Howland J. Comprehensive community interventions to promote health: implications for college-age drinking problems. *J Stud Alcohol.* 2002(suppl 14): 226–240; and Holder HD, Gruenewald PJ, Ponicki WR, et al. Effect of community-based interventions on high-risk drinking and alcohol-related injuries. *JAMA.* 2000;284:2341–2347.

18 Larimer ME, Cronce JM. Identification, prevention, and treatment: a review of individual-focused strategies to reduce problematic alcohol consumption by college students. *J Stud Alcohol.* 2002(suppl 14):148–163.

19 Wagenaar AC, Toomey TL. Effects of minimum drinking age laws: review and analyses of the literature from 1960 to 2000. *J Stud Alcohol.* 2002(suppl 14): 206–225.

20 Wagenaar A, O'Malley P, LaFond L. Lowered legal blood alcohol limits for young drivers: effects on drinking, driving, and driving-after-drinking behaviors in 30 states. *Am J Pub Health.* 2001;91(5):801–804.

21 Cook PJ, Moore MJ. The economics of alcohol abuse and alcohol-control policies. *Health Affairs* 2002; 21(2):120–133.

22 Toomey TL, Wagenaar AC. Op cit.

The acute effect of a large alcohol intake—swallowed accidentally by children, for example—is hypoglycemia (low blood sugar) severe enough to kill.[37] Binge drinking, especially following several days of little food, also can be deadly. The lack of food depletes glycogen stores, and heavy drinking suppresses gluconeogenesis. The resulting severe hypoglycemia is a medical emergency with the potential for coma and death.

A person who drinks heavily over a long period of time may have brain deficits that persist well after he or she achieves sobriety. Exactly how alcohol affects the brain and the likelihood of reversing the impact of heavy drinking on the brain remain hot topics in alcohol research today.[38] Chronic alcoholism produces many different mental disorders. Malnutrition is a probable factor in most of these, even when diet appears adequate. After years of drinking, brain cells become permanently damaged and unable to metabolize nutrients properly.

Alcohol's Effect on the Gastrointestinal System

Years of heavy drinking and ongoing contact with alcohol and acetaldehyde eventually damage the gastrointestinal system, which in turn discourages eating, affects absorption of protective nutrients, and leaves the digestive lining even more vulnerable to damage as the vicious cycle continues.

Chronic irritation from alcohol and acetaldehyde erodes protective mucosal linings, causing inflammation and release of destructive free radicals. **Esophagitis** (inflammation of the esophagus), esophageal stricture (closing), and swallowing difficulties are common among alcoholics. When the stomach is exposed repeatedly to alcohol at high concentrations, **gastritis** (inflammation of the stomach) often develops. Alcoholics frequently have diarrhea and malabsorption, evidence of intestinal damage. The mouth, throat, esophagus, stomach, and small and large intestines are all at greatly increased risk of cancer.[39] Smoking dramatically multiplies this risk.

Alcohol and the Liver

Metabolizing and detoxifying alcohol are almost entirely the responsibility of the liver. So it's not surprising that too much drinking hurts the liver more than any other site in the body. In the United States, heavy alcohol use is considered the most important risk factor for chronic liver disease. During the 1980s, alcoholic fatty liver, acute alcoholic hepatitis, and alcoholic cirrhosis together accounted for 46 percent of deaths from chronic liver disease and 49 percent of hospitalizations for liver disease.[40]

The earliest evidence of liver damage is fat accumulation, which can appear after only a few days of heavy drinking. Fatty liver (see **Figure SA.12**) recedes with abstinence but persists with continued drinking. Is fatty liver in and of itself harmful? The answer is controversial among liver researchers, with some experts suggesting it's a benign condition. However, studies show that 5 to 15 percent of people with alcoholic fatty liver who continue to drink develop liver fibrosis (excessive fibrous tissue) or cirrhosis (scarring) in only 5 to 10 years.[41] The abundance of accumulated fat is vulnerable to the production of unstable lipid molecules that contain excess oxygen (peroxidation) and of other destructive compounds, including free radicals.

Fat accumulation is one of several factors resulting in alcoholic liver disease; accumulation of NADH may be another. With regular high intakes of alcohol, alcohol and acetaldehyde continually irritate and inflame the liver, producing alcoholic hepatitis (persistent inflammation of the liver) in 10 to 35 percent of heavy drinkers. The inflammatory process also generates free radicals that batter away at liver cells.[42] The destruction of liver cells

esophagitis Inflammation of the esophagus.
gastritis Inflammation of the stomach.

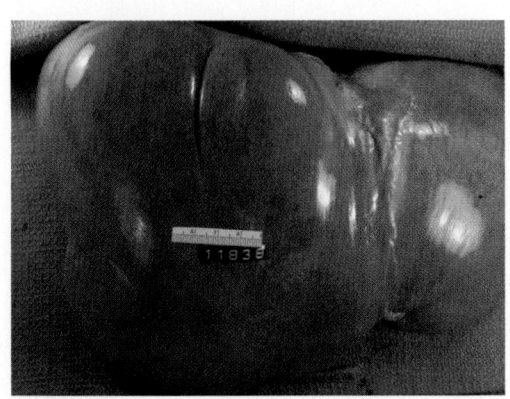

Figure SA.12 Fatty liver.

becomes self-perpetuating, especially if antioxidant nutrients are unavailable to help break the cycle. If the intestines also have been damaged, toxins, including those produced by the gut's microorganisms, may be able to cross the intestinal barrier into circulation, worsening the inflammation.[43]

Alcoholic hepatitis may be treatable, but it's often fatal. Alcoholic hepatitis also predisposes a person to liver cancer and cirrhosis, conditions that are usually fatal. With continued inflammation, the liver makes excessive collagen and becomes fibrous (fibrotic liver disease) and scarred (cirrhosis). This ultimately kills liver cells by choking off the tiny blood vessels that nourish them. About 10 to 20 percent of heavy drinkers develop cirrhosis.[44]

Dietary changes may be helpful in treating liver disease, but abstinence is essential. Reducing dietary fats somewhat reduces fat accumulation in the liver. Consuming adequate micronutrients and a healthful balance of macronutrients probably speeds recuperation from liver diseases in their earlier stages.[45] In late-stage liver disease, dietary restrictions, often of proteins, may slow disease progression or improve symptoms. One thing is clear, however: At any stage of alcoholic liver disease, popping nutrient supplements will not substitute for abstinence and may be detrimental.

Fetal Alcohol Syndrome

Fetal alcohol syndrome is perhaps the saddest result of alcohol consumption. Victims of this syndrome suffer a variety of congenital defects: mental retardation, coordination problems, and heart, eye, and genitourinary malformations, as well as low birth weight and slowed growth rate. Most apparent are characteristic facial abnormalities. Severe cases of fetal alcohol syndrome are rare, but subtle damage with one or two abnormalities,

Quick Bites

Are Alcoholics More Likely to Get Food Poisoning?

When alcohol inhibits the breakdown of another toxin, the effect can be dramatic. Consider seafood toxins, for example. The alcoholic who sits down for a good fish dinner should be extra careful about seafood because alcoholic liver disease makes him 200 times more likely to die from *Vibrio vulnificus*, a bacterium found in raw oysters. Alcohol also accentuates the symptoms of *ciguatera*, or "fish poisoning," a relatively common food poisoning in tropical areas where people eat large fish from infected waters.

fetal alcohol syndrome A set of physical and mental abnormalities observed in infants born to women who abuse alcohol during pregnancy. Affected infants exhibit poor growth, characteristic abnormal facial features, limited hand–eye coordination, and mental retardation.

Fyi Myths About Alcohol

FOR YOUR INFORMATION

Myths and misunderstandings just keep circulating about alcohol. Some of these statements are partly true, but most are completely false. Here are a few you may have heard:

- *Drinking isn't all that dangerous.* Wrong! One in three 18- to 24-year-olds admitted to emergency rooms for serious injuries is intoxicated. And alcohol use is associated with homicides, suicides, and drownings.
- *I can manage to drive well enough after a few drinks.* No. About one-half of all fatal traffic crashes among 18- to 24-year-olds involve alcohol.
- *I can sober up quickly if needed.* No. It takes about three hours to eliminate the alcohol content of two drinks, depending on your weight and other factors.

Nothing can speed up this process—not even coffee or cold showers.
- *Alcohol is a stimulant.* No. It's actually a depressant, but its initial depressing effect on inhibitions and judgment may make it seem stimulating.
- *Alcohol keeps you warm.* Partly true. It dilates blood vessels near the body's surface, giving a feeling of warmth. But as body heat escapes, alcohol cools the inner body.
- *Alcohol is an aphrodisiac.* Partly true. By suppressing inhibitions, it may loosen behavior. However, sexual function is often compromised by alcohol.
- *Most alcoholics live on skid row.* No. The highly visible skid-row alcoholic represents only a minority of alcoholics.

- *Beer is a source of vitamins.* Partly true. Beer does contain a fair amount of niacin. But you'd need about 1 liter to fulfill niacin requirements. Levels of other vitamins are much lower.
- *Alcohol helps you sleep.* No. Alcohol disrupts sleep patterns, leading to a restless, unsatisfying sleep.
- *Laboratory animals love to drink.* No. Alcohol is usually given by tube feeding because most animals refuse to drink it willingly.
- *It's good to have a beer before breastfeeding.* No. Alcohol may be relaxing and allow milk to flow more readily, but alcohol concentrations in breast milk are similar to those in the mother's blood. Alcohol reduces milk production by reducing the intensity of the infant's suckling.

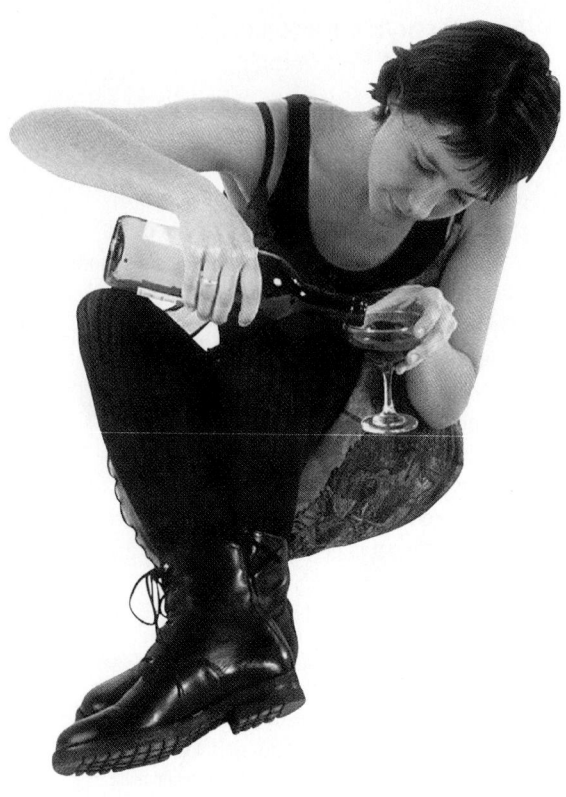

sometimes called "fetal alcohol effects," is probably much more wide-spread. Symptoms of the syndrome may not emerge until months after birth and are apt to go undiagnosed.[46] This disorder, a major cause of mental retardation in the United States, is preventable.

Alcohol is especially damaging in the early weeks of pregnancy, before a woman may know she's pregnant. It crosses the placenta into the tiny body of the fetus, where its effects are grossly magnified. Both the congeners in alcoholic beverages and the associated disturbed metabolism of vitamin A and folic acid, nutrients clearly required for fetal growth and development, can interfere with embryonic development.[47]

Relatively small amounts of alcohol may cause fetal alcohol syndrome. A safe level during pregnancy is not known; therefore, pregnant women should abstain from alcohol consumption. Unlike most other alcohol-related diseases, fetal alcohol damage does not require chronic intake. A binge—even having several drinks at a party—at the wrong moment of pregnancy can cause serious problems. However, population studies show that babies with neurodevelopmental problems are more common among women who drink more frequently during pregnancy.[48]

Official health advisories warn women against drinking alcohol if they are pregnant or considering becoming pregnant. Labels on alcoholic beverages must carry a warning for pregnant women. In 2002, 10.1 percent of pregnant women consumed alcohol, and 1.9 percent did so frequently.[49] **Figure SA.13** shows the prevalence of alcohol consumption by women of childbearing age.

Key Concepts: *Alcohol affects every organ system of the body. In the brain and nervous system, alcohol impairs coordination, judgment, reaction time, and vision. In the GI tract, alcohol damages cells of the esophagus and stomach and increases the risk for GI cancers. The liver is most severely affected by alcohol consumption, with damage culminating in alcoholic hepatitis and cirrhosis after years of alcohol abuse. Alcohol intake during pregnancy can have devastating effects on fetal development.*

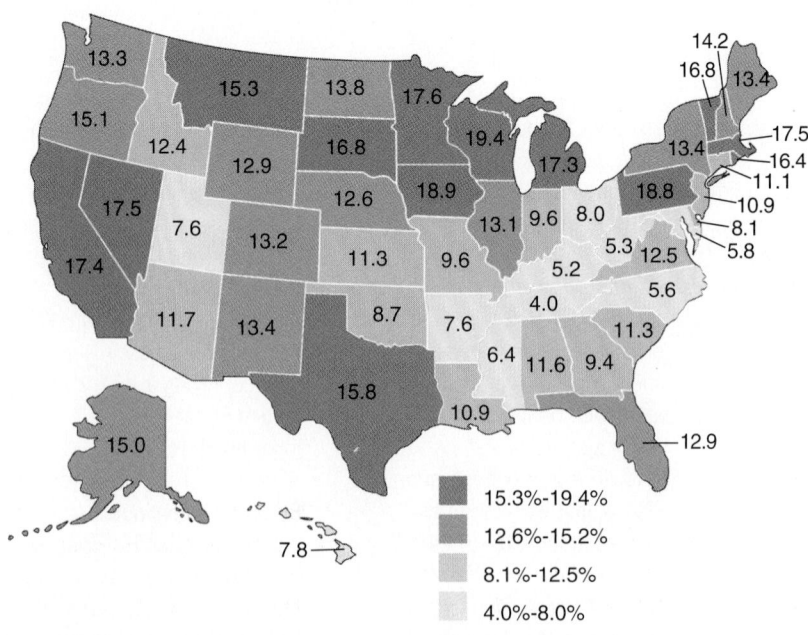

Figure SA.13 **Prevalence of frequent alcohol consumption among women of childbearing age (18–44 years).** Alcohol is especially damaging to the fetus during the early weeks of pregnancy—before a woman may know she is pregnant. **Source:** Alcohol consumption among pregnant and childbearing-aged women. *MMWR.* 1997;46:346–350.

* Consumption of an average of seven or more drinks per week or five or more drinks on at least one occasion during the preceding month.

Alcoholics and Malnutrition

In the United States, where food is plentiful and fortification of foods with vitamins and minerals is common, overt nutrient deficiencies are rare—except among alcoholics. The results of their poor diet interact with the results of alcohol's toxicity—which include diarrhea, malabsorption, liver malfunction, bleeding, bone marrow changes, and hormonal changes—to worsen malnutrition. In general, the more a person drinks, the worse the malnutrition. (See **Figure SA.14**.)

Poor Diet

A nationally representative study found that as alcohol quantity increased, diet quality worsened. As alcohol frequency increased, diet quality improved. Diet quality was poorest among the highest-quantity, lowest-frequency drinkers and best among the lowest-quantity, higher-frequency drinkers.[50]

Disordered eating is common among heavy drinkers, especially among alcoholic women.[51] Factors responsible for the poor diet of alcoholics are much easier to identify than to correct. Economic factors include poverty, lack of cooking facilities, and homelessness. Anxiety, depression, loneliness, and isolation are all characteristic of alcoholism, and all contribute to loss of appetite. So can physical pain. Lack of interest in food is common. There may be an aversion to many specific foods or to eating in general, especially after the experience of diarrhea, painful indigestion, or difficulty swallowing.

Heavy drinkers who get about half their calories from alcohol cannot eat enough to obtain adequate vitamins and minerals. Severely malnourished alcoholics often have multiple deficiencies.

Vitamin Deficiencies

Inadequate intake, poor absorption, increased vitamin destruction in the body, and urinary losses all contribute to vitamin deficiencies in the alcoholic. Alcohol also interferes with conversion of vitamin precursors to active forms.

Folate, thiamin, and vitamin A are most often affected by alcoholism. Folate deficiency contributes to malabsorption, anemia, and nerve damage—all of which worsen malnutrition. Vitamin A deficiency also creates a vicious cycle by damaging gastrointestinal lining and by impairing immunity, leaving the victim susceptible to infections. Thiamin deficiency contributes to classic diseases of alcoholism: the brain damage of Wernicke-Korsakoff syndrome, polyneuropathy (nerve inflammation), and cardiomyopathy (heart inflammation). Alcoholics can have overt scurvy from vitamin C deficiency. Vitamin B_6 and vitamin B_{12} deficiencies are less common.

Alcohol metabolism competes with the normal metabolism of vitamins and other nutrients. For example, metabolism of ethanol uses up the dehydrogenase enzyme that is also used for metabolism of retinol.[52] Retinol (vitamin A) uses that enzyme for its conversion to other active forms of vitamin A, and the disruption of its metabolism is probably one way that alcohol increases cancer risk. The same disruption may produce fetal birth defects when pregnant women drink.

Alcohol-induced fat malabsorption and metabolic abnormalities contribute to the depletion of fat-soluble vitamins A, D, E, and K. Blood-clotting factors drop with depleted vitamin K, increasing the risk of bleeding and anemia. Vitamin E deficiency is not generally recognized as a complication of alcoholism, but depletion of vitamin E due to fat malabsorption is possible. Optimal vitamin E is necessary to quench free radicals generated during alcohol metabolism.[53]

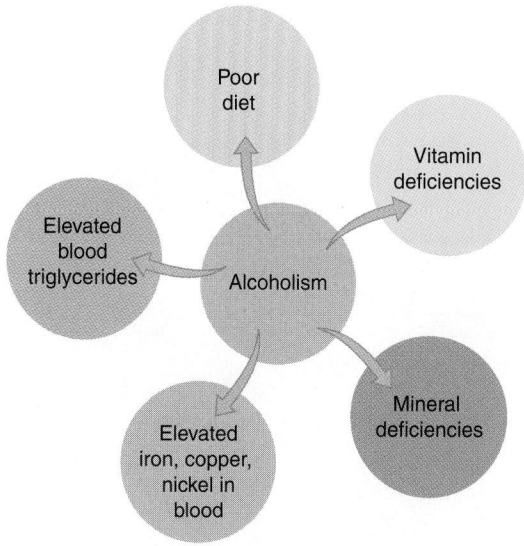

Figure SA.14 **Alcoholism and malnutrition.** Alcoholics' poor diets interact with alcohol's toxicity to worsen their malnutrition.

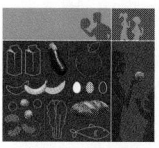

Dietary Guidelines for Americans, 2005
key recommendations

- Those who choose to drink alcoholic beverages should do so sensibly and in moderation—defined as the consumption of up to one drink per day for women and up to two drinks per day for men.
- Alcoholic beverages should not be consumed by some individuals, including those who cannot restrict their alcohol intake, women of childbearing age who may become pregnant, pregnant and lactating women, children and adolescents, individuals taking medications that can interact with alcohol, and those with specific medical conditions.
- Alcoholic beverages should be avoided by individuals engaging in activities that require attention, skill, or coordination, such as driving or operating machinery.

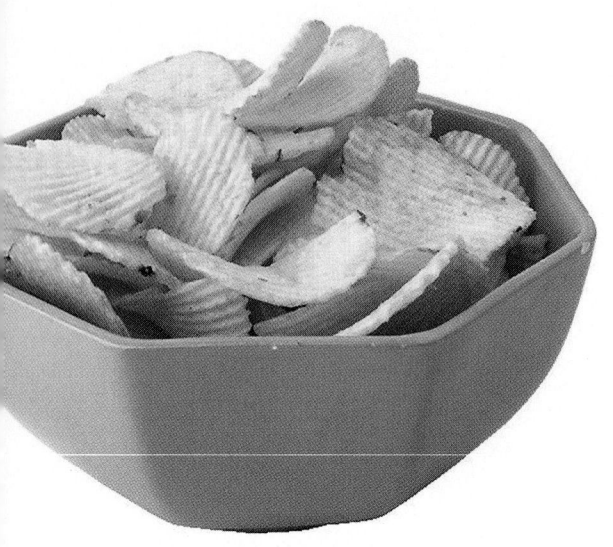

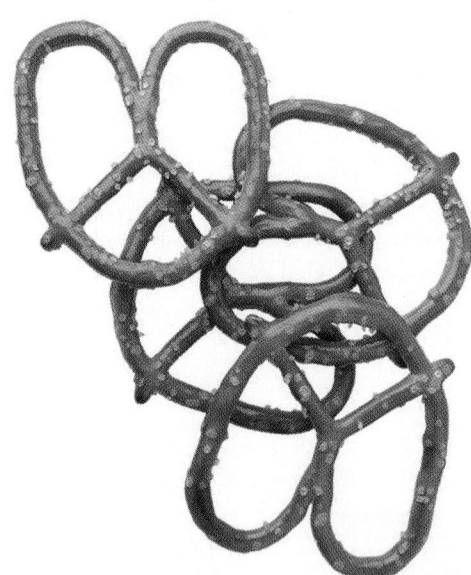

Mineral Deficiencies

Alcoholics are commonly deficient in minerals such as calcium, magnesium, iron, and zinc. Alcohol itself does not seem to affect their absorption. Rather, fluid losses and an inadequate diet are the primary culprits. Magnesium deficiency causes "shakes" similar to that seen in alcohol withdrawal. Chronic diarrhea and loss of epithelial tissue (caused by skin rashes or sloughing off of the digestive lining) may seriously deplete zinc, a mineral needed for immune function. In cases of bleeding, especially gastrointestinal blood loss, iron levels fall.

Not all minerals are lower in heavy drinkers than in nondrinkers. If there is no bleeding, a heavy drinker's iron levels tend to be higher than normal in the blood and liver, potentially contributing to harmful lipid peroxidation. Copper and nickel levels also may be elevated in advancing disease, but the reason and the effects are unclear.[54]

Macronutrients

Animal experiments can demonstrate a number of ways that alcohol alters digestion and metabolism of carbohydrate, fat, and protein, but the relevance to humans at the usual levels of intake is not certain. Alcohol interferes with amino acid absorption, but its overall effect on protein balance appears minimal. It inhibits gluconeogenesis and lowers blood sugar, probably contributing to hangovers and, at the most extreme, causing acute, potentially lethal hypoglycemia if a person who drinks heavily neglects to eat.[55]

Alcohol's most dramatic effect is on fats. You have seen that alcohol causes fatty liver. On the one hand, excess alcohol has the undesirable effect of raising blood triglyceride levels, often significantly. Hyperlipidemia (high blood fats) is common among heavy drinkers. Abstinence and a balanced diet can usually return blood lipids to normal.[56] On the other hand, moderate alcohol use increases protective high-density lipoproteins (HDL, or "good cholesterol"), an important factor in alcohol's relationship to the reduced risk for coronary artery disease.

Body Weight

Although alcoholic beverages provide minimal nutrient value, they do provide calories; alcohol contains 7 kilocalories per gram. Does alcohol consumption contribute to obesity? It appears likely. In an analysis of data collected from more than 37,000 people, researchers found that overweight drinkers consumed more drinks than leaner drinkers on the days that they drank.[57] Men and women who infrequently consume the greatest quantity of alcohol weigh more than those who frequently drink small amounts. Because smoking and drinking interact to influence body weight, the researchers looked only at current drinkers who had never smoked.

Drinking patterns are important. Alcohol consumption consists of two components: (1) the amount consumed on drinking days (quantity) and (2) how often drinking days occur (frequency). Although previous studies of the relation between drinking alcohol and body weight have been inconsistent, these studies looked at average consumption. A given average volume, however, can result from widely varying drinking patterns. An average volume of 2 drinks per day, for example, may result from consuming 2 drinks every day, 4 drinks every other day, 14 drinks on one day per week, or 30 drinks on two days per month. Body weight is more sensitive to drinking patterns than average volume.

Key Concepts: *Alcohol interferes with normal nutrition by reducing the intake of nutrient-dense foods and by affecting the absorption, metabolism, and excretion of many vitamins and minerals. Alcohol contains a significant number of calories (7 kilocalories per gram), and heavy episodic drinkers tend to weigh more than light drinkers.*

Does Alcohol Have Benefits?

Can a potentially harmful drink such as alcohol play a role in a healthful diet? The consensus of health experts is that it can—but not for everyone. The question continues to arouse much debate, however, and even those supporting alcohol's usefulness often have reservations. Public health statements on alcohol are typically accompanied by plenty of "ifs" and "buts."

Consistent epidemiological evidence suggests that low to moderate drinking reduces mortality among some groups.[58] (**Table SA.3** gives the official definitions of levels of drinking.) Compared with nondrinkers or heavy drinkers, middle-aged and older adults who drink moderate amounts of alcohol have a lower risk of mortality from all causes.[59] This includes people with heart disease,[60] diabetes,[61] high blood pressure,[62] or prior heart attack.[63] Consistent and growing evidence shows that alcohol reduces insulin resistance and may protect against heart disease by improving "good" cholesterol levels and reducing blood clotting.[64]

No evidence has suggested that moderate drinking harmed the people in the studies. In fact, analysis of data from the Nurses' Health Study, which involves more than 12,000 participants, suggests that in women, up to one drink per day does not impair mental functioning and may actually decrease the risk of mental decline with age.[65]

Tracked against alcohol intake, death rates typically follow what statisticians describe as a "U-shaped curve." Compared with people who rarely or never drink, total mortality rates are lower for people who drink slightly or moderately. The lowest rate is seen in people who consume one drink per week. Increasing the number of drinks confers no additional benefit. In fact, as the number of drinks increases, the mortality rate rises. People who consume two drinks per day have about the same mortality rate as nondrinkers.[66] Beyond three drinks per day, the death rate rises dramatically.[67] Heavy alcohol consumption increases the risk of stroke, for example, whereas light or moderate drinking appears to reduce that risk.[68] Alcohol's primary benefit is to raise protective HDL cholesterol levels. It may also inhibit formation of blood clots, but this connection is less clear.[69] In addition, alcohol may have subjective benefits such as stress relief and relaxation.

In most studies, wine, beer, and spirits appear equal in offering protection against heart disease. Findings of reduced rates of nonfatal heart attacks among moderate drinkers support the view that protective benefits are due to alcohol itself rather than other substances in alcoholic beverages.[70] However, international comparisons that highlight unexpectedly low rates of heart disease in France, despite a high-fat diet (the **French paradox**), suggest that red wine may have a unique protective effect. The apparent benefits of red wine may result from overall healthier behavior of people who drink red wine. As yet, a direct connection between red wine and health benefits remains unproved.[71] Nevertheless, recognizing that alcohol generally confers moderate protection, and noting the possibility that wine has a particular benefit, the Bureau of Alcohol, Tobacco, and Firearms

Quick Bites

First Wine?

Wine residue has been found on pottery shards that were dated back to about 3,000 B.C.E. They came from the ancient village of Godin Tepe in the Zagros Mountains of western Iran.

French paradox The phenomenon observed in the French, who have a lower incidence of heart disease than people whose diets contain comparable amounts of fat. Part of the difference has been attributed to the regular and moderate drinking of red wine.

in 1999 granted permission for wine labels to include one of the following statements:[72]

> The proud people who made this wine encourage you to consult your family doctor about the health effects of wine consumption.

> To learn the health effects of wine consumption, send for the Federal Government's Dietary Guidelines for Americans. . .

Table SA.3 **How Much Is Too Much?**

Term	Criterion
Moderate drinking (NIAAA)	Men: ≤ 2 drinks per day Women: ≤ 1 drink per day Over 65: ≤ 1 drink per day
At-risk drinking (NIAAA)	Men: > 14 drinks per week or > 4 drinks per occasion Women: > 7 drinks per week or > 3 drinks per occasion
Alcohol abuse (APA)	Maladaptive pattern of alcohol use leading to clinically significant impairment or distress, manifested within a 12-month period by one or more of the following: • Failure to fulfill role obligations at work, school, or home • Recurrent use in hazardous situations • Legal problems related to alcohol • Continued use despite alcohol-related social or interpersonal problems • Symptoms have never met criteria for alcohol dependence
Alcohol dependence (APA)	Maladaptive pattern of alcohol use leading to clinically significant impairment or distress, manifested within a 12-month period by three or more of the following: • Tolerance (either increasing amounts used or diminished effects with the same amount) • Withdrawal (withdrawal symptoms or use to relieve or avoid symptoms) • Use of larger amounts over a longer period than intended • Persistent desire or unsuccessful attempts to cut down or control use • Great deal of time spent obtaining or using or recovering from use • Important social, occupational, or recreational activities given up or reduced • Use despite knowledge of alcohol-related physical or psychological problems
Hazardous use (WHO)	Person at risk for adverse consequences
Harmful use (WHO)	Use resulting in physical or psychological harm

Note: NIAAA = National Institute on Alcohol Abuse and Alcoholism; APA = American Psychiatric Association; WHO = World Health Organization.
Source: O'Connor PG, Schottenfeld RS. Patients with alcohol problems. *N Engl J Med.* 1998;338(9):593. Copyright © 1998 Massachusetts Medical Society. All rights reserved. Reprinted with permission.

Because of the many harmful effects of alcohol (see **Figure SA.15**), public health agencies and organizations caution against inappropriate drinking. Although low to moderate alcohol use may offer some benefit, these groups advise people to discuss their alcohol intake with their doctors, and they urge moderation. The U.S. Preventive Services Task Force recommends that primary care doctors routinely screen patients for unhealthy alcohol use and, when appropriate, intervene with a brief counseling session to reduce alcohol misuse.[73] Public health officials also point out that numerous groups should not drink any alcohol:[74]

- People who cannot restrict their alcohol intake to moderate levels
- Children and adolescents
- People taking medications that can interact with alcohol

American Heart Association

Alcohol

If you drink alcohol, do so in moderation. This means an average of one to two drinks per day for men and one drink per day for women. Drinking more alcohol increases such dangers as alcoholism, high blood pressure, obesity, stroke, breast cancer, suicide and accidents. Also, it's not possible to predict in which people alcoholism will become a problem. Given these and other risks, the American Heart Association cautions people NOT to start drinking ... if they do not already drink alcohol. Consult your doctor on the benefits and risks of consuming alcohol in moderation.

Reproduced with permission. www.americanheart.org. © 2006, American Heart Association, Inc.

Figure SA.15 **Harmful effects of alcohol.** Because excess alcohol reaches all parts of the body, it causes a wide array of physical problems. Here are some of the ways alcohol can harm.

Addiction
Alcohol addiction destroys lives, families, and communities. Researchers are trying to learn why some people, and not others, become addicted.

Accidents and violence
These result from impairment of mental function and coordination.

Birth defects
Fetal alcohol syndrome can occur when pregnant women drink.

Emotional and social
Emotional, social, and economic problems are associated with heavy drinking.

Cardiomyopathy
Inflammation of the heart muscle is much more common in heavy drinkers.

Brain
Acute effects are drunkenness. Long-term effects of chronic alcohol excess are dementia, memory loss, and generalized impairment of mental function.

Liver disease
Heavy drinking can lead to alcoholic fatty liver, alcoholic hepatitis, cirrhosis, and liver cancer.

Gastritis
Continued contact with excess alcohol irritates and inflames the stomach lining.

Pancreatitis
Both chronic and acute pancreatitis are increased by alcoholism.

Cancer
Excess alcohol increases the risk of gastrointestinal, liver, and breast cancers. Smoking further increases these risks.

Anemia
Heavy drinkers often have poor diets and may bleed from the digestive tract.

Osteoporosis
Heavy drinking contributes to bone loss, especially in older women.

Peripheral neuropathy
Painful nerve inflammation in hands, arms, feet, and legs is common in long-time heavy alcohol users.

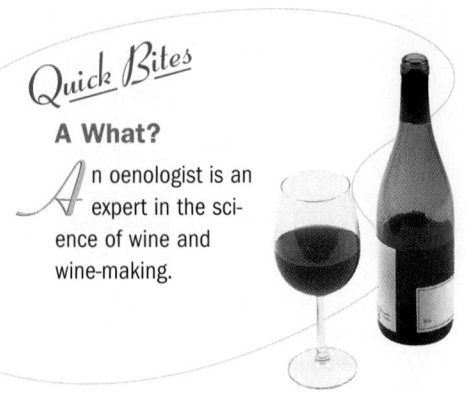

- People who have an alcohol-related illness or another illness that will be worsened by alcohol

- People who plan to drive, operate machinery, or take part in other activities that require attention, skill, or coordination

- Women who are pregnant or may become pregnant

- Women who are breastfeeding

- People with a personal or strong family history of alcoholism

Key Concepts: *Although alcohol has the potential to reduce risk for heart disease, most health organizations recommend moderate to no drinking. It is too early in the scientific investigation of alcohol's benefits to recommend alcohol intake for all adults. Some people, such as pregnant women, should not drink any alcohol.*

Label [to] **Table**

Have you ever wondered how much protein, carbohydrate, and fat are in a can of beer? If you've ever looked at a beer label, you know it's quite different from a food label. Look at the following information from a can of light beer and see if you can calculate the calories from carbohydrate, fat, and protein.

Serving size = 12 fl oz

Calories = 103 (kcal)

Carbohydrate = 5 g

Protein = 1 g

Fat = 0 g

First, to figure out how many calories come from the three macronutrients, multiply the number of grams by their respective calorie contribution per gram:

5 g carbohydrate × 4 kcal/g = 20 kcal from carbohydrate

1 g protein × 4 kcal/g = 4 kcal from protein

0 g fat × 9 kcal/g = 0 kcal from fat

Uh oh. Is this adding up correctly? So far we have accounted for only 24 of the 103 kilocalories in this beer. Where are the other 79 kilocalories? Don't forget that many of the calories in beer come from alcohol, and it's easy to calculate just how many grams are in this can of light beer. Remember alcohol has 7 kcalories per gram, so the remaining 79 kilocalories come from 11 grams of alcohol (79 ÷ 7 = 11.3).

So, for the 103 kilocalories this beer provides, you get very little (if any) protein, carbohydrate, or fat. Instead, a majority of the calories come from alcohol. This holds true for the micronutrients as well—beer contains negligible amounts of vitamins or minerals.

This is why people say alcoholic beverages have only "empty calories." They provide calories, but almost no nutrient value!

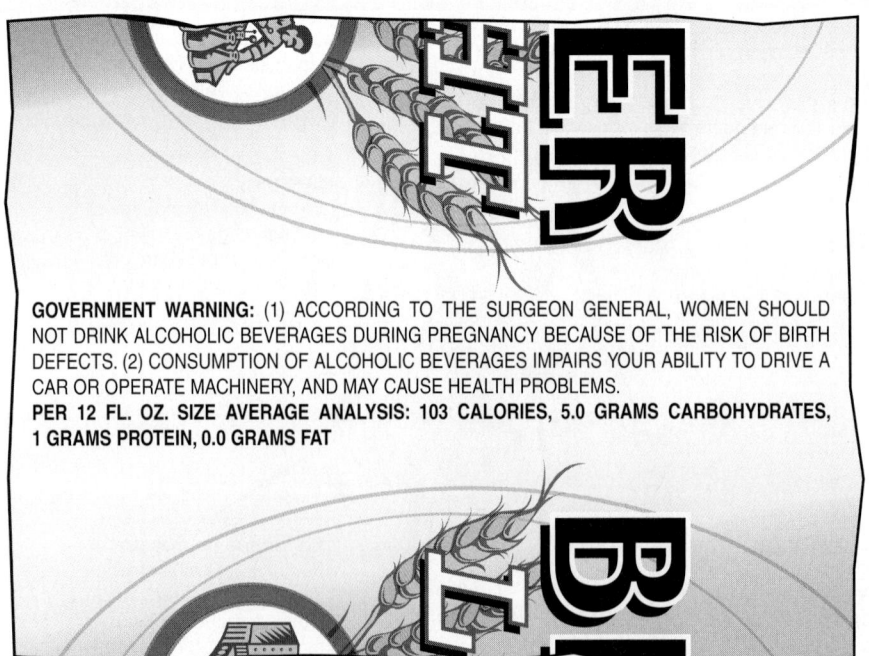

GOVERNMENT WARNING: (1) ACCORDING TO THE SURGEON GENERAL, WOMEN SHOULD NOT DRINK ALCOHOLIC BEVERAGES DURING PREGNANCY BECAUSE OF THE RISK OF BIRTH DEFECTS. (2) CONSUMPTION OF ALCOHOLIC BEVERAGES IMPAIRS YOUR ABILITY TO DRIVE A CAR OR OPERATE MACHINERY, AND MAY CAUSE HEALTH PROBLEMS.
PER 12 FL. OZ. SIZE AVERAGE ANALYSIS: 103 CALORIES, 5.0 GRAMS CARBOHYDRATES, 1 GRAMS PROTEIN, 0.0 GRAMS FAT

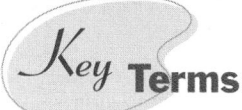

LEARNING *Portfolio*

Key Terms

	page		page
acetaldehyde	306	fatty liver	306
alcohol	302	fermentation	304
alcohol dehydrogenase (ADH)	306	fetal alcohol syndrome	317
		French paradox	321
alcohol poisoning	309	gastritis	316
aldehyde dehydrogenase (ALDH)	306	hangover	310
		methanol	302
binge drinking	306	methyl alcohol	302
blood–brain barrier	302	microsomal ethanol-oxidizing system (MEOS)	306
congeners	304		
esophagitis	316	standard drink	306
ethanol	302	wood alcohol	302
ethyl alcohol	302		

Study Points

➤ Alcohol, or ethyl alcohol, is a small organic compound with one hydroxyl (alcohol) group attached to two carbons.

➤ As an organic solvent, alcohol can dissolve fats and other lipids.

➤ Alcohol provides 7 kilocalories per gram but no essential function for the body; therefore, alcohol is not a nutrient.

➤ Alcohol requires no digestion and is absorbed easily all along the gastrointestinal tract.

➤ Most of the acetyl CoA produced from alcohol is routed to the synthesis of fatty acids; fatty liver is apparent even after one night of binge drinking.

➤ Different rates of alcohol metabolism can be attributed to different levels of the alcohol-metabolizing enzymes; these differences are due to genetic and gender variations.

➤ Alcohol affects all organs in the body, but the most obvious effects are in the brain and the nervous system, the GI system, and the liver.

➤ Malnutrition among alcoholics is common due to poor food choices and alcohol's interference with the absorption, metabolism, and excretion of nutrients.

➤ Fetal alcohol syndrome is one of the most devastating consequences of alcohol consumption, and it is preventable.

➤ Moderate alcohol consumption has been linked to reduced risk of heart disease.

➤ The potential benefits of moderate alcohol consumption may be related to effects on lipoprotein levels and the antioxidant components of beverages such as wine.

➤ Health organizations recommend moderate to no alcohol consumption.

Study Questions

1. What is a standard serving of beer, wine, and liquor?

2. List the ways food helps to delay or avoid inebriation.

3. Where does alcohol metabolism take place?

4. What are the three stages of alcohol metabolism?

5. What causes "fatty liver" in an alcoholic?

6. What causes a hangover? Is there any way to relieve one?

7. Among health authorities, what is the consensus about drinking alcohol?

8. List some factors that affect our ability to metabolize alcohol.

9. Why do health care professionals advise pregnant women not to drink alcohol?

10. List the positive and the negative effects of alcohol.

☞ [*Try*] This

Cruising Through the Medicine Cabinet

This exercise will increase your awareness of the amounts of alcohol in over-the-counter medications. Look through your medicine cabinet and check the ingredient lists of all the products there. In particular, take a close look at any mouthwash or cough syrup. Which products contain alcohol? How much? What do you think its purpose is in these medicines?

References

1 US Department of Health and Human Services and US Department of Agriculture. *Dietary Guidelines for Americans, 2005.* 6th ed. Washington, DC: US Government Printing Office, 2005.

2 Maimi TS, Brewer RD, Mokdad A, et al. Binge drinking among US adults. *JAMA.* 2003;289:70–75.

3 Foster WE, Vaughan RD, Foster WH, et al. Alcohol consumption and expenditures for underage drinking and adult excessive drinking. *JAMA.* 2003;289:989–995.

4 National Institute on Alcohol Abuse and Alcoholism (NIAAA). *Underage Drinking: A Major Public Health Problem.* Rockville, MD: NIAAA, April 2003. Alcohol Alert, No. 59.

5 Mokdad AH, Marks JS, Stroup DF, et al. Actual causes of death in the United States, 2000. *JAMA.* 2004;291:1238–1245.

6 Roe DA. *Alcohol and the Diet.* Westport, CT: AVI Publishing, 1979.

7 Ibid.

8 Mittal BV, Desai AP, Khade KR. Methyl alcohol poisoning: an autopsy study of 28 cases. *J Postgrad Med.* 1991;37:9–13.

9 Roe DA. Op. cit.

10 Vallee BL. Alcohol in the Western world. *Scientific American.* June 1998;80–85.

11 Swift R, Davidson D. Alcohol hangover: mechanisms and mediators. *Alcohol Health Res World.* 1998;22:54–60.

12 US Department of Health and Human Services and US Department of Agriculture. Op. cit.

13 USDA Center for Nutrition Policy and Promotion. *Does Alcohol Have a Place in a Healthy Diet?* Washington, DC: Center for Nutrition Policy and Promotion, 1997. Nutrition Insights, No. 4.

14 Seitz HK, Oneta CM. Gastrointestinal alcohol dehydrogenase. *Nutr Rev.* 1998;56:52–60.

15 Ibid.

16 Swift R, Davidson D. Op. cit.

17 Seitz HK, Oneta CM. Op. cit.

18 Ibid.

19 Swift R, Davidson D. Op. cit.

20 Wiese JG, Slipak MG, Browner WS. The alcohol hangover. *Ann Intern Med.* 2000;132:897–902.

21 Ibid.

22 Ibid.

23 Ibid.

24 Ibid.

25 Swift R, Davidson D. Op. cit.

26 Nordenberg T. "An aspirin a day. . .": just another cliché? *FDA Consumer.* March–April 1999;15–17.

27 Steinmetz CG, Xie P, Weiner H, et al. Structure of mitochondrial aldehyde dehydrogenase: the genetic component of ethanol aversion. *Br J Psychiatry.* 1996;168:762–767.

28 Vallee BL. Op. cit.

29 NIAAA. *Alcohol and Aging.* Rockville, MD: NIAAA, April 1998. Alcohol Alert, No. 40.

30 NIAAA. *Moderate Drinking.* Rockville, MD: NIAAA, April 1992. Alcohol Alert, No. 16.

31 USDA Center for Nutrition Policy and Promotion. Op. cit.

32 NIAAA. *Alcohol—An Important Women's Health Issue.* Rockville, MD: NIAAA, July 2004. Alcohol Alert, No. 62.

33 Swift R, Davidson D. Op. cit.

34 Baraona E, Abbittan CS, Dohmen K, et al. Gender differences in pharmacokinetics of alcohol. *Alcohol Clin Exp Res.* 2001; 25:502–507.

35 Valenzuela CF. Alcohol and neurotransmitter interactions. *Alcohol Health Res World.* 1997;21:108–148.

36 NIAAA. *Alcohol and Transportation Safety.* Rockville, MD: NIAAA, April 2001. Alcohol Alert, No. 52.

37 Bradford DE. Alcohol and the young child. *Alcohol Alcoholism.* 1984;19:173–175.

38 NIAAA. *Alcohol's Damaging Effects on the Brain.* Rockville, MD: NIAAA, October 2004. Alcohol Alert, No. 63.

39 Boffetta P, Hashibe M. Alcohol and cancer. *Lancet Oncol.* 2006;7(2):149–156.

40 Centers for Disease Control and Prevention. Deaths and hospitalizations from chronic liver disease and cirrhosis—United States, 1980–1989. *MMWR.* 1993;41:969–973.

41 Teli MR, Day CP, Burt AD, et al. Determinants of progression to cirrhosis or fibrosis in pure alcoholic fatty liver. *Lancet.* 1995;346:987–990.

42 Dey A, Cederbaum AI. Alcohol and oxidative liver damage. *Hepatology.* 2006;43(2 suppl):S63–S74.

43 NIAAA. *Alcohol and the Liver: Research Update.* Rockville, MD: NIAAA, 1998. Alcohol Alert, No. 42.

44 Ibid.

45 Teli MR, Day CP, Burt AD, et al. Op. cit.

46 Centers for Disease Control and Prevention. Identification of children with fetal alcohol syndrome and opportunity for referral of their mother for primary prevention, Washington, 1993–1997. *MMWR.* 1998;47:861–864.

47 Roe DA. Op. cit.

48 Centers for Disease Control and Prevention. Alcohol consumption among pregnant and childbearing-aged women—United States, 2002. *MMWR.* 2004;53:1178–1181.

49 Ibid.

50 Breslow RA, Guenther PM, Smothers BA. Alcohol drinking patterns and diet quality: the 1999–2000 National Health and Nutrition Examination Survey. *Am J Epidemiol.* 2006; 163(4):359–366.

51 Lilenfeld LR, Kaye WH. The link between alcoholism and eating disorders. *Alcohol Health Res World.* 1996;20:94–99.

52 Seitz HK, Oneta CM. Op. cit.; and Wang XD. Chronic alcohol intake interferes with retinoid metabolism and signaling. *Nutr Rev.* 1999;57:51–59.

53 Lieber CS. Nutrition in liver disorders and the role of alcohol. In: Shils ME, Shike M, Ross AC, Cabellero B, Cousins RJ, eds. *Modern Nutrition in Health and Disease.* 10th ed. Philadephia: Lippincott Williams & Wilkins, 2006:1235–1259.

54 Ibid.

55 Ibid.

56 Ibid.

57 Breslow RA, Smothers BA. Drinking patterns and body mass index in never smokers. *Am J Epidemiol.* 2005;161:368–376.

58 Klatsky AL. Should patients with heart disease drink alcohol? *JAMA.* 2001;285:2004–2006; and Doll R, Peto R, Boreham J, Sutherland I. Mortality in relation to alcohol consumption: a prospective study among male British doctors. *Int J Epidemiol.* 2005;34(1):199–204.

59 NIAAA. *State of the Science Report on the Effects of Moderate Drinking.* Bethesda, MD: NIAAA, 2003; and US Department of Health and Human Services and US Department of Agriculture. Op. cit.

60 Klatsky AL. Op. cit.

61 Ajani UA, Gaziano JM, Lotufo PA, et al. Alcohol consumption and risk of coronary heart disease by diabetes status. *Circulation.* 2000;102:500–505; and Solomon CG, Hu FB, Stampfer MJ, et al. Moderate alcohol consumption and risk of coronary heart disease among women with type 2 diabetes mellitus. *Circulation.* 2000;102:494–499.

62 Malinksi MK, Sesso HD, Lopez-Jimenez F, Buring JE, Gaziano JM. Alcohol consumption and cardiovascular disease mortality in hypertensive men. *Arch Intern Med.* 2004;164(6):623–628.

63 Muntwyler J, Hennekens CH, Buring JE, et al. Mortality and light to moderate alcohol consumption after myocardial infarction. *Lancet.* 1998;352:1882–1885.

64 Fagrell B, De Faire U, Bondy S, et al. The effects of light to moderate drinking on cardiovascular diseases. *J Intern Med.* 1999;246:331–340; and Paoletti R, Klatsky AL, Poli A, Zahari S, eds. *Moderate Alcohol Consumption and Cardiovascular Disease.* Dordrecht, The Netherlands: Kluwer, 2000.

65 Stampfer MJ, Kang JH, Chen J, et al. Effects of moderate alcohol consumption on cognitive function in women. *N Engl J Med.* 2005;352:245–253.

66 Gazino JM, Gaziano TA, Glynn RJ, et al. Light-to-moderate alcohol consumption and mortality in the Physicians' Health Study enrollment cohort. *J Am Coll Cardiol.* 2000;35(1):96–105.

67 Pearson TA. Alcohol and heart disease. *Circulation.* 1996;94:3023–3025.

68 Reynolds K, Lewis BL, Nolen JD, et al. Alcohol consumption and risk of stroke. *JAMA.* 2003;289:579–588.

69 Klatsky AL. Op. cit.

70 Bobak M, Skodova Z, Marmot M. Effect of beer drinking on risk of myocardial infarction: population based case-control study. *BMJ.* 2000;320:1378–1379; and Mukamal KJ, Conigrave KM, Mittleman MA, et al. Roles of drinking pattern and type of alcohol consumed in coronary heart disease in men. *N Engl J Med.* 2003;348:109–118.

71 Tjonneland A, Gronbaek M, Stripp C, Overvad K. Wine intake and diet in a random sample of 48763 Danish men and women. *Am J Clin Nutr.* 1999;69:49–54.

72 Treasury announces actions concerning labeling of alcoholic beverages. Bureau of Alcohol Tobacco and Firearms press release; February 5, 1999.

73 Saitz R. Unhealthy alcohol use. *N Engl J Med.* 2005;352:596–607.

74 Pearson TA. Op. cit.; and US Department of Health and Human Services and US Department Agriculture. Op. cit.

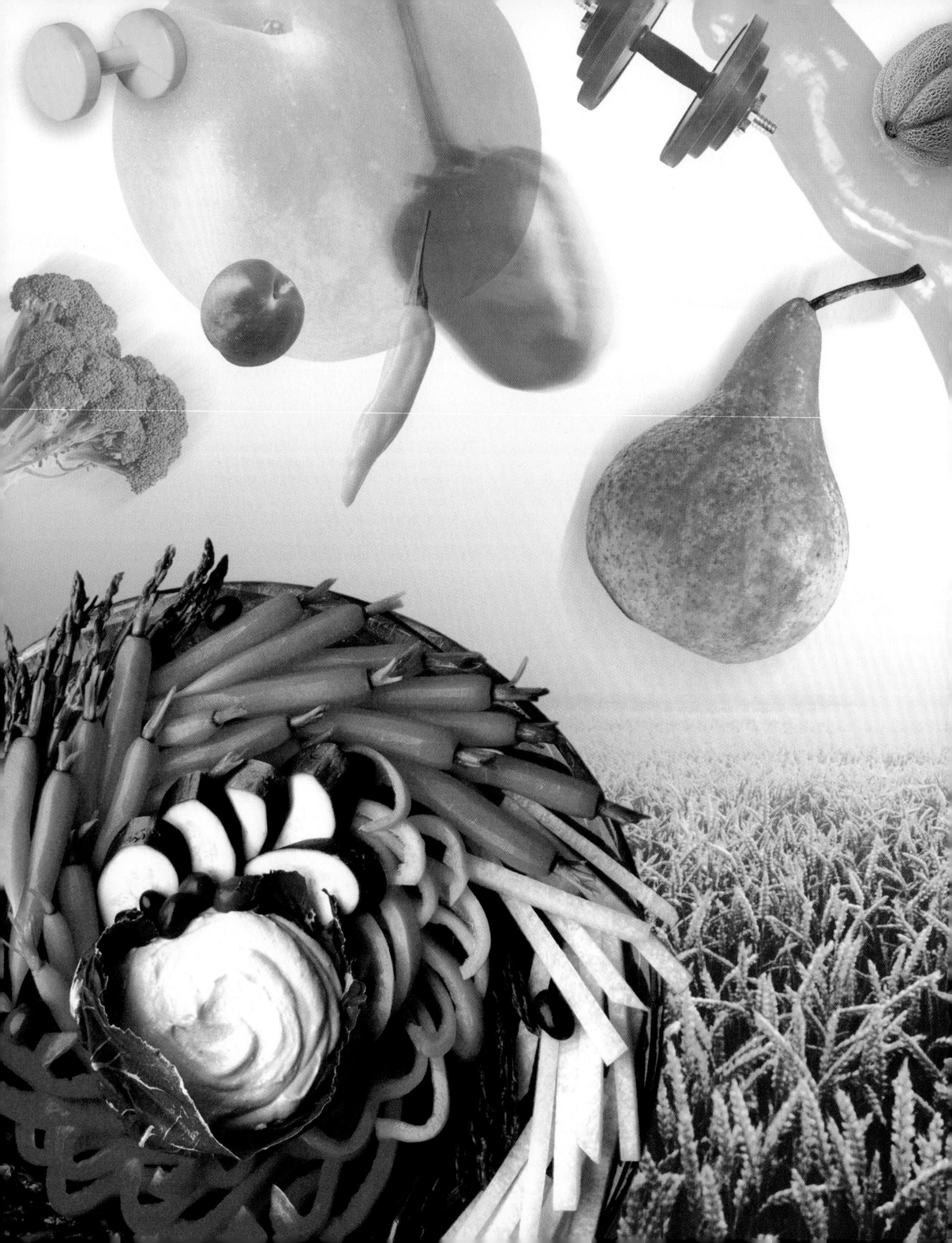

Chapter 8

Energy Balance, Body Composition, and Weight Management

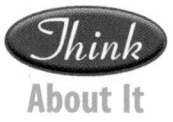
Think About It

1 How often do you reject dessert after a big meal?

2 When it comes to body fat distribution, are you an apple or a pear?

3 What does it mean to be metabolically fit?

4 How much time do you spend talking with your friends about weight?

Fyi **for your Information**

This chapter's FYI boxes include practical information on the following topics:
- What's Neat About NEAT?
- How Many Calories Do I Burn?
- High-Protein, Low Carbohydrate Diets for Weight Loss: Helpful or Harmful?
- Behaviors That Will Help You Manage Your Weight

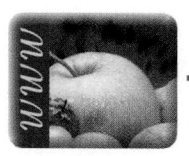

The Web site for this book offers many useful tools and is a great source for additional nutrition information for both students and instructors. Visit the site at **nutrition.jbpub.com** for information on energy balance, body composition, and weight management. You'll find exercises that explore the following topics:
- Leptin in Mice and Humans
- BMI Calculator
- Childhood Obesity
- Weighing In

Key **to Illustrations**

 Carbon Dioxide (CO_2)

 Water (H_2O)

What About *Bobbie?*

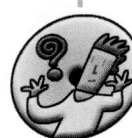

Track the choices Bobbie is making with Nutritionist Pro or EatRight Analysis software.

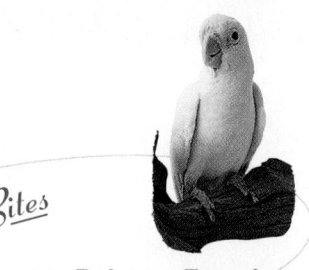

Quick Bites

Early Energy Balance Experiments

Erasistraus of Chios performed the first recorded experiment on energy balance in 280 B.C.E. Seeking to balance intake with output, he used a jar to fashion a kind of respiration apparatus. He then put two birds in the jar, weighing them and their excreta before and after feeding.

Your body is in the energy exchange business. Here's how it works. You balance the energy you expend with energy from the food in your diet. If you do a fairly good job of equalizing input and output, your body does the rest—maintaining energy equilibrium and keeping your weight steady. But what happens if you bring in more energy than your body can handle? It banks the excess energy as fat, and you gain weight. If your "account" grows too big, you become obese. Losing that extra weight—withdrawing the fat from your account—is not always easy.

Energy intake is the amount of fuel (calories) you take in through consumption of carbohydrate, protein, fat, and alcohol. **Energy output** is the amount you expend—primarily for basic body functions, physical activity, and the processing of food. An average adult consumes 1,800 to 3,000 kilocalories per day. In one year, that adds up to 657,000 to 1,095,000 kilocalories! Amazingly, despite such a huge intake of energy over time, most people maintain roughly the same weight during their working lives.

People who maintain a relatively constant weight are in **energy equilibrium**. Within limits, your body automatically regulates your weight, thanks to its ability to balance intake and expenditure. Your body can be in energy equilibrium even if your energy intake is very high, as long as your expenditure also is high. Conversely, your body can be in energy equilibrium when you don't expend much energy, as long as your intake also is low.

When you take in more energy than you need, you have a **positive energy balance**. You store the surplus as fat—the major energy reserve—and as glycogen, the short-term carbohydrate energy reserve. Pregnant women and growing children need a positive energy balance to increase energy stores. But the positive energy balance that results from overeating and inactivity, a common occurrence around major holidays, leads to unneeded weight gain.

When you take in less energy than you need, you have a **negative energy balance**. Reduced energy intake can be the result of illness, or it can be an intentional change for weight loss. To obtain fuel, your body uses stores of glycogen and fat (and breaks down body protein too, if the deficit is extreme), and body weight goes down. Thus, body weight change reflects overall **energy balance**. **Figure 8.1** shows different ratios of energy intake to energy expenditure.

Key Concepts: *Energy balance is the relationship between energy intake and energy output. Energy intake comes from the calories in food and beverages. Energy output is the amount of fuel used mainly for basic body functions, the processing of food, and physical activity.*

Energy In

We can measure the energy content of a food with a **bomb calorimeter**, like that shown in **Figure 8.2**. Inside a sealed chamber, the food is completely burned and sensors measure the amount of heat produced by its combustion. Your body is not as efficient as a bomb calorimeter. It does

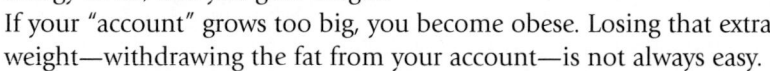

Energy Equilibrium

Energy Intake
• Carbohydrate
• Fat
• Protein

Energy Output
• Physical activity
• Food processing
• Basic body functions

Energy Input

Energy Output

Energy Input

Energy Output

Negative Energy Balance

Positive Energy Balance

Figure 8.1 **Energy balance.** Most people balance energy intake and output and stay in energy balance. People in negative energy balance lose weight, and those in positive energy balance gain weight.

not completely digest all food and is unable to oxidize nitrogen. When calculating the amount of energy your body can extract from food, the number of kilocalories released by complete combustion in a bomb calorimeter is adjusted downward as follows:

4 kilocalories per gram pure carbohydrate

4 kilocalories per gram pure protein

9 kilocalories per gram pure fat

7 kilocalories per gram pure alcohol

If we know a food's carbohydrate, fat, and protein content, we can use these numbers to estimate its calorie content.

Regulation of Food Intake

Internal and external cues help the body regulate food consumption and thus maintain energy equilibrium. Internal cues involve interactions and feedback mechanisms among hormones and hormonelike compounds and organ systems. External cues are stimuli in the eating environment and include the sight, smell, and taste of food. Internal and external cues work together to ensure that we eat enough to survive. However, the complex interplay of these cues makes it difficult to identify specific factors that cause overeating and obesity or disordered eating.

Hunger, Satiation, and Satiety

We experience internal cues as three different sensations that influence our eating behaviors. (See **Figure 8.3**.) The first, **hunger**, prompts eating ("I'm hungry"). Hunger is a physical sensation that includes the gnawing feeling in your stomach and signals the physiological need to eat. The second, **satiation**, tells you to stop eating ("I'm full"). The third, **satiety**, determines the interval between meals ("I'm not ready to eat again"). Satiety means not being hungry; it is influenced in part by how many calories you ate at your last meal.

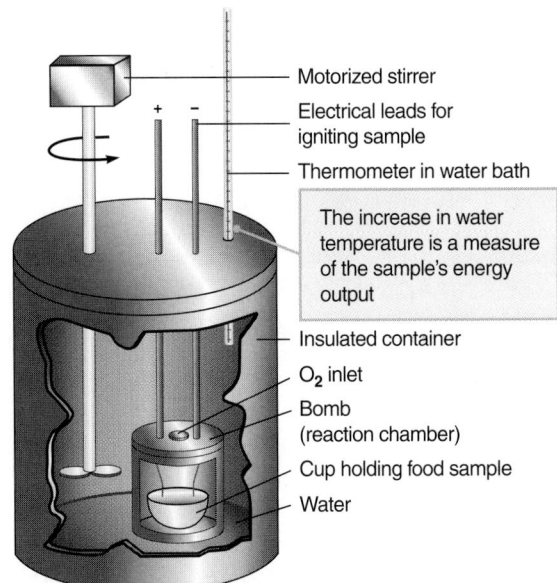

Figure 8.2 **Bomb calorimeter.** When a sample of food is completely burned inside the sealed chamber of a bomb calorimeter, it causes the temperature of the water surrounding the chamber to rise. This rise in temperature is a measure of the energy content of the food.

energy intake The caloric or energy content of food provided by the sources of dietary energy: carbohydrate (4 kcal/g), protein (4 kcal/g), fat (9 kcal/g), and alcohol (7 kcal/g).

energy output The use of calories or energy for basic body functions, physical activity, and processing of consumed foods.

energy equilibrium A balance of energy intake and output that results in little or no change in weight over time.

positive energy balance Energy intake exceeds energy expenditure, resulting in an increase in body energy stores and weight gain.

negative energy balance Energy intake is lower than energy expenditure, resulting in a depletion of body energy stores and weight loss.

energy balance The balance in the body between amounts of energy consumed and expended.

bomb calorimeter A device that uses the heat of combustion to measure the energy content of a food.

hunger The internal, physiological drive to find and consume food. Unlike appetite, hunger is usually experienced as a negative sensation, often manifesting as an uneasy or painful sensation.

satiation Feeling of satisfaction and fullness that terminates a meal.

satiety The effects of a food or meal that delay subsequent intake. Feeling of satisfaction and fullness following eating that quells the desire for food.

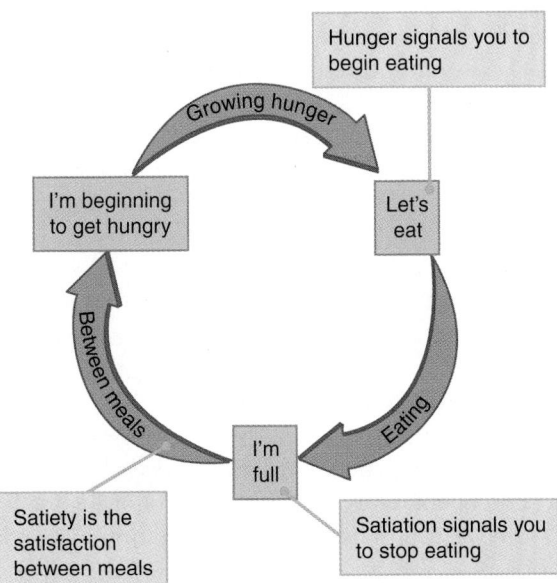

Figure 8.3 **Hunger, satiation, and satiety.** Hunger helps initiate eating. Satiation brings eating to a halt. Satiety is the state of nonhunger that determines the amount of time until eating begins again.

appetite A psychological desire to eat that is related to the pleasant sensations often associated with food.

Appetite

Internal and external cues can stimulate **appetite**, which complicates the workings of hunger, satiation, and satiety. To ensure adequate nourishment, appetite and hunger work in tandem. Appetite is the psychological desire to eat and is related to pleasant sensations associated with food. Hunger is the physiological need for food. In this sense, while appetite reflects our eating experiences, hunger is a basic drive. When you are truly hungry, any food will do, but appetite can trigger your desire for a specific food or type of food, even though you may not be hungry. For example, after a big meal of steak, potato, salad, and bread, you probably wouldn't want a second helping. But you might be tempted by the dessert cart! That's appetite. Even when we are hungry, illness and medication can cause loss of appetite and a lack of interest in food.

Key Concepts: *Food intake is regulated by sensations of hunger, a physiological drive to eat; satiation, feelings of satisfaction that lead to ending a meal; and satiety, continued feelings of fullness that delay the start of the next meal. Appetite is the psychological urge to eat and often has no relation to hunger.*

Control by Committee

What, then, stimulates hunger, satiation, satiety, and appetite? As you will see, there are multiple players involved. What you eat, the amount that you eat, and responses in the digestive tract, central nervous system, and general circulation influence your eating behavior. Sites throughout the body monitor energy status and send reports to the brain. Even the temperature of our environment affects how much we eat.

Diet Composition

The energy density (kcal/g), balance of energy sources (carbohydrates, lipids, and protein), and the form (liquid vs. solid) of your foods affect the amount you eat. Because people tend to eat a fairly constant amount of food, energy-dense diets (typical of high-fat, low-fiber diets) tend to result in excess energy consumption, at least in the short term.[1] Some researchers speculate, however, that over time (and especially outside the laboratory settings of most consumption research) some mechanism must compensate for changes in energy density.[2]

Protein appears to have a stronger satiating effect than fats or carbohydrates and also makes a stronger contribution to satiety.[3] In a small study comparing two breakfast meals, subjects ate less for lunch when their breakfast had more protein (20 percent of calories versus 14 percent of calories).[4] However, it is not clear what role protein plays in long-term energy balance. Bulkier foods, those with higher amounts of fiber and water, also have a higher satiety value.[5] Some types of fiber enhance satiation by slowing the rate at which the stomach empties, whereas others seem to enhance satiation by creating bulk.[6]

Liquid sources of calories (e.g., juices, soft drinks) generally have low satiety value. When people consume liquid or solid snacks with similar amounts of carbohydrates, subsequent food intake is greater following the liquid carbohydrate snacks.[7] However, soups, despite their liquid form, have relatively high satiety value.[8]

Sensory Properties

The aroma of freshly baked bread or the warmth and chewiness of chocolate chip cookies right out of the oven encourage us to eat more than our

Quick Bites

Why Do We Have Hunger Pangs?

When the stomach has been without food for at least three hours, intense stomach contractions can begin, sometimes lasting two to three minutes. Healthy young people have the strongest contractions, due to good muscle tone in the GI tract. After 12 to 24 hours, contractions of an empty stomach can cause painful hunger pangs.

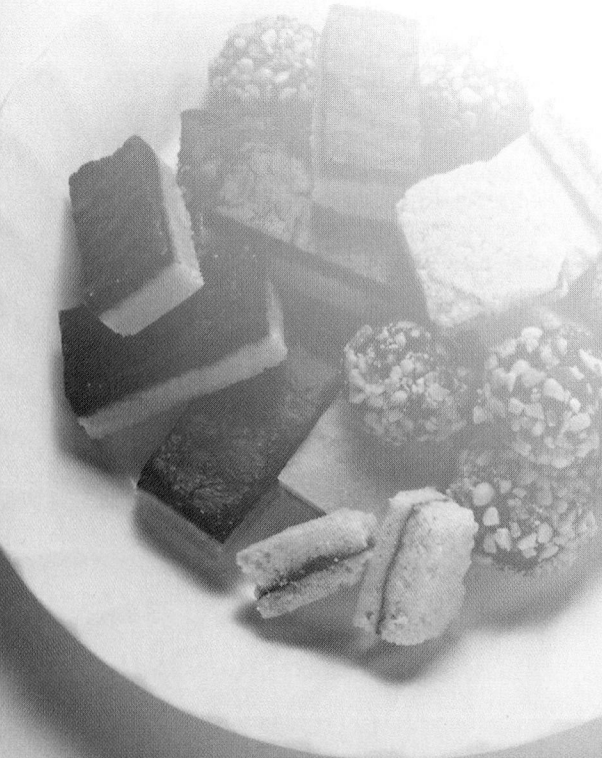

hunger dictates. Food's sensory properties—flavor, texture, color, temperature, and presentation—influence its appeal, and such external cues affect food intake.[9] (See **Figure 8.4**.) Taste is usually the reason why people choose a particular food. But foods that are pleasant to eat are often high in fat and are energy dense—properties that can lead to overeating.[10]

Portion Size

Portion size plays a role in how much we eat. In a controlled study of adults, people served a 1,000-gram portion (approximately 33 ounces) of macaroni and cheese for lunch ate 30 percent more than when they were served 500 grams (approximately 17 ounces).[11] It didn't matter whether the portions were served on individual plates or whether people served themselves from a serving dish.

When people select their own portions, the size of the serving bowl may affect the amount consumed. In a study of snack food consumption, adults presented with food in a large serving bowl took more food (and consumed about 140 more kilocalories) than when an equal amount of food was presented in a smaller bowl.[12] Children also are susceptible to the temptation of big portions, eating 25 percent more when served a double portion, but consuming less when they serve themselves.[13] We tend to respond visually to the amount of food on a plate or the size of a serving utensil and consider that "normal" rather than paying attention to internal feelings of satiation.[14] The dramatic increase in portion sizes eaten both at home and at restaurants[15] may be a major contributing factor to excess energy intake and weight gain.

Environmental and Social Factors

We tend to eat more in cold weather and less in hot weather. Systems in the **hypothalamus** that regulate body temperature and food intake probably interact to link temperature and eating behavior. In cold temperatures,

Quick Bites

Supersize Me!

Morgan Spurlock wrote, directed, produced, and is the lead character in *Supersize Me*, a film that documents Spurlock's consumption of a 30-day McDonald's-only diet. Whenever offered the option to "supersize" his order, Spurlock always selected the larger portion size. Starting at 185 pounds, the 6-foot, 2-inch Spurlock packed on 25 pounds and weighed 210 by the end of his experiment. His total cholesterol shot up from 165 to 230, his libido flagged, and he suffered headaches and depression.

hypothalamus [high-po-THAL-ah-mus] A region of the brain involved in regulating hunger and satiety, respiration, body temperature, water balance, and other body functions.

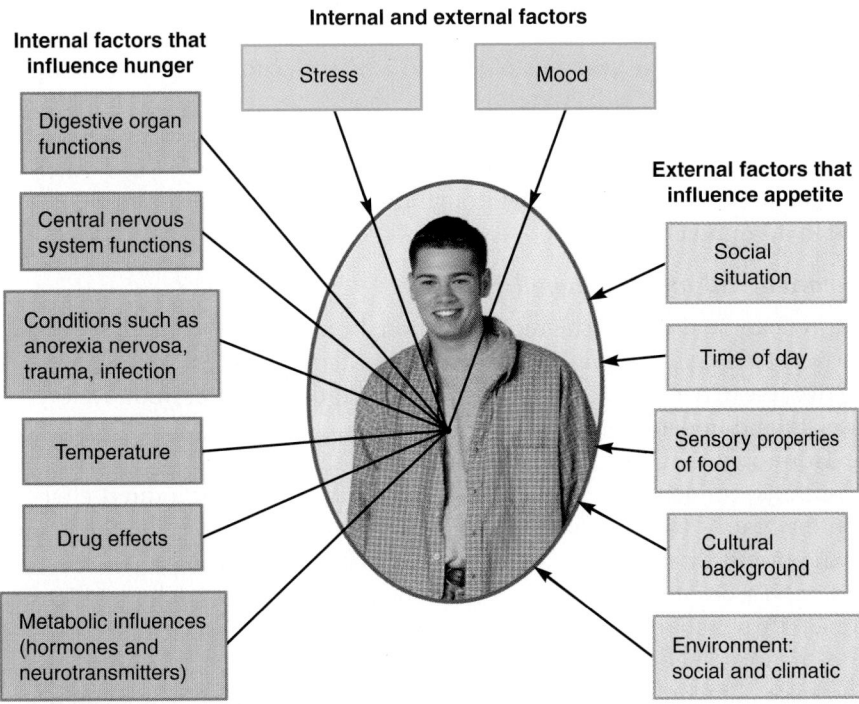

Figure 8.4 Internal and external influences on hunger and appetite.

increased food intake helps us survive by increasing the metabolic rate, which helps generate heat, and increasing fat stores, which provide insulation to reduce heat loss.[16]

Plate size, lighting, and socializing are other factors that influence consumption.[17] Any change in our surroundings that inhibits our self-monitoring of consumption tends to increase the volume that we eat. Larger plates and bowls encourage larger servings. We tend to eat more in dimly lit situations than when the lights are brighter, perhaps because we are less inhibited and self-conscious.[18] The best predictor of the amount of food that will be eaten at a given time is the number of people present. Studies show that meals eaten with other people last longer and tend to increase consumption by at least one-third compared with eating alone.[19]

When we are forced to pay attention to how much we are eating, we tend to eat less. A study demonstrated that college students and supermarket shoppers ate less in front of a mirror, spreading less full-fat cream cheese on baguettes and less full-fat margarine on bread than when a mirror was absent.[20] The researchers speculated that the mirror decreased food consumption by increasing self-awareness, providing an external reality check on the amount of food being consumed.

Emotional Factors

Many people use food to cope with stress and negative emotions. Eating can provide a powerful distraction from loneliness, anger, boredom, anxiety, shame, sadness, and inadequacy. To combat low moods, low energy levels, and low self-esteem, people often turn to the refrigerator. When we use food and eating to cope with our emotions, binge eating or other disturbed eating patterns can develop.

Gastrointestinal Sensations

As food fills your stomach and small intestine, they stretch and trigger signals to the brain. Your sense of fullness suppresses your urge to eat.[21]

Just passing a reasonable amount of food through the mouth can satisfy hunger temporarily—even if the food never reaches the stomach. When researchers fed large amounts of food to a person with a hole in the esophagus, hunger decreased, even though the food never reached the stomach. As we taste, salivate, chew, and swallow, the brain probably measures the passage of food, much as a water meter measures the flow of water. After a certain amount of food passes through the mouth, hunger diminishes for 20 to 40 minutes.[22]

Neurological and Hormonal Factors

More than 50 different chemicals are thought to be involved in the regulation of feeding. Determining the way these chemical factors work is an active research area that may lead to improved therapies for both overweight and underweight.

Hormones, hormonelike factors, and some drugs (including appetite suppressants) influence eating behavior through their direct or indirect effects on the brain.[23] **Neuropeptide Y (NPY)** is a hormonelike factor in the brain that powerfully stimulates appetite.[24] Although a number of signals can affect NPY activity, opposing signals from the hormones **ghrelin** and **leptin** link NPY secretion to daily feeding patterns.[25]

Ghrelin, sometimes called the "hunger hormone," is produced in the stomach. Ghrelin levels rise prior to a meal and fall quickly after food is

neuropeptide Y (NPY) A neurotransmitter widely distributed throughout the brain and peripheral nervous tissue. NPY activity has been linked to eating behavior, depression, anxiety, and cardiovascular function.

ghrelin A peptide hormone produced by the stomach that stimulates feeding; sometimes called the "hunger hormone."

leptin A hormone produced by adipose cells that signals the amount of body fat content and influences food intake; sometimes called the "satiety hormone."

consumed. The rise in ghrelin levels appears to stimulate NPY, thus encouraging feeding.

Leptin, sometimes called the "satiety hormone," is produced in fat cells. Leptin tells the central nervous system how much fat the body is storing. A rise in leptin levels appears to inhibit NPY, thus suppressing appetite.[26] Leptin also appears to signal pathways that enhance energy production to keep body weight in a normal range. Administering leptin to obese experimental animals lacking the hormone causes them to become normal weight.

Unfortunately, when body weight is high, these regulators act inconsistently. Common human obesity is associated with increased, not decreased, leptin levels,[27] and a trial of leptin in obese people produced variable amounts of weight loss.[28] Although obese people tend to have lower fasting ghrelin levels (suggesting that they would experience lower levels of hunger before a meal), they also have smaller reductions of ghrelin levels after a meal (suggesting that overeating may be due to lower levels of satiation).[29]

Key Concepts: *Diet composition and factors in the digestive tract and central nervous system influence eating behavior. The brain, especially the hypothalamus, receives signals from all over the body about energy status. External factors, such as portion size, social circumstances, and environmental conditions, as well as the food itself, can enhance or suppress appetite.*

Energy Out: Fuel Uses

Our bodies use fuel (expend energy) for three primary purposes:

1. To maintain basic physiological functions such as breathing and blood circulation

2. To process the food we eat

3. To power physical activity

We also expend energy to support growth, stay warm in cold environments, metabolize drugs, and deal with physical trauma, fever, and psychological stress. The sum of all energy expended is the **total energy expenditure (TEE)**. **Figure 8.5** illustrates the major components of energy expenditure.

Major Components of Energy Expenditure

Energy Expenditure at Rest

We generally expend most of our energy on the basic body functions needed to sustain life. This **basal energy expenditure (BEE)**, or **resting energy expenditure (REE)**, maintains heartbeat, respiration, nervous function, muscle tone, body temperature, and so on. Resting energy expenditure accounts for 60 to 75 percent of total energy expenditure.[30] The rate of energy expended at rest (kcal/hour) is measured as either the **basal metabolic rate (BMR)** or the **resting metabolic rate (RMR)**. BEE or REE refers to energy

total energy expenditure (TEE) The total of the resting energy expenditure (REE), energy used in physical activity, and energy used in processing food (TEF); usually expressed in kilocalories per day.

basal energy expenditure (BEE) The basal metabolic rate (BMR) extrapolated to 24 hours. Often used interchangeably with REE.

resting energy expenditure (REE) The minimum energy needed to maintain basic physiological functions (e.g., heart beat, muscle function, respiration). The resting metabolic rate (RMR) extrapolated to 24 hours. Often used interchangeably with BEE.

basal metabolic rate (BMR) A clinical measure of resting energy expenditure performed upon awakening, 10 to 12 hours after eating, and 12 to 18 hours after significant physical activity. Often used interchangeably with RMR.

resting metabolic rate (RMR) A clinical measure of resting energy expenditure performed three to four hours after eating or performing significant physical activity. Often used interchangeably with BMR.

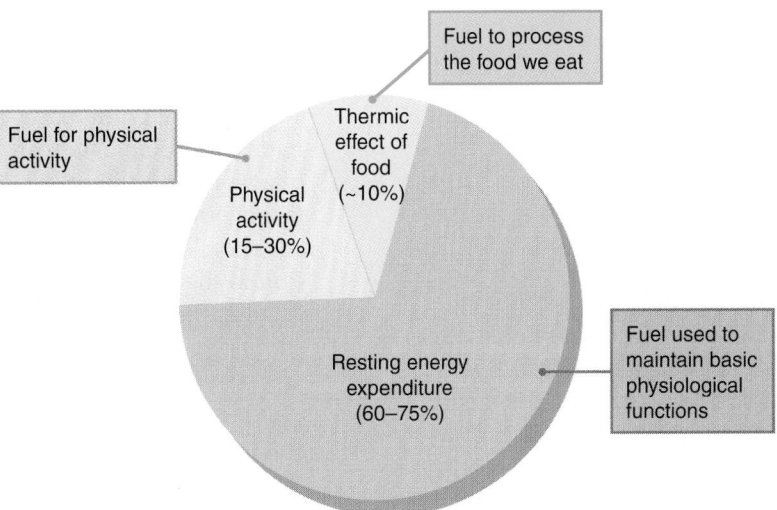

Figure 8.5 **Major components of energy expenditure.** You expend most of your energy to maintain basic body functions. Energy expended in physical activity can be significant and is the most variable component of total energy expenditure. The thermic effect of food is the energy needed to digest, absorb, transport, metabolize, and store ingested food.

Table 8.1 Approximate Energy Expenditure of Organs in Adults

Organ	Percentage of RMR
Liver	29
Brain	19
Heart	10
Kidney	7
Skeletal muscles (at rest)	18
Remainder (including bone)	17
	100

Source: Mahan LK, Escott-Stump S. *Krause's Food, Nutrition and Diet Therapy.* 10th ed. Philadelphia: WB Saunders, 2000:20. Reprinted by permission of Elsevier.

lean body mass The portion of the body exclusive of stored fat, including muscle, bone, connective tissue, organs, and water.

Quick Bites

Brrr! Shivering Away Calories

Cold weather increases energy needs. Shivering alone can increase the RMR by 2.5 times. Although shivering bodies use both fat and carbohydrate, carbohydrates are the preferred fuel. In addition, people with less body fat shiver more in the cold.

expended in a 24-hour period.[31] Researchers measure BMR under the following conditions:

1. The person is lying at rest.
2. The person has just awoken from a normal overnight sleep.
3. Ten to 12 hours have elapsed since the person's last meal.
4. No physical activity has taken place—usually for 12 to 18 hours.

The RMR differs slightly from the BMR. Researchers usually measure RMR three to four hours after a person eats or does significant physical work. RMR tends to be somewhat higher than BMR[32] and is a more practical concept because the ideal conditions for measuring BMR are more difficult to meet. For this reason, in the remainder of this text we will use the terms *resting metabolic rate* and *resting energy expenditure*.

Factors That Affect Resting Metabolic Rate. Over time, your RMR varies less than 5 percent. However, among different people, RMR can vary by as much as 25 percent. Individual differences in muscle and organ mass account for most of this variation. Resting muscles and organ tissue make the greatest contribution to RMR because they have greater metabolic activity than other tissue such as fat. (See **Table 8.1.**) Muscles, organs, bones, and fluids make up most of what is known as the **lean body mass**—the total mass of the body that isn't fat. Differences in lean body mass explain 70 to 80 percent of the variation in resting metabolic rate among individuals.[33] As a result, an extremely muscular person with a large lean body mass would have a higher resting energy expenditure than someone who weighs the same but has a higher proportion of body fat.

Age, gender, degree of muscle development, and, of course, body size are the primary influences on a person's lean body mass. In the aging adult, lean body mass tends to decrease while body fatness rises, resulting in an RMR reduction of about 2 to 3 percent per decade.[34] However, declining lean body mass does not account fully for the age-related decline in RMR, which also may reflect declining organ function.[35] Keeping physically active as we age helps slow loss of lean tissue and discourages accumulation of fat, thus maintaining a higher RMR.

Women usually have lower RMRs than men. Women tend to be smaller than men, and pound for pound they generally have less lean body mass. Yet even when differences in lean body mass are taken into account, a man's metabolic rate is still about 50 kilocalories per day higher than that of a woman.[36] The reason is unclear, but this difference is consistent throughout the lives of men and women. RMR also varies during the menstrual cycle, fluctuating from the low point about one week before ovulation to the high point just before the onset of menstruation.[37]

Other factors that influence metabolic rate may be less consistent, of shorter duration, or limited to individual situations. During sleep, RMR falls about 10 percent. RMR relative to lean body mass rises during periods of rapid growth, such as in infancy and adolescence. Hormones, especially thyroxine (thyroid hormone) and norepinephrine, help regulate metabolic rate. Inadequate thyroxine production (hypothyroidism) can slow the metabolic rate; excess thyroxine (hyperthyroidism) can increase the metabolic rate. Physical stress increases the metabolic rate, probably in response to changes in norepinephrine levels. Fever increases RMR by about 7 percent for each degree of temperature over 98.6°F. Environmental temperature also affects the metabolic rate. During exposure to cold, RMR increases.

As ambient temperatures rise above normal, RMR first decreases and then plateaus. At much higher temperatures, RMR increases. During starvation, the metabolic rate declines as the body slows basic functions to conserve energy and prolong survival. Finally, some variation in RMR has been attributed to unknown genetic factors.[38] **Figure 8.6** shows the factors that affect RMR.

Key Concepts: *We use energy to fuel basic body functions, process the food we eat, and support physical activity. The energy used in these basic functions is called the resting energy expenditure, or REE. Factors that affect resting energy expenditure include body composition, age, gender, fitness, genetics, stage of growth, hormone levels, fever, and environmental temperatures.*

Energy Expenditure for Physical Activity

Physical activity is more than just exercise and sport. It includes work, leisure activities, and other everyday activities—even fidgeting. Depending on whether a person is mostly sedentary or a top athlete in training, energy expended on physical activity accounts for 15 to 30 percent of total energy expenditure.[39] The energy cost of an activity depends on its type (whether it is walking, running, or typing, for example), duration, and intensity. **Table 8.2** shows the amounts of energy expended in specific activities.

Body size affects energy cost, too—it takes more energy to move a bigger mass, so a large person expends more calories per minute than a smaller person doing the same activity. Fitness level has an effect as well. A fit person exercises more efficiently, with lower energy costs. However, fit people also can exercise with greater intensity and duration, burning more calories overall.

Mental activity—such as studying for an exam—uses little energy. But if you fidget when you study, you may expend a significant amount of energy. The acronym **NEAT** stands for **nonexercise activity thermogenesis**, which is the energy associated with activities other than exercise, including fidgeting, maintenance of posture, and similar contributors to energy expenditure.[40] (See the FYI feature "What's Neat About NEAT?" and the Nutrition Science in Action entitled "NEAT Energy.")

Energy Expenditure to Process Food

Our bodies expend energy to digest, absorb, and metabolize the nutrients we take in, and these processes generate heat. This energy output is collectively called the **thermic effect of food (TEF)**. TEF peaks about one hour after eating and normally dissipates within five hours. It is lowest for fat and highest for protein. Converting excess protein and carbohydrate to energy stores (fat and glycogen) requires more energy than the efficient process of simply storing excess dietary fat as body fat. For a typical mixed diet, TEF accounts for approximately 10 percent of total energy expenditure,[41] but research suggests that TEF may be reduced in obese individuals[42] and may be reduced by irregular eating habits.[43] It's possible to increase the TEF by altering the macronutrient composition of the diet, but not by much—only about 50 kilocalories or so daily.

Key Concepts: *An individual's fitness level, weight, and the type, duration, and intensity of activity affect the amount of energy expended in physical activity. The thermic effect of food is the energy needed to process the food we eat and is influenced by the amount and mix of nutrients in the diet.*

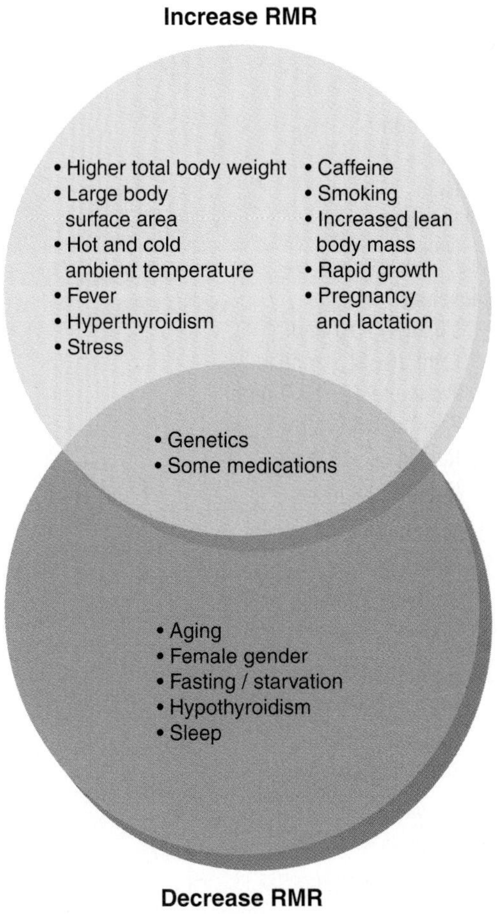

Increase RMR

- Higher total body weight
- Large body surface area
- Hot and cold ambient temperature
- Fever
- Hyperthyroidism
- Stress
- Caffeine
- Smoking
- Increased lean body mass
- Rapid growth
- Pregnancy and lactation

- Genetics
- Some medications

- Aging
- Female gender
- Fasting / starvation
- Hypothyroidism
- Sleep

Decrease RMR

Figure 8.6 **Factors that affect RMR.** Inherited traits determine whether you have a generally high or low RMR. Many environmental and physiological factors may temporarily raise RMR, and other factors may temporarily lower it.

nonexercise activity thermogenesis (NEAT) The output of energy associated with fidgeting, maintenance of posture, and other minimal physical exertions.

thermic effect of food (TEF) The energy used to digest, absorb, and metabolize energy-yielding foodstuffs. It constitutes about 10 percent of total energy expenditure but is influenced by various factors.

Quick Bites

Magic Underwear

James Levine, the endocrinologist and professor of medicine at the Mayo Clinic who coined the term "NEAT," uses what he calls "magic underwear," which contains sensors to measure the research subject's movements and body postures 120 times each minute.

Table 8.2 Amount of Energy Expended in Specific Activities

Description	kcal/h/kg	kcal/h/lb	50 kg / 110 lb	57 kg / 125 lb	68 kg / 150 lb	80 kg / 175 lb	91 kg / 200 lb
Aerobics							
Light	3.0	1.36	150	170	205	239	273
Moderate	5.0	2.27	250	284	341	398	455
Heavy	8.0	3.64	400	455	545	636	727
Bicycling							
Leisurely <10 mph	4.0	1.82	200	227	273	318	364
Light 10–11.9 mph	6.0	2.73	300	341	409	477	545
Moderate 12–13.9 mph	8.0	3.64	400	455	545	636	727
Fast 14–15.9 mph	10.0	4.55	500	568	682	795	909
Racing 16–19 mph	12.0	5.45	600	682	818	955	1091
BMX or mountain	8.5	3.86	425	483	580	676	773
Daily Activities							
Sleeping	1.2	0.55	60	68	82	95	109
Studying, reading, writing	1.8	0.82	90	102	123	143	164
Cooking, food preparation	2.5	1.14	125	142	170	199	227
Home Activities							
House painting, outside	4.0	1.82	200	227	273	318	364
General gardening	5.0	2.27	250	284	341	398	455
Shoveling snow	6.0	2.73	300	341	409	477	545
Running							
Jogging	7.0	3.18	350	398	477	557	636
Running 5 mph	8.0	3.64	400	455	545	636	727
Running 6 mph	10.0	4.55	500	568	682	795	909
Running 7 mph	11.5	5.23	575	653	784	915	1045
Running 8 mph	13.5	6.14	675	767	920	1074	1227
Running 9 mph	15.0	6.82	750	852	1023	1193	1364
Running 10 mph	16.0	7.27	800	909	1091	1273	1455
Sports							
Frisbee, ultimate	3.5	1.59	175	199	239	278	318
Hacky sack	4.0	1.82	200	227	273	318	364
Wind surfing	4.2	1.91	210	239	286	334	382
Golf	4.5	2.05	225	256	307	358	409
Skateboarding	5.0	2.27	250	284	341	398	455
Rollerblading	7.0	3.18	350	398	477	557	636
Soccer	7.0	3.18	350	398	477	557	636
Field hockey	8.0	3.64	400	455	545	636	727
Swimming, slow to moderate laps	8.0	3.64	400	455	545	636	727
Skiing downhill, moderate effort	6.0	2.73	300	341	409	477	545
Skiing cross country, moderate effort	8.0	3.64	400	455	545	636	727
Tennis, doubles	6.0	2.73	300	341	409	477	545
Tennis, singles	8.0	3.64	400	455	545	636	727
Walking							
Strolling <2 mph, level	2.0	0.91	100	114	136	159	182
Moderate pace ~3 mph, level	3.5	1.59	175	199	239	278	318
Moderate pace ~3 mph, uphill	6.0	2.73	300	341	409	477	545
Brisk pace ~3.5 mph, level	4.0	1.82	200	227	273	318	364
Very brisk pace ~4.5 mph, level	4.5	2.05	225	256	307	358	409

Source: Adapted from Nieman DC. *Exercise Testing and Prescription.* 4th ed. Mountain View, CA: Mayfield Publishing, 1999.

NUTRITION SCIENCE IN ACTION

NEAT Energy

Background: Nonexercise activity thermogenesis (NEAT) is a component of total energy expenditure and includes energy expended in daily activities such as sitting, standing, fidgeting, walking, and talking. To investigate NEAT, investigators have developed and validated a sensitive and reliable technology for measuring body position and motion 120 times per minute.

Hypothesis: Obese people expend less energy for NEAT than lean people.

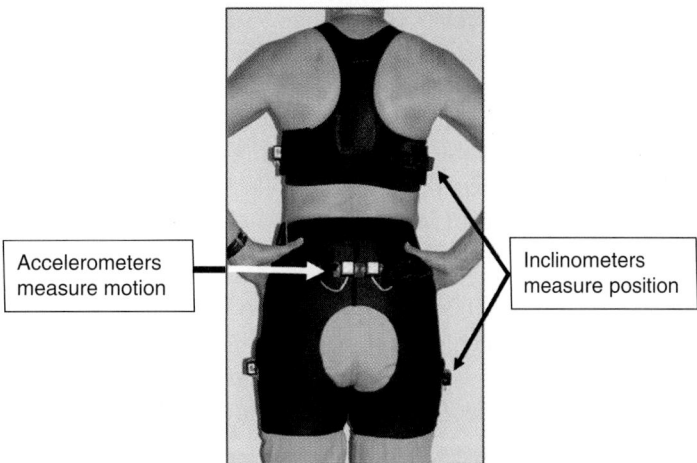

Accelerometers measure motion

Inclinometers measure position

Experimental Plan: Recruit 20 healthy volunteers who are self-proclaimed "couch potatoes." Ten participants are lean, and 10 are mildly obese with no complications of obesity. Monitor their total NEAT expenditure for 10 days as they continue their usual daily activities and occupations.

Results: The hypothesis is confirmed. Obese participants remained seated for about 2.5 hours per day longer than lean participants, for an average energy savings of 352 kcal/day.

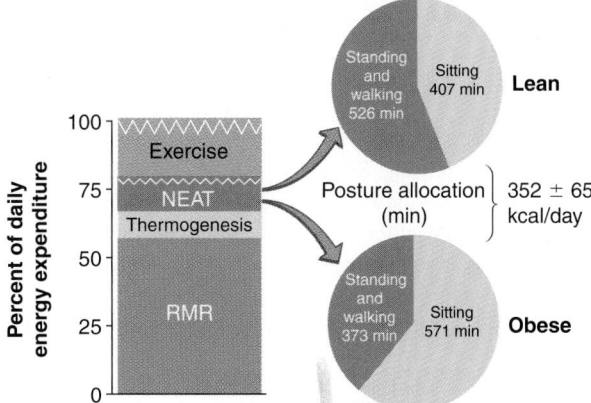

Conclusion and Discussion: Weight gain is a dynamic process that results from a long-term sustained imbalance between energy intake and energy expenditure. The "energy gap" required to explain the increased prevalence of obesity is only 100 to 200 kcal/day—less than the observed differences in NEAT between lean and obese people. Obesity might be prevented by simply increasing NEAT expenditures—limiting sedentary activities or increasing active behaviors such as standing, walking, and fidgeting. The underlying mechanisms for an individual's propensity to fidget are unknown and may be investigated by additional studies.

Source: Based on Levine JA, Lanningham-Foster LM, McCrady SK, et al. Interindividual variation in posture allocation: possible role in human obesity. *Science.* 2005;307:584–586. Photo used with permission from AAAS.

calorimetry [kal-oh-RIM-eh-tree] The measurement of the amount of heat given off by an organism. It is used to determine total energy expenditure.

calorimeter A device used to measure quantities of heat generated by various processes.

direct calorimetry Determination of energy use by the body by measuring the heat released from an organism enclosed in a small insulated chamber surrounded by water. The rise in the temperature of the water is directly related to the energy used by the organism.

indirect calorimetry Determination of energy use by the body without directly measuring the production of heat. Methods include gas exchange, the measurement of oxygen uptake and/or carbon dioxide output, and the doubly labeled water method.

doubly labeled water A method for measuring daily energy expenditure over extended time periods, typically 7 to 14 days, while subjects are living in their usual environments. Small amounts of water that is isotopically labeled with deuterium and oxygen-18 (^2H_2O and $H_2^{18}O$) are ingested. Energy expenditure can be calculated from the difference between the rates at which the body loses each isotope.

isotopes [EYE-so-towps] Forms of an element in which the atoms have the same number of protons but different numbers of neutrons.

The Measurement of Energy Expenditure

Calorimetry, the measurement of energy expenditure, helps us understand individual differences in energy expenditure and the effects of environmental conditions, as well as age, gender, exercise, and other factors.

A Brief History of Calorimetry

Antoine Lavoisier, an eighteenth-century French chemist, was the first to study food combustion in the body.[44] He theorized that just as a burning candle needs oxygen and releases heat, organisms need oxygen to live and release heat as they combust food.

Lavoisier built the first **calorimeter**, quite an achievement at that time. A calorimeter consists of a chamber within a chamber. The inner chamber is large enough to house an animal or human; the outer chamber is sensitive to temperature changes that occur in the inner one. Lavoisier packed ice into a sealed pocket around the inner chamber (his studies were possible only in winter, when ice was plentiful) and then placed it inside the outer chamber, which was insulated to shield it from the outside environment. As the animal in the inner chamber used energy, it produced heat that melted the ice. By collecting the resulting water and measuring its volume, Lavoisier could accurately calculate the amount of heat produced by the animal.

Direct and Indirect Calorimetry

Lavoisier's technique illustrates the principles of **direct calorimetry**. When your body combusts food, it captures some energy while losing the rest as heat. This heat loss is proportional to the body's total energy use and can

Fyi What's Neat About NEAT?

FOR YOUR INFORMATION

It seems Jan only has to look at food to gain weight. Yet her friend Molly doesn't seem to gain weight no matter what she eats. Both have the same height and frame, eat about the same amount of calories, and get about the same amount of exercise. So what's missing? Recent research suggests that fidgeting and movements such as posture adjustments may be part of the answer.

Studies in the early 1900s first suggested that weight gained in response to overeating wasn't proportional to the extra calories ingested. Following experiments on himself, the German scientist R. O. Neumann coined the term "luxuskonsumption" to describe his observation that excess calories did not result in weight gain and therefore must be lost as heat.[1] Further studies supported this idea,

showing wide individual variation in response to overfeeding. Some suggest that the ease of weight gain is genetically based.[2]

A study at the Mayo Clinic attributes differences in weight gain in response to overfeeding to a mechanism described as NEAT: nonexercise activity thermogenesis.[3] According to the researchers, NEAT is "the thermogenesis [heat production] that accompanies physical activities other than volitional [intentional] exercise, such as the activities of daily living, fidgeting, spontaneous muscle contraction, and maintaining posture when not recumbent."

In the NEAT study, 16 volunteers (12 men and 4 women) were given an extra 1,000 kilocalories per day—roughly equivalent to two double cheeseburgers—for a period of eight

weeks. Before the study began, careful measurements were made over a two-week period to determine each participant's maintenance energy requirements. Physical activity during the study was controlled, and meals were provided only through the Mayo Clinic General Clinical Research Center. Questionnaires and interviews were done to ensure compliance.

The average weight gained by the study participants was 4.7 kilograms (10.3 lb), but some gained as much as 7.2 kilograms (15.8 lb), whereas others added only 1.4 kilograms (3.1 lb). The theoretical expected weight gain from an eight-week excess of 56,000 kilocalories would be 7.3 kilograms (16.0 lb) to 9.1 kilograms (20.0 lb)—more than the maximum weight gain of any participant!

After accounting for RMR, TEF, and energy

be measured directly using a chamber like that constructed by Lavoisier. Modern chambers dispense with the ice and instead measure the temperature change in a surrounding layer of water.

Direct calorimetry is expensive and complex. The chamber must be large enough to accommodate a person, yet maintain the precision to measure the relatively small changes in temperature. Since the advent of alternative methods, direct calorimetry is no longer widely used.

Indirect calorimetry is easier and less expensive than direct calorimetry. It is "indirect" because energy production (as heat) is not measured directly. Instead, energy expenditure is estimated from a person's oxygen consumption and carbon dioxide production. Burning (oxidizing) fuel consumes oxygen and produces carbon dioxide in proportion to the amount of fuel burned and the amount of energy released.

For indirect calorimetry, a technician collects respiratory gases. During short periods of rest or exercise, expired air can be collected using a face mask, mouthpiece, or canopy system. (See **Figure 8.7**.) This cumbersome apparatus makes indirect calorimetry impractical for use during physically demanding activities or normal living conditions.

Doubly Labeled Water

A relatively new and easier technique to measure total energy expenditure is **doubly labeled water**. (See **Figure 8.8**.) Rather than measuring respiratory gases, this indirect calorimetry technique relies on measuring the **isotopes** (typically a form of an element with a higher than usual atomic mass but the same characteristics as the usual element) of hydrogen and oxygen in excreted water and carbon dioxide. A person swallows a small quantity of

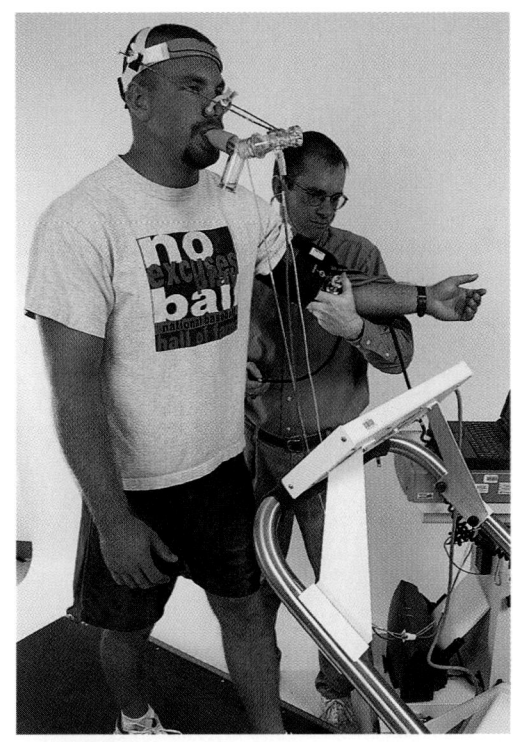

Figure 8.7 **Indirect calorimetry.** A technician collects respiratory gases and then calculates energy expenditure.

used in physical activity, the remaining energy expenditure was attributed to NEAT. The amount of energy expended as NEAT varied among the participants by nearly 800 kilocalories per day. Participants with higher NEAT resisted weight gain, suggesting that people who can effectively activate NEAT tend not to gain weight, even with overeating. Further, this suggests that obese people may not effectively activate NEAT.

In another study, the Mayo Clinic researchers found that obese individuals sat for two hours longer than lean individuals.[4] This pattern of activity (or lack thereof) didn't change when obese individuals lost weight or lean individuals gained weight.

So is the take-home message "fidget more, stand up straight, and you won't gain weight?" Not exactly. The researchers did not account for factors such as the extra energy needed to move a higher body weight in activity. In addition, in the first study they relied on self-reports and pedometers that lack precision and accuracy.[5] However, in the comparison of obese and lean individuals, a physical activity monitoring system was used to capture posture and movement data 120 times per minute. Attributing the entire difference in energy expenditure to NEAT ignores heat production by brown adipose tissue, a type of fat tissue that tends to "waste" energy.[6] Clearly, though, some individuals are able to resist weight gain, even when overeating, while others cannot. Further studies to better understand NEAT and the factors that regulate it may help to better understand

conditions of energy imbalance—not only obesity, but also anorexia nervosa.[7]

1 Neumann RO. Experimentalle Beitrage zur Lehre von dem taglichen Nahrungsbedarf der Menschen unter besonder Berucksichtigung der notwendigen Eisewissmenge. *Arch Hyg.* 1902;45:1–2.

2 Bouchard C, Tremblay A, Despres JP, et al. The response to long-term overfeeding in identical twins. *N Engl J Med.* 1990;322:1477–1482.

3 Levine JA, Eberhardt NL, Jensen MD. Role of nonexercise activity thermogenesis in resistance to fat gain in humans. *Science.* 1999;283:212–214.

4 Levine JA, Lanningham-Foster LM, McCrady SK, et al. Interindividual variation in posture allocation: possible role in human obesity. *Science.* 2005;307:584–586.

5 Ravussin E, Danforth E. Beyond sloth—physical activity and weight gain. *Science.* 1999;283:184–185.

6 Klaus S. Adipose tissue as a regulator of energy balance. *Curr Drug Targets.* 2004;5:241–250.

7 Levine JA. Nonexercise activity thermogenesis (NEAT): environment and biology. *Am J Physiol Endocrinol Metab.* 2004;286:E675–E685.

two kinds of water, one labeled with the hydrogen isotope deuterium (^{2}H) and the other labeled with an isotope of oxygen (oxygen-18, or ^{18}O). Both isotopes occur naturally and are nonradioactive. The body excretes oxygen-18 as part of water ($H_2^{18}O$) and carbon dioxide ($C^{18}O_2$). It excretes deuterium only as part of water (^2H_2O). Scientists use the difference between the rate of deuterium loss and oxygen-18 loss to calculate carbon dioxide output and determine the total energy expenditure.

The doubly labeled water technique is noninvasive and unobtrusive. Subjects can stay in their normal environment and perform normal activities during the testing period, which typically lasts 7 to 14 days or longer. This method is emerging as the gold standard against which other energy expenditure measurement methods are compared. For best accuracy, doubly labeled water studies should last at least 14 days. Unfortunately, the doubly labeled water technique is not widely available, and it's expensive—the ^{18}O isotope costs about $500 for a 70-kg adult, and the analytic equipment is costly. Therefore, the technique is not suited to large-scale studies. It has other limitations as well: It cannot give information about individual days, individual activities, or day-to-day variability.

Estimating Total Energy Expenditure

Directly measuring a person's total energy expenditure requires sophisticated equipment that is inaccessible to all but a few people in research settings. To determine the energy needs of most people, nutritionists must rely on calculated estimates.

An adult's REE can be estimated using an abbreviated method (see margin). The 1.0 and 0.9 factors for kilocalories per kilogram reflect the differences in body composition between men and women. Men have proportionally more lean body mass and therefore burn more calories per kilogram of body weight. This abbreviated method dramatically underestimates children's REE, however, and somewhat overestimates the REE of elders.

Abbreviated Method to Estimate REE

For adult men

REE = weight (kg) × 1.0 kcal/kg x 24 hr/day

REE = weight (kg) × 1.0 × 24

For adult women

REE = weight (kg) × 0.9 kcal/kg × 24 hr/day

REE = weight (kg) × 0.9 × 24

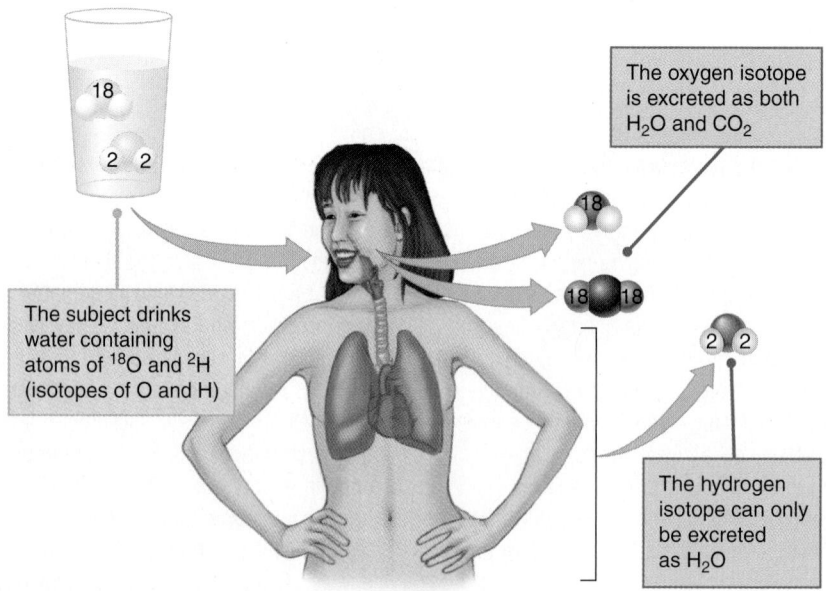

The oxygen isotope is excreted as both H_2O and CO_2

The subject drinks water containing atoms of ^{18}O and ^{2}H (isotopes of O and H)

The hydrogen isotope can only be excreted as H_2O

Figure 8.8 **Doubly labeled water.** When using doubly labeled water, scientists measure the excretion rates of the two isotopes to calculate carbon dioxide output and determine total energy expenditure.

The abbreviated method estimates only REE. To determine total energy expenditure (TEE), energy for physical activity and the thermic effect of food must be included. Energy expended in physical activity can be estimated as a percentage of REE based on a person's general activity level (see **Table 8.3**). Most adults in the United States and Canada have a light or moderate activity level. The thermic effect of food can be estimated as roughly 10 percent of the sum of REE plus energy expended in physical activity. Summing the three estimated components—REE, physical activity, and TEF—delivers the estimated total energy expenditure. See the FYI feature "How Many Calories Do I Burn?" for an example of these estimates in action.

DRIs for Energy: Estimated Energy Requirements

Just as there are Dietary Reference Intakes (DRIs) for nutrients, there are also DRIs for energy, called Estimated Energy Requirements (EERs).[45] The EER is defined as the energy intake predicted to maintain energy balance in a healthy person of normal weight. The EER equations for adults (see **Table 8.4**) predict total energy expenditure from age, height, weight,

---

Table 8.3 **Estimating Energy Expended in Physical Activity**

Percentage of REE	Activity Level	Description
20–30%	Sedentary	Mostly resting with little or no activity
30–45%	Light	Occasional unplanned activity, e.g., going for a stroll
45–65%	Moderate	Daily planned activity, such as brisk walks
65–90%	Heavy	Daily workout routine requiring several hours of continuous exercise
90–120%	Exceptional	Daily vigorous workouts for extended hours; training for competition

---

Table 8.4 **Estimated Energy Requirements (EER) for Adults**

Males

$EER = 662 - 9.53 \times Age\ [yr] + PA \times (15.91 \times Weight\ [kg] + 539.6 \times Height\ [m])$

PA = 1.0 Sedentary
    1.11 Low active
    1.25 Active
    1.48 Very active

Females

$EER = 354 - 6.91 \times Age\ [yr] + PA \times (9.36 \times Weight\ [kg] + 726 \times Height\ [m])$

PA = 1.0 Sedentary
    1.12 Low active
    1.27 Active
    1.45 Very active

Source: Institute of Medicine, Food and Nutrition Board. *Dietary Reference Intakes for Energy, Carbohydrate, Fiber, Fat, Fatty Acids, Cholesterol, Protein, and Amino Acids.* Washington, DC: National Academy Press, 2005. Reprinted with permission.

body composition The chemical or anatomical composition of the body. Commonly defined as the proportions of fat, muscle, bone, and other tissues in the body.

gender, and physical activity level. Separate equations have been developed for infants, children, and teens, and adjustments are made for pregnancy and lactation.

Key Concepts: *Energy expenditure can be measured using direct or indirect calorimetry. Direct calorimetry measures heat production by the body, whereas indirect calorimetry measures oxygen consumption and carbon dioxide production. The doubly labeled water method is becoming accepted as the gold standard for determining energy expenditure. In most situations, measuring energy expenditure is not practical, so a variety of equations have been developed for predicting energy expenditure.*

Body Composition: Understanding Fatness and Weight

Stepping onto a scale provides quick and easy feedback about your body weight. Yet many people have a distorted notion of their weight—thinking they're too fat when they aren't or thinking their weight is just fine when it isn't. In terms of your health risks, **body composition** is more important than body weight.

Body composition is the relative amount of fat and lean body mass. Excess body fatness is linked with increased risk for heart disease, hypertension, cancer, diabetes, and other chronic diseases. Two people with the same height and high weight may have very different health risks. Whereas one may be obese and have many weight-related health risks, the other could be very fit and muscular, with no increased disease risk.

[*Fyi*] How Many Calories Do I Burn?

FOR YOUR INFORMATION

You can estimate the amount of energy you use each day by using some simple equations. Remember that there will be quite a lot of individual variation in actual energy output, and so these calculated values are just estimates.

1. Convert your weight in pounds to weight in kilograms. For example, Carol is a 120-pound female. Her weight is 54.5 kilograms ($54.5 = 120 \div 2.2$).

$$\underline{\hspace{3cm}} \div 2.2 = \underline{\hspace{3cm}}$$
weight (lbs) \quad\quad weight (kg)

2. Estimate your personal REE.

For adult women:

$$REE = \underline{\hspace{2cm}} \times 0.9 \times 24$$
weight (kg)

For adult men:

$$REE = \underline{\hspace{2cm}} \times 1.0 \times 24$$
weight (kg)

For example, Carol has an estimated REE of 1,177 kilocalories ($1,177 = 54.5 \times 0.9 \times 24$).

3. Estimate your energy expended in physical activity (see Table 8.2).

$$Energy_{physical\ activity} = \underline{\hspace{2cm}} \times REE$$
From Table 8.2

For example, Carol has a light to moderate physical activity level. She expends about 530 kilocalories in physical activity ($530 = 0.45 \times 1,177$).

4. Estimate your thermic effect of food (TEF).

$$TEF = 0.1 \times \left(\underline{\hspace{1.5cm}} + \underline{\hspace{1.5cm}} \right)$$
$energy_{physical\ activity}$ \quad REE

For our example, Carol's thermic effect of food is about 171 kilocalories ($171 = 0.1 \times [530 + 1,177]$).

5. Estimate your personal total energy expenditure (TEE).

$$TEE = \underline{\hspace{1cm}} + \\ REE \\ \underline{\hspace{2cm}} + \underline{\hspace{2cm}} \\ energy_{physical\ activity} \quad TEF$$

For our example, Carol's total energy expenditure is about 1,878 kilocalories ($1,177 + 530 + 171$).

You may want to calculate your REE using the equations on page 342 and compare that result to this simplified method.

Assessing Body Weight

Body mass index (BMI) has become the accepted method for assessing body weight for height. This index, which is a ratio of weight to height squared, correlates reasonably well with body fatness and health risks.[46] To determine your BMI, accurately measure your height without shoes and your weight with minimal clothing. Then plug these numbers into the BMI equations in the margin. For adults, the National Heart, Lung, and Blood Institute (NHLBI) defines **underweight**, normal weight, **overweight**, and **obesity** as follows.[47]

- *Underweight:* BMI < 18.5 kg/m^2
- *Normal weight:* 18.5 kg/m^2 ≤ BMI < 25 kg/m^2
- *Overweight:* 25 kg/m^2 ≤ BMI < 30 kg/m^2
- *Obese:* BMI ≥ 30 kg/m^2

Table 8.5 can help you determine whether your weight is a healthy weight according to the *Dietary Guidelines for Americans.*

To calculate BMI

$$BMI = \frac{weight\ (kg)}{height\ (m)^2},\ or$$

$$BMI = \frac{weight\ (lb)}{height\ (in)^2} \times 704.5.$$

body mass index (BMI) Body weight (in kilograms) divided by the square of height (in meters), expressed in units of kg/m^2. Also called Quetelet index.

underweight BMI less than 18.5 kg/m^2.

overweight BMI at or above 25 kg/m^2 and less than 30 kg/m^2.

obesity BMI at or above 30 kg/m^2.

Table 8.5 Adult BMI Chart

BMI	19	20	21	22	23	24	25	26	27	28	29	30	31	32	33	34	35
Height							**Weight in Pounds**										
4'10"	91	96	100	105	110	115	119	124	129	134	138	143	148	153	158	162	167
4'11"	94	99	104	109	114	119	124	128	133	138	143	148	153	158	163	168	173
5'	97	102	107	112	118	123	128	133	138	143	148	153	158	163	158	174	179
5'1"	100	106	111	116	122	127	132	137	143	148	153	158	164	169	174	180	185
5'2"	104	109	115	120	126	131	136	142	147	153	158	164	169	175	180	186	191
5'3"	107	113	118	124	130	135	141	146	152	158	163	169	175	180	186	191	197
5'4"	110	116	122	128	134	140	145	151	157	163	169	174	180	186	192	197	204
5'5"	114	120	126	132	138	144	150	156	162	168	174	180	186	192	198	204	210
5'6"	118	124	130	136	142	148	155	161	167	173	179	186	192	198	204	210	216
5'7"	121	127	134	140	146	153	159	166	172	178	185	191	198	204	211	217	223
5'8"	125	131	138	144	151	158	164	171	177	184	190	197	203	210	216	223	230
5'9"	128	135	142	149	155	162	169	176	182	189	196	203	209	216	223	230	236
5'10"	132	139	146	153	160	167	174	181	188	195	202	209	216	222	229	236	243
5'11"	136	143	150	157	165	172	179	186	193	200	208	215	222	229	236	243	250
6'	140	147	154	162	169	177	184	191	199	206	213	221	228	235	242	250	258
6'1"	144	151	159	166	174	182	189	197	204	212	219	227	235	242	250	257	265
6'2"	148	155	163	171	179	186	194	202	210	218	225	233	241	249	256	264	272
6'3"	152	160	168	176	184	192	200	208	216	224	232	240	248	256	264	272	279
	Healthy Weight						**Overweight**					**Obese**					

Locate the height of interest in the leftmost column and read across the row for that height to the weight of interest. Follow the column of the weight up to the top row that lists the BMI. BMI of 19 to 24 is the healthy weight range, BMI of 25 to 29 is the overweight range, and BMI of 30 and above is in the obese range. Due to rounding, these ranges vary slightly from the NHLBI values.

Source: US Departments of Agriculture and Health and Human Services. *Dietary Guidelines for Americans.* 6th ed. Washington, DC: US Government Printing Office, 2005.

Is Shaq Too Fat?

Although BMI has become the standard reference for determining overweight and obesity, it has limitations at the extremes of body size and composition. Consider Shaquille O'Neal, the talented center for the Miami Heat. At 7 feet, 1 inch, and 325 pounds, Shaq has a BMI of 32.7—well into the range for obesity. LaDainian Tomlinson, star running back for the NFL's San Diego Chargers, could also be considered obese based on his BMI of 31.8 kg/m² (5 feet, 10 inches, 221 pounds)!

densitometry A method for estimating body composition from measurement of total body density.

underwater weighing Determining body density by measuring the volume of water displaced when the body is fully submerged in a specialized water tank. Also called hydrostatic weighing.

hydrostatic weighing See *underwater weighing*.

BodPod A device used to measure the density of the body based on the volume of air displaced as a person sits in a sealed chamber of known volume.

dual energy x-ray absorptiometry (DEXA) A body composition measurement technique originally developed to measure bone density.

total body water All of the water in the body, including intracellular and extracellular water, and water in the urinary and GI tracts.

Figure 8.9 **BMI and mortality.** People with a high or very low BMI have a higher relative mortality rate.
Source: Flegal KM, Graubard BI, Williamson DF, Gail MH. Excess deaths associated with underweight, overweight, and obesity. *JAMA.* 2005;293:1861–1867. Reprinted with permission from Bull Publishing. All rights reserved.

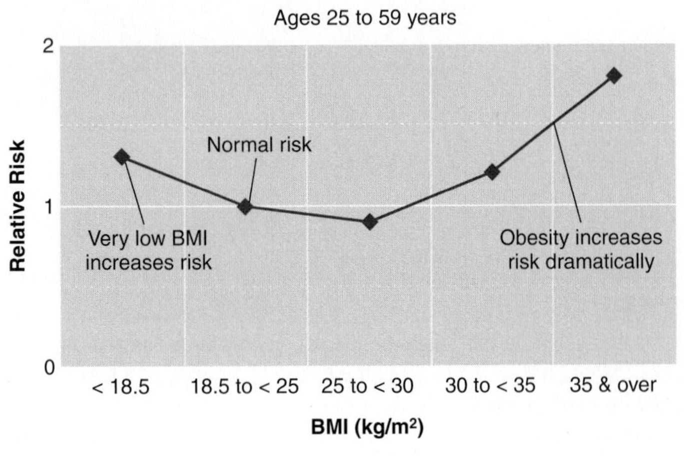

Ages 25 to 59 years

As **Figure 8.9** shows, correlating BMI with mortality produces a J-shaped curve. Studies indicate that underweight (BMI less than 18.5 kg/m²) is associated with increased mortality, as is obesity (BMI greater than or equal to 30 kg/m²). Normal weight and overweight are not associated with excess overall mortality.[48]

Although your BMI can give you a general idea of your overall health risks, it still doesn't tell you enough about whether you are carrying muscle weight or excess fat. A classic example is the heavy football player or bodybuilder with a large muscle mass who has a BMI greater than 30 kg/m² but is not overfat. For someone who has lost muscle mass, perhaps an older adult, BMI can underestimate health risks associated with excess body fat. BMI measurements should be interpreted cautiously when used for people who are petite, who have large body frames, or who are highly muscular.[49]

For children and teens, height and weight measurements can be compared to standard growth charts to see if the child is growing and gaining weight at the appropriate rate. (See Chapter 15 for more on growth charts.) For children and teens (2 to 20 years old), pediatric growth charts include age- and sex-specific percentile curves for BMI.[50] A BMI-for-age at or above the 95th percentile indicates overweight and the need for further evaluation and possible treatment. Further evaluation may also be indicated if the child's BMI-for-age is at or above the 85th percentile and is accompanied by other risk factors such as high blood pressure, high blood cholesterol, diabetes, and family history of obesity-related disease.[51] A BMI-for-age below the 5th percentile suggests that the child is underweight.

Key Concepts: *Body composition is a key element in determining energy expenditure and is an important factor in disease risk. Weight and height measures can be used to calculate BMI, which is correlated with body fatness and health risks. Elevated BMI in adults or children can increase health risks.*

Assessing Body Fatness

Fat is stored in the adipose tissue that lies directly under the skin. Fat tissue also surrounds internal organs. Healthy adult females typically have 20 to 35 percent body fat; for men, the range is 8 to 24 percent. Risk of chronic disease rises dramatically when body fat exceeds these levels.

Densitometry is the measure of body density (body mass divided by body volume). Because fat and lean tissues have different densities, if we know the person's volume and weight, we can calculate the ratio of fat to lean body mass. The density of fat doesn't vary, but hydration status, age, gender, and ethnicity all influence the density of lean body mass. For example, bone loss in the elderly leads to a lower density of lean body mass.

Densitometry and Underwater Weighing

Underwater weighing, also called **hydrostatic weighing**, is an accurate densitometry method that is used in research settings and some sports programs. Because fat is less dense than muscle, a person with more body fat will have a lower underwater weight than a person with the same body weight but less fat. With this technique, a seated person is submerged fully in water and weighed as **Figure 8.10** illustrates. Body density is calculated using the above-water weight, the submerged weight, and the quantity of water displaced during submersion. Underwater weighing often is impractical because it requires a special water tank and other nonportable, expensive equipment. The subject must exhale completely, submerge without taking a breath, and remain motionless until the water is still and the scale is steady—clearly not a welcome experience for everyone!

Densitometry and Air Displacement

The **BodPod** measures displacement of air to determine relative amounts of fat and fat-free mass for calculating body density. With this technique, a person sits in a sealed chamber of known volume and displaces a certain volume of air. Air displacement uses the same principles as underwater weighing, but it is much faster and easier. **Figure 8.11** shows an air displacement chamber.

Dual Energy X-Ray Absorptiometry

Dual energy x-ray absorptiometry (DEXA), a technique used to measure bone density, can also be used to analyze body composition by differentiating bone, other lean tissue, and fat.[52] A person undergoing a DEXA scan lies on a padded table while an x-ray detector above scans from head to foot, producing a two-dimensional image of tiny dots, or pixels. (See **Figure 8.12**.) Although the DEXA scan is an excellent technique, its accuracy in obese people and the effects of tissue thickness and hydration status on scan accuracy are unclear. Furthermore, the instrument is expensive and not practical for everyday use in the field.

Isotope Dilution

Researchers can directly measure **total body water** and use this quantity to estimate lean body mass. With this technique, the subject swallows a known quantity and concentration of isotopically labeled water. Unlike the doubly labeled water method, which compares two isotopes, this technique uses a single isotope to label the water. After three or four hours, it is assumed that the labeled water is fully mixed

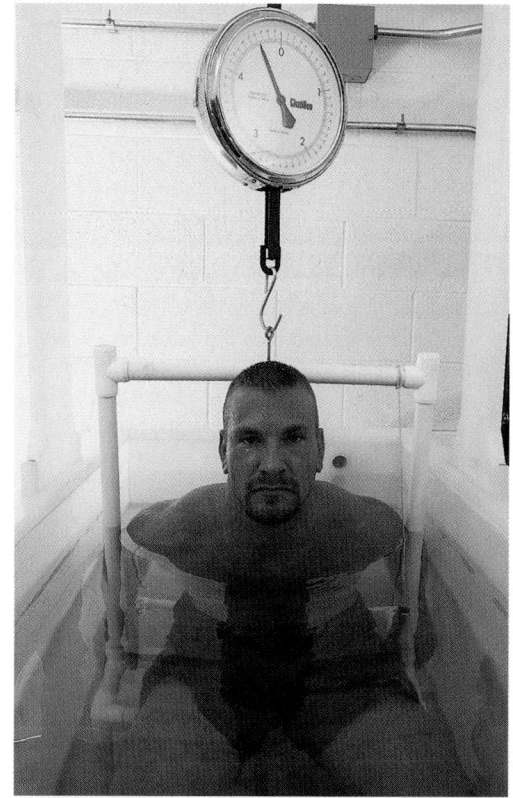

Figure 8.10 **Underwater weighing.** During underwater weighing, the subject must exhale completely, submerge without taking a breath, and remain motionless until the water is still and the scale is steady.

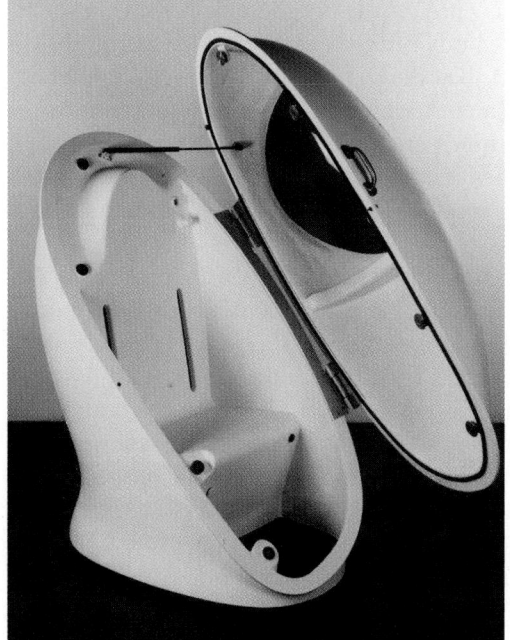

Figure 8.11 **BodPod.** By using air displacement, the BodPod provides an alternative to underwater weighing that is easier, cheaper, and of similar accuracy.

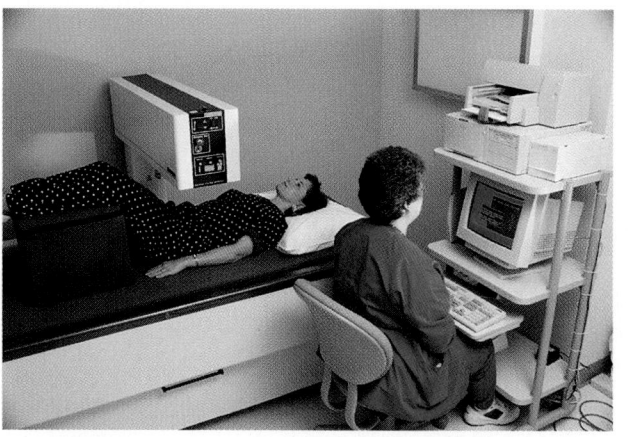

Figure 8.12 **DEXA (dual-energy x-ray absorptiometry scan).** The two-dimensional image produced from a DEXA scan can be used to assess body composition.

bioelectrical impedance analysis (BIA) Technique to estimate amounts of total body water, lean tissue mass, and total body fat. It uses the resistance of tissue to the flow of an alternating electric current.

computed tomography (CT) The gathering of anatomical information from cross-sectional images generated by a computer synthesis of x-ray data.

magnetic resonance imaging (MRI) Medical imaging technique that uses a magnetic field and radio-frequency radiation to generate anatomical information.

near-infrared interactance The measurement of body composition using infrared radiation. It is based on the principle that substances of different densities absorb, reflect, or transmit infrared light at different rates.

body fat distribution The pattern of fat distribution on the body.

gynoid obesity Excess storage of fat located primarily in the buttocks and thighs. Also called gynecoid obesity.

android obesity [AN-droyd] Excess storage of fat located primarily in the abdominal area.

waist circumference The waist measurement, as a marker of abdominal fat content, can be used to indicate health risks.

Quick Bites

Where's the Fat?

*T*he location of excess abdominal fat may hold information about health risks. Within the abdomen, visceral fat (fat surrounding the organs) may be more harmful than subcutaneous fat (fat under the skin). Only sophisticated imaging techniques, such as CT scans and MRI, can distinguish between the two.

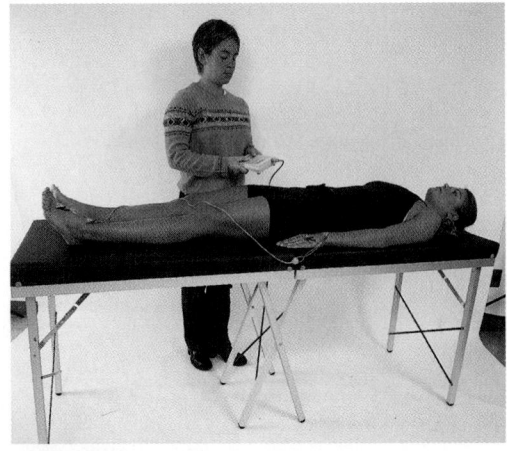

Figure 8.13 **Bioelectrical impedance analysis (BIA).** The measured resistance to a small electrical current passed through the body is used to estimate body composition.

in the body's water pool. The researcher takes a sample of body water (e.g., from plasma, saliva, or urine), measures the concentration of the isotope, and calculates the total volume of body water. Based on the assumption that lean body mass is 73 percent water, researchers can estimate the total lean body mass. Unfortunately, this assumption does not hold true for all people; the amount of water in lean body mass can vary, especially in the elderly. Obesity and dehydration from severe exercise and use of diuretics or laxatives also may influence the results.

Skinfold Thickness

As you learned in Chapter 2, "Nutrition Guidelines and Assessment," skinfold thicknesses often are used to measure body fatness. Typically, more than half of body fat is located just under the skin, and the percentage increases as body weight increases.[53]

Skinfold measurements are a low-tech method for assessing body fatness. A special caliper is used to measure skinfold thicknesses at several sites on the body—typically over the triceps muscles on the back of the upper arm, just below the shoulder blade, near the navel, and over the hips. Predictive equations then estimate regional and total body fatness.

Because of its simplicity and relatively low cost (less than $500 for calipers), skinfold anthropometry is popular in health clubs and weight-control programs. Skinfold measures also are widely used in large population studies. When done correctly, body composition estimates from skinfolds correlate well with those from underwater weighing, but an inexperienced or careless measurer can easily make large errors. Skinfold thicknesses are especially useful in tracking changes in subcutaneous fat distribution in an individual over time. They usually work better for assessing malnutrition than for identifying overweight and obesity.

Bioelectrical Impedance Analysis

Bioelectrical impedance analysis (BIA) measures the rate at which a small electric current flows through the body between electrodes placed on the wrist and ankle. (See **Figure 8.13**.) Fat doesn't conduct electricity well; it resists, or impedes, the current. In contrast, electrolyte-containing fluids readily conduct a current. These fluids are found mostly in lean body tissues, so the leaner the person, the less the resistance. From the impedance reading, the researcher calculates total body water and then estimates total lean body mass and body fatness.

Compared to underwater weighing, the results of BIA usually are as good as, and often slightly better than, skinfold measurements in assessing body fatness.[54] Just as in the isotope dilution method, age, obesity, and altered hydration can affect the accuracy of BIA results. Despite its limitations, bioelectrical impedance is accepted as a valuable tool for measuring body composition in field studies. The equipment is easily portable and only moderately expensive ($2,500–$8,000), making the technique popular at upscale health clubs and weight-loss centers. Similar to BIA, total body electrical conductivity (TOBEC) is an acceptably accurate measure of conductivity, but is less widely used because the equipment is expensive.

Computed Tomography and Magnetic Resonance Imaging

Although **computed tomography (CT)** and **magnetic resonance imaging (MRI)** are primarily medical diagnostic techniques, researchers can use them to distinguish and quantify body tissues. CT scans use x-ray beams to produce highly detailed cross-sectional images of body tissues (see

Figure 8.14). MRI technology uses a magnetic field and radio-frequency waves to both produce cross-sectional images and perform chemical analysis of body tissues. However, CT and MRI are costly techniques limited to research settings, and CT scans entail exposure to radiation.

Near-Infrared Interactance

Near-infrared interactance uses the principle that materials of different composition absorb, reflect, or transmit infrared light at different rates. With this technique, a probe acts as an infrared transmitter and detector. Placed on the biceps muscle, it transmits infrared light through the skin and detects the amount reflected. Analysis of the transmitted and reflected values can estimate body composition. The method, which became instantly popular in health clubs and athletic departments, has not yet been validated and appears to overestimate body fat in lean subjects and underestimate fatness in the obese. Experts do not currently recommend it for body composition assessment.[55]

Body Fat Distribution

Measurements of body fatness tell you more about your health risks than your weight does, but they still don't tell the whole story. Where the fat is located—**body fat distribution**—can be an independent risk factor.[56] The "pear shape," or **gynoid obesity**, more common in women has excess fat distributed predominantly around the hips and thighs. The "apple shape," or **android obesity**, typical of men has extra fat distributed higher up, around the abdomen. **Figure 8.15** shows the gynoid and android distributions of body fat.

Excess abdominal fat appears to raise blood lipid levels, which in turn interferes with insulin function. Consequently, android obesity has been linked to high blood lipids, glucose intolerance and insulin resistance, and high blood pressure; it increases the risk of heart disease and diabetes mellitus. These risks exist for both men and women who have excess abdominal fat. In fact, android obesity may indicate an increased breast cancer risk for women.[57]

If your **waist circumference** increases, you are probably gaining abdominal fat. National Institutes of Health (NIH) clinical guidelines suggest that for people with a BMI of 25 kg/m² to 34.9 kg/m², a waist circumference greater than 40 inches (102 centimeters) in men or greater than 35 inches (88 centimeters) in women is a sign of increased health risk. Combining measures of BMI and waist circumference is more predictive of cardiovascular disease risk than either measure alone.[58] When BMI is 35 kg/m² or higher, however, waist circumference measures do not predict health risks accurately.

Key Concepts: *Excess body fatness is associated with increased risk for chronic diseases, including heart disease and diabetes. Researchers use a number of different methods to assess body fatness. High cost may limit the usefulness of more sophisticated techniques. Distribution of body fat is important in evaluating risk of disease. Excess body fat around the abdomen is associated with higher disease risk than is excess fat around the hips and thighs. Waist circumference can be used to assess body fat distribution.*

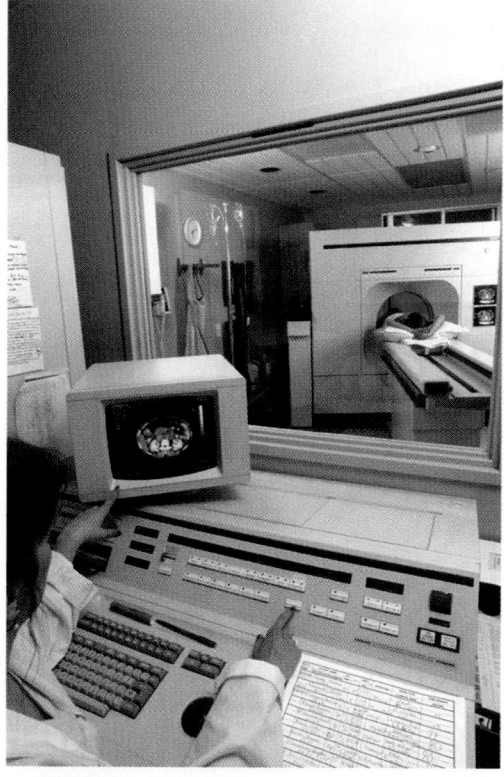

Figure 8.14 **Computed tomography (CT).** CT scans produce detailed cross-sectional images that can be used to quantify body composition.

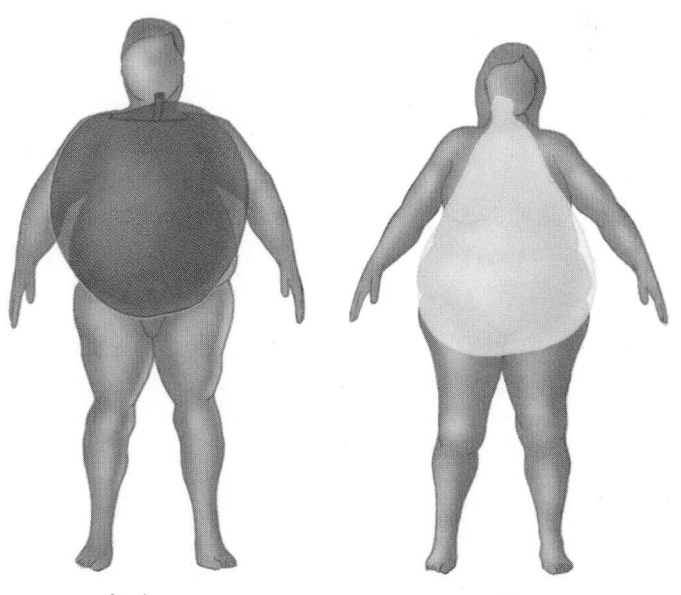

Apple
(android)

Pear
(gynoid)

Figure 8.15 **Differences in body fat distribution.** Men tend to carry excess fat around their abdomen (android obesity). Women tend to accumulate excess fat in their hips and thighs (gynoid obesity).

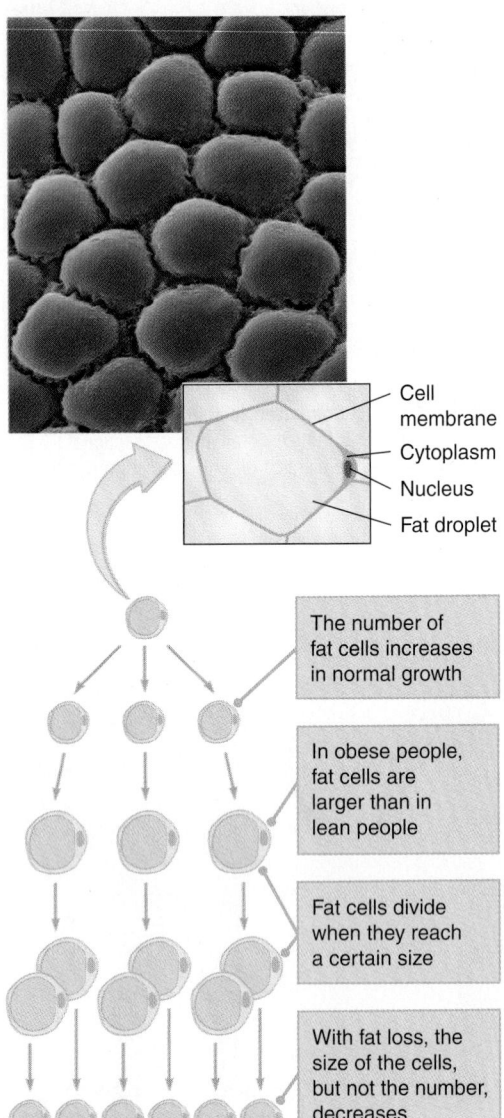

Cell membrane
Cytoplasm
Nucleus
Fat droplet

The number of fat cells increases in normal growth

In obese people, fat cells are larger than in lean people

Fat cells divide when they reach a certain size

With fat loss, the size of the cells, but not the number, decreases

Figure 8.16 **The formation of fat cells.** As body fat accumulates, fat cells enlarge and divide. Fat loss reduces the size of fat cells, but not their number.

Overweight and Obesity

Obesity has become a global problem[59] and has emerged as the most important contributor to ill health, displacing undernutrition and infectious diseases.[60] Not only is obesity prevalent in Europe and the Americas,[61] but it is also on the rise in Southeast Asia, where Japan and China have seen a marked increase. In North Africa, more than half the women in Morocco and Tunisia are overweight or obese,[62] and in the Middle East, the United Arab Emirates now recognizes obesity as a major public health problem.[63]

In the United States, the prevalence of overweight and obesity has increased dramatically, jumping from one of every four Americans to nearly two of every three![64] Nearly one of six children and teens (ages 6 to 19) are overweight (double the rate from 20 years earlier), and a similar number are at risk of becoming overweight.[65] This escalating problem is blamed on overconsumption of plentiful, tasty, and energy-dense foods, along with decreased physical activity. The goal of Healthy People 2010 is to cut the prevalence of obesity to no more than 15 percent in adults and 5 percent in children and adolescents.[66]

As overweight and obesity have increased, so has society's emphasis on thinness, as well as efforts at weight management. Every year, the diet industry rakes in $40 billion to $50 billion from weight-loss programs, diet books, pills, videos, and supplements. In 2000, 38 percent of adults surveyed said they were trying to lose weight.[67]

Children and adolescents also are concerned about weight. In studies of grade-school girls from various socioeconomic backgrounds, 28 to 40 percent reported that they sometimes dieted or were very often worried about being fat.[68]

Key Concepts: *Worldwide, the number of overweight or obese people has increased markedly in recent years. The rising rates among children are especially disturbing. At the same time, more people are engaging in weight-control efforts and starting to do so at younger ages.*

Factors in the Development of Obesity

At its simplest, obesity results from a chronic positive energy balance—energy intake regularly exceeds energy output, and weight is gained. But why? As we learn more about the factors that regulate feeding behavior and energy metabolism, scientists are beginning to unravel the specific mechanisms at work and, from there, to determine what may go wrong in people who are obese. Obesity is a complex disorder that probably involves several regulatory mechanisms and the way they interact and respond to biological factors such as heredity, age, and sex; to social and environmental factors; and to behavior and lifestyle choices.

Biological Factors

Heredity and Genetics. Researchers have long recognized hereditary patterns of obesity. When both parents are morbidly obese (body weight 100 percent above normal), the probability that their children will be obese is high (80 percent); when neither parent is obese, the probability that their children will be obese is relatively low (less than 10 percent). However, about 25 to 30 percent of obese individuals have normal-weight parents.[69]

To what extent are family patterns of obesity caused by the environment rather than heredity? Studies in twins confirm that the response to diet is mediated by a person's genetic makeup.[70] Researchers estimate that genes alone generally account for 50 to 90 percent of variations in the amount of stored body fat.[71]

Fat Cell Development. The number and size of fat cells in the body help determine how easily a person gains or loses fat. People with **hypercellular obesity**, an above-average number of fat cells, may have been born with them or may have developed them at certain critical times because of overeating. In **hypertrophic obesity**, fat cells are larger than normal. Fat cells continue to expand as they fill with more fat; when their capacity is reached, the body generates more cells. (See **Figure 8.16**.) Once body fat reaches three to five times the normal amount, fat tissue is likely to have both bigger fat cells *and* more of them, a condition called **hyperplastic obesity (hyperplasia)**.

Even with weight loss, the number of fat cells does not decline (though presumably some could be removed by liposuction). Fat cells do become smaller, but beyond a certain point, they resist further shrinking and the body strives to refill them with fat, making it difficult to maintain weight loss.

Sex and Age. In general, males and females set different weight standards for themselves. Beginning in grade school, boys are less likely than girls to consider themselves overweight; in fact, males of all ages accept some degree of overweight. Boys typically are more concerned about becoming taller and more muscular. As adolescents and young adults, most of us worry about body weight and appearance. A survey of college students aspiring to become registered dietitians, for example, found that most dieters in this group wanted to lose weight to improve appearance and increase self-esteem.[72]

By early adulthood, about the same number of men want to lose or gain weight, whereas almost all women want to lose weight. As adults, men tend to see themselves as overweight at higher weights, whereas women describe themselves as overweight when they are closer to a healthy body weight. (See **Figure 8.17**.) Adult women feel thin only when they weigh less than 90 percent of desirable body weight, whereas men rate themselves as thin even when they are above a healthy body weight.[73]

As we age, we become more concerned with our weight as it relates to health. Both men and women gain the most weight between 25 and 34 years of age. After that, we gain weight more slowly and then start to lose it after we reach age 55.[74] However, it's often important for seniors to maintain weight.

Although women try harder than men to avoid overweight or to slim down,[75] they frequently become obese after pregnancy and at menopause. In pregnancy, fat stores increase to meet the energy demands of breastfeeding. Many women retain this extra weight after they give birth, and become heavier with each child.

Race and Ethnicity. In the United States, the prevalence of obesity and attitudes about weight differ among racial and ethnic groups. Black and Hispanic women are more likely to be overweight than white women.[76] Rates of overweight are similar for black, Hispanic, and white men. Because of cultural factors, African Americans, Hispanic Americans, Native Americans, and Pacific Islanders typically value thinness less than white Americans do.[77]

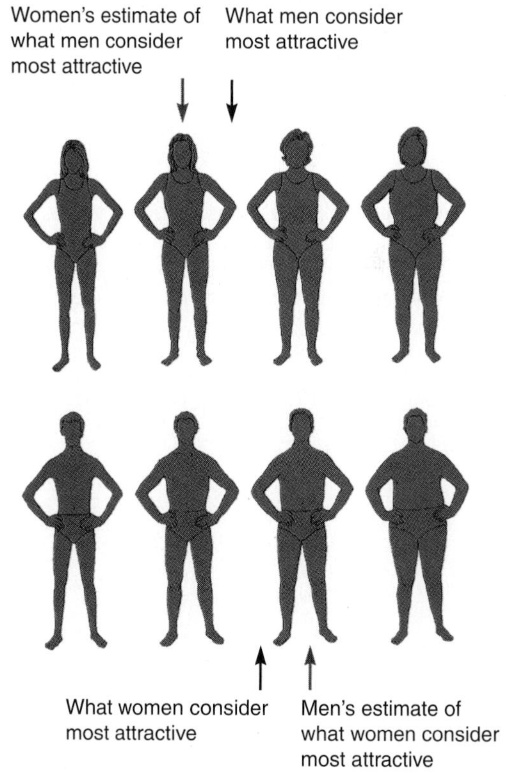

hypercellular obesity Obesity due to an above-average number of fat cells.

hypertrophic obesity Obesity due to an increase in the size of fat cells.

hyperplastic obesity (hyperplasia) Obesity due to an increase in both the size and number of fat cells.

Women's estimate of what men consider most attractive   What men consider most attractive

What women consider most attractive   Men's estimate of what women consider most attractive

Figure 8.17 **What men and women consider attractive.** Compared to men, women perceive attractive shapes to be slimmer.
Source: Data compiled from Fallon A, Rozin P. Sex differences in perceptions of desirable body shape. *Abnorm Psychol.* 1985;94:102–105; and Kalat J. *Introduction to Psychology.* 5th ed. Belmont, CA: Wadsworth, 1999.

Social and Environmental Factors

Socioeconomic Status. Americans are more likely to be obese if they have low socioeconomic status, and the stigma of obesity can impede their upward mobility. But obesity rates are rising among the affluent as well. Statistics show that in the early 1970s, 22.5 percent of low-income adults were obese; this value had risen to 32.5 percent in 2002. In contrast, only 9.7 percent of upper-income adults were obese in the 1970s; now that figure is over 26 percent.[78] Rural women tend to be heavier than women living in metropolitan areas, and southern women are the most likely to be overweight.[79]

Some studies suggest that employed women are thinner than those not in the labor force.[80] Employers tend to hire people of normal weight rather than those who are overweight or obese. Women who work outside the home also have extra income that can be used for healthier food choices, physical activity programs, and health care; on the other hand, they have less time to prepare healthful meals and get routine exercise. Changing jobs, losing a job, or retiring often changes eating patterns and subsequently body weight.

Education is another factor associated with body weight, but mainly for women. The prevalence of overweight among women ranges from 60 percent of those with less than a high school education to 29 percent of those with postgraduate college degrees.[81] A recent analysis has shown that race and education interact in their effects on women's body weights.[82] At the lowest level of education, average BMI (approximately 31 kg/m^2) is similar for middle-aged black and white women. But at higher education levels, black women were significantly heavier (BMI = 31.5 kg/m^2) than white women (BMI = 27.8 kg/m^2).

The Built Environment. Our immediate surroundings influence our behaviors, and researchers have begun to link aspects of the **built environment** with obesity. The built environment, which can be defined as "human formed, developed, or structured areas," includes buildings, roads, parks, and transportation systems.[83] These environments in which we live and work can either encourage or hinder physical activity and healthful eating.[84]

People who live in neighborhoods with sidewalks and safe streets are more physically active. But when neighborhoods have low "walkability" or are considered unsafe, BMIs tend to be higher. Socioeconomic factors are at work too—lower-income neighborhoods have fewer recreational facilities and healthful eating options. Fast food restaurants and convenience stores are more prevalent in low-income neighborhoods, whereas the number of supermarkets triples in wealthier neighborhoods.[85]

Social Factors. Social factors also influence the development of obesity. Abundant high-calorie, highly palatable foods, pervasive advertising promoting their consumption, and the social enjoyment of eating all create pressures to overeat. At the same time, our culture tells us that we should be thin, and we feel unhealthy pressures to diet. **Table 8.6** summarizes social characteristics that are key predictors of obesity.

Lifestyle and Behavior Factors

Physical Activity. Lack of exercise is a major contributing factor to weight gain and obesity. Only 22 percent of U.S. adults get the recommended amount of regular physical activity; more than 60 percent are not active on a regular basis, and 25 percent are not active at all. Inactivity is more common among women, older adults, less affluent adults, and black or

built environment Any human-formed, developed, or structured areas, including the urban environment that consists of buildings, roads, fixtures, parks, and all other human developments that form its physical character.

Hispanic adults.[86] In both children and adults, research links excessive television viewing to obesity.[87] For all ages, obesity itself may lead to physical inactivity, although the strength of this relationship is unclear.

Psychological Factors. Some people adopt eating as a strategy for dealing with the stresses and challenges of life. (Others use drugs, alcohol, smoking, shopping, gambling, and so on.) Eating also can provide entertainment and alleviate boredom. Some people use eating as a pick-me-up when fatigued, and some use eating to distract themselves from difficult problems or as a means of punishing themselves or others for real or imagined transgressions.

Certain obese people may be more prone to emotional eating than others. These subgroups include **restrained eaters** and **binge eaters**.[88] Restrained eaters try to reduce their calorie intake by fasting or avoiding food as long as possible. They skip meals, delay eating, or severely restrict the types of food they eat. Then, like a dam that bursts, they overeat when environmental or emotional stress triggers a complete release of inhibitions toward eating. Although not all obese binge eaters follow this pattern, the

restrained eaters Individuals who routinely avoid food as long as possible, and then gorge on food.

binge eaters Individuals who routinely consume a very large amount of food in a brief period of time (e.g., two hours) and lose control over how much and what is eaten.

Table 8.6 Sociocultural Influences on Obesity

Social Contexts

Culture	People in developed societies have more body fat than those in developing societies.
History	Fatness is increasing in the United States, but idealized weights are decreasing.

Social Characteristics

Age and lifestyle	Fatness increases during adulthood, declines in the elderly.
Gender	Obesity is more prevalent in women than in men.
Race and ethnicity	Obesity is more prevalent in African American, Hispanic, Native American, and Pacific Islander women.

Socioeconomic Status

Income	Obesity is more prevalent in lower-income women.
Education	Less-educated women have a higher incidence of obesity.
Occupational prestige	Obesity is more prevalent in women (people) in less prestigious jobs.
Employment	Women who are not employed have a higher incidence of obesity.
Household composition	Older people who live with others have a higher incidence of obesity.
Marriage	Married men have a higher incidence of obesity.
Residence	Rural women have a higher incidence of obesity.
Region	People residing in the South have a higher incidence of obesity.

Source: Adapted with permission from Dalton S. Body weight terminology, definitions, and measurements. In: Dalton S, ed. *Overweight and Weight Management: The Health Professional's Guide to Understanding and Practice.* Sudbury, MA: Jones and Bartlett Publishers. 1997:314.

"fast, then binge" behavior is common in obese people who chronically attempt to lose weight.[89] This pattern also occurs in women of normal weight who perceive themselves as fat. These restrained eating patterns appear to be passed on from mother to daughter.[90]

Binge eaters compulsively overeat, sometimes for days. Some people binge only at night, taking in most of their excess calories between 6 P.M. and the time they go to sleep. Binge eating is common among people enrolled in weight-loss programs—estimates of its prevalence range from 23 to 46 percent.[91] People who binge are more likely to be emotional eaters or to have psychological problems than those who do not binge. For more information about binge eating, see the "Spotlight on Eating Disorders."

People with a healthy lifestyle have more effective ways to meet their needs. They communicate assertively and manage interpersonal conflict effectively, so they don't shrink from problems or overreact. The person with a healthy lifestyle knows how to create and maintain relationships with others and has a solid network of friends and loved ones. Food is used appropriately—to fuel life's activities and gain personal satisfaction, not to manage stress.

Key Concepts: *Obesity tends to run in families. Sex, age, and environmental factors such as socioeconomic status, employment status, and having children are related to weight. Lifestyle choices and behavioral factors also affect weight. Overly restrained eating may result in episodes of overeating and weight gain. Binge eating is common among people in weight-loss programs.*

Health Risks of Overweight and Obesity

Overweight and obesity are major public health challenges. Obese people are at higher risk for heart disease, the leading cause of death in the United States and Canada, and for stroke, diabetes, hypertension, some forms of cancer, gallbladder and joint diseases,[92] and psychosocial problems. The longer obesity persists, the higher the risks. **Table 8.7** lists the effects that excess weight can have on your health. Scientists speculate that rising rates of obesity will soon reverse the increases in life expectancy that occurred throughout the twentieth century as a result of improved living conditions, advances in public health, and medical interventions.[93] The costs of obesity-related diseases are staggering—an estimated $75 billion annually.[94]

The blood lipid levels that typically accompany obesity—high serum triglycerides, low HDL, and a high LDL/HDL ratio—increase the risk for atherosclerosis. A person who is only mildly to moderately obese has an elevated risk of coronary heart disease. However, even modest weight loss (about 10 percent of body weight) reduces risk.[95]

Type 2 diabetes, the most common form of diabetes in the United States and Canada, is three times more likely to develop in people who are obese, especially if they have abdominal (android) obesity. Obesity increases insulin resistance and compromises the ability of body cells to take up glucose. Diabetes, in turn, is a risk factor for heart disease, kidney disease, and vascular problems. Again, even modest levels of weight reduction can improve glucose tolerance.

Overweight people are two to six times more likely to develop hypertension,[96] probably due to increased resistance in the peripheral blood vessels, changes in the way the kidneys handle sodium, and other changes in kidney function. Weight loss lowers blood pressure in overweight people with hypertension.

Although the exact reason is unknown, obesity increases the risk of cancer. The same food pattern that contributes to obesity (a diet high in calories and fat, plus low in fiber, fruits, and vegetables) also may be a cancer risk. Inactivity not only encourages obesity but also increases cancer risk. For example, women who are physically active have a lower risk of breast cancer than do sedentary women.[97] People who are obese have increased levels of hormones that influence development of some cancers. Obese women, for example, have more endometrial, gallbladder, cervical, and ovarian cancers.[98]

Obese people are more likely to have obstructive **sleep apnea**, in which the airway collapses during sleep and breathing stops for a short spell. As the body struggles for air, blood pressure spikes upward. Typically, the individual wakes up, gasps for air, begins breathing again, and then falls asleep until the airway collapses again and the cycle repeats. This pattern not only interrupts and prevents a good night's sleep, it also increases the risk of heart attack and stroke. Modest weight loss can alleviate sleep apnea, improve sleep quality, and reduce daytime drowsiness.[99]

sleep apnea Periods of absence of breathing during sleep.

Table 8.7 What Are the Risks of Being Overweight?

Heart Disease and Stroke

Hypertension and very high blood levels of cholesterol and triglycerides (blood fats) can lead to heart disease and often are linked to being overweight. Being overweight also contributes to angina (chest pain caused by decreased oxygen to the heart) and sudden death from heart disease or stroke without any signs or symptoms.

Diabetes

Overweight people are twice as likely to develop type 2 diabetes as people who are not overweight. Type 2 diabetes is a major cause of early death, heart disease, kidney disease, stroke, and blindness.

Cancer

Several types of cancer are associated with being overweight. In women, these include cancer of the uterus, gallbladder, cervix, ovary, breast, and colon. Overweight men are at greater risk for developing cancer of the colon, rectum, and prostate. For some types of cancer, such as colon or breast, it is not clear whether the increased risk is due to the extra weight or consumption of a high-fat and high-calorie diet.

Sleep Apnea

Sleep apnea is a serious condition that is closely associated with being overweight. Sleep apnea can cause a person to stop breathing for short periods during sleep and to snore heavily. Sleep apnea may cause daytime sleepiness and even heart failure. The risk for sleep apnea increases with higher body weights. Weight loss usually improves sleep apnea.

Osteoarthritis

Extra weight appears to increase the risk of osteoarthritis by placing extra pressure on weight-bearing joints and wearing away the cartilage (tissue that cushions the joints) that normally protects them. Weight loss can decrease stress on the knees, hips, and lower back and may improve the symptoms of osteoarthritis.

Gallbladder Disease

Gallbladder disease and gallstones are more common if you are overweight. Your risk of disease increases as your weight increases. It is not clear how being overweight may cause gallbladder disease.

Weight loss itself, particularly rapid weight loss or loss of a large amount of weight, can actually increase your chances of developing gallstones. Modest, slow weight loss of about one pound a week is less likely to cause gallstones.

Fatty Liver Disease

Fatty liver disease occurs when fat builds up in the liver cells and damages the liver. It can lead to liver failure. Fatty liver disease is linked to higher than normal blood glucose levels, which are more common in people who are overweight. Weight loss can help with blood glucose control and reduce the build-up of fat in the liver. Also, people who have fatty liver disease should avoid alcohol.

Source: NIDDK Weight Control Information Network. Do you know the health risks of being overweight? http://win.niddk.gov/publications/health_risks.htm. Accessed 12/30/06.

Weight Cycling

Weight cycling is a pattern of losing and regaining weight over and over again. You might expect this behavior to be harmful, perhaps harder on the body than overweight itself. However, research suggests that the potential benefits of weight loss for obese individuals still outweigh the potential risks of weight cycling.[100]

Researchers have found that women who repeatedly gain and lose weight, especially obese women, have significantly lower levels of HDL, the "good" cholesterol. Although low HDL levels are a significant risk factor for coronary artery disease (CAD), the investigators did not observe a direct link between weight cycling and CAD.[101] More research is necessary to observe the health and behaviors of these women over time. Another study has linked weight cycling with an increased risk for hypertension,[102] and research has suggested that weight cycling impairs immune function.[103]

Key Concepts: Obesity is a risk factor for many chronic diseases, including heart disease, cancer, hypertension, and diabetes. In many cases, a modest amount of weight loss (about 10 percent of initial body weight) can improve symptoms and disease management.

Weight Management

Each person has a unique set of interrelated factors that lead to weight gain. Approaches to weight management are just as complex, and to be effective, they must be tailored to the individual. As you continue reading, keep in mind the following definition of **weight management** from the American Dietetic Association; note that there is no mention of weight loss or ideal weight:

Weight management is the adoption of healthful and sustainable eating and exercise behaviors indicated for reduced disease risk and improved feelings of energy and well-being.[104]

The Perception of Weight

The weights of celebrity models often mold popular notions about desirable weight. In the early 1960s, as today, thin was "in." (In the 1960s, the trendsetter was supermodel Twiggy, who at 5 feet, 7 inches weighed only

weight cycling Repeated periods of gaining and losing weight. Also called yo-yo dieting.

weight management The adoption of healthful and sustainable eating and exercise behaviors that reduce disease risk and improve well-being.

Figure 8.18 **Society's changing standards of beauty.** Over time, society has increasingly valued thinness. (a) Ruben's *The Three Graces*, 1639. (b) Degas's *After the Bath*, 1896. (c) Celebrity Nicole Richie.

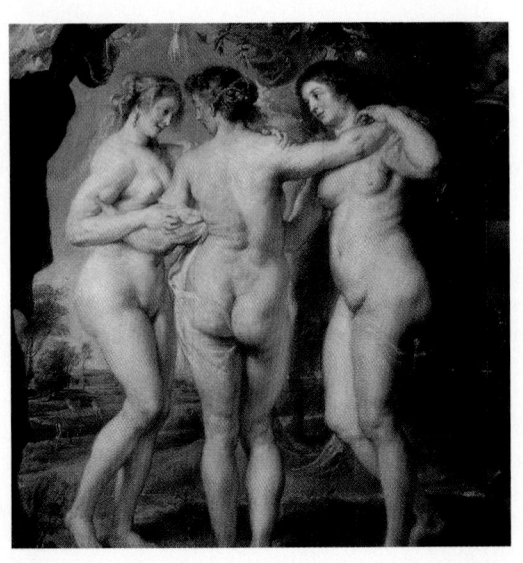

(a)

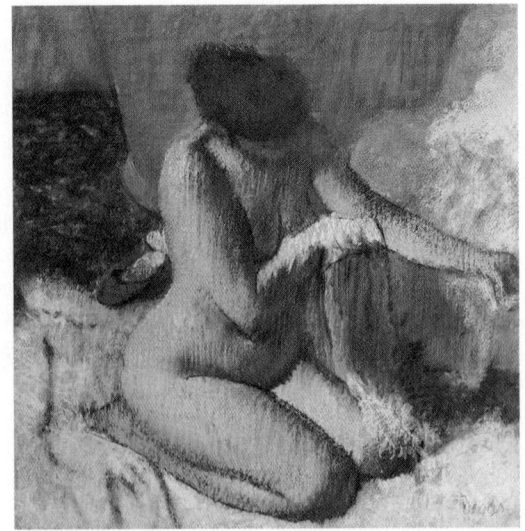

(b)

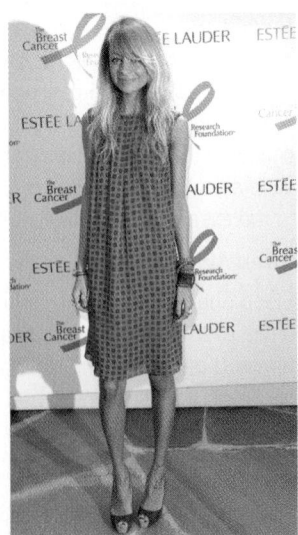

(c)

98 pounds; her BMI was a mere 15.4 kg/m²!) Since then, the number of diet and exercise articles in women's magazines has escalated, and diet books have become best-sellers. Dieting has become an institution with its own magazines, television shows, camps and resorts, and weight-loss gurus. However, the images in **Figure 8.18** show that beauty has not always been associated with thinness.

Despite obesity's link to health risks, a backlash against dieting has emerged. The antidiet advocates' rallying cry is "Diets don't work!" While acknowledging that severe obesity is dangerous, they argue for size acceptance and challenge the notion that mild obesity is unhealthful. In fact, data from the Centers for Disease Control and Prevention show that people who are overweight (BMI 25 to < 30 kg/m²) had no higher risk of mortality than people of normal weight.[105]

Health professionals now treat obesity as a complex disorder with multiple contributing factors. (See **Figure 8.19**.) They emphasize overall health and fitness rather than a number on the bathroom scale. Dietary recommendations emphasize moderation and a balanced diet that promotes consumption of healthful foods such as fruits, vegetables, and whole grains. Behavior change is still an important part of weight management, but change is seen as an ongoing process that requires new skills for maintaining a healthy lifestyle over the long run. Although vigorous exercise isn't required, substantial increases in moderate exercise are needed for long-term weight management.[106]

There are limitations as to what each of us can look like or what we can weigh. Although we shouldn't abandon efforts to achieve good health, we should balance our desire to lose weight with self-acceptance. If we engage in futile attempts to achieve an "ideal" body shape and weight, we may undermine our self-esteem and be harmed emotionally or even physically.

Key Concepts: *Many factors contribute to the complex disorder of obesity. Currently, experts suggest that the best way to manage weight is to improve health by establishing healthy eating and exercise patterns and accepting the limitations of heredity.*

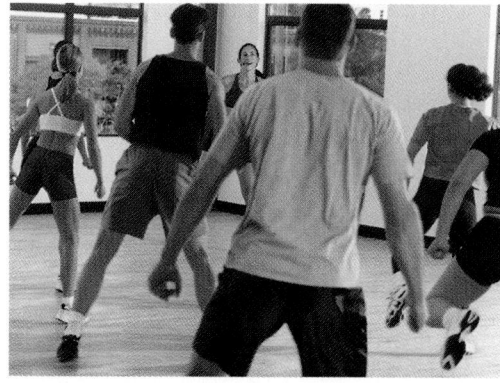

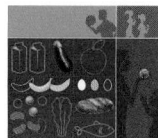

Dietary Guidelines for Americans, 2005
key recommendations

- To maintain body weight in a healthy range, balance calories from foods and beverages with calories expended.
- To prevent gradual weight gain over time, make small decreases in food and beverage calories and increase physical activity.

Key Recommendations for Specific Population Groups

- *Those who need to lose weight.* Aim for a slow, steady weight loss by decreasing calorie intake while maintaining an adequate nutrient intake and increasing physical activity.
- *Overweight children.* Reduce the rate of body weight gain while allowing growth and development. Consult a health care provider before placing a child on a weight-reduction diet.
- *Pregnant women.* Ensure appropriate weight gain as specified by a health care provider.
- *Breastfeeding women.* Moderate weight reduction is safe and does not compromise weight gain of the nursing infant.
- *Overweight adults and overweight children with chronic diseases and/or on medication.* Consult a health care provider about weight-loss strategies prior to starting a weight-reduction program to ensure appropriate management of other health conditions.

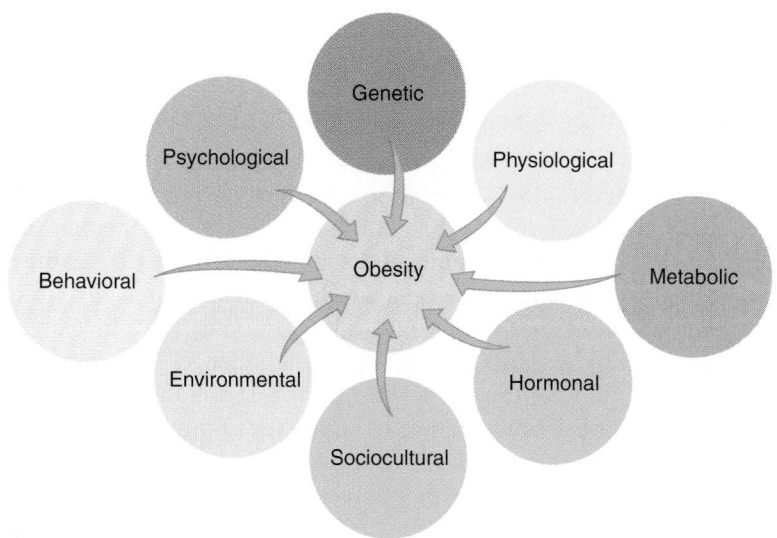

Figure 8.19 **Multiple factors contribute to obesity.** Obesity is a complex disorder that is not easy to treat.

metabolic fitness The absence of all metabolic and biochemical risk factors associated with obesity.

What Goals Should I Set?

What is a reasonable goal for weight management? According to the *Dietary Guidelines for Americans*, adults should aim to achieve and maintain a body weight that optimizes their health.[107] It doesn't take major weight loss to improve health; a modest weight loss of roughly 10 percent is enough to produce health benefits and perhaps to encourage continued success. A key initial goal is to prevent or stop weight gain. Small changes in energy intake and expenditure—for example, an intake reduction of 100 kilocalories per day—may be all that is needed to prevent weight gain.[108] Goals must be realistic and attainable. (See **Figure 8.20**.)

Many health experts suggest that people should aim for **metabolic fitness** rather than a specific weight,[109] especially if they have difficulty achieving or maintaining recommended BMI levels. If you are metabolically fit, you don't have any of the metabolic or biochemical risk factors associated with obesity—such as high LDL cholesterol, low HDL cholesterol, high levels of triglycerides, elevated blood glucose, insulin resistance, and high blood pressure. Other risk factors include excess abdominal fat.[110] If these risk factors are at normal levels, a person is considered metabolically fit, even if BMI is elevated. If not, the person has an increased risk for coronary heart disease, diabetes, gout, hypertension, and associated conditions. You can reduce these risk factors or even bring them within normal ranges through modest weight loss (5 to 10 percent of initial body weight) achieved by a small reduction in calorie intake and a moderate increase in physical activity (e.g., walking 30 minutes per day, no fewer than five days per week). In fact, researchers estimate that most of the weight gain seen in the U.S. population could be eliminated by as little as a 100 kilocalorie per day shift in intake and expenditure.[111] You also can improve metabolic fitness just by increasing physical activity levels.[112]

Don't focus on a particular weight as your goal. Instead, focus on living a lifestyle that includes eating moderate amounts of healthful foods, getting plenty of exercise, thinking positively, and learning to cope with stress. Learn to use your body's hunger and satiation signals to regulate eating and then let the pounds fall where they may. Most people who follow this advice will approach the healthy BMI ranges discussed earlier. Some will still weigh more than societal standards call for—but their weight will be right for them. By letting a healthy lifestyle determine your weight, you can avoid developing unhealthy patterns of eating and a negative body image.

Adopting a Healthy Weight-Management Lifestyle

Most weight problems are lifestyle problems. Even though more and more young people are developing weight problems, most arrive at early adulthood with the advantage of having a "normal" body weight—neither too fat nor too thin. In fact, many young adults get away with terrible eating and exercise habits and don't develop a weight problem. But as the rapid growth of adolescence slows and family and career obligations increase, maintaining a healthy weight becomes a greater challenge. If you develop a lifestyle for successful weight management during early adulthood, healthy behavior patterns have a better chance of taking firm hold.

Permanent weight management is not something you start and stop. You need to adopt healthful behaviors that you can maintain throughout your life. People who have long-term success share common behavioral strategies that include eating a diet low in fat, frequent self-monitoring of body weight and food intake, and high levels of regular physical activity.[113]

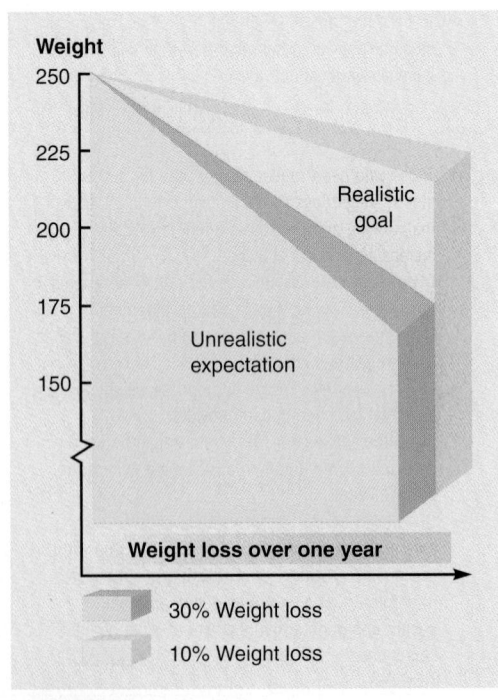

Weight

250
225
200 Realistic goal
175
150 Unrealistic expectation

Weight loss over one year

30% Weight loss
10% Weight loss

Figure 8.20 **Expectations and reasonable weight goals.** People who establish moderate rather than aggressive goals are more likely to succeed in their weight-loss program.

To maintain your weight over the long term, focus on healthy behaviors and develop coping strategies to deal with the stresses and challenges in your life. **Figure 8.21** shows the necessary components of an effective weight-management program.

Key Concepts: *Healthy weight management means focusing on metabolic fitness— healthy levels of blood lipids and blood pressure—rather than on achieving a specific weight. Permanent healthy behaviors are necessary for a long-term weight-management lifestyle.*

Diet and Eating Habits

In contrast to "dieting," which involves some form of food restriction, "diet" refers to your daily food choices. Everyone has a diet, but not everyone is dieting. You need to develop a balanced diet of moderate caloric intake that includes foods you enjoy and that enables you to maintain a healthy body composition.

Total Calories

If you want to lose weight, you must take in fewer calories than you expend. Over the long term, you are more likely to control your weight successfully by cutting 200 to 300 kilocalories per day rather than drastically restricting your diet to only 1,000 to 1,200 kilocalories per day. Simply eliminating one can of regular soda from your daily routine would reduce your energy intake by about 150 kilocalories. Eating a half-serving of fries instead of a whole serving would save another 100 kilocalories. You don't need to make major diet changes; just make small, sustainable changes and focus on the balance of food groups suggested by MyPyramid. The MyPyramid Tracker feature on the MyPyramid Web site (http://mypyramid.gov) can help you evaluate your intake and find small changes that you can make.

Overconsumption of total calories is closely tied to portion sizes. Most of us significantly underestimate the amount of food we eat; at the same time, the size of portions served as single servings in restaurants and convenience stores has increased.[114] Limiting portion sizes to those recommended in MyPyramid is critical for weight management. You'll probably find it easier to monitor and manage your total food intake if you concentrate on portion sizes rather than counting calories.

Crash Diets Don't Work

Don't go on a "crash diet" that contains only minimal calories. You need to consume enough food to meet your need for essential nutrients. Very low calorie intake promotes rapid loss of water, reduced RMR, and potential nutrient deficiencies Once you lose weight, you probably won't maintain it unless you continue some degree of calorie restriction. So it is important that you adopt a level of food intake that you can live with. A highly restricted diet just won't work over the long term.

Balancing Energy Sources: Fat

In addition to balancing energy intake with energy output, achieving a balanced intake of energy sources is important for successful weight management. Although we all need some dietary fat, you should avoid overeating fatty foods. Because fat is the most concentrated source of calories, limiting fat in the diet can help you limit your total calories. Research suggests that fat calories are more easily converted to body fat than calories from protein or carbohydrate.[115] In a study of older men (ages 55 to 79), higher energy

American Dietetic Association

Weight Management

It is the position of the American Dietetic Association that successful weight management to improve overall health for adults requires a lifelong commitment to healthful lifestyle behaviors emphasizing sustainable and enjoyable eating practices and daily physical activity.

J Am Diet Assoc. 2002;102:1145–1155.
Reprinted with permission.

Quick Bites

Double-Checking Dietary Recall

When researchers checked the validity of food diaries and self-reports, they found that obese people underreport their energy intake by 20 to 50 percent and lean people underreport by 10 to 30 percent. Energy expenditure in the obese subjects was normal relative to their body size.

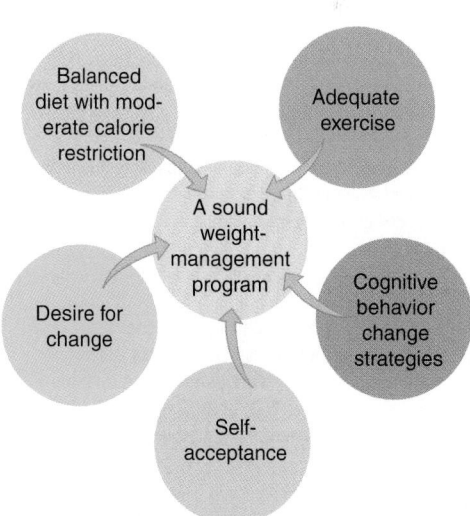

Figure 8.21 **Components of a sound weight-management program.** Recognizing the need for change, establishing reasonable goals, adopting goal-directed activities and self-monitoring them, and rewarding goal attainment can help successfully implement the components of a sound weight-management program.

intake from fat was associated with higher BMI levels.[116] Fat should supply about 20 to 35 percent of your average total daily calories, which translates into 45 to 75 grams of fat each day in a 2,000-kilocalorie diet.

Some people are better fat burners than others; that is, they burn more of the fat they take in and therefore have less fat to store. People who burn fat at a relatively slow rate convert more dietary fat to stored body fat. For these people, the tendency to hoard fat may be an important part of the genetic tendency toward obesity, so restricting fat calories may help them manage their weight.

Several large surveys of the relationship between what we eat and how much we weigh have found that eating more fat and fewer complex carbohydrates is associated with excess body fat.[117] High-fat, low-fiber diets tend to delay satiation and encourage overeating. If you eat a diet with lots of whole grains, fresh fruits, and vegetables and reduce your reliance on meats and processed foods, you will reduce fat consumption and increase dietary fiber. Watch out for processed foods labeled "fat-free" or "reduced-fat"; they can be high in calories despite their lower fat content.

Balancing Energy Sources: Carbohydrates

To lose weight, dieters often cut back on bread, pasta, and potatoes. But these foods, along with vegetables, legumes, and other grain products, are rich in the complex carbohydrates and fiber that can help you achieve and maintain a healthy body weight. Fiber-rich foods help provide a feeling of satiation, or fullness, that can keep you from overeating. Carbohydrates should make up 45 to 65 percent of your total daily calories. Avoid mixing your carbohydrate sources with high-fat toppings and sauces, however. Experiment with lower-fat alternatives. Instead of sour cream on your baked potato, try plain yogurt, or even salsa! Rather than cream sauces on your pasta, use tomato-based sauces.

High-sugar foods usually provide calories but few nutrients. You should consume them sparingly, so choose fresh fruits and whole grains instead of candy and sugary cereals.

Balancing Energy Sources: Protein

Many popular diet books promote a high-protein, low-carbohydrate intake. They often proclaim their plan to be a "scientific breakthrough," although most contain speculations that have been recycled since the 1800s. Even though they promise "all you can eat," such diets typically involve significant calorie restriction. This lower energy intake is what actually causes any weight loss that occurs. A high-protein, low-carbohydrate, low-calorie diet does not conform to the *Dietary Guidelines for Americans* and is difficult to maintain. Most authorities recommend diets high in complex carbohydrates and moderate in protein consumption. (See the FYI feature "High-Protein, Low-Carbohydrate Diets for Weight Loss: Helpful or Harmful?")

Although protein promotes a sense of fullness, foods high in protein often are high in fat. Including some lean protein in each meal is a good idea, but stick to the recommended intake: 10 to 35 percent of total daily calories.

Eating Habits

Equally important to weight management is eating small, frequent meals—three or more per day plus snacks—on a dependable, regular schedule. If you skip meals, you are apt to feel excessively hungry and deprived, and you will be more likely to snack or binge on high-calorie, high-fat, or sugary foods. A person who eats on a regular schedule is more likely to reduce total energy intake and improve lipid levels than a person who eats irregularly.[118] Also, a

---

American Heart Association

Commercial Weight Reduction Programs

Being overweight, even by just 10 to 15 pounds, can lead to health problems. And obesity is a risk factor for cardiovascular disease. That's why the American Heart Association encourages people to achieve and maintain a healthy weight. Effective weight loss programs should include

- informed consent (participant or patient information)
- appropriate health risk screening
- guidelines for who needs to be evaluated by a physician
- individualized nutrition, physical activity and behavioral components
- counseling by qualified health professionals
- identification of reasonable weight-loss goals
- a maintenance program that lasts for at least two years
- evaluation of the long-term effectiveness and safety of the program

Reproduced with permission. www.americanheart.org. © 2006, American Heart Association, Inc.

regular meal pattern usually includes breakfast—a benefit when trying to manage weight. Research shows that morning intake is much more satiating than late-night eating and will help reduce overall energy intake.[119] Also, in a study of healthy, lean women, skipping breakfast lowered insulin sensitivity, raised LDL and total cholesterol, and led to higher energy intake.[120]

If you follow a regular pattern of eating and set up some "decision rules" that govern your food choices, you will be able to handle the many details that go into a healthful diet. Decision rules governing breakfast, for example, might be as follows:

- Most of the time, choose a low-sugar, high-fiber cereal with nonfat milk.
- Once in a while, have an egg that's prepared without added fat (e.g., hard-boiled or scrambled).
- Save pancakes and waffles for special occasions.

When you proclaim some foods "off limits," you are setting up a rule to be broken. Instead, adopt the principle of "everything in moderation." Troublesome foods might be placed off limits temporarily until you regain control. If you can learn to eat in moderation, you can achieve a healthy diet and manage your weight successfully; no foods need to be entirely off limits, though some should be eaten prudently. Making the healthier choice more often than not is the essence of moderation.

Key Concepts: *Balancing energy sources and controlling portion sizes can help reduce overall energy consumption. Reducing fat intake is a major step toward lowering calorie intake. Fiber-rich foods provide a feeling of fullness that can help prevent overeating. When planning a diet, aim for a caloric intake of 20 to 35 percent fat, 10 to 35 percent protein, and 45 to 65 percent carbohydrate.*

Physical Activity

Regular physical activity is a vital component of weight management and promotes fitness and good health. At the same time, it discourages overeating by reducing stress; it produces positive feelings that reinforce self-worth and a sense of accomplishment; and it often includes pleasant socialization. To prevent weight gain and maximize health benefits, adults should aim for 60 minutes of moderate-intensity physical activity each day.[121]

Look for ways to incorporate more physical activity into your daily life. (See **Figure 8.22.**) You may not think you have an hour each day to devote to moderate-intensity physical activity, but you don't have to get this exercise all at once; you can break it up throughout the day.[122] Walk the dog for an extra half-hour daily, for example. Use a stairway instead of an elevator. Walk briskly instead of using transportation. Take up an active hobby such as bicycling.

Increasing your activity level by just a small amount can help you maintain your current weight or lose a moderate amount of weight. "Going for the burn" and "no pain, no gain" were the mottos of the aerobics movement during the 1970s and 1980s, but such intense activity is neither necessary nor desirable. Instead, regular exercise of moderate intensity—any activity that expends 4 to 7 kilocalories per minute (240 to 420 kilocalories per hour; see Table 8.2)—provides substantial health benefits.

Once you have increased your everyday activity level, consider beginning a formal exercise program that includes cardiorespiratory endurance exercise, resistance training, and stretching exercises. Regular, moderate cardiorespiratory endurance exercise, sustained for 45 minutes to 1 hour, can help trim body fat permanently. Strength training helps increase fat-free mass, which results in more calorie burning even outside of exercise periods.

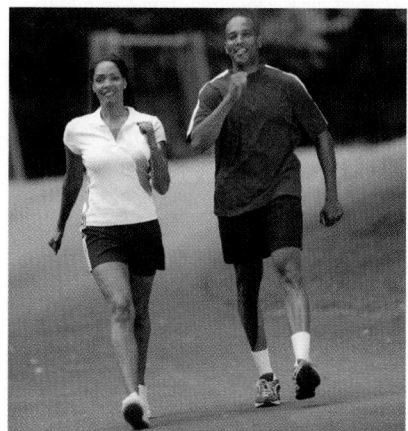

Figure 8.22 **Weight management through lifetime habits.** To achieve long-term weight management, healthy habits must become part of one's daily routine.

positive self-talk Constructive mental or verbal statements made to one's self to change a belief or behavior.

negative self-talk Mental or verbal statements made to one's self that reinforce negative or destructive self perceptions.

ABC model of behavior A behavioral model that includes the external and internal events that precede and follow the behavior. The "A" stands for antecedents, the events that precede the behavior ("B"), which is followed by consequences ("C") that positively or negatively reinforce the behavior.

One thing is clear: Regular exercise, maintained throughout life, makes weight management easier. The sooner you establish good habits, the better. You will succeed in maintaining your weight if you make exercise an integral part of the lifestyle you enjoy now and will enjoy in the future.

Key Concepts: Successful weight management involves regular physical activity as well as healthful food choices. Small increases in activity have significant health benefits and help weight loss and maintenance. To prevent weight gain and maximize health benefits, you should include at least 60 minutes of moderate physical activity in your daily routine.

Thinking and Emotions

What goes on in your head is another factor in a healthy lifestyle and successful weight management. The way you think about yourself and your world influences, and is influenced by, how you feel and how you act. Certain kinds of thinking produce negative emotions, which can undermine a healthy lifestyle.

When we compare ourselves to an internally held picture of an "ideal self," we are more likely to have low self-esteem and feel negative emotions. The "ideal self" we envision is often the result of having adopted perfectionistic goals and beliefs about how we "should" be. You might know

Fyi High-Protein, Low-Carbohydrate Diets for Weight Loss: Helpful or Harmful?

FOR YOUR INFORMATION

High-protein, low-carbohydrate weight-loss diets are in style. Browse through the weight-loss section of any major bookstore, and you will find books such as *Dr. Atkins' New Diet Revolution, The South Beach Diet, Sugar Busters,* and *Enter the Zone.* All these books promote various high-protein diets for weight loss.

These diets revisit the idea, popular in the 1970s (and with historical roots dating back nearly 200 years), that carbohydrates (starches and sugars) make us fat. Proponents of high-protein diets point to the fact that throughout the high-carb, low-fat 1980s and early 1990s and with the explosion of fat-free foods, Americans got fatter. They fail to note that although the percentage of calories from fat in U.S. diets has decreased, Americans are eating more total fat and total calories (and therefore more total grams of fat) and exercising less—a recipe for weight gain.

Do High-Protein, Low-Carbohydrate Diets Work?

The Atkins diet made headlines in November 2002 when researchers from Duke University presented results of a study comparing the

Atkins diet to the American Heart Association's (AHA) low-fat diet at the AHA's annual scientific meeting. Headlines of "Atkins diet meets with success," "Vindication for the Atkins diet?" and "Atkins diet beats low-fat fare" had meat-lovers cheering and dietitians cringing. Skeptics argued that the study, funded by the Atkins Center for Complementary Medicine, included too few people and failed to monitor participants' actual food intake and exercise levels.

Since this report, several studies of low-carbohydrate diets have been published, some of which were funded by government sources. One study compared a low-carbohydrate ($\leq$30 grams per day) diet to a calorie-restricted, low-fat diet ($\leq$30 percent of calories from fat; caloric restriction of 500 kcal per day) for severely obese adults.[1] The study lasted six months and included 132 total subjects. In the other study, 63 obese adults were randomly assigned to either a low-carbohydrate, high-protein, high-fat diet (based on the Atkins diet) or a low-calorie, high-carbohydrate, low-fat diet (60 percent carbohydrate, 25 percent fat, 15 percent protein).[2] Subjects were followed for a one-year period.

At the six-month time point in both studies, people on the low-carbohydrate diets had lost more weight (about 8 pounds more on average). When the subjects were followed for one year, however, difference in weight loss became nonsignificant. Overall weight loss was relatively small compared with the participants' starting weights. Improvements in blood cholesterol levels initially seen on the low-carbohydrate diet also became nonsignificant as time progressed. In both studies, drop-out rates were high—about 60 percent of those who began the studies. This attrition rate makes interpretation of the results difficult, if not impossible.[3] A review of published studies concluded that participant weight loss on low-carbohydrate diets was mainly associated with decreased calorie intake rather than reduced carbohydrate content.[4]

In another study that compared four different types of popular weight-loss diets, overall weight loss at one year was similar regardless of diet.[5] Heart disease risk factors improved for each diet group, but in different ways. The very low fat vegetarian Ornish diet was best for lowering LDL cholesterol, whereas other

someone who believes "If I don't do things perfectly, I'm a failure" or "It's terrible if I'm not thin." When we accept these irrational beliefs, we may actually cause ourselves stress and emotional conflict. The remedy is to challenge such beliefs and replace them with more realistic ones.

The beliefs and attitudes you hold give rise to self-talk, an internal dialogue you carry on with yourself about events that happen to and around you. When you talk yourself through the steps of a job and then praise yourself when it's successfully completed, you are engaging in **positive self-talk**. When you make self-deprecating remarks or angry and guilt-producing comments and when you blame yourself unnecessarily, you are engaging in **negative self-talk**. Negative self-talk can undermine efforts at self-control and lead to feelings of anxiety and depression.

Your beliefs and attitudes influence how you interpret what happens to you and what you can expect in the future, as well as how you feel and react. Realistic beliefs and goals combined with positive self-talk and problem-solving efforts support a healthy lifestyle.

Stress Management

Stress management can be an important part of weight management.[123] You can use the **ABC model of behavior (Figure 8.23)** to help you cope with daily stresses and their effects on eating behavior.

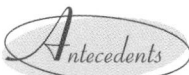

Antecedents

Her mouth starts watering as she passes by a bakery with delicious sights and aromas.

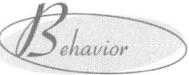

Behavior

She purchases many pastries, intending some for later. Despite this resolve, she succumbs to the need for instant gratification, immediately eating them all.

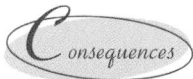

Consequences

She regrets her behavior and feels guilty. Overeating may leave her feeling ill and nauseated.

Figure 8.23 **The ABC model of eating behavior.** Conquering overeating often requires a psychological strategy for changing ingrained habits and other behaviors.

---

diets, including Atkins and the Zone, were better at raising HDL cholesterol.

So what explains reports of dramatic weight loss and no hunger while eating pork rinds, bacon, sausage, and steak? Removing carbohydrates from the diet causes the body to deplete glycogen stores, which results in a rapid loss of water. The ketosis that results from low carbohydrate intake can also enhance fluid loss. High protein intake tends to be satiating, and the monotony of the diet also blunts the appetite. Although the effects are small, an increase in protein intake (e.g., 30 to 35 percent of calories) causes a slight increase in energy expenditure, possibly from the extra energy needed to convert protein to glucose.[6]

Are High-Protein, Low-Carbohydrate Diets Safe?

In a review of research on low-carbohydrate diets, Levine and colleagues found insufficient evidence to recommend for or against this approach to weight loss.[7] They note that common concerns include accumulation of ketones, abnormal insulin metabolism, impaired liver and kidney function, salt and water depletion, impaired renal function, and

hyperlipidemia resulting from high fat intake. Their analysis of weight outcomes and complications was limited by small sample sizes, high drop-out rates, short study durations, and high variability in measured outcomes. It is likely, though, that people who start a low-carbohydrate diet do not stay on it long enough to develop serious complications, although constipation, nausea, weakness, dehydration, and fatigue are common side effects.

The Best Diet to Follow

Is there a "best" diet? If there were, we wouldn't have so many diet books vying for our attention and money! What we know about our nutrient needs still points to the *Dietary Guidelines for Americans* for guidance: The best diet emphasizes fruits, vegetables, and grains—not high-protein foods. From what we have seen in research studies, it is very difficult for individuals to stick to a particular diet, especially those diets that are most restrictive.[8] And although weight *loss* may be the goal of many, weight *maintenance* is the key to reducing the health risks of obesity. Weight maintenance requires permanent changes to eating habits and, more

important, increased physical activity. The specific strategies for making those changes, and making them permanent, will vary from person to person. So, instead of a walk through the diet book aisle, save your money and improve your health with a *fitness* walk through the mall.

1 Samaha FF, Iqbal N, Seshadri P, et al. A low-carbohydrate as compared with a low-fat diet in severe obesity. *N Engl J Med.* 2003;348:2074–2081.

2 Foster GD, Wyatt HR, Hill JO, et al. A randomized trial of a low-carbohydrate diet for obesity. *N Engl J Med.* 2003;348:2082–2090.

3 Ware JH. Interpreting incomplete data in studies of diet and weight loss. *N Engl J Med.* 2003;348:2136–2137.

4 Bravata DM, Sanders L, Huang J, et al. Efficacy and safety of low-carbohydrate diets: a systematic review. *JAMA.* 2003;289(14):1837–1850.

5 Dansinger ML, Gleason JA, Griffith JL, Selker HP, Schaefer EJ. Comparison of the Atkins, Ornish, Weight Watchers, and Zone diets for weight loss and heart disease risk reduction: a randomized trial. *JAMA.* 2005;293:43–53.

6 Buchholz AC, Schoeller DA. Is a calorie a calorie? *Am J Clin Nutr.* 2004;79(suppl):899S–906S.

7 Levine MJ, Jones JM, Lineback DR. Low-carbohydrate diets: assessing the science and knowledge gaps, summary of an ILSI North America workshop. *J Am Diet Assoc.* 2006;106:2086–2094.

8 Dansinger ML, Gleason JA, Griffith JL, Selker HP, Schaefer EJ. Op. cit.

The ABC model helps you manage the events that trigger behaviors and the factors that reinforce them. *Antecedents,* the "A" part of the model, are the events that precede the behavior and trigger it. Overeating is one possible *behavior,* the "B" part of the model. The *consequences,* or "C," follow and reinforce the "B." The "C" may be desirable, such as relief from stress, or undesirable, such as guilt or weight gain. Consequences may be immediate or, like weight gain, occur in the future; consequences that occur immediately have the greatest influence.

Identifying the cues (A) that trigger overeating is the first step to changing or avoiding these triggers. You might remove problem foods from the house or avoid the grocery store's candy aisle. You can sometimes manipulate antecedents to trigger positive behaviors (for example, putting exercise clothes by the door to prompt exercise).

You can change the behavior of overeating (B) by using positive self-talk to encourage a new behavior and avoiding excuses and rationalizations to eat something inappropriate.

Positive consequences (C) help to reinforce new behaviors. You could sign a contract with a friend that rewards you for deciding not to overeat. Rewards such as time for physical activity not only reinforce behavior but also develop fitness. **Table 8.8** summarizes cognitive-behavioral tools for changing habits and behavior patterns.

Table 8.8 Cognitive-Behavioral Tools for Changing Behavior

Tool	Description
Self-monitoring	Prospectively recording information about behavior to identify the antecedents (what precedes and elicits a particular action), the behaviors of interest (usually eating behavior), and the consequences (the thoughts, feelings, and reactions that accompany the behavior of interest).
Environmental management	Avoiding or changing cues that trigger undesirable behavior (e.g., not driving by the doughnut shop, putting the cookie jar out of sight), or instituting new cues to elicit new behaviors (e.g., putting your walking shoes by the door as a reminder to exercise); also called "stimulus control."
Alternate behaviors	Learning new ways of responding to old cues or circumstances that can't be changed or avoided (e.g., taking a walk when you get upset instead of getting something to eat).
Reward	Giving yourself, or arranging to be given, rewards for engaging in desired behaviors.
Negative reinforcement	Arranging to give up something desirable (e.g., money) or to endure something undesirable (e.g., wash your friend's car) for engaging in unwanted behaviors.
Social support	Getting others to participate in or otherwise provide emotional and physical support of your weight-management efforts.
Cognitive coping	Reducing negative self-talk, increasing positive self-talk, and challenging beliefs that undermine your resolve and contribute to negative emotions; setting reasonable goals and avoiding "thinking traps."
Managing emotions	Using reframing, disengagement, imagery, and self-soothing to reduce or manage negative emotions.
Relapse prevention and recovery	Identifying high-risk situations that pose a hazard for relapsing, and learning to recover from small indiscretions before they become major relapses.

Source: Adapted from Nash JD. *The New Maximize Your Body Potential.* Palo Alto, CA: Bull Publishing Company, 1997. Used with permission.

Balancing Acceptance and Change

It's not enough to change your behavior to manage obesity. Self-acceptance is equally necessary. (See **Table 8.9.**) Accepting yourself as you are will help your self-esteem and improve your general satisfaction with life. It is destructive to be overly concerned with the importance of body weight and shape or to have unattainable goals of idealized physical appearance. But don't confuse self-acceptance with complacency or a do-nothing attitude that ignores health risks.

If you must diet, do so in combination with exercise, and avoid very low calorie diets. Don't try to lose more than one-half to one pound per week. Realize that most low-calorie diets cause a rapid loss of body water at first. When this phase passes, weight loss declines. As a result, dieters often are misled into believing that their efforts are not working. They then give up, not realizing that smaller losses later in the diet actually are better than the initial big losses. In fact, the later loss is mostly fat loss, whereas the initial loss is primarily fluid loss.

Key Concepts: Identifying cues that precede overeating can help a person make behavior changes. Long-term weight management should include self-acceptance and enhanced self-esteem. Goals of idealized body size and shape should be replaced with goals that promote good health and a lifetime of fitness.

Weight-Management Approaches

Do certain weight-loss diets have adverse health consequences? Is it unhealthy to lose weight quickly? Will the weight stay off? What motivates people to lose weight and to maintain weight? What are the barriers to losing weight and/or to maintaining weight?

In a study of popular weight-loss diets, 160 participants with an average BMI of 35 kg/m^2 were randomly assigned to one of four weight-loss diets: Weight Watchers (restriction of portion sizes and calories; 1,200 to 1,600 calories daily), Atkins (low carbohydrate—less than 20 grams daily at onset, gradual increase to 50 grams), Zone (40–30–30 balance of percentage calories from carbohydrate, fat, and protein, respectively), and Ornish (vegetarian, less than 10 percent of calories from fat).[124] Subjects lost weight on all four diets, but no one diet was more effective than any of the others. Compliance was a key factor—only about 25 percent of subjects in each group maintained the diet at a level of 6 on a 10-point scale (1 = no adherence, 10 = perfect adherence), but dietary adherence was strongly associated with weight loss. Those who stuck to the diets best lost on average 7 percent of body weight, a meaningful start in reducing health risks.

A wide range of weight-management approaches is available to the consumer. It's important to investigate your options thoroughly to find the approach best suited to your personal needs.

Self-Help Books and Manuals

Some people respond well to simple information provided in an easy-to-understand format. They are able to change their behavior by referring to good, well-researched self-help manuals and books,[125] and even Internet-based resources. The proliferation of diet books is nothing short of phenomenal,

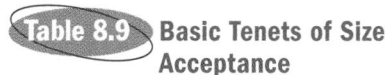

Table 8.9 **Basic Tenets of Size Acceptance**

- Human beings come in a variety of sizes and shapes. We celebrate this diversity as a positive characteristic of the human race.
- There is no ideal body size, shape, or weight that every individual should strive to achieve.
- Every body is a good body, whatever its size or shape.
- Self-esteem and body image are strongly linked. Helping people feel good about their bodies and about who they are can help motivate and maintain healthy behaviors.
- Appearance stereotyping is inherently unfair to the individual because it is based on superficial factors over which the individual has little or no control.
- We respect the bodies of others even though they might be quite different from our own.
- Each person is responsible for taking care of his/her body.
- Good health is not defined by body size; it is a state of physical, mental, and social well-being.

People of all sizes and shapes can reduce their risk of poor health by adopting a healthy lifestyle.

Source: Excerpted from *Basic Tenets of Health at Every Size*, developed by dietitians and nutritionists who are advocates of size acceptance; their efforts coordinated by Joanne P. Ikeda, MA, RD, Nutrition Education Specialist, Department of Nutritional Sciences, University of California, Berkeley.

however, and each year dozens of dubious weight-loss diet books reach the market. When evaluating a diet book or Web site diet plan, be alert to the following warning flags:

- Unbalanced diet patterns. The recommended pattern should not stray too far from that of MyPyramid (see Chapter 2, "Nutrition Guidelines and Assessment").

- Claims of a "scientific breakthrough" or promises of "quick and easy" weight loss. There is no "quick fix" when it comes to weight management.

- Irrational food instructions, such as food restrictions (e.g., no fruits), illogical overemphasis of some foods (e.g., five grapefruits daily), and irrational food patterns (e.g., don't eat meat and bread at the same meal). Such restrictions set the stage for feelings of deprivation and binge eating.

- The promise of a cure for some disease along with weight loss. That's not only a waste of money, but also potentially dangerous.

Should you decide on the "do-it-yourself" route, develop specific goals for your diet, exercise, and maintenance plans. (See the FYI feature "Behaviors That Will Help You Manage Your Weight.") Keep tabs on your habits and become more involved in activities other than eating, especially fitness activities. Long-term success depends on maintaining the lifestyle changes that helped you lose the weight in the first place.

Meal Replacements

Some people turn to meal replacements—shakes and bars, for example—to help lose weight. Meal replacements are convenient, often contain added vitamins and minerals, and reduce the choices and temptations available at mealtime. When compared with traditional, reduced-calorie diet programs, people using meal replacements lost slightly more weight and were less likely to stop the program.[126] The challenge is to learn long-term eating strategies that will allow weight management without reliance on special products.

Self-Help Groups

Self-help groups, often led by laypeople, help many people cope with their weight. Such groups can share experiences, reduce the isolation and alienation felt by many obese people, and provide an understanding and accepting community.

Commercial Programs

Commercial weight-loss programs provide group or individual counseling and group support. Some sell prepackaged foods or nutritional supplements. Some companies employ dietitians, health educators, psychologists, or physicians to develop and guide the program at the corporate level. The Federal Trade Commission (FTC) encourages commercial programs to release the following information to potential clients:

- Staff training and education
- Risks of overweight and obesity

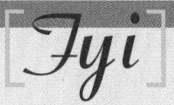

Behaviors That Will Help You Manage Your Weight

FOR YOUR INFORMATION

Set the Right Goals

Setting the right goals is an important first step. Most people trying to lose weight focus just on weight loss. However, you'll be more successful if you focus on dietary and exercise changes that lead to long-term weight change. Successful weight managers select no more than two or three goals at a time.

Effective goals are (1) specific, (2) attainable, and (3) forgiving. "Exercise more" is a commendable ideal, but it's not specific. "Walk five miles every day" is specific and measurable, but is it attainable if you're just starting out? "Walk 30 minutes every day" is more attainable, but what happens if you're held up at work or there's a thunderstorm? "Walk 30 minutes, five days each week" is specific, attainable, and forgiving. In short, a great goal!

Nothing Succeeds Like Success

Select a series of short-term goals that get you closer and closer to the ultimate goal (for example, consider reducing fat intake from 40 percent of calories to 35 percent and later to 30 percent). Nothing succeeds like success. This strategy employs two important behavioral principles: (1) consecutive goals that move you ahead in small steps are the best way to reach a distant point, and (2) consecutive rewards keep the overall effort invigorated.

Reward Success (But Not with Food)

You're more likely to keep working toward your goal if you are rewarded—especially when goals are difficult to reach. An effective reward is something that is desirable, timely, and contingent on meeting your goal. Your rewards may be tangible (e.g., a movie or music CD or a payment toward buying a more costly item) or intangible (e.g., an afternoon off from studying or just an hour of quiet time away from the daily demands of school). As you meet small goals, give yourself numerous small rewards; don't wait to meet your ultimate goal for a single reward. The long, difficult effort might lead you to give up.

Balance Your (Food) Checkbook

Keeping track of your behavior—observing and recording calorie intake, servings of fruits and vegetables, exercise frequency and duration, or any other wellness behavior—can help alter that behavior. Self-monitoring usually changes a behavior in the desired direction and can produce "real-time" records for you and your health care provider. For example, you can track your exercise progress. A record of increasing exercise encourages you to keep up the good work. If the record shows little or no progress, you know that a change of strategy is needed. Some people find that specific self-monitoring forms make it easier, while others prefer to use their own recording system.

Although you don't need to step on the scale every day, monitoring your weight regularly (once a week) can help you maintain your lower weight. Use a graph rather than a list or calendar notations so that you have a picture of cumulative progress. Changes in your body's water content, rather than fat content, are responsible for most of the up and down fluctuations from day to day. A long-term downward trend reflects fat losses.

Avoid a Chain Reaction

Identify the social or environmental cues that seem to encourage undesirable eating, and then change those cues. For example, you may learn from reflection or self-monitoring that you're more likely to overeat while watching television, when treats are on display at the campus café, or when you're around a certain friend. You might then try to break the association between eating and the cue (don't eat while watching television), avoid or eliminate the cue (avoid sitting near the display counter), or change the circumstances surrounding the cue (plan to meet with your friend in nonfood settings). In general, visible and accessible food items often are cues for unplanned eating.

Get the (Fullness) Message

Changing the way you go about eating can make it easier to eat less without feeling deprived. It takes 15 or more minutes for your brain to get the message you've been fed. Slowing the rate of eating can allow satiation (fullness) signals to begin by the end of the meal. Eating lots of vegetables also can make you feel fuller. Another trick is to use smaller plates so that moderate portions do not appear meager. Changing your eating schedule, or setting one, can be helpful, especially if you tend to skip or delay meals and overeat later.

The Backsliding Phenomenon

You've just signed a contract with yourself to avoid high-fat desserts for one month when you're presented with an array of your favorite "to die for" desserts. You say to yourself, "just this once" and satisfy your craving. Most of us have experienced the "backsliding phenomenon" in which we have lost our resolve and slipped back into a former bad habit. When it happens, be prepared for it and move on with your resolve. You're most apt to backslide when you're tempted by something unexpected and your self-control is threatened. You can remove high-fat snacks from your home, but not from other places you eat. Imagine tempting situations in your mind's eye and practice coping with them successfully. If you do slip, don't waste time with self-blame. Learn from the experience and get back on track.

Source: Adapted from National Heart, Lung, and Blood Institute. *Guide to Behavior Change.* http://www.nhlbi.nih.gov/health/public/heart/obesity/lose_wt/behavior.htm. Accessed 06/20/06.

very low calorie diets (VLCD) Diets supplying 400 to 800 kilocalories per day, which include adequate high-quality protein, little or no fat, and little carbohydrate.

- Risks of their products or program
- Cost
- Program outcomes: success and failure rates

Be sure to obtain this information before you register for a weight-loss program, and think twice about any program that does not willingly provide it. In a comparison of a structured commercial program (food plan + activity plan + cognitive restructuring behavior modification plan + weekly meetings) to a self-help strategy, the commercial program supported modest levels of weight loss, but more than the self-help strategy achieved over a two-year period.[127]

Several commercial programs, such as Optifast and Health Management Resources (HMR), use **very low calorie diets (VLCD)** containing only 400 to 800 kilocalories per day as the initial phase of treatment. When such diets were first introduced in the 1970s, several deaths resulted from cardiac abnormalities. As a result, VLCD should be undertaken only with close medical supervision.

Professional Private Counselors

Private counselors can be physicians, psychotherapists, nutritionists, or registered dietitians. They provide individualized approaches to weight management and the support and attention that some obese people may need. Some programs use the Internet rather than face-to-face counseling sessions. Regular e-mail behavioral counseling and feedback from a trained counselor can improve weight loss.[128] However, a comparison of a commercial Internet-based weight-loss program to a self-help weight-loss manual found higher weight loss at one year in the self-help group (4 percent of initial body weight versus 1 percent).[129]

Carefully scrutinize the training and credentials of private counselors before committing to any program. Effective weight-loss counselors should do the following:[130]

1. Assess obesity risk
2. Ask about readiness to lose weight
3. Advise in designing a weight-control program
4. Assist in establishing appropriate intervention
5. Arrange for follow-up

Antiobesity Prescription Drugs

The pharmaceutical industry has long searched for a "magic bullet" to battle obesity, but a cure has failed to emerge. Two popular antiobesity drugs, fenfluramine (one component of a combination called fen-phen) and dexfenfluramine (Redux), were withdrawn from the market after research found that they were the likely cause of life-threatening lung disease and heart valve problems.[131] With the recognition that obesity involves multiple factors, the focus is shifting to drugs with multiple mechanisms and drugs to be used in conjunction with proper diet and exercise.[132]

Antiobesity prescription drugs approved for short-term use include Dexedrine, other amphetamines, and amphetamine derivatives. For long-term use, only two prescription drugs—Xenical and Meridia—are presently approved for treating obesity. Xenical (orlistat) interferes with pancreatic lipase and reduces fat digestion and absorption. Because Xenical blocks fat absorption by as much as 30 percent, it must be accompanied by a low-fat diet; otherwise, the unabsorbed fat can produce diarrhea and flatulence. The

Quick Bites

Antiobesity Munchies

Sometimes, ideas for new drugs come from unusual places. Take "rimonabant," an antiobesity drug in the clinical trial phase. Rimonabant blocks a receptor in the central nervous system that responds to the active ingredient in marijuana, THC (delta-9-tetra-hydrocannabinol). Once these receptors were discovered, scientists wondered whether they played a role in the "munchies" experienced by marijuana smokers. Studies so far have been positive—obese mice lost weight when fed a cannabinoid receptor inhibitor.

drug also blocks fat-soluble nutrient absorption, so it's necessary to take a vitamin supplement as well.[133] Sales of Xenical fell in 2002 amid research showing that the drug improved weight loss by only 2 to 3 percent.[134]

Meridia (sibutramine) is an appetite suppressant that affects the balance of chemicals in the brain. Meridia was believed to be safer than earlier antiobesity drugs, but like all prescription drugs, it can have side effects—in this case increased blood pressure and heart rate.[135] With questions about its safety, public-interest groups in the United States have asked the FDA to withdraw it from the market, and authorities in Italy have banned it from sale.[136]

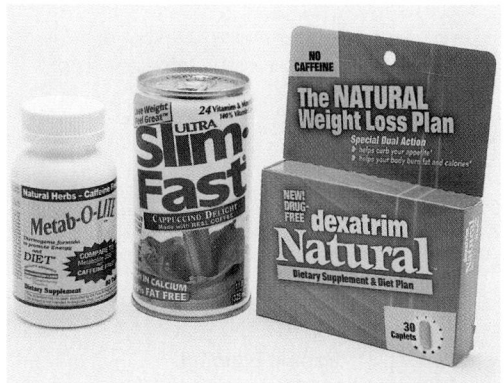

The FDA has approved the use of antiobesity drugs only in combination with calorie-restricted diets. Aside from Xenical, antiobesity drugs are addictive and have the potential for abuse. Antiobesity agents shouldn't be used in combination with each other or with other drugs for appetite control, because the safety of such combinations has not been evaluated. The drugs should be used only in people who are obese—not people looking to lose just a few pounds. Are they effective? A review of numerous clinical trials suggests that the benefits of drug therapy over behavioral interventions are modest at best.[137]

With recent advances in the understanding of hormones and other factors that regulate appetite and satiety, scientists have new targets for the development of weight-loss medications. Leptin was a major focus of research until it became clear that leptin therapy is effective only for those with genetic defects in synthesis of leptin or its receptors. Current efforts are exploring compounds that may block the action of ghrelin and suppress NPY production.

Over-the-Counter Drugs and Dietary Supplements

Nonprescription (over-the-counter, or OTC) weight-loss pills may contain caffeine, benzocaine, or fiber. Caffeine is a stimulant and diuretic. Benzocaine numbs the tongue, which reduces taste sensations and discourages eating. Pills with fiber are designed to fill the stomach and provide a feeling of fullness. Although moderately effective, fiber pills can lead to dehydration; much of the lost weight is water, which is easily regained when the pills are stopped.

Numerous dietary supplements are marketed for weight loss, with names such as "Weight Away." Common ingredients include chromium picolinate, chitosan, hydroxycitric acid (HCA), glucomannan, and pyruvate. Few studies have evaluated these products for weight loss, and what little evidence exists is not convincing enough to recommend their use.[138]

In 2004, following years of study and an accumulation of reported adverse effects, the FDA banned the use of ephedra in dietary supplements—the government's first ban of a dietary supplement. Ephedra was an ingredient in many supplements marketed for weight loss and enhanced sports performance. Although it promotes modest short-term weight loss,[139] ephedra (also known as ma huang) is dangerous to people with hypertension, heart disease, or diabetes. Safety data from 50 different research studies found two- to threefold increases in risk for adverse events,[140] and the FDA's evidence linked ephedra to 155 deaths and dozens of heart attacks and strokes. The ban was overturned in federal court in 2005, a ruling that the FDA successfully appealed in 2006.

Over-the-counter medicines and dietary supplements are no substitute for exercise and healthful eating. There is no quick, easy way to effectively lose weight.

extreme obesity Obesity characterized by body weight exceeding 100 percent of normal; a condition so severe it often requires surgery.

morbid obesity See *extreme obesity*.

Surgery

Sometimes, surgery can successfully treat **extreme obesity** (also called **morbid obesity**), defined as a BMI of 40 kg/m² or higher. Surgery should be a last-ditch effort, taken only when all legitimate, less-invasive methods have failed. The two most common procedures are gastric banding and gastric bypass. Gastric banding reduces stomach size by creating a smaller upper stomach, or "pouch," thus limiting intake to only a few calories at one time.[141] Gastric bypass also creates a smaller stomach pouch and then connects that pouch to a shortened section of small intestine. (See **Figure 8.24**.) Reducing the size of the stomach reduces food intake, and bypassing the upper part of the small intestine reduces digestion and absorption of caloric foods. The absorption of some micronutrients is also reduced—an obvious drawback. Such surgeries are growing in popularity: In 1998, more than 13,300 procedures were performed. By 2003, the number of procedures was expected to be nearly 103,000.[142]

The results are impressive. Patients lose substantially more weight than those who try diet and exercise, or even weight-loss medications. Although weight loss tends to plateau by 18 to 24 months after surgery, it is not unusual for patients to have maintained a 50 percent loss of initial body weight after five years.[143]

The long-term effectiveness of gastric surgery depends on how patients manage their eating. They can defeat the procedure by consuming high-calorie drinks or semisolid foods that overcome stomach size. With time the pouch stretches, allowing more solid foods, but by then, doctors hope that the patient has established healthy eating habits. Also, RMR can decline significantly after gastric surgery, making weight loss more difficult; thus, exercise is important along with diet modifications.[144] Studies show that gastric bypass leads to dramatically lower levels of ghrelin, the gastric hormone that increases food intake.[145] Lower levels of ghrelin likely contribute to the effectiveness of the procedure.

Liposuction is a cosmetic surgical procedure that reshapes the body by removing fat. Although the procedure removes some fat cells, the body still has billions of other fat cells ready to store extra fat. Thus, liposuction is not effective for significant or long-term weight loss. It should not be undertaken casually. Risks include blood clots, perforation injuries, skin and nerve damage, and unfavorable drug reactions.

Summary of Weight-Management Strategies

For best effect, weight-management strategies need to be individualized. Until the science of nutrigenomics advances far enough to match an individual's genetics to the right diet plan, dietary strategies that reduce chronic disease risks (more fruits and vegetables, whole grains, and fish)[146] should be combined with physical activity to achieve a modest but persistent reduction in calories.[147] For individuals who are morbidly obese, consultation with a physician is essential to determine the right approach for managing weight and improving health.

Key Concepts: *Books, Internet resources, and commercial programs can help some individuals lose weight. However, consumers should always proceed with caution before spending money. Drugs have potential side effects and must be used with caution and medical supervision. For those who are extremely obese, surgical intervention is an aggressive, last-resort approach to weight management. Liposuction removes fat cells from specific parts of the body but is not considered an effective approach to weight control.*

Gastric Banding

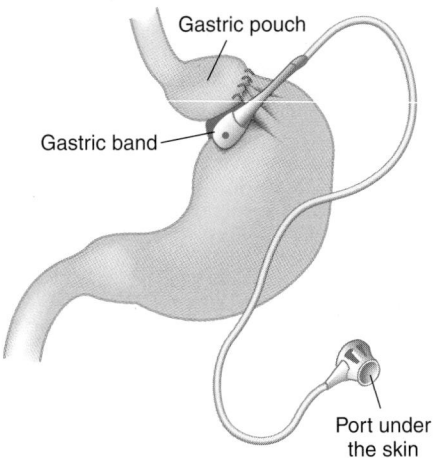

Gastric pouch

Gastric band

Port under the skin

Gastric Bypass

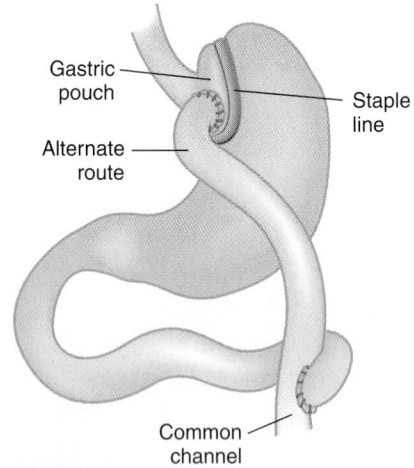

Gastric pouch

Staple line

Alternate route

Common channel

Figure 8.24 **Gastric surgery in obesity treatment.** In gastric banding, surgery reduces the size of the stomach. The band can be adjusted by an infusion of saline through a port that lies just beneath the skin. In gastric bypass, an alternate route carries food to the jejunum, bypassing the duodenum and most of the stomach.

Source: Steinbrook R. Surgery for severe obesity. *N Engl J Med.* 2004;350:1075–1079. Copyright © 2004 Massachusetts Medical Society. All rights reserved. Reprinted by permission.

Underweight

From a public health standpoint, underweight is much less of a problem than obesity, but those who are underweight can find it troublesome and frustrating. Underweight is usually defined as a BMI below 18.5 kg/m². When low BMI is simply an inherited pattern, there is no need to worry about health risks as long as diet and other health behaviors are appropriate. But your health is at risk if your underweight results from undernutrition; deficits in protein, vitamins, and minerals, as well as energy, can cause health problems ranging from fatigue to compromised immune function. Underweight women are more likely to suffer amenorrhea, low fertility, and poor pregnancy outcome.

Causes and Assessment

The causes of underweight are as diverse as those of overweight and include the following:

- Altered response to hunger, appetite, satiation, satiety, and external cues (described earlier in this chapter)
- Factors in eating disorders such as distorted body image, compulsive dieting, and compulsive overexercising
- Metabolic and hereditary factors
- Prolonged psychological and emotional stress
- Addiction to alcohol and street drugs
- Bizarre diet patterns or otherwise inadequate diets

Underweight can be a sign of underlying disease, such as cancer. Illness can speed up metabolic rate, spoil the appetite, or interfere with digestion. Correcting underweight helps improve the quality of life.

Weight-Gain Strategies

The way to gain weight is to create a positive energy balance. Here are some strategies:

- Have small, frequent meals consisting of nutrient-dense and energy-dense foods and beverages.
- Drink fluids at the end of the meal or, better yet, between meals to avoid filling the stomach with liquids of low nutrient density.
- Try high-calorie weight-gain beverages and foods.
- Use timers or other cues (similar to the ABC model in Figure 8.23, but with a different goal) to prompt eating.
- Take a balanced vitamin/mineral supplement to ensure that poor appetite isn't a result of nutritional deficiency.

Sometimes prescription drugs, such as appetite stimulants, are helpful. Medication also can speed stomach emptying, improving appetite for the next meal. Digestive enzyme replacements help people who are underweight due to poor digestion or absorption.

Exercise has a role in weight gain as well. Simple anaerobic or isometric exercise encourages weight gain as lean body mass rather than fat.

Key Concepts: *Underweight is not as common as overweight. Gaining weight can be difficult, but the basic concepts of energy balance apply. Changes in diet along with regular physical activity are important strategies for gaining weight.*

Label [to] **Table**

Do you believe that by choosing cookies or chips labeled "low-fat" or sticking with certain brand names associated with "diet foods" you are automatically making the right decisions? It may surprise you to know that many low-fat or fat-free products have nearly the same amount of calories as the full-fat versions! After reading this chapter you now know that when it comes to weight loss, total calories are just as important as calories from fat. If you eat a fat-free food, but eat so much of it that your calories are excessive, you will still gain weight. To illustrate this point, let's compare the nutrition labels from some leading cookie manufacturers. The lower-fat cookie label (on right) claims they are "better for you" and have "50% less fat" compared to the regular cookies. Here are the labels:

Regular Cookie	Lower-Fat Cookie
Serving 2 cookies (29g)	*Serving 2 cookies (26g)*
Calories 140	*Calories 110*
Calories from fat 50	*Calories from fat 25*
Total Fat 6g	*Total Fat 3g*

True, there is a 50 percent reduction in fat content (6g vs. 3g), which is an important part of the picture. However, take a look at the Total Calories. The lower-fat cookies only have 30 fewer kilocalories than the regular cookies, which may be a surprise to those who think they are saving more.

There is another interesting piece of information on these labels: the serving size. At first glance, you may think the serving size of the cookies are the same, two cookies. However after further inspection you can see that the lower-fat cookies are slightly smaller. A 10 percent reduction in size/weight is certainly worth noting when you are trying to explain how a product can have fewer calories.

The next time you are in the cookie aisle debating whether you should settle a craving with a low-fat product or its full-fat version, be a smart consumer and read the label before you buy!

Nutrition Facts

Serving Size: 2 cookies (29g)
Servings Per Container about 16

Amount Per Serving

Calories 140   Calories from fat 50

% Daily Value*

Total Fat 6g	9%
Saturated Fat 1.5g	8%
Trans Fat 0.5g	
Cholesterol 0mg	0%
Sodium 105mg	4%
Total Carbohydrate 21g	7%
Dietary Fiber less than 1g	3%
Sugars 8g	

Protein 2g

Vitamin A 0%	•	Vitamin C 0%
Calcium 0%	•	Iron 4%

* Percent Daily Values are based on a 2,000 calorie diet. Your daily values may be higher or lower depending on your calorie needs:

		Calories: 2000	2,500
Total Fat	Less Than	65g	80g
Sat Fat	Less Than	20g	25g
Cholesterol	Less Than	300mg	300mg
Sodium	Less Than	2,400mg	2,400mg
Total Carbohydrate		300g	375g
Dietary Fiber		25g	30g

Regular cookie

Nutrition Facts

Serving Size: 2 cookies (26g)
Servings Per Container: 18

Amount Per Serving

Calories 110   Calories from fat 25

% Daily Value*

Total Fat 3g	5%
Saturated Fat 0.5g	3%
Polyunsaturated Fat 0g	
Monounsaturated Fat 1g	
Trans Fat 0g	
Cholesterol 0mg	0%
Sodium 130mg	5%
Total Carbohydrate 20g	7%
Dietary Fiber 0g	0%
Sugars 10g	

Protein 1g

Vitamin A 0%	•	Vitamin C 0%
Calcium 0%	•	Iron 2%

* Percent Daily Values are based on a 2,000 calorie diet. Your daily values may be higher or lower depending on your calorie needs:

		Calories: 2000	2,500
Total Fat	Less Than	65g	80g
Sat Fat	Less Than	20g	25g
Cholesterol	Less Than	300mg	300mg
Sodium	Less Than	2,400mg	2,400mg
Total Carbohydrate		300g	375g
Dietary Fiber		25g	30g

Lower-fat cookie

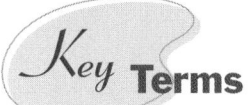 LEARNING *Portfolio* c h a p t e r 8

Key Terms

Study Points

➤ Energy balance is the relationship between energy intake and energy output.

➤ The energy content in food can be measured directly using a bomb calorimeter or estimated using the following factors: 4 kilocalories per gram for carbohydrate and protein, 9 kilocalories per gram for fat, and 7 kilocalories per gram for alcohol.

➤ Food intake is regulated by hunger, satiation, satiety, and appetite, which are influenced by complex factors. Hunger is the physiological need to eat. Satiation is the feeling of fullness that leads to termination of a meal. Satiety is the feeling of satisfaction and lack of hunger that determines the interval until the next meal. Appetite is a desire to eat that is influenced by external factors such as flavors and smells, and environmental and cultural factors.

➤ Gastrointestinal stimulation, circulating nutrients, neurotransmitters, and hormones signal the brain to regulate food intake.

➤ The major components of energy expenditure are resting energy expenditure, the thermic effect of food, and energy for physical activity.

➤ Calorimetry is the measurement of energy use, either directly by measuring heat production or indirectly by determining oxygen intake and carbon dioxide production.

➤ Body composition, age, gender, genetics, and hormonal activity affect the amount of energy used for resting metabolism.

➤ The energy cost of physical activity is affected by a person's size and the intensity and duration of the activity.

➤ Body composition—the relative amounts of fat and lean body mass—has a major influence on energy expenditure and risk of chronic disease.

➤ Body mass index—a ratio correlated with total body fatness and risk of chronic disease—is calculated with height and weight measurements.

➤ The prevalence of obesity and overweight is escalating worldwide, contributing to chronic disease.

➤ Health risks associated with obesity are more pronounced when excess body fat is located in the abdominal region of the body.

➤ The factors that cause obesity are not completely understood, but a complex interaction of hormonal and metabolic factors is believed to play a role, along with genetic, sociocultural, and psychological factors.

➤ Rather than focus on ideal body weight, many professionals now promote health and fitness goals.

➤ Physical activity improves fitness and helps achieve the negative energy balance needed for weight reduction.

➤ Abandoning unrealistic ideas of thinness and accepting body weight and shape are important elements in weight management.

➤ Long-term weight management includes a balanced diet of moderately restricted calorie intake, adequate exercise, cognitive-behavioral strategies for changing habits and behavior patterns, and attention to balancing self-acceptance and the desire for change.

➤ Surgical approaches to weight control should be considered only as a last resort for the morbidly obese.

➤ If the cause is not hereditary, being underweight can pose health problems.

➤ Gaining weight can be difficult for individuals who are underweight.

Study Questions

1. Explain the concept of energy balance.

2. List and describe the three main components of energy expenditure.

3. Explain the three main factors that determine energy expenditure in activity.

4. List the techniques for measuring body composition.

5. Obesity is seen as a complex disorder with multiple contributing factors. List the types of factors involved in the development and maintenance of obesity.

6. What body mass index (BMI) values are associated with being underweight, overweight, and obese? Do these vary for men and women?

7. Describe the concept of metabolic fitness.

8. What is the difference between hyperplastic and hypertrophic obesity?

9. What are the components of a sound approach to weight management?

10. Explain how the ABCs of behavior modification can assist with weight control.

11. Define "underweight."

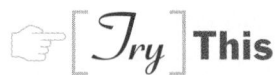 **This**

A One-Week Energy Balance Check

The purpose of this exercise is to see if you're in energy balance by monitoring your body weight for one week. Measure your weight on a Monday morning soon after you wake up. Record your weight. Don't change your normal routine of exercise and food intake. One week later weigh yourself again (on a Monday morning just after waking). Did your weight change? If not, your energy intake closely matched your energy output. If so, did you gain or lose weight? What factors do you think contributed to your body weight change? Try repeating this exercise over a longer period of time. Measure and record your weight every Monday morning for six months. What happens?

Increasing Your Energy Output

Physical activity is the part of your energy output that varies the most. The purpose of this exercise is to increase your energy expenditure by committing to daily exercise for one week. Make each exercise session about 30 minutes long, and remember that the longer the duration, the harder the intensity, and the larger the muscle groups involved, the greater the energy expenditure. Choose an exercise you enjoy—such as walking, jogging, cycling, swimming, or rollerblading. Once your week is complete, ask yourself these questions: How did this week's daily exercise affect my energy balance? Have I gained or lost weight during the week? Did I compensate for the extra energy expenditure by increasing my calorie intake?

Changing Your Energy Input

Would you like to change your weight by a pound or two? The purpose of this exercise is to increase or decrease your energy input (calorie intake) so that you gain or lose 1 pound by the end of a week. How? Make only minor adjustments in your usual diet but try to change the energy content for each of your meals by a small amount. Keep a food log and use Appendix A, EatRight Analysis Software, or Nutritionist Pro software to estimate your calorie total for each of the days. Your goal is to change your calorie total by approximately 500 kilocalories per day. You should not consume fewer than 1,500 kilocalories (for women) or 1,800 kilocalories (for men) per day. Weigh yourself at the start of your week and at the end. What change, if any, do you see?

What About Bobbie?

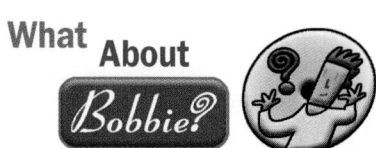

Remember, Bobbie is a 20-year-old college sophomore who weighs 155 pounds and is 5 feet, 4 inches tall. She gained 10 pounds her freshman year and would like to lose it because she feels healthier when her weight is closer to 145 pounds. She exercises infrequently but likes to walk with her friends and occasionally goes to an aerobics class. How would you suggest she lose the extra 10 pounds? First, let's start by reducing her calorie intake slightly. Here is Bobbie's typical day of eating and some small changes in portion sizes that will save some calories.

Typical Day	Alternative	Kcal
BREAKFAST		
1 cinnamon-raisin bagel		
3 Tbsp. light cream cheese	1 Tbsp. light cream cheese	70 saved
Coffee, 2 Tbsp. 2% milk, 2 tsp. sugar		
SNACK		
1 banana		
LUNCH		
2 slices sourdough bread		
2 ounces turkey lunch meat 2 tsp. regular mayo, 2 tsp. mustard, 1 slice tomato, dill pickle, lettuce leaf		
12 oz. diet coke		
Salad		
2 C iceberg lettuce with 2 Tbsp. each: shredded carrot, chopped egg, croutons, kidney beans, Italian dressing	1 Tbsp. Italian dressing	55 saved
1 chocolate chip cookie		
SNACK		
1 ½ oz. tortilla chips, ½ C salsa	1 oz. tortilla chips	70 saved
2 C water		
DINNER		
1 ½ C pasta	1 C pasta	100 saved
3 oz. meatballs, 3 oz. spaghetti sauce, 2 Tbsp. parmesan cheese		
1 slice garlic bread	delete garlic bread	185 saved
½ C green beans	1 C green beans	25 added
1 tsp. butter	delete butter	30 saved
12 oz. diet cola		
SNACK		
1 slice cheese pizza		
	Total	**500 saved**

As you can see, small changes in Bobbie's diet can result in a 500-kilocalorie deficit, which will translate to approximately 1 pound per week of weight loss. This doesn't take into account any extra exercise she might do. So if she starts to work out more regularly, she can make fewer changes in her calorie intake and still lose 1 pound per week.

References

1 Devitt AA, Mattes RD. Effects of food unit size and energy density on intake in humans. *Appetite.* 2004;42:213–220; and Rolls BJ, Drewnowski A, Ledikwe JH. Changing the energy density of the diet as a strategy for weight management. *J Am Diet Assoc.* 2005;105:S98–S103.

2 de Castro JM. Dietary energy density is associated with increased intake in free-living humans. *J Nutr.* 2004;134:335–341.

3 Anderson GH, Moore SE. Dietary proteins in the regulation of food intake and body weight in humans. *J Nutr.* 2004; 134:974S–979S; Gerstein DE, Woodward-Lopez G, Evans AE, et al. Clarifying concepts about macronutrients' effects of satiation and satiety. *J Am Diet Assoc.* 2004;104:1151–1153; and Mattes RD, Hollis J, Hayes D, Stunkard AJ. Appetite: measurement and manipulation misgivings. *J Am Diet Assoc.* 2005; 105:S87–S97.

4 Vander Wal JS, Marth JM, Khosla P, Jen C, Dhurandhar NV. Short-term effect of eggs on satiety in overweight and obese subjects. *J Am Coll Nutr.* 2005;24(6):510–515.

5 Gerstein DE, Woodward-Lopez G, Evans AE, et al. Op. cit.; and Rolls BJ, Drewnowski A, Ledikwe JH. Op. cit.

6 Burton-Freeman B. Dietary fiber and energy regulation. *J Nutr.* 2000;130:272S–275S.

7 DiMeglio DP, Mattes RD. Liquid versus solid carbohydrate: effects on food intake and body weight. *Int J Obes.* 2000; 24:794–800.

8 Mattes R. Soup and satiety. *Physiol Behav.* 2004;83:739–747.

9 Stubbs RJ, Johnstone AM, Mazalan N, et al. Effect of altering the variety of sensorially distinct foods, of the same macronutrient content, on food intake and body weight in men. *Eur J Clin Nutr.* 2001;55:19–28.

10 Gerstein DE, Woodward-Lopez G, Evans AE, et al. Op. cit.

11 Rolls BJ, Morris EL, Roe LS. Portion size of food affects energy intake in normal-weight and overweight men and women. *Am J Clin Nutr.* 2002;76:1207–1213.

12 Wansink B, Cheney MM. Super Bowls: serving bowl size and food consumption. *JAMA.* 2005;293:1727–1728.

13 Orlet Fisher J, Rolls BJ, Birch LL. Children's bite size and intake of an entrée are greater with large portions than with age-appropriate or self-selected portions. *Am J Clin Nutr.* 2003;77(5):1164–1170.

14 Wansink B, Painter JE, North J. Bottomless bowls: why visual cues of portion size may influence intake. *Obes Res.* 2005; 13:93–100; and Geier AB, Rozin P, Doros G. Unit bias. *Psychol Sci.* 2006;17(6):521–525.

15 Nielsen SJ, Popkin BM. Patterns and trends in food portion sizes, 1977–1998. *JAMA.* 2003;289(4):450–453.

16 Guyton, AC, Hall JE. *Textbook of Medical Physiology.* 10th ed. Philadephia: WB Saunders; 2000.

17 Wansink B. Environmental factors that increase the food intake and consumption volume of unknowing consumers. *Ann Rev Nutr.* 2004;24:455–479.

18 Ibid.

19 Wansink, Op. cit.; and de Castro JM, Brewer E. The amount eaten in meals by humans is a power function of the number of people present. *Physiol Behav.* 1992;51:121–125.

20 Sentyrz SM, Bushman BJ. Mirror, mirror on the wall, who's the thinnest one of all? Effects of self-awareness on consumption of full-fat, reduced-fat, and no-fat products. *J Appl Psychol.* 1998;83:944–949.

21 Guyton AC, Hall JE. *Textbook of Medical Physiology.* 10th ed. Philadelphia: WB Saunders, 2000.

22 Ibid.

23 Schwartz MW, Woods SC, Porter D Jr., et al. Central nervous system control of food intake. *Nature.* 2000;404(6):661–671.

24 Kalra SP, Kalra PS. Neuropeptide Y: a physiological orexigen modulated by the feedback action of ghrelin and leptin. *Endocrine.* 2003;22(1):49–56.

25 Kalra SP, Kalra PS. NPY and cohorts in regulating appetite, obesity and metabolic syndrome: beneficial effects of gene therapy. *Neuropeptides.* 2004;38(4):201–211.

26 Schwartz MW, Baskin DG, Kaiyala KJ, Woods SC. Model for the regulation of energy balance and adiposity by the central nervous system. *Am J Clin Nutr.* 1999;69:584–596.

27 Brodsky IG. Hormones and growth factors. In: Shils ME, Shike M, Ross AC, Cabellero B, Cousins RJ, eds. *Modern Nutrition in Health and Disease.* 10th ed. Philadephia: Lippincott Williams & Wilkins, 2006:636–654.

28 Bowles L, Kopelman P. Leptin: of mice and men? *J Clin Pathol.* 2001;54:1–3.

29 le Roux CW, Patterson M, Vincent RP, et al. Postprandial plasma ghrelin is suppressed proportional to meal calorie content in normal-weight but not obese subjects. *J Clin Endocrinol Metab.* 2004;90:1068–1071.

30 Wilmore JH, Costill DL. *Physiology of Sport and Exercise.* 2nd ed. Champaign, IL: Human Kinetics, 1999.

31 Institute of Medicine, Food and Nutrition Board. *Dietary Reference Intakes for Energy, Carbohydrate, Fiber, Fat, Fatty Acids, Cholesterol, Protein, and Amino Acids.* Washington, DC: National Academy Press, 2005.

32 Ibid.

33 Ibid.

34 Poehlman ET, Berke EM, Joseph JR, Gardner AW, Goran MI. Influence of aerobic capacity, body composition and thyroid hormones on the age-related decline in resting metabolic rate. *Metabolism.* 1992;41:915–921.

35 Mahan LK, Escott-Stump S. *Krause's Food, Nutrition and Diet Therapy.* 10th ed. Philadelphia: WB Saunders, 2005.

36 Bouchard C, ed. *The Genetics of Obesity.* Boca Raton, FL: CRC Press, 1994:135–145.

37 Mahan LK, Escott-Stump S. Op. cit.

38 Arciero PJ, Goran MI, Poehlman ET. Resting metabolic rate is lower in women compared to men. *J Appl Physiol.* 1993; 75:2514–2520.

39 Wilmore JH, Costill DL. Op. cit.

40 Levine JA, Eberhardt NL, Jensen MD. Role of nonexercise activity thermogenesis in resistance to fat gain in humans. *Science.* 1999;283:212–214; and Levine JA. Nonexercise activity thermogenesis (NEAT): environment and biology. *Am J Physiol Endocrinol Metab.* 2004;286:E675–E685.

41 Wilmore JH, Costill DL. Op. cit.

42 Granata GP, Brandon LJ. The thermic effect of food and obesity: discrepant results and methodological variations. *Nutr Rev.* 2002;60:223–233; and de Jonge L, Bray GA. The thermic effect of food is reduced in obesity. *Nutr Rev.* 2002;60:295–297.

43 Farshchi HR, Taylor MA, Macdonald IA. Decreased thermic effect of food after an irregular compared with a regular meal pattern in healthy lean women. *Int J Obes.* 2004;28:653–660.

44 Carpenter KJ. A short history of nutritional science: part 1 (1785–1885). *J Nutr.* 2003;133:638–645.

45 Institute of Medicine, Food and Nutrition Board. Op. cit.

46 Rippe JM, Crossley S, Ringer R. Obesity as a chronic disease: modern medical and lifestyle management. *J Am Diet Assoc.* 1998(suppl):S9–S15. Theme issue.

47 National Heart, Lung, and Blood Institute. *The Practical Guide: Identification, Evaluation and Treatment of Overweight and Obesity in Adults.* October 2000. NIH publication 00-4084. http://www.nhlbi.nih.gov/guidelines/obesity/prctgd_c.pdf. Accessed 7/5/06.

48 Flegal KM, Graubard BI, Williamson DF, Gail MH. Excess deaths associated with underweight, overweight, and obesity. *JAMA.* 2005;293:1861–1867.

49 USDA Center for Nutrition Policy and Promotion. *Body Mass Index and Health.* Washington, DC: Center for Nutrition Policy and Promotion, 2000. Nutrition Insights, No. 16.

50 National Center for Health Statistics. *2000 CDC Growth Charts: United States.* http://www.cdc.gov/growthcharts. Accessed 7/5/06.

51 Barlow, SE, Dietz WH. Obesity evaluation and treatment: expert committee recommendations. *Pediatrics.* 1998;102, E29. http://www.pediatrics.org/cgi/content/full/102/3/e29. Accessed 7/5/06.

52 Pietrobelli A, Formica C, Wang Z, Heymsfield SB. Dual-energy x-ray absorptiometry body composition model: a review of physical concepts. *Am J Physiol.* 1996;34:E941–E951.

53 Pi-Sunyer FX. Obesity. In: Shils ME, Olson JA, Shike M., eds. *Modern Nutrition in Health and Disease.* 9th ed. Philadelphia: Williams & Wilkins, 1999:1395–1418.

54 Lee RD, Nieman DC. *Nutritional Assessment.* 2nd ed. St. Louis: Mosby-Year Book, 1996.

55 Ibid.

56 Heymsfield SB, Baumgartner RN. Body composition and anthropometry. In: Shils ME, Shike M, Ross AC, Cabellero B, Cousins RJ, eds. *Modern Nutrition in Health and Disease.* 10th ed. Philadephia: Lippincott Williams & Wilkins, 2006: 751–770.

57 Ziegler RG. Anthropometry and breast cancer. *J Nutr.* 1997; 127(suppl 5):924S–928S.

58 Zhu S, Heshka S, Wang Z, et al. Combination of BMI and waist circumference for identifying cardiovascular risk factors in whites. *Obes Res.* 2004;12:633–645.

59 Friedman JM. Obesity in the new millennium. *Nature.* 2000; 404:632–634.

60 Kopelman PG. Obesity as a medical problem. *Nature.* 2000; 404:635–643.

61 Uauy R, Albala C, Kain J. Obesity trends in Latin America: transitioning from under- to overweight. *J Nutr.* 2001; 131:893S–899S.

62 Mokhatar N, Elati J, Chabir R, et al. Diet culture and obesity in northern Africa. *J Nutr.* 2001;131:887S–892S.

63 Kopelman PG. Op. cit.

64 Hedley AA, Ogden CL, Johnson CL, et al. Overweight and obesity among US children, adolescents, and adults, 1999–2002. *JAMA.* 2004;291:2847–2850.

65 Ibid.

66 US Department of Health and Human Services. Leading health indicators. In: *Healthy People 2010: Understanding and Improving Health.* 2nd ed. Washington, DC: US Government Printing Office, 2000.

67 National Center for Chronic Disease Prevention and Health Promotion. *Behavioral Risk Factor Surveillance System.* http://www.cdc.gov/brfss/. Accessed 7/5/06.

68 Gustafson-Larson AM, Terry RD. Weight-related behaviors and concerns of fourth-grade children. *J Am Diet Assoc.* 1992; 92:818–822.

69 Bouchard, C. Genetic factors and body weight regulation. In: Dalton S, ed. *Overweight and Weight Management: The Health Professional's Guide to Understanding and Practice.* Sudbury, MA: Jones and Bartlett Publishers, 1997:161–186.

70 Loos RJ, Rankinen T. Gene-diet interactions on body weight changes. *J Am Diet Assoc.* 2005;105:29–34.

71 Barsh GS, Faroogi S, O'Rahilly S. Genetics of body-weight regulation. *Nature.* 2000;404:644–651.

72 McArthur LH, Howard AB. Dietetics majors' weight-reduction beliefs, behaviors, and information sources. *J Am Coll Health.* 2001;49:175–181.

73 Anderson AE. Eating disorders in males. In: Brownell KD, Fairburn CG, eds. *Eating Disorders and Obesity.* New York: Guilford, 1995:177–182.

74 Williamson DF, Kahn HS, Remington PL, Anda RF. The 10-year incidence of overweight and major weight gain in US adults. *Arch Intern Med.* 1990;150:665–672.

75 Pliner P, Chaiken S, Flett GL. Gender differences in concern with body weight and physical appearance over the life span. *Personal Soc Psychol Bull.* 1990;16:262–273.

76 Kopelman PG. Op. cit.

77 James W. The epidemiology of obesity. In: Chadwick D, Cardew G, eds. *The Origins and Consequences of Obesity.* Chichester, England: Wiley, 1996:1–16.

78 Maheshwari N, Robinson J, Kohatsu N, Zimmerman B. Obesity spreading out to all income levels. Paper presented at: American Heart Association's 45th Annual Conference on Cardiovascular Disease Epidemiology and Prevention; May 2, 2005. Abstract 26. http://www.americanheart.org /presenter.jhtml?identifier=3030596. Accessed 7/5/06.

79 Sobal J, Troiano R, Frongillo E. Rural-urban differences in obesity. *Rural Sociol.* 1996;61:289–305.

80 Sobal J, Rauschenbach B, Frongillo E. Marital status, fatness, and obesity. *Social Sci Med.* 1992;35:915–923.

81 National Center for Health Statistics. Prevalence of overweight and obesity among adults in the United States. http://www.cdc.gov/nchs/products/pubs/pubd/hestats/3and4/overweight.htm. Accessed 7/5/06.

82 Lewis TT, Everson-Rose SA, Sternfeld B, et al. Race, education, and weight change in a biracial sample of women at midlife. *Arch Intern Med.* 2005;165:545–551.

83 Centers for Disease Control and Prevention. *Healthy Places Terminology.* http://www.cdc.gov/healthyplaces/terminology.htm. Accessed 7/5/06.

84 Booth KM, Pinkston MM, Poston WSC. Obesity and the built environment. *J Am Diet Assoc.* 2005;105:S110–S117.

85 Morland K, Wing S, Diez Roux A, Poole C. Neighborhood characteristics associated with the location of food stores and food service places. *Am J Prev Med.* 2002;22:23–29.

86 Keim NL, Blanton CA, Kretsch MJ. America's obesity epidemic: measuring physical activity to promote an active lifestyle. *J Am Diet Assoc.* 2004;104:1398–1409.

87 Hu FB, Li TY, Colditz GA, Willett WC, Manson JE. Television watching and other sedentary behaviors in relation to risk of obesity and type 2 diabetes in women. *JAMA.* 2003;289:1785–1791; and Andersen RE, Crespo CJ, Barlett SJ, Cheskin LC, Pratt M. Relationship of physical activity and television watching with body weight and level of fatness among children. *JAMA.* 1998;282:1561–1567.

88 Faith M S, Allison DB, Geliebter A. Emotional eating and obesity. In: Dalton S, ed. *Overweight and Weight Management: The Health Professional's Guide to Understanding and Practice.* Sudbury, MA: Jones and Bartlett Publishers, 1997:439–465.

89 Arnow B, Kenardy J, Agras WS. The emotional eating scale: the development of a measure to assess coping with negative affect by eating. *Int J Eating Dis.* 1995;18:79–90.

90 Cutting TM, Fisher JO, Grimm-Thomas K, Birch LL. Like mother, like daughter: familial patterns of overweight are mediated by mothers' dietary disinhibition. *Am J Clin Nutr.* 1999;69:608–613.

91 Marcus MD. Binge eating in obesity. In: Fairburn CG, Wilson GT, eds. *Binge Eating: Nature, Assessment, and Treatment.* New York: Guilford, 1993:77–96.

92 Bray GA, Champagne CM. Beyond energy balance: there is more to obesity than kilocalories. *J Am Diet Assoc.* 2005;105:S17–S23.

93 Olshansky SJ, Passaro DJ, Hershow RC. A potential decline in life expectancy in the United States in the 21st century. *N Engl J Med.* 2005;352:1138–1145.

94 Finkelstein EA, Fiebelkorn IC, Wang G. State-level estimates of annual medical expenditures attributable to obesity. *Obes Res.* 2004;12:18–24.

95 Blackburn GL. Effects of weight loss on weight-related risk factors. In: Brownell KD, Fairburn CG, eds. *Eating Disorders and Obesity.* New York: Guilford, 1995:406–410.

96 National High Blood Pressure Education Program (NHBPEP) Working Group. Report on primary prevention of hypertension. *Arch Intern Med.* 1993;153:186.

97 Rockhill B, Willett WC, Hunter DJ, et al. A prospective study of recreational physical activity and breast cancer. *Arch Intern Med.* 1999;59(19):2290–2296.

98 Pi-Sunyer XF. Medical complications of obesity. In: Brownell KD, Fairburn CG, eds. *Eating Disorders and Obesity.* New York: Guilford, 1995.

99 Blackburn GL. Op. cit.

100 Kirschenbaum DS, Fitzgibbon ML. Controversy about the treatment of obesity: criticisms or challenges? *Behav Ther.* 1995;26:43–68.

101 Olson MB, Kelsey SF, Bittner V, et al. Weight cycling and high-density lipoprotein cholesterol in women: evidence of an adverse effect. A report from the NHLBI-sponsored WISE study. *J Am Coll Cardiol.* 2000;36(5):1565–1571.

102 Schulz M, Liese AD, Boeing H, et al. Associations of short-term weight changes and weight cycling with incidence of essential hypertension in the EPIC-Potsdam Study. *J Hum Hypertens.* 2005;19:61–67.

103 Shade ED, Ulrich CM, Wener MH, et al. Frequent intentional weight loss is associated with lower natural killer cell toxicity in postmenopausal women. *J Am Diet Assoc.* 2004;104:903–912.

104 Position of the American Dietetic Association: weight management. *J Am Diet Assoc.* 2002;102:1145–1155.

105 Flegal KM, Graubard BI, Williamson DF, Gail MH. Op. cit.

106 Hill JO, Thompson H, Wyatt H. Weight maintenance: what's missing? *J Am Diet Assoc.* 2005;105:S63–S66.

107 US Department of Health and Human Services and US Department of Agriculture. *Dietary Guidelines for Americans, 2005.* 6th ed. Washington, DC: US Government Printing Office, 2005.

108 Hill JO, Thompson H, Wyatt H. Op. cit.

109 Campfield LA. Treatment options and the maintenance of weight loss. In: Allison DB, Pi-Sunyer FX, eds. *Obesity Treatment: Establishing Goals, Improving Outcomes, and Reviewing the Research Agenda.* New York: Plenum, 1995:93–95.

110 Grundy SM, Cleeman JI, Daniels SR, et al. AHA scientific statement: diagnosis and management of metabolic syndrome. *Circulation.* 2005;112:e285–e290.

111 Hill JO, Wyatt HR, Reed GW, Peters JC. Obesity and the environment: where do we go from here? *Science.* 2003;299:853–855.

112 Irwin ML, Mayer-Davis EJ, Addy CL, et al. Moderate-intensity physical activity and fasting insulin levels in women: the Cross-Cultural Activity Participation Study. *Diabetes Care.* 2000;23(4):449.

113 Wing RR, Hill JO. Successful weight loss maintenance. *Annu Rev Nutr.* 2001;21:323–341.

114 Young LR, Nestle M. The contribution of expanding portion sizes to the US obesity epidemic. *Am J Public Health.* 2002;92:246–249.

115 Stubbs RJ, Prentice AM, James WP. Carbohydrates and energy balance. *Ann N Y Acad Sci.* 1997;819:44–69.

116 Satia-About AJ, Patterson RE, Schiller RN, Kristal AR. Energy from fat is associated with obesity in US men: results from the prostate cancer prevention trial. *Prev Med.* 2002;34:493–501.

117 Miller WC, Niederpruem MG, Wallace JP, Lindeman AK. Dietary fat, sugar, and fiber predict body fat content. *J Am Diet Assoc.* 1994;94:612–615.

118 Farshchi HR, Taylor MA, Macdonald IA. Beneficial metabolic effects of regular meal frequency on dietary thermogenesis, insulin sensitivity, and fasting lipid profiles in healthy obese women. *Am J Clin Nutr.* 2005;81:16–24.

119 de Castro JM. The time of day of food intake influences overall intake in humans. *J Nutr.* 2004;134:104–111.

120 Farshchi HR, Taylor MA, Macdonald IA. Deleterious effects of omitting breakfast on insulin sensitivity and fasting lipid profiles in healthy lean women. *Am J Clin Nutr.* 2005; 81:388–396.

121 Institute of Medicine, Food and Nutrition Board. Op. cit.

122 Ibid.

123 Christiano B, Mizes S. Appraisal and coping deficits associated with eating disorders: implications for treatment. *Cognitive Behav Pract.* 1997;4:263–290.

124 Dansinger ML, Gleason JA, Griffith JL, Selker HP, Schaefer EJ. Comparison of the Atkins, Ornish, Weight Watchers, and Zone diets for weight loss and heart disease risk reduction: a randomized trial. *JAMA.* 2005;293:43–53.

125 Carter JC, Fairburn CG. Cognitive-behavioral self-help for binge eating disorder: a controlled effectiveness study. *J Consult Clin Psychol.* 1998;66:616–623.

126 Berkel LA, Poston WSC, Reeves RS. Behavioral interventions for obesity. *J Am Diet Assoc.* 2005;105:S35–S43.

127 Heshka S, Anderson JW, Atkinson RL, et al. Weight loss with self-help compared with a structured commercial program: a randomized trial. *JAMA.* 2003;289(14):1792–1798.

128 Tate DF, Jackvony EH, Wing RR. Effects of Internet behavioral counseling on weight loss in adults at risk for type 2 diabetes: a randomized trial. *JAMA.* 2003;289(14):1833–1836.

129 Womble LG, Wadden TA, McGuckin BG, et al. A randomized controlled trial of a commercial Internet weight loss program. *Obes Res.* 2004;12:1011–1018.

130 Serdula MK, Kahn LK, Dietz WH. Weight loss counseling revisited. *JAMA.* 2003;289(14):1747–1750.

131 Weissman NJ. Appetite suppressants and valvular heart disease. *Am J Med Sci.* 2001;32:285–291.

132 Campfield LA. The role of pharmacological agents in the treatment of obesity. In: Dalton S, ed. *Overweight and Weight Management: The Health Professional's Guide to Understanding and Practice.* Sudbury, MA: Jones and Bartlett Publishers, 1997:466–485.

133 Lucas KH, Kaplan-Machlis B. Orlistat—a novel weight loss therapy. *Ann Pharmacother.* 2001;35:314–328.

134 Gura T. Obesity drug pipeline not so fat. *Science.* 2003; 299:849–852.

135 Aronne LJ. Modern medical management of obesity: the role of pharmaceutical intervention. *J Am Diet Assoc.* 1998; 10(suppl 2):S23–S26.

136 Ibid.

137 Haddock CK, Poston WSC, Dill PL, Foreyt JP, Ericsson M. Pharmacotherapy for obesity: a quantitative analysis of four decades of published randomized clinical trials. *Int J Obes.* 2002;226:262–273.

138 Pittler MH, Ernst E. Dietary supplements for body-weight reduction: a systematic review. *Am J Clin Nutr.* 2004; 79:529–536; and Dwyer JT, Allison DB, Coates PM. Dietary supplements in weight reduction. *J Am Diet Assoc.* 2005; 105:S80–S86.

139 Shekelle OG, Mardy ML, Morton SC, et al. Efficacy and safety of ephedra and ephedrine for weight loss and athletic performance: a meta-analysis. *JAMA.* 2003;289:1537–1545.

140 Fontanarosa PB, Rennie D, DeAngelis CD. The need for regulation of dietary supplements—lessons from ephedra. *JAMA.* 2003;289:1568–1570.

141 Wadden TA, Byrne KJ, Krauthamer-Ewing S. Obesity: management. In: Shils ME, Shike M, Ross AC, Cabellero B, Cousins RJ, eds. *Modern Nutrition in Health and Disease.* 10th ed. Philadelphia: Lippincott Williams & Wilkins, 2006:1029–1042.

142 Heena P, Santry MD, Gillen DL, Launderdale DS. Trends in bariatric surgical procedures. *JAMA.* 2005;294:1909–1917.

143 Ibid.

144 NIDDK Weight-control Information Network. Gastrointestinal surgery for severe obesity. http://www.win.niddk .nih.gov/publications/gastric.htm. Accessed 12/30/06.

145 Cummings DE, Weigle DS, Frayo S, et al. Ghrelin-leptin tango in body-weight regulation. *Gastroenterology.* 2003; 124(5):1532–1544.

146 Eyre H, Kahn R, Robertson RM, et al. Preventing cancer, cardiovascular disease, and diabetes: a common agenda for the American Cancer Society, the American Diabetes Association, and the American Heart Association. *Circulation.* 2004; 109:3244–3255.

147 Eckel RH. The dietary approach to obesity: is it the diet or the disorder? *JAMA.* 2005;293:96–97.

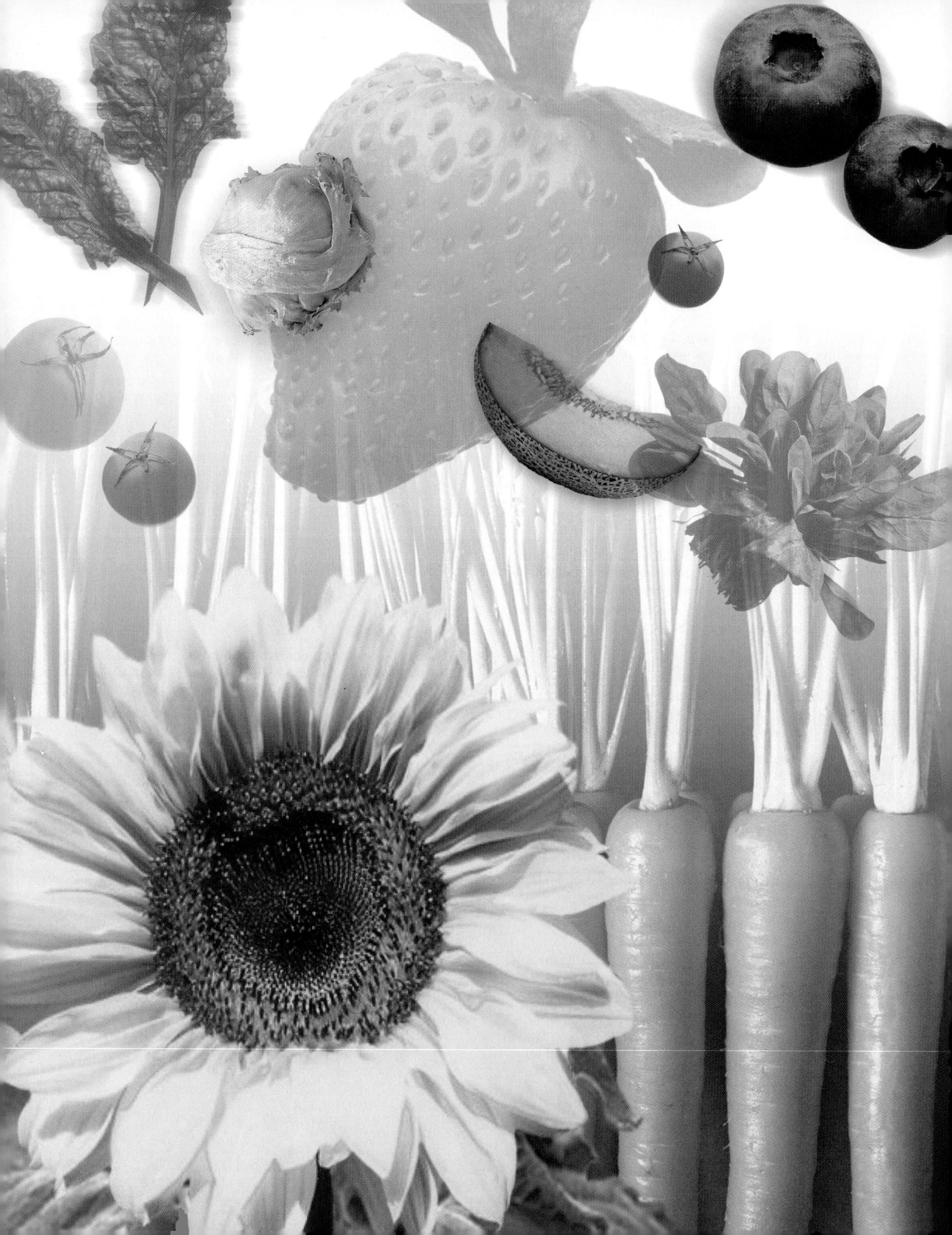

Chapter 9

Fat-Soluble Vitamins

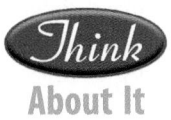

Think About It

1 How do you feel about taking vitamin supplements?

2 Which food group, if any, supplies most of your vitamin needs?

3 From a well-lighted area, you step into a dark room. Over time, you see details. What's going on?

4 Your grandmother is a strict vegetarian and she seldom goes outdoors. What can you tell her about vitamin D intake?

Fyi for your Information

This chapter's FYI box includes practical information on the following topic:
• A Short History of Vitamins

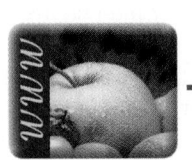

The Web site for this book offers many useful tools and is a great source for additional nutrition information for both students and instructors. Visit the site at **nutrition.jbpub.com** for information on fat-soluble vitamins. You'll find exercises that explore the following topics:
• New Roles for Vitamin A?

• Vitamin D

• Vitamin E in 3-D

• "K" Is for Clotting

Key to Illustrations

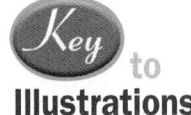

  Chylomicrons

  Fat-Soluble Vitamins

  Free Radicals

  Lipids/Fats

  Minerals

  Water-Soluble Vitamins

What About Bobbie?

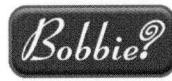

Track the choices Bobbie is making with Nutritionist Pro or EatRight Analysis software.

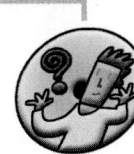

𝒴ou get a panicky call from your sister-in-law—her 6-month-old baby is turning orange! She and her husband have done everything the pediatrician told them to do about feeding; just last month they started giving the baby infant cereal, and now they have started him on strained baby food. They introduced just one food at a time. In fact, they have only fed him one food other than cereal—carrots. Yes, the baby liked them, so much that he eats two to three jars at each meal! Do you think that could be the problem? But aren't vegetables supposed to be good for you?

Vegetables are healthful foods, and carrots are an important source of many nutrients. Carrots are probably best known as a source of beta-carotene, a vitamin A precursor and the pigment that gives carrots their orange color. Your sister-in-law's baby is eating large quantities of carrots, and the excess beta-carotene circulating in his blood gives the skin a yellow-orange cast. This condition is known as **carotenodermia** and is completely harmless. But it has probably given at least one or two new parents a scare!

carotenodermia A harmless yellow-orange cast to the skin due to high levels of carotenoids in the bloodstream resulting from consumption of extremely large amounts of carotenoid-rich foods, such as carrot juice.

Understanding Vitamins

Vitamins. Just the word probably makes you think of health and well-being! Children can quickly tell you that fruits and vegetables are good sources of vitamins and can recite some of the best food sources: oranges for vitamin C, carrots for vitamin A, and so on. For many people, however, vitamins have become something to purchase and take in supplement form, not a criterion for choosing foods. Americans spend huge amounts of money, billions of dollars each year, on vitamin supplements. Their reasons for taking vitamins are almost as varied as the vitamins themselves—some people take supplements because they "don't eat right." Some take them for extra "insurance," whereas others look to vitamins to prevent and cure a whole host of conditions, from colds to cancer. Is all this money well spent?

To answer this question, you need to consider several aspects of vitamin supplementation. First, survey data indicate few widespread nutrient deficiencies in the United States. From that perspective, people are probably taking many supplements unnecessarily. A second aspect is the common sentiment that "if a little is good, more must be better." This misguided belief can lead to problems when applied to vitamin supplementation. Although high doses of some vitamins cause no ill effects, others can have serious, life-long consequences. A third consideration is that research continues to identify relationships between vitamins and reduced risk of some diseases, so some supplementation may be warranted. These two chapters on vitamins will help you explore some of the implications of too much or too little of a vitamin in the diet and understand the facts about vitamins: what they are, what they do in the body, and which foods contain them. Armed with this information, you will be able to make wise decisions about food and whether to take supplements.

Think About It 1

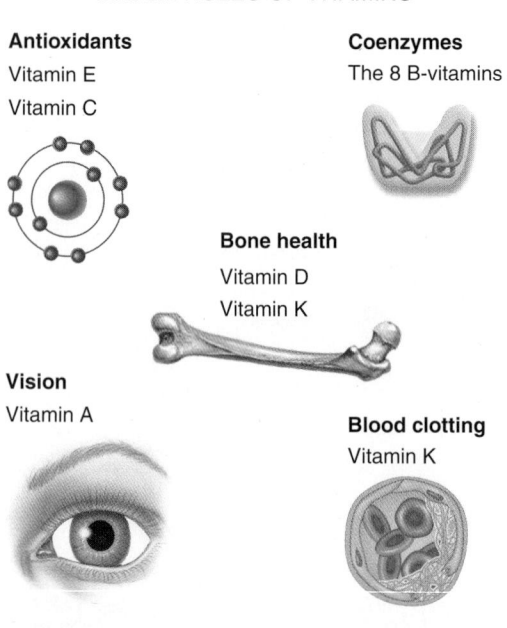

MAJOR ROLES OF VITAMINS

Antioxidants
Vitamin E
Vitamin C

Coenzymes
The 8 B-vitamins

Bone health
Vitamin D
Vitamin K

Vision
Vitamin A

Blood clotting
Vitamin K

Figure 9.1 **Major roles of vitamins.** Vitamins are crucial for normal functioning, growth, and maintenance of body tissues. Compared to carbohydrate, fat, and protein, the body needs tiny amounts of vitamins.

Anatomy of the Vitamins

Vitamins differ from fat, protein, and carbohydrate in many important ways. For one, the body requires large amounts of carbohydrates, proteins, and fats—amounts measured in grams. By comparison, the daily needs for vitamins are small—a mere microgram or two in some cases. In addition, unlike fat, protein, and carbohydrate, vitamins are not an energy source. However, many vitamins play crucial roles in regulating the chemical reactions that allow us to extract energy from those nutrients. Another difference is structural: Vitamins are individual units rather than long chains of smaller units.

Like fat, carbohydrate, and protein, however, vitamins are organic (carbon-containing) compounds essential for normal functioning, growth, and maintenance of the body. The functions of vitamins are often interrelated (see **Figure 9.1**), so a deficiency of just one can cause profound health problems.

Fat-Soluble Versus Water-Soluble Vitamins

Scientists classify vitamins as "fat-soluble" and "water-soluble." Vitamins A, D, E, and K are lipidlike molecules that are soluble in fat. The B vitamins and vitamin C, on the other hand, are soluble in water. This difference in solubility affects the way the body absorbs, transports, and stores vitamins. **Figure 9.2** illustrates the body's absorption of vitamins.

Figure 9.2 **Absorption of vitamins.** Water-soluble vitamins are absorbed in the intestinal cells and delivered directly to the bloodstream. Fat-soluble vitamins are absorbed with fat.

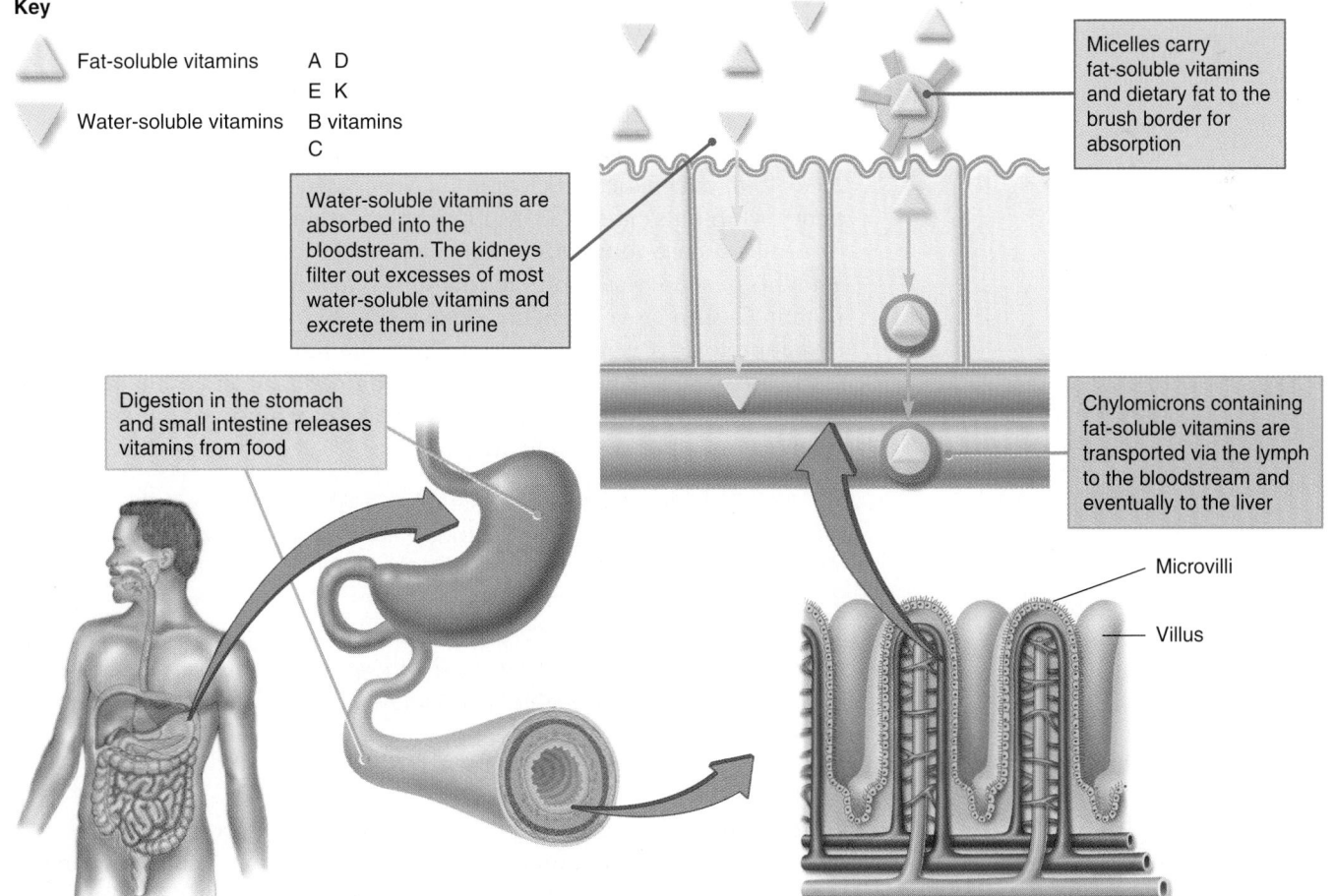

Key

△ Fat-soluble vitamins   A D E K

▽ Water-soluble vitamins   B vitamins C

Water-soluble vitamins are absorbed into the bloodstream. The kidneys filter out excesses of most water-soluble vitamins and excrete them in urine

Micelles carry fat-soluble vitamins and dietary fat to the brush border for absorption

Digestion in the stomach and small intestine releases vitamins from food

Chylomicrons containing fat-soluble vitamins are transported via the lymph to the bloodstream and eventually to the liver

Microvilli

Villus

provitamins Inactive forms of vitamins that the body can convert into active useable forms. Also referred to as vitamin precursors.

vitamin precursors See *provitamins*.

retinoids Compounds in foods that have chemical structures similar to vitamin A. Retinoids include the active forms of vitamin A (retinol, retinal, and retinoic acid) and the main storage forms of retinol (retinyl esters).

retinol The alcohol form of vitamin A; one of the retinoids; thought to be the main physiologically active form of vitamin A; interconvertible with retinal.

retinal The aldehyde form of vitamin A; one of the retinoids; the active form of vitamin A in the photoreceptors of the retina; interconvertible with retinol.

retinoic acid The acid form of vitamin A; one of the retinoids; formed from retinal but not interconvertible; helps growth, cell differentiation, and the immune system; does not have a role in vision or reproduction.

carotenoids A group of yellow, orange, and red pigments in plants, including foods. Many of these compounds are precursors of vitamin A.

provitamin A Carotenoid precursors of vitamin A in foods of plant origin, primarily deeply colored fruits and vegetables.

Intestinal cells absorb fat-soluble vitamins along with dietary fat. The amount absorbed typically varies from 40 to 90 percent of the amount consumed; efficiency of absorption generally falls as the dietary intake rises above the body's needs. Just like triglycerides and other dietary lipids, lipoproteins carry absorbed fat-soluble vitamins on their journey through the lymph and bloodstream. As chylomicrons move through the blood, cells take up most of the triglycerides and leave behind chylomicron remnants that contain the fat-soluble vitamins. The liver picks up these remnants and either stores the vitamins for future use or repackages them for delivery via the bloodstream to other tissues.

Water-soluble vitamins are dissolved in the watery compartments of foods. Once absorbed, these nutrients travel directly into the bloodstream and then move independently in and around the cells of the body. Unlike fat-soluble vitamins, water-soluble vitamins do not need lipoprotein carriers. Their storage and excretion differ too. Whereas most fat-soluble vitamins accumulate and can be stored indefinitely, the kidneys filter out excess amounts of most water-soluble vitamins and excrete them in urine. Two vitamins are exceptions to this general rule: Water-soluble vitamin B_{12} is stored more readily than the other water-soluble vitamins, and fat-soluble vitamin K is excreted more readily than the other fat-soluble vitamins.

Storage and Toxicity

Fat-soluble vitamins accumulate in the liver and adipose tissues, where they can be drawn upon in times of need. Once these vitamin stores are established, you can go for days, weeks, or even months without consuming more and suffer no ill effects. On the other hand, excessive intake of the fat-soluble vitamins A or D can exceed the body's storage capacity, with toxic effects.

Your body does not store most water-soluble vitamins in appreciable amounts, so they should be a part of your daily diet. Small variations in daily intake typically do not cause problems, however. For example, it takes 20 to 40 days of a diet deficient in the water-soluble vitamin C before deficiency symptoms emerge. Consuming excess water-soluble vitamins usually is harmless, since your body simply excretes the surplus. However, large amounts of some water-soluble vitamins—vitamin B_6, folate, niacin, even vitamin C—can be problematic, often seriously so.

Vitamin toxicity is rarely linked to high vitamin intakes from food or to the use of supplements that contain 100 to 150 percent of the recommended amounts. However, people who take megadoses of one or more vitamins run a high risk of toxicity.

Key Concepts: *Vitamins are organic substances needed in minuscule amounts for various roles in regulation of body processes. Two classes of vitamins have been identified: fat-soluble vitamins (A, D, E, and K) and water-soluble vitamins (the B vitamins and vitamin C). Fat-soluble vitamins, which are stored in the liver and fatty tissues of the body, are generally excreted much more slowly than water-soluble vitamins. Because they are stored for long periods, fat-soluble vitamins generally pose a greater risk of toxicity than water-soluble vitamins when consumed in excess.*

Provitamins

Certain vitamins in foods are in inactive forms that the body cannot use directly. These substances are known as **provitamins**, or **vitamin precursors**. Once a provitamin is ingested, the body converts it to the active vitamin form. One familiar provitamin in many fruits and vegetables is beta-carotene (**Figure 9.3**). Once beta-carotene is absorbed, the body converts it to an active form of vitamin A. In fact, beta-carotene is a major source of vitamin A in the diet. When experts calculate vitamin requirements or monitor consumption, they must take provitamins into account.

Vitamins in Foods

What foods do you think of as good sources of vitamins? As mentioned, even very young children know that fruits and vegetables are important in the diet because "they give you vitamins." In fact, vitamins are found in every food group, including the fats and oils that most of us are trying to eat less of. One more reason to include variety in your diet is that no one food group, or one choice within a food group, is a good source of all vitamins.

The amounts of specific vitamins in a food depend on several factors. For plant foods—whether fruits, vegetables, or grains—sunlight, growing conditions, and the plant's maturity at harvest all affect the vitamin content. Although an animal's diet can have some impact on animal-derived food, its capacity for absorption and storage keeps the vitamin content fairly consistent.

Generally, the more a food is processed and cooked, the more vitamins it loses. Most food processing (e.g., cooking, milling grain, canning vegetables, and drying fruit) reduces vitamin content. For more information on how to preserve the vitamin content of your foods, see the FYI feature "Fresh, Frozen, or Canned? Raw or Cooked?" in Chapter 10, "Water-Soluble Vitamins."

Key Concepts: *All types of foods contain vitamins. Provitamins are vitamin precursors that the body can convert to the active vitamin form. Growing conditions, storage, processing, and cooking all affect the amounts of vitamins in foods.*

Vitamin A: The Retinoids

Vitamin A is best known for its role in vision, but it is also crucial for proper growth, reproduction, immunity, and cell differentiation. It helps maintain healthy bones as well as skin and mucous membranes. Vitamin A deficiency not only can destroy vision, but also disrupts numerous functions throughout the body.

Forms of Vitamin A

The body uses three active forms of vitamin A, known collectively as the **retinoids**. These compounds include **retinol**, the alcohol form of vitamin A; **retinal**, the aldehyde form of vitamin A; and **retinoic acid**, the acid form of vitamin A (see **Figure 9.4**). Although all three forms have essential functions, retinol is the key player in the vitamin A family. In fact, the standard unit for quantifying the biologic activity of the various forms of vitamin A and its precursors is known as a retinol activity equivalent (RAE).

Your body can easily convert retinol, which is required for reproduction and bone health, to retinal, the form of vitamin A essential for night and color vision. In turn, retinal can re-form retinol or it can irreversibly form retinoic acid, which is important for cell growth and differentiation. The interconvertible nature of retinol and retinal allows them to support all the activities of the vitamin A family.

Colorful plant pigments called **carotenoids** are precursors of vitamin A. The body converts some carotenoids, the **provitamin A** compounds, to vitamin A with varying degrees of efficiency. The yellow-orange pigment

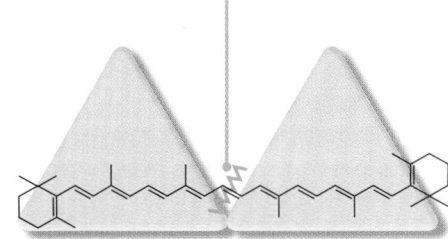

Once beta-carotene is absorbed, it can be cleaved in the middle to yield two molecules of vitamin A

Beta-carotene, a vitamin A precursor

Figure 9.3 **Beta-carotene.** Beta-carotene may be cleaved at different locations, so it may yield less than two molecules of vitamin A. Other provitamin A carotenoids yield less vitamin A than beta-carotene.

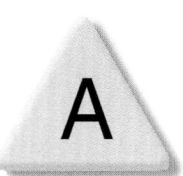

Retinol

Retinal

Retinoic acid

Figure 9.4 **Forms of vitamin A.** Retinol is the alcohol form of vitamin A, retinal is the aldehyde form, and retinoic acid is the acid form.

retinyl esters The main storage form of vitamin A; one of the retinoids. Retinyl esters are retinol combined with fatty acids, usually palmitic acid. Also known as preformed vitamin A.

retinol-binding protein (RBP) A carrier protein that binds to retinol and transports it in the bloodstream from the liver to destination cells.

cornea The transparent outer surface of the eye.

retina A paper-thin tissue that lines the back of the eye and contains cells called rods and cones.

rods Light-sensitive cells in the retina that react to dim light and transmit black-and-white images.

cones Light-sensitive cells in the retina that are sensitive to bright light and translate it into color images.

beta-carotene can be cleaved into two molecules of retinal and thus has the highest potential vitamin A activity of the provitamin A family. Of all the provitamin A carotenoids, beta-carotene yields the most vitamin A. **Figure 9.5** shows the interconversions of the three active forms of vitamin A.

Storage and Transport of Vitamin A

In well-nourished people, the liver stores more than 90 percent of the body's vitamin A; the remainder is deposited in adipose tissue, lungs, and kidneys.[1] The body stores vitamin A primarily as **retinyl esters**—retinol linked to a fatty acid, usually palmitic acid. Your liver gradually accumulates vitamin A reserves, which reach their peak in adulthood. The liver releases retinol in just the right amounts to maintain normal retinol blood levels. A healthy liver can store up to a year's supply of vitamin A, but taking large doses of vitamin A supplements can exceed this capacity and lead to toxicity.

Many fat-soluble vitamins need carrier proteins to ferry them in the blood to where the body needs them. For instance, **retinol-binding protein (RBP)** carries retinol released by the liver. Once the RBP drops off the retinol to a target cell, the cell can convert retinol to retinal or retinoic acid as needed. Continued production of RBP requires zinc and adequate intake of protein.

Key Concepts: *Vitamin A occurs in three forms in the body: retinol, retinal, and retinoic acid. Each form of the vitamin has specific roles in the body. Most vitamin A is stored by the liver in the form of retinyl esters. Retinol-binding protein carries vitamin A in the bloodstream.*

Functions of Vitamin A

Vitamin A is crucial for vision, for maintaining healthy cells (particularly skin cells) for fighting infections and bolstering immune function, and for promoting growth and development. (See **Figure 9.6**.) In addition, the provitamin A carotenoids may play a role in prevention of cancer and other chronic diseases.

Vitamin A and Vision

When light enters the eye, it passes through the **cornea**, a transparent membrane, and hits the **retina**, the paper-thin tissues that line the back of the eye. The retina contains millions of light-sensitive cells called **rods** and **cones**. The rods react to dim light and process black-and-white images. The cones respond to bright light and translate it into color images. Within both rods and cones, a cascade of reactions converts light into a nerve signal the brain can process so we experience sight.

VITAMIN A INTERCONVERSIONS

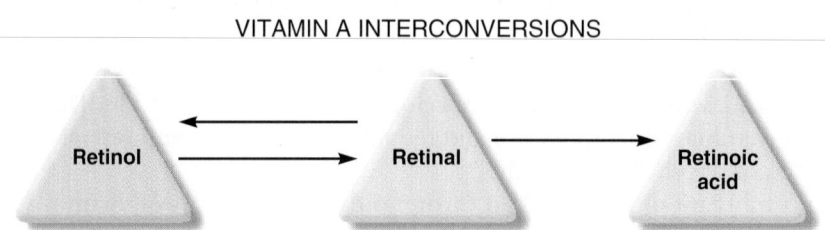

Figure 9.5 **Vitamin A interconversions.** Whereas retinol and retinal are interconvertible, the reaction that forms retinoic acid is irreversible.

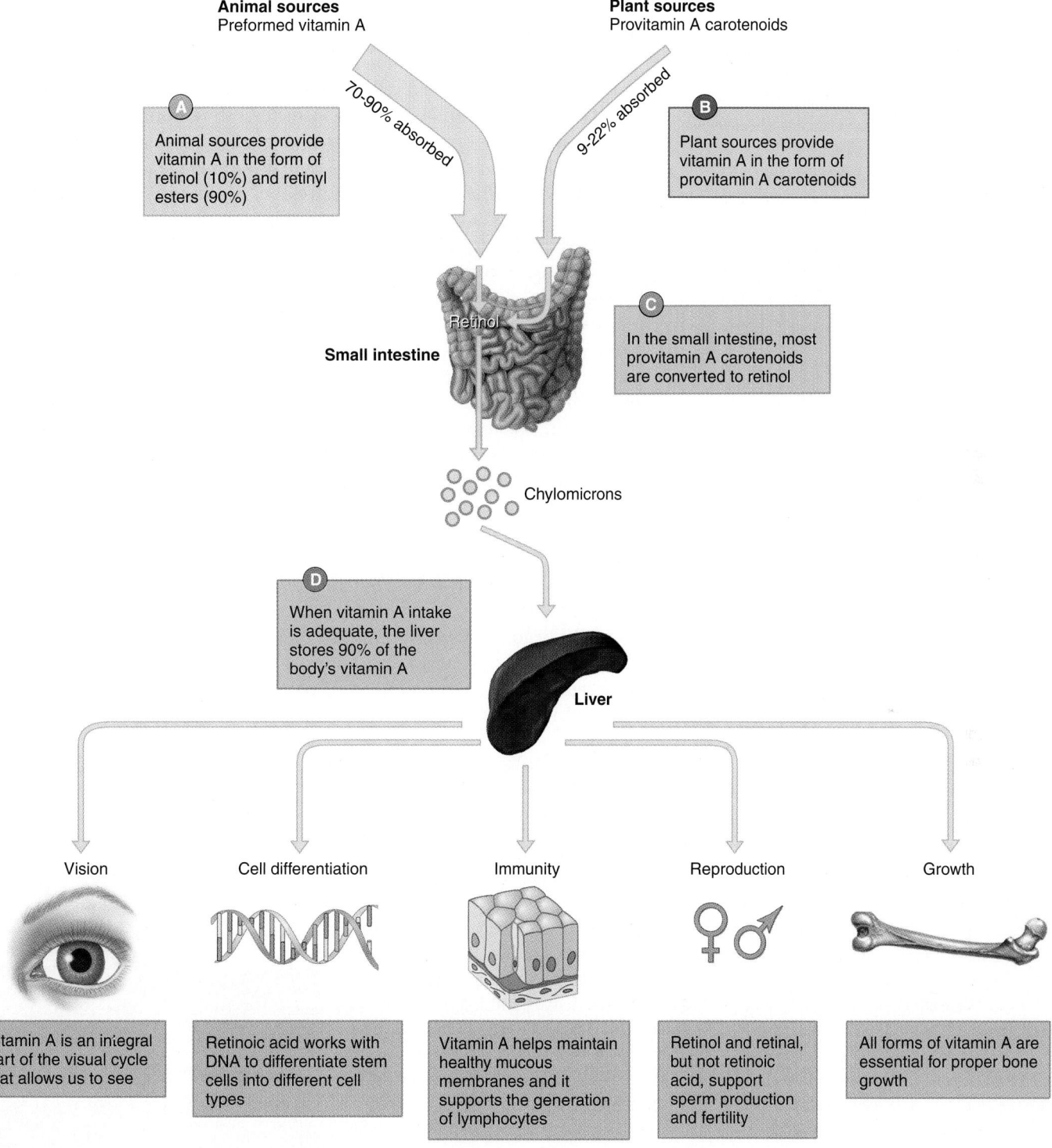

VITAMIN A: FROM SOURCE TO DESTINATION

Animal sources
Preformed vitamin A

Plant sources
Provitamin A carotenoids

70-90% absorbed

9-22% absorbed

A Animal sources provide vitamin A in the form of retinol (10%) and retinyl esters (90%)

B Plant sources provide vitamin A in the form of provitamin A carotenoids

Retinol

Small intestine

C In the small intestine, most provitamin A carotenoids are converted to retinol

Chylomicrons

D When vitamin A intake is adequate, the liver stores 90% of the body's vitamin A

Liver

Vision

Cell differentiation

Immunity

Reproduction

Growth

Vitamin A is an integral part of the visual cycle that allows us to see

Retinoic acid works with DNA to differentiate stem cells into different cell types

Vitamin A helps maintain healthy mucous membranes and it supports the generation of lymphocytes

Retinol and retinal, but not retinoic acid, support sperm production and fertility

All forms of vitamin A are essential for proper bone growth

Figure 9.6 **Vitamin A: from source to destination.** Retinoids from animal foods and carotenoids from plant foods are absorbed from the small intestine and carried by chylomicrons to the liver. Vitamin A plays a crucial role in vision and is essential for proper cell synthesis, reproduction, and bone growth.

opsin A protein that combines with retinal to form rhodopsin in rod cells.

rhodopsin Found in rod cells, a light-sensitive pigment molecule that consists of a protein called opsin combined with retinal.

bleaching process A complex light-stimulated reaction in which rod cells lose color as rhodopsin is split into retinal and opsin.

dark adaptation The process that increases the rhodopsin concentration in your eyes, allowing them to detect images in the dark better.

night blindness The inability of the eyes to adjust to dim light or to regain vision quickly after exposure to a flash of bright light.

How does retinol become a functioning part of the retina? (See **Figure 9.7.**) Retinol is carried in the blood to the retina, where it is converted to retinal. Retinal in turn combines with the protein **opsin** to form a pigment known as **rhodopsin**. Rhodopsin is abundant in rod cells and makes it possible to see in dim light. When light strikes the retina, rod cells undergo a **bleaching process**, causing the color of the rod cells to fade. In this transformation, retinal separates from the opsin and undergoes a structural shift, from a "bent," or *cis*, configuration, to a "straightened," or *trans*, configuration. As the retinal detaches, the opsin changes shape as well, disrupting the activities in the cell membrane and generating an electrical impulse. This impulse is relayed to the brain, and you see a black-and-white image. Most of the retinal released in this process is quickly converted back to *trans*-retinol, and then to *cis*-retinal, which spontaneously recombines with opsin. The re-formed rhodopsin can respond to light again and begin another cycle.

You've probably had the experience of stepping into a dark room and being unable to see until your eyes adjust. The familiar explanation for this, that you must wait for your pupils to dilate and let in more light, is only part of the story. Your eyes also adapt by changing the amount of available rhodopsin. If you awaken in the middle of the night and turn on a bright light, the light level is blinding until your eyes adjust. Rhodopsin breaks down quickly in bright light, and the reduced supply makes the rod cells less light sensitive. Conversely, when you enter a dark room, your eyes produce rhodopsin to increase their sensitivity to light. Known as **dark adaptation**, the speed of adjustment to dim light is related directly to the amount of vitamin A available to regenerate rhodopsin. People with a vitamin A deficiency experience **night blindness**, the inability of the eyes to adjust to dim light or to regain vision quickly after exposure to a flash of bright light. Due to the lack of vitamin A, rhodopsin regeneration slows dramatically. Although the eyes contain only 0.01 percent of the body's vitamin A, they

Fyi A Short History of Vitamins

FOR YOUR INFORMATION

From roughly 1500 B.C.E. to 1900 C.E. there was an empirical understanding that some diseases (which we now call vitamin deficiency diseases) could be cured by eating certain foods. About 400 B.C.E. the Greek physician Hippocrates, following the practice of Arab and Egyptian physicians, prescribed beef liver to people who were unable to see certain stars in the night sky. His maxim was "Let food be thy medicine," but he did not know that beef liver is a rich source of vitamin A, a fat-soluble vitamin necessary for vision.

Similarly, Native Americans knew empirically that extracts of pine needles could prevent or cure scurvy, a condition that includes bleeding gums and loss of energy. In 1753 James Lind, a Scottish surgeon, urged the British navy to include lemon juice in the diet of sailors to prevent scurvy. The navy finally adopted this practice 40 years later. In 1865 they substituted limes, which gave British sailors their nickname "limeys." We now know that the pine needles and citrus fruits provide vitamin C, a water-soluble vitamin whose deficiency causes scurvy.

Many scientists began systematically studying deficiency diseases in the late nineteenth century. They induced "deficiency states" in animals or humans by depriving them of certain foods. The subjects were restored to health when they ate the withheld food. In 1880 the Dutch scientist Christiaan Eijkman, for instance, produced beriberi in chickens by feeding them only polished (white) rice. When

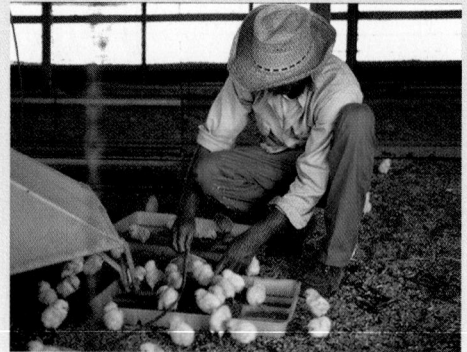

he restored their normal food of unpolished (brown) rice, the chickens quickly recovered. We now know that thiamin, which is removed during polishing, is essential for the health of both man and bird.

STRUCTURE OF RETINA   VISUAL CYCLE IN RETINA

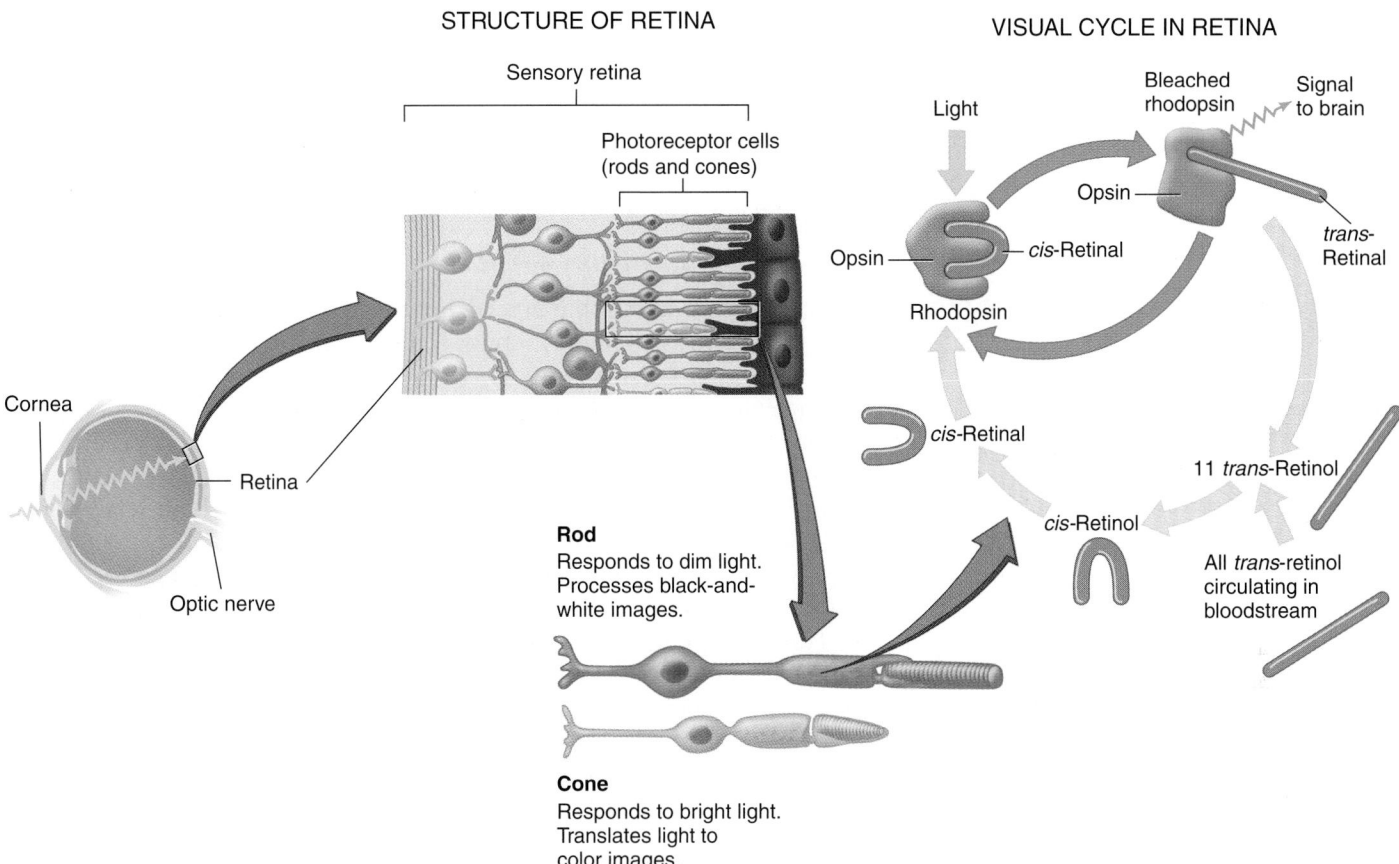

Figure 9.7 **Vitamin A and the visual cycle.** Rhodopsin is the combination of the protein opsin and vitamin A (retinal). When stimulated by light, opsin changes shape and vitamin A changes from its bent *cis* form to a straighter *trans* form. This sends a signal to the brain and you see an image in black and white. A similar process using a different protein called iodopsin provides color.

In the early twentieth century, scientists began to use chemistry to isolate and identify the critical factors in food that relieved "deficiency states." In 1912, for instance, Casimir Funk isolated a nitrogen-containing compound (an amine) in rice hulls. When given to thiamin-deprived chickens in its pure form, this amine restored the birds to health. Because this compound was required for life (vita) and was nitrogen-containing (amine), Funk coined the term *vitamines* to describe these essential growth factors. Other vitamines, or vitamins, as they later came to be called, continued to be discovered, purified, and eventually synthesized.

The discovery and naming of vitamins did not proceed without false starts. Some candidate substances did not meet the test of time, and thus we have no vitamins F, G, H, I, or J. On the other hand, vitamin B turned out to be a group of water-soluble vitamins rather than a single vitamin, so today we have eight "B vitamins." The last vitamin to be discovered was vitamin B_{12} and it was not completely synthesized until 1972.

As the vitamins were being isolated and characterized, it became clear that many Americans were not getting enough vitamins, so the National Academy of Sciences established recommended vitamin intakes. Many foods, especially flour and breads, are now fortified or enriched with vitamins.

Today we are exploring the health effects of vitamins beyond simply preventing deficiency diseases. This phase started in 1955, when large doses of niacin were found to lower cholesterol levels. Intense research is exploring the potential of the antioxidant vitamins C and E to slow aging and reduce risks for cancer, heart disease, and cataract formation. Several B vitamins are under investigation for their role in heart disease. Vitamins B_6, folate, and vitamin B_{12} affect the body's levels of the amino acid homocysteine, which was identified as an independent risk factor for coronary heart disease.

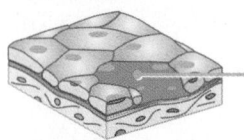

Retinoic acid helps maintain the integrity of cells in the mucous membrane

Inadequate retinoic acid impairs the structure and function of these cells

Figure 9.8 **Mucous membrane integrity.** Mucous membranes contain a higher percentage of goblet cells. Without retinoic acid, fewer stem cells become goblet cells and these surfaces become hard and scaly.

iodopsin Color-sensitive pigment molecules in cone cells that consist of opsin-like proteins combined with retinal.

stem cells A formative cell whose daughter cells may differentiate into other cell types.

epithelial cells The millions of cells that line and protect the external and internal surfaces of the body. Epithelial cells form epithelial tissues such as skin and mucous membranes.

epithelial tissue A closely packed layer of epithelial cells that covers the body and lines its cavities.

goblet cells One of the many types of specialized cells that produce and secrete mucus. These cells are found in the stomach, intestines, and portions of the respiratory tract.

Quick Bites

Vitamin A Isn't Just for Eyes

A study conducted in Nepal showed that women who took vitamin A supplements during pregnancy had a much lower risk of maternal mortality than those who took a placebo. The researchers concluded that regular and adequate intake of vitamin A or beta-carotene can reduce the risk of pregnancy-related death in areas where vitamin A deficiency is common.

are so sensitive to vitamin A levels that one injection of the vitamin can relieve night blindness within minutes.[2]

Vitamin A is also involved in color vision, as part of the pigment iodopsin in cone cells. During color vision, **iodopsin** undergoes a transformation cycle similar to that of rhodopsin. A lack of vitamin A affects rod cells before it affects cone cells, so as a vitamin A deficiency worsens, night blindness emerges before color blindness.

Vitamin A in Cell Differentiation

Vitamin A's role in vision is crucial, but this function uses only a small fraction of the body's vitamin A supply. A much larger proportion, in the form of retinoic acid, is put to work in normal cell differentiation, the process through which **stem cells** develop into highly specific types of cells with unique functions. Retinoic acid interacts with receptor sites on a cell's DNA—the genetic material that spurs production of particular proteins. When retinoic acid helps activate these receptors in the cell nucleus, stem cells begin transforming into mature differentiated cells.

This retinoic acid–dependent differentiation can be seen in **epithelial cells**, the millions of cells that cover and protect the external and internal surfaces of the body. (See **Figure 9.8**.) Epithelial cells form **epithelial tissue**, the largest of which is the skin. The epithelial tissue that lines internal organs includes the mucous membranes of the mouth, nose, stomach, intestine, and eyelids. When epithelial cells differentiate, some develop into mucus-secreting cells (**goblet cells**), and others become different types of mature cells, such as skin cells.[3]

Vitamin A and Immune Function

Vitamin A influences the immune system in important ways. It helps maintain the health of epithelial tissues, the first line of defense against bacterial, parasitic, and viral attack. Vitamin A also supports the generation of T lymphocytes, important immune cells, maintaining the body's ability to mount an immune response against infectious invaders.[4]

Vitamin A and Reproduction

Although the exact biochemical mechanism is unknown, vitamin A affects both male and female reproductive processes. Both retinol and retinal support reproduction, but retinoic acid does not. In men, vitamin A supports the production of sperm; in women, it helps maintain fertility, possibly by supporting the production of reproductive tract secretions.

Vitamin A and Bone Health

Vitamin A (retinol, retinal, and retinoic acid) is essential for bone growth. As with the reproductive system, the exact mechanism is unclear, but a lack of vitamin A causes bones to weaken, although they also become thicker than normal. This may be due to a disruption of the bone remodeling process and the failure of immature bone cells to develop properly.

Key Concepts: *Vitamin A plays a crucial role in vision as part of the compound rhodopsin in the rod cells of the retina. When light hits the retina, rhodopsin separates, changes shape, and sends a nerve impulse to the brain. When vitamin A is inadequate, the lack of rhodopsin makes it difficult to see in dim light. Vitamin A is also involved in cell differentiation, growth and development, immune function, reproduction, and bone health.*

Dietary Recommendations for Vitamin A

Similar amounts of dietary retinoids and carotenoids do not provide the same amount of vitamin A. To develop dietary recommendations, scientists reconciled this difference by creating a standardized measurement based on retinol, called **retinol activity equivalents (RAE)**. One retinol activity equivalent is the amount of a given form of vitamin A equal to the activity of 1 microgram (1/1,000,000 of a gram) of retinol. Using this standard, 12 micrograms (μg) of beta-carotene equals 1 RAE, and 24 micrograms of other carotenoids yields 1 RAE. (See **Figure 9.9**.)

You may also see the vitamin A content of dietary supplements expressed as **international units (IU)**. IU is an inexact, outdated measure of vitamin A that was derived using research that did not account for the poor bio-availability, or absorption efficiency, of carotenoids. One IU of vitamin A activity is equal to about 0.3 microgram of retinol from animal foods and 3.6 micrograms of beta-carotene from plant foods.

Most Americans take in adequate amounts of vitamin A and have large stores of the vitamin in their livers. The RDA for vitamin A for males aged 14 years and older is 900 micrograms RAE. For females aged 14 years and older, the vitamin A RDA is 700 micrograms RAE. Pregnant women should consume slightly more vitamin A (770 micrograms), while lactating women are advised to consume 1,300 micrograms RAE.[5]

Sources of Vitamin A

About half the dietary vitamin A intake comes from animal food sources as **preformed vitamin A**, the retinoids (including retinyl esters, which are the main storage form of vitamin A). The other half of dietary vitamin A intake comes from fruits and vegetables in the form of provitamin A carotenoids, especially beta-carotene. **Figure 9.10** shows foods that are good sources of vitamin A.

Retinoids are found naturally only in animal foods. About 10 percent of vitamin A content is in the form of retinol, and the remaining 90 percent is retinyl esters. Liver and fish liver oils (e.g., cod liver oil) are among the top sources. Milk fat (as in whole milk, butter, and other dairy products) also contains vitamin A. Foods fortified with vitamin A (in the form of retinyl palmitate or retinyl acetate) include margarine, some breakfast cereals, and reduced-fat milks. Reduced-fat milks that are not fortified vary greatly in vitamin A content (e.g., unfortified nonfat milk contains no vitamin A). Products that are made from reduced-fat or skim milk, such as yogurt, are not generally fortified with vitamin A. The body absorbs about 75 percent of dietary retinol and retinyl esters.

The best sources of provitamin A carotenoids are dark-green and yellow-orange vegetables, such as carrots, spinach, broccoli, squash, sweet potatoes, and some orange-colored fruits such as cantaloupes, peaches, apricots, and mangos. In a varied diet, beta-carotene supplies about one-third the total

1 retinol activity equivalent (RAE) = 1 μg retinol

= 2 μg supplemental beta-carotene

= 12 μg dietary beta-carotene

= 24 μg dietary carotenoids

Figure 9.9 Retinol equivalents conversion.

retinol activity equivalents (RAE) A unit of measurement of the vitamin A content of a food. One RAE equals 1 μg of retinol.

international units (IU) An outdated system to measure vitamin activity. This measurement does not consider differences in bioavailability.

preformed vitamin A Retinyl esters, the main storage form of vitamin A. About 90 percent of dietary retinol is in the form of esters, mostly found in foods from animal sources.

VITAMIN A

Daily Value = 5000 IU

Exceptionally good sources		
Beef liver, cooked	85 g (3 oz)	26,957 IU
Sweet potato	110 g (1 small)	21,140 IU
Carrots, cooked	85 g (~1/2 cup)	14,622 IU
Chicken liver, cooked	85 g (3 oz)	11,329 IU
Spinach, cooked	85 g (~1/2 cup)	8,909 IU
Spinach, raw	85 g (~3 cups)	7,970 IU
Collards, cooked	85 g (~1/2 cup)	6,897 IU
Romaine lettuce, raw	85 g (~1 1/2 cups)	4,936 IU
Cantaloupe, fresh	140 g (1/4 med. melon)	4,735 IU
Peppers, red, cooked	85 g (~1/2 cup)	4,672 IU
Apricot, dried	40 g (~3 Tbsp)	1,412 IU
Broccoli, cooked	85 g (~1/2 cup)	1,316 IU
Wheat bran flakes cereal	30 g (3/4 cup)	1,293 IU
Oatmeal, instant, fortified, cooked	1 cup	1,252 IU
Tomato juice, canned	240 ml (1 cup)	1,111 IU
Mango, fresh	140 g (~1 cup)	1,071 IU
Watermelon, fresh	280 g (1/16 melon)	913 IU
Black-eyed peas, cooked	90 g (~1/2 cup)	712 IU
Prunes, dried	40 g (~5 prunes)	705 IU
Green beans, cooked	85 g (~3/4 cup)	595 IU
Corn flakes cereal	30 g (1 cup)	537 IU
All-bran cereal	30 g (1/2 cup)	510 IU
Milk, 1%, 2%, nonfat	240 ml (1 cup)	500 IU

High: 20% DV or more

Good: 10–19% DV

Figure 9.10 **Food sources of vitamin A.** Vitamin A is found as retinol in animal foods and as beta-carotene and other carotenoids in plant foods. Some of the best sources are liver, orange and deep-yellow vegetables, and dark-green leafy vegetables. This figure, and others like it in the vitamin and mineral chapters, references the Daily Value standard used on food labels. By law, a food may be labeled a "Good Source" of a nutrient if it contains 10–19% of the Daily Value for that nutrient, and it is a "High Source" if it contains ≥20% of the DV. Units are IU to be consistent with Daily Value definitions.
Source: U.S. Department of Agriculture, Agricultural Research Service. USDA National Nutrient Database for Standard Reference, Release 18. 2005. http://www.ars.usda.gov/nutrientdata.

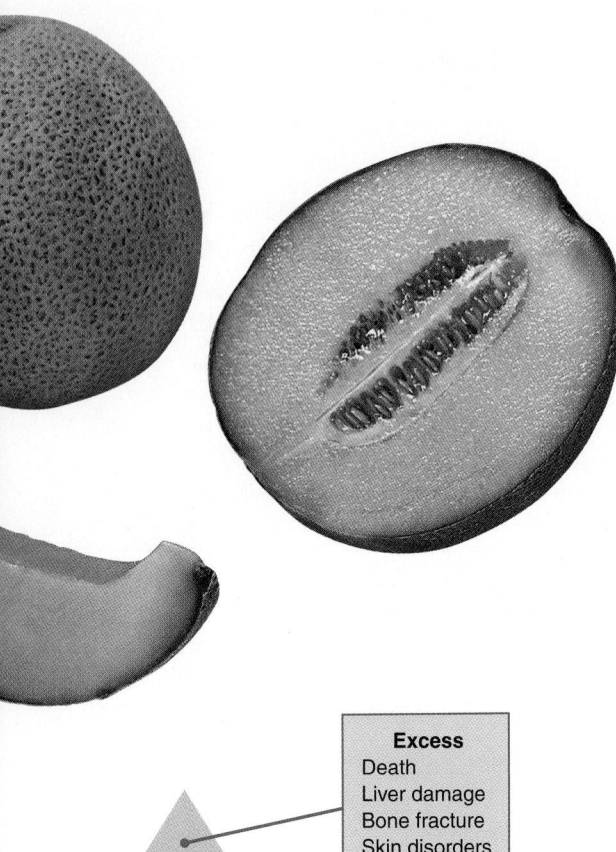

Excess
Death
Liver damage
Bone fracture
Skin disorders
Birth defects

Vitamin A

A
Adequate

Deficiency
Night blindness
Xerophthalmia
Hyperkeratosis
Infection
Death

Figure 9.11 **Vitamin A intake.** A broad range of vitamin A intake is adequate and provides for normal function. Too much or too little vitamin A can have serious consequences.

xerophthalmia A condition caused by vitamin A deficiency that dries the cornea and mucous membranes of the eye.

vitamin A, even though the body absorbs this provitamin less efficiently than retinol or retinyl esters. For more information about carotenoids, see "The Carotenoids" section later in this chapter.

Key Concepts: *Intake recommendations for vitamin A are expressed in RAEs (retinol activity equivalents) to account for the differences in bioavailability between retinoids and carotenoids. Current recommendations suggest that adult men consume 900 micrograms RAE each day; the recommendation for adult women is 700 micrograms RAE. Retinol is available from a few animal foods such as liver, fish liver oils, milk fat, and egg yolks. Vitamin A can also be formed from precursor compounds called carotenoids, which are found in some yellow-orange fruits and in dark-green and yellow-orange vegetables.*

Vitamin A Deficiency

Although dietary deficiency of vitamin A is rare in North America and western Europe, it is the leading cause of childhood blindness worldwide, especially in Southeast Asia, parts of Africa, and Central and South America. In these regions, vitamin A deficiency typically results from general protein-energy malnutrition in infants and young children. It is estimated that 500,000 preschool children worldwide become blind each year as a result of vitamin A deficiency. (See **Figure 9.11**.) Vitamin A deficiency retards growth and development and leads to bone deformities.

Although few Americans suffer from a vitamin A deficiency, certain groups are at risk. Newborns, especially premature infants, are at risk because their liver stores of vitamin A are low. Because their diets lack vitamin A–rich foods, impoverished people, particularly children and older adults, may suffer marginal vitamin A status. People with alcoholism or liver disease are at risk because their damaged livers may be incapable of storing much vitamin A. Medicines that alter lipid absorption inhibit vitamin A absorption too. People who have chronic diarrhea, celiac disease, Crohn's disease, cystic fibrosis, or pancreatic insufficiency and other fat-malabsorption conditions may develop vitamin A deficiency over time. In the United States, vitamin A deficiency occurs most often in people who suffer from fat-malabsorption syndromes or severely restricted diets as seen in anorexia nervosa. Inadequate intake of zinc also can cause symptoms of vitamin A deficiency because zinc is required for the body to use vitamin A efficiently.

Eyes

Night blindness is an early symptom of vitamin A deficiency, and can be corrected completely with early treatment. As the deficiency worsens, the lack of retinoic acid interferes with the normal differentiation of epithelial cells and reduces the formation of mucus-secreting goblet cells. As mucus production drops, the cornea and conjunctiva (the outer surface of the eye) and the mucous membrane lining the inner surface of the eyelid become extremely dry. The lack of mucus prevents the eye from washing away dirt and bacteria, thus increasing the likelihood of infection. As the cornea deteriorates, foamy, white triangular patches known as Bitot's spots develop. Eventually, irreversible scars form on the cornea, which also develops ulcers and sometimes liquefies during the final stages of deterioration. Collectively, these symptoms that progress toward total blindness are known as **xerophthalmia**. Unlike night blindness, which can be reversed with a single dose of vitamin A, corneal drying and scarring usually is permanent.

Skin

A lack of retinoic acid shifts the differentiation of epithelial cells toward the production of skin cells. This increased supply packs the skin with extra cells, increasing the density and making the skin hard and scaly. An early symptom of vitamin A deficiency is follicular **hyperkeratosis**, or "goose flesh." In this condition, the hair follicles on the skin become plugged with keratin, a protein normally present only on the outermost surface of the skin. As a result, the skin becomes rough and bumpy. Sweat glands lose their ability to secrete perspiration. Typically, hyperkeratosis causes thickening of the palms and soles, as well as attacking the flexure areas (elbows, knees, wrists, and ankles) of the skin. In advanced stages the entire body can be involved. Usually, the appearance of hyperkeratotic symptoms in the skin lags behind the development of other symptoms of vitamin A deficiency. When vitamin A is restored, the skin is slower to recover than other affected tissues.[6]

Other Epithelial Cells

Hyperkeratosis affects other types of epithelial cells and disrupts their ability to secrete mucus. This particularly affects the mouth, respiratory tract, urinary tract, female genital tract, seminal vesicles of the testes, and glands of the eyes, making them vulnerable to infection. In men, a vitamin A deficiency halts the production of sperm. Women can become infertile, possibly due to disruptions in the production of reproductive tract secretions.

Hyperkeratinization near sensory receptors causes a loss of taste and smell, which in turn can cause loss of appetite and weight.

Immune Function

When lack of vitamin A leads to dry and dysfunctional epithelial tissues, microorganisms easily can breach the body's defenses. The respiratory tract, mucous membranes, and skin become especially vulnerable to infection. To make things worse, insufficient vitamin A reduces the number of T lymphocytes, which are important immune cells, and compromises their ability to mount an immune response. Vitamin A deficiency thus leaves a person highly susceptible to bacterial, parasitic, and viral infections. Children with mild vitamin A deficiencies run a high risk of diarrhea, respiratory tract infections, and measles. People with severe vitamin A deficiencies have such impaired immune systems that simple infections may be fatal.[7]

Vitamin A Toxicity

The Tolerable Upper Intake Level (UL) for vitamin A is 3,000 micrograms RAE as retinol. Vitamin A toxicity occurs infrequently, but as more people take megadoses of nutritional supplements, the potential for toxic overdoses increases. With the exception of a sustained diet of large amounts of liver or fish oils, food alone generally cannot supply massive amounts of vitamin A. Children tend to be more vulnerable to toxicity, and overenthusiastic supplementation of children's diets with vitamin A can be dangerous. Vitamin A toxicity has a wide range of symptoms, both subtle and overt, including fatigue, vomiting, abdominal pain, bone and joint pain, loss of appetite, skin disorders, headache, blurred or double vision, and liver damage, which in turn leads to jaundice. (See Figure 9.11.) High

hyperkeratosis Excessive accumulation of the protein keratin that produces rough and bumpy skin, most commonly affecting the palms and soles, as well as flexure areas (elbows, knees, wrists, ankles). It can affect moist epithelial tissues and impair their ability to secrete mucus. Also called hyperkeratinization.

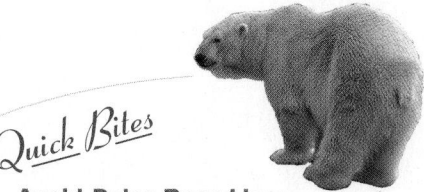

Quick Bites

Avoid Polar Bear Liver

Liver and onions may be your favorite meal, but do not use polar bear liver. Polar bear liver is so rich in vitamin A that a single serving can be toxic for humans.

teratogen Any substance that causes birth defects.

retinol intake and serum retinol levels have been linked to an increased risk of fractures.[8] Vitamin A toxicity can be fatal!

Preformed vitamin A, taken in excess, is a known **teratogen**. Birth defects associated with vitamin A toxicity include cleft palate, heart abnormalities, and brain malfunction.[9] Excess vitamin A is most hazardous when taken during the two weeks prior to conception and the first two months of pregnancy. The embryo is undergoing a great deal of cell differentiation, and excess amounts of vitamin A appear to interfere with the vitamin's normal support of this process. An acute excess intake of vitamin A as retinol during pregnancy also can cause spontaneous abortions. Pregnant women should avoid prenatal supplements that contain retinol and instead use those that have beta-carotene as the vitamin A source. Pregnant women should get the approval of their doctor before taking retinol-containing supplements.

Although large doses of beta-carotene (provitamin A) may cause the harmless condition carotenodermia, they do not seem to cause any serious side effects. Conversion of beta-carotene to retinol occurs relatively slowly, and its absorption decreases as dietary intake increases.

Acne Treatment

Up to 90 percent of boys and up to 80 percent of girls experience acne during adolescence, making it the most common skin ailment seen by physicians. The disease has a wide spectrum, ranging from just a few transient pimples to large, chronic, painful nodules that scar when healing.[10]

Retinoic acid is the most commonly prescribed treatment to reduce the formation of blackheads and whiteheads. Retin-A (all-*trans*-retinoic acid) is available for topical use (applied to the skin). Accutane (13-*cis*-retinoic acid) is taken orally. Both Retin-A and Accutane increase one's sensitivity to the sun, so sun exposure must be limited to avoid sunburn. More important, these medications, like any large dose of vitamin A, cause birth defects, so any woman who may become pregnant should not take them. Since retinoids accumulate in fat stores, even from topical administration, these medications should be discontinued at least two years before becoming pregnant.

Key Concepts: *Deficiency of vitamin A results in progressive vision loss from temporary night blindness, then reversible blindness, and finally permanent blindness. In addition, the lack of mucus secretions and reduced immune function make the person with vitamin A deficiency vulnerable to infections. Vitamin A toxicity can result from the use of supplements, even with dosages just a few times higher than the RDA. The consequences of vitamin A toxicity during pregnancy are potentially devastating, and pregnant women should avoid both retinol-containing supplements and medications made from retinoids, such as Accutane and Retin-A.*

The Carotenoids

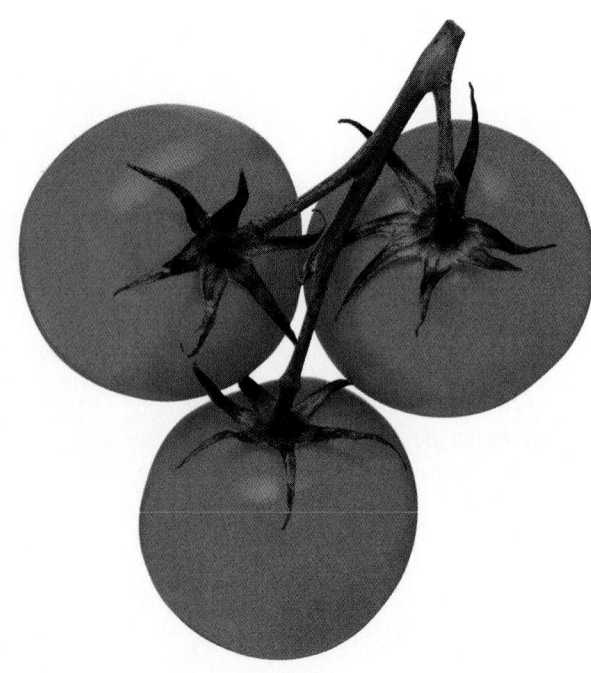

Carotenoids are naturally occurring compounds that give the deep yellow, orange, and red colors to fruits and vegetables such as apricots, carrots, and tomatoes. Carotenoids also are abundant in dark-green vegetables, such as spinach, but the carotenoid colors are hidden by the plentiful green pigment chlorophyll. Researchers have identified about 600 carotenoids, 50 of which are typically found in the U.S. diet, but they have identified only 34 in blood samples and human milk.[11] The major carotenoids are alpha-carotene, beta-carotene, lutein, zeaxanthin, cryptoxanthin, and lycopene. The yellow-orange pigment beta-carotene, which lends its color to cantaloupe, carrots, and squash, is the most common carotenoid.[12] The body can convert alpha-carotene, beta-carotene, and beta-cryptoxanthin to retinol, so they are called provitamin A carotenoids. Lycopene, lutein, and zeaxanthin have no vitamin A activity, so they are called nonprovitamin A carotenoids.

Functions of Carotenoids

Although carotenoids have diverse biological functions independent of their conversion to vitamin A, there is no evidence that carotenoids are essential nutrients in the technical sense. Because no other specific nutrient functions have been identified for any of the carotenoids, the Food and Nutrition Board has not established Dietary Reference Intakes (DRIs) for carotenoids.[13] Yet carotenoids have roles in fighting free radicals, bolstering immune function, enhancing vision, and preventing cancer.

Carotenoids as Antioxidants

Beta-carotene and other carotenoids function as potent antioxidants—substances that can interfere with the damaging effects of free radicals, which are highly unstable, reactive compounds. Free radicals can damage both the structure and function of cell membranes, nucleic acids, and electron-dense regions of proteins.[14] This damage may form the biological basis of several acute medical problems, such as premature aging, cancer, atherosclerosis, cataracts, age-related macular degeneration, and an array of degenerative diseases.[15] For more information about free radicals and antioxidants, see the "Vitamin E" section later in this chapter.

Carotenoids and the Immune System

Carotenoids can boost the immune response. Beta-carotene has been shown to enhance certain measures of immune function when taken as a supplement by elderly males[16] and healthy male nonsmokers.[17] Carotenoids also help protect skin from redness and damage following exposure to ultraviolet (UV) radiation.[18]

Carotenoids and Vision

In the eye, lutein and its close relative zeaxanthin are found in the macula, the central portion of the retina that is responsible for sharp and detailed vision. Scientists believe these carotenoids filter harmful blue light in the macula and scavenge free radicals in retinal tissues.[19] Epidemiological studies suggest that increased intake of lutein lowers risk for age-related macular degeneration.[20] People with the highest intakes of lutein and zeaxanthin also have a decreased risk of cataracts.[21] However, beta-carotene supplementation seems to have no influence.[22]

Carotenoids and Cancer

Certain carotenoids, including lycopene and beta-carotene, can strengthen growth-regulatory signals between cells. Growth-inhibiting signals from normal cells can help prevent damaged cells from reproducing, especially cells damaged by chemical carcinogens.[23] People with the highest intakes of carotenoid-rich fruits and vegetables and/or high blood levels of specific carotenoids usually have the lowest risk for certain types of cancer. Animal and human studies associate foods rich in specific carotenoids with reduced risks of specific cancers:[24]

- Lycopene may lower the risk of prostate cancer.
- Lutein, zeaxanthin, alpha-carotene, and lycopene may lower the risk of lung cancer.
- Alpha-carotene, beta-carotene, lutein, and zeaxanthin may lower the risk of breast cancer.

Quick Bites

And They Called It Cantaloupe

The word *cantaloupe* comes from a papal garden in a small town near Rome named Cantaloupo. One-half of a medium cantaloupe has 466 RAE as beta-carotene.

Generally, studies show stronger effects from fruits and vegetables in the diet than from isolated carotenoid supplementation.

Absorption and Storage of Carotenoids

In foods, fibrous proteins tightly bind carotenoids, so your body absorbs only 20 to 40 percent of what you consume. (See **Figure 9.12**.) This proportion drops even further—to 10 percent or less—as the amount of carotenoids you eat increases. Olestra, the fat substitute in some snack foods, and dietary fiber also reduce carotenoid absorption. Conversely, dietary fat, protein, and vitamin E enhance carotenoid absorption. When dietary fat enters the small intestine, bile is secreted, which helps emulsify the fat and enhances the absorption of carotenoids. In fact, when there is a lack of bile, carotenoids are not absorbed.[25] Intestinal cells convert most absorbed carotenoids to vitamin A and deliver the remaining absorbed and unchanged carotenoids to the lymph and eventually the bloodstream, where they circulate bound to lipoproteins.

Although the liver and adipose tissue are the primary carotenoid storage depots, the kidneys, adrenal glands, and other fatty tissues throughout the body also contain carotenoids.[26] Extremely large intakes of carotenoid-rich foods have not been associated with toxic effects, but they can have disconcerting results. Carotenoids are strong coloring agents, and people who regularly drink carrot juice, for example, may suddenly discover that their skin has acquired an orange tinge! They have the harmless condition carotenodermia, just like the baby in the introduction to this chapter.

Sources of Carotenoids

Orange and yellow fruits and vegetables generally contain beta-carotene, alpha-carotene, and cryptoxanthin. Good sources of beta-carotene include carrots, pumpkins, winter squash, sweet potatoes, and some orange-colored fruits such as cantaloupes, apricots, and mangos. Carrots and pumpkins are rich in alpha-carotene too. Because of its yellow-orange color, beta-carotene is added to margarine, gelatin, soft drinks, cake mixes, cereals, and other products. Dark-green vegetables also contain abundant carotenoids; however, they produce less vitamin A than ripe orange-colored fruit.[27]

Surprisingly, oranges and tangerines have little beta-carotene, but they are rich in cryptoxanthin. Lycopene has a more reddish color; you will find it in tomatoes and tomato products, pink grapefruit, guava, and watermelon. Lutein and zeaxanthin are in leafy green vegetables, pumpkin, and red pepper. Cryptoxanthin is found in mangos, nectarines, oranges, papaya, and tangerines.[28] Since it's hard to identify carotenoids in food just by looking, and because we know all of the major carotenoids are important, eating a wide variety of fruits and vegetables, and plenty of them, ensures a good intake of all.

A few minutes of cooking breaks some of the chemical bonds in food. This helps release carotenoids and makes them easier to absorb. In a study of healthy females, daily consumption of processed carrots and spinach over a four-week period tripled their beta-carotene blood levels compared to their blood levels when they consumed these vegetables raw.[29] Cooked tomato products yield more lycopene than raw tomatoes because heat ruptures plant cell walls, releasing the carotenoid.

Quick Bites

The Production Continues

Compared to freshly picked fruit, watermelon stored for 14 days at 70°F gained up to 40 percent more lycopene and 50 percent to 139 percent extra beta-carotene. Study findings showed that watermelons continue to produce these nutrients after they are picked and that chilling slows this process.

Quick Bites

Pizza Versus Tomato Juice

One U.S. study linked intake of tomato sauce, tomatoes, and pizza to lowered risk of prostate cancer. Tomato juice, however, was not protective. That's not surprising. According to John Erdman, Ph.D., of the University of Illinois in Urbana, the cancer-fighting carotenoid found in tomatoes (lycopene) is a fat-soluble substance, so it needs some fat like that found in pizza and most pasta sauces to be absorbed. The lycopene in tomato juice, however, seems to be especially poorly absorbed.

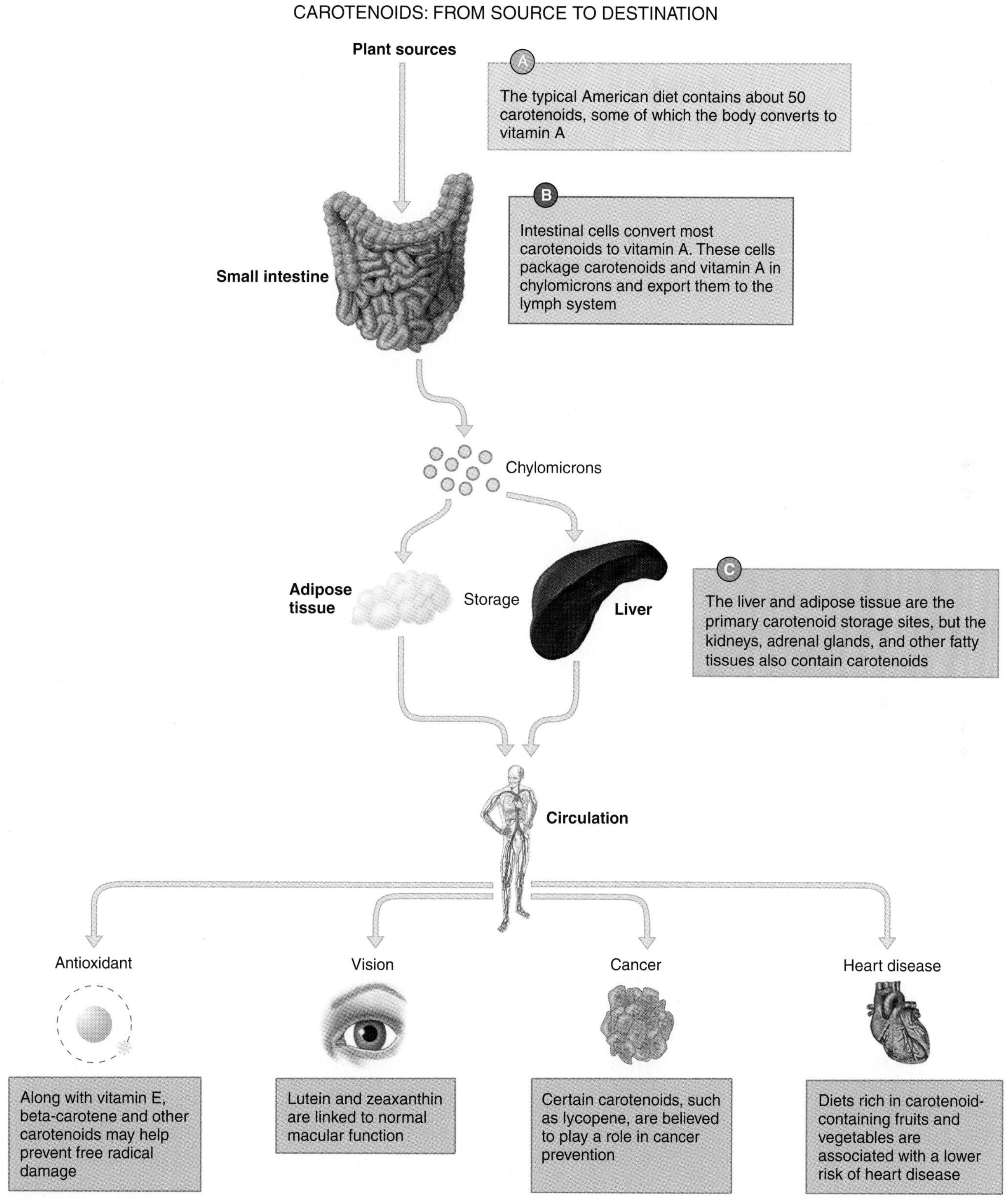

CAROTENOIDS: FROM SOURCE TO DESTINATION

Plant sources

A
The typical American diet contains about 50 carotenoids, some of which the body converts to vitamin A

Small intestine

B
Intestinal cells convert most carotenoids to vitamin A. These cells package carotenoids and vitamin A in chylomicrons and export them to the lymph system

Chylomicrons

Adipose tissue   Storage   **Liver**

C
The liver and adipose tissue are the primary carotenoid storage sites, but the kidneys, adrenal glands, and other fatty tissues also contain carotenoids

Circulation

Antioxidant

Vision

Cancer

Heart disease

Along with vitamin E, beta-carotene and other carotenoids may help prevent free radical damage

Lutein and zeaxanthin are linked to normal macular function

Certain carotenoids, such as lycopene, are believed to play a role in cancer prevention

Diets rich in carotenoid-containing fruits and vegetables are associated with a lower risk of heart disease

Figure 9.12 **Carotenoids: from source to destination.** In the body, the provitamin A carotenoids alpha-carotene, beta-carotene, and beta-cryptoxanthin can be converted to retinol. The nonprovitamin A carotenoids lycopene, lutein, and zeaxanthin have no vitamin A activity. Independent of vitamin A activity, carotenoids can function as antioxidants, and may be involved in normal macular function and reduced risk of heart disease and cancer.

antirachitic Pertaining to activities of an agent used to treat rickets.

Carotenoid Supplementation

More and more people are taking carotenoid supplements. Mixed carotenoid supplements derived from sea algae or palm oil contain a variety of carotenoids, including the six major ones. A UL has not been set for beta-carotene or carotenoids. Instead, the Food and Nutrition Board advises against supplementation for the general population and supports existing recommendations for increased consumption of carotenoid-rich fruits and vegetables.

Many scientists have searched for a connection between beta-carotene supplementation and a reduced risk of heart disease and cancer, but a consistent association has not emerged.[30] Beta-carotene supplements actually may cause harm to current smokers and people exposed to asbestos.[31] On the other hand, there is a strong link between eating fruits and vegetables rich in carotenoids and reduced disease rates.[32] In foods there may be beneficial interactions among naturally occurring beta-carotene, other carotenoids, and other phytochemicals. Additional carotenoids, such as lycopene, lutein, and cryptoxanthin, are now being studied. Although eating carotenoid-rich fruits and vegetables is clearly linked to reduced disease rates, the use of carotenoid supplements is not recommended.

Vitamin D

Sometimes called the sunshine vitamin, vitamin D is unique because, given sufficient sunlight, your body can synthesize all it needs of this fat-soluble nutrient. In fact, it could be argued that vitamin D is technically not a nutrient—it is synthesized and functions like a hormone, and it is not always necessary in the diet. When the ultraviolet rays of the sun strike the skin, they alter a precursor derived from cholesterol, converting it into vitamin D. Although fortified milk and other foods supply vitamin D, your body can make plenty as long as it gets regular exposure to sunlight.

Vitamin D is essential for bone health and may help reduce cancer risk. In children, it promotes bone development and growth. In adults, it is necessary for bone maintenance. In the elderly, vitamin D helps prevent osteoporosis and fractures. In addition, supplemental vitamin D can reduce the risk of falls in the elderly.[33] Although severe vitamin D deficiency in children and adults is rare, vitamin D deficiency is widespread among sick people and the elderly.[34]

Forms and Formation of Vitamin D

Vitamin D can be considered either a vitamin or a hormone. Like other vitamins, a lack of dietary vitamin D (coupled with minimal sun exposure) will cause a deficiency. The active form of vitamin D is like a hormone because it is made in one part of the body and regulates activities in other parts. (See **Figure 9.13**.)

Ten compounds, called vitamin D_1 through D_{10}, exhibit **antirachitic** properties; that is, they prevent a childhood bone disease called rickets. The most important of these compounds are D_2 (ergocalciferol) and D_3 (cholecalciferol). Ergocalciferol is found exclusively in plant foods. Cholecalciferol is found in animal foods (eggs and fish oils), but most is synthesized in the skin.

In the skin, UV radiation from the sun converts a cholesterol derivative (7-dehydrocholesterol) to cholecalciferol, which then enters the bloodstream and travels to the liver. The liver also receives dietary cholecalciferol

VITAMIN D: FROM SOURCE TO DESTINATION

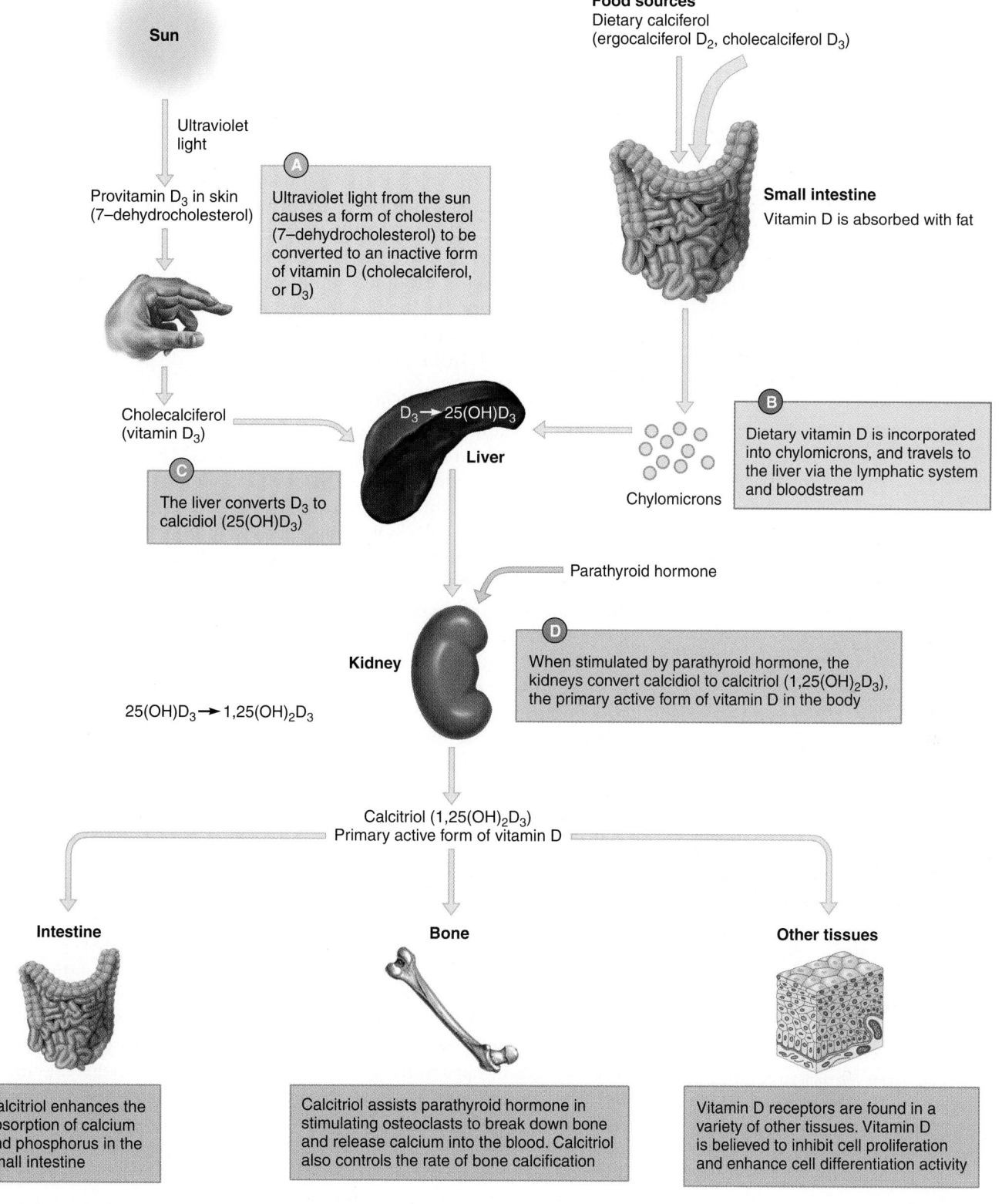

Sun

Ultraviolet light

Provitamin D_3 in skin (7–dehydrocholesterol)

Ⓐ Ultraviolet light from the sun causes a form of cholesterol (7–dehydrocholesterol) to be converted to an inactive form of vitamin D (cholecalciferol, or D_3)

Cholecalciferol (vitamin D_3)

Ⓒ The liver converts D_3 to calcidiol (25(OH)D_3)

Food sources
Dietary calciferol
(ergocalciferol D_2, cholecalciferol D_3)

Small intestine
Vitamin D is absorbed with fat

$D_3 \rightarrow 25(OH)D_3$
Liver

Chylomicrons

Ⓑ Dietary vitamin D is incorporated into chylomicrons, and travels to the liver via the lymphatic system and bloodstream

Parathyroid hormone

Kidney

Ⓓ When stimulated by parathyroid hormone, the kidneys convert calcidiol to calcitriol (1,25(OH)$_2$D$_3$), the primary active form of vitamin D in the body

$25(OH)D_3 \rightarrow 1,25(OH)_2D_3$

Calcitriol (1,25(OH)$_2$D$_3$)
Primary active form of vitamin D

Intestine

Calcitriol enhances the absorption of calcium and phosphorus in the small intestine

Bone

Calcitriol assists parathyroid hormone in stimulating osteoclasts to break down bone and release calcium into the blood. Calcitriol also controls the rate of bone calcification

Other tissues

Vitamin D receptors are found in a variety of other tissues. Vitamin D is believed to inhibit cell proliferation and enhance cell differentiation activity

Figure 9.13 **Vitamin D: from source to destination.** Vitamin D is unique because, given sufficient sunlight, your body can synthesize all it needs. Both dietary and endogenous vitamin D must be activated by reactions in the kidneys and liver. Active vitamin D [1,25(OH)$_2$D$_3$, or calcitriol] is important for calcium balance and bone health, and may have a role in cell differentiation.

and ergocalciferol from chylomicrons. In the liver, cholecalciferol and ergocalciferol are converted into calcidiol and then sent to the kidneys. The kidneys perform the final step—the formation of **1,25-dihydroxyvitamin D₃** **[1,25(OH)₂D₃]**, also called **calcitriol**. $1,25(OH)_2D_3$ is the active form of vitamin D, and the body derives about 90 percent of its $1,25(OH)_2D_3$ from the cholecalciferol synthesized in the skin.[35]

Functions of Vitamin D

Vitamin D is a regulatory compound. Although its primary role is to regulate blood calcium levels,[36] it also is important for regulating cell differentiation and growth. Research shows that vitamin D may be protective against colorectal cancer.[37] (See the Nutrition Science in Action feature "Vitamin D and Colon Cancer.") Investigators also are looking for ways vitamin D and its derivatives might treat other conditions of abnormal cell growth, such as psoriasis and cancers of the blood, lung, and cervix. Vitamin D deficiency has been linked to increased risk for cardiovascular disease, multiple sclerosis, rheumatoid arthritis, and type 1 diabetes.[38]

Regulation of Blood Calcium Levels

The liver and adipose tissues store vitamin D. In times of need, the liver and kidneys convert stored vitamin D to $1,25(OH)_2D_3$, the biologically active form in the body. $1,25(OH)_2D_3$ helps maintain calcium and phosphorus blood levels within a normal range. $1,25(OH)_2D_3$ acts directly and in concert with two other hormones: **parathyroid hormone** (parathormone) from the parathyroid gland, and **calcitonin** from the thyroid gland. (See Figure 11.21 in Chapter 11.) These hormones regulate activity in the bone, kidneys, and small intestine to adjust blood calcium levels. Much as a thermostat monitors temperature, receptors in the parathyroid gland monitor the blood levels of calcium.

When blood calcium levels drop, the parathyroid gland releases parathyroid hormone (PTH). PTH stimulates the activity of **osteoclasts** (bone cells that digest the bone matrix), releasing calcium ions from bone into the bloodstream. Parathyroid hormone also raises blood calcium levels by signaling the kidneys to slow calcium excretion. In addition, PTH stimulates the kidneys to activate vitamin D. $1,25(OH)_2D_3$ is released by the kidneys and enhances the action of PTH on bone cells. $1,25(OH)_2D_3$ then stimulates the intestinal cells to make more carrier proteins for calcium transport, enhancing the absorption of calcium from food and thereby helping to elevate blood levels of calcium.

When blood calcium levels are too high, the thyroid gland releases calcitonin and the parathyroid gland decreases its release of PTH. Calcitonin inhibits the activity of osteoclasts, shifting the balance toward the activity of **osteoblasts** (bone-building cells). This net bone-building activity removes calcium ions from the bloodstream and deposits them in new bone. Calcitonin promotes bone growth in children and helps maintain bone health during pregnancy and lactation. Since high levels of calcium in the blood inhibit release of parathyroid hormone, the kidneys continue to excrete calcium. In the absence of PTH, the kidneys activate little or no $1,25(OH)_2D_3$. In the small intestine, lower $1,25(OH)_2D_3$ levels reduce the production of protein carriers for calcium transport, thus reducing calcium absorption.

Even if calcium and phosphorus intakes are adequate, teeth and bones do not calcify normally without $1,25(OH)_2D_3$. Conversely, calcification progresses

---

1,25-dihydroxyvitamin D₃ [1,25(OH)₂D₃] The active form of vitamin D. It is an important regulator of blood calcium levels.

calcitriol See *1,25-dihydroxyvitamin D₃*.

parathyroid hormone A hormone secreted by the parathyroid glands in response to low blood calcium. It stimulates calcium release from bone and calcium absorption by the intestines, while decreasing calcium excretion by the kidneys. It acts in conjunction with 1,25(OH)₂D₃ to raise blood calcium. Also called parathormone.

calcitonin A hormone secreted by the thyroid gland in response to elevated blood calcium. It stimulates calcium deposition in bone and calcium excretion by the kidneys, thus reducing blood calcium.

osteoclasts Bone cells that promote bone resorption and calcium mobilization.

osteoblasts Bone cells that promote bone deposition and growth.

Quick Bites

"Children's Disease of the English"

*I*n the seventeenth century, vitamin D deficiency was so common in British children that rickets was called the "children's disease of the English." Diets provided little vitamin D and the lack of sun during many months of the year inhibited vitamin D synthesis in the skin.

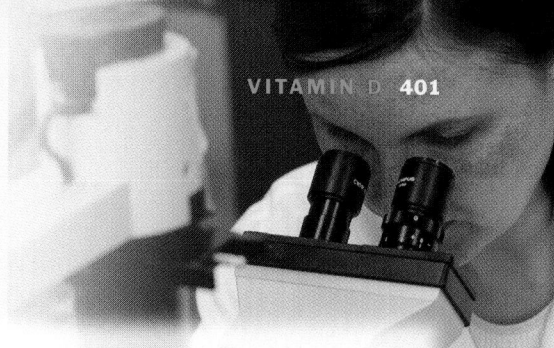

NUTRITION SCIENCE IN ACTION

Vitamin D and Colon Cancer

Background: Studies of mice fed a diet rich in vitamin D have shown that vitamin D lowers the risk of colon cancer. Studies of humans link calcium and reduced colon cancer risk. Because vitamin D increases the absorption of calcium, high vitamin D intake may reduce colon cancer risk.

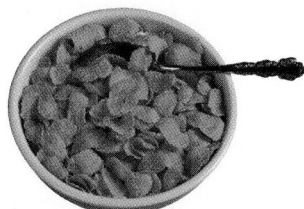

Hypothesis: People who have high vitamin D intakes will have a lower risk of colon cancer than people with low vitamin D intakes.

Experimental Plan: Recruit subjects aged 50 to 75 years from 13 Veterans Administration medical centers. Obtain complete medical histories and dietary information. Exclude subjects who are currently participating in other studies, have a history of colon disease, or have had prior colonic surgery or colonic examination. Follow and collect data for three years.

Results: The hypothesis is confirmed. Analyses of the data from 1,770 participants showed significant reductions in the relative risk of cancer with increased intake of vitamin D. Total calcium and total folate intake also showed significant risk reduction, but vitamin D dominated both. Participants who consumed more than 645 IU (16 micrograms) of vitamin D daily were 40 percent less likely to have advanced polyps.

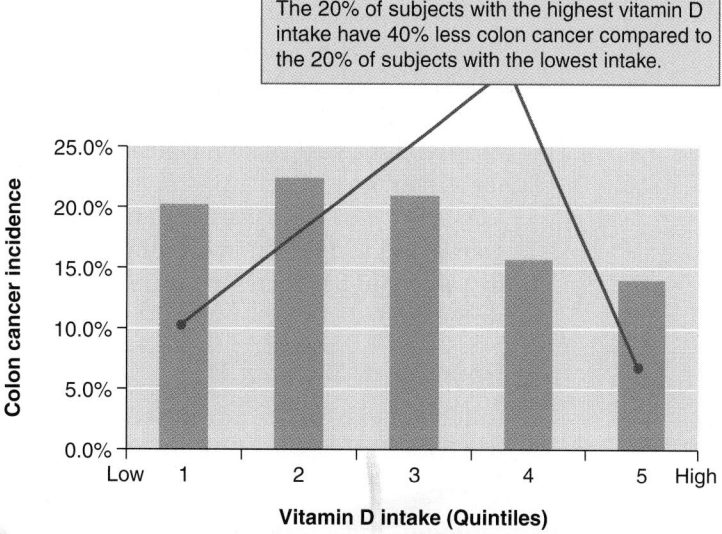

The 20% of subjects with the highest vitamin D intake have 40% less colon cancer compared to the 20% of subjects with the lowest intake.

Conclusion and Discussion: Consuming vitamin D plus calcium may be a low-risk preventive strategy for colon cancer. This study also showed that smoking and moderate to heavy alcohol use increased the risk of colon cancer. Although men accounted for 96.8 percent of the study subjects, other studies confirmed these results in women. Scientists suggest that future studies will also compare the effects of vitamin D supplements with those obtained from diets rich in vitamin D.

Source: Based on Lieberman D, Prindiville S, Weiss D, Willett W, for VA Cooperative Study Group 380. Risk factors for advanced colonic neoplasia and hyperplastic polyps in asymptomatic individuals. *JAMA.* 2003;290(22):2959–2967.

normally when 1,25(OH)$_2$D$_3$ status is adequate even if calcium and phosphorus levels are low. 1,25(OH)$_2$D$_3$ controls the rate of calcification independent of the absolute blood levels of calcium and phosphorus.

Key Concepts: *The best-known function of vitamin D, in the active form of 1,25(OH)$_2$D$_3$, is to help regulate blood calcium levels. 1,25(OH)$_2$D$_3$ works with two other hormones, parathyroid hormone and calcitonin, to alter the amount of calcium in the bone, the amount excreted from the kidneys, and the amount absorbed from the intestine to keep blood levels in a normal range. It is known that 1,25(OH)$_2$D$_3$ has effects on other tissues, but these functions have not been well studied.*

Dietary Recommendations for Vitamin D

Although the body can synthesize vitamin D, scientists still recognize vitamin D as an essential nutrient for most people. Because of the variability of sunlight throughout the year, and some people's limited sun exposure, intake recommendations have been developed. Dietary recommendations are given as Adequate Intake (AI) levels that assume no available vitamin D from skin synthesis.[39]

Infants are born with stores of vitamin D that last about nine months. Beyond that, they must obtain vitamin D via exposure to sunlight, formula, or a supplement administered under the guidance of a physician. Breast milk contains very little vitamin D and is unlikely to meet a baby's needs beyond infancy. Exclusively breastfed infants who receive little exposure to sunlight need supplemental vitamin D. The AI for infants and children from birth to 18 years is 5 micrograms per day.

In later adulthood, the intake recommendations for vitamin D increase because vitamin D synthesis decreases with aging. For men and women aged 19 through 50 years, the AI for vitamin D is 5 micrograms per day. For people aged 51 through 70, the AI increases to 10 micrograms per day, and for people older than 70, the AI rises to 15 micrograms per day.

A recent review evaluated vitamin D in relation to bone mineral density, lower extremity function, dental health, and risk of falls, fractures, and colorectal cancer.[40] This study found that most people do not reach optimal blood vitamin D levels with currently recommended intakes. The researchers suggest that recommended vitamin D intakes should be increased to 25 micrograms for all adults.

As is the case with vitamin A, International Units (IU) rather than micrograms (μg) will be found on supplement labels. The conversion works out to 1 μg = 40 IU. Therefore, 200 IU is the equivalent of the AI for ages 19 through 50.

Sources of Vitamin D

In theory, all of our required vitamin D could be synthesized in the skin when it is exposed to UV light. In fact, the diet may supply only about 10 percent of our needs.[41]

Sunlight and Vitamin D Synthesis

How much exposure to the sun is needed for an adequate supply of vitamin D? It depends on several factors, including the following:

- *Time of day.* The sun's rays are most intense between 10:00 A.M. and 2:00 P.M.

- *Season.* The sun is higher in the sky and delivers more radiation during the summer months.

- *Environment.* Eighty percent or more of the sun's UV rays penetrate clouds,[42] but ordinary window glass blocks UV radiation.

- *Location.* Sunlight is less intense in the northern and southern latitudes than near the equator. A sun worshipper in Florida receives 50 percent more radiation than one in Maine. (See **Figure 9.14**.)

- *Use of sunscreen.* Sunscreen protects the skin against sun damage, but it also blocks the ultraviolet light necessary for vitamin D synthesis.

- *Skin type.* Light-skinned people absorb UV rays more quickly than dark-skinned people.

A rule of thumb is to expose your hands, face, and arms to the sun for about one-third to one-half the time it would take you to burn.[43] Repeat this exposure two to three times per week to get adequate vitamin D.

Dietary Sources of Vitamin D

Few foods naturally contain vitamin D, so the major dietary sources of the nutrient are vitamin D–fortified milk and other fortified foods, such as breakfast cereal. In the United States, milk is fortified with 10 micrograms of vitamin D (400 IU) per quart. In the early 1990s, three surveys of the vitamin D content of fortified milk in the United States and Canada suggested that as many as 70 percent of the milk samples did not contain vitamin D in the range of 8 to 12 micrograms. Some samples of nonfat milk contained no vitamin D.[44] Because of this variability, the U.S. Food and Drug Administration now monitors dairies' compliance with vitamin D fortification.

Vitamin D is found in oily fish (e.g., herring, salmon, and sardines) as well as in cod liver oil and other fish oils. Egg yolk, butter, and liver supply various amounts of vitamin D depending on the vitamin D content of the foods consumed by the source animals. Plants are a poor source, so strict vegetarians must get their vitamin D through exposure to sunlight. If sun exposure is not possible, nutritionists may recommend dietary supplements. **Figure 9.15** shows some foods that are sources of vitamin D.

Key Concepts: *Intake recommendations for vitamin D are very small: only 5 micrograms per day for young adults. Needs from the diet increase with age as the ability of the skin to synthesize vitamin D declines. Few foods are naturally good sources of vitamin D, and so most of the dietary intake comes from fortified milk and other fortified foods.*

Vitamin D Deficiency

Long-term deficiency of vitamin D takes a profound toll on the skeleton. When vitamin D is in short supply, the intestines absorb only about 10 to 15 percent of dietary calcium, so bones don't get enough of this bone-building mineral.

Rickets and Osteomalacia

In children with vitamin D deficiency, the bones weaken and the skeleton fails to harden. This condition is called **rickets** and is characterized by "bow legs," "knock-knees," and other skeletal deformities. In the United States and Canada, nutritional rickets has been all but eliminated by vitamin D–fortified milk, infant vitamin supplements, and vitamin supplements for children with fat-malabsorption conditions. Scattered cases of

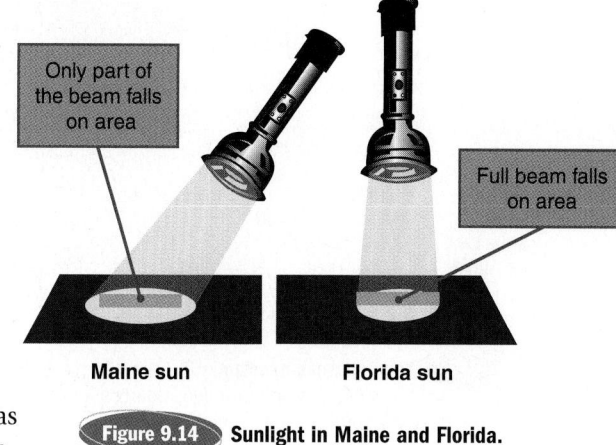

Only part of the beam falls on area

Full beam falls on area

Maine sun   Florida sun

Figure 9.14 **Sunlight in Maine and Florida.**

Quick Bites

Do You Know Vitamin D When You See It?

The general terms *vitamin D* and *calciferol* are used to refer to both vitamin D_2 (ergocalciferol) and vitamin D_3 (cholecalciferol), and to any combination of these two compounds.

rickets A bone disease in children that results from vitamin D deficiency.

Think About It **4**

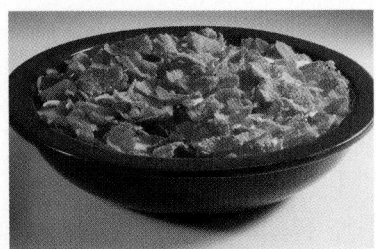

VITAMIN D

Daily Value = 400 IU

Exceptionally good sources

Cod liver oil	1 Tbsp	1,360 IU
Salmon, canned, solids + bones	55 g (2 oz)	420 IU
Sardines, canned, solids + bones	55 g (2 oz)	150 IU
Milk, 1% milkfat	240 ml (1 cup)	129 IU
Milk, nonfat	240 ml (1 cup)	103 IU
Milk, whole, 3.25% milkfat	240 ml (1 cup)	99 IU
Fortified, ready-to-eat cereals	30 g	40–50 IU

**High:
20% DV
or more**

Figure 9.15 **Food sources of vitamin D.** Only a few foods are naturally good sources of vitamin D. Therefore, fortified foods such as milk and ready-to-eat cereals are important, especially for people with limited exposure to the sun. Units are IU to be consistent with Daily Value definitions. **Source:** U.S. Department of Agriculture, Agricultural Research Service. USDA National Nutrient Database for Standard Reference, Release 18. 2005. http://www.ars.usda.gov/nutrientdata.

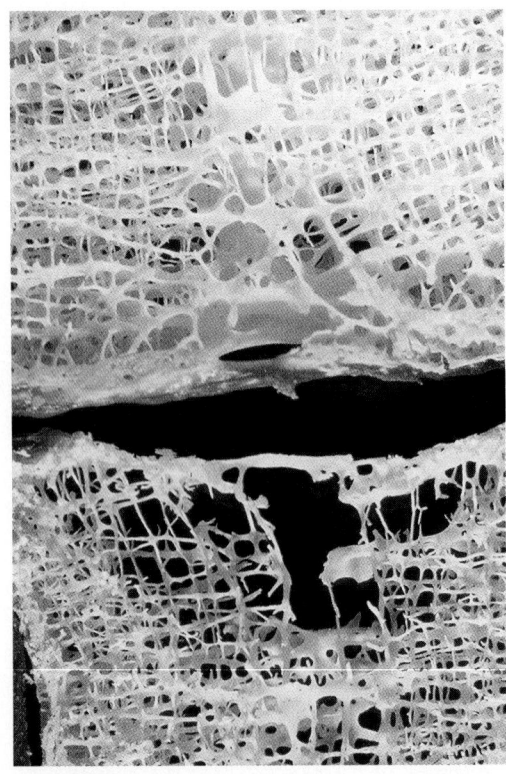

Figure 9.16 **Osteoporosis.** Normal (top) and osteoporotic bone (bottom). The osteoporotic bone is noticeably less dense.

rickets, however, have been seen in infants allergic to cow's milk and dark-skinned infants who were breastfed, drank nonfortified soy milk, or in some cases had metabolic disorders.[45] Although severe vitamin D deficiency in children and adults is rare, deficiency does exist among sick people and the elderly.[46]

In adults, vitamin D deficiency causes a similar skeletal problem called **osteomalacia**, or "soft bones." Osteomalacia increases the risk for fractures in the hip, spine, and other bones. In addition to preventing adequate calcium absorption, osteomalacia alters the function of the parathyroid gland, boosting calcium losses from the bones. Risk of osteomalacia is high in people who have diseases that affect the stomach, kidneys, gallbladder, liver, or intestine—organs that are involved with the absorption or activation of vitamin D.

Osteoporosis

Along with osteomalacia, vitamin D deficiency is associated with **osteoporosis**, increased bone turnover, and an increased risk of bone fractures.[47] (See **Figure 9.16**.) Vitamin D supplementation of elderly women slows bone turnover, increases bone density, and decreases nonvertebral fractures.[48] In elders with low blood levels of cholecalciferol, vitamin D supplementation substantially reduces the risk of osteoporotic fractures, including hip fractures.[49] For more information on osteoporosis see Chapter 11, "Water and Major Minerals," and Chapter 14, "Diet and Health."

Who Is Most at Risk for Vitamin D Deficiency?

In 1998 a pivotal study was published suggesting that many more people are deficient in vitamin D than had been suspected. The investigation of nearly 300 patients hospitalized in Boston showed that almost three of five people had too little vitamin D to maintain optimal levels of calcium in their bones.[50]

One explanation for the vitamin D shortfall may be that more people are protecting their skin with sunscreen, which may help prevent skin cancer but reduces vitamin D synthesis. Any sunscreen with a sun protection factor (SPF) of 8 or more blocks vitamin D synthesis in the skin. The problem worsens with age. Adults older than 65 years have a fourfold decrease in their ability to produce vitamin D_3 via the sun, compared with adults 20 to 30 years old.[51] Among free-living adults, fewer than 10 percent of those aged 51 to 70 years and fewer than 2 percent of those over 70 years met the AI for vitamin D from food alone.[52]

Living in a northern region compounds the problem. During the dead of winter, daylight hours are so short and the sunlight is so weak that vitamin D synthesis halts. (See **Figure 9.17**.) Although the same is true for the southern latitudes, little of the world's population lives in this region. Fortunately, the skin of most people younger than 50 years can make sufficient amounts of vitamin D with just the amount of skin on the hands exposed for 10 to 15 minutes per day during warmer months. Most younger people make and store enough vitamin D during the summer to last through the winter months.

People over age 50 are advised to expose some skin to the sun for about 15 minutes each day during warm months. In the winter, many experts recommend a vitamin supplement. Most multivitamin/mineral supplements contain 10 micrograms (400 IU) of vitamin D. Healthy adults over age 70 should check with their physicians to determine whether more supplemental vitamin D is in order.

Vitamin D Toxicity

Sun exposure does not cause vitamin D toxicity, but high supplement doses can be highly toxic. The UL for adults older than 19 years is 50 micrograms (2,000 IU) per day. Before consuming supplements that contain more than the AI, people should consult a physician.

The hallmark of vitamin D toxicity is hypercalcemia—a high concentration of calcium in the blood. This condition affects numerous tissues in the body. Initially, it hampers the kidneys' ability to concentrate urine, causing excessive urination and thirst. Prolonged hypercalcemia can cause the excess calcium in the bloodstream to leave deposits in the soft tissues of the body, including the kidneys, blood vessels, heart, and lungs. Hypercalcemia also seems to affect the central nervous system, causing a severe depressive illness as well as nausea, vomiting, and loss of appetite.

Excess vitamin D can also promote loss of bone mass as the increased levels of $1,25(OH)_2D_3$ help pull calcium from the bones into the bloodstream. In one report of 40 cases of vitamin D toxicity in adults aged 50 and older, four people who were taking more than 30 micrograms (1,200 IU) of supplemental vitamin D per day were losing three times as much calcium through their urine as people who were taking less vitamin D.[53]

Key Concepts: Because vitamin D's primary function is to regulate the level of calcium in the blood, which affects storage of calcium in bone, a deficiency of the nutrient affects the skeletal system. In children, vitamin D deficiency leads to rickets; in adults, lack of the nutrient causes osteomalacia and contributes to osteoporosis. Vitamin D is toxic when consumed in excess and large doses should be taken only under a physician's supervision. Exposure to sun does not cause vitamin D toxicity.

Vitamin E

Consumers have long embraced the practice of taking large amounts of vitamin E, once touted as being able to boost sexual prowess and to prevent gray hair, wrinkles, and other signs of aging. Although many of these rumored benefits of vitamin E have never been supported by science, a growing body of research suggests that the nutrient may, in fact, be an important protector against chronic diseases associated with aging.

Forms of Vitamin E

In 1922 researchers discovered that an unknown substance in vegetable oils was necessary for reproduction in rats. It was given the chemical name **tocopherol**, from the Greek word *tokos*, meaning "childbirth," added to the verb *phero*, meaning "to bring forth." The ending *ol* reflects the alcohol nature of the molecule. It was a full 40 years after discovery, however, before scientists gathered evidence showing that humans also need this substance, which they labeled vitamin E. In 1968 the Food and Nutrition Board of the National Academy of Sciences officially recognized vitamin E as an essential nutrient.

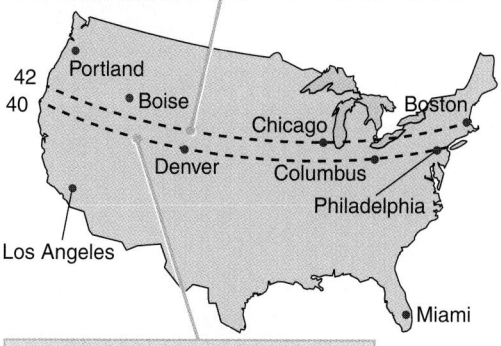

North of 42 degrees latitude, sunlight is too weak to synthesize vitamin D from late October through early March. The same effect occurs during the winter in the southern hemisphere south of 42 degrees latitude

At 40 degrees latitude, sunlight is too weak to synthesize vitamin D during January and February

Figure 9.17 **Mapping vitamin D synthesis.** Vitamin D synthesis halts for part of the winter if sunlight is too weak. In Los Angeles and Miami, the sunlight is strong enough to synthesize vitamin D year-round, even in January.

osteomalacia A disease in adults that results from vitamin D deficiency; it is marked by softening of the bones, leading to bending of the spine, bowing of the legs, and increased risk for fractures.

osteoporosis A bone disease characterized by a decrease in bone mineral density and the appearance of small holes in bones due to loss of minerals.

tocopherol The chemical name for vitamin E. There are four tocopherols (alpha, beta, gamma, delta), but only alpha-tocopherol is active in the body.

Quick Bites

Too Much Cover

Many Arab women are clothed so that only their eyes are exposed to sunlight. Even though these women live in sunny climates near the equator, many suffer from osteomalacia.

Vitamin E is not a single compound. It is actually two sets of four compounds each: the tocopherols (alpha, beta, gamma, and delta) and the chemically related **tocotrienols** (alpha, beta, gamma, and delta). Although all are absorbed, only alpha-tocopherol contributes toward meeting the human vitamin E requirement. Alpha-tocopherol is the most common form of vitamin E in food.

As with all fat-soluble vitamins, absorption of vitamin E requires adequate absorption of dietary fat. Like the other fat-soluble vitamins, it travels via chylomicrons and other lipoproteins for distribution throughout the body. (See **Figure 9.18.**) The GI tract absorbs 20 to 80 percent of dietary alpha-tocopherol, and the percentage declines as the amount of vitamin E consumed increases. Unabsorbed vitamin E is excreted in fecal matter.

Unlike the fat-soluble vitamins A and D, vitamin E does not accumulate in the liver. Adipose tissue contains about 90 percent of the vitamin E in the body. The remaining vitamin E is found in virtually every cell membrane in every tissue.

Functions of Vitamin E

Vitamin E is an antioxidant and its activity is enhanced by other nutrients involved in antioxidant pathways, such as vitamin C and selenium (a mineral). During normal metabolic processes, oxygen often reacts with other compounds to generate free radicals—highly unstable, toxic molecules that contain one unpaired electron. These unpaired electrons make free radicals highly reactive. Typically, a free radical attacks a nearby compound and steals an electron from it. Although that stabilizes the original free radical "thief," it turns the "robbed" molecule into a free radical, sparking a chain reaction capable of instantly producing a flood of free radicals.

Under normal circumstances, your body generates free radicals to help eliminate unwanted molecules. If various enzymes and antioxidants fail to control free radical activity, these highly reactive compounds attack cell membranes and cell constituents, including DNA. This unleashing of free radicals sets the stage for chronic diseases such as cancer and atherosclerosis.

A form of free radical damage that promotes atherosclerosis is **lipid peroxidation**—the production of unstable lipid molecules that contain an excess of oxygen. In this process, the cleavage of a carbon–carbon double bond in a fatty acid yields an intermediate compound that reacts with oxygen to form peroxides or free radicals. To stop lipid peroxidation, vitamin E acts as a potent antioxidant and interrupts the cascade of free radical formation. Vitamin E donates an electron to the electron-seeking free radical, thus preventing the free radical from finding an electron somewhere else and causing more damage. This makes vitamin E itself a free radical, but not a very reactive one. The body excretes some of this altered vitamin E and recycles the rest by adding an electron from another antioxidant, such as vitamin C. This vitamin C radical can regain its antioxidant form by swiping an electron from **glutathione**. The enzyme glutathione reductase restores glutathione to its antioxidant form and depends on the mineral selenium.

The polyunsaturated fatty acids (PUFAs) in cell membranes are especially vulnerable to assault by free radicals. Vitamin E resides in cell membranes and other phospholipid-rich tissues, where it serves as one of the body's chief defenses against damage by free radicals. (See **Figure 9.19.**)

tocotrienols Four compounds (alpha, beta, gamma, delta) chemically related to tocopherols. The tocotrienols and tocopherols are collectively known as vitamin E.

lipid peroxidation Production of unstable, highly reactive lipid molecules that contain excess amounts of oxygen.

glutathione A tripeptide of glycine, cysteine, and glutamic acid that is involved in protection of cells from oxidative damage.

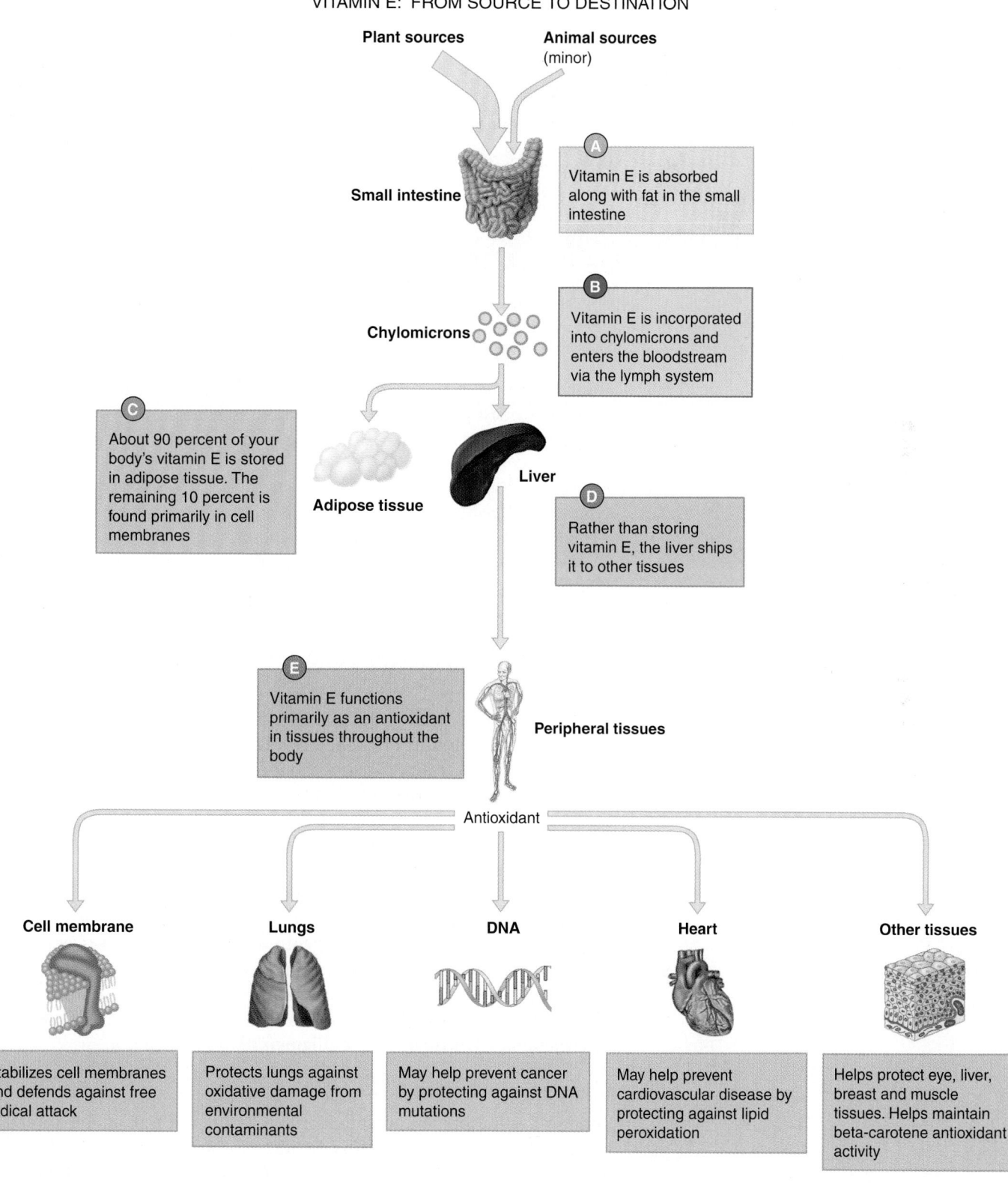

VITAMIN E: FROM SOURCE TO DESTINATION

Plant sources **Animal sources** (minor)

Small intestine

A Vitamin E is absorbed along with fat in the small intestine

Chylomicrons

B Vitamin E is incorporated into chylomicrons and enters the bloodstream via the lymph system

C About 90 percent of your body's vitamin E is stored in adipose tissue. The remaining 10 percent is found primarily in cell membranes

Adipose tissue

Liver

D Rather than storing vitamin E, the liver ships it to other tissues

E Vitamin E functions primarily as an antioxidant in tissues throughout the body

Peripheral tissues

Antioxidant

Cell membrane **Lungs** **DNA** **Heart** **Other tissues**

Stabilizes cell membranes and defends against free radical attack

Protects lungs against oxidative damage from environmental contaminants

May help prevent cancer by protecting against DNA mutations

May help prevent cardiovascular disease by protecting against lipid peroxidation

Helps protect eye, liver, breast and muscle tissues. Helps maintain beta-carotene antioxidant activity

Figure 9.18 **Vitamin E: from source to destination.** Vitamin E is absorbed in the small intestine and carried to the liver by chylomicrons. The antioxidant activity of vitamin E helps stabilize cell membranes, protects tissues from oxidative damage, and reduces the risk of cancer and heart disease.

Key

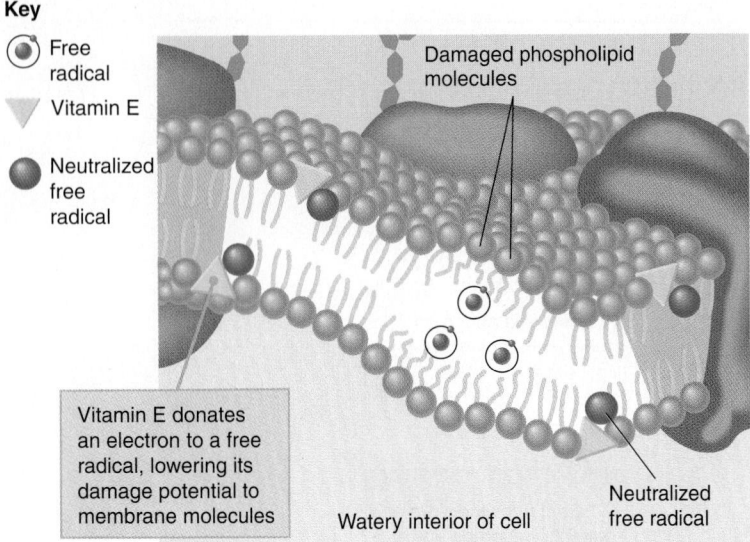

- Free radical
- Vitamin E
- Neutralized free radical

Damaged phospholipid molecules

Vitamin E donates an electron to a free radical, lowering its damage potential to membrane molecules

Watery interior of cell

Neutralized free radical

Figure 9.19 **Free radical damage.** Vitamin E helps prevent free radical damage to polyunsaturated fatty acids in cell membranes.

Observational studies have suggested that high intakes of antioxidant vitamins, including vitamin E, may lower the risk of some chronic diseases, especially heart disease.[54] However, only four published large-scale, randomized, double-blind clinical intervention studies have tested the ability of vitamin E to prevent heart attack. One was strongly positive, but the other three had neutral results. Currently, there are insufficient data to recommend supplemental vitamin E for heart disease prevention in the general population.[55]

What about other age-related diseases? In some people, supplemental vitamin E appears to reverse age-related declines in immune function. Results of a clinical trial showed that supplemental vitamin E reduced the incidence and duration of respiratory infections in nursing home residents.[56] Promising preliminary results suggest vitamin E may slow the progression of Alzheimer's disease, but it is still too early to draw any conclusions. Some evidence suggests vitamin E may protect against prostate cancer, but overall evidence supporting a role against cancer is weak.[57]

Key Concepts: *Vitamin E is really a set of compounds called tocopherols and tocotrienols. Alpha-tocopherol is the only form of vitamin E that meets the vitamin E requirement. Vitamin E functions as an antioxidant, protecting cell membranes in all parts of the body from the damaging effects of oxidation. Vitamin E has been connected to reduction of risk for many degenerative diseases, such as heart disease and cancer.*

Dietary Recommendations for Vitamin E

To prevent vitamin E deficiency, the intake requirement must be related to body size and to polyunsaturated fatty acid intake. When PUFA intake is minimal, small amounts of vitamin E will prevent symptoms of deficiency. As PUFA intake increases, the concentration of PUFA in tissues also rises and more vitamin E is needed to prevent oxidation. Since the vitamin E content of oils tends to parallel the PUFA concentration, balancing the two is usually not a problem; however, when people limit fat intake, they may also limit vitamin E intake.

The RDA for vitamin E accommodates generous PUFA intake. It is set at 15 milligrams per day of alpha-tocopherol for adults (including pregnant women) and 19 milligrams per day for women who are breastfeeding. Supplement labels may still list vitamin E content in outdated International Units. If the vitamin E in the supplement is from natural sources, 1 IU equals 0.67 milligrams alpha-tocopherol. If synthetic vitamin E is used, the conversion is 1 IU equals 0.45 milligrams alpha-tocopherol.

Sources of Vitamin E

Vitamin E is found in many different foods from both plant and animal sources. Wheat germ oil contains the highest concentration of usable vitamin E. Vegetable and seed oils, such as safflower, cottonseed, and sunflower seed oils, are also rich sources. Although soybean and corn oils contain much vitamin E, only about 10 percent is alpha-tocopherol, the active form of vitamin E.[58] Foods made from vegetable oils, such as margarine and salad dressings, as well as nuts and seeds, also are good sources. Although substantial amounts of vitamin E are found in strawberries and some green leafy vegetables, most fruits and vegetables contribute only small amounts. Animal products are medium to poor sources of vitamin E and vary widely in their content depending on the fat composition of the given animal's diet. **Figure 9.20** shows foods that are good sources of vitamin E.

In the typical U.S. diet, about 20 percent of vitamin E intake comes from salad oils, margarine, and shortening. Vegetables supply about 15 percent, and more than 12 percent comes from meat, poultry, and fish. Breakfast cereal supplies about 10 percent and fruit contributes about 9 percent of the dietary vitamin E.[59] NHANES III data suggest that American adults consume 8 to 12 milligrams of vitamin E per day from foods. However, this value is likely to be less than actual consumption due to typical underreporting of total fat and energy intake.[60]

Cooking, processing, and storage can reduce the vitamin E content of foods substantially. (See **Table 9.1.**) During the milling of wheat to make white flour, for instance, vitamin E–rich wheat germ is removed, and if chloride dioxide is used for the bleaching process, all vitamin E is lost. Refining and purifying vegetable oils takes a substantial toll on their vitamin E content. In fact, the by-products of the refining process contain so much vitamin E that they are used to make supplements. Oxygen is the destructive culprit that attacks vitamin E, and both light and heat accelerate oxidation. Safflower oils stored at room temperature for three months lose more than half of their vitamin E. Roasting destroys 80 percent of the vitamin E in almonds.

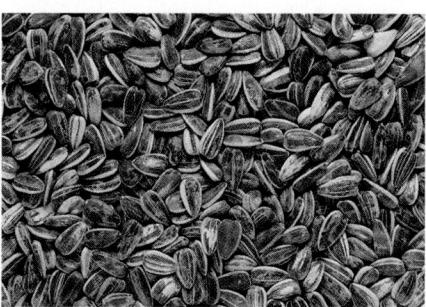

Figure 9.20 **Food sources of vitamin E.** Nuts and seeds, vegetable oil, and products made from vegetable oil, such as margarine, are among the best sources of vitamin E. Units are IU to be consistent with Daily Value definitions. **Note:** USDA tables list vitamin E in mg-alpha tocopherol equivalents. Conversion to IU was done using 1 mg-ATE=1.5 IU. The USDA Nutrient Database is not complete for vitamin E. **Source:** U.S. Department of Agriculture, Agricultural Research Service. USDA National Nutrient Database for Standard Reference, Release 18. 2005. http://www.ars.usda.gov/nutrientdata.

VITAMIN E

Daily Value = 30 IU

Exceptionally good source

Wheat germ oil	1 Tbsp	30.5 IU

High: 20% DV or more

Total cereal	30 g (~3/4 cup)	20.3 IU
Product 19 cereal	30 g (~1 cup)	20.3 IU
Sunflower seeds	30 g (~1 oz)	11.7 IU
Almonds	30 g (~1 oz)	11.6 IU
Tomato paste, canned	130 g (~1/2 cup)	8.4 IU
Cottonseed oil	1 Tbsp	7.2 IU
Safflower oil	1 Tbsp	7.0 IU
Special K cereal	30 g (~1 cup)	6.9 IU
Hazelnuts	30 g (~1 oz)	6.8 IU

Good: 10–19% DV

Spinach, frozen, cooked	85 g (~1/2 cup)	4.5 IU
Corn oil	1 Tbsp	4.2 IU
Peanuts	30 g (~1 oz)	3.8 IU
Turnip greens, cooked	85 g (~2/3 cup)	3.4 IU

Key Concepts: The RDA for vitamin E is 15 milligrams of alpha-tocopherol for both men and women. Vitamin E is found in wheat germ, vegetable and seed oils, and products made from these oils, such as salad dressing and margarine. Processing foods can reduce their vitamin E content.

Vitamin E Deficiency

Because of the widespread use of vegetable oils and other sources in the food supply, vitamin E deficiency is rare in North America. Most deficiencies occur in people with fat-malabsorption syndromes such as cystic fibrosis. One feature of vitamin E deficiency is premature **hemolysis**—the breakdown of red blood cells. Without vitamin E to protect the cells against oxidation, destruction of cell membranes is rampant, causing red blood cells to burst. Hemolysis, and the associated anemia (called hemolytic anemia), is most often seen in infants born prematurely, before vitamin E has been transferred from mother to fetus in the last weeks of pregnancy. Special formulas and supplemental vitamin E are administered to premature babies to help correct the problem.

In children and adults, fat-malabsorption disorders and subsequent vitamin E deficiency usually cause neurological problems that affect the spinal cord and peripheral nerves. In adults, malabsorption must be prolonged, from 5 to 10 years, before signs of deficiency surface.

Vitamin E Toxicity

Vitamin E is relatively nontoxic, especially compared with fat-soluble vitamins A and D. One hazard of large doses of vitamin E, however, is that the dose counters vitamin K's blood-clotting mechanism, described in the next section. People who take anticoagulant medications such as warfarin (Coumadin) or aspirin to prevent blood clots should confer with a physician before they self-prescribe large doses of vitamin E.

The antioxidant effects of vitamin E along with its inhibitory effects on platelet adhesion make it a logical choice for reducing heart disease risk. Observational studies support this theory, but results of clinical trials are limited and inconclusive.[61] It is not yet appropriate to recommend high vitamin E intake to reduce risk of chronic disease. For adults, the UL is 1,000 milligrams per day of any form of supplemental alpha-tocopherol.[62] Larger amounts can cause bleeding.[63] An analysis of 19 studies with more

hemolysis The breakdown of red blood cells that usually occurs at the end of a red blood cell's normal life span. This process releases hemoglobin.

Table 9.1 Reported Storage and Processing Losses of Vitamin E

Food	Test Conditions	Vitamin E Loss
Peanut oil	Frying at 347°F (175°C) 30 minutes	32%
Safflower oil	Stored at room temperature, 3 months	55%
Tortillas	Stored at room temperature, 12 months	95%
Almonds	Roasting	80%
Wheat germ	Storage at 39°F (4°C) 6 months	10%
Wheat	Processing to white flour	92%
Bread	Baking	5–50%

Source: *Vitamin E Factbook*, LaGrange, IL: VERIS, 1999. Reprinted with the written consent of Veris Research Information Services.

than 135,000 patients with chronic disease found that supplementation of 400 IU (approximately 270 milligrams) or more can increase mortality and should be avoided.[64]

Key Concepts: *Deficiencies of vitamin E are rare in adults, occurring primarily in people with fat-malabsorption syndromes. Preterm infants also run a high risk of vitamin E deficiency because they are delivered before the nutrient has a chance to move from the mother to the infant. Hemolysis is the hallmark of such a deficiency. Vitamin E is relatively nontoxic, though large doses interfere with blood clotting.*

Vitamin K

In 1929 Danish researcher Henrik Dam discovered a nutrient that plays a crucial role in blood clotting. He named it vitamin "K" for "koagulation." Although most people give little thought to consuming enough of this nutrient, vitamin K stands between life and death. Without vitamin K to promote blood clotting, a single cut would eventually lead to death by blood loss.

Vitamin K is a family of compounds known as quinones. It includes **phylloquinone** (K$_1$) from plant sources, **menaquinones** (collectively known as K$_2$) from animal sources and synthesized by our intestinal bacteria, and the synthetic substances **menadione**, Synkayvite, and Hykinone (collectively known as K$_3$). Phylloquinone is the major form in the diet and the most biologically active. Menaquinone is only 70 percent as active, and the synthetics drop to 20 percent. Phylloquinone, menaquinone, and the synthetic compound menadione are fat-soluble and primarily stored in the liver. These stores are relatively small and used up rapidly.

phylloquinone The form of vitamin K that comes from plant sources. Also known as vitamin K$_1$.

menaquinones Forms of vitamin K that come from animal sources. Also produced by intestinal bacteria, they are collectively known as vitamin K$_2$.

menadione A medicinal form of vitamin K that can be toxic to infants. Also known as vitamin K$_3$.

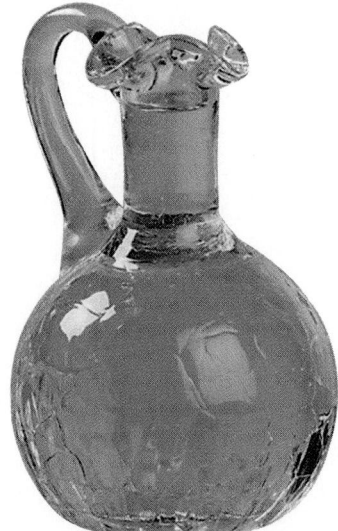

The synthetic compounds Synkayvite and Hykinone are water-soluble. These forms are well suited to the treatment of vitamin K deficiency caused by fat-malabsorption disorders. Menadione is considered an unsafe supplemental form of vitamin K.

Functions of Vitamin K

When you get a cut, small or large, and start to bleed, a series of reactions forms a clot that stops the flow of blood. This cascade of reactions involves the production of a series of proteins, and ultimately the protein fibrin. (See **Figure 9.21**.) Four of the procoagulation proteins in the cascade are vitamin K dependent, and all require calcium for activation. For example, vitamin K converts the precursor protein preprothrombin to prothrombin by adding carbon dioxide to glutamic acid (an amino acid) in the protein.

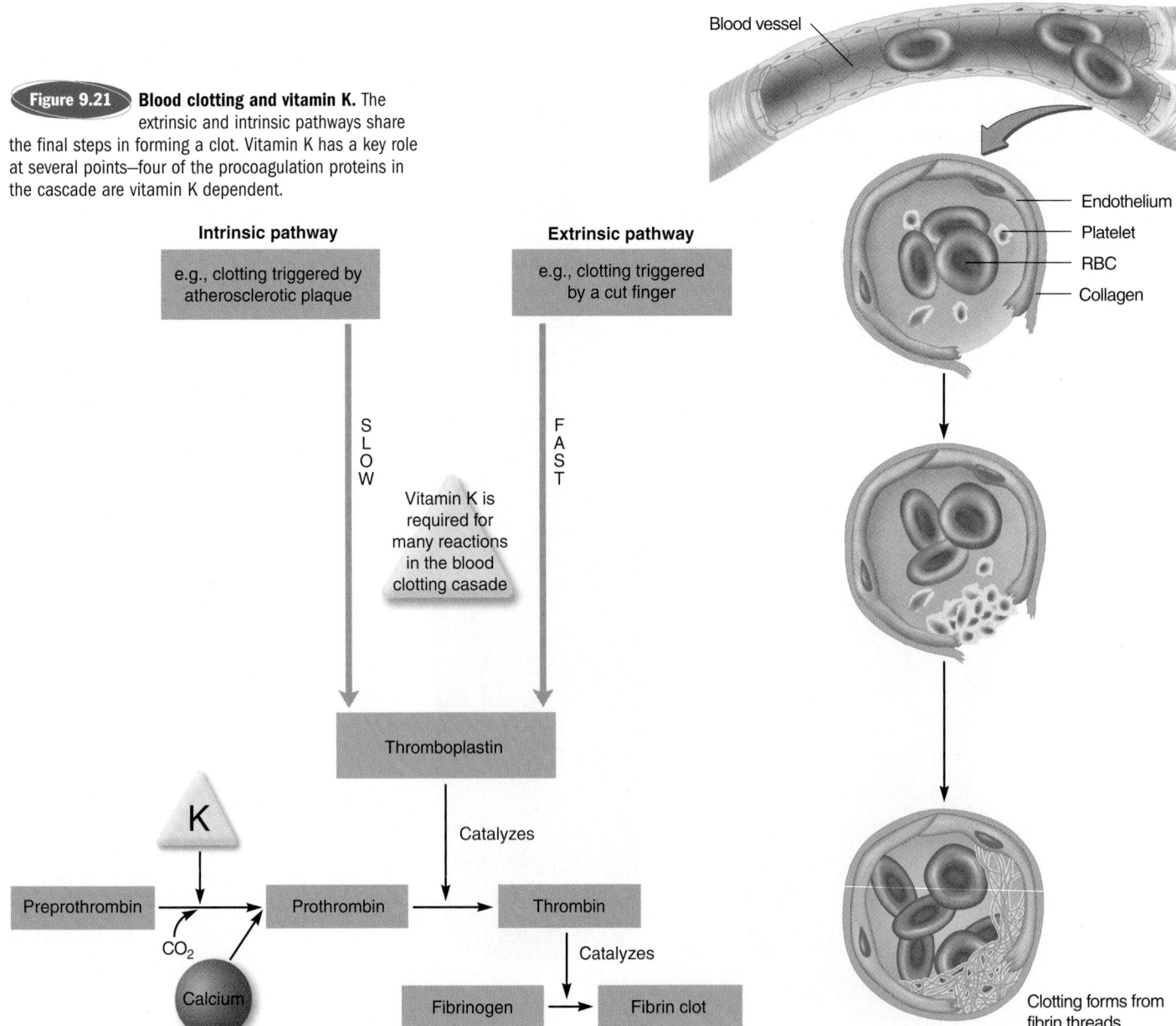

Figure 9.21 **Blood clotting and vitamin K.** The extrinsic and intrinsic pathways share the final steps in forming a clot. Vitamin K has a key role at several points—four of the procoagulation proteins in the cascade are vitamin K dependent.

Intrinsic pathway

e.g., clotting triggered by atherosclerotic plaque

Extrinsic pathway

e.g., clotting triggered by a cut finger

S L O W

F A S T

Vitamin K is required for many reactions in the blood clotting casade

Thromboplastin

Catalyzes

K

Preprothrombin → Prothrombin → Thrombin

CO_2

Calcium

Catalyzes

Fibrinogen → Fibrin clot

Blood vessel

Endothelium
Platelet
RBC
Collagen

Clotting forms from fibrin threads

This change imparts a calcium-binding capacity, which allows prothrombin to be changed to thrombin. These reactions are integral to the formation of a blood clot.

In addition to promoting the formation of blood clots, vitamin K assists bone formation.[65] The vitamin is thought to work by facilitating a process needed to allow the protein osteocalcin to strengthen the skeleton.

Vitamin K is important to the carboxylation of osteocalcin, which allows osteocalcin to become saturated with carboxyl groups. (See **Figure 9.22**.) Some research has shown a correlation between undercarboxylated osteocalcin and bone fractures; other evidence suggests an association between elevated risk of fractures and low levels of vitamin K in the blood.[66] At least two other bone proteins require vitamin K for carboxylation, underscoring the vitamin's importance to bone health.

Key Concepts: *Vitamin K was named for the Danish word "koagulation" because the nutrient works to promote the formation of blood clots. Vitamin K also is involved in bone health.*

Dietary Recommendations for Vitamin K

The AI for vitamin K for adult males is 120 micrograms. Recommendations for women are slightly lower: 90 micrograms per day. The AI doesn't change for pregnant and lactating women.

Dietary intake of vitamin K varies with age. In general, adults younger than 45 have intakes that range from 60 to 110 micrograms of phylloquinone per day. In contrast, intakes for adults older than 55 range from 80 to 210 micrograms of phylloquinone per day. Experts attribute this difference to the greater vegetable consumption of older adults compared with that of younger adults.[67]

As with other fat-soluble vitamins, vitamin K absorption depends on normal consumption and digestion of dietary fat. Absorption is poor in people with fat-malabsorption syndromes. Even under normal conditions, absorption of dietary vitamin K may be as low as 40 percent. (See **Figure 9.23**.)

Typical diets easily support vitamin K's role in blood clotting, but researchers have found preliminary evidence that more than 400 micrograms per day of dietary vitamin K may be necessary to support its role in bone health.[68]

Sources of Vitamin K

We obtain vitamin K from two sources: food (mostly plant food) and bacteria living in our colons. Dietary vitamin K is absorbed in the small intestine, and vitamin K produced by bacteria is absorbed in the colon.[69]

Phylloquinone is the primary form of dietary vitamin K. Green leafy vegetables, especially spinach, turnip greens, broccoli, and Brussels sprouts, supply substantial amounts of phylloquinone. Certain vegetable oils (soybean, cottonseed, canola, and olive) also are good sources.[70] Exposure to light degrades vitamin K, so the phylloquinone content of oils varies not only with brand and batch but also with storage time if the oils are bottled in transparent containers. Therefore, vegetable oils may not be a reliable source of vitamin K.

In general, animal products contain limited amounts of vitamin K. Small amounts of menaquinones are found in egg yolks and butter, and various cheeses contain moderate amounts. Soybean products such as tofu contain substantial amounts of menaquinones. Liver contains moderate amounts of

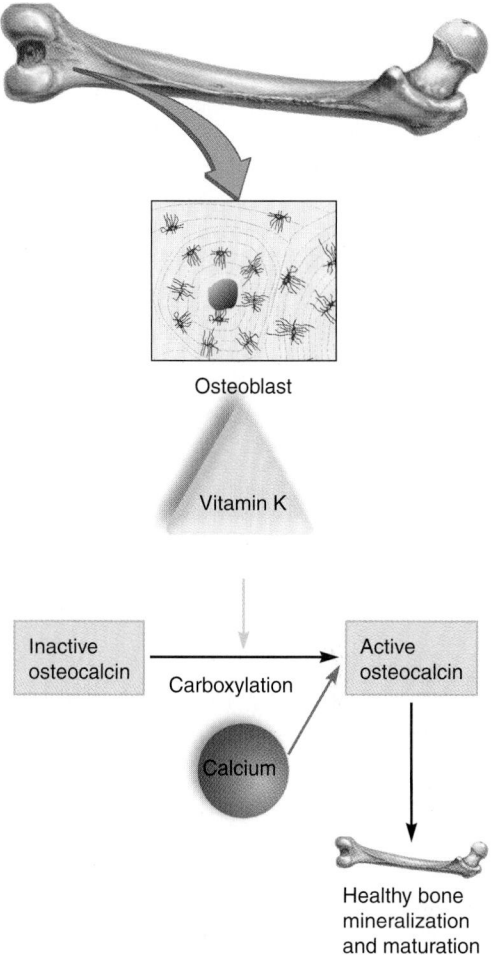

Figure 9.22 **Vitamin K and bone health**. Osteocalcin is an abundant bone protein that is required for bone mineralization and maturation. Vitamin K helps in the carboxylation of osteocalcin, greatly enhancing its calcium-binding properties.

menaquinones, but because most people rarely eat liver, it is unlikely to contribute much to the general consumption of vitamin K. The concentrations of menaquinones in other animal organs, such as kidney, heart, and muscle, are low and nutritionally insignificant.[71] **Figure 9.24** shows foods that contain vitamin K.

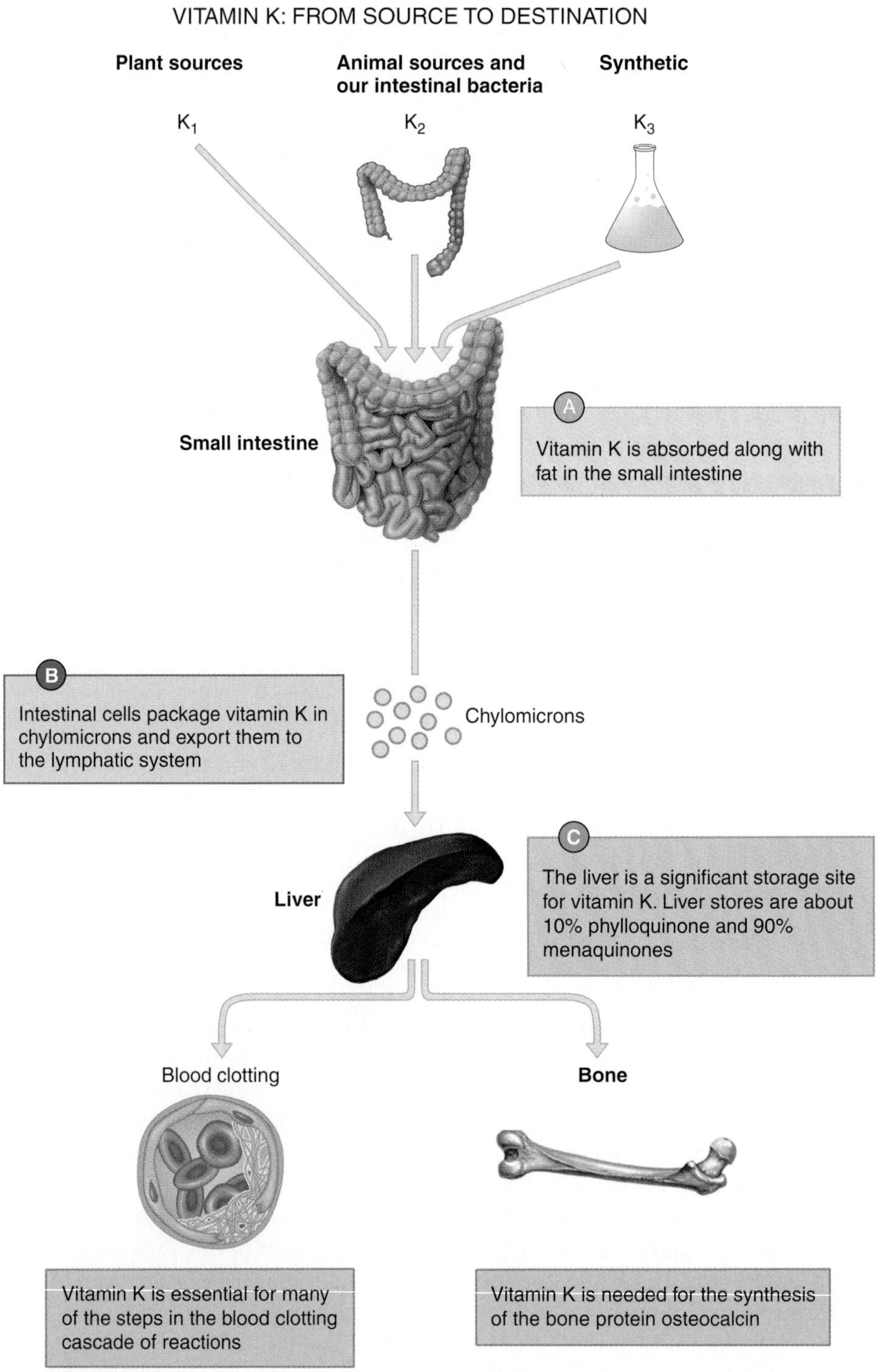

VITAMIN K: FROM SOURCE TO DESTINATION

Plant sources K_1

Animal sources and our intestinal bacteria K_2

Synthetic K_3

Small intestine

A Vitamin K is absorbed along with fat in the small intestine

B Intestinal cells package vitamin K in chylomicrons and export them to the lymphatic system

Chylomicrons

Liver

C The liver is a significant storage site for vitamin K. Liver stores are about 10% phylloquinone and 90% menaquinones

Blood clotting

Bone

Vitamin K is essential for many of the steps in the blood clotting cascade of reactions

Vitamin K is needed for the synthesis of the bone protein osteocalcin

Figure 9.23 **Vitamin K: from source to destination.** Green leafy vegetables are rich sources of vitamin K. Intestinal bacteria produce 10 to 15 percent of our vitamin K, much less than previously believed. Vitamin K is important in both blood clotting and bone health.

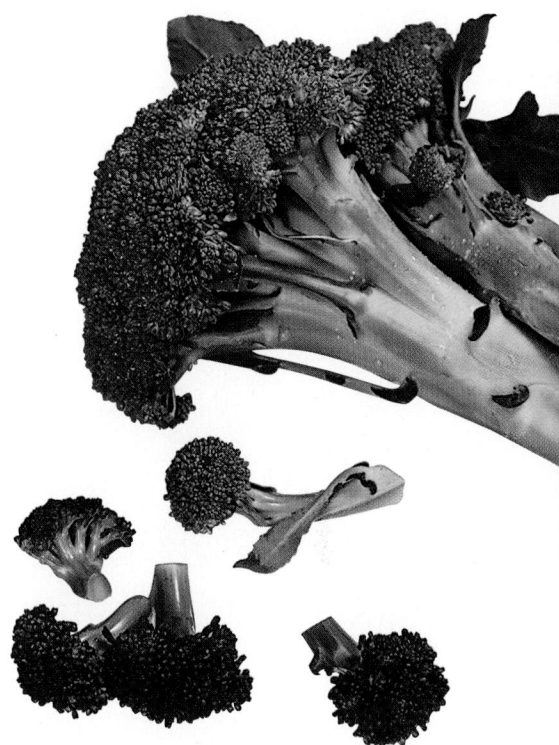

Key Concepts: *Dietary recommendations for vitamin K intake are small; the AI for adult men is 120 micrograms, and for adult women it is 90 micrograms. Vitamin K is found primarily in green vegetables and in some vegetable oils. Animal foods, in general, contain limited amounts of vitamin K.*

Vitamin K Deficiency

Although vitamin K has a crucial role in blood clotting, the body needs only small amounts. This makes vitamin K deficiency rare in healthy adults. On the other hand, preliminary research suggests that typical diets are supplying less than optimal amounts for bone health. Low dietary vitamin K intake is associated with reduced bone density in women[72] and also has been linked to increased fracture risk.[73]

People who suffer fat-malabsorption syndromes, such as celiac disease, sprue, cystic fibrosis, ulcerative colitis, and Crohn's disease, however, can develop vitamin K deficiency. Prolonged use of antibiotics may cause a deficiency because the drugs can destroy the intestinal bacteria that produce vitamin K. Prior to surgery, a patient's vitamin K status is often tested to assess the risk for hemorrhaging because antibiotics are frequently part of the treatment regimen.

Megadoses of vitamins A and E counteract the actions of vitamin K. Vitamin A appears to hamper intestinal absorption of vitamin K, and excess

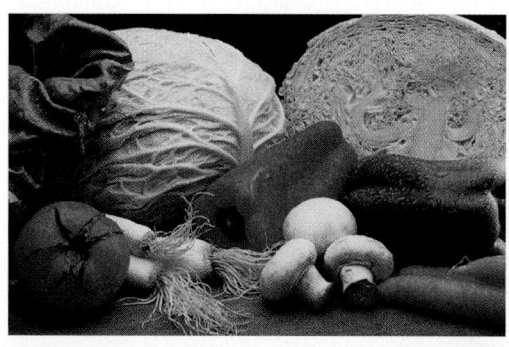

VITAMIN K

Daily Value = 80 μg

Exceptionally good sources

Food	Amount	Vitamin K
Kale, cooked	85 g (~1/2 cup)	694 μg
Spinach, raw	85 g (~3 cups)	410 μg
Turnip greens, raw	85 g (~3 cups)	213 μg
Broccoli, cooked	85 g (~1/2 cup)	120 μg
Romaine lettuce, raw	85 g (~1 1/2 cups)	87 μg
Cabbage, raw	85 g (~1 1/4 cups)	51 μg
Asparagus, cooked	85 g (~1/2 cup)	43 μg
Okra, cooked	85 g (~1/2 cup)	34 μg
Black-eyed peas, cooked	90 g (~1/2 cup)	33 μg
Blackberries, raw	140 g (~1 cup)	28 μg
Soybean oil	1 Tbsp.	27 μg
Blueberries, raw	140 g (~3/4 cup)	27 μg
Green beans, cooked	85 g (~2/3 cup)	14 μg
Cauliflower, raw	85 g (~3/4 cup)	13.6 μg
Artichokes, cooked	85 g (~1/2 cup)	13 μg
Tomato, green, raw	85 g (1 small)	8.6 μg

High: 20% DV or more

Good: 10–19% DV

Figure 9.24 **Food sources of vitamin K.** The best sources of vitamin K are vegetables, especially leafy greens and those in the cabbage family.

Source: U.S. Department of Agriculture, Agricultural Research Service. USDA National Nutrient Database for Standard Reference, Release 18. 2005. http://www.ars.usda.gov/nutrientdata.

vitamin E seems to decrease the vitamin K–dependent clotting factor, thus promoting bleeding.

Physicians prescribe anticoagulant medications, such as warfarin (Coumadin) to reduce the risk of internal blood clotting that could block blood vessels leading to the heart or brain. People who take anticoagulants should maintain a consistent pattern of vitamin K consumption, because large fluctuations can interfere with the effectiveness of these drugs.[74]

Newborn babies, especially those who are breastfed, also run a risk of vitamin K deficiency because at birth they lack the intestinal bacteria that produce the nutrient, and they don't receive much vitamin K via the diet. To prevent hemorrhaging, infants typically receive an injection of vitamin K at birth. This dose usually meets their needs for several weeks, until the vitamin K–producing bacteria begin to flourish.

Vitamin K Toxicity

Vitamin K is stored primarily in the liver and is also found in bone. Because the body excretes vitamin K much more rapidly than the other fat-soluble vitamins, toxicity from food is rare and no UL has been set for vitamin K. A vitamin K overdose can cause hemolytic anemia. This condition has been seen in newborns who receive vitamin K in the form of menadione, rather than the recommended form, phylloquinone.

Key Concepts: *Vitamin K deficiencies are extremely rare. Because it takes several weeks before the intestinal bacteria that produce vitamin K begin to flourish in the intestine, newborns are routinely given injections of vitamin K at birth. Vitamin K toxicity is rare because the body excretes the nutrient more readily than the other fat-soluble vitamins.*

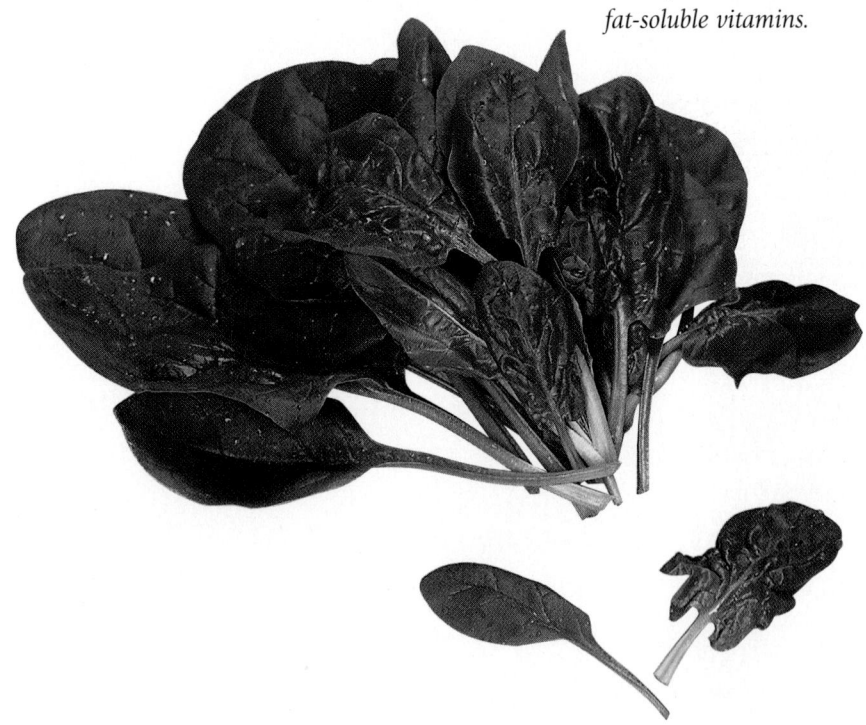

Label [to] **Table**

It is well known that milk is an excellent source of calcium, but did you know that milk also contains three of the four fat-soluble vitamins? Let's take a look at the Nutrition Facts from a carton of nonfat milk.

Nonfat milk	
Calories	90
Total Fat	0
Cholesterol	less than 5mg
Sodium	130mg
Total Carbohydrate	13g
Dietary Fiber	0g
Sugars	12g
Protein	9g
Vitamin A	10% DV
Vitamin C	4% DV
Calcium	30% DV
Iron	0% DV
Vitamin D	25% DV

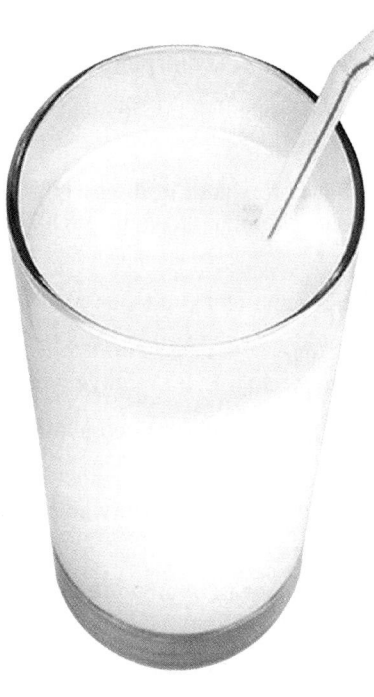

Milk contains the fat-soluble vitamins A and D. Vitamin A is found naturally in whole milk and is added to reduced-fat milks. All milks are fortified with vitamin D. Although it is true that fat-soluble vitamins can be toxic in large doses because they are stored in the body, the amounts added to milk are not of concern. Vitamin K is not listed on the label, but milk is a good source of this fat-soluble vitamin as well. (Each cup of milk provides 10 micrograms, which is 12.5% of the Daily Value.)

A one-cup serving of fortified milk provides 10 percent of the 5,000 IU Daily Value of vitamin A. If you drank three cups of milk per day, you would get about one-third of your recommended amount of vitamin A. That's good news because dietary vitamin A is not always easy to obtain. One form, retinol, is found mainly in liver and fish liver oil, which are not always staples of the typical American diet. The provitamin forms of vitamin A, the carotenoids, are found in green leafy and dark orange vegetables.

Vitamin D is important because it helps with the absorption of calcium and phosphorus, both important for bone health. Fish liver oil, sardines, and some fortified cereals are also good sources of vitamin D. As shown in the nutrition label, just one cup of milk gives you one-quarter of the vitamin D Daily Value. That's 25 percent of 10 µg, or 2.5 µg.

Keep in mind when selecting milk that nonfat (skim) milk contains vitamins A and D just like the higher-fat 2% and whole milk. Don't let the large banner "Vitamin A and D" printed on containers of whole milk trick you into thinking it contains more. It doesn't!

Nutrition Facts

Serving Size: 1 cup (240mL)
Servings Per Container about 8

Amount Per Serving

Calories 90   Calories from fat 0

	% Daily Value*
Total Fat 0g	0%
Saturated Fat 0g	0%
Trans Fat 0g	
Cholesterol less than 5mg	1%
Sodium 130mg	5%
Total Carbohydrate 13g	4%
Dietary Fiber 0g	0%
Sugars 12g	
Protein 9g	18%

Vitamin A 10%	•	Vitamin C 4%	
Calcium 30%	•	Iron 0%	
Vitamin D 25%			

* Percent Daily Values are based on a 2,000 calorie diet. Your daily values may be higher or lower depending on your calorie needs:

		Calories:	2,000	2,500
Total Fat	Less Than		65g	80g
Sat Fat	Less Than		20g	25g
Cholesterol	Less Than		300mg	300mg
Sodium	Less Than		2,400mg	2,400mg
Total Carbohydrate			300g	375g
Dietary Fiber			25g	30g
Protein			50g	65g

Calories per gram:
Fat 9 • Carbohydrate 4 • Protein 4

AMOUNTS PER 1 CUP SERVING:	FAT
WHOLE MILK	8g
FAT FREE MILK	0g

INGREDIENTS: GRADE A FAT FREE MILK, VITAMIN A PALMITATE, VITAMIN D₃.

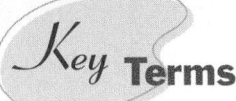

LEARNING *Portfolio* c h a p t e r 9

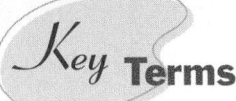

Key Terms

	page		page
antirachitic	398	osteoclasts	400
bleaching process	388	osteomalacia	405
calcitonin	400	osteoporosis	405
calcitriol	400	parathyroid hormone	400
carotenodermia	382	phylloquinone	411
carotenoids	384	preformed vitamin A	391
cones	386	provitamin A	384
cornea	386	provitamins	384
dark adaptation	388	retina	386
epithelial cells	390	retinal	384
epithelial tissue	390	retinoic acid	384
glutathione	406	retinoids	384
goblet cells	390	retinol	384
hemolysis	410	retinol activity equivalents	
hypercalcemia	405	(RAE)	391
hyperkeratosis	393	retinol-binding protein (RBP)	386
international units (IU)	391	retinyl esters	386
iodopsin	390	rhodopsin	388
lipid peroxidation	406	rickets	403
menadione	411	rods	386
menaquinones	411	stem cells	390
night blindness	388	teratogen	394
1,25-dihydroxyvitamin D_3		tocopherol	405
[1,25(OH)$_2$D$_3$]	400	tocotrienols	406
opsin	388	vitamin precursors	384
osteoblasts	400	xerophthalmia	392

Study Points

> Vitamins are organic substances the body needs in minuscule amounts.

> Two classes of vitamins exist: fat-soluble vitamins (A, D, E, K) and water-soluble vitamins (B vitamins and vitamin C).

> Vitamin A comes from preformed retinoids and the precursor carotenoids.

> Vitamin A functions in vision, cell differentiation, growth and development, and immune function.

> Sources of vitamin A include milk fat, liver, green leafy and yellow-orange vegetables, and yellow-orange fruits.

> Night blindness is an early symptom of vitamin A deficiency that, if not treated, can result in permanent blindness.

> Vitamin A is toxic when taken in large doses, causing liver damage and other problems.

> Vitamin D functions like a hormone and the body can synthesize it, but it is still considered a vitamin.

> A vitamin D precursor is produced from cholesterol when UV light hits the skin. Reactions in the liver and kidney are needed to produce a fully active vitamin D molecule.

> Vitamin D in foods is available mainly from fortified milk and other fortified products.

> The primary function of vitamin D is the regulation of blood levels of calcium.

> Vitamin D deficiency contributes to skeletal problems.

> Toxicity of vitamin D can develop with doses just a few times larger than the AI level.

> Vitamin E is an important antioxidant in the body and may help reduce the risk of chronic diseases such as heart disease and cancer.

> Vitamin E is found in vegetable oils and foods made from those oils.

> Deficiency and toxicity of vitamin E are relatively rare.

> Vitamin K is an important factor in blood coagulation.

> Although synthesized by intestinal bacteria, most of the vitamin K in the body comes from dietary sources, especially green vegetables.

> Vitamin K deficiency is rare, but newborns are susceptible if not given an injection of vitamin K at birth.

> Because the body excretes vitamin K easily, toxicity is unlikely.

Study Questions

1. **List at least three characteristics of fat-soluble vitamins.**

2. **List the four fat-soluble vitamins by their general names and specific active forms.**

3. **What are the main roles of vitamin A in the body?**

4. **What vitamin deficiency is associated with night blindness?**

5. **What antioxidant is responsible for the yellow-orange color of cantaloupes?**

6. **Which fat-soluble vitamin is considered a hormone? What organs do this hormone affect?**

7. **From what precursor can vitamin D be synthesized?**

8. **What are the toxicity and deficiency symptoms of vitamin E?**

9. **How does a vitamin K deficiency lead to the inability to form a blood clot?**

10. **Which two fat-soluble vitamins are most toxic? Least toxic?**

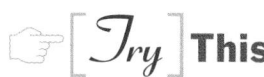 **This**

The PUFA Protection Challenge: Vitamin E Versus Oxygen

The object of this experiment is to see if vitamin E protects polyunsaturated fats (PUFAs) from oxidation. You'll need two glasses, one bottle of either safflower or corn oil, and some liquid vitamin E gel caps (can be purchased at any pharmacy). Pour equal amounts of oil in each of the glasses. Bite a hole in 10 of the vitamin E gel caps and squeeze their contents into ONE of the glasses. Mark this glass with tape and write the letter E on it. Let the glasses sit uncovered on a countertop for several days or weeks. Check the freshness or rancidity of the oils by smelling them and noting whether they look clear or cloudy. Over time, one will become more rancid than the other. Which glass container won the challenge—the one with or without vitamin E? Why?

What About Bobbie?

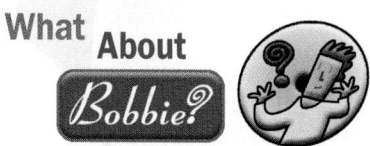

Let's check out Bobbie's intake of vitamin A. Refresh yourself with her day of eating in Chapter 1. How do you think Bobbie did in terms of this fat-soluble vitamin? Her intake of 493 μg RAE is about 70 percent of the RDA of 700 μg RAE, so Bobbie is likely meeting her needs for vitamin A. Here are her best vitamin A sources:

Food	Vitamin A (μg RAE)
Carrot (2 Tbsp)	193
Cream cheese (3 Tbsp)	97
Spaghetti sauce (3 oz)	83
Cheese pizza (1 slice)	83
Salsa (1/2 cup)	43

Bobbie's best sources of vitamin A were both preformed vitamin A sources (animal-origin foods such as cream cheese and pizza cheese) and foods with vitamin A precursors (e.g., beta-carotene from carrots.)

Here are some ways she could improve her vitamin A intake:

- Use spinach greens as the base of her salad instead of iceberg lettuce.
- Continue adding shredded carrots to her salad and consider adding them to her sandwich, too.
- Add a slice or two of tomato on top of the bagel with cream cheese.
- Alternate bagels (not high in vitamin A) and fortified cereals (high in vitamin A) for breakfast. This change would also add some milk to her diet, which would further increase her vitamin A intake (~140 μg RAE per cup).

References

1 Mahan KL, Escott-Stump S, eds. *Krause's Food, Nutrition, and Diet Therapy*. 11th ed. Philadelphia: WB Saunders, 2004.

2 Guyton AC, Hall JE. *Textbook of Medical Physiology*. 10th ed. Philadelphia: WB Saunders, 2000.

3 McCollough FS, Northrop-Clewes CA, Thurnham DI. The effect of vitamin A on epithelial integrity. *Proc Nutr Soc*. 1999;58(2):289–293.

4 Semba RD. The role of vitamin A and related retinoids in immune function. *Nutr Rev*. 1998;56(1 pt 2):S38–S48.

5 Institute of Medicine, Food and Nutrition Board. *Dietary Reference Intakes for Vitamin A, Vitamin K, Arsenic, Boron, Chromium, Copper, Iron, Manganese, Molybdenum, Nickel, Silicon, Vanadium, and Zinc*. Washington, DC: National Academy Press, 2001.

6 McCollough FS, Northrop-Clewes CA, Thurnham DI. Op. cit.

7 Semba RD. Op. cit.

8 Feskanich D, Singh V, Willett WC, Colditz GA. Vitamin A intake and hip fractures among postmenopausal women. *JAMA*. 2002;287:47–54; and Michaelsson K, Lithell H, Vessby B, Melhus H. Serum retinol levels and the risk of fracture. *N Engl J Med*. 2003;348:287–294.

9 Rothman KJ, Moore LL, Singer MR, et al. Teratogenicity of high vitamin A intake. *N Engl J Med*. 1995;333(21):1360–1373; and Oakley GP, Erickson JD. Vitamin A and birth defects. *N Engl J Med*. 1995;333(21):1414–1415.

10 Koo J. Acne: psychological effects are more than skin deep. *Skin Care Today*. 1998;4:4–5.

11 Institute of Medicine, Food and Nutrition Board. *Dietary Reference Intakes for Vitamin C, Vitamin E, Selenium, and Carotenoids*. Washington, DC: National Academy Press, 2000.

12 Olson JA, Krinsky NI. Introduction: the colorful, fascinating world of the carotenoids: important physiologic modulators. *FASEB J*. 1995;9:1547–1550.

13 Institute of Medicine, Food and Nutrition Board. 2000. Op. cit.

14 Jacob RA, Burri BJ. Oxidative damage and defense. *Am J Clin Nutr*. 1996;63:985S–990S.

15 Rock CL, Jacob RA, Bowen PE. Update on the biological characteristics of the antioxidant micronutrients: vitamin C, vitamin E, and the carotenoids. *J Am Diet Assoc*. 1996;96:693–702.

16 Santos MS, Meydani SN, Leka L, et al. Natural killer cell activity in elderly men is enhanced by beta-carotene supplementation. *Am J Clin Nutr*. 1996;64:772–777.

17 Hughes DA, Wright AJ, Finglas PM, et al. The effect of beta-carotene supplementation on the immune function of blood monocytes from healthy male nonsmokers. *J Lab Clin Med*. 1997;129:309–317.

18 Gollnick H, Hopfenmuller W, Hemmes C, et al. Systemic beta-carotene plus topical UV sunscreen are an optimal protection against harmful effects of natural UV sunlight: results of the Berlin-Eilath study. *Eur J Dermatol*. 1996;6:200–205; and Fuller CJ, Faulkner H, Bendich A, et al. Effect of beta-carotene supplementation on photosuppression of delayed-type hyperactivity in normal young men. *Am J Clin Nutr*. 1992;56:684–690.

19 Krinsky NI, Landrum JT, Bone RA. Biologic mechanisms of the protective role of lutein and zeaxanthin in the eye. *Annu Rev Nutr*. 2003;23:171–201.

20 Sies H, Stahl W. Non-nutritive bioactive constituents of plants: lycopene, lutein, and zeaxanthin. *Int J Vitam Nutr Res*. 2003:73(2):95–100.

21 Institute of Medicine, Food and Nutrition Board. 2000. Op. cit.

22 Christen WG, Manson JE, Glynn RJ, et al. A randomized trial of beta carotene and age-related cataract in US physicians. *Arch Ophthalmol*. 2003;121(3):372–378.

23 Rock CL, Jacob RA, Bowen PE. Op. cit.; and Zhang LX, Cooney RV, Bertram JS. Carotenoids up-regulate connexin-43 gene expression independent of their provitamin A or antioxidant properties. *Cancer Res*. 1992;52:5707–5712.

24 Fairfield KM, Fletcher RH. Vitamins in chronic disease prevention in adults: scientific review. *JAMA*. 2002;287:3116–3126.

25 Rock CL, Jacob RA, Bowen PE. Op. cit.

26 Institute of Medicine, Food and Nutrition Board. 2000. Op. cit.

27 Institute of Medicine, Food and Nutrition Board. 2001. Op. cit.

28 Mangels AR, Holden JM, Beecher GR, et al. Carotenoid content of fruits and vegetables: an evaluation of analytic data. *J Am Diet Assoc*. 1993;93:284–296.

29 Rock CL, Lovalo JL, Emenhiser C, et al. Bioavailability of beta-carotene is lower in raw than in processed carrots and spinach in women. *J Nutr*. 1998;128(5):913–916.

30 Hinds TS, West WL, Knight EM. Carotenoids and retinoids: a review of research, clinical, and public health applications. *J Clin Pharmacol*. 1997;37:551–558.

31 Institute of Medicine, Food and Nutrition Board. 2000. Op. cit.

32 Fairfield KM, Fletcher RH. Op. cit.; and Wright ME, Mayne ST, Swanson CA, Sinha R, Alavanja MC. Dietary carotenoids, vegetables, and lung cancer risk in women: the Missouri women's health study (United States). *Cancer Causes Control*. 2003;14(1):85–89.

33 Bischoff-Ferrari HA, Dawson-Hughes B, Willett WC, et al. Effect of vitamin D on falls: a meta-analysis. *JAMA*. 2004;291:1999–2006.

34 Fairfield KM, Fletcher RH. Op. cit.

35 Eastell R, Riggs BL. Vitamin D and osteoporosis. In: Feldman D, Glorieux FH, Piek JW, eds. *Vitamin D*. San Diego: Academic Press, 1997:695–711.

36 Holick MF. Vitamin D: a millennium perspective. *J Cell Biochem*. 2003;88(2):296–307.

37 Lieberman D, Prindiville S, Weiss D, Willett W, for VA Cooperative Study Group 380. Risk factors for advanced colonic neoplasia and hyperplastic polyps in asymptomatic individuals. *JAMA*. 2003;290(22):2959–2967; and Bouillon R, Moody T, Sporn M, Barrett JC, Norman AW. NIH deltanoids meeting on Vitamin D and cancer. Conclusion and strategic options. *J Steroid Biochem Mol Biol*. 2005;97:3–5.

38 Holick MF. Sunlight and vitamin D for bone health and prevention of autoimmune diseases, cancers, and cardiovascular disease. *Am J Clin Nutr*. 2004;80(suppl):1678S–1688S.

39 Institute of Medicine, Food and Nutrition Board. *Dietary Reference Intakes for Calcium, Phosphorus, Magnesium, Vitamin D, and Fluoride*. Washington, DC: National Academy Press, 1997.

40 Bischoff-Ferrari HA, Giovannucci E, Willett WC, et al. Estimation of optimal serum concentrations of 25-hydroxy-vitamin D for multiple health outcomes. *Am J Clin Nutr*. 2006;84(1):18–28.

41 Vitamin D deficiency deemed widespread. *Tufts University Health & Nutrition Letter*. May 1998;16(3):1.

42 American Academy of Dermatology. The sun and your skin. http://www.aad.org/NR/exeres/B1BBACE1-A0D0-4565-AA74-63B7E6957239.htm?NRMODE=Published. Accessed 7/30/06.

43 Vitamin D deficiency: the silent epidemic. *Nutr Action*. 1997; 24(8):4.

44 Chen TC, Shao A, Heath H, Holick MF. An update on the vitamin D content of fortified milk from the United States and Canada. *N Engl J Med*. 1993;329:1507; and Holick MF, Shao Q, Liu WW, Chen TC. The vitamin D content of fortified milk and infant formula. *N Engl J Med*. 1992;326:1178–1181.

45 Gessner BD, de Schweinitz E, Petersen KM, Lewandowski C. Nutritional rickets among breast-fed black and Alaska Native children. *Alaska Med*. 1997;39:72–74, 87; Centers for Disease Control and Prevention. Severe malnutrition among young children—Georgia, January 1997–June 1999. *MMWR*. 2001;50:224–227; Rowe P. Why is rickets resurgent in the USA? *Lancet* 2001;357:1100; and Yu JW, Pekeles G, Legault L, et al. Milk allergy and vitamin D deficiency rickets: a common disorder associated with an uncommon disease. *Ann Allergy Asthma Immunol*. 2006;96(4):615–619.

46 Gessner BD, de Schweinitz E, Petersen KM, Lewandowski C. Op. cit.

47 Eastell R, Riggs BL. Vitamin D and osteoporosis. In: Feldman D, Glorieux FH, Piek JW, eds. *Vitamin D*. San Diego: Academic Press, 1997:695–711; and Chapuy M-C, Meunier PJ. Vitamin D insufficiency in adults and the elderly. In: Feldman D, Glorieux FH, Piek JW, eds. Op. cit., 679–693.

48 Malabanan AO, Holick MF. Vitamin D and bone health in postmenopausal women. *J Women's Health*. 2003;12(2): 151–156.

49 Chapuy MC, Arlot ME, Duboeuf F, et al. Vitamin D3 and calcium to prevent hip fractures in elderly women. *N Engl J Med*. 1992;327:1637–1642; and Chapuy MC, Arlot ME, Delmas PD, Meunier PJ. Effect of calcium and cholecalciferol treatment for three years on hip fractures in elderly women. *BMJ*. 1994; 308:1081–1082.

50 Thomas MK, Lloyd-Jones DM, Thadhani RF, et al. Hypovitaminosis D in medical inpatients. *N Engl J Med*. 1998; 338:777–783.

51 Need AG, Morris HA, Horowitz M, Nordin C. Effects of skin thickness, age, body fat, and sunlight on serum 25-hydroxyvitamin D. *Am J Clin Nutr*. 1993;58:882–885; and Holick MF, Matsuoka LY, Wortsman J. Age, vitamin D, and solar ultraviolet [letter]. *Lancet*. 1989;2(8671):1104–1105.

52 Moore C. Vitamin D intake in the United States. *J Am Diet Assoc*. 2004;104:980–983.

53 Adams JS, Lee G. Gains in bone mineral density with resolution of vitamin D intoxication. *Ann Intern Med*. 1997;127(3): 203–206; and Marriott BM. Vitamin D supplementation: a word of caution. *Ann Intern Med*. 1997;127(3):231–233.

54 Jialal I, Traber M, Devaraj S. Is there a vitamin E paradox? *Curr Opin Lipidol*. 2001;12:49–53; and Kaul N, Devaraj S, Jialal I. Alpha-tocopherol and atherosclerosis. *Exp Biol Med*. 2001; 226:5–12.

55 Institute of Medicine, Food and Nutrition Board. 2000. Op. cit.

56 Meydani SN, Han SN, Hamer DH. Vitamin E and respiratory infection in the elderly. *Ann N Y Acad Sci*. 2004;1031:214–222.

57 Institute of Medicine, Food and Nutrition Board. 2000. Op. cit.

58 Ibid.

59 Ibid.

60 Ibid.

61 Fairfield KM, Fletcher RH. Op. cit.

62 Institute of Medicine, Food and Nutrition Board. 2000. Op. cit.

63 Horwitt MK. Critique of the requirement for vitamin E. *Am J Clin Nutr*. 2001;73:1003–1005.

64 Miller ER III, Pastor-Barriuso R, Dalal D, et al. Meta-analysis: high-dosage vitamin E supplementation may increase all-cause mortality. *Ann Intern Med*. 2005;142:37–46.

65 Niemeier A, Kassem M, Toedter K, et al. Expression of LRP1 by human osteoblasts: a mechanism for the delivery of lipoproteins and vitamin K(1) to bone. *J Bone Miner Res*. 2005; 20:283–293.

66 Sokoll LJ, Booth SL, O'Brien ME, et al. Changes in serum osteocalcin, plasma phylloquinone, and urinary gamma-carboxyglutamic acid in response to altered intakes of dietary phylloquinone in human subjects. *Am J Clin Nutr*. 1997;65:779–784.

67 Booth SL, Suttie JW. Dietary intake and adequacy of vitamin K. *J Nutr*. 1998;128(5):785–788.

68 "Special K" takes on new meaning. *Tufts University Health & Nutrition Letter*. 1997;15(5):1, 7.

69 Institute of Medicine, Food and Nutrition Board. 2001. Op. cit.

70 Booth SL, Davidson KW, Lichtenstein AH, Sadowski JA. Plasma concentrations of dihydro-vitamin K1 following dietary intake of a hydrogenated vitamin K1-rich vegetable oil. *Lipids*. 1996;31:709–713; and Fenton ST, Price RJ, Bolton-Smith C, Harrington D, Shearer MJ. Nutrient sources of phylloquinone (vitamin K1) in Scottish men and women [abstract]. *Proc Nutr Soc*. 1997;56:301.

71 Shearer MJ, Bach A, Kohlmeier M. Chemistry, nutritional sources, tissue distribution and metabolism of vitamin K with special reference to bone health. *J Nutr*. 1996;126(suppl): 1181S–1186S.

72 Booth SL, Broe KE, Gagnon DR, et al. Vitamin K intake and bone mineral density in women and men. *Am J Clin Nutr*. 2003;77(2):512–516.

73 Fairfield KM, Fletcher RH. Op. cit.

74 Booth SL, Charnley JM, Sadowski JA, et al. Dietary vitamin K1 and stability of oral anticoagulation: proposal of a diet with constant vitamin K1 content. *Thrombosis Haemostasis*. 1997; 77:504–509.

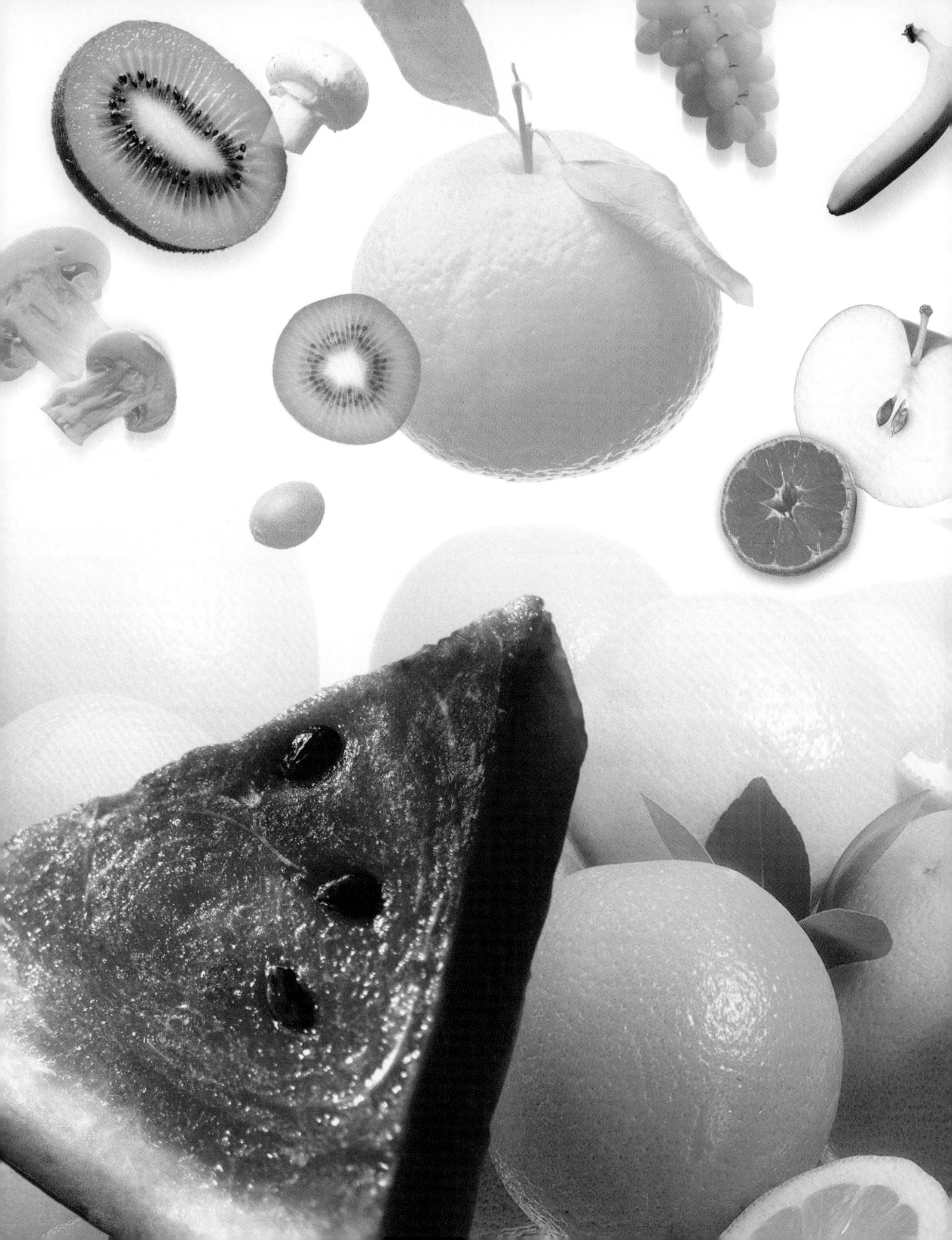

Chapter 10

Water-Soluble Vitamins

Think About It

1 When cooking vegetables, how often do you think about vitamin loss?

2 Because of a friend's suggestion, you take a vitamin pill, and it causes intense flushing and itching. What has she probably given you, and what does your reaction tell you?

3 You decide to follow a vegetarian lifestyle. What vitamin deficiency should you watch out for?

4 Do you know anyone who takes vitamin C to prevent colds? What do you think of this strategy?

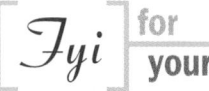

Fyi for your Information

This chapter's FYI boxes include practical information on the following topics:
- Fresh, Frozen, or Canned? Raw or Cooked?
- The B Vitamins and Heart Disease

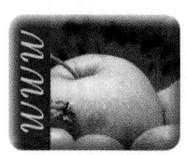

The Web site for this book offers many useful tools and is a great source for additional nutrition information for both students and instructors. Visit the site at nutrition.jbpub.com for information on water-soluble vitamins. You'll find exercises that explore the following topics:
- Safe Supplements
- Harmful Supplements
- Exercise and Water-Soluble Vitamins
- Overdosing on Niacin

Key to Illustrations

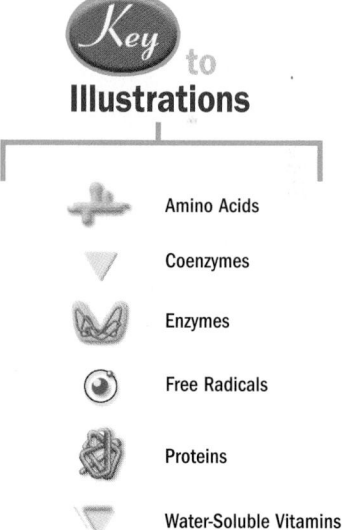

- Amino Acids
- Coenzymes
- Enzymes
- Free Radicals
- Proteins
- Water-Soluble Vitamins

What About Bobbie?

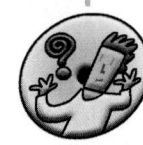

Track the choices Bobbie is making with Nutritionist Pro or EatRight Analysis software.

*F*eeling tired, run down, stressed out? Burning the candle at both ends? Too many workouts wearing you out? You've heard that vitamins give you energy. So a lack of energy must be a signal that you need more vitamins, right? Well, probably not.

First the facts: Because the body does not metabolize vitamins to yield ATP, they are not a source of energy. However, many of the B vitamins (water-soluble vitamins) facilitate the metabolic reactions that release energy from carbohydrate, fat, and protein. So in a sense, vitamins help you get energy by allowing carbohydrate, fat, and protein to become cellular fuel.

In times of stress, you need more energy than normal and therefore more vitamins, so a supplement is in order, right? Well, not really. First we need to define stress. Certainly physical stress (e.g., injury and illness) increases the body's need for energy, protein, and many vitamins and minerals to aid healing. But emotional stress (e.g., anxiety and fear) does not. It may seem that you expend a lot of mental energy studying for finals, but studying requires no more energy than sitting and chatting with your friends.

But surely if you do more physical exercise, you should take a vitamin, right? Again, not necessarily. Physical activity requires energy and therefore vitamins to help extract energy from food. But the food you consume to meet your energy needs for physical activity contains vitamins too, unless you meet your extra energy needs with chips and sodas! In most cases, healthful food choices—plenty of whole grains, fruits, vegetables, lean meats or meat alternatives, and low-fat dairy products—provide all the vitamins you need. So, check out your diet before you check out the vitamin supplements.

The Water-Soluble Vitamins: Eight Bs and a C

Water-soluble vitamins consist of the eight B vitamins and vitamin C. Scientists first viewed vitamin B as a single compound. However, after further study, they discovered that "it" was actually several vitamins. To differentiate the various B vitamins, scientists initially added numbers to the letter B—vitamins B_6 and B_{12}, for example. Today, with the exception of B_6 and B_{12}, we usually refer to the B vitamins by their names: thiamin (B_1), riboflavin (B_2), niacin (B_3), pantothenic acid, biotin, and folate.

Although fat-soluble vitamins tend to accumulate in the body, the kidneys readily remove and excrete excess water-soluble vitamins, with the exception of B_{12}. Also in contrast to fat-soluble vitamins, water-soluble vitamins are particularly susceptible to destruction by heat or alkalinity, which can break the chemical bonds between atoms. Some cooking practices are particularly harmful to vitamins in foods. Prolonged heat, such as

Quick Bites

What Do You Believe?

*T*hirty-five percent of Americans surveyed in 1997 said that they believed vitamin supplements were necessary to ensure good health. Women were more likely than men to believe they needed supplements.

Quick Bites

Is It a Fruit or a Vegetable?

*I*n the eighteenth century, botanists defined fruits as the organ surrounding the seeds. This definition considers cucumbers, eggplants, peppers, pea pods, and corn kernels as fruits. Legally, though, they are all vegetables. In the late 1800s, the U.S. Supreme Court, while trying the case of a tomato importer, established a definition based on linguistic custom and usage. The importer had to pay the vegetable tax.

beriberi Thiamin-deficiency disease. Symptoms include muscle weakness, loss of appetite, nerve degeneration, and edema in some cases.

that used to bake a vegetable casserole, tends to destroy the chemical bonds. Many cooks add baking soda, which is alkaline, to cooking water to reduce cooking time and intensify the vegetable's color. Vitamin C, thiamin, and riboflavin are especially vulnerable to heat and alkalinity. Water-soluble vitamins are hydrophilic by nature, and water will leach them from vegetables during cooking. Cooking only partially destroys the vitamin content of a food, and some cooking methods are less destructive than others. The best cooking methods—steaming, stir-frying, and microwaving—use minimal amounts of water.

Think About It 1

The B Vitamins

B vitamins act primarily as coenzymes, or as parts of coenzymes (compounds that enable specific enzymes to function). (See **Figure 10.1**.) The B vitamin part of a coenzyme helps catalyze the workings of metabolic pathways in cells. All B vitamins function in energy-producing metabolic reactions, and some also participate in other aspects of cellular metabolism.

Varied diets contain significant amounts of many vitamins, and vitamins often are added to foods such as cereals and other grain products. In the 1940s, the U.S. government mandated enrichment of bread and cereal products made from milled grains. During the milling process, much of the B vitamin content is removed along with the germ, bran, and husk. The addition of the B vitamins thiamin, riboflavin, and niacin helps restore the lost vitamins. Now, because of a 1998 FDA requirement, all enriched bread, flour, corn meal, pasta, rice, and other grains products must be fortified with folic acid.[1]

During the production of highly refined grain products, processing also removes vitamin B_6, magnesium, and zinc. Enrichment does not replace these nutrients. To ensure a good balance of nutrients, experts recommend that people regularly eat whole-grain products such as whole-wheat bread, brown rice, and oatmeal.

Thiamin

Although mentioned in ancient Chinese writings from 2,600 B.C.E., the thiamin deficiency disease **beriberi** remained largely unknown until the nineteenth century, when milling and refining grains became popular. In 1885 Dr. K. Takaki, Director General of the Japanese Naval Medical Services, demonstrated beriberi's dietary origins when he cured afflicted sailors by supplementing their diets with meat, milk, and whole grains.[2] Some years later, Christian Eijkman, a Dutch medical officer, induced beriberi in birds by feeding them only white rice, and then cured them by adding bran to their diet.[3] This led to the discovery of an "anti-beriberi" factor—thiamin.

Isolated in 1926, thiamin (also known as vitamin B_1) gets its name from *thio*, meaning "sulfur," and *amine*, the nitrogen-containing group in the vitamin. As **Figure 10.2** shows, thiamin consists of a sulfur-containing ring and a nitrogen-containing ring attached to a carbon atom. Heat easily breaks the bonds between the two rings and the carbon atom, so cooking reduces a food's thiamin content. Alkaline solutions (those with a pH of 8 or higher) also break these bonds.

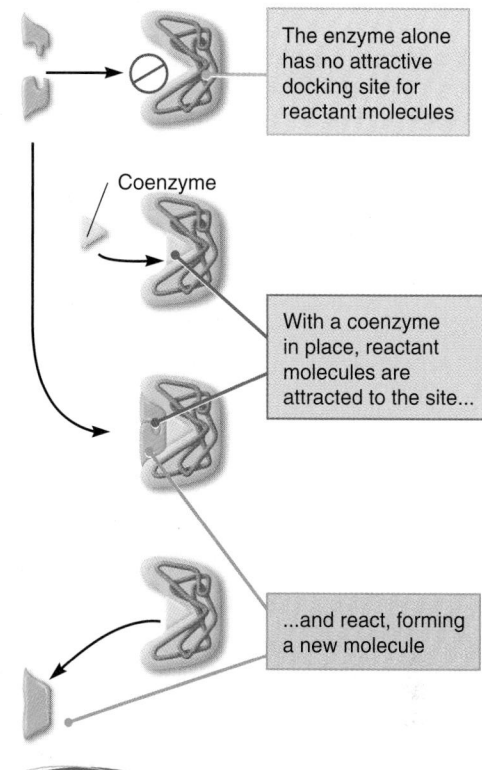

The enzyme alone has no attractive docking site for reactant molecules

Coenzyme

With a coenzyme in place, reactant molecules are attracted to the site...

...and react, forming a new molecule

Figure 10.1 **The coenzyme–enzyme partnership.** The B vitamins form coenzymes that enable specific enzymes to catalyze reactions.

THIAMIN

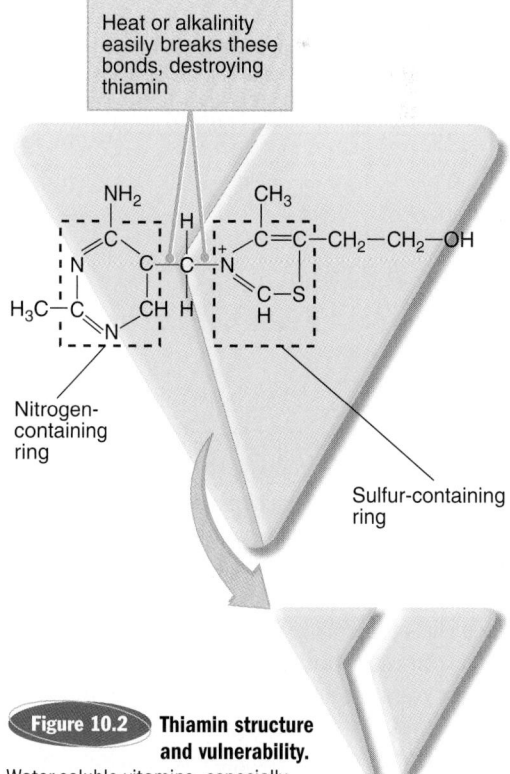

Heat or alkalinity easily breaks these bonds, destroying thiamin

Nitrogen-containing ring

Sulfur-containing ring

Figure 10.2 **Thiamin structure and vulnerability.** Water-soluble vitamins, especially thiamin, riboflavin, and vitamin C, are vulnerable to heat and alkalinity.

thiamin pyrophosphate (TPP) A coenzyme of which the vitamin thiamin is a part. It plays a key role in decarboxylation and helps drive the reaction that forms acetyl CoA from pyruvate during metabolism.

decarboxylation Removal of a carboxyl group (–COOH) from a molecule. The carboxyl group is then released as carbon dioxide (CO_2).

Functions of Thiamin

Like the other B vitamins, thiamin is an important participant in many energy-yielding reactions. Specifically, thiamin is the vitamin portion of the coenzyme **thiamin pyrophosphate (TPP)**, shown in **Figure 10.3**. TPP participates in a vital reaction known as **decarboxylation**, which removes a carboxyl group (–COOH) and releases it as carbon dioxide (CO_2). During glucose metabolism, for example, decarboxylation removes one carbon from the three-carbon substance pyruvate to form the two-carbon molecule acetyl CoA. (See **Figure 10.4**.) TPP is also involved in a decarboxylation step in the citric acid cycle.

Cells also use TPP in the pentose phosphate pathway, an alternative pathway to glycolysis. This series of reactions metabolizes glucose to make, among other products, the five-carbon monosaccharide deoxyribose for DNA synthesis, the five-carbon monosaccharide ribose for RNA synthesis, and the energy-rich molecule NADPH to help power biosynthesis.

Thiamin pyrophosphate also plays a role in nerve function, though the mechanism is still under investigation. Scientists suspect that TPP helps synthesize and regulate neurotransmitters—chemicals involved in the transmission of messages throughout the nervous system. TPP also may help produce energy to fuel nerve tissue.

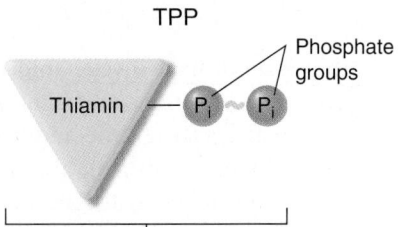

TPP

Thiamin pyrophosphate (TPP)

Figure 10.3 **Thiamin pyrophosphate (TPP).** Thiamin pyrophosphate contains the B vitamin thiamin and two phosphate groups.

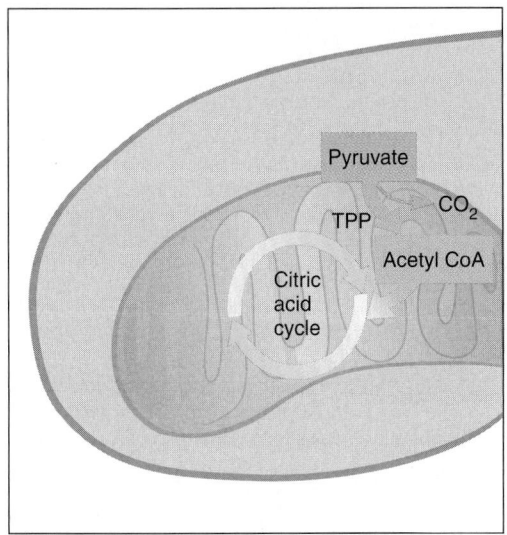

Figure 10.4 **TPP helps convert pyruvate to acetyl CoA.** In addition to coenzyme A and NAD⁺, three other catalytic cofactors—TPP, α-lipoic acid, and FAD—help convert pyruvate to acetyl CoA.

Dietary Recommendations for Thiamin

The small difference in the RDA for adult men and women reflects the differences in their average size and energy use. The RDA for adult men aged 19 years and older is 1.2 milligrams; for adult women of the same age, the RDA is 1.1 milligrams per day. Pregnancy and lactation increase energy requirements, so thiamin requirements rise during these life stages. Thiamin intake recommendations are 1.4 milligrams per day during pregnancy and

---

[*Fyi*] Fresh, Frozen, or Canned? Raw or Cooked?

FOR YOUR INFORMATION

Selecting and Preparing Foods to Maximize Vitamin Content

A food's vitamin content depends first on the original amount in the plant or animal while it is alive and growing. Although grazing materials and feed may have a minor impact on vitamin content, animal products tend to have fairly consistent levels. This reflects the animal's ability to concentrate and store vitamins. The vitamin content of plants, however, depends more on soil and growing conditions such as available moisture and sunlight. The maturity of a fruit or vegetable at the time it is harvested also influences its vitamin content.

Light, heat, air, acid, alkali, and cooking fluids can attack vitamins, so proper storage, processing, and cooking are important. Ideally, you should shop for produce as the Europeans do: choose fresh fruits and vegetables daily to minimize nutrient losses associated with prolonged storage. Barring that, choose clean, undamaged produce at each of your regular shopping trips. When storing foods, avoid temperature extremes, and minimize exposure to light and air with refrigeration or covered storage. It's best to eat fruits and vegetables soon after purchase; normal storage can decrease their vitamin content. The vitamin C content of

fresh green beans, for example, drops by half after six days at home.

What about frozen and canned foods? The heat processing used in canning fruits and vegetables does deplete small amounts of vitamins. Researchers at the University of Illinois determined, however, that most of what is lost ends up in the liquid in which the food is packed.[1] In addition, the vitamin content of canned foods is shelf stable and remains constant even after two years. The thiamin content of canned meats and beans is comparable to home-prepared versions. Vegetable sources of folate, such as spinach,

1.5 milligrams per day during lactation. If a person's diet supplies adequate energy and includes thiamin-rich foods, it generally contains adequate amounts of thiamin.

Sources of Thiamin

Thiamin is found throughout the food supply, though most foods contain only small amounts. Pork is one of the richest food sources of thiamin. Legumes (mature beans and peas), some nuts and seeds, and some types of fish and seafood are good sources. Most thiamin in the U.S. diet, however, comes from enriched or whole-grain products such as bread, pasta, rice, and ready-to-eat cereals.[4] **Figure 10.5** shows some foods that provide thiamin.

Meat (except pork and organ meats), dairy products, seafood, and most fruits contain very little thiamin. Eating a wide variety of foods is the best way to ensure adequate thiamin consumption.

There are few data from studies of humans on the bioavailability of thiamin from food.[5] See the section on thiamin toxicity for details about absorption of thiamin from supplements.

Thiamin Deficiency

In industrialized countries, thiamin deficiency usually is related to heavy alcohol consumption combined with limited food consumption. Alcoholics are at risk for thiamin deficiency for two reasons: (1) Alcohol contributes calories without contributing nutrients, and (2) alcohol interferes with absorption of thiamin and many other vitamins. The poor and the elderly also may be at risk of deficiency due to inadequate energy intake or consumption of nutrient-poor foods. Eating

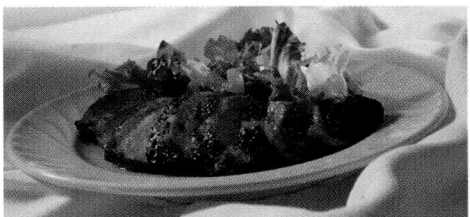

THIAMIN

Daily Value = 1.5 mg

High: 20% DV or more

Exceptionally good source

Total cereal	30 g (³/4 cup)	2.1 mg
Pork, loin roast, lean only, cooked	85 g (3 oz)	0.80 mg
Corn flakes cereal	30 g (1 cup)	0.64 mg
Ham, extra lean, cooked	85 g (3 oz)	0.59 mg
Cheerios cereal	30 g (1 cup)	0.54 mg
Bagel, plain	90 g (1 4" bagel)	0.48 mg
Fish, tuna, cooked	85 g (3 oz)	0.43 mg
White bread, enriched	50 g (2 slices)	0.41 mg
Fiber One cereal	30 g (¹/2 cup)	0.38 mg
Spaghetti, enriched, cooked	140 g (1 cup)	0.38 mg
Oatmeal, instant, fortified, cooked	1 cup	0.34 mg
Navy beans, cooked	90 g (~¹/2 cup)	0.34 mg

Good: 10–19% DV

Wheat germ	15 g (¹/4 cup)	0.28 mg
Orange juice, chilled	240 ml (1 cup)	0.28 mg
Sesame seeds	30 g (~1 oz)	0.24 mg
Rice, white, enriched, cooked	140 g (~ ³/4 cup)	0.23 mg
Salmon, cooked	85 g (3 oz)	0.23 mg
Soybeans, cooked	90 g (~¹/2 cup)	0.23 mg
Black beans, cooked	90 g (~¹/2 cup)	0.22 mg
Pecans	30 g (~1 oz)	0.20 mg
Grits, corn, enriched, cooked	1 cup	0.20 mg
Brazilnuts	30 g (~1 oz)	0.19 mg
Baked beans, canned	130 g (~¹/2 cup)	0.19 mg
Whole wheat bread	50 g (2 slices)	0.18 mg
Oysters, cooked	85 g (3 oz)	0.16 mg
Lentils, cooked	90 g (~¹/2 cup)	0.15 mg
Soy milk	240 ml (1 cup)	0.15 mg

Figure 10.5 **Food sources of thiamin.** Pork, whole and enriched grains, and fortified cereals are rich in thiamin. Most animal foods contain little thiamin. **Source:** U.S. Department of Agriculture, Agricultural Research Service. USDA National Nutrient Database for Standard Reference, Release 18. 2005. http://www.ars.usda.gov/nutrientdata.

retain most of their folate content when canned or frozen. The carotenes in vegetables and fruits are stable during the canning process. In fact, current research suggests the lycopene in tomatoes is a more effective antioxidant (it has been linked to reducing prostate cancer[2]) after tomatoes have been heated or canned.[3] Ready-to-drink orange juice loses about 2 percent of its vitamin C content each day once opened.[4]

Once fruits and vegetables are home and stored carefully, what is the best way to cook them? To maximize the vitamin content, think minimal—minimal amounts of heat, minimal

amounts of cooking water, and minimal exposure to air. Try to minimize handling the food before and during cooking. While dicing a food such as a potato reduces cooking time, it also exposes more surface area to vitamin-destroying influences. So, cut if you must, but not too small.

Steaming and microwaving are the best cooking methods for preserving vitamin content, because they minimize cooking time and water use. If you boil foods, try to use the cooking water for sauces, stews, or soups, because it contains many of the water-soluble vitamins lost from the food during cooking.

To retain the most vitamins in your food, be gentle with storage and handling, and kind with cooking. Minimize (heat, water, air exposure) to maximize!

1 University of Illinois, Department of Food Science and Human Nutrition. *Nutrient Conservation in Canned, Frozen, and Fresh Foods.* Urbana, IL: Oct 1997.

2 Giovannucci E, Ascherio A, Rimm EB, et al. Intake of carotenoids and retinol in relation to risk of prostate cancer. *J Natl Cancer Inst.* 1995;87:1767–1779.

3 Tonucci LH, Holden JM, Beecher GR, et al. Carotenoid content of thermally processed tomato-based food products. *J Agr Food Chem.* 1995;43:579–583.

4 Johnston CS, Bowling DL. Stability of ascorbic acid in commercially available orange juice. *J Am Diet Assoc.* 2002;102:525–529.

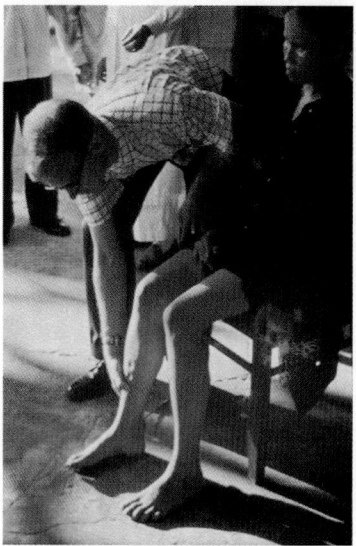

Figure 10.6 Edema, especially in the feet and legs, is a symptom of wet beriberi.

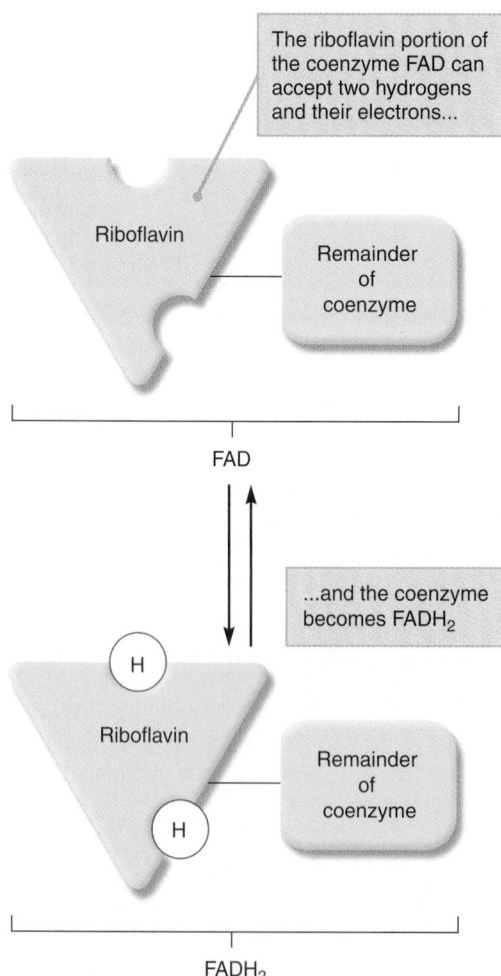

The riboflavin portion of the coenzyme FAD can accept two hydrogens and their electrons...

Riboflavin

Remainder of coenzyme

FAD

...and the coenzyme becomes FADH₂

Riboflavin

Remainder of coenzyme

FADH₂

Figure 10.7 **Riboflavin coenzymes easily transfer hydrogens.** The riboflavin coenzyme flavin adenine dinucleotide (FAD) accepts hydrogens and electrons to become FADH₂.

mostly highly processed but unenriched foods and empty-calorie items such as alcohol, sugar, and fat can lead to a deficiency.

Beriberi

Beriberi is a term from the Singhalese language (spoken in Sri Lanka) that means "I can't, I can't." This is a perfect description of beriberi, the hallmarks of which include muscle weakness, loss of appetite, and nerve degeneration. This deficiency disease occurs in people whose major source of energy is polished rice, which is common in Southeast Asia. Polishing removes the rice hulls and thus their major source of thiamin.

An inadequate supply of this essential nutrient affects the cardiovascular, muscular, nervous, and gastrointestinal systems, which all rely on thiamin to help fuel their activities. The brain and nervous system rely on glucose for energy, and thiamin, as part of TPP, is crucial in glucose metabolism. The first signs of thiamin deficiency are weakness, irritability, headache, fatigue, and depression—functions associated with the brain and nervous system. These disturbances may appear after only 10 days on a thiamin-free diet.

As symptoms progress, "dry" beriberi (beriberi without edema) causes nerve degeneration, loss of nerve transmission leading to tingling sensations throughout the body, muscle wasting, poor arm and leg coordination, and deep pain in the calf muscles. "Wet" beriberi has additional symptoms, including an enlarged heart, heart failure, and severe edema (**Figure 10.6**). Because many B vitamins are in the same foods as thiamin, thiamin deficiency and other B vitamin deficiencies often go hand in hand.

Wernicke-Korsakoff Syndrome

Alcohol-induced malnutrition is the most common cause of Wernicke-Korsakoff syndrome, another thiamin-deficiency disease. Symptoms include mental confusion, staggering, and constant rapid eye movements or paralysis of the eye muscles.

Thiamin Toxicity

To date, there are no reports of thiamin toxicity from either food or supplements. Supplements, which are cheap to produce, often include up to 200 times the Daily Value for thiamin. The Food and Nutrition Board has not set a Tolerable Upper Intake Level (UL) for this nutrient. Because thiamin absorption declines rapidly when a person consumes five or more milligrams at once, large doses of thiamin appear to be relatively innocuous. In addition, the kidneys rapidly excrete excess thiamin via urine.[6]

Riboflavin

Scientists discovered that heating the "anti-beriberi factor" destroyed its anti-beriberi properties but left its growth-promoting properties unscathed. The factor actually contained two active compounds—heat-vulnerable thiamin and a heat-stable component. In 1917, scientists identified the heat-stable component as another vitamin—called vitamin B₂ in England and vitamin G in the United States. This naming confusion ended when the new vitamin was finally dubbed riboflavin.

Riboflavin is named for its yellow color (*flavin* means "yellow" in Latin). The vitamin accepts and donates electrons with ease, so it participates in many oxidation-reduction reactions.

Functions of Riboflavin

Riboflavin is a part of two coenzymes: flavin mononucleotide (FMN) and flavin adenine dinucleotide (FAD). These coenzymes participate in numerous metabolic pathways, including the citric acid cycle and the beta-oxidation pathway that breaks down fatty acids. FMN and FAD act first as electron and hydrogen acceptors. In the citric acid cycle, for instance, FAD accepts hydrogen and electrons, forming the reduced form, $FADH_2$ (**Figure 10.7**). Later, this coenzyme delivers its high-energy electrons to the mitochondrial electron transport chain to produce ATP. Another riboflavin coenzyme, FMN, also accepts hydrogen and electrons, forming $FMNH_2$. FMN works in the electron transport chain to move electrons. Both coenzymes are crucial in energy metabolism.

Riboflavin-containing coenzymes also participate in reactions that remove ammonia during the deamination of some amino acids.[7] Riboflavin also is associated with the antioxidant activity of **glutathione peroxidase** enzyme.

Dietary Recommendations for Riboflavin

For adults aged 19 and older, the RDA is 1.1 milligrams per day for women and 1.3 milligrams per day for men. Intake recommendations for riboflavin, like those for thiamin, reflect the higher energy needs of males. Pregnancy and lactation increase energy needs, so the RDA for women rises to 1.4 milligrams per day during pregnancy and to 1.6 milligrams per day during lactation.

Sources of Riboflavin

Although most plant and animal foods contain some riboflavin, milk, milk drinks, and yogurt supply about 15 percent of the riboflavin in the U.S. diet. Bread and bread products contribute approximately 10 percent, and ready-to-eat cereals add nearly as much.[8] Riboflavin is one of the four vitamins (thiamin, riboflavin, niacin, and folic acid) and one mineral (iron) that are added to enriched grain products. Organ meats such as liver and kidney are good sources of riboflavin, as are mushrooms and cottage cheese. **Figure 10.8** shows foods that provide riboflavin.

Riboflavin is more stable than thiamin and is resistant to acid, heat, and oxidation. On the other hand, light easily breaks it down. Riboflavin-rich foods should be stored in opaque packages. For example, packaging milk in paper or plastic cartons rather than clear glass better protects milk's riboflavin content.[9] (See **Figure 10.9**.)

About 95 percent of the riboflavin in food is bioavailable, and the body can absorb large amounts from a single meal or supplement.[10]

Riboflavin Deficiency

Riboflavin deficiencies are rare. Several large surveys suggest that in the United States men take in about 2 milligrams of riboflavin per day, and women consume about 1.5 milligrams per day. Some people, however, consume only marginal amounts. Because people with alcoholism tend to have poor diets, for example, they risk riboflavin deficiency. Long-term use of barbiturate drugs such as phenobarbital also may lead to riboflavin deficiency. Repeated exposure to these drugs activates enzymes in the liver that

RIBOFLAVIN

Daily Value = 1.7 mg

Exceptionally good sources

Beef liver, cooked	85 g (3 oz)	2.9 mg
Wheat bran flakes cereal	30 g (³/4 cup)	1.77 mg
Chicken liver, cooked	85 g (3 oz)	1.69 mg

High: 20% DV or more

Corn flakes cereal	30 g (1 cup)	0.79 mg
Yogurt, plain, nonfat	225 g (1 8-oz container)	0.53 mg
Cheerios cereal	30 g (¹/2 cup)	0.50 mg
Yogurt, plain, lowfat	225 g (1 8-oz container)	0.49 mg
Milk, 1%, 2%, whole (3.25%)	240 ml (1 cup)	0.46 mg
Milk, nonfat	240 ml (1 cup)	0.45 mg
Fiber One cereal	30 g (¹/2 cup)	0.43 mg
Oatmeal, instant, fortified, cooked	1 cup	0.40 mg
Squid, cooked	85 g (3 oz)	0.39 mg
Buttermilk, low-fat	240 ml (1 cup)	0.38 mg
Clams, cooked	85 g (3 oz)	0.36 mg
Pork, loin chops, lean only, cooked	85 g (3 oz)	0.34 mg

Good: 10–19% DV

Ham, extra lean, cooked	85 g (3 oz)	0.30 mg
Bagel, plain	90 g (1 4" bagel)	0.28 mg
Egg, hardcooked	50 g (1 large)	0.26 mg
Mushrooms, cooked	85 g (~¹/2 cup)	0.26 mg
White bread, enriched	50 g (2 slices)	0.26 mg
Herring, cooked	85 g (3 oz)	0.25 mg
Almonds	30 g (~1 oz)	0.24 mg
Turkey, dark meat, cooked	85 g (3 oz)	0.21 mg
Beef, porterhouse steak, cooked	85 g (3 oz)	0.21 mg
Spinach, cooked	85 g (~¹/2 cup)	0.20 mg
Cottage cheese, 2% milkfat	110 g (~¹/2 cup)	0.20 mg
Tomato paste, canned	130 g (~¹/2 cup)	0.20 mg
Chicken, dark meat, cooked	85 g (3 oz)	0.19 mg

Figure 10.8 **Food sources of riboflavin.** The best sources of riboflavin include milk, liver, whole and enriched grains, and fortified cereals.
Source: U.S. Department of Agriculture, Agricultural Research Service. USDA National Nutrient Database for Standard Reference, Release 18. 2005. http://www.ars.usda.gov/nutrientdata.

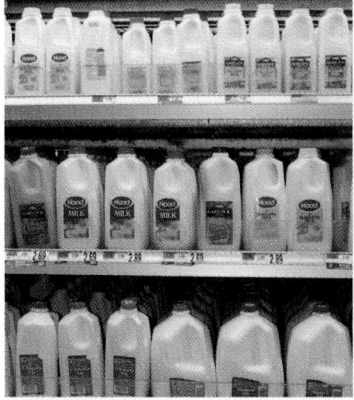

Figure 10.9 **Packaging affects riboflavin content in milk.** Light breaks down riboflavin easily, so foods high in riboflavin (e.g., milk) are best stored in opaque containers.

glutathione peroxidase A selenium-containing enzyme that promotes the breakdown of fatty acids that have undergone peroxidation.

ariboflavinosis Riboflavin deficiency.

glossitis Inflammation of the tongue; a symptom of riboflavin deficiency.

angular stomatitis Inflammation and cracking of the skin at the corners of the mouth; a symptom of riboflavin deficiency.

cheilosis Inflammation and cracking of the lips; a symptom of riboflavin deficiency.

seborrheic dermatitis Disease of the oil-producing glands of the skin; a symptom of riboflavin deficiency.

Figure 10.10 **Niacin is part of the coenzymes NAD$^+$ and NADP$^+$.** Niacin, as nicotinamide, is an integral part of coenzymes critical to several metabolic reactions. NAD$^+$ is crucial to the formation of ATP, and NADP$^+$ is crucial to biosynthesis.

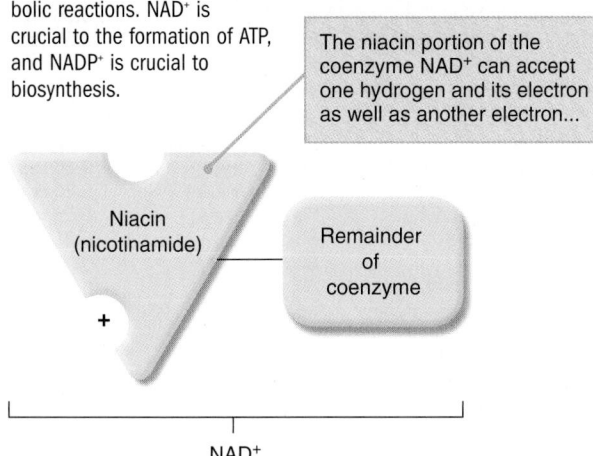

The niacin portion of the coenzyme NAD$^+$ can accept one hydrogen and its electron as well as another electron...

NAD$^+$

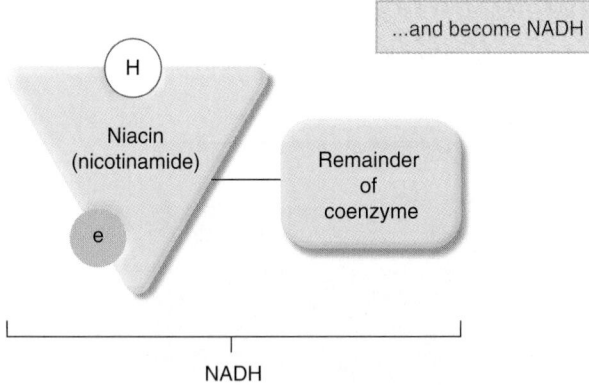

...and become NADH

NADH

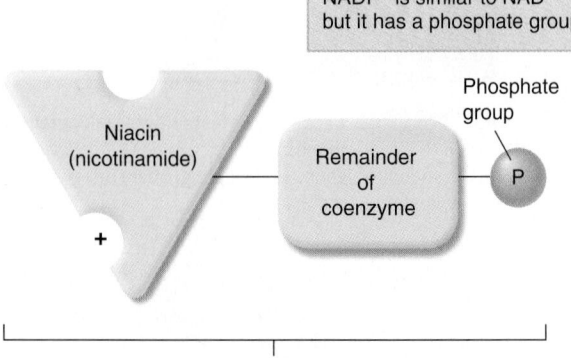

NADP$^+$ is similar to NAD$^+$ but it has a phosphate group

NADP$^+$

accelerate the metabolism of riboflavin. Cancer, heart disease, and diabetes may also cause or worsen a riboflavin deficiency.[11]

Riboflavin deficiency (**ariboflavinosis**) shows up first around the mouth. The tongue gets shiny, smooth, and inflamed (**glossitis**); the mouth becomes painful and sore; the skin at the corners of the mouth cracks (**angular stomatitis**); and the lips become inflamed and split (**cheilosis**). The oil-producing glands of the skin become clogged (**seborrheic dermatitis**); and as the deficiency becomes severe, a characteristic anemia develops. Riboflavin deficiency usually goes hand in hand with other nutrient deficiencies. In addition, riboflavin deficiency may lead to vitamin B$_6$ deficiency by interfering with vitamin B$_6$ metabolism.[12]

Riboflavin Toxicity

No cases of riboflavin toxicity have been reported. Because the body readily excretes excess riboflavin, even large doses appear to pose no risk of harm. A UL has not been set for riboflavin.

Niacin

In 1867 scientists first produced a substance called nicotinic acid by oxidizing the nicotine from tobacco. Nicotinic acid is not, however, the same as or even closely related to the nicotine molecule. Seventy years later, Conrad Elvehjem at the University of Wisconsin demonstrated that nicotinic acid cured dogs of a canine version of the human niacin-deficiency disease pellagra. In the early 1940s, the vitamin was renamed "niacin," an acronym of "nicotinic acid vitamin," so that people would not confuse it with nicotine.

Niacin actually is the name for two similarly functioning compounds: nicotinic acid and nicotinamide (also known as niacinamide). Like the other B vitamins, niacin is a coenzyme component (see **Figure 10.10**) and participates in at least 200 metabolic pathways.

Functions of Niacin

The niacin coenzymes, nicotinamide adenine dinucleotide (NAD$^+$) and nicotinamide adenine dinucleotide phosphate (NADP$^+$), play key roles in oxidation-reduction reactions. NAD$^+$ accepts electrons and hydrogen (i.e., is reduced) to form NADH. Under aerobic conditions, NADH carries high-energy electrons to the electron transport chain to help produce ATP. When you need energy in anaerobic conditions (say, during vigorous activity that pushes the body beyond its aerobic capacity), NADH powers the conversion of pyruvate to lactate as it loses electrons and a hydrogen (i.e., is oxidized) to become NAD$^+$. (See **Figure 10.11**.) This regenerated NAD$^+$ helps power the continued operation of glycolysis. Without it, glycolysis would halt, shutting off the supply of energy from glucose.

Many metabolic pathways that promote the synthesis of new compounds, such as fatty acids, rely on NADPH, the reduced form of NADP$^+$. NADPH is concentrated in cells (such as liver cells) that make large amounts of fatty acids.

Dietary Recommendations for Niacin

Niacin is unique among the B vitamins because your body can make it from the amino acid **tryptophan** as well as obtain it from foods. Intake recommendations are expressed as **niacin equivalents (NE)**, a measure that includes both preformed dietary niacin and niacin derived from tryptophan. The RDA for adult men of all ages is 16 milligrams of NE per day, and the RDA for adult women of all ages is 14 milligrams of NE. It increases to 18 milligrams of NE for pregnancy and 17 milligrams of NE for lactation.

Sources of Niacin

Most of the preformed niacin in the U.S. diet comes from meat, poultry, fish, enriched and whole-grain breads and grain products, and fortified ready-to-eat cereals. In a typical U.S. diet, beef and processed meats are substantial contributors.[13] Other good sources of niacin include mushrooms, peanuts, liver, and seafood. **Figure 10.12** shows foods that provide niacin. Because the vitamin is stable when heated, little niacin is lost during cooking.

The niacin precursor tryptophan is found in protein-rich animal foods, with the exception of gelatin. To convert tryptophan to niacin, your body needs other nutrients: riboflavin, vitamin B$_6$, and iron. Sixty milligrams of

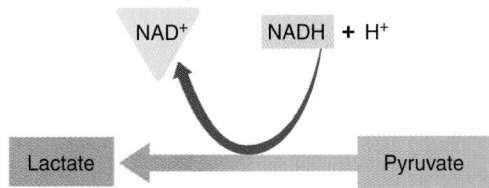

Figure 10.11 **Niacin helps convert pyruvate to lactate.** As a component of the coenzymes NAD$^+$ and NADH, niacin participates in many metabolic reactions.

tryptophan An amino acid that serves as a niacin precursor in the body. In the body, 60 milligrams of tryptophan yields about 1 milligram of niacin, or 1 niacin equivalent (NE).

niacin equivalents (NE) A measure that includes preformed dietary niacin as well as niacin derived from tryptophan; 60 milligrams of tryptophan yields about 1 milligram of niacin.

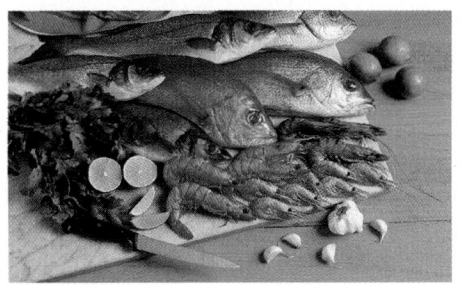

NIACIN

Daily Value = 20 mg

High: 20% DV or more	Beef liver, cooked	85 g (3 oz)	14.9 mg
	Chicken, light meat, cooked	85 g (3 oz)	11.4 mg
	Chicken liver, cooked	85 g (3 oz)	9.4 mg
	Salmon, cooked	85 g (3 oz)	8.6 mg
	Tuna, canned	55 g (2 oz)	7.3 mg
	Halibut, cooked	85 g (3 oz)	6.1 mg
	Turkey, light meat, cooked	85 g (3 oz)	5.8 mg
	Corn flakes cereal	30 g (1 cup)	5.8 mg
	Chicken, dark meat, cooked	85 g (3 oz)	5.6 mg
	Beef, ground, extra lean, cooked	85 g (3 oz)	5.1 mg
	All Bran cereal	30 g (1/2 cup)	5.1 mg
	Fiber One cereal	30 g (1/2 cup)	5.0 mg
	Oatmeal, instant, fortified, cooked	1 cup	4.8 mg
	Peanut butter	2 Tbsp	4.3 mg
	Ham, extra lean, cooked	85 g (3 oz)	4.2 mg
	Pork, loin roast, lean only, cooked	85 g (3 oz)	4.0 mg
	Tomato paste, canned	130 g (~1/2 cup)	4.0 mg
Good: 10–19% DV	Beef, T-bone steak, cooked	85 g (3 oz)	3.9 mg
	Beef, porterhouse steak, cooked	85 g (3 oz)	3.9 mg
	Mushrooms, cooked	85 g (~1/2 cup)	3.8 mg
	White bread, enriched	50 g (2 slices)	3.8 mg
	Salmon, canned, solids + bones	55 g (2 oz)	3.6 mg
	Bagel, plain	90 g (1 4" bagel)	3.6 mg
	Turkey, dark meat, cooked	85 g (3 oz)	3.1 mg
	Barley, cooked	140 g (~1 cup)	2.9 mg
	Sardines, canned, solids + bones	55 g (2 oz)	2.9 mg
	Clams, cooked	85 g (3 oz)	2.9 mg
	Spaghetti, enriched, cooked	140 g (1 cup)	2.4 mg
	Shrimp, cooked	85 g (3 oz)	2.2 mg
	Cod, cooked	85 g (3 oz)	2.1 mg
	Rice, white, enriched, cooked	140 g (~3/4 cup)	2.1 mg

Quick Bites

Are You Smoking That Bread?

In the 1940s, anti-tobacco forces were confused about the differences between niacin and nicotine. They mistakenly warned that niacin-enriched bread could cause an addiction to cigarettes!

Figure 10.12 **Food sources of niacin.** Niacin is found mainly in meats and grains. Enrichment adds niacin as well as thiamin, riboflavin, folic acid, and iron to processed grains.
Source: U.S. Department of Agriculture, Agricultural Research Service. USDA National Nutrient Database for Standard Reference, Release 18. 2005. http://www.ars.usda.gov/nutrientdata.

CALCULATION OF NE FOR AN 80-KG (176-LB) MAN

> **His protein RDA is**
>
> 80 kg × 0.8 g/kg = 64 g protein

Let us assume his diet contains 94 g of high-quality protein so that

> 94 g dietary protein
> − 64 g protein (his protein RDA)
> _____
> 30 g protein in excess of needs

Tryptophan makes up about 1% of the protein so that

> 30 g protein × 0.01 = 0.3 g tryptophan
> (300 mg tryptophan)

60 mg tryptophan ≐ 1 mg niacin (1 NE) so that

> 300 mg tryptophan ÷ 60 =
> 5 mg niacin (5 NE)

> **Shortcut Method**
> 30 g excess protein ÷ 6 = 5 mg niacin (5 NE)

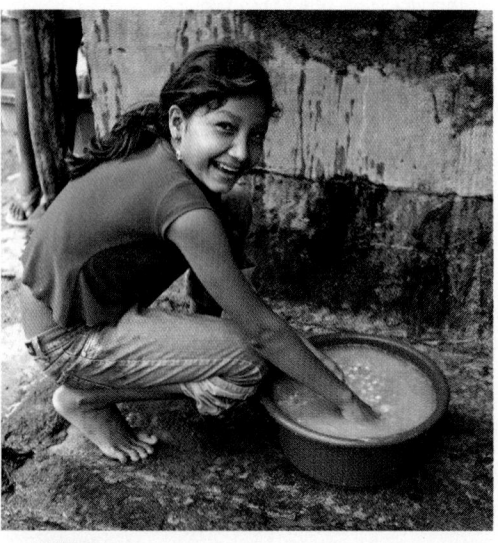

Figure 10.13 Soaking corn in a solution of lime (calcium hydroxide) releases bound niacin.

tryptophan yield about 1 milligram of niacin, or 1 niacin equivalent (NE). To quickly determine the number of milligrams of niacin derived from tryptophan, divide the grams of high-quality dietary protein that exceed protein needs by 6. For instance, 30 grams of excess protein, divided by 6, yields 5 milligrams of niacin.

Because riboflavin, vitamin B_6, and iron affect the conversion of tryptophan to niacin, a deficiency of any one of these nutrients decreases tryptophan conversion. Certain rare metabolic disorders disrupt tryptophan conversion pathways. Pregnancy, on the other hand, increases the efficiency of converting tryptophan to niacin.

Tryptophan supplies about half of the average American's niacin intake. When estimating niacin consumption, remember that tables of food composition list only preformed niacin and therefore underestimate the amount of niacin some foods contribute via tryptophan.

Niacin Deficiency

First documented in 1735 by a Spanish physician named Gaspar Casal, the niacin-deficiency disease pellagra was originally named *mal de la rosa*, or "red sickness," for the telltale redness that appears around the necks of people with the disease. Severely roughened skin is another hallmark, and the condition was later dubbed pellagra for the Italian *pelle*, or "skin," and *agra*, or "rough." Because the niacin coenzymes NAD^+ and $NADP^+$ are involved in just about every metabolic pathway, niacin deficiency wreaks havoc throughout the body. The primary symptoms of pellagra are known as the three Ds: dementia, diarrhea, and dermatitis. In severe cases, a fourth D—death—is the final outcome. Deficiencies of iron and vitamin B_6 may also contribute to pellagra.

During the early 1900s, as corn became a staple in the southwestern United States, pellagra emerged in epidemic proportions. A protein in corn tightly binds niacin, so only about 30 percent is bioavailable.[14] We now know, however, that soaking corn in a solution of lime (calcium hydroxide) releases that bound niacin, as **Figure 10.13** shows. This disease also was common among the rural poor in the Southeast, who subsisted on a diet of corn (maize), molasses, and salt pork, which is mostly fat. Between the end of World War I and the end of World War II, pellagra afflicted some 200,000 Americans. The incidence of pellagra started to decline during World War II because of the mandatory enrichment of bread flour and other cereal grains with niacin. After World War II, the enrichment program, combined with the postwar affluence that allowed people to purchase more protein-rich meat, poultry, and fish, finally curbed the disease. Sadly, pellagra continues to plague people living in Southeast Asia and Africa, whose diets lack sufficient niacin and protein.

Niacin Toxicity and Medicinal Uses of Niacin

Niacin, in the form of nicotinic acid, has long been known to lower blood levels of LDL cholesterol while raising HDL cholesterol levels when taken in doses of 1,300 to 3,000 milligrams per day. However, adverse effects can be seen at much lower doses. Consuming as little as 250 milligrams of nicotinic acid at one time—about 15 to 17 times the RDA for adults—can cause flushing of the face, arms, and chest; itching; headaches; rash; nausea; glucose intolerance; and blurred vision.[15] Moreover, liver abnormalities sometimes show up within a week in people who take high-dose nicotinic acid supplements. Based on these complications, the established adult UL for niacin is 35 milligrams per day from fortified foods, supplements, and/or medications. Niacin supplements containing more than the RDA should be taken only under medical supervision.

Thin About

2

Sustained-release nicotinic acid supplements deliver the dose throughout the day rather than all at once. This may alleviate flushing and some of the other immediate side effects, but sustained-release supplements can be toxic to the liver when taken for months or years.[16]

Researchers became interested in the potential of nicotinamide to prevent type 1 diabetes based on a study showing that nicotinamide protects insulin-secreting cells from inflammation and improves their function after the onset of diabetes.[17] However, a prospective clinical trial, the European Nicotinamide Diabetes Intervention Trial (ENDIT), showed that nicotinamide supplementation did not stop the development of diabetes.[18]

Key Concepts: *Thiamin, riboflavin, and niacin are all incorporated into coenzymes that catalyze energy-yielding reactions. All three B vitamins participate in pathways that metabolize carbohydrate, protein, and fat. Enriched grains are a major source of these B vitamins, with pork ranking as a good source of thiamin, milk as a major source of riboflavin, and high-protein foods as sources of niacin. Deficiencies of these vitamins are rare in the United States. People with alcoholism have the highest risk of deficiencies. High doses of thiamin and riboflavin appear to be harmless, but megadoses of niacin should be taken only under medical supervision.*

Pantothenic Acid

In the 1930s a chemist named Roger J. Williams discovered that yeast require a certain nutrient, which he called pantothenic acid. He suggested that if yeast needed this nutrient, humans might need it, too. First isolated in 1938, the chemical structure of pantothenic acid was identified by scientists in 1940.

The name pantothenic acid is derived from the Greek word *pantothen,* meaning "from every side." This B vitamin is widespread in the food supply, so it is well named.

Functions of Pantothenic Acid

Pantothenic acid is a component of coenzyme A (CoA), which in turn is a component of acetyl CoA. (See **Figure 10.14.**) Acetyl CoA sits at the crossroads of a number of metabolic pathways—both energy-generating pathways and biosynthetic pathways. It is formed from pyruvate (see **Figure 10.15**), starts the citric acid cycle, is a key building block of fatty acids, and is a precursor of ketone bodies.

Fatty acids also are known as acyl groups, and pantothenic acid is a component of the acyl carrier protein. During fatty acid synthesis, the acyl carrier protein binds fatty acids and carries them through a series of reactions that increases their chain length.

Dietary Recommendations for Pantothenic Acid

There are few data upon which to base dietary recommendations for pantothenic acid. As you learned in Chapter 2, when the data are insufficient to set an Estimated Average Requirement (EAR) for a nutrient, an RDA cannot be established. In these cases, and thus for pantothenic acid, an Adequate Intake (AI) level is set instead. For adults aged 19 to 50, the AI for pantothenic acid is 5 milligrams per day.

Sources of Pantothenic Acid

Pantothenic acid is widespread in the food supply. Although data on the specific pantothenic acid content of foods are sparse, food sources known to contain this vitamin include chicken, beef, potatoes, oats, tomato products,

PANTOTHENIC ACID AND COENZYME A

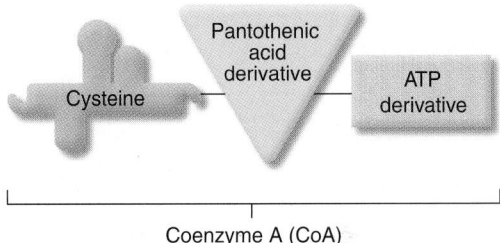

Figure 10.14 **Pantothenic acid and coenzyme A.** Pantothenic acid forms part of coenzyme A, which in turn is a component of acetyl CoA. Through coenzyme A, pantothenic acid is involved in many metabolic reactions.

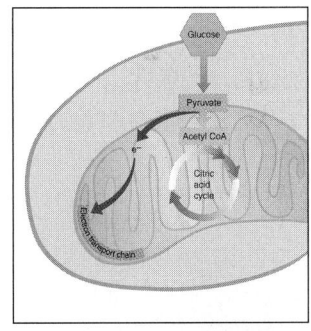

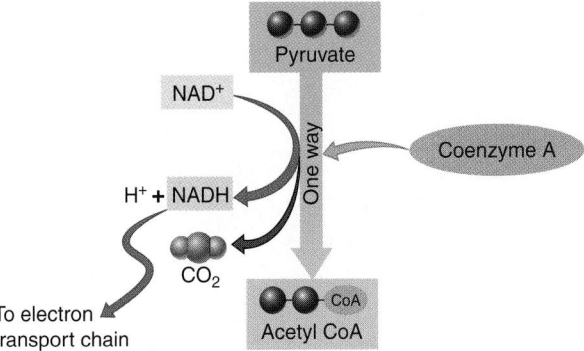

Figure 10.15 **Pantothenic acid helps convert pyruvate to acetyl CoA.** As part of coenzyme A, pantothenic acid helps form acetyl CoA from pyruvate. Niacin participates in this reaction as part of the coenzyme NAD⁺.

PANTOTHENIC ACID

Daily Value = 10 mg

High: **20% DV** **or more**	Beef liver, cooked	85 g (3 oz)	6.0 mg
	Chicken liver, cooked	85 g (3 oz)	5.7 mg
	Sunflower seeds	30 g (~1 oz)	2.1 mg
Good: **10–19%** **DV**	Mushrooms, cooked	85 g (~1/2 cup)	1.8 mg
	Yogurt, plain, nonfat	225 g (1 8-oz container)	1.5 mg
	Yogurt, plain, low-fat	225 g (1 8-oz container)	1.3 mg
	Turkey, dark meat, cooked	85 g (3 oz)	1.1 mg
	Chicken, dark meat, cooked	85 g (3 oz)	1.0 mg

Figure 10.16 **Food sources of pantothenic acid.** Pantothenic acid is found widely in foods, but is abundant in only a few sources such as liver.
Source: U.S. Department of Agriculture, Agricultural Research Service. USDA National Nutrient Database for Standard Reference, Release 18. 2005. http://www.ars.usda.gov/nutrientdata.

liver, kidney, yeast, egg yolk, broccoli, and whole grains.[19] **Figure 10.16** shows foods that are good sources of pantothenic acid.

Pantothenic acid is damaged easily. Freezing and canning appear to decrease the pantothenic acid content of vegetables, meat, fish, and dairy products. Processing and refining grains can reduce their pantothenic acid content by nearly 75 percent.[20]

Scientists do not have clear information about the bioavailability of pantothenic acid. We assume that the nutrient is well absorbed.

Pantothenic Acid Deficiency

Pantothenic acid deficiencies are virtually nonexistent in the general population. The only observed cases of pantothenic acid deficiency are in people who were fed diets that completely lacked the nutrient or who were given a substance that prevents metabolism of pantothenic acid. These people suffered symptoms that included irritability, restlessness, fatigue, apathy, malaise, sleep disturbances, nausea, vomiting, numbness, tingling, muscle cramps, staggering gait, and hypoglycemia.

Pantothenic Acid Toxicity

High intakes of pantothenic acid have not caused adverse effects. Risk of toxicity appears to be extremely low, and therefore a UL has not been established.

Biotin

In 1924 three factors were identified as necessary for the growth of microorganisms. They were called "bios II," "vitamin H," and "coenzyme R." It soon became clear that all three were the same water-soluble, sulfur-containing vitamin—biotin.

In food, biotin is found both free and bound to protein. When proteins are digested, a biotin–lysine complex called **biocytin** is released.

Functions of Biotin

Biotin-containing enzymes mainly catalyze **carboxylation** reactions, in which carbon dioxide is added to a substrate. (See **Figure 10.17**.) Some of the reactions that rely on biotin-containing enzymes include the following:

- Adding carbon dioxide to three-carbon pyruvate to yield four-carbon oxaloacetate. This process is one of the first steps in gluconeogenesis

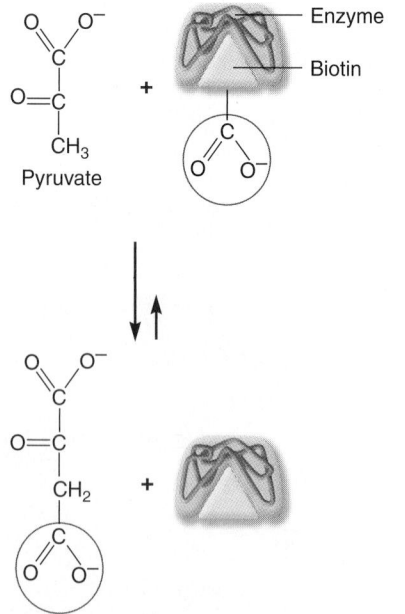

Pyruvate

Enzyme

Biotin

Oxaloacetate

Figure 10.17 **Biotin aids carboxylation reactions.** Biotin is a coenzyme for several carboxylase enzymes. These enzymes transfer carboxyl groups, such as in the conversion of pyruvate to oxaloacetate.

- Entry of three-carbon fatty acids into the citric acid cycle to yield energy
- Elongating fatty acid chains during fatty acid synthesis
- Breaking down leucine to the ketone body acetoacetate
- Breaking down isoleucine, methionine, threonine, and valine for entry into the citric acid cycle
- Synthesizing DNA

Dietary Recommendations for Biotin

Just like pantothenic acid, there are not enough data on biotin to establish an EAR or an RDA. In fact, we know so little about human biotin requirements that the Adequate Intake value for adults is mathematically determined from the AI level for infants.[21] The infant value is based on the amount of biotin in human milk. The AI for biotin for adult men and women of all ages is 30 micrograms per day.

Sources of Biotin

Most tables of food composition do not list biotin content because it hasn't been determined for many foods. Good sources of biotin include cauliflower, liver, peanuts, and cheese. Most fruits and meats rank as poor sources. The enzyme **biotinidase** readily releases biotin from biocytin. Egg yolks are also a good source of biotin, but a protein called **avidin** in raw egg whites binds biotin and prevents its absorption from raw eggs. Heat destroys avidin, so it is unlikely to cause a biotin deficiency unless you eat a lot of raw eggs—at least a dozen daily. Of course, you should avoid eating anything that contains raw eggs because they might harbor *Salmonella* bacteria and cause foodborne illness.

Biotin Deficiency

Eating raw egg whites over a long period—months or years—can cause biotin deficiency. Because some anticonvulsant drugs break down biotin, people who take them for long periods also risk a deficiency. Infants born with biotinidase deficiency suffer from a rare genetic defect that leads to biotin depletion. Symptoms progress from initial hair loss and rash to convulsions and other neurological disorders. The deficiency also can delay growth and development. Early diagnosis and daily high doses of biotin (e.g., 10 milligrams per day) usually clear up symptoms. If not treated, biotin deficiency causes changes in blood pH that can lead to coma and death.

Biotin Toxicity

Biotin does not appear to be toxic at high doses. Children with biotinidase deficiency have been given as much as 200 milligrams of biotin daily without adverse side effects. A UL for biotin has not been established.

Vitamin B$_6$

Vitamin B$_6$ is a group of six compounds: pyridoxal (PL), pyridoxine (PN), pyridoxamine (PM), and their phosphorylated forms (PLP, PNP, and PMP), in which a phosphate group has been added (see **Figure 10.18**). Food contains the phosphorylated forms, PLP, PNP, and PMP, but digestion strips off the phosphate groups. PL, PN, and PM then travel to the liver, which converts them to PLP (pyridoxal phosphate), the primary active coenzyme form.[22]

biocytin A biotin–lysine complex released from digested protein.

carboxylation A reaction that adds a carboxyl group (–COOH) to a substrate, replacing a hydrogen atom.

biotinidase An enzyme in the small intestine that releases biotin from biocytin.

avidin A protein in raw egg whites that binds biotin, preventing its absorption. Avidin is destroyed by heat.

Quick Bites

Busy Bacteria

You may be aware that bacteria in the colon synthesize vitamin K, but did you know that colonic bacteria also make some biotin? Then again, when synthesizing this B vitamin these busy microbes may be pursuing a futile effort. Since the colon is downstream from the small intestine, the site of most biotin absorption, the bacteria's biotin may not be absorbed efficiently. Bacterial synthesis of biotin probably does not make an important contribution to your body's supply of biotin.

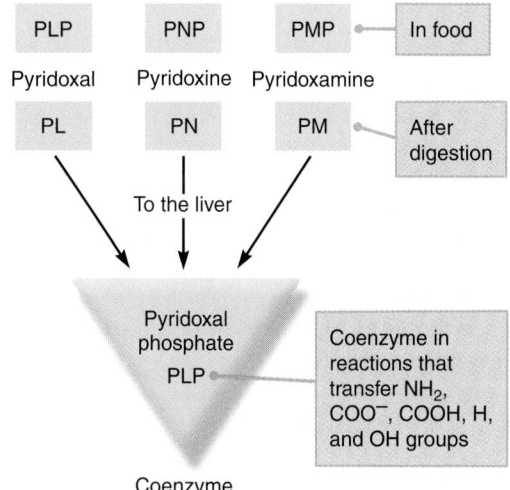

Figure 10.18   **The vitamin B$_6$ family and coenzyme form.** Vitamin B$_6$ is a group of six compounds: pyridoxal (PL), pyridoxine (PN), pyridoxamine (PM), and their phosphorylated forms PLP, PNP, and PMP. Digestion removes the phosphate groups and the liver converts PL, PN, and PM to PLP (pyridoxal phosphate), the active coenzyme form.

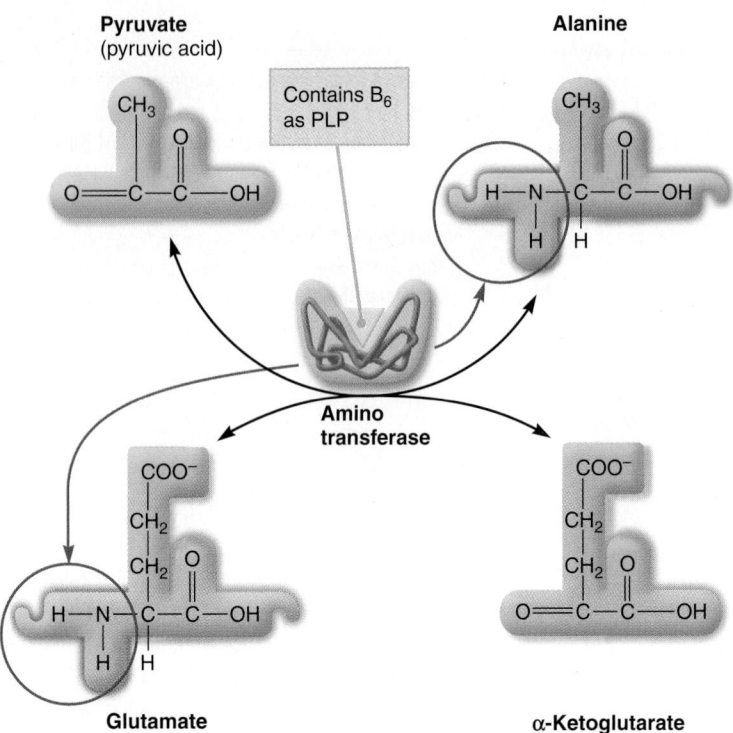

Figure 10.19 Vitamin B_6 aids transamination reactions. Vitamin B_6, as part of PLP, helps transfer an amino group from an amino acid to a ketoacid and produce a new amino acid.

microcytic hypochromic anemia Anemia characterized by small, pale red blood cells that lack adequate hemoglobin to carry oxygen; can be caused by deficiency of iron or vitamin B_6.

anemia Abnormally low concentration of hemoglobin in the bloodstream; can be caused by impaired synthesis of red blood cells, increased destruction of red cells, or significant loss of blood.

homocysteine An amino acid precursor of cysteine and a risk factor for heart disease.

Functions of Vitamin B_6

The vitamin B_6 coenzyme PLP supports more than 100 different enzymes involved in reactions that include the transfer of amino groups (NH_2), carboxyl groups (COO^- or COOH), or water (as H and OH). These enzymes support protein metabolism, blood cell synthesis, carbohydrate metabolism, and neurotransmitter synthesis.

Protein Metabolism

One of the primary tasks of PLP is to help metabolize amino acids and other nitrogen-containing compounds. As **Figure 10.19** shows, PLP plays a key role in transamination reactions, helping transfer an amino group from an amino acid to a keto acid and produce a new amino acid. Transamination, catalyzed by PLP, enables the body to make the 11 nonessential amino acids. Without adequate supplies of vitamin B_6, all amino acids become "indispensable," meaning the body cannot synthesize them and must obtain them from the diet (see the discussion of amino acids in Chapter 6, "Proteins and Amino Acids"). Over time, vitamin B_6 deficiency impairs protein synthesis and cell metabolism.

Blood Cell Synthesis

PLP supports the synthesis of the white blood cells of the immune system and is crucial for the synthesis of the red blood cells' hemoglobin rings, which carry oxygen. PLP also helps bind oxygen to hemoglobin. Inadequate vitamin B_6 disturbs this binding process, causing **microcytic hypochromic anemia**. In this type of **anemia**, red blood cells are smaller than normal and lack sufficient hemoglobin to carry oxygen. Iron deficiency also can cause microcytic hypochromic anemia.

Carbohydrate Metabolism

Through its role in transamination reactions, PLP participates in gluconeogenesis—producing glucose from amino acids. In addition, PLP facilitates glycogen breakdown.

Neurotransmitter Synthesis

PLP helps produce a number of neurotransmitters, including serotonin, gamma-amino butyric acid (GABA), dopamine, and norepinephrine. A vitamin B_6 deficiency can cause neurological symptoms—depression, headaches, confusion, and convulsions.

Vitamin B_6, Folate, and Heart Disease

Moderately high blood levels of the amino acid **homocysteine** are associated with fatal cardiovascular events. Homocysteine blood levels are influenced by dietary intake of B_6, folate, and vitamin B_{12}. Low intake of B_6 or folate can result in high homocysteine levels. Because the body accumulates large vitamin B_{12} stores to draw on when needed, variations in B_{12} intake seldom affect homocysteine levels. The body lowers homocysteine levels in one of two ways: (1) Two PLP-dependent enzymes help convert homocysteine to cysteine, or (2) folate and vitamin B_{12}–dependent enzymes help convert homocysteine to methionine. An increase in fruit and vegetable intake also can affect homocysteine levels. In a Dutch study, subjects who consumed a "high" fruit and vegetable diet (500 g fruits and vegetables plus 200 mL of juice per day; approximately 1.5 mg B$_6$ and 170 μg folate per 2,000 kcal) had significantly lower plasma homocysteine concentrations that those who consumed a "low" fruit and vegetable diet (100 g of fruits and vegetables per day; approximately 1.2 mg B$_6$ and 100 μg folate per 2,000 kcal).[23] Because the differences in vitamin B$_6$ and folate content between the diets were so small, the authors suggest that other components in fruits and vegetables also may influence homocysteine.

Another study found that women with the highest intakes of B$_6$ and folate have about half the risk of a heart attack as women with the lowest intakes. Vitamin B$_6$ may have beneficial effects independent of homocysteine levels. Researchers have found that low B$_6$ status increased risk for stroke, whereas increased homocysteine levels were not associated with risk.[24] Furthermore, when intakes were considered separately, B$_6$ and folate had similar disease-reduction effects.[25]

Other Functions

The vitamin B$_6$ coenzyme also helps convert tryptophan to the B vitamin niacin, as described earlier.

Dietary Recommendations for Vitamin B$_6$

The RDA for vitamin B$_6$ for men and women aged 19 to 50 is 1.3 milligrams per day. For men 51 years and older, the RDA is 1.7 milligrams per day; for women 51 years and older, the RDA is 1.5 milligrams per day. Due to the role of vitamin B$_6$ in amino acid metabolism, people on very-high-protein diets may need higher intakes.[26]

Sources of Vitamin B$_6$

In the United States, the primary sources of vitamin B$_6$ are fortified, ready-to-eat cereals; mixed foods (including sandwiches) that contain primarily meat, fish, or poultry; white potatoes and other starchy vegetables; and noncitrus fruits.[27] Highly fortified cereals, beef liver and other organ meats, and fortified soy-based meat substitutes are especially rich sources. Other good sources of vitamin B$_6$ include bananas, potatoes, and sunflower seeds. Although whole grains contain vitamin B$_6$, refining removes B$_6$, and enrichment does not replace it. **Figure 10.20** shows foods that provide vitamin B$_6$.

Vitamin B$_6$ is not particularly stable and is especially sensitive to temperature. Heat can destroy as much as 50 percent of a food's vitamin B$_6$ content. About 75 percent of the vitamin B$_6$ in a varied diet is bioavailable, and vitamin B$_6$ taken without food is almost completely absorbed, even when taken in megadoses.[28]

Vitamin B$_6$ Deficiency

Vitamin B$_6$ deficiencies are rare. When one does occur, the deficiency leads to microcytic hypochromic anemia, seborrheic dermatitis, and neurological symptoms such as depression, confusion, and convulsions.

Alcoholism boosts the risk of vitamin B$_6$ deficiency because alcohol decreases absorption of the nutrient and hampers synthesis of the coenzyme PLP. A breakdown product of alcohol metabolism also interferes with

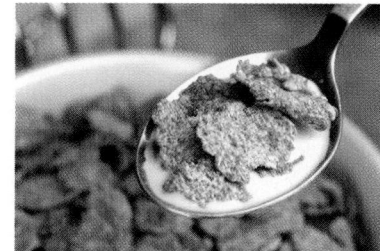

VITAMIN B$_6$

Daily Value = 2 mg

Exceptionally good sources

Wheat bran flakes cereal	30 g (³/4 cup)	2.1 mg
All Bran cereal	30 g (¹/2 cup)	2.0 mg

High: 20% DV or more

Corn flakes cereal	30 g (1 cup)	1.0 mg
Beef liver, cooked	85 g (3 oz)	0.9 mg
Cheerios cereal	30 g (1 cup)	0.7 mg
Chicken liver, cooked	85 g (3 oz)	0.6 mg
Garbanzo beans, canned	130 g (~¹/2 cup)	0.6 mg
Chicken, light meat, cooked	85 g (3 oz)	0.5 mg
Banana, fresh	140 g (1 9" banana)	0.5 mg
Fiber One cereal	30 g (¹/2 cup)	0.5 mg
Turkey, light meat, cooked	85 g (3 oz)	0.5 mg
Pork, loin roast, lean only	85 g (3 oz)	0.4 mg
Beef, ground, extra lean, cooked	85 g (3 oz)	0.4 mg
Ham, extra lean, cooked	85 g (3 oz)	0.4 mg

Good: 10–19% DV

Halibut, cooked	85 g (3 oz)	0.3 mg
Potato, baked, w/skin	110 g (1 small)	0.3 mg
Turkey, dark meat, cooked	85 g (3 oz)	0.3 mg
Chicken, dark meat, cooked	85 g (3 oz)	0.3 mg
Beef, porterhouse steak, cooked	85 g (3 oz)	0.3 mg
Herring, cooked	85 g (3 oz)	0.3 mg
Tomato juice, canned	240 ml (1 cup)	0.3 mg
Sweet potato, cooked	110 g (1 small)	0.3 mg
Sesame seeds	30 g (~1 oz)	0.2 mg
Sunflower seeds	30 g (~1 oz)	0.2 mg

Figure 10.20 **Food sources of vitamin B$_6$.** Meats are generally good sources of vitamin B$_6$ along with certain fruits (e.g., bananas) and vegetables (e.g., potatoes, carrots).
Source: U.S. Department of Agriculture, Agricultural Research Service. USDA National Nutrient Database for Standard Reference, Release 18. 2005. http://www.ars.usda.gov/nutrientdata.

the functioning of vitamin B_6 coenzymes. In addition, two conditions frequently suffered by people with alcoholism—cirrhosis and hepatitis—damage liver tissue, preventing the liver from metabolizing vitamin B_6 to its coenzyme form.

Vitamin B_6 Toxicity and Medicinal Uses of Vitamin B_6

Megadoses of supplemental vitamin B_6—2,000 milligrams or more per day—can cause irreversible nerve damage that affects the ability to walk and causes numbness in the extremities.[29] Side effects have been noted at levels of 1,000 milligrams per day as well.

Some women self-prescribe large doses of vitamin B_6 to treat premenstrual syndrome (PMS)—the headache, bloating, irritability, and depression that may occur during the week or so before the onset of menstruation. Although vitamin B_6 has long been reputed to be an antidote for PMS, research has failed to prove its effectiveness.[30]

Despite the risk of toxicity, some people have recommended high doses of vitamin B_6 as a treatment for carpal tunnel syndrome—a repetitive strain injury characterized by painful tingling in the wrist and fingers. Most well-designed scientific studies carried out in recent years, however, have failed to find a link between vitamin B_6 and improvement of carpal tunnel syndrome.[31]

The reasons for the nerve damage associated with B_6 excess are unclear, but modification of proteins by PLP may be involved. The UL for vitamin B_6 intake is 100 milligrams per day, a common amount in over-the-counter

[*Fyi*] The B Vitamins and Heart Disease

FOR YOUR INFORMATION

In 1968, pathologist Kilmer McCully examined the body of a 2-month-old boy who had died of the rare genetic disease homocystinuria—a condition with sky-high levels of the amino acid homocysteine in the urine. The child's arteries were so hardened and clogged that they resembled those of an adult with severe heart disease. This case was similar to one of an 8-year-old child.

These two cases led Dr. McCully to postulate that high blood levels of homocysteine may be linked to increased risk of heart disease. For the next decade, Dr. McCully held fast to his controversial theory despite the skepticism of his colleagues, who found only scant and largely unsubstantiated supporting evidence. In 1978, his outspoken defense of homocysteine as a risk factor for heart disease cost him his job.[1]

In the 1990s, a landmark report from the Physicians' Health Study sparked renewed interest in Dr. McCully's theory linking homocysteine and heart disease. In this ongoing study of a large group of physicians, Harvard University researchers found that those with the highest blood levels of homocysteine had more than triple the heart disease risk of their counterparts with lower homocysteine blood levels.[2] This suggests that homocysteine is an independent risk factor for cardiovascular disease that may be on a par with high blood cholesterol and smoking.

In 1993 a research team from the Jean Mayer USDA Human Nutrition Research Center on Aging at Tufts University showed that high homocysteine levels go hand in hand with low blood levels of vitamins B_6, B_{12}, and especially folate.[3] This association makes sense, since these three nutrients participate in metabolic pathways that convert homocysteine to other compounds in the body. When one or more of these vitamins is lacking, homocysteine builds up in the blood over time. Based on the Tufts study, one in five older adults may have homocysteine levels high enough to put them at risk.

During the 1990s scores of studies clearly linked elevated homocysteine to heart attacks, as well as to strokes, blood clots in the legs, and damage to arteries throughout the rest of the body.[4] Homocysteine may contribute to clogged arteries by triggering the proliferation of smooth muscle cells just beneath the innermost layer of the artery wall. These excess cells add to the plaque and other debris that line the arteries and promote blood clots.

In 1998 a report from the Nurses' Health Study examined whether B vitamin intake affects heart disease risk. In this ongoing study, Harvard researchers have been monitoring the health and eating habits of more than 80,000 female nurses since 1980. They found that women who took in the most folate—from either foods or supplements—were 31 percent less likely to suffer a heart attack than the

vitamin supplements. Because of the potential hazards, vitamin B_6 megadoses should be taken only under medical supervision.

Key Concepts: *Pantothenic acid and biotin are widespread in the food supply. Deficiencies of these B vitamins are rare because most people consume adequate amounts. Like the other B vitamins, pantothenic acid and biotin are parts of coenzymes involved in the metabolism of fat, carbohydrate, and protein. Vitamin B_6 is found in animal and plant foods and participates in protein metabolism, synthesis of neurotransmitters, and other metabolic pathways. Prolonged megadoses of vitamin B_6 can cause nerve damage.*

Folate

Eating raw liver, unappetizing though that may be, has long been known to cure a degenerative type of anemia. In 1945 a search for liver's curative component led to the discoveries of folate and vitamin B_{12}. Because folate and B_{12} work together to perform a number of biochemical functions, a deficiency of either one produces the same abnormalities in red blood cells.

As **Figure 10.21** shows, folate has three parts: pteridine, *para*-aminobenzoic acid (PABA), and at least one molecule of glutamic acid (glutamate). About 90 percent of the folate molecules found naturally in foods contain 3 to

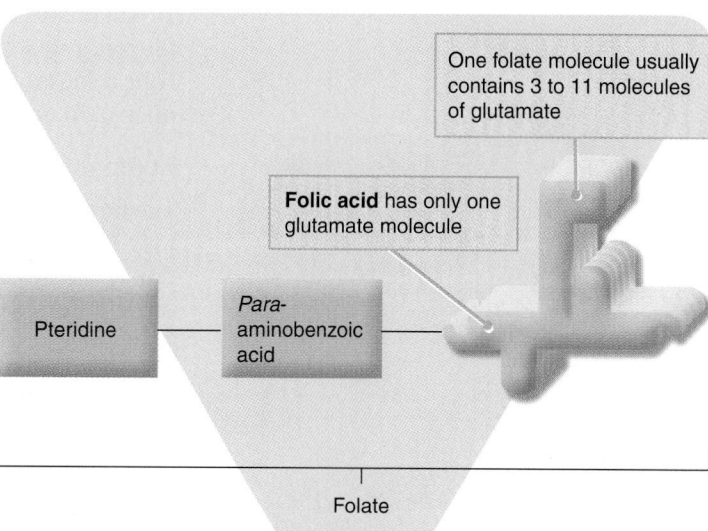

One folate molecule usually contains 3 to 11 molecules of glutamate

Folic acid has only one glutamate molecule

Pteridine

Para-aminobenzoic acid

Folate

Figure 10.21 **Folate and its major components.** Folate is made up of pteridine, *para*-aminobenzoic acid (PABA), and at least one molecule of glutamic acid (glutamate).

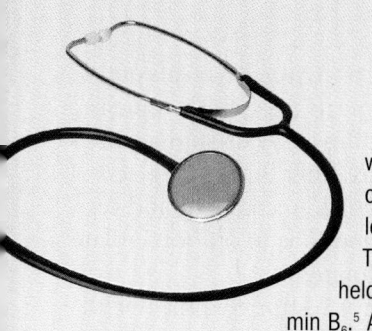

women who consumed the least folate. The same held true for vitamin B_6.[5] A study in Australia, however, did not find an association between risk of fatal cardiovascular disease in the general public and lower folate and B_{12} status.[6] A prospective study in the Netherlands found no increased heart disease risk in healthy adults with elevated homocysteine levels.[7] Lowering of homocysteine levels through supplementation with folic acid, vitamin B_{12}, and vitamin B_6 did reduce risk of future coronary events in people with preexisting heart disease.[8]

In 2006, two large prospective studies of patients with preexisting vascular disease failed to find clinical benefit (with the possible exception of stroke reduction) from using folic acid and vitamin B_{12}—with or without the addi-

tion of vitamin B_6—to lower homocysteine levels.[9] The preexisting vascular disease in these study populations may have overwhelmed any beneficial effects of B vitamin supplementation. Critics of these studies have suggested that we need longer prospective studies of normal populations to definitively identify the benefits of lowering homocysteine levels.

At this time, no major health organization recommends across-the-board testing for homocysteine. Some physicians, however, do advise testing for people with a strong family history of heart disease and those who have suffered a heart attack or other coronary event in the absence of high blood cholesterol or other risk factors. A simple blood test can measure homocysteine levels at a cost between $50 and $120. When ordered by a physician, many insurers, including Medicare, will cover the expense.

1 McCully KS. *The Homocysteine Revolution*. New Canaan, CT: Keats Publishing, 1997.

2 Stampfer MJ, Malinow MR, Willett WC, et al. A prospective study of plasma homocyst(e)ine and risk of myocardial infarction in US physicians. *JAMA*. 1992;268:877–881.

3 Selhub J, Jacques PF, Wilson PW, et al. Vitamin status and intake as primary determinants of homocysteinemia in an elderly population. *JAMA*. 1993;270:2693–2698.

4 McCully KS. Homocysteine, folate, vitamin B_6, and cardiovascular disease. *JAMA*. 1998;279:392–393.

5 Rimm E, Willett WC, Hu FB, et al. Folate and vitamin B_6 from diet and supplements in relation to risk of coronary heart disease among women. *JAMA*. 1998;279:359–364.

6 Hung J, Beilby JP, Knuiman MW, Divitini M. Folate and vitamin B-12 and risk of fatal cardiovascular disease: cohort study from Brusselton, Western Australia. *BMJ*. 2003;326:131–136.

7 de Bree A, Verschuren MM, Blom HJ, Nadeau M, Trijbels FJM, Kromhout D. Coronary heart disease mortality, plasma homocysteine, and B-vitamins: a prospective study. *Atherosclerosis*. 2003;166:369–377.

8 Schnyder G, Roffi M, Flammer Y, Pin R, Hess OM. Effect of homocysteine-lowering therapy with folic acid, vitamin B_{12}, and vitamin B_6 on clinical outcome after percutaneous coronary intervention. The Swiss Heart Study: a randomized controlled trial. *JAMA*. 2002;288:973–979.

9 Bonaa KH, Njolstad I, Ueland PM, et al. Homocysteine lowering and cardiovascular events after acute myocardial infarction. *N Engl J Med*. 2006;354:1578–1588; and The Heart Outcomes Prevention Evaluation (HOPE) 2 Investigators. Homocysteine lowering with folic acid and B vitamins in vascular disease. *N Engl J Med*. 2006;354:1567–1577.

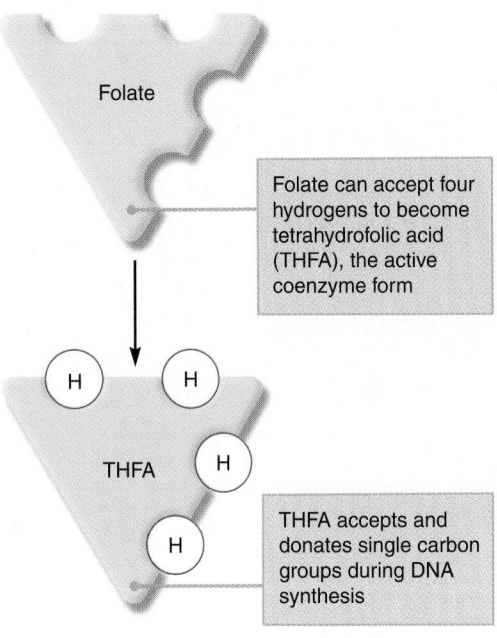

Figure 10.22 **Folate, THFA, and DNA.** Five forms of tetrahydrofolic acid (THFA) are the active coenzyme forms of folate.

dietary folate equivalents (DFE) A measure of folate intake used to account for the high bioavailability of folic acid taken as a supplement compared with the lower bioavailability of the folate found in foods.

DRI Values and Bioavailability of Folate

1 μg DFE = 1 μg food folate

= 0.5 μg folic acid taken on an empty stomach

= 0.6 μg folic acid consumed with meals

11 glutamates. All but one of these glutamates is removed in the small intestine prior to absorption. The folic acid form of folate has only one glutamate. Folic acid is the most stable form of folate and is the form used for supplementation and fortification.

Functions of Folate

The body converts folate to a coenzyme called tetrahydrofolic acid (THFA). (See **Figure 10.22.**) THFA has five active forms, all of which accept and donate one-carbon units during DNA synthesis, amino acid metabolism, cell division, and the maturation of red blood cells and other cells.

Dietary Recommendations for Folate

The bioavailability of folate varies depending on stomach contents and the folate source. The body absorbs nearly 100 percent of folic acid in supplements taken on an empty stomach. Some research suggests, however, that the presence of even a small portion of food reduces the absorption of supplemental folic acid to about 85 percent—the same as the bioavailability of folic acid in fortified breads and cereals.[32] The bioavailability of folate naturally present in food is lower—about 50 to 67 percent of intake.[33] To account for these differences, DRI values are expressed as **dietary folate equivalents (DFE)**.

The RDA for folate for males and females aged 19 years and older is 400 micrograms of DFE per day. The folate RDA for women increases significantly during pregnancy and lactation: 600 micrograms of DFE per day for pregnant women and 500 micrograms DFE per day while a woman is breastfeeding. To reduce the risk of bearing a child with certain birth defects, especially neural tube defects, the Institute of Medicine and the U.S. Public Health Service advise women of childbearing age to take in 400 micrograms of synthetic folic acid daily, from fortified foods or supplements, as well as to eat folate-containing foods.[34]

Sources of Folate

Most folate in the U.S. diet comes from fortified ready-to-eat cereals and various vegetables. Spinach and other dark-green leafy vegetables, asparagus, broccoli, orange juice, wheat germ, liver, sunflower seeds, and legumes are particularly good sources. Although vegetables other than dark-green leafy ones are less rich in folate, we eat foods such as green beans and vegetable soup so often that they make major contributions to our total folate intake.[35] **Figure 10.23** shows foods that provide folate.

Folate status during the early stages of pregnancy is strongly linked with birth defects, specifically neural tube defects. Studies consistently show that folic acid supplementation around the time of conception reduces risk of these birth defects by nearly 70 percent. This link prompted the U.S. government to mandate folate fortification of enriched cereal grains, including bread, pasta, flour, breakfast cereal, and rice.[36] This 1998 mandate called for a fortification level of 1.4 milligrams of folic acid per kilogram of grain.

Scientists estimate that folate fortification increases folic acid intake by about 100 micrograms per day (an amount provided by slightly more than one-half cup of enriched pasta or one slice of bread) and boosts daily consumption by women of childbearing age to 400 micrograms of folic acid. When food survey data were adjusted to reflect folic acid supplementation and correct for differences in bioavailability, folate intakes met or surpassed the EAR in 67 to 95 percent of the population groups. However, 68 to 87 percent of women of childbearing age had synthetic folic acid intakes below 400 micrograms per day.[37]

Folate is extremely vulnerable to heat, ultraviolet light, and exposure to oxygen. Cooking and other food-processing and preparation techniques can destroy 50 to 90 percent of a food's folate. Experts recommend eating folate-rich fruits and vegetables raw, or cooking them quickly in minimal amounts of water via steaming, stir-frying, or microwaving. Vitamin C in foods also helps protect folate from oxidation.

Folate Deficiency

Many scientists believe that folate deficiency is the most prevalent of all vitamin deficiencies. Studies suggest that up to 10 percent of the U.S. population have insufficient folate stores. Deficiency may stem from the following conditions:

- *Inadequate folate consumption.* General malnutrition, often due to famine or poverty, causes folate deficiency. Cultural cooking methods that destroy folate, eating habits that avoid raw folate-rich vegetables, alcoholism, excessive dieting, and anorexia nervosa and bulimia nervosa can severely limit folate intake. The infirm or neglected elderly and institutionalized psychiatric patients also are at risk.

- *Inadequate folate absorption* due to abnormalities in the mucosal cells lining the GI tract.

Quick Bites

Can Folate Prevent Cancer?

When women took multivitamins containing folate for at least 15 years, they had a 75 percent reduction in colon cancer risk, according to the Harvard Nurses' Health Study. Folate intakes of more than 600 micrograms per day reduced breast cancer risk by 50 percent.

FOLATE

Daily Value = 400 μg

Exceptionally good sources

Chicken liver, cooked	85 g (3 oz)	491 μg
Wheat bran flakes cereal	30 g (1 cup)	417 μg
All Bran cereal	30 g (1/2 cup)	404 μg
Product 19 cereal	30 g (1 cup)	400 μg

High: 20% DV or more

Beef liver, cooked	85 g (3 oz)	215 μg
Cheerios cereal	30 g (1 cup)	200 μg
Spinach, raw	85 g (~3 cups)	165 μg
Lentils, cooked	90 g (~1/2 cup)	163 μg
Pinto beans, cooked	90 g (~1/2 cup)	155 μg
Corn flakes cereal	30 g (1 cup)	144 μg
Black beans, cooked	90 g (~1/2 cup)	134 μg
Asparagus, cooked	85 g (~1/2 cup)	127 μg
Spinach, cooked	85 g (~1/2 cup)	124 μg
Romaine lettuce, raw	85 g (~11/2 cups)	116 μg
Blackeyed peas, cooked	90 g (~1/2 cup)	114 μg
Spaghetti, enriched, cooked	140 g (1 cup)	102 μg
Oatmeal, instant, fortified, cooked	1 cup	101 μg
Turnip greens, cooked	85 g (~2/3 cup)	100 μg
Soybeans, cooked	90 g (~1/2 cup)	100 μg
Broccoli, cooked	85 g (~1/2 cup)	92 μg
White bread, enriched	50 g (2 slices)	92 μg
Rice, white, enriched, cooked	140 g (~3/4 cup)	81 μg

Good: 10–19% DV

Collards, cooked	85 g (~1/2 cup)	79 μg
Sunflower seeds	30 g (~ 1 oz)	71 μg
Beets, cooked	85 g (~1/2 cup)	68 μg
Mustard greens, cooked	85 g (~2/3 cup)	62 μg
Tomato juice, canned	240 ml (1 cup)	49 μg
Kidney beans, canned	85 g (~1/2 cup)	47 μg
Orange juice, chilled	240 ml (1 cup)	45 μg
Crab, Alaska king, cooked	85 g (3 oz)	43 μg
Artichokes, cooked	85 g (~1/2 cup)	43 μg
Wheat germ	15 g (1/4 cup)	42 μg
Orange, fresh	140 g (1 medium)	42 μg

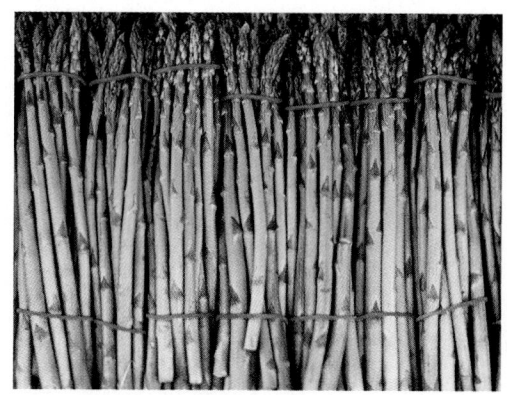

Figure 10.23 **Food sources of folate.** Good sources of folate are a diverse collection of foods: liver, legumes, leafy greens, and orange juice. Enriched grains and fortified cereals are other ways to include folic acid in the diet.
Source: U.S. Department of Agriculture, Agricultural Research Service. USDA National Nutrient Database for Standard Reference, Release 18. 2005. http://www.ars.usda.gov/nutrientdata.

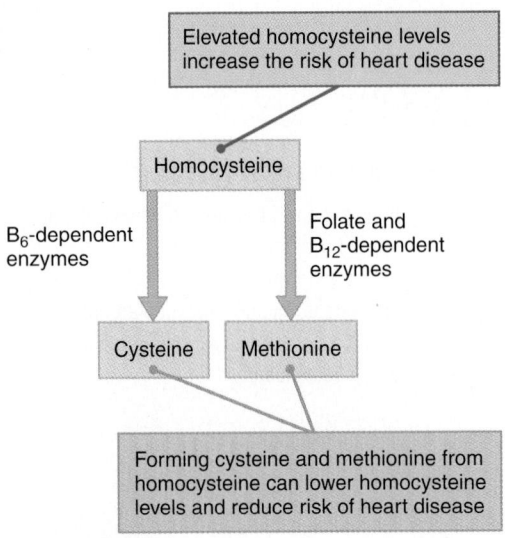

Figure 10.24 **Homocysteine and heart disease.** Elevated homocysteine levels are linked to an increased risk of heart disease. B$_6$-, B$_{12}$-, and folate-dependent enzymes help lower the amount of homocysteine by converting it to cysteine and methionine.

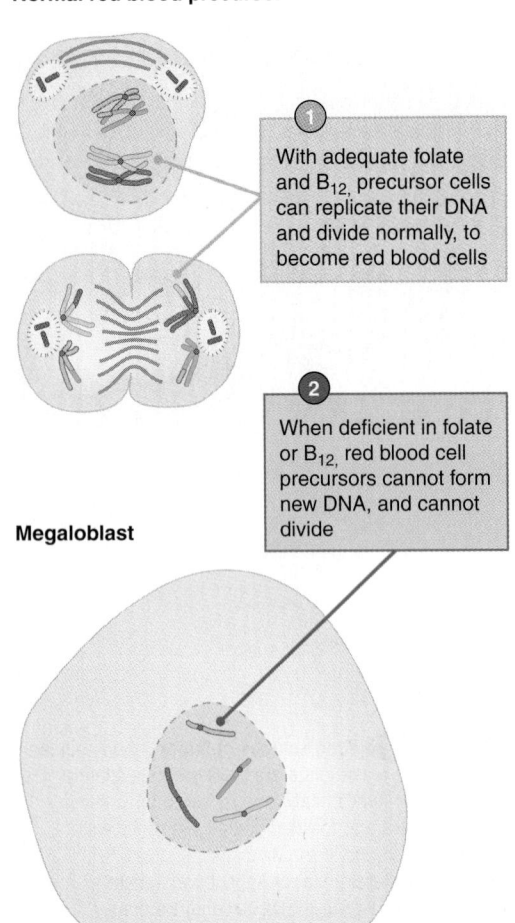

- *Increased folate requirements* due to pregnancy and lactation, or other conditions. Certain diseases, such as blood disorders, leukemia, lymphoma, and psoriasis, can increase folate needs.
- *Impaired folate utilization,* typically associated with a vitamin B$_6$ deficiency.
- *Altered folate metabolism* arising from use of alcohol or certain prescription drugs such as barbiturates. Sulfa drugs and anticonvulsants probably impair folate absorption.
- *Excessive folate excretion* due to prolonged diarrhea.

Folate and Heart Disease

Recent research suggests that folate has an important role in preventing heart disease. Folate works with vitamin B$_{12}$ and vitamin B$_6$ to reduce elevated homocysteine, which is a risk factor for heart attacks.[38] (See **Figure 10.24**.) When folate intake is inadequate, homocysteine levels rise; during a folate deficiency, homocysteine levels are markedly elevated. As folate intake increases, homocysteine levels drop. The Food and Nutrition Board used homocysteine levels as a primary factor in estimating the folate RDA, and the recommended folate intakes help maintain homocysteine at reduced levels. A daily intake of 400 micrograms of supplemental folic acid was adequate for reducing plasma homocysteine levels in older adults.[39]

Megaloblastic Anemia

A cellular deficiency of either folate or vitamin B$_{12}$ can impair DNA synthesis in proliferating cells without significant alterations in RNA and protein synthesis. The lack of DNA first affects red blood cells, which are rapidly dividing cells that typically turn over every 120 days. When red blood cell precursors in the bone marrow cannot form new DNA, they cannot divide normally to become red blood cells. As these precursor cells continue to synthesize protein and other cell components, they grow into large, bizarre shapes. (See **Figure 10.25**.) These large, fragile, immature cells, called **megaloblasts**, displace red blood cells and are a hallmark of **megaloblastic anemia.**

Megaloblasts may mature into **macrocytes**—abnormally large red blood cells with short life spans. As megaloblasts and macrocytes proliferate and the number of normal red blood cells decreases, the blood's ability to carry oxygen drops, causing weakness and fatigue. Folate-deficiency anemia commonly causes depression, irritability, forgetfulness, and disturbed sleep.

Impaired DNA synthesis also affects the rapidly dividing cells lining the gastrointestinal tract. As a result, large, immature GI cells multiply and accumulate along the absorptive surface of the digestive tract, where they interfere with absorption, causing chronic diarrhea. In the mouth, these defective cells cause the tongue to appear beefy red. A lack of folate also impairs the synthesis of white blood cells, which are vital to the immune response.

Depending on their magnitude, the body's folate stores can sustain normal functioning for two to four months after folate intake stops. Appropriate vitamin replacement restores normal cell reproduction within 24 hours.

Neural Tube Defects

A large body of evidence links poor folate status during the early stages of pregnancy to an increased risk of a birth defect known as a

Figure 10.25 **Megaloblastic anemia.** When red blood cell precursors in the bone marrow cannot form new DNA, they cannot divide normally. These precursor cells continue to grow and become large, fragile, immature cells called megaloblasts. Megaloblasts displace red blood cells, resulting in megaloblastic anemia.

neural tube defect (NTD). In this type of birth defect, the neural tube fails to encase the spinal cord during early fetal development. This causes a number of disorders, including **spina bifida** and **anencephaly**. (See **Figure 10.26**.) Worldwide, NTDs afflict one to nine of every 1,000 infants born. The FDA's mandate to fortify enriched grains with folic acid has been estimated to have reduced the incidence of spina bifida by 20 percent.[40] Interestingly, one study suggests that both Down syndrome and spina bifida may result from the same genetic abnormality in folate metabolism.[41] Studies also show that women deficient in folate are more likely to have low-birth-weight babies[42] and premature deliveries.[43]

Folate Toxicity

Because folate works so closely with vitamin B$_{12}$, it can mask a vitamin B$_{12}$ deficiency. Older adults have increased risk of B$_{12}$ deficiency, and consuming excess folate can prevent the formation of altered red blood cells that signals a lack of B$_{12}$. Some evidence also suggests that high intakes of folic acid may prompt or exacerbate the neurological problems associated with vitamin B$_{12}$ deficiency.

Although rare, when hypersensitive people take folic acid supplements, they may suffer hives or respiratory distress. The UL for adults is 1,000 micrograms per day of folic acid from supplements and fortified foods. Researchers have found that folate intake in elders did not generally exceed the UL; however, 20 to 30 percent of children exceed the UL for their age groups (UL for ages 1–3 years = 300 μg/d; UL for ages 4–6 years = 400 μg/d).[44]

Vitamin B$_{12}$

Vitamin B$_{12}$ is also called cobalamin, a generic term that describes a group of cobalt-containing compounds. Scientists usually use the term *vitamin B$_{12}$* to refer to the free vitamin compound called cyanocobalamin. In the United States, it is the only form of vitamin B$_{12}$ commercially available in supplements.

Functions of Vitamin B$_{12}$

Vitamin B$_{12}$ plays a key role in folate metabolism by transferring a methyl group (–CH$_3$) from the folate coenzyme THFA, as **Figure 10.27** shows. Without vitamin B$_{12}$, THFA cannot change into its methylene form—the

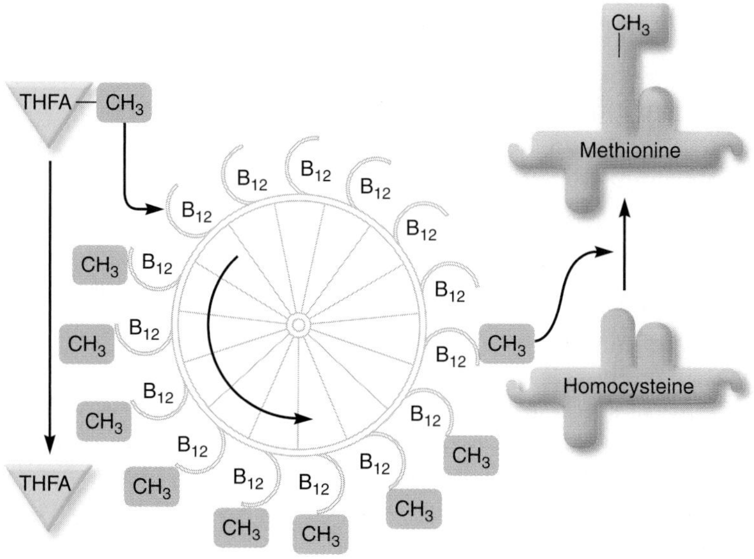

megaloblasts Large, immature red blood cells produced when precursor cells fail to divide normally due to impaired DNA synthesis.

megaloblastic anemia Excess amounts of megaloblasts in the blood caused by deficiency of folate or vitamin B$_{12}$.

macrocytes Abnormally large red blood cells with short life spans.

neural tube defect (NTD) A birth defect resulting from failure of the neural tube to develop properly during early fetal development.

spina bifida A type of neural tube birth defect.

anencephaly A type of neural tube birth defect in which part or all of the brain is missing.

SPINE AFFECTED BY SPINA BIFIDA

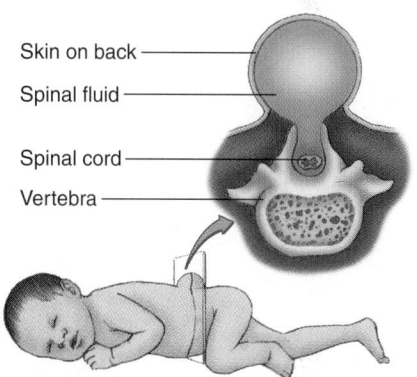

Skin on back
Spinal fluid
Spinal cord
Vertebra

Figure 10.26 **Neural tube defects.** Poor folate status during the early stages of pregnancy, even before a woman may realize she is pregnant, increases the risk of a neural tube defect.

CH$_3$

Methionine

THFA — CH$_3$

B$_{12}$

CH$_3$

CH$_3$

CH$_3$

THFA

CH$_3$

CH$_3$

CH$_3$

CH$_3$

CH$_3$

CH$_3$

CH$_3$

Homocysteine

Figure 10.27 **Vitamin B$_{12}$ helps transfer methyl groups.** Vitamin B$_{12}$ helps transfer a methyl group (–CH$_3$) from the folate coenzyme THFA. One destination for the methyl group is the reaction that converts homocysteine to methionine. This conversion reduces homocysteine blood levels, thereby lowering the risk of heart disease.

myelin sheath The protective coating that surrounds nerve fibers.

R-protein A protein produced by the salivary glands that may protect vitamin B_{12} as it travels through the stomach and into the small intestine.

atrophic gastritis An age-related condition in which the stomach loses its ability to secrete acid. In severe cases, ability to make intrinsic factor is also impaired.

active form in many important metabolic pathways. For instance, a deficiency of the methylene form of THFA inhibits DNA synthesis. The partnership between B_{12} and folate coenzyme THFA means that a vitamin B_{12} deficiency can lead to a folate deficiency, and a lack of either B_{12} or folate can precipitate megaloblastic anemia. Vitamin B_{12}–dependent enzymes also work with THFA to convert homocysteine to methionine, thereby reducing homocysteine blood levels and lowering the risk of heart disease.

Vitamin B_{12} also helps maintain the **myelin sheath**, the protective coating that surrounds nerve fibers. In addition, by helping to rearrange carbon atoms in fatty acid chains, vitamin B_{12} helps prepare them to enter the citric acid cycle.

Absorption of Vitamin B_{12}

The absorption of vitamin B_{12} is a complex process that requires several factors. (See **Figure 10.28**.) In the stomach, vitamin B_{12} binds with **R-protein**, a protein produced by the salivary glands that may protect vitamin B_{12} as it travels through the stomach and into the small intestine. Once there, pancreatic proteases such as trypsin cleave vitamin B_{12} from R-protein. Vitamin B_{12} then binds to intrinsic factor, a substance produced by the parietal cells of the stomach, the same cells that produce hydrochloric acid. Together, the two substances journey to the ileum of the small intestine and attach to receptor cells on the organ's brush border. The receptor cells absorb vitamin B_{12} and transfer it to transcobalamin II, a protein carrier in the blood. Transcobalamin II enters the bloodstream and delivers vitamin B_{12} to the liver, bone marrow, and developing blood cells.

A defect at any point in this process can cause a vitamin B_{12} deficiency. Factors that can impair vitamin B_{12} absorption include the following:

- Lack of R-protein, pancreatic enzymes, or intrinsic factor
- Absence or removal of the ileum or stomach
- Overgrowth of bacteria in the stomach
- Tapeworm
- Reduction of gastric acid production due to prolonged use of acid-inhibiting medications or an age-related condition called **atrophic gastritis**

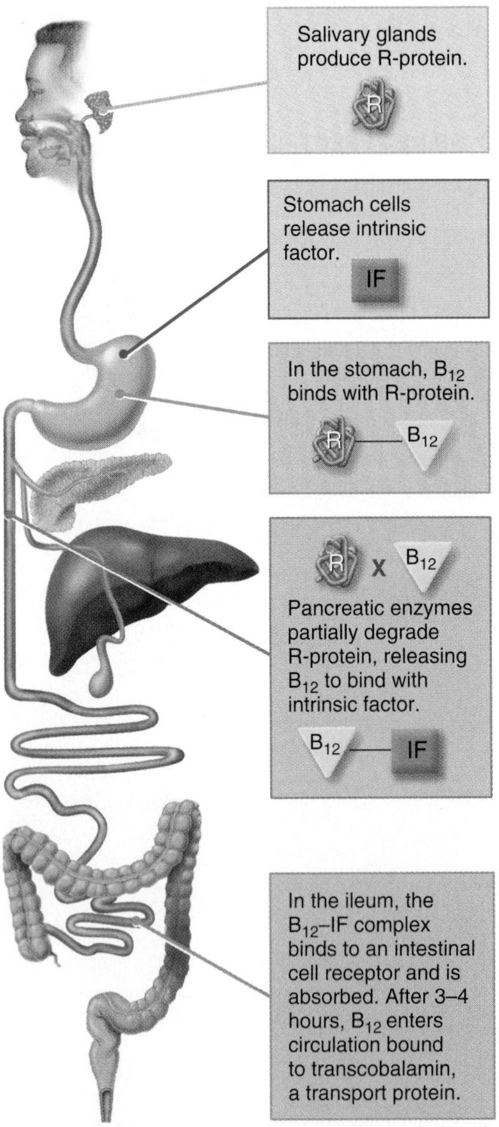

Dietary Recommendations for Vitamin B_{12}

The RDA for men and women aged 19 to 50 is 2.4 micrograms per day. Although the value for adults 51 and older is the same, up to 30 percent of these older adults have atrophic gastritis, which decreases the bioavailability of vitamin B_{12} naturally found in animal foods. People with atrophic gastritis should focus on fortified foods and dietary supplements for most of their B_{12} intake. The form of vitamin B_{12} in these sources is well absorbed—even by people with atrophic gastritis.[45]

Sources of Vitamin B_{12}

Except for fortified foods such as ready-to-eat cereals or some soy milks, animal-derived foods are the only good sources of vitamin B_{12}. Bacteria in animal stomachs synthesize B_{12}, and B_{12} is in the soil that animals consume when eating and grazing. Animals store excess B_{12} in their tissues, especially their livers. Unlike the other B vitamins, B_{12} is not normally present in plant foods. Although products made from soy paste and sea algae list vitamin B_{12} as an ingredient, they contain only an inactive and biologically unavailable form.

Salivary glands produce R-protein.

Stomach cells release intrinsic factor.
IF

In the stomach, B_{12} binds with R-protein.
R—B_{12}

R X B_{12}
Pancreatic enzymes partially degrade R-protein, releasing B_{12} to bind with intrinsic factor.
B_{12}—IF

In the ileum, the B_{12}–IF complex binds to an intestinal cell receptor and is absorbed. After 3–4 hours, B_{12} enters circulation bound to transcobalamin, a transport protein.

Figure 10.28 **Absorption of vitamin B_{12}.** Absorption of B_{12} is a complex process that involves many factors and sites in the GI tract. Defects in this process, especially a lack of intrinsic factor, impair B_{12} absorption and can lead to B_{12} deficiency.

Mixed foods, including sandwiches whose main ingredient is meat, fish, or poultry, contribute most of our dietary B$_{12}$. The next most important sources are milk and milk products for women and beef for men. Although shellfish, liver and other organ meats, some game meat, and some kinds of fish are the richest sources of B$_{12}$, few people regularly eat these foods.[46] Figure 10.29 shows foods that provide vitamin B$_{12}$.

Although definitive data are lacking, scientists conservatively estimate that about 50 percent of dietary B$_{12}$ is bioavailable. That percentage may drop when a person consumes foods particularly high in vitamin B$_{12}$.

Vitamin B$_{12}$ Deficiency

Whereas a folate deficiency has several causes, often in combination, a vitamin B$_{12}$ deficiency is almost always due to impaired absorption, especially in older people. To circumvent malabsorption, vitamin B$_{12}$ injections deliver the vitamin directly to the bloodstream. Because the liver stores a substantial amount of B$_{12}$, monthly shots usually are sufficient. Other treatments include taking megadoses of vitamin B$_{12}$ supplements (300 times the RDA) that overwhelm impaired absorption, and using a vitamin B$_{12}$–containing nasal gel.

Vegetarians who eat neither meat nor dairy products are at risk of vitamin B$_{12}$ deficiency unless they take vitamin B$_{12}$ supplements or regularly eat fortified cereals. Adult livers store large amounts (3–5 milligrams) of vitamin B$_{12}$, so deficiencies develop slowly—over 3 to 12 years. Strict vegetarian (vegan) mothers who breastfeed may put their infants at risk of long-term neurological problems unless they include supplemental vitamin B$_{12}$ in their diets.

Symptoms of Vitamin B$_{12}$ Deficiency

The major outcome of impaired vitamin B$_{12}$ absorption is vitamin B$_{12}$–deficiency anemia. As in folate-deficiency anemia, lack of B$_{12}$ causes the formation of megaloblasts and macrocytes rather than normal red blood cells. But there are important differences. Folate deficiency may lead to cognitive defects and depression, but B$_{12}$ deficiency causes the myelin sheath to swell and break down, leading to brain abnormalities and spinal cord degeneration.

Neurological symptoms include tingling and numbness in the extremities, abnormal gait, and cognitive changes ranging from loss of concentration to memory loss, disorientation, and dementia.[47] If the megaloblastic anemia is inappropriately treated with folate, red blood cell production normalizes, but neurological damage worsens. Neurological effects may or may not be reversible, depending on their duration.

Pernicious Anemia

Pernicious anemia is the result of an autoimmune disorder in which the body destroys the parietal cells in the stomach.[48] Loss of parietal cells means a loss of intrinsic factor, which in turn reduces vitamin B$_{12}$ absorption. Pernicious anemia is a major cause of vitamin B$_{12}$ deficiency, although in the elderly, malabsorption of food-bound B$_{12}$ causes the majority of B$_{12}$ deficiency cases.[49] Pernicious anemia can affect people of all ages, races, and ethnic origins. Without treatment, nerve degeneration from vitamin B$_{12}$ deficiency becomes

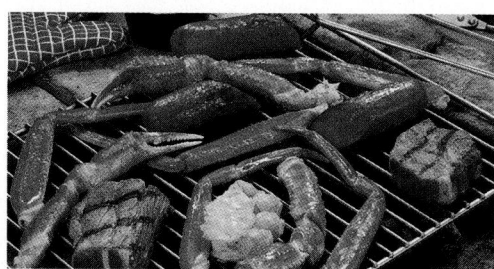

VITAMIN B$_{12}$

Daily Value = 6 µg

High: 20% DV or more

Good: 10–19% DV

Exceptionally good sources

Clams, cooked	85 g (3 oz)	84.1 µg
Beef liver, cooked	85 g (3 oz)	60.0 µg
Oysters, cooked	85 g (3 oz)	29.8 µg
Chicken liver, cooked	85 g (3 oz)	14.3 µg
Herring, cooked	85 g (3 oz)	11.2 µg
Crab, Alaska King, cooked	85 g (3 oz)	9.8 µg
Crab, blue, cooked	85 g (3 oz)	6.2 µg
Wheat bran flakes cereal	30 g (3/4 cup)	6.2 µg
All Bran cereal	30 g (1/2 cup)	6.0 µg
Sardines, canned, solids + bones	55 g (2 oz)	4.9 µg
Salmon, cooked	85 g (3 oz)	2.6 µg
Lobster, cooked	85 g (3 oz)	2.6 µg
Beef, ground, extra lean, cooked	85 g (3 oz)	2.1 µg
Beef, T-bone steak, cooked	85 g (3 oz)	1.9 µg
Tuna, canned	55 g (2 oz)	1.6 µg
Yogurt, plain, nonfat	225 g (8-oz container)	1.4 µg
Shrimp, cooked	85 g (3 oz)	1.3 µg
Yogurt, plain, lowfat	225 g (8-oz container)	1.3 µg
Milk, nonfat	240 ml (1 cup)	1.3 µg
Halibut, cooked	85 g (3 oz)	1.2 µg
Milk, 2% milkfat	240 ml (1 cup)	1.1 µg
Milk, whole 3.25% milkfat	240 ml (1 cup)	1.1 µg
Squid, cooked	85 g (3 oz)	1.1 µg
Milk, 1% milkfat	240 ml (1 cup)	1.1 µg
Frankfurter, beef	55 g (1 each)	1.0 µg
Cod, cooked	85 g (3 oz)	0.9 µg
Cottage cheese, 2% milkfat	110 g (~1/2 cup)	0.8 µg
Bologna, beef	55 g (2 slices)	0.7 µg
Pork, loin chops, lean only, cooked	85 g (3 oz)	0.7 µg

Figure 10.29 **Food sources of vitamin B$_{12}$.** Vitamin B$_{12}$ is found naturally only in foods of animal origin such as liver, meats, and milk. Some cereals are fortified with vitamin B$_{12}$. **Note:** The DV for vitamin B$_{12}$ is substantially higher than the current (1998) RDA of 2.4 micrograms for those age 14 and older. **Source:** U.S. Department of Agriculture, Agricultural Research Service. USDA National Nutrient Database for Standard Reference, Release 18. 2005. http://www.ars.usda.gov/nutrientdata.

pernicious anemia A form of anemia that results from an autoimmune disorder that damages cells lining the stomach and inhibits vitamin B$_{12}$ absorption, leading to vitamin B$_{12}$ deficiency.

reducing agent A compound that donates electrons or hydrogen atoms to another compound.

connective tissues Tissues composed primarily of fibrous proteins such as collagen, and which contain few cells. Their primary function is to bind together and support various body structures.

Quick Bites

Chili Peppers Are Hot Stuff

An estimated one-quarter of the world's adults eat chili peppers every day. By weight, chili peppers are one of the richest sources of vitamins A and C. In addition, capsaicin, the substance that causes your mouth to burn, jump-starts the digestive process by stimulating salivation.

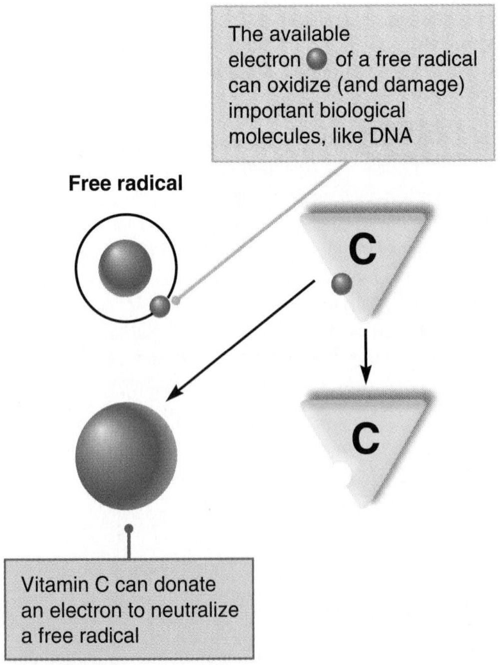

The available electron ● of a free radical can oxidize (and damage) important biological molecules, like DNA

Free radical

Vitamin C can donate an electron to neutralize a free radical

Figure 10.30 Vitamin C is an antioxidant. Vitamin C minimizes free radical damage by donating an electron. Vitamin C also indirectly activates many enzymes. Although essential to enzyme activity, unlike the B vitamins, vitamin C is not a coenzyme.

irreversible and ultimately proves fatal. In fact, *pernicious* means "leading to death." Fortunately, timely vitamin B_{12} injections usually reverse the blood abnormalities and other signs of pernicious anemia within a matter of days. People with pernicious anemia are at a higher risk for stomach cancer.

Vitamin B_{12} Toxicity

High levels of vitamin B_{12} from food or supplements have not been shown to cause harmful side effects in healthy people. Doses of 1 milligram are routinely used to treat pernicious anemia with no ill effects. A UL for vitamin B_{12} has not been determined.

Key Concepts: *Folate and vitamin B_{12} work closely together. Fruits, vegetables, enriched grains, and fortified cereals contain folate, but only animal foods and fortified cereals contain bioavailable vitamin B_{12}. A deficiency of folate causes megaloblastic anemia and has been associated with neural tube defects. Deficiency of B_{12} causes a form of megaloblastic anemia and irreversible nerve damage. Vitamin B_{12} deficiency usually results from poor absorption, either due to pernicious anemia or other GI problems, such as atrophic gastritis. Because vitamin B_{12} is found only in animal foods, strict vegetarians must find an alternative source. Folate, vitamin B_{12}, and vitamin B_6 all play roles in the metabolism of the amino acid homocysteine, which has been implicated in heart disease.*

Vitamin C

For centuries, the insidious disease scurvy dogged humankind. Explorers and seafaring men especially feared this mysterious ailment that inflicted aching pain and made each journey a gamble with death. Writings that date back as far as 1,500 B.C.E. describe their suffering in detail.

Though they did not know why, some travelers avoided this scourge. Unknowingly, they had eaten foods that contained vitamin C. The mystery began to be solved in 1746 by James Lind, a 30-year-old ship's surgeon in the British navy. In a controlled human nutrition clinical trial (see Figure 1.12 in Chapter 1, "Nutrients and Nourishment"), he carefully evaluated six different therapies for scurvy and showed that only those patients who received lemons or oranges recovered.[50] In the mid-1800s in Great Britain it was known that when potatoes were scarce, outbreaks of scurvy occurred.[51] When neither potatoes nor fruit were available, green vegetables were found to prevent scurvy. It was not until 1930 that scientists isolated the substance responsible for curing scurvy, the "antiascorbutic" factor, and named it vitamin C.

Vitamin C comes in two interchangeable, biologically active forms: a reduced form called ascorbic acid and an oxidized form called dehydroascorbic acid. Although most animals manufacture their own vitamin C, humans cannot, sharing this dubious distinction with fruit-eating bats, guinea pigs, and a few other isolated species. For some unknown reason, humans also appear to require much less vitamin C than most other animals.

Functions of Vitamin C

Vitamin C is an antioxidant—it acts as a **reducing agent** and participates in many reactions by donating electrons or hydrogen ions. It also is essential to the activity of many enzymes. But unlike the B vitamins, it is not a coenzyme, and only indirectly activates enzymes.

Collagen Synthesis

Vitamin C plays an important role in the formation of collagen, a fibrous protein that helps reinforce the **connective tissues** that hold together the structures of the body. Collagen is made up of individual, linear proteins that wrap around one another like a cord of rope, forming a triple helix that imparts strength and flexibility. It is the most abundant protein in our bodies and the main fibrous component of skin, bone, tendons, cartilage, and teeth. It also is the major protein in connective tissue, which binds cells and tissues together, and in scar tissue.

Antioxidant Activity

Like vitamin E and beta-carotene (see Chapter 9), vitamin C works as an antioxidant and minimizes free radical damage in cells. As an antioxidant, vitamin C has been hypothesized to reduce risk of chronic diseases such as heart disease, certain forms of cancer, and cataracts. Current evidence does not support a strong link between vitamin C and cardiovascular disease. Evidence is more convincing for a role in cancer risk reduction, although it is still not clear whether the protective effects are due to vitamin C or to fruit and vegetable consumption in general.[52] In addition to working independently as an antioxidant (**Figure 10.30**), vitamin C helps recycle oxidized vitamin E for reuse in the cells.[53] Finally, vitamin C stabilizes the reduced form of the folate coenzyme.

Iron Absorption

As a reducing agent, vitamin C enhances the absorption of nonheme iron, which comes mainly from plant foods (the small intestine absorbs nonheme iron better when it is reduced).

Synthesis of Vital Cell Compounds

Vitamin C helps synthesize carnitine, a compound that carries fatty acids from the cytosol to the mitochondria for energy production. Vitamin C also helps synthesize norepinephrine, epinephrine, the neurotransmitter serotonin, the thyroid hormone thyroxine, bile acids, steroid hormones, and purine bases used in DNA synthesis.

Immune Function

Vitamin C enables lymphocytes and other cells of the immune system to function properly. This explains why people may need more vitamin C during an illness. Because chemical-detoxifying systems in cells use vitamin C, drug use also can boost vitamin C requirements.

Dietary Recommendations for Vitamin C

For adults aged 19 and older, the RDA for vitamin C is 90 milligrams per day for men and 75 milligrams per day for women. For women, the RDA rises to 85 milligrams per day during pregnancy and 120 milligrams per day during lactation. Because smoking increases the metabolic turnover of vitamin C, the Food and Nutrition Board estimates that smokers require 35 milligrams per day more than nonsmokers.[54]

Sources of Vitamin C

Particularly good sources of vitamin C include potatoes, citrus fruits, tomatoes, fortified juice drinks, broccoli, strawberries, kiwi fruit, cabbage, spinach and other leafy greens, and green peppers. Because vitamin C is highly vulnerable to heat and oxygen, fresh fruits and vegetables are the optimal sources. **Figure 10.31** shows some foods that provide vitamin C.

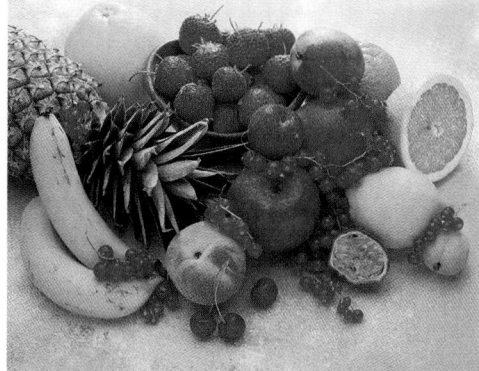

VITAMIN C

Daily Value = 60 mg

Exceptionally good sources

Orange juice, chilled	240 ml (1 cup)	83.1 mg
Strawberries, fresh	140 g (~1 cup)	82.3 mg
Orange, fresh	140 g (1 medium)	74.5 mg
Wheat bran flakes	30 g (³/4 cup)	62.1 mg
Broccoli, cooked	85 g (~1/2 cup)	55.2 mg
Cantaloupe, fresh	140 g (1/4 medium melon)	51.4 mg
Tomato juice, canned	240 ml (1 cup)	45.2 mg
Mango, fresh	140 g (~3/4 cup)	38.8 mg
Cauliflower, cooked	85 g (~3/4 cup)	37.7 mg
Spinach, raw	85 g (~3 cups)	23.9 mg
Pineapple, fresh	140 g (~1 cup)	23.7 mg
Sweet potato, cooked	110 g (1 small)	21.6 mg
Mustard greens, cooked	85 g (~2/3 cup)	21.5 mg
Romaine lettuce, raw	85 g (~1 1/2 cups)	20.4 mg
Clams, cooked	85 g (3 oz)	18.8 mg
Watermelon, fresh	280 g (1/16 melon)	18.5 mg
Cabbage, cooked	85 g (~1/2 cup)	17.1 mg
Kiwi fruit, fresh	140 g (2 medium)	16.0 mg
Collards, cooked	85 g (~1/2 cup)	15.5 mg
Soybeans, cooked	90 g (~1/2 cup)	15.3 mg
Swiss chard, cooked	85 g (~1/2 cup)	15.3 mg
Okra, cooked	85 g (~1/2 cup)	13.9 mg
Blueberries, fresh	140 g (~3/4 cup)	13.6 mg
Banana, fresh	140 g (1 9" banana)	12.2 mg
Potato, baked	110 g (1 small)	10.6 mg
Peach, fresh	140 g (2 small)	9.2 mg
Acorn squash, cooked	85 g (~1/2 cup)	9.2 mg
Spinach, cooked	85 g (~1/2 cup)	8.3 mg
Green beans, cooked	85 g (~3/4 cup)	8.2 mg
Corn flakes cereal	30 g (1 cup)	6.6 mg
Asparagus, cooked	85 g (~1/2 cup)	6.5 mg
Cheerios cereal	30 g (1 cup)	6.0 mg

High: 20% DV or more

Good: 10–19% DV

Figure 10.31 **Food sources of vitamin C.** Vitamin C is found mainly in fruits and vegetables. Although citrus fruits are notoriously good sources, many other popular fruits and vegetables are rich in vitamin C. **Source:** U.S. Department of Agriculture, Agricultural Research Service. USDA National Nutrient Database for Standard Reference, Release 18. 2005. http://www.ars.usda.gov/nutrientdata.

When people take in 30 milligrams to 120 milligrams daily, the intestine absorbs about 80 to 90 percent of vitamin C. However, when vitamin C consumption exceeds 6,000 milligrams daily, absorption drops to about 20 percent. Most of the residual vitamin C is excreted in the urine.

Vitamin C Deficiency

Scurvy is the well-known vitamin C–deficiency disease. Its first symptoms surface after about a month on a vitamin C–free diet. As the body loses its ability to synthesize collagen, connective tissue starts breaking down and gums and joints begin to bleed. Weakness develops, and small hemorrhages appear around the hair follicles on the arms and legs. As the disease progresses, previously healed wounds reopen, and bone pain, fractures, diarrhea, and psychological problems such as depression commonly emerge.

Scurvy is rare in developed countries, but possible among those who eat few fruits and vegetables, follow extremely restricted diets, or abuse alcohol or drugs.[55] Less severe vitamin C deficiency can impair cellular functions without causing overt scurvy. The most common symptoms are inflammation of the gums and fatigue.

Vitamin C Toxicity

Although megadoses of vitamin C do not appear to be acutely toxic to most healthy people, taking more than 2,000 milligrams daily for a prolonged period may lead to nausea, abdominal cramps, diarrhea, and nosebleeds.[56] The UL for vitamin C is 2,000 milligrams per day. In people with kidney disease, excess vitamin C also may contribute to oxalate-containing kidney stones. In healthy people, epidemiological studies do not support an association between excess vitamin C intake and kidney stones.[57] High vitamin C intakes also may bolster iron absorption—useful for some, but problematic for people with **hemochromatosis**, a metabolic disease that causes excess iron accumulation.

hemochromatosis A metabolic disorder that results in excess iron deposits in the body.

Finally, some experts suspect that large amounts of vitamin C may stimulate free radical damage by enhancing oxidation (a pro-oxidant effect), the opposite of its usual antioxidant activity. This suspicion is based on test-tube experiments that show vitamin C acting as a pro-oxidant when it comes into contact with iron or another metal.[58]

As for vitamin C's notoriety as a purported cure for the common cold, reviews of relevant research show no significant effect on the incidence of colds. At best, in some people, high doses may reduce the severity and duration of cold symptoms.[59]

Key Concepts: *Vitamin C, which is found in many fruits and vegetables, functions mainly in collagen synthesis. It also acts as an antioxidant. Vitamin C helps boost iron absorption and plays a part in hormone and neurotransmitter synthesis. A deficiency of vitamin C leads to scurvy, although this is rare today. Megadoses of vitamin C can cause gastrointestinal disturbances.*

Vitamin-like Compounds

The body synthesizes a number of vitamin-like compounds that play essential roles in maintaining metabolism. These include choline, carnitine, inositol, taurine, and lipoic acid. Although the risk of a deficiency is minimal in healthy people, it is unclear whether certain diseases cause deficiencies of these compounds and whether they should be added to infant formulas. Currently, many manufacturers of infant formula do add some of these compounds to their products.

Choline

Choline helps maintain the structural integrity of cell membranes and accelerates the production of acetylcholine, an important neurotransmitter involved in memory, muscle control, and other functions. Choline also is a component of lecithins and bile (choline was named after the French word for bile, *chole*). Likewise, it is a source of methyl groups needed for DNA methylation. Metabolic pathways link choline, methionine, folate, and vitamins B_6 and B_{12}. Low choline intake appears to increase folate requirements; conversely, low folate intake increases choline requirements.[60]

With the help of vitamin B_{12} and folate, the liver forms choline from the amino acids serine and methionine. If you eat enough protein to provide the essential amino acid methionine, your body can manufacture choline. Insufficient data are available to determine whether choline is truly essential in the human diet. The research that exists suggests that people on diets devoid of choline develop fatty liver and liver damage.

Because choline is widespread in the food supply, the risk of a deficiency is minimal in healthy people. Liver, eggs, beef, cauliflower, and peanuts are especially rich in choline. An AI for choline has been set at 550 milligrams per day for adult men, and 425 milligrams per day for adult women.

High doses of choline can cause hypotension (low blood pressure), sweating, diarrhea, and fishy body odor. The UL for adults is 3,500 milligrams of choline per day.

Carnitine

Carnitine carries fatty acids from the cytosol into the mitochondria for entry into the citric acid cycle. In the mitochondria, carnitine also helps dispose of excess organic acids produced via metabolic pathways. The liver synthesizes carnitine from the amino acids lysine and methionine.

Meat and dairy products are the major dietary sources of carnitine. Carnitine does not appear to be an essential compound for healthy people, because strict vegetarians often eat diets virtually lacking carnitine without suffering ill effects. Low blood levels of carnitine have been observed in malnourished children and adults. Diets deficient in the amino acids needed to make carnitine may cause abnormal fatty acid metabolism.

Carnitine in large doses has been helpful in removing toxic compounds in people with certain inborn errors of metabolism. In addition, high doses of carnitine have been successful in treating progressive muscle disease, deterioration of the heart muscle, and most recently, carnitine depletion in kidney dialysis patients.[61]

Inositol

Inositol is part of cell membrane phospholipids. Inositol phospholipids, a family of lipids containing inositol derivatives, are precursors of eicosanoids, substances that work like hormones in the body (for more on eicosanoids, see Chapter 5, "Lipids"). Inositol participates in a chain of reactions that ultimately increases the concentration of intracellular calcium, which in turn elicits a number of cell responses such as the relaying of messages by nerve cells. This may explain why inositol phospholipids are concentrated in brain tissue.

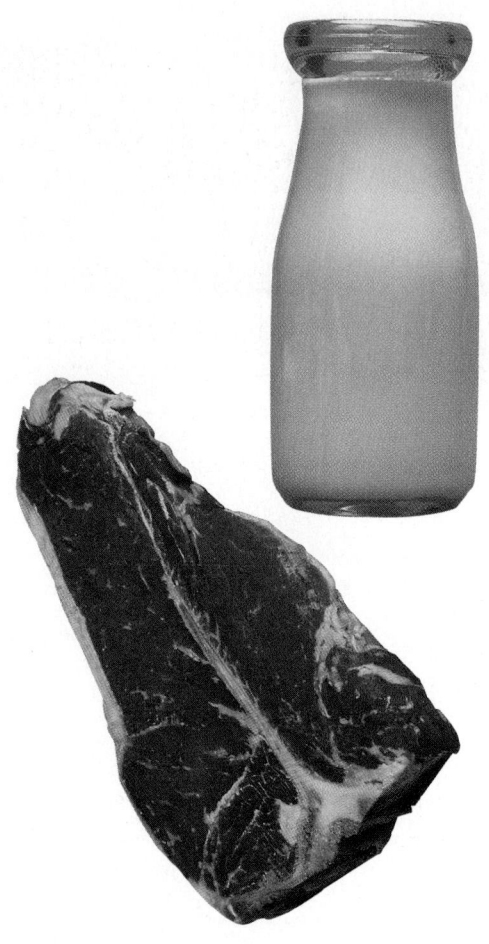

The body synthesizes inositol from glucose, and these two molecules have similar structures. Although there are nine forms of inositol, myo-inositol is the only one involved in human nutrition.

Although some plant foods contain inositol, animal-derived foods supply most dietary inositol. There is no reason to suspect inositol deficiency in the general population, and the Food and Nutrition Board has not set recommended intake levels. Inositol seems to become essential only for people with impaired inositol metabolism. Animal studies suggest that abnormal inositol metabolism may be associated with certain medical conditions such as diabetes, multiple sclerosis, kidney failure, and some cancers.

Taurine

Taurine seems to play a role in photoreceptor activity in the eye, antioxidant activity in white blood cells and pulmonary tissue, central nervous system function, platelet aggregation, heart muscle contraction, insulin activity, and cell growth and differentiation. Derived from the amino acids methionine and cysteine, taurine is concentrated in muscle, platelets, and nerve tissue and is attached to bile acids.

There is no evidence of taurine deficiency in the general population. Although it is found naturally only in foods from animal sources, strict vegetarians are not deficient. Apparently, people are able to synthesize all the taurine they need.

Taurine supplements may be useful for children with cystic fibrosis and preterm infants who absorb fat poorly. In these children, the taurine attached to bile acids may help increase fat absorption. Taurine is one of several amino acids that have become popular additives to so-called smart drinks designed to assist in mental activities. However, no solid scientific evidence links taurine to improved mental abilities.

Lipoic Acid

Lipoic acid is a necessary cofactor in energy-producing reactions in mitochondria. For instance, lipoic acid helps convert pyruvate to acetyl CoA, the major linking step between glycolysis and the citric acid cycle. It is a potent antioxidant and is unique because it can neutralize both fat-soluble and water-soluble free radicals. Although health food stores sell lipoic acid supplements, no evidence supports their use by healthy people.

Bogus Vitamins

Many dietary supplements contain unnecessary substances. Yet hucksters often call these substances vitamins and tout their supposed benefits as health enhancers and disease treatments. Despite ample scientific evidence to the contrary, quacks still hawk laetrile ("vitamin B_{17}") as a cancer cure. Some supplements contain hesperidin, *para*-aminobenzoic acid (PABA), pangamic acid, or rutin, even though these substances are not essential for human health. Think twice before you pay a premium price for supplements that contain these bogus vitamins.

Key Concepts: *The body contains a number of vitamin-like compounds synthesized from glucose and amino acids and found in the food supply. Although deficiencies of these substances are unlikely, some people with certain medical conditions may benefit from supplemental amounts of some of these compounds. Of course, supplements should be taken only with a physician's recommendation. Researchers are examining the needs for these substances and their effects on the body.*

Label [to] **Table**

The FDA requires all manufacturers to add folic acid to enriched grain products such as bread, flour, rice, and pasta. Folic acid, the synthetic form of folate, has been shown to decrease risk of neural tube defects. Folic acid or folate (its natural form) may also be important in reducing risk of heart disease and colon cancer. Prior to the fortification of enriched grains, it was difficult for some people to get enough of this B vitamin, in part because it is destroyed easily during cooking and storage. The purpose of folic acid fortification is to ensure most people, especially women of childbearing age, can meet their needs for this B vitamin. Look at the Nutrition Facts label on a pasta package. Note how much folic acid is in a serving of pasta!

Nutrition Facts

Serving Size: 1/2 cup (56g)
Servings Per Container: 8

Amount Per Serving

Calories 200   Calories from fat 10

	% Daily Value*
Total Fat 1g	2%
Saturated Fat 0g	0%
Trans Fat 0g	
Cholesterol 0mg	0%
Sodium 0mg	0%
Total Carbohydrate 41g	14%
Dietary Fiber 2g	8%
Sugars 1g	
Protein 7g	

Vitamin A 0%	•	Vitamin C 0%
Calcium 0%	•	Iron 10%
Thiamin 35%	•	Riboflavin 15%
Niacin 20%	•	Folic acid 30%

* Percent Daily Values are based on a 2,000 calorie diet. Your daily values may be higher or lower depending on your calorie needs:

		Calories:	2000	2,500
Total Fat	Less Than		65g	80g
Sat Fat	Less Than		20g	25g
Cholesterol	Less Than		300mg	300mg
Sodium	Less Than		2,400mg	2,400mg
Total Carbohydrate			300g	375g
Dietary Fiber			25g	30g

Calories per gram:
Fat 9   Carbohydrate 4   Protein 4

Calories	200
Total fat	2% (1g)
Saturated fat	0%
Cholesterol	0%
Sodium	0%
Total carbohydrate	14%
Vitamin A	0%
Vitamin C	0%
Calcium	0%
Iron	10%
Folic acid	30%
Thiamin	35%
Niacin	20%
Riboflavin	15%

Some vegetables and legumes also contain folate, so combining pasta with vegetables, or enriched rice with black beans, would provide substantial amounts of folate. The next time you are at the grocery store, pay close attention to the food labels on grain products to see just how much folate you could consume from different grain products.

Looking again at this food label, what other water-soluble vitamins do you see? In addition to folic acid, this pasta contains substantial amounts of thiamin, niacin, and riboflavin. These are the "enrichment" vitamins, and one serving of pasta provides 15 to 35 percent of the Daily Value of each.

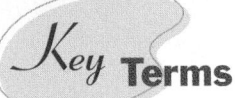

LEARNING *Portfolio*   c h a p t e r   1 0

Key Terms

	page		page
anemia	436	homocysteine	436
angular stomatitis	430	macrocytes	443
anencephaly	443	megaloblastic anemia	443
ariboflavinosis	430	megaloblasts	443
atrophic gastritis	444	microcytic hypochromic anemia	436
avidin	435		
beriberi	424	myelin sheath	444
biocytin	435	neural tube defect (NTD)	443
biotinidase	435	niacin equivalents (NE)	431
carboxylation	435	pernicious anemia	445
cheilosis	430	R-protein	444
connective tissues	446	reducing agent	446
decarboxylation	426	seborrheic dermatitis	430
dietary folate equivalents (DFE)	440	spina bifida	443
glossitis	430	thiamin pyrophosphate (TPP)	426
glutathione peroxidase	429	tryptophan	431
hemochromatosis	448		

Study Points

> The water-soluble vitamins include the eight B vitamins and vitamin C.

> Thiamin (vitamin B$_1$) functions as the coenzyme thiamin pyrophosphate (TPP) in energy metabolism.

> Thiamin deficiency results in the classic disease beriberi. In industrialized countries, thiamin deficiency most often is associated with alcoholism. There is no known danger of toxicity related to high intakes of thiamin.

> Riboflavin (vitamin B$_2$) forms part of the coenzymes FAD and FMN, which function in energy metabolism as hydrogen and electron carriers.

> Ariboflavinosis (riboflavin deficiency) is characterized by inflammation of the mouth and tongue.

> Niacin (vitamin B$_3$) participates in energy metabolism as part of the coenzymes NAD$^+$ and NADP$^+$.

> Niacin deficiency results in pellagra, a disease characterized by diarrhea, dermatitis, dementia, and death.

> High doses of niacin, such as in the treatment of high blood cholesterol, can have toxic side effects including liver damage.

> Pantothenic acid is a part of coenzyme A, a critical player in energy metabolism.

> Biotin-containing enzymes catalyze carboxylation reactions, which are important in many pathways involving energy-yielding nutrients.

> Biotin deficiency is rare, but may be induced by regularly consuming large quantities of raw egg whites.

> The coenzyme form of vitamin B$_6$ (pyridoxine) is called pyridoxal phosphate (PLP); it participates in a variety of reactions, primarily involving amino acid metabolism.

> Megadoses of vitamin B$_6$ can cause permanent nerve damage.

> Folate and vitamin B$_{12}$ work closely together in a number of metabolic pathways, including reactions in cell division and DNA synthesis.

> Deficiency of either folate or vitamin B$_{12}$ will result in megaloblastic anemia, but vitamin B$_{12}$ deficiency also causes irreversible nerve damage.

> Poor folate status is associated with development of neural tube defects during pregnancy. Therefore, women of childbearing age are advised to take in 400 micrograms of folic acid each day from fortified foods or supplements in addition to other dietary folate.

> Vitamin C (ascorbic acid) functions in the synthesis of collagen and other vital compounds, and also works as an antioxidant.

> Vitamin C deficiency can cause scurvy, which is characterized by bleeding gums and small hemorrhages on the skin.

> A number of vitamin-like compounds have been identified, including choline, inositol, and taurine. These compounds are synthesized by the body and are not dietary essentials.

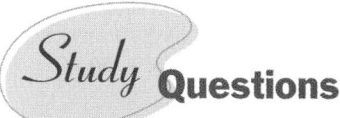

Study Questions

1. **List the nine water-soluble vitamins and give one main function for each.**

2. **Which water-soluble vitamin can be made from an amino acid?**

3 **Name the diseases and/or characteristic symptoms of deficiency of each water-soluble vitamin.**

4. **A lack of which three B vitamins can cause anemia? Describe the differences among these anemias.**

5. **List the water-soluble vitamins demonstrated to be toxic in large doses. What signs indicate toxic levels of each vitamin?**

☞ [Try] **This**

The Antioxidant and the Apple

This experiment will help you see how vitamin C acts as an antioxidant. You will need an apple and a lemon. Slice the apple into eight pieces. Put four on one plate and four on another. Slice open the lemon and squeeze its juices over the apple slices on one plate. Leave the lemon on this plate to remind you which apple slices have been sprayed with lemon juice. Let both plates sit for 30 minutes. Do the apple slices look any different after 30 minutes? What is the difference? Why? 👆

Supplemental Income

The object of this exercise is to critically review vitamin supplements. Go to the drug store and look at a few multivitamin supplements and "stress" formulas. Look at the %DV for the water-soluble vitamins. Do you see any that have more than 1000% of the DV? Compare prices. Is it more expensive to buy supplements with more of these vitamins? Considering what you learned in this chapter, would it benefit you to take supplements that contain such a high amount of these vitamins? Why do you think supplements contain such large quantities of these vitamins? 👆

What About Bobbie?

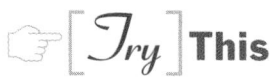

Let's take a look at Bobbie's intake of five water-soluble vitamins: thiamin, riboflavin, niacin, vitamin B_{12}, and vitamin C. Let's examine her day of eating (see Chapter 1) using the guidelines you've learned in this chapter. How did Bobbie do in terms of these water-soluble vitamins? She did well; she consumed ample amounts of most due to her varied food choices. Here is a summary of each of the vitamins.

Thiamin

Bobbie consumed 2.0 milligrams of thiamin, which is more than the RDA of 1.1 milligrams. Most of the foods Bobbie ate this day contributed to her thiamin intake, but the ones that contributed the most were the enriched grains from the bread, bagel, and spaghetti.

Riboflavin

Bobbie consumed 2.2 milligrams of riboflavin on this day, or more than the RDA of 1.1 milligrams. As with thiamin, a variety of foods contributed to her riboflavin intake, but the enriched grains (bread, bagel, and pasta) were among the best contributors. The meatballs Bobbie ate at dinner also contributed riboflavin.

Niacin

Bobbie's intake of niacin was also above her RDA. She consumed 27.5 milligrams this day compared to her RDA of 14 milligrams. If you remember from the protein chapter that Bobbie's intake of protein was quite high, it shouldn't surprise you that her niacin intake is high, too. Meat, poultry, fish, and other protein-containing foods, along with enriched grains, are some of the best sources of niacin. In this case, Bobbie's turkey sandwich, spaghetti with meatballs, and cheese pizza contributed niacin.

Vitamin B_{12}

Bobbie's intake of vitamin B_{12} (3.7 µg), like her intake of the other B vitamins, was above the RDA (2.4 µg). The foods that contributed to Bobbie's vitamin B_{12} intake were the animal products (turkey, egg, meatballs, parmesan cheese, and cheese pizza).

Vitamin C

Although Bobbie enjoys tomato products such as salsa, spaghetti sauce, and pizza sauce, her intake of vitamin C (42 milligrams) was less than the RDA of 75 milligrams. Here are some other ways Bobbie could have included more vitamin C in her diet:
- Have some orange or grapefruit juice with breakfast.
- Choose spinach, broccoli, or Brussels sprouts instead of green beans for dinner.
- Use spinach as the base of her salad instead of iceberg lettuce.
- Add some sliced red pepper to her salad at lunch.
- Have an orange as a snack instead of the tortilla chips.

References

1 US Department of Health and Human Services. FDA announces name changes for lower-fat milks and folic acid fortification for bakery products. *HHS News*. December 31, 1997.

2 Carpenter KJ. A short history of nutritional science: part 2 (1885–1912). *J Nutr*. 2003;133:975–984.

3 Ibid.

4 Institute of Medicine, Food and Nutrition Board. *Dietary Reference Intakes for Thiamin, Riboflavin, Niacin, Vitamin B6, Folate, Vitamin B12, Pantothenic Acid, Biotin, and Choline*. Washington, DC: National Academy Press, 1998.

5 Ibid.

6 Ibid.

7 Murray RK, Granner DK, Mayes PA, Rodwell VW. *Harper's Biochemistry*. 24th ed. Stamford, CT: Appleton & Lange, 1996.

8 Institute of Medicine, Food and Nutrition Board. Op. cit.

9 Mestdagh F, De Meulenaer B, De Clippeleer J, et al. Protective influence of several packaging materials on light oxidation of milk. *J Dairy Sci*. 2005;88:499–510.

10 Zempleni J, Galloway JR, McCormick DB. Pharmacokinetics of orally and intravenously administered riboflavin in healthy humans. *Am J Clin Nutr*. 1996;63:54–66.

11 Institute of Medicine, Food and Nutrition Board. Op. cit.

12 McCormick DB. Two interconnected B vitamins: riboflavin and pyridoxine. *Physiol Rev*. 1989;69:1170–1198.

13 Institute of Medicine, Food and Nutrition Board. Op. cit.

14 Carpenter KJ, Lewin WJ. A reexamination of the composition of diets associated with pellagra. *J Nutr*. 1985;115:543–552.

15 McKenney JM, Proctor JD, Harris S, Chinchili VM. A comparison of the efficacy and toxic effects of sustained- vs. immediate-release niacin in hypercholesterolemic patients. *JAMA*. 1994;271:672–677.

16 Ibid.; and Gibbons LW, Gonzalez V, Gordon N, Grundy S. The prevalence of side effects with regular and sustained-release nicotinic acid. *Am J Med*. 1995;99:378–385.

17 Visalli N, Cavallo MG, Signore A, et al. A multi-centre randomized trial of two different doses of nicotinamide in patients with recent-onset type 1 diabetes (the IMDIAB VI). *Diabetes Metab Res Rev*. 1999;15:181–185.

18 Gale EA, Bingley PJ, Emmett CL, et al. European Nicotinamide Diabetes Intervention Trial (ENDIT). *Lancet*. 2004; 63(9413):910.

19 Trumbo PR. Pantothenic acid. In: Shils, ME, Shike M, Ross AC, Cabellero B, Cousins RJ, eds. *Modern Nutrition in Health and Disease*. 10th ed. Philadelphia: Lippincott Williams & Wilkins, 2006:426–469.

20 Institute of Medicine, Food and Nutrition Board. Op. cit.

21 Ibid.

22 Ibid.

23 Broekmans WMR, Klöpping-Ketelaars IAA, Schuurman CRWC, et al. Fruits and vegetables increase plasma carotenoids and vitamins and decrease homocysteine in humans. *J Nutr*. 2000;130:1578–1583.

24 Kelly PJ, Shih VE, Kistler JP, et al. Low vitamin B6 but not homocyst(e)ine is associated with increased risk of stroke and transient ischemic attack in the era of folic acid grain fortification. *Stoke*. 2003;34(6):e51–e54.

25 Rimm EB, Willett WC, Hu FB, et al. Folate and vitamin B6 from diet and supplements in relation to risk of coronary heart disease among women. *JAMA*. 1998;279:359–364.

26 Institute of Medicine, Food and Nutrition Board. Op. cit.

27 Ibid.

28 Gregory JF. Bioavailability of vitamin B6. *Eur J Clin Nutr*. 1997;51:S54–S59.

29 Schaumberg H, Kaplan J, Windebank A, et al. Sensory neuropathy from pyridoxine abuse. *N Engl J Med*. 1983; 309:445–448.

30 Kurzer MS. Women, food and mood. *Nutr Rev*. 1997;55:268.

31 Franzblau A. The relationship of vitamin B6 status to median nerve function and carpal tunnel syndrome among active industrial workers. *J Occupation Environment Med*. 1996; 38:485–491; and Aufiero E, Stitik TP, Foye PM, Chen B. Pyridoxine hydrochloride treatment of carpal tunnel syndrome: a review. *Nutr Rev*. 2004;62(3):96–104.

32 Pfeiffer CM, Rogers LM, Bailey LB, et al. Absorption of folate from fortified cereal-grain products and of supplemental folate consumed with or without food determined by using a dual-label stable-isotope protocol. *Am J Clin Nutr*. 1997; 66:1388–1397.

33 Institute of Medicine, Food and Nutrition Board. Op. cit.; and Suitor CW, Bailey LB. Dietary folate equivalents: interpretation and application. *J Am Diet Assoc*. 2000;100:88–94.

34 Mills JL. Fortification of foods with folic acid: how much is enough? *N Engl J Med*. 2000;342:1442–1445.

35 Institute of Medicine, Food and Nutrition Board. Op. cit.

36 US Department of Health and Human Services. Op. cit.

37 Lewis CJ, Crane NT, Wilson DB, Yetley EA. Estimated folate intakes: data updated to reflect food fortification, increased bioavailability, and dietary supplement use. *Am J Clin Nutr*. 1999;70:198–207.

38 Institute of Medicine, Food and Nutrition Board. Op. cit., 260–264; and Jacques PF, Selhub J, Bostom AG, et al. The effect of folic acid fortification on plasma folate and total homocysteine concentrations. *N Engl J Med*. 1999; 340:1449–1454.

39 Van Oort FV, Melse-Boonstra A, Brouwer IA, et al. Folic acid and reduction of plasma homocysteine concentrations in older adults: a dose–response study. *Am J Clin Nutr*. 2003; 77(5):1318–1323.

40 Green NS. Folic acid supplementation and prevention of birth defects. *J Nutr*. 2002;132(8 suppl):2356S–2360S.

41 James SJ, Pogribna M, Pogribny IP, et al. Abnormal folate metabolism and mutation in the methylenetetrahydrofolate reductase gene may be maternal risk factors for Down syndrome. *Am J Clin Nutr*. 1999;70:495–501.

42 Relton CL, Pearce MS, Parker L. The influence of erythrocyte folate and serum vitamin B12 status on birth weight. *Br J Nutr*. 2005;93(5):593–599.

43 Siega-Riz AM, Savitz DA, Zeisel SH, et al. Second trimester folate status and preterm birth. *Am J Obstet Gynecol.* 2004; 191(6):1851–1857.

44 Lewis CJ, et al. Op. cit.

45 Hurwitz A, Brady DA, Schaal SE, et al. Gastric acidity in older adults. *JAMA.* 1997;278:659–662.

46 Institute of Medicine, Food and Nutrition Board. Op. cit.

47 Ibid.

48 Ibid.

49 Dharmarajan TS, Adiga GU, Norkus EP. Vitamin B_{12} deficiency: recognizing subtle symptoms in older adults. *Geriatrics.* 2003; 58(3):30–38.

50 Carpenter KJ. A short history of nutritional science: part 1 (1785–1885). *J Nutr.* 2003;133:638–645.

51 Ibid.

52 Fairfield KM, Fletcher RH. Vitamins for chronic disease prevention in adults: scientific review. *JAMA.* 2002;287:3116–3126.

53 Sauberlich HE. Pharmacology of vitamin C. *Ann Rev Nutr.* 1994;14:371.

54 Institute of Medicine, Food and Nutrition Board. *Dietary Reference Intakes for Vitamin C, Vitamin E, Selenium, and Carotenoids.* Washington, DC: National Academy Press, 2000.

55 Ibid.

56 Johnston CS, Retrum KR, Srilakshmi JC. Antihistamine effects and complications of supplemental vitamin C. *J Am Diet Assoc.* 1992;8:988–989.

57 Institute of Medicine, Food and Nutrition Board. 2000. Op. cit.

58 Halliwell B. Antioxidants: sense or speculation? *Nutr Today.* 1994;29:15–19.

59 Institute of Medicine, Food and Nutrition Board. 2000. Op. cit.

60 Niculescu MD, Zeisel SH. Diet, methyl donors and DNA methylation: interactions between dietary folate, methionine, and choline. *J Nutr.* 2002;132:2333S–2335S.

61 Bellinghieri G, Santoro D, Calvani M, Mallamace A, Savica V. Carnitine and hemodialysis. *Am J Kidney Dis.* 2003;41 (3 suppl 1):S116–S122.

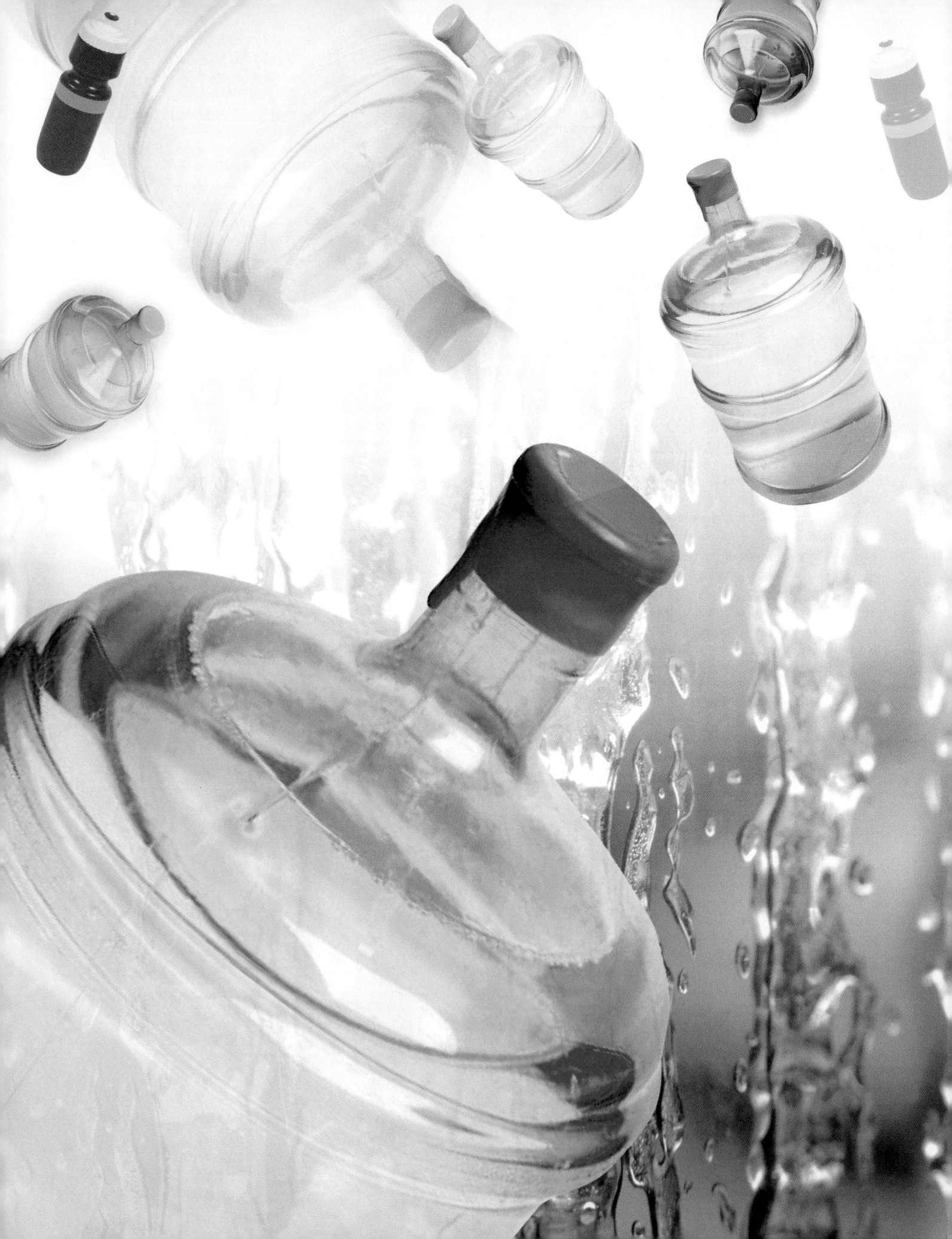

Chapter **11**

Water and Major Minerals

Think About It

1 How much water does it usually take to quench your thirst?
2 Does drinking caffeinated beverages make you feel dehydrated?
3 How often do you salt your food before tasting it?
4 What's your primary source of calcium?

Fyi for your Information

This chapter's FYI boxes include practical information on the following topics:
- Tap, Filtered, or Bottled: Which Water Is Best?
- Calcium Supplements: Are They Right for You?

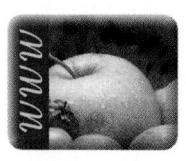

The Web site for this book offers many useful tools and is a great source for additional nutrition information for both students and instructors. Visit the site at **nutrition.jbpub.com** for information on water and major minerals. You'll find exercises that explore the following topics:
- The Water in Your State
- Calcium
- Making Hard Water Soft

Key to Illustrations

 Minerals

 Water

What About Bobbie?

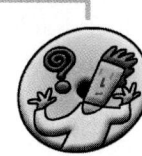

Track the choices Bobbie is making with Nutritionist Pro or EatRight Analysis software.

hydrogen bonds Noncovalent bonds between hydrogen and an atom, usually oxygen, in another molecule.

electrolytes [ih-LEK-tro-lites] Substances that dissociate into charged particles (ions) when dissolved in water or other solvents and thus become capable of conducting an electrical current. The terms *electrolyte* and *ion* often are used interchangeably.

heat capacity The amount of energy required to raise the temperature of a substance 1°C.

An adult male is approximately 62% water, 17% protein, 15% fat, and 6% minerals and glycogen

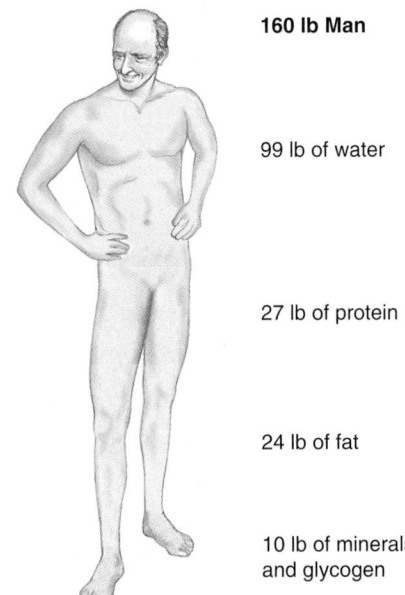

160 lb Man

99 lb of water

27 lb of protein

24 lb of fat

10 lb of minerals and glycogen

Figure 11.1 **Body composition.** The main constituent of the body is water. Adult males have more lean tissue and less fat than adult females, and therefore have more body water.

On your coast-to-coast flight with your father and your brother, you observe your father drink water frequently throughout the flight, whereas your brother alternates between Coke and beer. When you arrive at your destination, your brother complains of feeling utterly exhausted. In contrast, your father is lively and ready for a night on the town. How do you explain this?

First, it's important to know that the familiar beverage cart is not a random gesture of kindness by the airlines: Regular fluid intake on flights is necessary for health! Although you are unaware of it, water evaporates from the skin at an accelerated rate in the low-humidity, high-altitude, pressurized cabin of an airplane. Thus, drinking fluids during the flight helps prevent dehydration. But you must choose the fluids carefully. Alcoholic and caffeinated beverages are diuretics. This means that they may increase fluid loss as urine, and therefore in the short-term may not replace fluid losses as effectively as water, juice, and other caffeine-free beverages.

Your brother's lack of energy may be a symptom of mild dehydration. Although he has been drinking fluids, the diuretic effect of alcohol and caffeine may have limited fluid replacement. Dad, however, had the right idea—plenty of water along the way—and he's ready for action!

Water: The Essential Ingredient for Life

Water is absolutely essential. You could probably survive for weeks without food. But you can live only a few days without water. Humans have no capacity to store "spare" water, so we must quickly replace any that's lost.

Overall, water makes up between 45 and 75 percent of a person's weight. (See **Figure 11.1**.) Leaner people have proportionately more water because muscle tissue is nearly three-fourths water by weight, whereas adipose tissue is only about 10 percent water.

The one bit of chemistry that almost everyone can rattle off is the chemical formula for water: H_2O. Water is such a simple molecule (**Figure 11.2**) that people often do not appreciate its extraordinary physical and chemical properties. Water's strong surface tension, high heat capacity, and ability to dissolve many substances result from **hydrogen bonds** between a hydrogen atom of one water molecule and the oxygen atom of another water molecule.

Water in your body contains numerous dissolved minerals, called **electrolytes**, that are kept in constant balance. To live, each cell must have just the right mix of water and electrolytes. Although intracellular and extracellular fluids have different mixes, the proportions in each must stay within a narrow range. Despite a continuous flow of molecules between intracellular fluid, extracellular fluid, and the outside environment, the body maintains its electrolyte balance through the intake and excretion of water and the movement of ions.

Functions of Water

Water performs a wide variety of tasks in the body. (See **Figure 11.3**.) Water is the highway that moves nutrients and wastes between cells and organs. In the intestines, water solubilizes and moves nutrients to your cells and tissues, and it also carries waste out of your body in urine. What about nutrients and wastes that are not water-soluble? Your body either modifies them chemically so that they dissolve in water or packages them with proteins (e.g., lipoproteins). Your body's watery fluids, such as the bloodstream, can easily transport these protein packages throughout the body.

Heat Capacity

The **heat capacity** of a substance is the amount of energy required to raise its temperature 1 degree Celsius. Raising the temperature of a substance with a high heat capacity requires more energy than raising the temperature of a substance with a low one. Water, for instance, has about three times the heat capacity of iron. Warming or cooling a substance with a high heat capacity requires a relatively large amount of energy. You may have noticed this property when heating items in a microwave oven. Watery foods such as soup take much longer to heat than foods that contain little water, such as pizza and butter. Because of water's high heat capacity, it takes a lot of heat to change the temperature of the body; body water dampens the effects of extreme environmental temperatures on conditions in cells.

Cooling Ability

A rise in body temperature, whether due to exercise, environmental conditions, or illness, triggers the body's cooling system. If you get too warm, blood vessels dilate and you begin to sweat. The perspiration evaporates on the skin, thereby cooling your body. Moisture readily evaporates in dry air, so perspiring is most effective for cooling when the humidity is low. When the humidity is high, such as in humid, tropical environments, sweat does not evaporate readily, so even profuse sweating may not cool the body effectively.

Participation in Metabolism

Nearly all the chemical reactions of metabolism involve water. Water is the solvent for many biologically essential molecules (e.g., glucose, vitamins, minerals, and amino acids), and it is a product or reactant in many biochemical reactions.

pH Balance

Water is also an essential component of the body's mechanisms to maintain pH (acid–base) balance in the narrow range necessary for life. One of the major buffer systems involves carbonic acid and bicarbonate. Carbonic acid forms when dissolved carbon dioxide reacts with water ($CO_2 + H_2O \rightarrow H_2CO_3$). Carbonic acid can then dissociate to form H^+ and HCO_3^- (bicarbonate). The resulting H^+ helps increase acidity, lowering pH.

Body Fluids

Water is the major component of all body fluids. These fluids serve essential mechanical functions such as shock absorption, lubrication, cleansing, and protection. For example, amniotic fluid provides a gentle cushion that protects the fetus, synovial fluid allows joints to move smoothly, tears lubricate and cleanse the eyes, and saliva moistens food and makes swallowing possible.

Water is a polar molecule. Although its net charge is zero, oxygen's strong attraction of the hydrogens' electrons makes it positive at one end and negative at the other

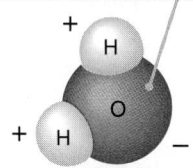

The more positive end of each water molecule is attracted to the more negative end of another – these weak attractions are called hydrogen bonds

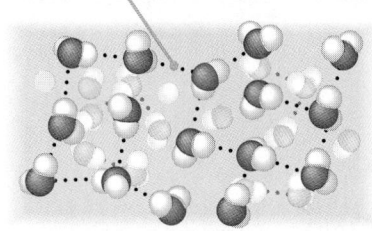

The millions of weak hydrogen bonds between water molecules are strong enough to support this water strider

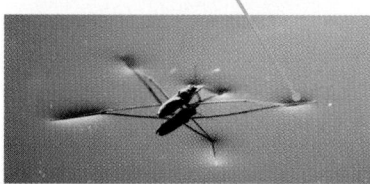

Figure 11.2 **Water—a simple, yet powerful, molecule.** Water has a strong surface tension and high heat capacity. Because dissolved molecules are more likely to come together and react with one another, water's ability to dissolve substances makes chemical reactions more efficient.

Resistance to temperature change (heat capacity)

Cooling

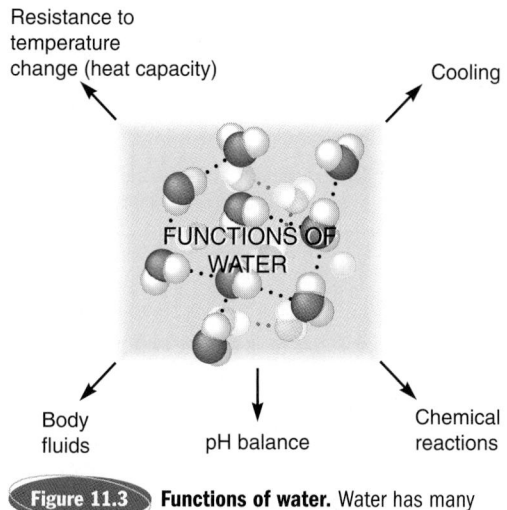

FUNCTIONS OF WATER

Body fluids

pH balance

Chemical reactions

Figure 11.3 **Functions of water.** Water has many critical functions in the body.

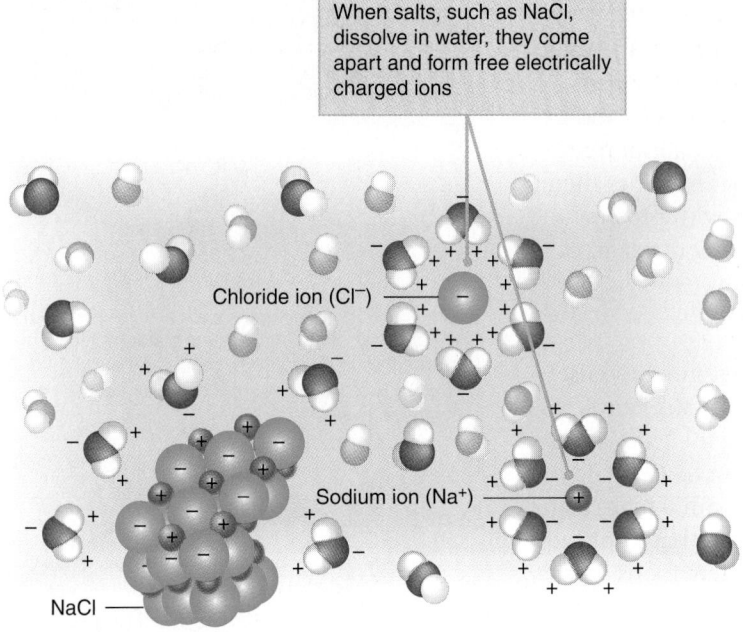

When salts, such as NaCl, dissolve in water, they come apart and form free electrically charged ions

Chloride ion (Cl⁻)

Sodium ion (Na⁺)

NaCl

Figure 11.4 **Dissolving salt in water.** When dissolving salt, the oxygen atoms of the water molecules are attracted to the negatively charged chloride ions. Water's hydrogen atoms are attracted to the positively charged sodium ions.

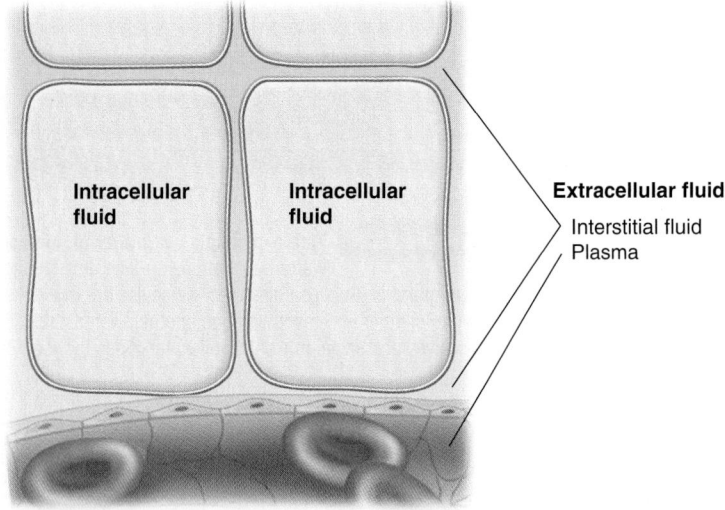

Intracellular fluid

Intracellular fluid

Extracellular fluid
Interstitial fluid
Plasma

Figure 11.5 **Intracellular and extracellular fluid.** Extracellular fluids and their solutes (except for proteins) move across capillary membranes easily. Plasma (the fluid portion of the blood) has a higher concentration of proteins than interstitial fluid. Excluding protein, their compositions are roughly the same.

Electrolytes and Water: A Delicate Equilibrium

Your body precisely controls and balances the concentration of electrolytes dissolved in its watery fluids. When **salts**, such as sodium chloride, dissolve in water (**Figure 11.4**), they come apart and form free **ions**, which are positively (e.g., Na⁺) and negatively (e.g., Cl⁻) charged particles. In an electrolyte solution, the number of positive charges always equals the number of negative charges. The main positively charged ions (**cations**) in the body are sodium and potassium, and the main negatively charged ions (**anions**) are chloride and phosphate.

There are two major fluid compartments in the body. About two-thirds of body water is in intracellular fluid, and one-third is in extracellular fluid. The major components of extracellular fluid are interstitial fluid (the fluid between cells) and blood **plasma** (the fluid portion of blood). (See **Figure 11.5**.)

Sodium is the main cation in extracellular fluid, whereas potassium is the predominant cation in intracellular fluid. To maintain the balance of sodium and potassium, all cell membranes incorporate **sodium-potassium pumps** (**Figure 11.6**) that actively pump sodium out of the cell while allowing potassium back in. If solutes are more concentrated on one side of a **semipermeable membrane** (through which water, but not **solutes**, can pass easily), water flows to the side of higher concentration until the concentrations on both sides are the same. This movement is called **osmosis**; **osmotic pressure** is the force that causes water to flow across a membrane to the side with a higher concentration of ions. (See **Figure 11.7**.)

Key Concepts: *Water is the most essential nutrient; we can survive much longer without food than without water. Water's functions in the body include temperature regulation, metabolism, acid–base regulation, lubrication, and protection. The balance of body fluids and the amount of electrolytes dissolved in the body's water are controlled precisely. Potassium is the main intracellular cation, and sodium is the main extracellular cation.*

salts Compounds that result from the replacement of the hydrogen of an acid with a metal or a group that acts like a metal.

ions Atoms or groups of atoms with an electrical charge resulting from the loss or gain of one or more electrons.

cations Ions that carry a positive charge.

anions Ions that carry a negative charge.

plasma The fluid portion of the blood that contains blood cells and other components.

sodium-potassium pumps Mechanisms that pump sodium ions out of a cell, allowing potassium ions to enter the cell.

semipermeable membrane Membrane that allows passage of some substances but blocks others.

solutes Substances that are dissolved in a solvent.

osmosis The movement of a solvent, such as water, through a semipermeable membrane from the low-solute to the high-solute solution until the concentrations on both sides of the membrane are equal.

osmotic pressure The pressure exerted on a semipermeable membrane by a solvent, usually water, moving from the side of low-solute to the side of high-solute concentration.

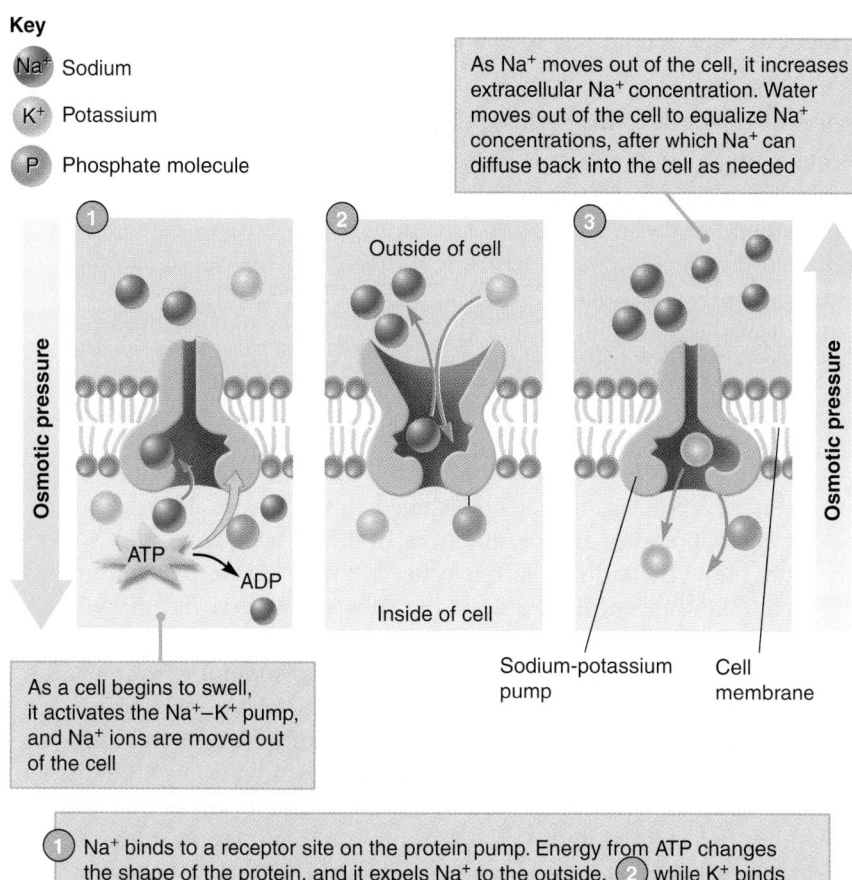

Key
Na+ Sodium
K+ Potassium
P Phosphate molecule
As Na+ moves out of the cell, it increases extracellular Na+ concentration. Water moves out of the cell to equalize Na+ concentrations, after which Na+ can diffuse back into the cell as needed
1
2
3
Outside of cell
Osmotic pressure
ATP
ADP
Inside of cell
Osmotic pressure
Sodium-potassium pump
Cell membrane
As a cell begins to swell, it activates the Na+–K+ pump, and Na+ ions are moved out of the cell
1 Na+ binds to a receptor site on the protein pump. Energy from ATP changes the shape of the protein, and it expels Na+ to the outside, 2 while K+ binds to a newly formed receptor site, causing another shape change that expels the K+ to the cell's interior 3

Figure 11.6 **Sodium-potassium pump.** The movement of sodium and potassium in and out of cells helps maintain the proper volume of fluid in the cell.

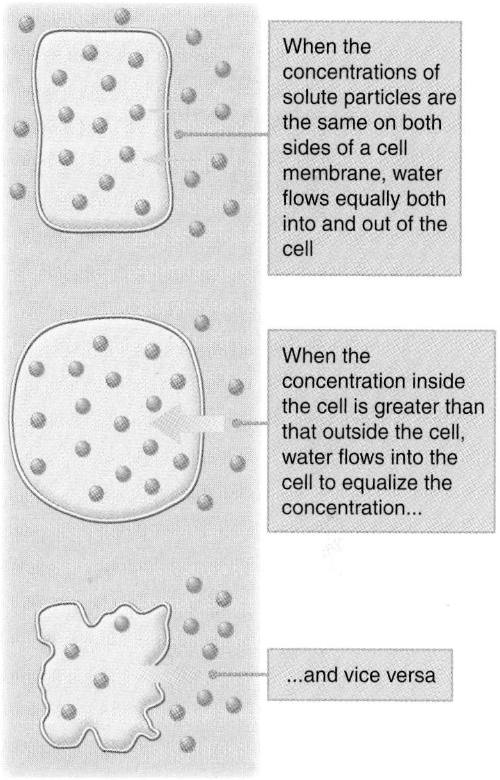

When the concentrations of solute particles are the same on both sides of a cell membrane, water flows equally both into and out of the cell
When the concentration inside the cell is greater than that outside the cell, water flows into the cell to equalize the concentration...
...and vice versa

Figure 11.7 **Osmosis.** Water moves across cell membranes to equalize concentrations of dissolved particles.

Intake Recommendations: How Much Water Is Enough?

There is no one answer to the question of how much water is sufficient. We each need a different amount, depending on our size, body composition, and activity level, as well as the temperature and humidity of the environment. Over the course of a few hours, body water deficits can occur due to reduced intake or increased water losses from physical activity and environmental (e.g., heat) exposure. However, on a day-to-day basis, fluid intake, driven by the combination of thirst and the consumption of food and beverages at meals, allows maintenance of hydration status and total body water at normal levels.

The Adequate Intake (AI) for total water is 3.7 liters per day for men and 2.7 liters per day for women.[1] Intake recommendations are higher during pregnancy (3.0 liters per day) and lactation (3.8 liters per day). Activity and sweating increase water needs, so athletes and active people need much more water, especially if they work and train in warm, humid climates.

Water intake comes from a combination of drinking water, beverages, and the water in foods. Survey data suggest that about 75 to 80 percent of our total water intake comes from beverages, with the remaining 20 to 25 percent from foods. Some foods, such as fruits and vegetables, contain a substantial amount of water, whereas others—grain products, for example—provide very little. (See **Figure 11.8**.) Our bodies also produce a small

Water content (%)
100
50
0
96
87
75
64
50
37
36
16
3
Lettuce
Orange
Baked potato
Roasted chicken
Cooked beef
Cheddar cheese
Bread
Butter
Cereal

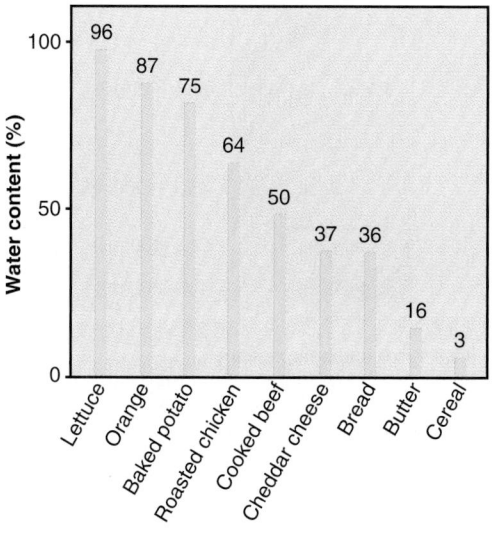

Figure 11.8 **Water content of various foods.** As you might expect, crunchy vegetables contain more water than dry cereal. But did you know that potatoes contain a high percentage of water?

amount of water (about 250 to 350 milliliters per day) in metabolic reactions. (See Chapter 7, "Metabolism.")

Sports Drinks and Water Absorption

Drinking plenty of plain water and eating a healthful diet easily replaces the fluid and electrolytes a person loses during moderate exercise in pleasant weather. But if you are involved in endurance activities or strenuous exercise in hot weather, consider using sports drinks instead of just plain water. Sports drinks contain glucose and electrolytes that improve the drink's taste, help maintain blood glucose levels, and enhance absorption.[2] (See Chapter 13, "Sports Nutrition.")

Water Excretion: Where Does the Water Go?

We continuously lose water from our bodies through various routes. In the lungs, water evaporates and exits in exhaled air. Water also departs through the skin by evaporation and perspiration. In the GI tract, feces carry water out of the body. The kidneys excrete water in urine. **Figure 11.9** summarizes sources and amounts of fluid output and shows how these balance with fluid intake.

Depending on the amount of water, protein, and sodium consumed, the body loses about 1 to 2 liters of water each day through urine. During exercise, urine production declines and fluid losses from the skin and lungs increase. **Insensible water loss**—the continuous evaporation of water from the lungs and skin—typically accounts for about one-fourth to one-half of daily fluid loss. High altitude, low humidity, and high temperatures increase these losses. During a coast-to-coast airplane flight, the low cabin humidity can cause insensible fluid losses of 4 to 6 cups (about 1,000 to 1,500 mL).[3]

Insensible losses rise, sometimes dramatically, during illness. Fever, coughing, rapid breathing, and watery nasal secretions all significantly increase water loss. This is one of the reasons that doctors recommend increasing your fluid intake when you are sick.

Water plays a critical role in the elimination of wastes. Urea, a breakdown product of protein metabolism, is a major component of urine. If we overconsume protein and salt (a common situation with the typical American diet), the kidneys have to work harder to eliminate excess urea and sodium from the body. This task requires water, so unless kidney function is impaired, the more protein and sodium you consume, the more fluid you need to consume and the more urine you are likely to produce.

Key Concepts: *The AI for fluid intake is 3.7 liters per day for men and 2.7 liters per day for women. Water intake comes from a combination of foods, fluids, and water produced in normal metabolism. The main method of water excretion is in urine. In addition, fluid is lost through the skin and lungs, and in the feces. Losses are higher when a person perspires heavily or is ill. Water is critical in eliminating the body's waste products.*

Water Balance

Our bodies maintain water balance by mechanisms that control water intake (e.g., thirst) and water excretion. Because of water's critical roles, the body works not only to balance fluid between compartments, but also to closely regulate total body water.

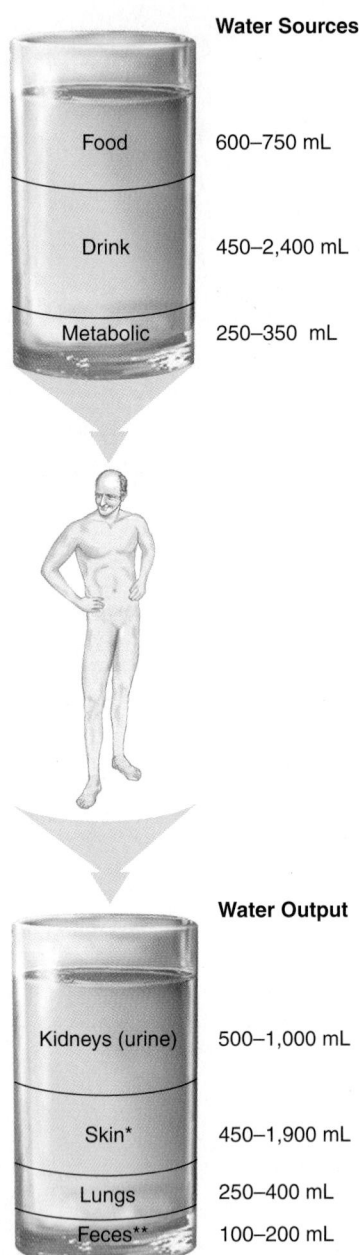

Water Sources

Food	600–750 mL
Drink	450–2,400 mL
Metabolic	250–350 mL

Water Output

Kidneys (urine)	500–1,000 mL
Skin*	450–1,900 mL
Lungs	250–400 mL
Feces**	100–200 mL

* (Insensible and perspiration)
The volume of perspiration is normally about 100 mL per day. In very hot weather or during heavy exercise, a person may lose 1 to 2 liters per hour.

** People with severe diarrhea can lose several liters of water per day in feces.

Figure 11.9 **Typical daily fluid intake and output.** To maintain fluid balance, your body regulates its fluid intake and output.

Regulation of Fluid Excretion

Our kidneys adjust the amount and concentration of urine in response to the body's hydration status. The kidneys can excrete a small volume of concentrated urine or a large volume of dilute urine while maintaining a relatively constant excretion of solutes such as sodium and potassium. This ability to regulate water excretion without major changes in solute excretion is an important survival mechanism, especially when water is in short supply.

When water intake is low, the kidneys conserve water. While continuing to excrete solutes, they reabsorb water, thus decreasing urine volume and concentrating the urine. When the body has an excess of water, the kidneys form and excrete a large volume of dilute urine.

How do the kidneys know when to conserve water? **Osmoreceptors**, special cells in the hypothalamus of the brain, are exquisitely sensitive to very small increases in extracellular sodium concentration and thus sense the body's need for water. If the sodium concentration rises, these receptors signal the pituitary gland to release **antidiuretic hormone (ADH)**. ADH decreases water loss by causing the kidneys to reabsorb water rather than excrete it in the urine. (See **Figure 11.10**.)

In minute concentrations, ADH signals the kidney to conserve water. In higher concentrations ADH is a potent **vasoconstrictor**, which is why it also is called **vasopressin**. Although ADH is far less sensitive to blood volume than to plasma **osmolarity** (concentration of electrolytes), a severe loss of blood also triggers its release. A loss of 15 to 25 percent of blood volume will cause up to a 50-fold increase in ADH levels. Nausea is a potent trigger. ADH levels increase 100-fold after vomiting. Some drugs (e.g., nicotine and morphine) stimulate the release of ADH, but others (e.g., alcohol and caffeine) inhibit it.[4]

Regulation of Blood Volume and Pressure

The kidneys themselves have sensors that detect falling blood pressure. (See **Figure 11.11**.) In response, the kidneys release **renin**, an enzyme that splits off a small protein, **angiotensin I**, from the blood protein **angiotensinogen**. Within seconds, enzymes in the small blood vessels of the lungs convert nearly all angiotensin I to **angiotensin II**. Although angiotensin II is a

insensible water loss The continual loss of body water by evaporation from the respiratory tract and diffusion through the skin.

osmoreceptors Neurons in the hypothalamus that detect changes in the fluid concentration in blood and regulate the release of antidiuretic hormone.

antidiuretic hormone (ADH) A peptide hormone secreted by the pituitary gland. It increases blood pressure and prevents fluid excretion by the kidneys. Also called vasopressin.

vasoconstrictor A substance that causes blood vessels to constrict.

vasopressin See *antidiuretic hormone*.

osmolarity The concentration of dissolved particles (e.g., electrolytes) in a solution expressed per unit of volume.

renin An enzyme, produced by the kidney, that affects blood pressure by catalyzing the conversion of angiotensinogen to angiotensin I.

angiotensin I [an-jee-oh-TEN-sin one] A 10-amino-acid peptide that is a precursor of angiotensin II.

angiotensinogen A circulating protein produced by the liver from which angiotensin I is cleaved by the action of renin.

angiotensin II In the lungs, the 8-amino-acid peptide angiotensin II is formed from angiotensin I. Angiotensin II is a powerful vasoconstrictor that rapidly raises blood pressure.

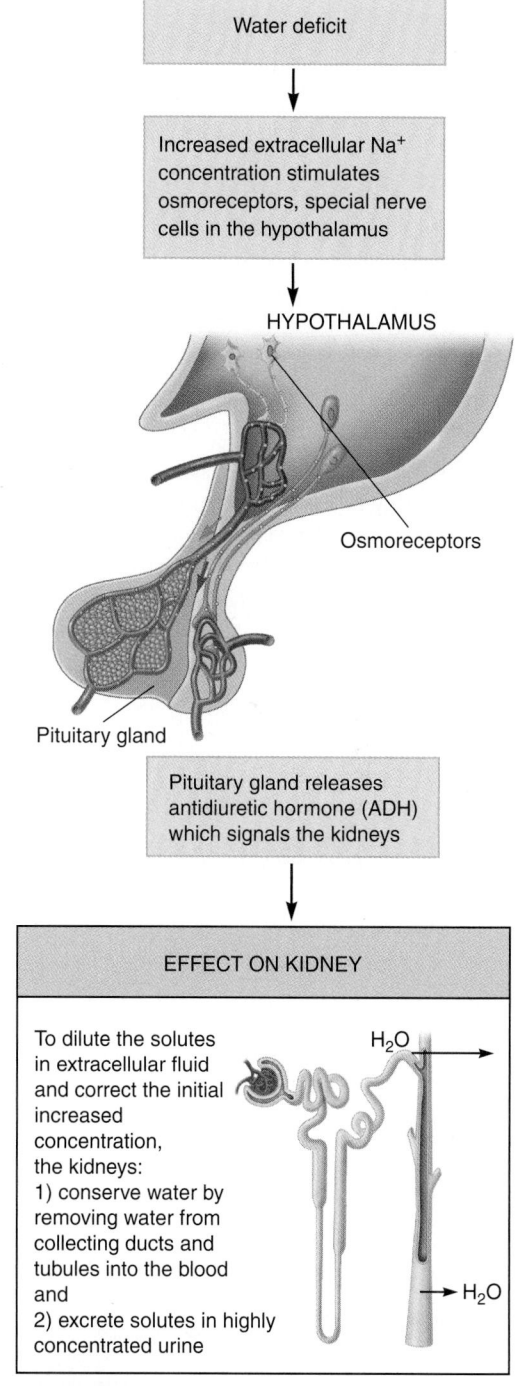

Figure 11.10 **Antidiuretic hormone regulates excretion.** In response to a water deficit, the osmoreceptor-ADH feedback system regulates solute concentrations in extracellular fluid.

aldosterone [al-DOS-ter-own] A steroid hormone secreted from the adrenal glands that acts on the kidneys to regulate electrolyte and water balance. It raises blood pressure by promoting retention of sodium (and thus water) and excretion of potassium.

powerful vasoconstrictor, it also acts directly on the kidneys to decrease excretion of sodium and water. In addition, this protein causes the release of **aldosterone**, a hormone from the adrenal glands. Aldosterone also causes the kidneys to retain sodium, and since water follows sodium, water retention increases as well. All of these processes work to restore blood pressure and volume.

The ability of angiotensin II to act as a vasoconstrictor and increase blood pressure is a life-saving measure. This acute short-term action helps

Quick Bites

How Do Desert-Dwelling Animals Avoid Dehydration?

Some desert animals can concentrate their urine to nearly 100 times the maximum concentration of human urine. This allows such animals to survive on water obtained from food and their own metabolic reactions. Aquatic animals, on the other hand, minimally concentrate their urine. Beavers concentrate their urine to only about half that of humans.

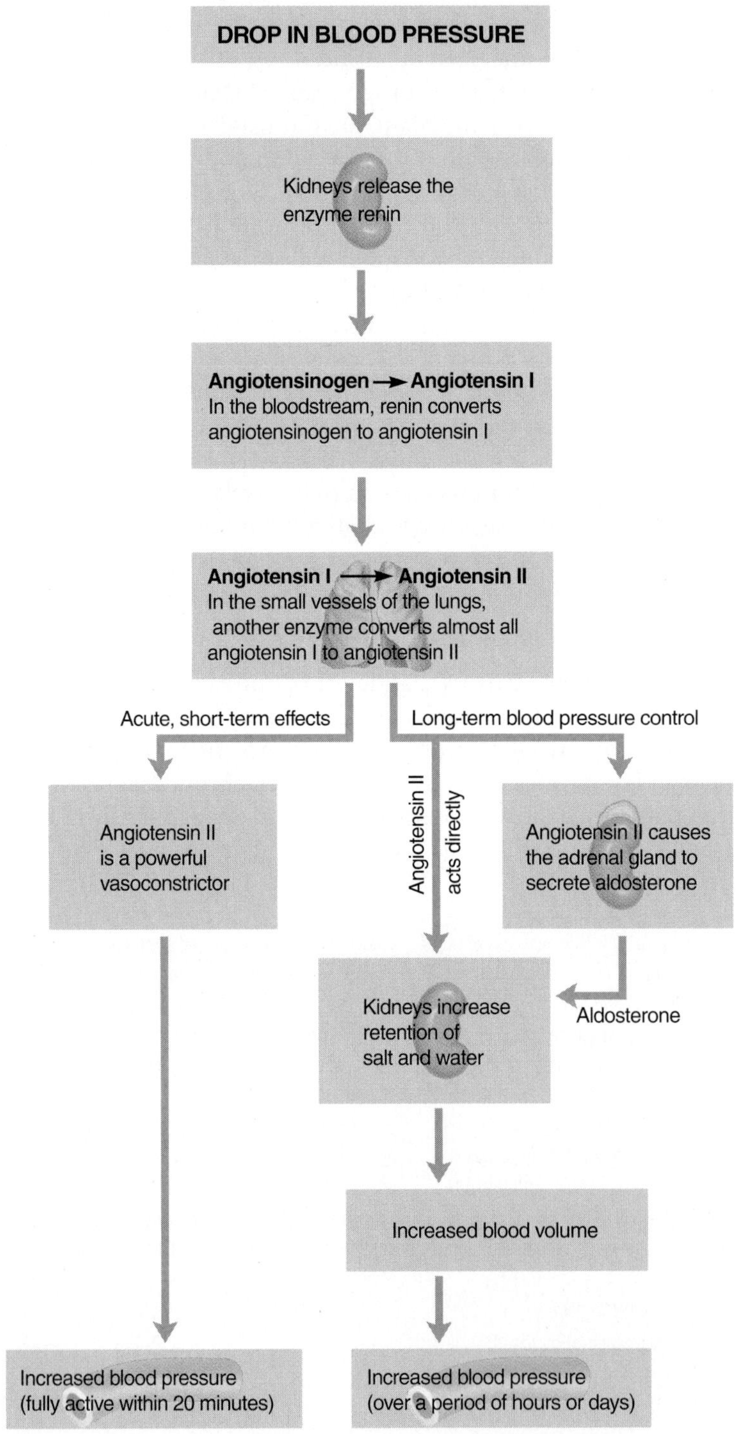

Figure 11.11 **Regulating blood volume and pressure.** Within minutes after severe hemorrhage, the renin-angiotensin-vasoconstrictor mechanism is powerful enough to cause a life-saving rise in blood pressure. Malfunctions in the long-term blood pressure control mechanism can cause persistently high blood pressure (hypertension).

compensate for a severe loss of blood, such as occurs during a hemorrhage. Angiotensin II's effect on the kidney increases extracellular fluid volume and arterial blood pressure over a period of hours or days. Although slower, this long-term action is more powerful than acute vasoconstriction in returning blood pressure to normal.

Perhaps the most important role of the renin-angiotensin system is its response to dietary sodium. It allows a person to consume either very small or very large amounts of sodium without causing major changes in extracellular fluid volume or blood pressure. Since water follows sodium, increased sodium intake increases extracellular fluid volume and blood pressure. This reduces the secretion of renin and production of angiotensin, leading to decreased retention of sodium and water by the kidneys. The resulting excretion of water and sodium returns extracellular volume and blood pressure to normal. A low sodium intake triggers the opposite effects.

Thirst

Although taste, availability, cultural patterns, and personal habits affect the amount of fluids we consume, thirst is our most important stimulus for drinking. Why do we become thirsty? The four major stimuli for thirst are as follows:[5]

1. Increased osmolarity of the fluid surrounding the osmoreceptors in the hypothalamus

2. Reduced blood volume and blood pressure

3. Increased angiotensin II

4. Dryness of the mouth and mucous membranes lining the esophagus

Drinking fluids temporarily alleviates thirst, so we stop our fluid intake and do not overhydrate. Remarkably, studies show that animals drink almost precisely the amount of water necessary to return their blood volume and electrolyte concentrations to normal.[6]

Nevertheless, thirst is not always a reliable guide to avoiding dehydration. Hot weather or heavy exercise can cause fluid losses of up to 1 to 2 liters per hour and deplete our fluids before we feel thirsty.[7] After you drink water, your body can take 30 to 60 minutes to absorb and distribute it throughout the body. For example, imagine you are roller blading in the hot sun and after an hour you pause momentarily to quench your thirst with a 0.5-liter bottle of water. That's not enough—you still have a deficit of 0.5 to 1.5 liters of water, and you'll continue to lose water while your body absorbs and distributes the water you just drank. To avoid dehydration in hot weather or when exercising, you need to drink fluids early and often.

Because heavy activity easily can cause dehydration, athletes also must be careful to drink adequate amounts of fluid. Athletic performance improves if athletes anticipate their water needs well before they begin to feel thirst. (See Chapter 13, "Sports Nutrition," for more on water recommendations for athletes.)

Older people and infants are particularly vulnerable to dehydration. The sensitivity of the thirst response declines with age, putting the elderly at high risk. Infants need to take in a large amount of water relative to their size because a large proportion of their body weight is water. Breast milk or infant formula provides an appropriate amount of fluid for infants. People who care for children and elders must remember to give them fluids often.

Quick Bites

Water, Water Everywhere and Not a Drop to Drink!

When shipwrecked sailors drink seawater, they quickly become severely dehydrated. This is because the concentration of salt in seawater is about double the maximum concentration of salt in urine. Thus, it takes 2 liters of urine to rid the body of the solutes ingested by drinking 1 liter of seawater.

Quick Bites

Why Do Salty Foods Make You Thirsty?

The thirst mechanism is highly sensitive to extracellular sodium concentration. Even a tiny rise in sodium crosses the thirst threshold and triggers the desire to drink.

Quick Bites

Is Airline Drinking Water Tainted?

About one-sixth of the drinking water samples taken in 2004 from airplane galley water taps were contaminated with bacteria. The findings prompted the Environmental Protection Agency to advise passengers with compromised immune systems or other health concerns to request canned or bottled beverages and avoid drinking coffee or tea made with tap water.

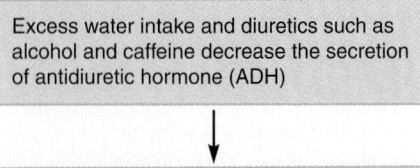

Excess water intake and diuretics such as alcohol and caffeine decrease the secretion of antidiuretic hormone (ADH)

↓

A fall in ADH levels signals the kidney to concentrate solutes in extracellular fluid by excreting water

↓

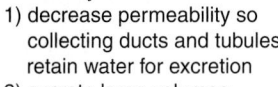

EFFECT ON KIDNEY

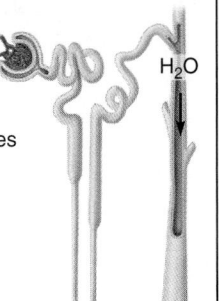

To concentrate solutes in extracellular fluid and correct the initial decreased concentration, the kidneys:
1) decrease permeability so collecting ducts and tubules retain water for excretion
2) excrete large volumes of dilute urine

H₂O

Figure 11.12 **Effects of decreased ADH level on kidney output.** Alcohol and caffeine increase water excretion by slowing the release of antidiuretic hormone (ADH).

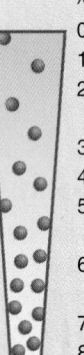

% Body weight loss

0
1 Thirst
2 Increased thirst, loss of appetite, discomfort
3 Impatience, decreased blood volume
4 Nausea, slowing of physical work
5 Difficulty concentrating, apathy, tingling extremities
6 Increasing body temperature, pulse and respiration rate
7 Stumbling, headache
8 Dizziness, labored breathing
9 Weakness, mental confusion
10 Muscle spasms, indistinct speech
11 Kidney failure, poor circulation due to decreased blood volume

Figure 11.13 **Effects of progressive dehydration.**

Water Reabsorption in the Gastrointestinal Tract

The operation of the gastrointestinal tract requires many liters of fluid each day. If all the secretions from the salivary glands, stomach, small intestine, pancreas, and gallbladder passed through the GI tract and out in the feces, we would dehydrate very rapidly! Fortunately, the small and large intestines reabsorb almost all of the water that enters them, so little water actually is lost in feces.

Key Concepts: *The body has mechanisms that balance water among compartments and regulate total body water. Antidiuretic hormone (ADH) stimulates water reabsorption in the kidneys, while aldosterone stimulates the kidneys to reabsorb sodium. Thirst is not a reliable indicator to avoid dehydration when fluid losses are high, such as during hot weather or heavy exercise.*

Alcohol, Caffeine, and Common Medications Affect Fluid Balance

Anyone who regularly consumes alcohol probably realizes that it is a diuretic—a substance that increases fluid loss through increased urination. Alcohol suppresses ADH production (see **Figure 11.12**), and excessive alcohol consumption can cause dehydration with symptoms of thirst, weakness, dryness of mucous membranes, dizziness, and light-headedness—all common effects of a hangover.

A cup of coffee can provide a morning pick-me-up, but the caffeine is a mild diuretic. A typical pattern of many busy Americans is a few cups of coffee in the morning, a caffeinated soda with lunch, another in the afternoon, and maybe a glass of wine or a beer with dinner. Studies of the effects of caffeinated beverages on overall hydration status have produced inconsistent results, however.[8] Although some suggest that a fondness for caffeinated beverages can cause chronic mild dehydration, the DRI committee examining water and electrolyte requirements concluded that caffeinated beverages contribute to the total water intake in a manner similar to noncaffeinated beverages.[9] Most Americans seem to consume a sufficient quantity and variety of beverages to maintain fluid balance.[10]

Doctors often prescribe diuretic medications to help lower blood pressure or decrease swelling caused by fluid retention. Because these medications can disrupt sodium and potassium balance, doctors typically monitor the patient's blood electrolyte levels and may prescribe potassium supplements to maintain a proper balance.

Dehydration

Dehydration, or too little water, is a major killer worldwide—infants and the frail elderly are especially vulnerable. Gastrointestinal infections are primarily responsible. These infections cause diarrhea and prolonged vomiting, leading to excessive water loss. Unless treated rapidly, a person who loses an amount of water equal to 20 percent of body weight is likely to become comatose and die. Burns also can cause deadly dehydration. Extensively damaged skin cannot protect the body and prevent excessive fluid loss.

Dehydration diminishes physical and mental performance. (See **Figure 11.13**.) Early signs of dehydration include fatigue, dry mouth, headache, and dark urine with a strong odor. Change in urine color reflects the body's attempt to conserve water by increasing water reabsorption in the kidney. You probably have noticed that your urine becomes darker when you haven't had much to drink, whereas your urine is almost colorless when you've had plenty to drink. Low fluid intake increases the risk of kidney stones, and some experts believe it also increases the risk of urinary tract, breast, and colon cancers.[11]

Seniors and infants are particularly vulnerable to dehydration. The sense of thirst often diminishes with age, and seniors often take diuretic medications. For a variety of reasons, seniors may stop eating and drinking. The resulting physical and mental deterioration creates a vicious cycle, with food and fluid intake continuing to worsen.

Because infants can lose water rapidly through their skin, they need ample fluid relative to their size. Breast milk or infant formula generally provides all the fluid a baby needs. Severe diarrhea can cause swift and deadly dehydration, especially in seniors and infants. Normally, the intestines reabsorb nearly all the fluid secreted by digestive organs. But when intestinal disease causes diarrhea or prolonged vomiting, dehydration can occur. Worldwide, dehydration is a major killer of babies and young children, with infection the underlying culprit.

Water consumption, of course, is the primary treatment for dehydration. Oral rehydration solutions also can be used; typically these consist of simple ingredients including clean water, sugar, and table salt. Oral rehydration may be sufficient for mild dehydration, but intravenous fluids and hospitalization may be necessary for moderate to severe dehydration. Diarrhea and prolonged vomiting, which cause heavy fluid and electrolyte losses, can be fatal unless the person is rapidly rehydrated with electrolyte solutions.

Water Intoxication

Because drinking fluids temporarily alleviates thirst, we rarely drink to the point of overhydration and dilution of body fluids. However, replacement of fluid losses following intensive or prolonged exercise with plain water (and no electrolytes) can result in overhydration and hyponatremia (low blood sodium) in athletes.[12] (See Chapter 13, "Sports Nutrition," for more on fluid balance for athletes.) Acute water toxicity has been reported due to rapid consumption of large quantities of fluids that greatly exceeded the kidney's maximal excretion rate of approximately 0.7 to 1.0 liters per hour.[13] A fraternity hazing ritual, for example, caused fatal water intoxication in a California State University student who was forced to drink large quantities of water while exercising vigorously.[14]

Overhydration can occur in people with untreated glandular disorders that cause excessive water retention. However, in some psychiatric cases, overhydration has been fatal.[15] People with certain mental disorders have a compulsion to drink huge quantities of water, but their kidneys usually are able to keep up, since normal kidneys can excrete 15 to 20 liters of urine per day. Several years ago, some dieters overenthusiastically followed a fad weight-reduction diet calling for massive water intake and suffered seizures from overhydration.

Key Concepts: *Diuretic medications increase urinary fluid losses. Alcohol and caffeine have mild diuretic effects. Dehydration occurs when fluid loss exceeds fluid intake; it is a potential consequence of gastrointestinal disease, burns, and heavy sweating. Treatment involves replacing fluids, along with electrolytes if the condition is severe. Water intoxication is rare; normal kidneys can excrete many liters of fluid each day.*

major mineral A major mineral is required in the diet and present in the body in large amounts compared with trace minerals.

Major Minerals

Unlike the nutrient molecules you have studied so far, minerals are inorganic elemental atoms or ions. Unlike carbohydrate, protein, and fat, minerals are not changed during digestion or when the body uses them. Unlike many vitamins, minerals are not destroyed by heat, light, or alkalinity. Calcium remains calcium, be it in seashells, milk, or bones. Iron remains iron, whether it is part of a cast-iron skillet or carried in the bloodstream as part of hemoglobin. This is true for all minerals.

Minerals play many essential roles in the body. Some minerals, such as magnesium, participate in the catalytic activity of enzymes. Others serve a structural function; for example, calcium and phosphorus are among the minerals that make our bones hard. Minerals are categorized as major or trace minerals based on the amount needed in the diet and the amount of the mineral in the body. The body requires more than 100 milligrams per day of each **major mineral**, whereas the dietary need for each trace mineral is less than 100 milligrams daily. **Figure 11.14** shows the relative amounts of the major and trace minerals in the body. This classification of minerals is unrelated to the mineral's biological importance. For example, iron is a trace mineral, but it plays a critical role in many major metabolic reactions. The trace minerals are discussed in Chapter 12.

Fyi Tap, Filtered, or Bottled: Which Water Is Best?

FOR YOUR INFORMATION

Everywhere you look, it seems like more and more people are carrying and sipping on bottles of water. Theme parks even sell shoulder holsters for you to carry your bottle around with you. What's with the water craze? And what's wrong with the good old water fountain?

During the mid to late 1980s, the growth in use of bottled water began. Initially, bottled mineral waters, like Perrier, were associated with wealth and glamour. But like many trends adopted by the wealthy (white bread, for instance), bottled water soon became desirable to a wider range of people. It is now estimated that Americans drink 7.5 billion gallons of bottled water each year![1] The U.S. per capita consumption of bottled water for 2005 was 26.1 gallons. U.S. residents now drink more bottled water annually than any other beverage except carbonated soft drinks. Major soft drink companies, such as Coca-Cola and PepsiCo, sell their own brands of bottled water.

There are probably several factors fueling the growth of the bottled-water industry.

Baby boomers are seeking natural, low-calorie beverages, and fitness consciousness has reemphasized the importance of hydration. Media reports of contamination of tap water in major metropolitan areas spark concerns about the safety and quality of tap water. Most Americans choose bottled water for what they think is *not* in it, rather than for what it contains.

From a nutritional perspective, it's important to drink plenty of fluids. Water is one of the best ways to replace lost fluids, and, at the simplest level, the source of water doesn't really matter. Standards for municipal water systems are enforced by the Environmental Protection Agency (EPA), which requires regular testing and monitoring. Tap water can be considered a safe, clean source of water. Many municipal water systems add fluoride to tap water, an important weapon in the prevention of tooth decay. However, home-installed filtration systems for removing chlorine may also remove added fluoride, and most bottled waters do not contain fluoride.

Some people don't like the taste of their local water supply, and don't want to bother with maintaining a filtration system. In this case, or if you want your water "to go," bottled water may be the choice. The bottled-water industry offers

- high-volume, returnable containers from suppliers who stock the "water coolers" for offices or supermarkets;
- the familiar brands (e.g., Evian, Zephyrhills, Dasani, Aquafina) that are sold as alternatives to soft drinks; and
- bottled water in vending machines.

The bottled-water industry is regulated by the Food and Drug Administration (FDA), which, in 1995, published Standards of Identity for bottled water, set maximum allowable standards for contaminants, and established Current Good Manufacturing Practices (CGMP) for bottling plants. Keep in mind that the FDA regulates bottled waters that are sold interstate, and not those sold only in a particular area or state. Individual states may have their own quality standards for locally distributed waters.

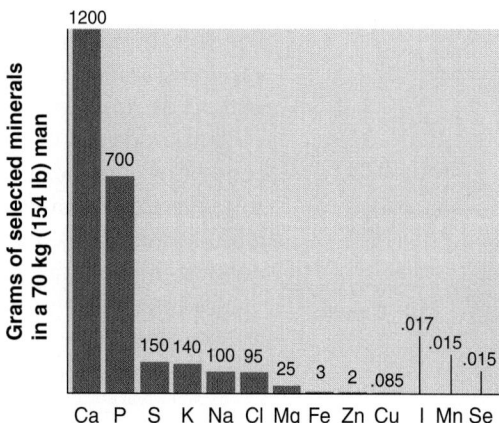

Key

■ Major minerals

■ Trace minerals

Figure 11.14 **Minerals in the human body.** Dietary minerals also are elements in the periodic table. Based on the amount of a mineral needed in the diet and the amount in the body, nutritionists categorize a mineral as major or trace.
Sources: Groff JL and Gropper SS. *Advanced Nutrition and Human Metabolism.* 3rd ed. Belmont CA: Wadsworth/Thomson Learning, 2000; and Stipanuk MH. *Biochemical and Physiological Aspects of Human Nutrition.* Philadelphia: WB Saunders, 2000.

Look beyond terms such as *artesian, mineral, spring,* or *purified* (see Table 1). The labels on most bottled water list the source of the water. Some consumers may be surprised to find that their favorite brand of water is really from a municipal source, not an underground spring! Nutrition Facts labels are required if the manufacturer makes a claim (e.g., sodium free) or adds minerals. These labels often do not show the natural mineral content of the water, which is really the only other nutritional aspect that could be expected.

Once again, the choice is up to the consumer—there is no clearly best choice of water. Cost, taste, convenience, and safety are all issues to consider.

[1] International Bottled Water Association. Bottled water: more than just a story about sales growth. April 13, 2006. http://www.bottledwater.org/public/2006_Releases /2006-04-13_bevmkt.htm. Access 7/13/06.

Table 1 **Definitions of Bottled Water Terms**

- *Mineral water* must contain at least 250 parts per million (ppm) of dissolved minerals and come from a geologically and physically protected underground water source.
- *Purified water* is tap or ground water that has been treated by distillation, deionization, or reverse osmosis. This may be labeled "distilled water" if produced by steam distillation and condensation.
- *Spring water* comes from an underground formation from which water flows naturally to the surface; it is collected either at the spring or from a bore hole to the underground formation.
- *Artesian water* comes from tapping a confined underground aquifer that is below the natural water table. Generally the artesian well is located in a depression where the water table of the surrounding hills is higher. The "head" of pressure from the water table forces the water up through the tap line.
- *Ground water* comes from a subsurface saturated zone and is not under the direct influence of surface water.
- *Well water* comes from a drilled hole that taps the water of an aquifer, and is pumped to the surface.

Source: International Bottled Water Association. Frequently asked questions. http://www.bottledwater.org/public /BWFactsHome_main.htm. Accessed 7/13/06; and US Food and Drug Administration. Bottled water regulation and the FDA. August/September 2002. http://www.cfsan.fda.gov/ ~ dms/botwatr.html. Accessed 7/13/06.

Minerals in Foods

Foods from both plants and animals are sources of minerals. Generally speaking, animal tissue contains minerals in the proportion that the animal needs, so animal-derived foods are more reliable mineral sources.

Plant foods can be excellent sources of several minerals, but the mineral content of plants can vary dramatically depending on the minerals in the soil where the plants are found. Even the maturity of a vegetable, fruit, or grain can influence its mineral content. Because actual mineral content varies so much, the values published in food composition tables can be misleading. Often these values are omitted. Like plant foods, drinking water has variable mineral content. Nevertheless, it sometimes can be a significant source of minerals such as sodium, magnesium, and fluoride.

Bioavailability

Your GI tract absorbs a much smaller proportion of minerals than vitamins—and probably for good reason. Once absorbed, excess minerals often are difficult for the body to flush out. In many cases, the body adjusts mineral absorption in relation to needs. For example, a calcium-deficient person absorbs calcium more readily than does a person with normal calcium status.

Megadosing with single mineral supplements can hamper the absorption of other minerals. Minerals such as calcium, iron, zinc, and magnesium, for example, all have similar chemical properties and compete for absorption.

Fiber and other components of food also affect mineral bioavailability. (See **Figure 11.15**.) High-fiber diets reduce absorption of iron, calcium, zinc, and magnesium. **Phytate** (a component of whole grains) binds minerals and carries them out of the intestine unabsorbed. **Oxalate** (found in spinach and rhubarb) binds calcium, markedly reducing calcium absorption.

Key Concepts: *Minerals are essential inorganic elements. Those that we need and store in larger amounts are called major minerals, and those that we need in very small quantities are called trace minerals. A wide variety of foods contain minerals. Physiological needs, competition with minerals, and the fiber content of food all affect mineral bioavailability.*

Sodium

Many people do not realize that sodium (Na) is an essential nutrient. We know sodium best as a component of sodium chloride (table salt), and we have heard for years that we shouldn't eat too much salt. The *Dietary Guidelines* suggest that we "choose and prepare foods with little salt."[16] Nevertheless, some sodium in the diet is essential for normal body function.

Functions of Sodium

Sodium is the major cation in extracellular fluid and a critical electrolyte in the regulation of body fluids. It acts in concert with potassium, the major cation in intracellular fluid, and chloride, the major anion in extracellular fluid, to maintain proper body water distribution and blood pressure. (See **Figure 11.16**.) Nerve transmission and muscle function require sodium. Sodium also helps control the body's acidity and aids the absorption of some nutrients, such as glucose.

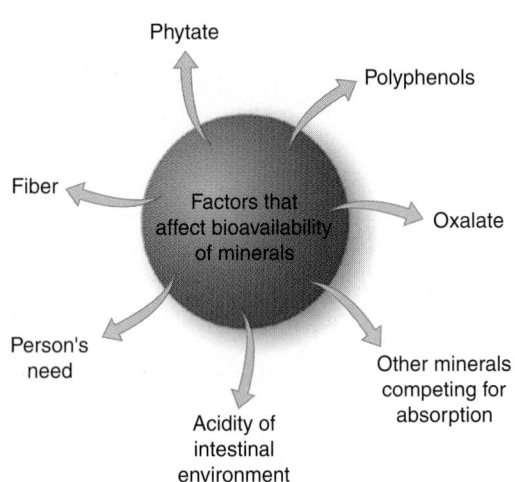

Figure 11.15 **Factors that affect the bioavailability of minerals.** A person's need and the dietary components of a meal can enhance or inhibit the absorption of a mineral.

Electrolytes	Extracellular* fluid concentration	Intracellular** fluid concentration
	meq/L	meq/L
Cations		
Sodium (Na⁺)	140	13
Potassium (K⁺)	5	140
Calcium (Ca²⁺)	5	Minimal
Magnesium (Mg²⁺)	2	7
Total	**151**	**160**
Anions		
Chloride (Cl⁻)	104	3
Bicarbonate (HCO₃⁻)	24	10
Sulfate (SO₄²⁻)	1	---
Phosphate (HPO₄²⁻)	2	107
Proteins	15	40
Organic anions	5	---
Total	**151**	**160**

* Values are for plasma. Interstitial fluid concentrations vary slightly (about 4 percent)

** Values are for cell water in muscle

Figure 11.16 **Cations and anions in intracellular and extracellular fluid.** Potassium, magnesium, phosphate, and proteins are the main solutes inside a cell. Sodium, chloride, and bicarbonate are the main solutes outside the cell.
Source: Oh MS, Uribarri J. Electrolytes, water, and acid–base balance. In: Shils ME, Shike M, Ross AC, Cabellero B, Cousins RJ, eds. *Modern Nutrition in Health and Disease.* 10th ed. Philadelphia: Lippincott Williams & Wilkins, 2006:149–193. Reprinted with permission.

Dietary Recommendations for Sodium

We rarely eat too little sodium; in fact, most of us eat substantially more than we need. Actual sodium *requirements* by the body are relatively small—only a few hundred milligrams daily. In order to make sure that the diet contains adequate amounts of all nutrients, however, the Food and Nutrition Board set the AI for sodium for adults at 1,500 milligrams per day.[17] The Tolerable Upper Intake Level (UL) for sodium is 2,300 milligrams per day. This suggested maximum level is echoed in the American Heart Association's Diet and Lifestyle Recommendations. The Daily Value on food labels is similar—2,400 milligrams per day (the amount in about one teaspoon of table salt).

Sources of Sodium

The typical American diet contains 3,000 to 6,000 milligrams of sodium daily. Not only do Americans consume more than the recommended amounts of sodium, but they also are poor judges of the amount of sodium in their diets.[18] Surprisingly, processed foods—not table salt—contribute the most sodium. (See **Table 11.1**.)

Figure 11.17 shows a breakdown of the sources of sodium in our diets. Soy sauce and other sauces; pickled foods; salty or smoked meats, cheese, and fish; salted snack foods; bouillon cubes; and canned and instant soups are all high-sodium foods. Seasonings based on salt (such as "lemon salt" and "seasoning salt") and those containing the flavor enhancer monosodium glutamate (MSG) also are high in sodium. If your diet is based on Asian foods that contain liberal amounts of soy sauce and MSG, you could be taking in 12,000 to 16,000 milligrams of sodium per day.

Your intestinal tract absorbs nearly all dietary sodium, which then travels throughout the body in the bloodstream. Your kidneys, those remarkable organs, retain the exact amount of sodium the body needs and excrete the excess sodium in the urine along with water.

Taking in too much sodium and not enough water can worsen dehydration. The old practice of giving athletes salt tablets before or after exercise is unnecessary and possibly harmful. On the other hand, radical sodium

phytate (phytic acid) A phosphorus-containing compound in the outer husks of cereal grains that binds with minerals and inhibits their absorption.

oxalate (oxalic acid) An organic acid in some leafy green vegetables, such as spinach, that binds to calcium to form calcium oxalate, an insoluble compound the body cannot absorb.

Quick Bites

Sacred Salt

The physiological need for salt played an important role in shaping human history. Population groups tended to congregate where salt can be found, and civilizations in Africa, India, the Middle East, and China developed around rich salt deposits. At times, salt was traded at a value twice that of gold.

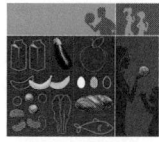

Dietary Guidelines for Americans, 2005
key recommendations

- Consume less than 2,300 mg (approximately 1 teaspoon of salt) of sodium per day.
- Choose and prepare foods with little salt. At the same time, consume potassium-rich foods, such as fruits and vegetables.

Key Recommendations for Specific Population Groups

- *Individuals with hypertension, blacks, and middle-aged and older adults.* Aim to consume no more than 1,500 mg of sodium per day, and meet the potassium recommendation (4,700 mg/day) with food.

Table 11.1 Sodium Content of Various Foods

Food	Serving Size	Sodium (mg)
Cucumber, fresh	1 large (8 ¼")	6
Dill pickle	1 large (4")	1,730
Roast pork	3 oz (85 g)	40
Ham, cured	3 oz (85 g)	1,275
Whole-wheat bread	1 slice	130
Biscuit from mix	1 (2oz)	540
Fresh tomato	1 medium	6
Spaghetti sauce, jar	½ C	600
Two-percent milk	1 C (240 mL)	100
American cheese	1 oz	420
Baked potato	1 medium	10
Potato chips	1 oz	150

As food becomes more processed, the sodium content increases

Source: U.S. Department of Agriculture, Agricultural Research Service. USDA National Nutrient Database for Standard Reference, Release 18. 2005. http://www.ars.usda.gov/nutrientdata.

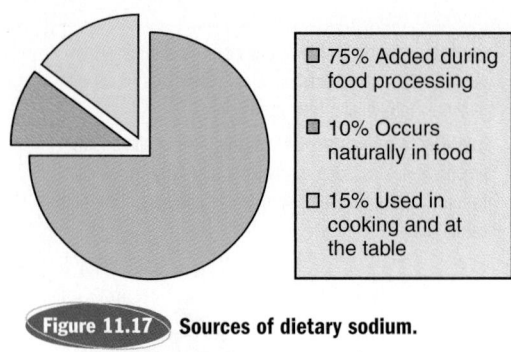

- ☐ 75% Added during food processing
- ☐ 10% Occurs naturally in food
- ☐ 15% Used in cooking and at the table

Figure 11.17 **Sources of dietary sodium.**

hyponatremia Abnormally low sodium concentrations in the blood due to excessive excretion of sodium (by the kidney), prolonged vomiting, or diarrhea.

hypernatremia Abnormally high sodium concentrations in the blood due to increased kidney retention of sodium or rapid ingestion of large amounts of salt.

hypervolemia An abnormal increase in the circulating blood volume.

restriction is not a good idea either. Even though most Americans consume too much sodium, severe sodium restriction can limit the availability of other essential nutrients such as vitamin B$_6$, calcium, iron, and magnesium.[19]

Hyponatremia

Blood sodium concentration sometimes can drop too low, usually as a result of severe diarrhea, vomiting, or intense prolonged sweating with replacement of water but not sodium. Consuming only water without food or other mineral sources also can depress blood sodium levels. The primary symptoms of low blood sodium, **hyponatremia**, resemble dehydration symptoms, and the treatment is similar—replacement of fluid and minerals through liquids and foods or intravenous solutions if necessary. If severe hyponatremia is not treated, extracellular fluid moves into cells, causing them to swell. As brain cells swell and malfunction, the afflicted person can experience headache, confusion, seizures, or coma. Many illnesses, including cancer, kidney disease, and heart disease, can cause low blood sodium concentration. In these situations, treatment usually targets the underlying condition that caused the electrolyte imbalance.[20]

Hypernatremia

Rapid intake of large amounts of sodium (e.g., drinking seawater) can cause the retention of sodium and water in the blood. This causes **hypernatremia**, abnormally high concentration of sodium in the blood, and **hypervolemia**, an abnormal increase in blood volume. This leads to edema (swelling) and a rise in blood pressure. A healthy person with normal kidneys and ample water intake rapidly excretes excess sodium, so hypernatremia usually is seen only in patients with congestive heart failure or kidney disease. Eating too much sodium over a long period of time can contribute to high blood pressure (hypertension) in some people. (See the Nutrition Science in Action feature "Exercise and Sodium Sensitivity.") Excess dietary sodium can also contribute to osteoporosis by increasing calcium loss in the urine.

Key Concepts: *Sodium is the major cation in the extracellular fluid; it plays a critical role in regulating proper water distribution and blood pressure. Nearly all of the sodium that people ingest is absorbed. Control of serum sodium is regulated by excretion. Our diets contain an overabundance of sodium, largely from processed foods. A typical American diet contains between 3,000 and 6,000 milligrams of sodium per day. The AI for sodium is 1,500 milligrams per day, and the UL is 2,300 milligrams. Abnormally low or high levels of sodium in the blood usually are associated with heart or kidney disease rather than dietary deficiency or excess.*

Potassium

Just as sodium is the major extracellular cation, potassium (K) is the key cation in cells. Potassium also can affect hypertension, but in a different way. If people with hypertension eat a diet rich in potassium-containing foods (such as fruits and vegetables), their blood pressure often improves.[21]

Functions of Potassium

Intracellular fluid contains about 95 percent of the body's potassium, with the highest amount in skeletal muscle cells. The flow of sodium and potassium in and out of cells is an important component of muscle contractions

Quick Bites

Versatile Potassium

During the Middle Ages, saltpeter (potassium nitrate) was discovered to be a useful substance. It was used to extract other minerals from rock, as a fertilizer, and as an ingredient in gunpowder. It wasn't used to cure meat until the sixteenth or seventeenth century. Saltpeter was a major ingredient in the curing mixture until 1940, about the time that refrigeration emerged. Today, food manufacturers use small amounts of nitrites rather than saltpeter to preserve foods such as bacon, ham, and some sausages.

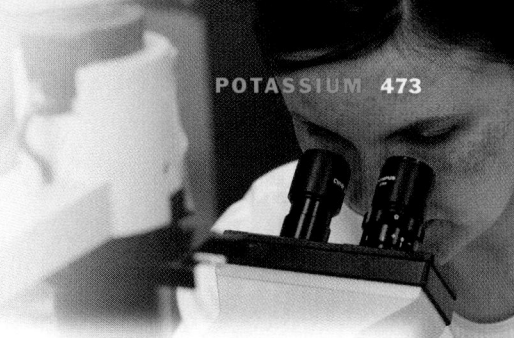

NUTRITION SCIENCE IN ACTION
Exercise and Sodium Sensitivity

Observations: Most people with hypertension (persistent high blood pressure) are sodium sensitive; that is, increasing or reducing intake of sodium alters blood pressure. Some hypertensive people are sodium resistant; that is, changes in sodium intake do not affect blood pressure. In older adults, aerobic exercise training has been shown to lower blood pressure. The effect of aerobic exercise on blood pressure sensitivity to dietary sodium (Na+) is unknown.

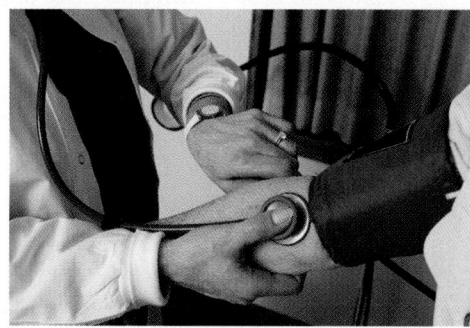

Hypothesis: Aerobic exercise training in older people with hypertension changes sodium sensitivity, with individuals switching from being sodium sensitive to sodium resistant.

Experimental Plan: Recruit 31 (12 male and 19 female) moderately overweight adults (ages 55–70 years) with mild hypertension but otherwise in good health. Design two diets—one high in sodium and the other low in sodium, but otherwise identical. Randomly have subjects consume one diet for eight days, eat regular food during a one-week washout, then consume the alternate diet for eight days. Measure blood pressure at baseline and on the eighth day of each sodium diet. Train subjects aerobically for six months with three 40-minute sessions per week of supervised treadmill walking. Measure subjects' blood pressures, repeat dietary crossover trial, and then measure blood pressures again.

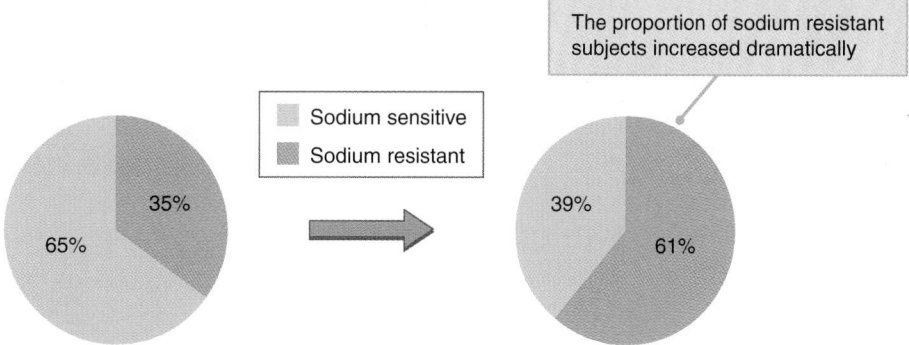

The proportion of sodium resistant subjects increased dramatically

Sodium sensitive
Sodium resistant

35%
65%

39%
61%

Baseline   **After aerobic training**

Results: The hypothesis is confirmed. At baseline, 20 subjects (65 percent) were sodium sensitive and 11 (35 percent) were sodium resistant. After six months of aerobic training, 9 sodium-sensitive individuals became sodium resistant, and one sodium-resistant individual became sodium sensitive. The net postexercise result was 12 (39 percent) sodium-sensitive and 19 (61 percent) sodium-resistant subjects.

Conclusion and Discussion: This study shows that aerobic training in older hypertensive people can alter blood pressure sensitivity to dietary sodium and increase the proportion of individuals who are sodium resistant. The precise mechanism responsible for this change is unknown. Future studies are needed to determine these underlying mechanisms and to examine the health implications of changing sodium sensitivity status.

Source: Dengel DR, Brown MD, Reynolds TH, Kuskowsk MA, Supiano MA. Effect of aerobic exercise training on blood pressure sensitivity to dietary sodium in older hypertensives. *J Hum Hypertens.* 2006;20:372–378. Reprinted by permission from Macmillan Publishers Ltd.: Journal of Human Hypertension, copyright 2006.

Key
- ■ Sodium
- ■ Potassium

Less processed → More processed

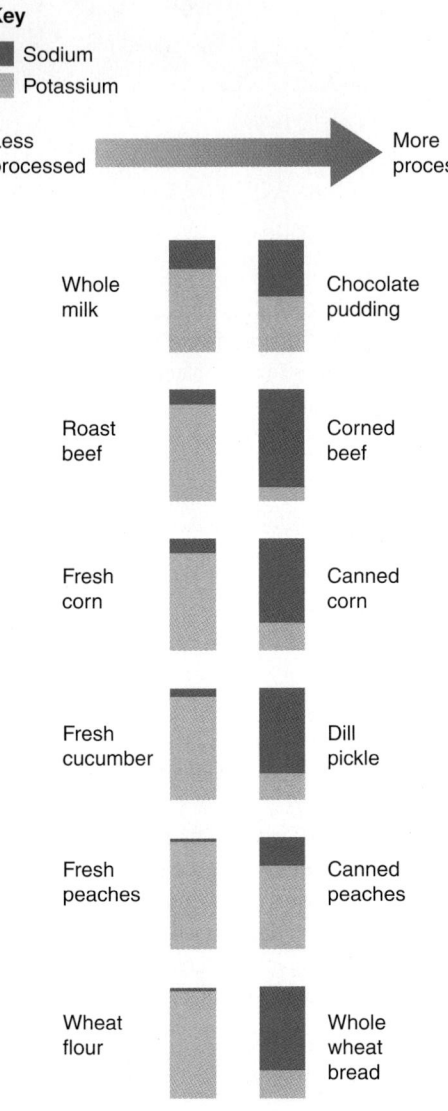

Whole milk — Chocolate pudding

Roast beef — Corned beef

Fresh corn — Canned corn

Fresh cucumber — Dill pickle

Fresh peaches — Canned peaches

Wheat flour — Whole wheat bread

Figure 11.18 **Effects of food processing on sodium and potassium content.** Food processing tends to remove potassium and add sodium. Even when potassium is not removed, adding sodium reduces the ratio of potassium to sodium.

Quick Bites

Banana Facts

You may know that bananas are high in potassium, but did you also know that they have an unusually high carbohydrate content? Before ripening, a banana is almost entirely starch. After ripening, certain varieties are almost entirely sugar—as much as 20 percent by weight.

and the transmission of nerve impulses. The central nervous system (CNS) zealously protects its potassium—CNS potassium levels remain constant even in the face of falling levels in the muscle and blood. Potassium also helps regulate blood pressure.

Dietary Recommendations for Potassium

Although food manufacturers often add sodium to processed foods, they do not routinely add potassium. If a person's diet includes a lot of processed foods, it may fail to meet the potassium recommendations. Based on studies showing that potassium blunts the blood-pressure-raising effects of salt, the DRI Committee suggested a target intake level (AI) of 4,700 milligrams per day for adults.[22] This is higher than the current Daily Value of 3,500 milligrams and substantially more than most Americans eat (2,000 to 3,000 milligrams per day). **Figure 11.18** shows the effects that food processing has on the sodium and potassium levels in foods.

Sources of Potassium

Fresh vegetables and fruits, especially potatoes, spinach, melons, and bananas, are major dietary sources of potassium. Fresh meat, milk, coffee, and tea also contain significant potassium. (See **Figure 11.19**.) Many but not all salt substitutes contain potassium chloride—check the label to be sure. Generous intakes of fruits and vegetables, as recommended by the MyPyramid food guidance system, will help increase potassium intake. Blacks may especially benefit from increased potassium intake—this population group typically has low intake of potassium and a high prevalence of hypertension and salt sensitivity.[23]

POTASSIUM

Daily Value = 3,500 mg

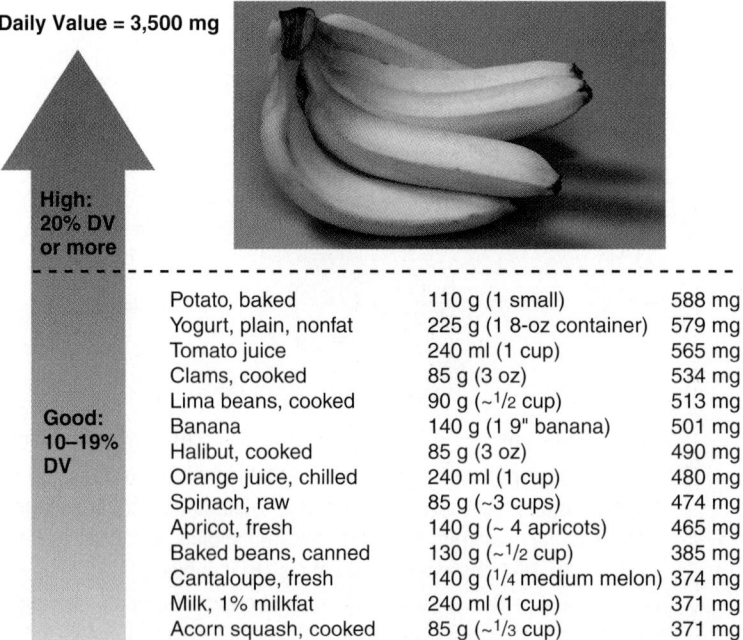

High: 20% DV or more

Good: 10–19% DV

Potato, baked	110 g (1 small)	588 mg
Yogurt, plain, nonfat	225 g (1 8-oz container)	579 mg
Tomato juice	240 ml (1 cup)	565 mg
Clams, cooked	85 g (3 oz)	534 mg
Lima beans, cooked	90 g (~1/2 cup)	513 mg
Banana	140 g (1 9" banana)	501 mg
Halibut, cooked	85 g (3 oz)	490 mg
Orange juice, chilled	240 ml (1 cup)	480 mg
Spinach, raw	85 g (~3 cups)	474 mg
Apricot, fresh	140 g (~ 4 apricots)	465 mg
Baked beans, canned	130 g (~1/2 cup)	385 mg
Cantaloupe, fresh	140 g (1/4 medium melon)	374 mg
Milk, 1% milkfat	240 ml (1 cup)	371 mg
Acorn squash, cooked	85 g (~1/3 cup)	371 mg

Figure 11.19 **Food sources of potassium.** The best food sources of potassium are fresh fruits and vegetables, and certain dairy products and fish.
Source: U.S. Department of Agriculture, Agricultural Research Service. USDA National Nutrient Database for Standard Reference, Release 18. 2005. http://www.ars.usda.gov/nutrientdata.

Hypokalemia

Hypokalemia, low blood potassium, results from potassium depletion. Moderate potassium deficiency is a likely factor in hypertension risk. Low potassium intake can also disrupt acid–base balance in the body and contribute to bone loss and kidney stones.[24] Severe potassium deficiency usually results from excessive losses. Prolonged vomiting, chronic diarrhea, laxative abuse, and use of diuretics are the most common causes of low blood potassium. Insufficient dietary potassium intake magnifies the effects of excess potassium loss. Symptoms include muscle weakness, loss of appetite, and confusion. Severe or rapid potassium depletion can disrupt heart rhythms—a potentially fatal problem.

People with poor diets, such as alcoholics and individuals who suffer from anorexia nervosa or bulimia nervosa, are at highest risk of potassium deficiency. Hypokalemia also is possible in people who overuse strong laxatives. Some diuretics prescribed for hypertension cause increased excretion of both water and potassium. People taking these diuretics are at increased risk for hypokalemia and must pay special attention to their potassium intake. Their doctors may prescribe potassium supplements to counter losses. Athletes and people doing physical labor in high temperatures have high water losses, so they also risk potassium deficiency.

Hyperkalemia

The kidneys effectively remove excess potassium, so the risk of toxicity from dietary intake is usually low. However, malfunctioning kidneys or an excess of intravenous potassium can cause **hyperkalemia**, or a high concentration of potassium in the blood. Because severe hyperkalemia can slow and eventually stop the heart, people who suffer from kidney failure must monitor their potassium intake carefully. The "cocktail" of drugs administered during execution by lethal injection sometimes includes potassium.

Key Concepts: *Potassium is the major cation in the intracellular fluid. With sodium, it regulates muscle contractions and nerve impulse transmissions. For healthy adults, the AI for potassium is 4,700 milligrams per day, substantially more than most Americans consume. The major sources of dietary potassium are vegetables and fruits. The symptoms of hypokalemia are loss of appetite, muscle cramps, and confusion. Severe hyperkalemia can cause cardiac arrest and death.*

Chloride

Chloride (Cl^-) and chlorine (Cl_2) are not the same. Chloride is a negatively charged atom that people commonly eat as a component of table salt (NaCl). Chlorine, a highly reactive molecule composed of two atoms, is a poisonous gas. Water treatment facilities commonly use chlorine to kill bacteria and other germs.

Functions of Chloride

Chloride is the major extracellular anion in the body. Although mostly found outside cells, chloride readily moves in and out of red blood cells. As these cells transport oxygen to body tissues or carbon dioxide to the lungs, the concentration of chloride ions shifts to sustain a neutral charge in the cell. This **chloride shift** maintains lower levels of chloride ions in arterial red blood cells than in venous red blood cells.

hypokalemia Inadequate levels of potassium in the blood.

hyperkalemia Abnormally high potassium concentrations in the blood.

chloride shift The movement of chloride ions in and out of red blood cells to maintain a lower level of chloride in red blood cells in the arteries than in the veins.

metabolic alkalosis An abnormal pH of body fluids usually caused by significant loss of acid from the body or increased levels of bicarbonate.

You have probably noticed the salty taste that sodium chloride (NaCl) imparts to blood, sweat, and tears. Both sodium and chloride help maintain the body's fluid balance. Chloride also readily combines with hydrogen ions (H^+) to form hydrochloric acid (HCl). In the stomach, hydrochloric acid kills many disease-causing bacteria that have been ingested and helps prepare protein for enzymatic digestion. In the large intestine, bacterial activity forms acid products. To neutralize these acid products, the cells lining the large intestine absorb chloride ions and secrete alkaline bicarbonate ions.[25] During an immune response, white blood cells use chloride ions to form a powerful chemical weapon to kill invading bacteria. In neurons, the coordinated movements of chloride and the cations sodium, potassium, and calcium help transmit nerve impulses.

Dietary Recommendations for Chloride

Most of us consume much more chloride than the 2,300 milligrams per day that is the adult AI. Consumption of excess sodium and chloride may aggravate hypertension in salt-sensitive people. Since most chloride is consumed with sodium, limiting sodium to 2,300 milligrams as recommended by the American Heart Association would result in a chloride intake of about 3,450 milligrams. The Daily Value for chloride is 3,400 milligrams, just under the adult UL for chloride, which is 3,600 milligrams per day.

Sources of Chloride

Although some fruits and vegetables naturally contain chloride, most of our chloride intake comes from salt (for dietary sources of salt, see the "Sodium" section earlier in this chapter). You usually can estimate the chloride content of processed foods from the sodium content by using this simple formula:

$$\text{chloride content} = 1.5 \times \text{sodium content.}$$

The average intake of chloride from salt is 4,500 milligrams per day (7.5 g of salt), which is much more than recommended. Reducing the use of salt, as recommended in the *Dietary Guidelines for Americans*, will reduce chloride intake. The kidneys excrete excess chloride, and some chloride also is lost in sweat. The only known cause of high blood chloride levels is severe dehydration.

Hypochloremia

Because vomiting removes hydrochloric acid along with other stomach contents, frequent vomiting can cause a chloride deficiency. People with bulimia nervosa often use self-induced vomiting as a way to compensate for binge eating, and thus may have low levels of chloride and other critical electrolytes, such as potassium. A person who combines repeated vomiting with inadequate consumption of fluid and minerals can suffer dehydration and **metabolic alkalosis** (high blood pH). Small variations in blood pH can have profound consequences—a 5 percent rise in pH can be fatal. Alkalosis can cause abnormal heart rhythm, a substantial drop in blood flow to the brain, decreased oxygen delivery to tissues, and abnormal metabolic activity. To treat this problem, doctors administer oral or intravenous fluids containing the deficient minerals. This replenishment of minerals and fluids restores pH balance.[26]

Key Concepts: *Chloride is involved in many important metabolic functions. It is used to form the hydrochloric acid secreted in the stomach and is important in the generation of nerve impulses as well as in immune function. For healthy adults, the AI for chloride is 2,300 milligrams per day; average chloride intake from salt is 4,500 milligrams per day. People with bulimia nervosa may develop chloride deficiency as a result of self-induced vomiting.*

Calcium

Our bodies contain more calcium (Ca) than any other mineral, about 1.5 to 2 percent of our total weight. Adequate calcium intake over one's lifetime is essential for healthy bones and teeth that will remain strong into old age. Although we associate calcium primarily with bones, it plays many important roles in the body. Getting enough calcium in your diet not only maintains healthy bones but also may help prevent hypertension, decrease your odds of getting colon or breast cancer, improve weight control, and reduce the risk of developing kidney stones.

Functions of Calcium

Bones and teeth contain more than 99 percent of the body's calcium. This mineral makes bones hard and strong, able to withstand tremendous force without breaking—most of the time. The other 1 percent of body calcium is in blood and soft tissues, where it plays many equally crucial roles in such vital functions as muscle contraction, nerve impulse transmission, blood clotting, and cell metabolism. **Figure 11.20** shows the functions of calcium.

Bone Structure

Most of us think of bone as a simple structural framework for our bodies. We forget that bone is living tissue that changes in response to physical stresses. Bone also encases the marrow, the source of many types of blood and immune cells, and serves as the reserve site for minerals such as calcium and phosphorus.

Bone is made up of cells and an extracellular matrix. Two types of cells, osteoblasts and osteoclasts, continually remodel our bones—building them up and tearing them down. Osteoblasts are the construction team, and osteoclasts are the demolition team. Osteoblasts first secrete the collagen protein matrix that forms the initial framework for new bone. Then these bone builders help move minerals from the extracellular fluid to the bone surface, where the minerals become a hard crystalline material that surrounds the collagen fibers. Most of the calcium in bone is in the form of **hydroxyapatite**—a crystalline mineral complex of calcium and phosphorus. By weight, bone is two-thirds mineral and one-third water and protein, primarily collagen. While osteoblasts continually deposit bone, osteoclasts perform the opposite function by resorbing bone. As they break down bone, they release calcium and phosphate, which enter the bloodstream.

The activities of osteoblasts and osteoclasts determine how bones grow and change over time. Mineralization of bone is favored during **linear growth** (growth in height) and for 5 to 10 years thereafter. It is thought that we achieve peak bone mass sometime around age 30.

Throughout life, our bones change in response to our activities. The dynamic nature of bone allows it to be strengthened and rebuilt in areas under repeated stress—bone thickens when repeatedly subjected to loads.

hydroxyapatite A crystalline mineral compound of calcium and phosphorus that makes up bone.

linear growth Increase in body length/height.

American Heart Association

Women and Calcium

Women should ask their physicians about how much calcium they need in their diets. Fat-free milk and low-fat dairy products are recommended. They're excellent sources of calcium.

Reproduced with permission. *www.americanheart.org.* © 2006, American Heart Association, Inc.

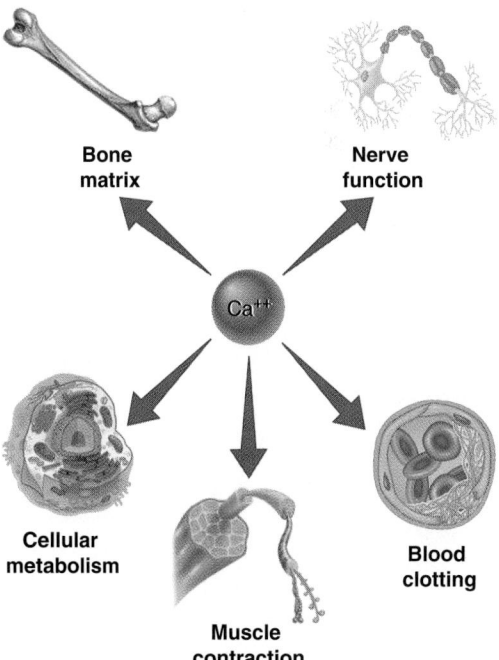

Bone matrix

Nerve function

Ca++

Cellular metabolism

Muscle contraction

Blood clotting

Figure 11.20 **Functions of calcium.** In addition to playing a key role in bone health, calcium in blood and soft tissues is essential for such diverse functions as blood clotting, muscle contractions, and nerve impulse transmission.

Even elderly adults can strengthen and rebuild their bones by performing weight-bearing exercise such as walking or weight lifting.[27]

The calcium in bones serves as a reservoir for calcium that is needed throughout the body. The body maintains a constant calcium blood level at all costs—at the expense of bone strength if necessary. Even if calcium intake is very low, the calcium concentration in the bloodstream remains steady because the body removes calcium from bone to sustain an adequate supply to other tissues. In the absence of kidney disease or hormonal abnormalities, your blood calcium level remains normal even if your diet is extremely deficient in calcium.

Nerve Function

Calcium is a key factor in normal transmission of nerve impulses. The movement of calcium into nerve cells triggers the release of neurotransmitters at the junction between nerves. The neuron releases neurotransmitters in direct proportion to the number of calcium ions that flow through the cell's calcium channels. Insufficient calcium can inhibit nerve transmissions.

Blood Clotting

Calcium is essential for the formation of **fibrin**, the fibrous protein that makes up the structure of blood clots. Calcium participates in nearly every step of the blood-clotting cascade. Blood will not clot in the absence of calcium, but calcium levels in the body seldom fall low enough to significantly impair blood clotting.

Muscle Contraction

Calcium has a central role in muscle contractions because the flow of calcium ions inside muscle cells is crucial for enabling muscles to contract and relax. Calcium sits at a critical location on the muscle fiber, facilitating the interaction of the muscle proteins myosin and actin. Stimulation of muscle fibers by nerve impulses, hormones, or stretch in the fiber increases the amount of calcium in the muscle cells and causes the muscle to contract. As the cells pump calcium ions back outside, the muscle relaxes. During exercise, one cause of muscle fatigue is the impaired activity of calcium in muscle cells.

Cellular Metabolism

Calcium is also a key player in regulation of cellular metabolism. When calcium enters a cell, it can bind to **calmodulin**, a regulatory protein. This binding activates calmodulin, which helps regulate a variety of enzymatic processes that affect cell secretions, **ciliary action**, cell division, and cell proliferation.

Regulation of Blood Calcium

Circulating calcium performs a myriad of functions that are so critical that the body will demineralize bone to prevent even minor dips in blood calcium levels. Three hormones—calcitriol (the active form of vitamin D), parathyroid hormone, and calcitonin—regulate calcium status. They control intestinal absorption of calcium, bone calcium release, and calcium excretion by the kidneys. (See **Figure 11.21**.) In people with inadequate calcium intakes, high sodium intake, excess caffeine, and other diuretics can affect calcium balance by increasing the rate of calcium excretion in the urine.[28]

fibrin A stringy, insoluble protein that is the final product of the blood-clotting process.

calmodulin A calcium-binding protein that regulates a variety of cellular activities, such as cell division and proliferation.

ciliary action Wavelike motion of small hairlike projections on some cells.

Vitamin D

Vitamin D increases calcium absorption by the intestine. Calcitriol, the active form of vitamin D, increases the production of calcium-binding proteins in the lining of the small intestine. The rate of calcium absorption seems to be directly proportional to the quantity of calcium-binding proteins.

Parathyroid Hormone

When plasma calcium levels are too low, the parathyroid gland secretes parathyroid hormone (PTH). PTH activates bone-resorbing osteoclasts that break down bone and release calcium and phosphorus into the blood. It also increases kidney reabsorption of calcium and stimulates calcitriol production, which then enhances intestinal calcium absorption. PTH greatly

LOW BLOOD CALCIUM		HIGH BLOOD CALCIUM	
Increase PTH secretion and calcitriol formation	**Thyroid/Parathyroid**	**Secrete calcitonin**	**Decrease PTH secretion and calcitriol formation**
Parathyroid gland secretes parathormone (PTH). Increased PTH levels stimulate calcitriol (vitamin D₃) production in the kidney	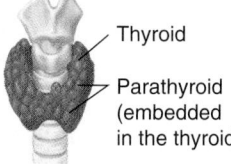 Thyroid / Parathyroid (embedded in the thyroid)	Thyroid gland secretes calcitonin	Parathormone formation slows and PTH levels drop. Decreased PTH levels slow calcitriol formation
Absorb more dietary calcium	**Small intestine**	**Absorb less dietary calcium**	
Calcitriol increases intestinal absorption of calcium and phosphorus	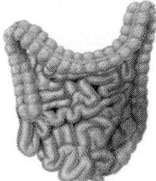	No major effect – calcitonin slightly inhibits calcium absorption	Decreased calcitriol slows intestinal absorption of calcium and phosphorus
Retain calcium	**Kidney**	**Excrete calcium**	
PTH and calcitriol increase calcium reabsorption in the kidney, thus decreasing calcium excretion	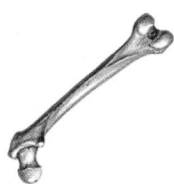	No major effect – calcitonin slightly increases calcium excretion	Decreased PTH and calcitriol levels increase calcium excretion
Move calcium from bone to bloodstream	**Bone**	**Move calcium from bloodstream to bone**	
PTH and calcitriol work together to stimulate osteoclast activity. The osteoclasts gobble up bone, releasing calcium into the bloodstream		Calcitonin inhibits the activity of osteoclasts, shifting the balance toward the deposition of calcium in bone	Decreased PTH and calcitriol levels slow osteoclast activity and breakdown of bone
RAISE BLOOD CALCIUM		**LOWER BLOOD CALCIUM**	

Figure 11.21 **Regulating blood calcium levels.** Calcitonin has only a weak effect on calcium ion concentration. It is fast acting, but any decrease in calcium ion concentration triggers the release of PTH, which almost completely overrides the calcitonin effect. In prolonged calcium excess or deficiency, the parathyroid mechanism is the most powerful hormonal mechanism for maintaining normal blood calcium levels.

increases phosphorus excretion, so phosphorus blood levels actually drop in response to PTH despite an initial increase in supply from the breakdown of bone.

Calcitonin

When plasma calcium is too high, the thyroid gland secretes calcitonin. Calcitonin has weak effects on plasma calcium levels and acts in opposition to PTH. Although it has no major effects in the small intestine and kidney, it inhibits the formation and activity of osteoclasts. This shifts the osteoclast–osteoblast balance toward bone deposition. High concentrations of calcium in the blood decrease PTH production, and thus calcitriol production, slowing processes that move calcium into the bloodstream.

Dietary Recommendations for Calcium

Optimal calcium intake throughout life is extremely important. Bones become stronger and denser as children and young adults develop. Later in life, bones gradually become less dense. If children and young adults fail to take in enough calcium, they are more likely to develop osteoporosis (fragile, porous bones that easily break) later in life. The Adequate Intake level for calcium is 1,000 milligrams per day for adults aged 19 to 50, although calcium intake recommendations vary slightly among public health organizations. Adolescents need more calcium to maximize peak bone mass (the AI for ages 9 to 18 is 1,300 mg per day). The AI for adults aged 51 and older increases to 1,200 milligrams per day.

Unfortunately, many of us fall far short of these recommended calcium intakes. Although average calcium intake has increased slightly (from 743 milligrams per day in 1977–1978 to 813 milligrams per day in 1995),[29] most Americans still fail to meet current recommendations. Population surveys of girls and young women aged 12 to 19 years show their average cal-

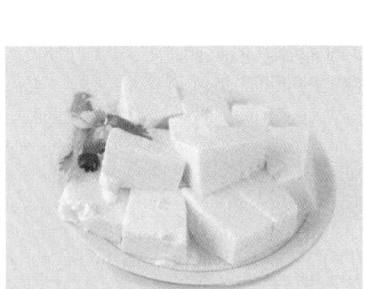

Figure 11.22 **Food sources of calcium.** Calcium is found in milk and dairy products, certain green leafy vegetables, and canned fish with bones.
Source: U.S. Department of Agriculture, Agricultural Research Service. USDA National Nutrient Database for Standard Reference, Release 18. 2005. http://www.ars.usda.gov/nutrientdata.

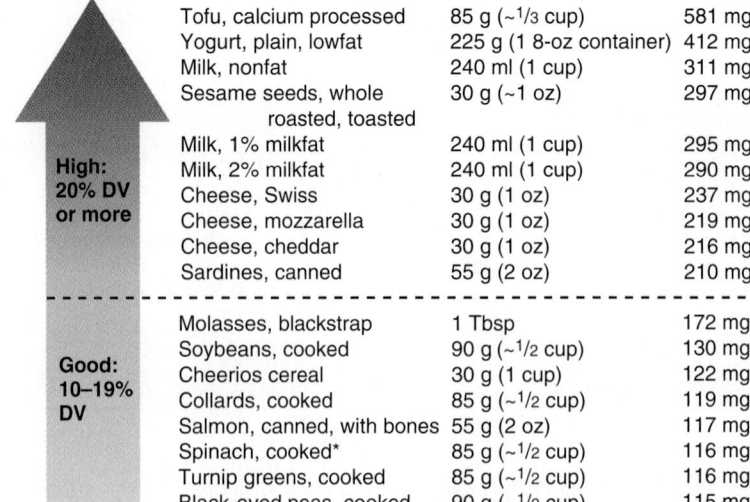

CALCIUM

Daily Value = 1,000 mg

High: 20% DV or more		
Tofu, calcium processed	85 g (~1/3 cup)	581 mg
Yogurt, plain, lowfat	225 g (1 8-oz container)	412 mg
Milk, nonfat	240 ml (1 cup)	311 mg
Sesame seeds, whole roasted, toasted	30 g (~1 oz)	297 mg
Milk, 1% milkfat	240 ml (1 cup)	295 mg
Milk, 2% milkfat	240 ml (1 cup)	290 mg
Cheese, Swiss	30 g (1 oz)	237 mg
Cheese, mozzarella	30 g (1 oz)	219 mg
Cheese, cheddar	30 g (1 oz)	216 mg
Sardines, canned	55 g (2 oz)	210 mg

Good: 10–19% DV		
Molasses, blackstrap	1 Tbsp	172 mg
Soybeans, cooked	90 g (~1/2 cup)	130 mg
Cheerios cereal	30 g (1 cup)	122 mg
Collards, cooked	85 g (~1/2 cup)	119 mg
Salmon, canned, with bones	55 g (2 oz)	117 mg
Spinach, cooked*	85 g (~1/2 cup)	116 mg
Turnip greens, cooked	85 g (~1/2 cup)	116 mg
Black-eyed peas, cooked	90 g (~1/2 cup)	115 mg

*In spinach, oxalate binds calcium and prevents absorption of all but about 5 percent of the plant's calcium.

cium intake to be less than 900 milligrams per day, which is well below recommended intake levels.[30] Many of these young women will attain a suboptimal peak bone mass and will be prone to osteoporosis as they age.

Sources of Calcium

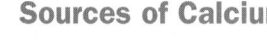

Dairy products provide more than half of the calcium in the typical American diet. Of all the dairy products, nonfat milk is the most nutrient dense because of its high calcium content and low fat and calorie content. Nonfat yogurt is another excellent source of calcium. Cottage cheese has the least calcium of the dairy foods because processing removes much of its calcium. Ice cream and cheese are good sources of calcium, but they should be eaten only in moderation because of their high fat content.

Green leafy vegetables such as spinach have high levels of calcium, but most of the calcium is bound to oxalate and therefore cannot be absorbed. Chinese cabbage, kale, turnip greens, and calcium-processed tofu contain significant amounts of bioavailable calcium. Canned fish with bones, such as sardines, provides lots of calcium as long as you eat the bones. **Figure 11.22** shows food sources of calcium.

Some brands of orange juice, cereal, bread, and yogurt products are now fortified with calcium, making them good sources. Check labels carefully, because only a few of the many products on grocery shelves are fortified with calcium. **Figure 11.23** shows the variation in bioavailability among various sources of calcium.

Although eating a variety of healthful foods is always the best way to obtain nutrients, some people, especially those with limited dairy intake, may need to take supplements to ensure adequate calcium intake. Flavored, chewable, calcium-containing antacids are an inexpensive and easy-to-take source of extra calcium. For more information, see the FYI feature "Calcium Supplements: Are They Right for You?"

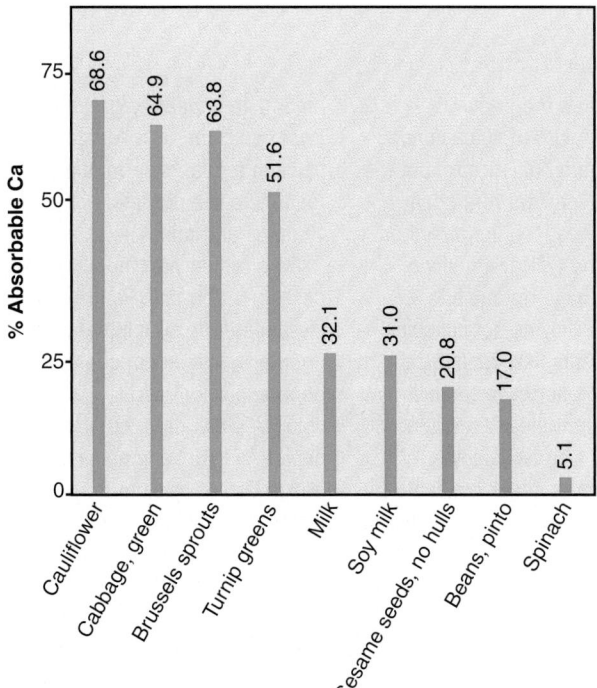

Figure 11.23 **Bioavailability of calcium from different sources.** Your body can absorb more than two-thirds of the calcium in cauliflower, but only about 5 percent of the calcium in spinach. Oxalate in spinich binds calcium and inhibits its bioavailability.
Source: Adapted from Weaver CM, Plawecki KL. Dietary calcium: adequacy of a vegetarian diet. *Am J Clin Nutr.* 1994;59(suppl):1238S–1241S.

Calcium Absorption

The body normally absorbs 25 to 75 percent of dietary calcium, depending on a variety of factors such as age, presence of adequate vitamin D, the body's need for calcium, and calcium intake. For example, if a child and a healthy elderly person eat the same meal, the child may absorb 75 percent of the calcium in the food, whereas the elderly person might absorb only 25 percent. Calcium absorption is particularly high during pregnancy and infancy and is at its lowest in old age.

Calcium absorption is inversely related to calcium intake. The body adjusts the percentage it absorbs based on the amount in the diet: An increase in dietary calcium reduces absorption, and a decrease in dietary calcium enhances absorption.[31] In the absence of vitamin D, calcium absorption can drop to less than 10 percent of dietary calcium.[32] Phytates (in nuts, seeds, and grains) depress calcium absorption, as do oxalates and high levels of phosphorus and magnesium from supplements.

Dietary fiber, except for wheat bran, has little effect on calcium absorption. High intakes of wheat bran have been found to depress calcium absorption from milk. Low estrogen levels, as seen in postmenopausal women, can lower calcium absorption to about 20 percent. Many women take estrogen supplements after menopause to maintain calcium absorption and lower the risk of osteoporosis. Calcium from supplements is absorbed most efficiently when taken between meals at individual doses of 500 milligrams or less.[33]

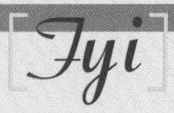

Calcium Supplements: Are They Right for You?

FOR YOUR INFORMATION

After reading the section on calcium, you may be wondering whether you need a calcium supplement. After all, calcium is critical for so many bodily functions, and getting enough calcium reduces the risk of osteoporosis later in life.

Before you head to the supplement aisle at the grocery store, take a critical look at your diet, especially your intake of milk and other dairy products. In the United States and Canada dairy foods are the major sources of dietary calcium; without them, it may be difficult to reach the AI for calcium. People who exclude dairy products, such as vegans and those with milk allergy, must choose foods carefully to find rich calcium sources.

Calcium sources vary widely in their bioavailability. Although labels are required to list the %DV for calcium, they don't indicate

how much of that calcium the body will absorb. For example, $\frac{1}{2}$ cup of spinach contains about 120 milligrams of calcium, but the body will absorb only 5 percent of that calcium! Intake recommendations are based on the mix of sources in the typical American diet. Other cultures manage on much lower intakes in part because they do not consume the many food constituents that deplete calcium or reduce its absorption. Vegetarians may, in fact, need less calcium than meat eaters. If you are considering spinach as your sole source of calcium, however, check out **Table 1.** It shows the amount of certain foods needed to equal the calcium available from 1 cup of milk (about 30 percent of the 300 milligrams of calcium in 1 cup of milk is bioavailable).

You can see from Table 1 that the amount of bioavailable calcium varies quite a bit

among green leafy vegetables! If your diet is low in calcium, try adding some of the higher-calcium foods. Incorporating calcium-rich foods into the diet adds other important vitamins and minerals.

Even armed with more information about calcium in the diet, you may still decide to investigate the supplement market. Again, there are a variety of choices: calcium carbonate, calcium citrate, calcium lactate, calcium phosphate, coral calcium . . . how to decide? First, it's important to know that the absorption of calcium from most supplements is about equal—roughly 30 percent. The calcium citrate malate that is used in some brands of fortified juice, and a limited number of supplements, is absorbed a little better—35 percent. However, a typical calcium citrate malate tablet has less calcium

Hypocalcemia

A lower than normal level of calcium in the blood is called **hypocalcemia**. Because the body uses bone calcium to maintain normal blood calcium levels, hypocalcemia is relatively uncommon. The causes of hypocalcemia include kidney failure, parathyroid disorders, and vitamin D deficiency. Significant hypocalcemia can cause muscle spasms, facial grimacing, and convulsions.

A chronic dietary calcium deficiency can result in osteoporosis either by suboptimal bone growth in childhood and adolescence or increased rate of bone loss after menopause. Studies also link low calcium intake to an increased risk of hypertension, colon cancer, and preeclampsia (a complication of pregnancy marked by high blood pressure, edema, and protein in the urine).[34]

Hypercalcemia

The two major causes of **hypercalcemia** are cancer and the overproduction of PTH by the parathyroid gland. Hypercalcemia can result in fatigue, confusion, loss of appetite, and constipation. Calcium may be deposited in the soft tissues, where it can impair organ function. Very high levels of blood calcium can lead to coma and cardiac arrest.

Excess calcium supplementation usually does not result in hypercalcemia, but may cause mineral imbalances by interfering with the absorption of other minerals, such as iron, magnesium, and zinc. Calcium supplements that contain citrate and ascorbic acid enhance iron absorption, but other forms can cut iron absorption in half. Calcium also may interfere with absorption of

hypocalcemia A deficiency of calcium in the blood.
hypercalcemia Abnormally high concentrations of calcium in the blood.

than a tablet of another type such as calcium carbonate. Calcium carbonate is usually the most concentrated per tablet, so taking fewer pills per day will supply enough; also, this type of supplement tends to be less expensive. Chelated calcium supplements can improve absorption a bit, but the extra expense is probably not worth it.

Other factors to consider are that calcium supplements may be absorbed better if taken between meals. Also, you need to get plenty of vitamin D, either through casual exposure to the sun, in fortified milk, or as part of a supplement (many calcium supplements have added vitamin D). Vitamin D is important for the absorption of calcium. In addition, bones get stronger with regular, weight-bearing exercise, so make sure to include that in your healthful lifestyle.

Table 1 **Foods That Provide the Calcium Equivalent of 1 Cup (8 fl oz) of Milk**

Food	Amount	Food	Amount
Almonds, dry roasted	6 oz	Mustard greens	1 ⅓ C
Beans, pinto	6 ⅓ C	Radish	4 ½ C
Beans, red	7 C	Rutabaga	2 ¼ C
Beans, white	2 ½ C	Sesame seeds, no hulls	12 oz
Broccoli	2 ½ C	Soy milk, unfortified	30 C
Brussels sprouts	4 C	Spinach	7 ¾ C
Cabbage, Chinese	1 C	Tofu, calcium set	½ C
Cabbage, green	3 C	Turnip greens	1 C
Calcium-fortified juices*	5 fl oz	Watercress	3 ½ C
Cauliflower	4 C		
Kale	1 ¾ C		
Kohlrabi	3 ½ C		

*Fortified with calcium as calcium citrate malate.
Source: Adapted from Weaver CM, Plawecki KL. Dietary calcium: adequacy of a vegetarian diet. *Am J Clin Nutr.* 1994;59(suppl):1238S–1241S.

phosphorylation The addition of phosphate to an organic (carbon-containing) compound. Oxidative phosphorylation is the formation of high-energy phosphate bonds (ADP + Pi → ATP) from the energy released by oxidation of energy-yielding nutrients.

some medications, such as tetracycline.[35] The Food and Nutrition Board has established a UL for calcium of 2,500 milligrams per day.

Key Concepts: *Calcium is a major component of bones and teeth. In addition, calcium is required for muscle contraction, nerve impulse transmission, blood clotting, and regulation of cell metabolism. For adults, 1,000 milligrams per day is recommended; a greater amount is suggested for adolescents and older adults. Dairy foods and fortified foods are major dietary sources of calcium. Calcium status is regulated by three hormones that control intestinal absorption, bone calcium release, and kidney excretion: calcitriol, parathyroid hormone, and calcitonin. Lack of dietary calcium contributes to the development of osteoporosis.*

Phosphorus

Phosphorus (P), like calcium, serves many roles in the biochemical reactions of cells and has a critical role in bone as part of the mineral complex hydroxyapatite. Phosphorus intake typically exceeds that of calcium because it is so widespread in the food supply. Most phosphorus in the body is in the form of the phosphate ion (PO_4^{3-}). In fact, phosphate is the most abundant intracellular anion.

Functions of Phosphorus

Bones are the major storehouse of phosphorus, holding nearly 85 percent of the body's supply. The remaining phosphorus is found in cells of soft tissues (~15 percent) and extracellular fluid (~0.1 percent). It helps activate and deactivate enzymes in a process called **phosphorylation**. Phosphorus is an essential component of ATP, the universal energy source for all cells. Phosphorus also is a component of DNA, RNA, and phospholipids in cell membranes and lipoproteins.

Dietary Recommendations for Phosphorus

The phosphorus RDA for adults is 700 milligrams per day. Adolescents need more, about 1,250 milligrams per day, to support growth. The average adult intake is between 1,000 and 1,500 milligrams per day, so phosphorus deficiencies due to dietary insufficiency are rarely seen.

Sources of Phosphorus

Phosphorus is abundant in our food supply. In general, foods rich in protein (milk, meat, and eggs) also are rich in phosphorus. Food additives, especially those in processed meat and soft drinks, supply up to 30 percent of our phosphorus. **Figure 11.24** shows selected food sources of phosphorus. Food manufacturers often add phosphate salts to processed foods to improve moisture retention and smoothness.

Because phosphorus density is higher in cow's milk than in most other foods, people with high dairy-product intakes have high-phosphorus diets. Soft drinks often contain phosphoric acid, although the phosphorus level is not high—about 50 milligrams in a 12-ounce cola, compared with 370 milligrams in 12 ounces of fat-free milk. However, among heavy cola drinkers who consume five or more per day, soda is an important contributor to phosphorus intake.[36] Dairy products have phosphorus plus calcium (460 milligrams in 12 ounces), whereas sodas have phosphorus but virtually no calcium (10 milligrams or less in a 12-ounce can)—an important distinction.

Our bodies directly absorb phosphorus from most food sources, with one major exception—plant seeds. All plant seeds (beans, peas, cereals, and nuts) contain phosphorus in a storage form, phytic acid. Our bodies do not produce the enzymes necessary to break down phytic acid. Still, we can absorb up to

50 percent of this phosphorus because other foods and bacteria in our large intestines contain the necessary enzymes. Yeasts also can break down phytic acid, so our bodies absorb more phosphorus from whole grains when part of leavened bread, for example, than from grains in unleavened bread and breakfast cereals. Although excess calcium interferes with phosphorus absorption—possibly because unabsorbed calcium binds with phytic acid and prevents bacterial breakdown—typical dietary calcium levels have no effect.

Generally, we absorb between 55 and 70 percent of dietary phosphorus, and the kidneys excrete any excess in the urine. Unlike calcium absorption, phosphorus absorption does not increase as dietary intake decreases.[37] On the other hand, the body's phosphorus needs can drive phosphorus absorption efficiency. Although the efficiency of phosphorus absorption, unlike calcium absorption, does not vary with increased dietary intake, it rises dramatically when the body has low phosphorus levels.

In the intestines, calcitriol enhances both calcium and phosphorus absorption. Parathyroid hormone, on the other hand, has opposite effects on calcium and phosphorus levels. PTH not only maintains calcium levels by stimulating the kidneys to reabsorb calcium, but also causes rapid loss of phosphorus in the urine. The two most important regulators of urinary phosphorus excretion are PTH and the amount of phosphorus in the diet.[38]

Hypophosphatemia

Phosphorus is so common in foods that only near-total starvation will cause a dietary phosphorus deficiency. Rather, an underlying disorder typically causes **hypophosphatemia**, low blood phosphate, either by restricting absorption or enhancing excretion. Physicians commonly encounter hypophosphatemia, and about 2 percent of patients admitted to general hospitals suffer from it.[39] Some of its more common causes include **hyperparathyroidism** (excessive secretion of PTH, often because of a parathyroid tumor), vitamin D deficiency, and overuse of aluminum-, magnesium-, or calcium-containing antacids that bind phosphate. Common symptoms of hypophosphatemia include anorexia, dizziness, bone pain, muscle weakness, and a waddling gait. Chronic hypophosphatemia affects primarily the

hypophosphatemia Abnormally low phosphate concentration in the blood.

hyperparathyroidism Excessive secretion of parathyroid hormone, which alters calcium metabolism.

PHOSPHORUS

Daily Value = 1,000 mg

Cheese, provolone	85 g (3 oz)	422 mg
Beef liver, cooked	85 g (3 oz)	422 mg
Yogurt, plain, nonfat	225 g (one 8 oz container)	356 mg
Sunflower seeds	30 g (~1 oz)	346 mg
Herring, cooked	85 g (3 oz)	258 mg
Milk, nonfat	240 ml (1 cup)	251 mg
Milk, 1% milkfat	240 ml (1 cup)	235 mg
Milk, 2% milkfat	240 ml (1 cup)	233 mg
Chicken, white meat, cooked	85 g (3 oz)	194 mg
Beef, ground, extra lean, cooked	85 g (3 oz)	175 mg
Oysters, cooked	85 g (3 oz)	173 mg
Lentils, cooked	90 g (~1/2 cup)	162 mg
Tofu, calcium processed	85 g (~1/3 cup)	162 mg
Chicken, dark meat, cooked	85 g (~3 oz)	152 mg
All Bran cereal	30 g (~1/2 cup)	150 mg
Almonds	30 g (1 oz)	142 mg
Soy milk	240 ml (1 cup)	137 mg
Black beans, cooked	90 g (~1/2 cup)	126 mg
Peanut butter	2 Tbsp	115 mg

High: 20% DV or more

Good: 10–19% DV

Figure 11.24 **Food sources of phosphorus.** Phosphorus is abundant in the food supply. Meats, legumes, nuts, dairy products, and grains tend to have more phosphorus than fruits and vegetables.
Source: U.S. Department of Agriculture, Agricultural Research Service. USDA National Nutrient Database for Standard Reference, Release 18. 2005. http://www.ars.usda.gov/nutrientdata.

hyperphosphatemia Abnormally high phosphate concentration in the blood.

musculoskeletal system, causing muscle weakness and damage, including respiratory problems due to poor diaphragm function. Long-standing hypophosphatemia can cause rickets and osteomalacia.

Hyperphosphatemia

Physicians also frequently see **hyperphosphatemia**, high blood phosphate, which most commonly is a consequence of kidney disease. Other causes include an underactive parathyroid gland, taking too many vitamin D supplements, and overuse of phosphate-containing laxatives. Excess phosphorus can bind calcium, and since low calcium concentrations can cause nerve fibers to discharge repeatedly without provocation, this can lead to severe muscle spasms and convulsions.

If your diet contains excessive phosphorus and not enough calcium, you may be at risk for increased bone loss. However, a high phosphorus intake alone is unlikely to have an adverse affect on bone health.[40] Replacing milk as a beverage with cola, a common practice among adolescents and Americans of all ages, increases phosphates in the diet (from cola) while reducing calcium intake. Some experts believe that this practice may be a significant factor in the development of osteoporosis later in life. The UL for phosphorus is 4,000 milligrams per day for people aged 9 to 70.

Key Concepts: *Phosphorus is common in many crucial metabolic systems. It is used to activate and deactivate enzymes and is an essential component of ATP, the energy source of the cell. Phosphorus is found in the phospholipids of cell membranes and is part of the hydroxyapatite in bone. About 85 percent of phosphorus is found in bone. Milk and meat are major sources of dietary phosphorus, and up to 30 percent of dietary intake comes from food additives. The RDA for adults is 700 milligrams per day, increasing to 1,250 milligrams per day for teens. Diets high in phosphorus and low in calcium can contribute to bone loss.*

Magnesium

Magnesium (Mg) is the fourth most abundant cation in the body and is about one-sixth as plentiful in cells as potassium. About 50 to 60 percent of the body's magnesium is in bone, with the remainder distributed equally between muscle and other soft tissue. The magnesium in bone provides a large reservoir in case deficiencies in soft tissue magnesium occur. Most magnesium resides in cells, with only 1 percent in extracellular fluid.

Functions of Magnesium

Magnesium participates in more than 300 types of enzyme-mediated reactions in the body, including those in DNA and protein synthesis. In the mitochondria, magnesium is essential for the production of ATP via the electron transport chain. Since ATP is the universal energy source for all cells, an absence of magnesium would quickly halt cellular activity. In the glycolysis pathway alone, seven key enzymes require magnesium. Magnesium also participates in muscle contraction and blood clotting.

Dietary Recommendations for Magnesium

Because of the large amount of magnesium in bone, blood magnesium levels may not be indicative of total body status. Therefore, assessing deficiency and setting intake recommendations is difficult. The RDA for magnesium in adults aged 19 to 30 years is 400 milligrams per day for men and 310 milligrams per day for women. This value rises slightly in adults aged 31 to 70, to 420 milligrams for men and 320 milligrams for women.

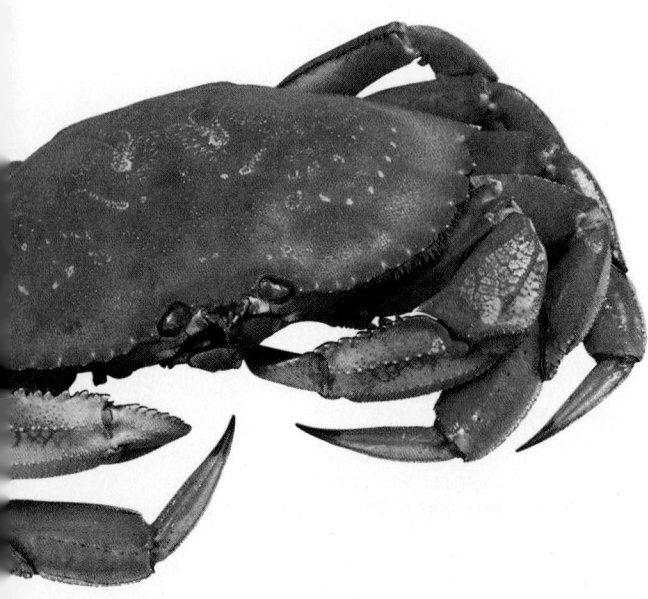

The average adult diet in the United States contains only about three-fourths of the magnesium RDA, and slightly less than the EAR (Estimated Average Requirement) for magnesium. Despite this, symptoms due to low magnesium are relatively uncommon in healthy people. This is because so much magnesium is stored in bone that levels in cells and body fluids remain constant even if intake is somewhat less than optimal.

Sources of Magnesium

Magnesium is ubiquitous in foods, but the amount varies widely depending on the food source. This mineral enters our diet mostly from plants. Whole grains and vegetables such as spinach and potatoes are good sources of magnesium, as are legumes, tofu, and some types of seafood. **Figure 11.25** shows food sources of magnesium.

Refined foods are low in magnesium content. Processed grains lose up to 80 percent of their magnesium, and enrichment does not replace it. Chocolate contains modest amounts of magnesium, but unfortunately not enough to compensate for its high fat and calorie content. Tap water can also be a significant source of the mineral in some communities with "hard" water. Total magnesium intake usually is proportional to calorie intake, so young people and adult men have higher intakes than women and the elderly.

We generally absorb about 50 percent of dietary magnesium. Although high-fiber diets often have a negative effect on mineral absorption, high-fiber foods containing fermentable carbohydrates (e.g., resistant starch, oligosaccharides, and pectin) actually improve magnesium absorption. High calcium intake, usually in the form of supplements, can interfere with magnesium absorption. This is another reason why food is a better source of nutrients than supplements. People who must take calcium supplements should be sure to regularly eat foods with high magnesium content.

Hypomagnesemia

Deficiency in any of the three major intracellular minerals—magnesium, potassium, and phosphorus—usually is associated with deficiencies in the other two. It is uncommon to see an isolated deficiency of any of the intracellular minerals.[41]

Hypomagnesemia, or magnesium deficiency, occurs with a variety of diseases, including kidney disease, and is associated with alcoholism and some types of diuretic drugs. People who have prolonged diarrhea can be at risk for magnesium deficiency. People who have chronically poor diets are also at risk, especially if they abuse alcohol. Nearly all chronic alcoholics have symptoms of hypomagnesemia because they often have poor diets and because alcohol increases urinary excretion of magnesium.

In research studies, healthy people whose diets are deficient in magnesium usually have no symptoms for a few weeks because of the large supply of magnesium stored in bone. Gradually, loss of appetite, nausea, and weakness develop. After more time, muscle cramps, irritability, and confusion occur. The heart rhythm may become disturbed. If hypomagnesemia becomes extreme, death can result, usually due to heart rhythm problems.

hypomagnesemia An abnormally low concentration of magnesium in the blood.

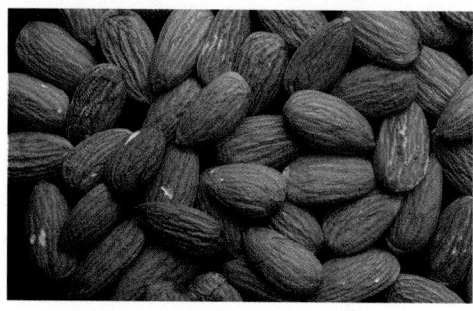

MAGNESIUM

Daily Value = 400 mg

	High: 20% DV or more		
	Sesame seeds	30 g (~1 oz)	107 mg
	Halibut, cooked	85 g (3 oz)	91 mg
	Cashews	30 g (~1/4 cup)	88 mg
	Almonds	30 g (~1 oz)	82 mg
	Oysters, cooked	85 g (3 oz)	81 mg
Good: 10–19% DV	Spinach, raw	85 g (~3 cups)	67 mg
	Black beans, cooked	90 g (~1/2 cup)	63 mg
	All Bran cereal	30 g (1/2 cup)	62 mg
	Rice, brown, cooked	140 g (~3/4 cup)	62 mg
	Crab, Alaska King, cooked	85 g (3 oz)	54 mg
	Soybeans, cooked	90 g (1/2 cup)	54 mg
	Peanut butter	2 Tbsp	49 mg
	Tofu, calcium processed	85 g (~1/3 cup)	49 mg
	Blackeyed peas, cooked	90 g (~1/2 cup)	47 mg
	Yogurt, plain, nonfat	225 g (1-8 oz container)	43 mg
	Whole-wheat bread	50 g (2 slices)	43 mg
	Molasses, blackstrap	1 Tbsp	43 mg
	Wheat bran flakes cereal	30 g (~3/4 cup)	42 mg

Figure 11.25 **Food sources of magnesium.** Most of the magnesium in the diet comes from plant foods such as grains, vegetables, and legumes.
Source: U.S. Department of Agriculture, Agricultural Research Service. USDA National Nutrient Database for Standard Reference, Release 18. 2005. http://www.ars.usda.gov/nutrientdata

hypermagnesemia An abnormally high concentration of magnesium in the blood.

Hypermagnesemia

Hypermagnesemia, an abnormally high concentration of magnesium in the blood, is uncommon in the absence of kidney disease. People with kidney failure, especially if they use magnesium-containing antacids or laxatives, are most likely to suffer hypermagnesemia. High blood magnesium leads to nausea and general weakness. The UL established by the Food and Nutrition Board recommends that healthy people not take more than 350 milligrams of magnesium per day as a supplement or in medicines. Physicians sometimes intentionally administer high doses of magnesium during pregnancy to stop premature labor. This requires frequent monitoring to avoid toxicity that can lead to respiratory paralysis and death.

Key Concepts: *Magnesium is a cofactor for more than 300 enzymes. Magnesium is required for cardiac and nerve function, and it helps form ATP. Sixty percent of magnesium is stored in bone. The RDA for magnesium in adults is 400 milligrams per day for men and 310 milligrams per day for women. Whole grains and vegetables are good sources of magnesium. People who suffer from chronic diarrhea or vomiting can be at risk for magnesium deficiency. Alcoholism is associated with magnesium deficiency because alcoholics are often malnourished and because alcohol stimulates urinary loss of magnesium.*

Sulfur

Sulfur (S) is different from the other minerals discussed in this chapter because it is not used alone as a nutrient. In the body, sulfur primarily is a component of organic compounds, such as the vitamins biotin and thiamin and the amino acids methionine and cysteine. Sulfur in these amino acids is especially important to protein structure. Disulfide bridges that form when sulfur atoms bind to each other cause proteins to fold in specific ways as sulfur atoms along the protein are pulled together. A protein's folding and shape are critical for its function. Sulfur is also important in some of the liver's drug detoxifying pathways. In its ionic form, sulfate (SO_4^{2-}), sulfur helps maintain acid–base balance.

Sulfur-containing amino acids provide ample sulfur for anyone who consumes adequate amounts of protein. Deficiency of sulfur is unknown in humans.

Key Concepts: *Sulfur is a component of the amino acids methionine and cysteine, as well as of the vitamins biotin and thiamin. Sulfur is important in drug detoxification and in maintaining acid–base balance. Since sulfur is a component of all proteins, a diet sufficient in protein contains adequate sulfur.*

Major Minerals and Health

Hypertension

Hypertension, or persistent high blood pressure, affects nearly 25 percent of adult Americans, and more than half of those older than 65. It is a major risk factor for heart disease, kidney disease, and stroke. Many experts believe that a major cause of hypertension is a genetic predisposition combined with a high-sodium diet. Epidemiological studies show that people from high-sodium-consuming countries have a higher incidence of hypertension than people from countries with lower sodium intakes. In addition, when primitive people adopt "modern" diets, their blood pressure rises and some develop hypertension.[42]

Sodium is not the only dietary factor associated with hypertension. Excess weight tends to raise blood pressure; regular exercise and weight loss

Quick Bites

Do Onions Make You Cry?

The cabbage and onion families have sulfur-based compounds that are transformed into odiferous compounds when their tissues are broken. Cutting into a raw onion mixes the contents of its cells, bringing enzymes into contact with an odorless precursor substance apparently derived from the sulfur-containing amino acid cysteine. The volatile result, a powerful sulfur-containing irritant, causes most people's eyes to water, apparently by dissolving in fluids that surround the eye and forming sulfuric acid.

help to reduce blood pressure. Reducing consumption of alcohol also tends to reduce blood pressure, and it improves the effectiveness of antihypertensive medications. Diets rich in calcium, magnesium, and potassium reduce blood pressure as well.[43] Dietary survey data show low intakes of potassium, magnesium, and calcium in the southeastern United States, a region known as the "stroke belt" because of its high rates of hypertension and stroke.[44] The mechanism by which these minerals act on hypertension may be due in part to their interrelationship with sodium metabolism. For more on hypertension, see Chapter 14, "Diet and Health."

Osteoporosis

Osteoporosis means "porous bone." It's a good description. In osteoporosis, bone mass or density declines and bone quality deteriorates, leaving the bones fragile and vulnerable to fractures. Osteoporosis affects more than 25 million Americans and is the major cause of bone fractures in older adults, primarily postmenopausal women.

Calcium is an important factor in bone health, but it is not the only nutritive factor. Normal development and mineralization of bone requires calcium, phosphorus, fluoride, magnesium, vitamin D, vitamin A, vitamin K, and protein. A study of postmenopausal women found significant relationships between bone mineral density and intake of energy, protein, calcium, magnesium, zinc, and vitamin C.[45] For more on osteoporosis and its risk factors, see Chapter 14, "Diet and Health."

Key Concepts: *Hypertension is a risk factor for heart disease, kidney disease, and stroke. High sodium intake is a risk factor for hypertension. Some evidence suggests that low intake of potassium, calcium, and possibly magnesium may also contribute to the development of hypertension. Osteoporosis is a progressive loss of bone mass, resulting in fragile bones that are susceptible to fracture. Several minerals, including calcium, phosphorus, magnesium, and fluoride, are important for bone health.*

Label [to] **Table**

After reading this chapter you should have a greater appreciation of the importance of calcium in your diet. If you don't consume dairy products, or consume them infrequently, getting enough calcium can be difficult. Today, soft drinks have become more popular than milk. To combat your potential lack of calcium, more and more food products are being fortified with this mineral. Did you know that many brands of orange juice now provide as much calcium per serving as a glass of milk? Check out the following Nutrition Facts label from a calcium-fortified orange juice.

This orange juice contains 35% of the Daily Value for calcium (1,000 mg). That's 350 milligrams of the 1,000 milligrams you need. That's a pretty good hit of calcium for just one 8-ounce glass of OJ. Surprisingly, it's slightly more calcium than an 8-ounce cup of milk. You can see from the comparison at the bottom of the label that this fortified juice increases the calcium %DV from 2% (in regular orange juice) to 35%.

Look at the label again. How much fiber can you get from this juice? That's right; fiber isn't listed on the label because most juices don't contain fiber. Since the majority of Americans need more fiber in their diets, it's a good idea not to go overboard on juices and choose whole pieces of fruit as well.

In addition to being a great source of calcium, this orange juice contains folate (another hard-to-get nutrient), lots of vitamin C, other B vitamins, and potassium. As part of a breakfast or even with a snack, this juice packs a lot of nutrients in its 110 calories.

Nutrition Facts

Serving Size: 8 fl oz (240 mL)
Servings Per Container: 8

Amount Per Serving

Calories 110   Calories from fat 0

	% Daily Value*
Total Fat 0g	
Sodium 0mg	0%
Potassium 450mg	13%
Total Carbohydrate 26g	9%
Sugars 22g	
Protein 2g	

Vitamin C 180%	•	Calcium 35%
Thiamin 10%	•	Niacin 4%
Vitamin B 6%	•	Folate 15%

Not a significant source of saturated fat, trans fat, cholesterol, dietary fiber, vitamin A, and iron.

* Percent Daily Values are based on a 2,000 calorie diet.

% of Daily Value of Calcium:

Calcium-Fortified Orange Juice	35%
Regular Orange Juice	2%

% of Daily Value of Viatmin C:

Calcium-Fortified Orange Juice	180%
Regular Orange Juice	120%

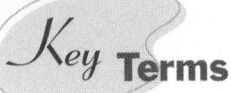

LEARNING *Portfolio* chapter 11

Key Terms

	page		page
aldosterone [al-DOS-ter-own]	464	hypokalemia	475
angiotensin I [an-jee-oh-TEN-sin one]	463	hypomagnesemia	487
		hyponatremia	472
angiotensin II	463	hypophosphatemia	485
angiotensinogen	463	insensible water loss	463
anions	460	ions	460
antidiuretic hormone (ADH)	463	linear growth	477
calmodulin	478	major mineral	468
cations	460	metabolic alkalosis	476
chloride shift	475	osmolarity	463
ciliary action	478	osmoreceptors	463
electrolytes [ih-LEK-tro-lites]	458	osmosis	460
fibrin	478	osmotic pressure	460
heat capacity	458	oxalate (oxalic acid)	471
hydrogen bonds	458	phosphorylation	484
hydroxyapatite	477	phytate (phytic acid)	471
hypercalcemia	483	plasma	460
hyperkalemia	475	renin	463
hypermagnesemia	488	salts	460
hypernatremia	472	semipermeable membrane	460
hyperparathyroidism	485	sodium-potassium pumps	460
hyperphosphatemia	486	solutes	460
hypervolemia	472	vasoconstrictor	463
hypocalcemia	483	vasopressin	463

Study Points

➤ Water is the most essential nutrient; we can live much longer without food than without water. The AI for water is 3.7 liters per day for men and 2.7 liters per day for women.

➤ Water is important for the movement of nutrients and waste, cellular reactions, temperature regulation, and acid–base balance. Moreover, fluids in the body lubricate and cushion joints, cleanse the eyes, and moisten the food we eat.

➤ Dissolved ions, or electrolytes, help to maintain normal fluid balance.

➤ Fluid is lost from the body via the urine, skin, feces, and lungs. The hormones ADH and aldosterone regulate fluid excretion from the kidneys.

➤ The thirst response stimulates fluid intake. Caffeine, alcohol, and diuretic medications increase fluid excretion. Dehydration results when fluid intake is less than losses; it can seriously impair physical and mental performance.

➤ Minerals are inorganic elements and are categorized as major or trace depending on the amount in the body and the amount needed in the diet.

➤ The bioavailability of minerals may be affected by excess intake of single-mineral supplements, phytate, oxalate, and fiber in plant foods, and mineral status in the body.

➤ Sodium, the major extracellular cation, helps regulate water distribution and blood pressure. The adult AI for sodium is 1,500 milligrams per day, and the UL is 2,300 milligrams—less than average intakes (3,000 mg to 6,000 milligrams per day).

➤ Potassium, the major cation in the intracellular fluid, is necessary for nerve and muscle function. It is provided in the diet mainly from unprocessed foods, including fruits and vegetables. The adult AI for potassium is 4,700 milligrams per day, substantially more than what most Americans eat (2,000 to 3,000 milligrams per day).

➤ Chloride is the major extracellular anion and a component of stomach acid. Chloride deficiency is most often associated with prolonged vomiting. Most Americans consume much more chloride than the AI, which is 2,300 milligrams per day.

➤ Calcium, the most abundant mineral in the body, is found in bones. It also functions in blood clotting, nerve and muscle function, and cellular metabolism. Major dietary sources of calcium are dairy products, calcium-fortified foods, and certain vegetables.

➤ Phosphorus is a key component of ATP, DNA, RNA, phospholipids, and lipoproteins. Because phosphorus is widespread in foods, dietary phosphorus intake is rarely inadequate.

➤ Plant foods such as whole grains and vegetables are important sources of magnesium, which is a cofactor for hundreds of enzymes. Low levels of magnesium are associated with kidney disease, alcoholism, and use of diuretics.

➤ Sulfur does not function alone as a nutrient, but as a component of certain amino acids and the vitamins biotin and thiamin.

➤ Hypertension increases risk for heart disease, stroke, and kidney disease. Sodium has long been linked to hypertension, but only some individuals are salt sensitive. Other dietary factors linked to hypertension include high chloride intake and low potassium, calcium, and magnesium intake.

➤ Osteoporosis results from excessive bone loss. Postmenopausal women are at highest risk for osteoporosis. Adequate dietary calcium, vitamin D, and physical activity throughout the life span reduce the risk for osteoporosis.

Study Questions

1. What are the two main factors that affect absorption of a mineral?

2. What functions does chloride perform in the human body?

3. What is the role of aldosterone in the body, and how is it released?

4. Name four of the main biological functions of water.

5. What is the recommended intake level for sodium?

6. What three major minerals affect bone health?

7. What are the major functions of calcium, other than its relation to bone health?

8. How does the body compensate for low calcium intake?

9. Which people have a high risk of hypo-magnesemia?

10. How does the body use sulfur? What is its role in protein function?

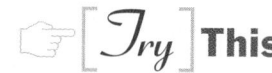 *Try* This

Calcium Food Diary

The purpose of this exercise is to see how much calcium you consume in a typical day. Start by keeping a food diary for three days (two weekdays and one weekend day). While keeping the diary, try not to change your eating habits. (Altering the way you eat would reduce the accuracy of your project.) After completing the diary, add up the amounts of calcium you consume using Appendix A in the back of your textbook or using the EatRight Analysis or Nutritionist Pro software. The calcium AI value for adults between the ages of 19 and 50 is 1,000 milligrams. How does your average calcium intake compare? If your calcium intake is not meeting the AI, how can you include more calcium in your diet?

Osmosis Experiment

Purchase some celery and let it sit for a week or two until it becomes limp. When the celery looks limp and lifeless, fill your sink with cold water and soak the celery. When it has soaked for several hours, take the celery out and examine its appearance. Notice anything different? Since the crispness of celery is due to osmotic pressure, when you soaked the limp celery, it absorbed water into its cells and became crisp again.

What About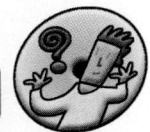

Let's take a look at Bobbie's intake of the major minerals calcium, magnesium, and sodium. Refer to Chapter 1 to refresh yourself with Bobbie's one-day intake. How do you think she did?

Calcium

Bobbie's calcium intake was low on the day she recorded her food intake. She consumed 710 milligrams, but the Adequate Intake (AI) for a 20-year-old woman is 1,000 milligrams. If this day reflects her usual intake, then she is at risk of poor bone mineralization and a lower than average peak bone mass. This increases her risk of osteoporosis.

Magnesium

Bobbie's intake of magnesium was 310 milligrams and the Recommended Dietary Allowance (RDA) for a woman her age is 320 milligrams. If this one-day record reflects her usual eating, she probably is consuming an adequate amount of magnesium and does not need to increase her intake of this mineral. Some of the best sources of magnesium in her diet were the banana, tortilla chips, and spaghetti noodles.

Sodium

Bobbie's intake of 4,820 milligrams of sodium was much higher than the AI of 1,500 milligrams and twice the UL of 2,300 milligrams per day! This should not be a surprise because most of Bobbie's meals are either convenience items or prepared by someone else (e.g., the school's cafeteria), which makes it hard to control sodium content. The biggest contributors to her high intake of sodium were the sourdough bread, salad dressing, salsa, spaghetti sauce, and pizza. Bobbie should try to eat fewer convenience foods and more fresh foods. She would also benefit from drinking extra water because her intake of sodium is so high.

References

1 Institute of Medicine, Food and Nutrition Board. *Dietary Reference Intakes for Water, Potassium, Sodium, Chloride, and Sulfate.* Washington, DC: National Academy Press, 2004.

2 Davis JM, Burgess WA, Slentz CA, Bartoli WP. Fluid availability of sports drinks differing in carbohydrate type and concentration. *Am J Clin Nutr.* 1990;51(6):1054–1057; and Millard-Stafford M, Rosskopf LB, Snow TK, Hinson BT. Water versus carbohydrate-electrolyte ingestion before and during a 15-km run in the heat. *Int J Sport Nutr.* 1997;7(1):26–38.

3 Johnson R, Tulin B. *Travel Fitness.* Champaign, IL: Human Kinetics, 1995.

4 Guyton AC, Hall JE. *Textbook of Medical Physiology.* 10th ed. Philadelphia: WB Saunders, 2000.

5 Ibid.

6 Ibid.

7 Ibid.

8 Institute of Medicine, Food and Nutrition Board. Op. cit.

9 Ibid.

10 Kleiner SM. Water: an essential but overlooked nutrient. *J Am Diet Assoc.* 1999;2:200–206.

11 Ibid.

12 Murray B, Stofan J, Eichner ER. Hyponatremia in athletes. *Gatorade Sports Science Institute, Sports Science Exchange.* 2003;16(1).

13 Institute of Medicine, Food and Nutrition Board. Op. cit.

14 Nevius CW. In hazing, dumb stunts can be fatal. *San Francisco Chronicle.* February 8, 2005. http://sfgate.com/cgi-bin/article.cgi?file=/c/a/2005/02/08/BAG61B7D341.DTL. Accessed 7/13/06.

15 Loas G, Mercier-Guidez E. Fatal self-induced water intoxication among schizophrenic inpatients. *Eur Psychiatry.* 2002;17:307–310.

16 US Department of Agriculture and US Department of Health and Human Services. *Dietary Guidelines for Americans.* 6th ed. Washington, DC: US Government Printing Office, 2005.

17 Institute of Medicine, Food and Nutrition Board. Op. cit.

18 Loria CM, Obarzanek E, Ernst ND. Choose and prepare foods with less salt: dietary advice for all Americans. *J Nutr.* 2001; 131(2S-1):536S–551S.

19 Morris CD. Effect of dietary sodium restriction on overall nutrient intake. *Am J Clin Nutr.* 1997;65(2 suppl):687S–691S.

20 Cogan MG. *Fluid and Electrolytes.* Englewood Cliffs, NJ: Appleton & Lange, 1991.

21 Kaplan NM. *Clinical Hypertension.* Baltimore, MD: Williams & Wilkins, 1998:48–51.

22 Institute of Medicine, Food and Nutrition Board. Op. cit.

23 US Departments of Agriculture and Health and Human Services. Op. cit.

24 Institute of Medicine, Food and Nutrition Board. Op. cit.

25 Guyton AC, Hall JE. Op. cit.

26 Fauci AS, Braunwald E, Isselbacher KJ, Wilson JD, Martin JB, Kasper D, Hauser SL, Longo DL. *Harrison's Principles of Internal Medicine*. 14th ed. New York: McGraw-Hill, 1997.

27 Waltzer KB. Simple, sensible preventive measures for managed care settings. *Geriatrics*. 1998;53(10):65–68, 75–77, 81; quiz 82.

28 National Institutes of Health. Osteoporosis prevention, diagnosis, and therapy. *NIH Consensus Statement* 2000, March 27–29;17(2):1–34.

29 Frazão E, ed. *America's Eating Habits: Changes and Consequences*. Washington, DC: US Department of Agriculture, Food and Rural Economics Division, April 1999. Agriculture Information Bulletin, No. 750 (AIB-750).

30 National Institutes of Health. Optimal calcium intake. *NIH Consensus Statement* 1994, June 6–8;12(4):1–31.

31 Institute of Medicine, Food and Nutrition Board. *Dietary Reference Intakes for Calcium, Phosphorus, Magnesium, Vitamin D, and Fluoride*. Washington, DC: National Academy Press, 1997.

32 National Institutes of Health. 1994. Op. cit.

33 Ibid.

34 Ibid.

35 Ibid.

36 Institute of Medicine, Food and Nutrition Board. 1997. Op. cit.

37 Ibid.

38 Ibid.

39 Stein JH. *Internal Medicine*. St. Louis: Mosby-Year Book, 1994.

40 Institute of Medicine, Food and Nutrition Board. 1997. Op. cit.

41 Fauci AS, et al. Op. cit.

42 Zemel MB. Dietary pattern and hypertension: the DASH study. *Nutr Rev*. 1997;55:303–308.

43 Kotchen TA, McCarron DA. Dietary electrolytes and blood pressure: a statement for healthcare professionals from the American Heart Association Nutrition Committee. *Circulation*. 1998;6:613–617.

44 Hajjar I, Kotchen T. Regional variations of blood pressure in the United States are associated with regional variations in dietary intakes: the NHANES-III data. *J Nutr*. 2003; 133:211–214.

45 Ilich JZ, Brownbill RA, Tamborini L. Bone and nutrition in elderly women: protein, energy, and calcium as major determinants of bone mineral density. *Eur J Clin Nutr*. 2003; 57(4):554–565.

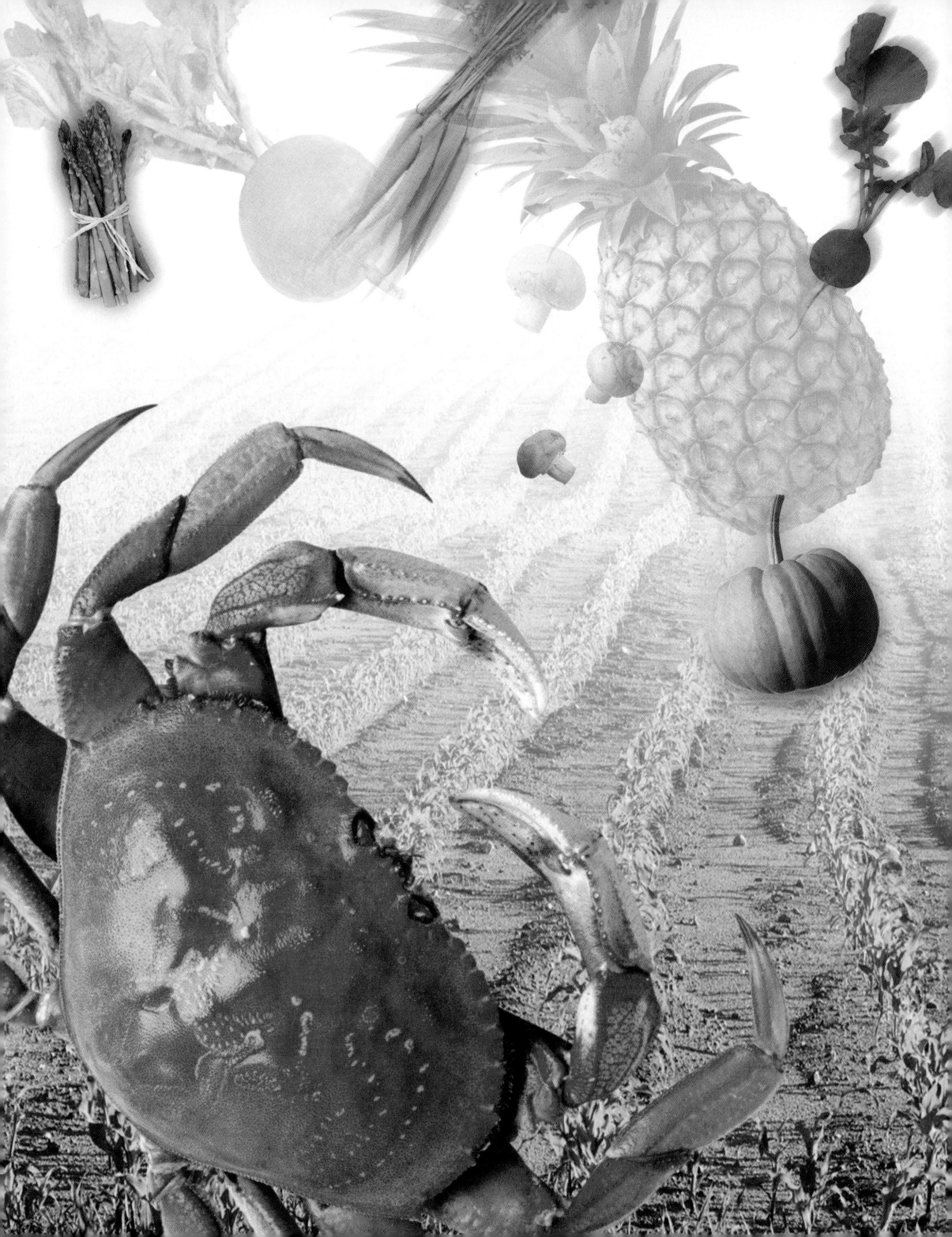

Chapter 12

Trace Minerals

Think About It

1 Do you think a person with an infection should take iron supplements?

2 You disclose to a friend that you tend to be low in iron. She knows you are a vegetarian and suggests you drink milk. What false assumption might she be making?

3 You know that a number of people in your family have had goiter or take thyroxine. You also notice that none of these people like fish. Any relationship?

4 Some people argue that fluoridation is overdone. What is your position? Would you vote for fluoridating all water supplies?

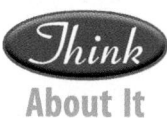

Fyi for your Information

This chapter's FYI boxes include practical information on the following topics:
- Zinc and the Common Cold
- Chromium, Exercise, and Body Composition

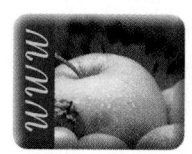

The Web site for this book offers many useful tools and is a great source for additional nutrition information for both students and instructors. Visit the site at nutrition.jbpub.com for information on trace minerals. You'll find exercises that explore the following topics:
- Highlighting Heme
- The ADA's Stand on Supplements
- What Food Labels Can Claim
- Glowing Thyroids!

Key to Illustrations

 Enzymes

 Fat-Soluble Vitamins

 Free Radicals

 Minerals

 Proteins

What About Bobbie?

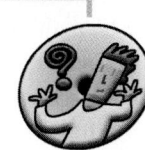

Track the choices Bobbie is making with Nutritionist Pro or EatRight Analysis software.

One of your "meat-and-potatoes" friends argues that animal foods are the best sources of minerals because animals concentrate the minerals they eat from plants. Your vegetarian friend disagrees, saying that minerals are plentiful in plant foods, but processing removes them. Another friend contends that American agricultural practices have stripped the mineral content from the soil, so supplements are really the only way to get adequate mineral intake. Who's right?

As you saw in Chapter 11, protein-rich animal foods are good sources of some minerals such as calcium, phosphorus, and sulfur. Other major minerals (e.g., potassium and magnesium) are plentiful in plant foods. This chapter focuses on trace minerals—that is, minerals present in the body in small quantities, and therefore needed by the body in small amounts. Meats are the best food sources for some of these minerals—iron and zinc, for instance. Whole grains are also good sources of several minerals, including iron, copper, selenium, and manganese. And water is a major source of fluoride, a mineral that often occurs naturally in water or is added during municipal water treatment.

But what about the mineral content of soil? (See **Figure 12.1**.) The mineral content of soil certainly influences the nutrient value of the plants that grow in it. This is especially true for the trace minerals selenium and iodine. How important is this to our dietary intake? Is the soil's mineral content depleted, as some supplement suppliers claim? Adequate nutrition is as important for healthy plants as it is for healthy livestock and people. If soil lacks a nutrient the plant needs, the plant will not grow. Fertilization adds nutrients to the soil, and so does the natural degradation of rocks, plants, and animals. There is little evidence for specific nutritional claims based on the mineral content of the soil. In addition, few people consume only foods grown locally. A varied diet typically includes foods from many different locales and thus from a wide variety of soils.

What Are Trace Elements?

Trace elements are essential minerals found in a large variety of animal and plant foods; these nutrients have both regulatory and structural functions in the body. Trace elements differ from the major minerals (e.g., calcium, phosphorus, magnesium) in two ways. First, the dietary requirements for each of the trace elements are less than 100 milligrams per day. For example, iron and zinc intake recommendations for adults range from 8 milligrams to 18 milligrams per day, whereas the adult daily calcium recommendation is 1,000 milligrams per day. Second, the total amount of each trace element found in the body is small, less than 5 grams. For example, the total amount of iron in the body is 2 to 4 grams, or about the

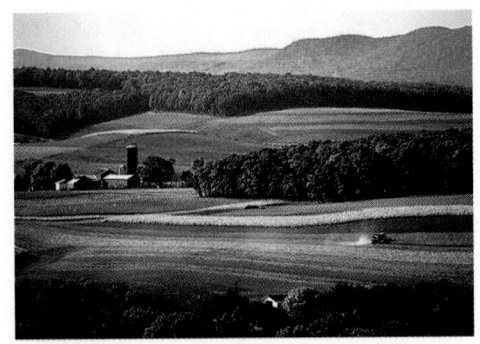

Figure 12.1 **Mineral content of soil influences the nutrient value of plants.** The mineral content of plants reflects the mineral content of the soil in which they are grown.

amount of iron in a small nail. In contrast, a typical adult body contains more than 1,000 grams of calcium. **Figure 12.2** shows the trace elements on the periodic table.

Why Are Trace Elements Important?

Despite the minuscule amounts in the body, trace elements are crucial to many body functions, including metabolic pathways. Trace elements serve as cofactors for enzymes, components of hormones, and participants in oxidation-reduction reactions. They are essential for growth and for normal functioning of the immune system. Deficiencies may cause delayed sexual maturation, poor growth, mediocre work performance, faulty immune function, tooth decay, and altered hormonal function.

Technological advances in recent years have triggered an explosion of exciting new research because scientists can now track trace elements throughout the body more effectively. Working together, nutritionists, biochemists, biologists, immunologists, geneticists, and epidemiologists are uncovering the mysteries behind many of these fascinating elements and finding new links between trace elements and a variety of diseases and genetic disorders.

Other Characteristics of Trace Elements

Foods from animal sources, particularly liver, are good sources of many trace minerals. Amounts in plant foods can differ dramatically from region to region, depending on the soil's mineral content. Even the maturity of a vegetable, fruit, or grain can influence its mineral content. Since actual mineral content is so variable, the values published in food composition tables can be misleading. Food tables, even many of the popular computerized

Quick Bites

Hair Analysis Is a Misguided Measure

Although discredited as a measure of trace mineral status in individuals, hair analysis is promoted with the claim that it can reveal mineral deficiencies. This measure lacks sensitivity and is unreliable. The color, diameter, and rate of growth of a person's hair, the season of the year, the geographic location, and the person's age and sex can affect the levels of minerals in hair. It is possible for hair concentration of an element (zinc, for example) to be high even though deficiency exists in the body. Hair dyes, perming agents, and certain shampoos also alter the mineral content of hair.

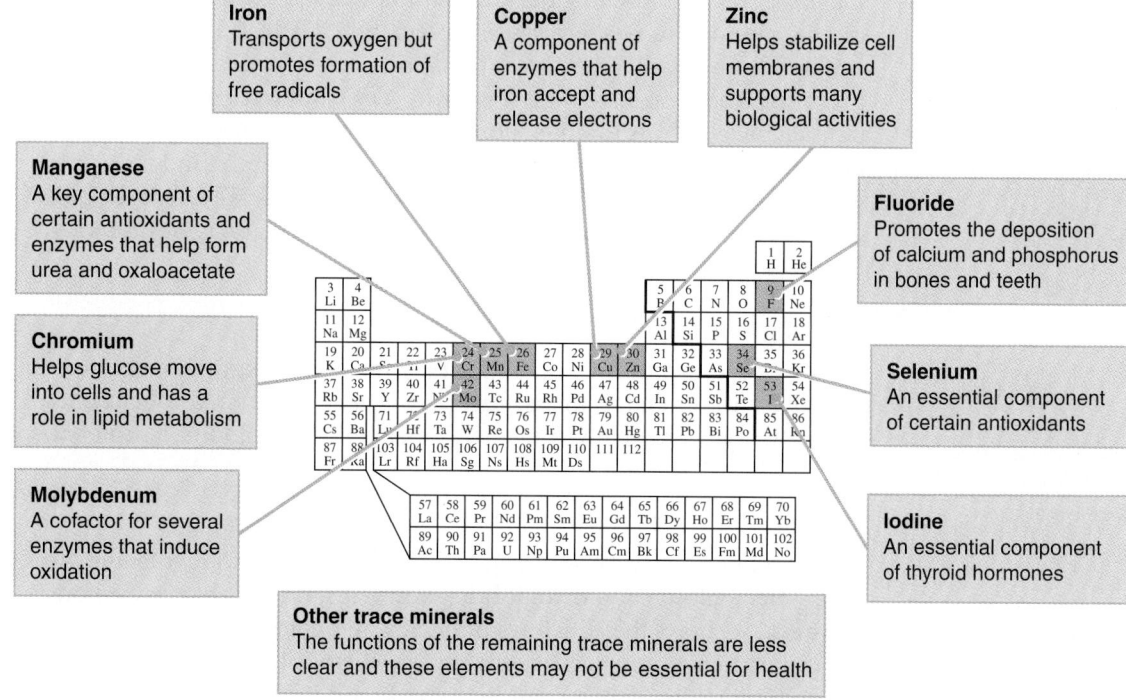

Iron
Transports oxygen but promotes formation of free radicals

Copper
A component of enzymes that help iron accept and release electrons

Zinc
Helps stabilize cell membranes and supports many biological activities

Manganese
A key component of certain antioxidants and enzymes that help form urea and oxaloacetate

Fluoride
Promotes the deposition of calcium and phosphorus in bones and teeth

Chromium
Helps glucose move into cells and has a role in lipid metabolism

Selenium
An essential component of certain antioxidants

Molybdenum
A cofactor for several enzymes that induce oxidation

Iodine
An essential component of thyroid hormones

Other trace minerals
The functions of the remaining trace minerals are less clear and these elements may not be essential for health

Figure 12.2 **Trace elements on the periodic table.** Trace minerals are found in the body and required in the diet in small amounts, but they play important roles in the body.

ferrous iron (Fe²⁺) The reduced form of iron most commonly found in food.

ferric iron (Fe³⁺) The oxidized form of iron able to be bound to transferrin for transport.

heme A chemical complex with a central iron atom (ferric iron Fe³⁺) that forms the oxygen-binding part of hemoglobin and myoglobin.

myoglobin The oxygen-transporting protein of muscle that resembles blood hemoglobin in function.

nutrient databases, often have incomplete information about trace mineral content.

Even if we are fairly sure of the amount of a particular mineral in a food, other components of the diet can affect the mineral's bioavailability. Trace minerals are affected by the same factors that affect bioavailability of the major minerals (see **Figure 12.3**), including fiber, phytate, polyphenols, oxalate, the acidity of the intestinal environment, and the person's need for that mineral. High doses of other minerals can compete with trace minerals and inhibit their absorption. Treatment for mineral toxicity sometimes exploits these antagonistic interactions between minerals. For example, high doses of zinc may be given to patients with a genetic disorder of copper overload (Wilson's disease) because zinc inhibits copper absorption.

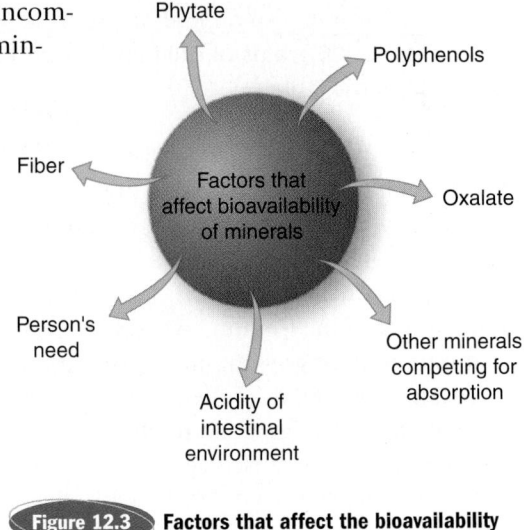

Figure 12.3 **Factors that affect the bioavailability of minerals.**

Iron

Iron (Fe) is the fourth most abundant mineral in the earth's crust, yet iron deficiency is the most common nutrient deficiency in the world; from 500 to 600 million people suffer from iron-deficiency anemia.[1] On the other hand, hemochromatosis, a disease of excess iron absorption, is one of the most common inherited disorders. If not detected early, this disorder can damage organs severely, causing premature death.

Why is iron useful? Iron has a special property. It easily changes between two of its oxidation states—**ferrous iron (Fe²⁺)** and **ferric iron (Fe³⁺)**—by transferring electrons to other atoms. This property makes iron essential for numerous oxidation-reduction reactions, and allows it to bind reversibly with oxygen, nitrogen, and sulfur. The ability to shift easily between oxidative states also endows iron with its "dark side"—the ability to promote formation of destructive free radicals.

Functions of Iron

Iron is well known for its role in the body's use of energy; it is required for oxygen transport and is an essential component of hundreds of enzymes, many of which are involved in energy metabolism. In addition, iron plays a role in brain development and in the immune system.

Oxygen Transport

Iron's ability to carry oxygen is crucial. As a component of two **heme** proteins—hemoglobin and **myoglobin**—iron transports oxygen in the body. **Figure 12.4** shows the structures of heme and hemoglobin. With iron at the center, heme proteins have the unique chemical property of easily loading and unloading oxygen, and they give blood its red color. Hemoglobin in red blood cells transports oxygen in the blood, delivering it through the capillary beds to the tissues. Myoglobin in muscle facilitates the movement of oxygen into muscle cells.

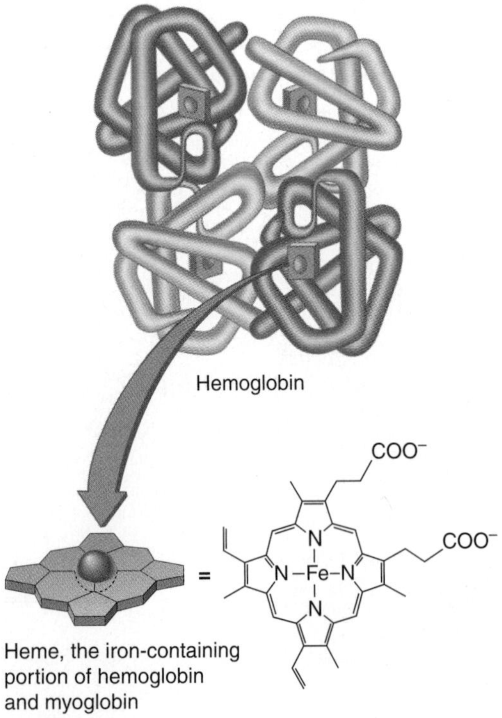

Hemoglobin

COO⁻

COO⁻

=

Heme, the iron-containing portion of hemoglobin and myoglobin

Figure 12.4 **Heme in hemoglobin.** Iron in the heme portion of hemoglobin and myoglobin binds and releases oxygen easily. Hemoglobin in red blood cells transports oxygen in the blood and gives blood its red color.

Enzymes

Hundreds of enzymes have iron as a constituent or need it as a cofactor in reactions. One of iron's best-known roles is as a component of enzymes involved in energy metabolism. **Cytochromes**, for example, are heme-containing compounds critical to the electron transport chain.

The rate-limiting enzyme in gluconeogenesis requires iron. Iron also is a cofactor for antioxidant enzymes that protect against damaging free radicals. Interestingly, excess iron can also catalyze the formation of these highly reactive and potentially destructive substances.

Immune Function

Although iron is necessary for optimal immune function, it also serves as a nutrient for bacteria. Because iron supplementation can worsen an infection, this poses a dilemma for treating iron deficiencies in areas of the world with rampant infectious diseases. In the absence of an infection, however, current research indicates that iron supplementation is safe for treating iron deficiency.[2]

Brain Function

Iron is essential for synthesizing neurotransmitters and for optimal brain growth.[3] Evidence also supports a role for iron in **myelinization**—the development of the myelin sheath around nerve fibers.[4] Iron's participation in brain development is an active area of research, since numerous studies report an association between iron-deficiency anemia in children and deficits in their behavioral and cognitive development. **Figure 12.5** summarizes the functions of iron.

Regulation of Iron in the Body

Total body iron averages approximately 3.8 grams in men and 2.3 grams in women. When the body has sufficient iron to meet its needs, most iron (greater than 70 percent) can be classified as functional iron; the remainder is storage or transport iron. More than 80 percent of the body's functional iron is found in the red blood cells as hemoglobin, and the rest is found in myoglobin and enzymes (e.g., cytochromes).[5] The body regulates its iron status by balancing absorption, transport, storage, and losses.[6] **Table 12.1** shows the normal distribution of iron in men and women.

cytochromes Heme proteins that transfer electrons in the electron transport chain through the alternate oxidation and reduction of iron.

myelinization Development of the myelin sheath, a substance that surrounds nerve fibers.

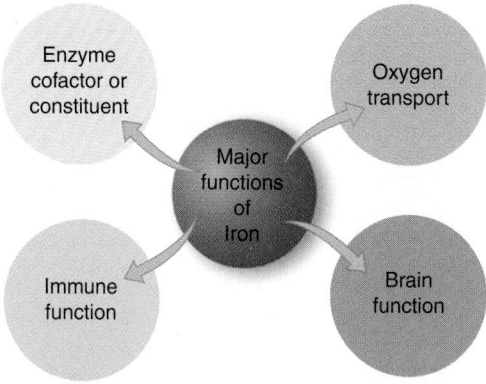

Figure 12.5 **Major functions of iron.** Well known for its role in transporting oxygen in the blood, iron also is essential for optimal immune function and nerve health. In addition, it is a cofactor in numerous reactions.

Table 12.1 **Normal Distribution of Iron-Containing Compounds (mg iron per kg body weight)**

Compound	Men	Women
Storage Complexes		
Ferritin	9	4
Hemosiderin	4	1
Transport Protein		
Transferrin	<1	<1
Functional Compounds		
Hemoglobin	31	31
Myoglobin	4	4
Enzymes	2	2
TOTAL	50	42

Source: Centers for Disease Control and Prevention. Recommendations to report and control iron deficiency in the United States. *MMWR.* 1998;(RR–3):7.

Quick Bites

But It Worked in the Lab...

The evidence is clear from carefully conducted clinical trials that supplements reduce iron deficiency during pregnancy. However, public health supplementation programs in communities often are unsuccessful. Why the discrepancy? Although the clinical trials support the distribution and consumption of iron pills, programs in the "real world" have several limiting factors: inadequate supply of iron tablets, limited access to care, poor or nonexistent nutrition counseling, lack of knowledge, and the uncomfortable side effects experienced by some women. These factors are important causes of noncompliance.

transferrin A protein synthesized in the liver that transports iron in the blood to the erythroblasts for use in heme synthesis.

ferritin A complex of iron and apoferritin that is a major storage form of iron.

heme iron The iron found in the hemoglobin and myoglobin of animal foods.

nonheme iron The iron in plants and the iron in animal foods that is not part of hemoglobin or myoglobin.

Iron Absorption

Iron absorption in the gastrointestinal tract is the primary regulator of iron levels. When the absorptive mechanism operates normally, a person maintains functional iron and tends to establish iron stores. The body's capacity to absorb dietary iron depends on the body's iron status and need, normal GI function, the amount and type of iron in the diet, and dietary factors that enhance or inhibit iron absorption.

Process of Iron Absorption. To avoid iron toxicity, the body regulates its absorption of iron. (See **Figure 12.6**.) Intestinal cells act as gatekeepers, forming an initial barrier that turns away excess (and potentially harmful) iron. Once admitted into the intestinal cell, iron has three potential fates:

- It can be used by the cell itself.
- It can be released into the blood and carried to other tissues by **transferrin**, the major iron-transporting protein in the body.
- It can be stored as **ferritin**.

The body's need for iron determines its fate: The greater the need, particularly for synthesis of red blood cells, the more transferrin binds iron and transports it to bone marrow and other tissues. If iron stores are high, the extra iron remains in the cell and is excreted along with mucosal cells that are sloughed off at the end of their life cycle. Some scientists propose that intestinal ferritin acts as an "iron sink," which prevents the accumulation of iron to toxic levels.[7]

Effect of the Body's Iron Status on Iron Absorption. Depending on the size of the body's iron stores, absorption of dietary iron (i.e., iron bioavailability) can vary from less than 1 percent to greater than 50 percent. The GI tract

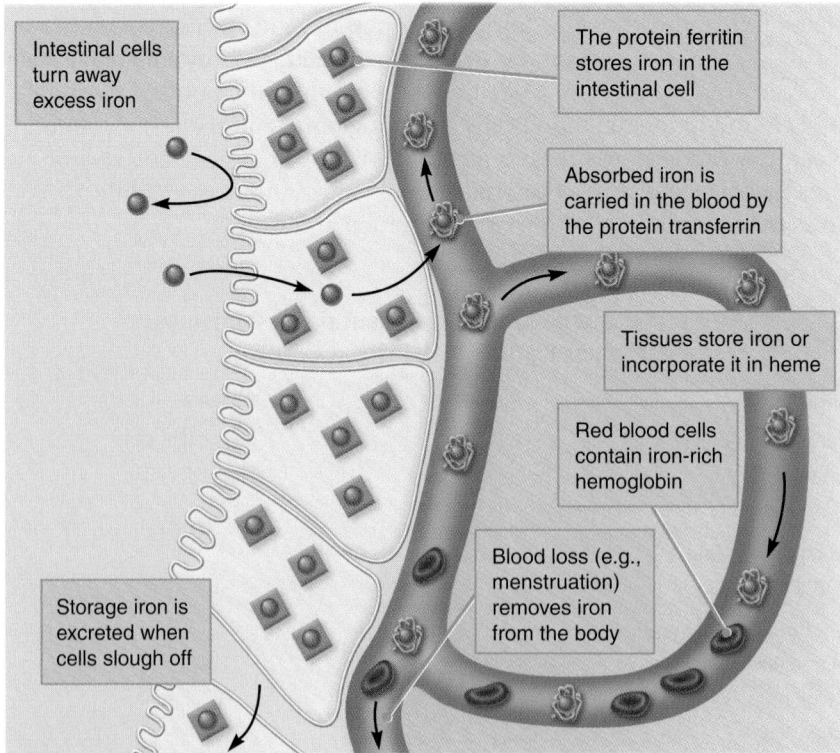

Intestinal cells turn away excess iron

The protein ferritin stores iron in the intestinal cell

Absorbed iron is carried in the blood by the protein transferrin

Tissues store iron or incorporate it in heme

Red blood cells contain iron-rich hemoglobin

Blood loss (e.g., menstruation) removes iron from the body

Storage iron is excreted when cells slough off

Figure 12.6 **Iron absorption.** The amount of iron absorbed depends on several factors—normal GI function, need for iron, the amount and kind of iron consumed, and dietary factors that enhance or inhibit iron absorption.

increases iron absorption when the body's iron stores are low and decreases absorption when stores are sufficient. The body also gives priority to red blood cell production; an increased production rate, such as during pregnancy or after blood loss, can trigger a several-fold increase in iron uptake.[8]

Among adults, men absorb approximately 6 percent of dietary iron, and nonpregnant women of childbearing age absorb approximately 13 percent. Women's higher absorption rate primarily reflects their lower iron intake and higher iron losses as a result of menstruation. Iron absorption also is high among iron-deficient persons.

Effect of GI Function on Iron Absorption. Although most iron absorption occurs in the duodenum and jejunum of the small intestine, the stomach also has an important role. Gastric acid facilitates the solubilization of iron and promotes the conversion of ferric iron (Fe^{3+}) to ferrous iron (Fe^{2+}), the form that most easily enters the absorptive intestinal cells. The stomach's retention and mechanical mixing of food also maximize iron's bioavailability. Gastric acid production generally declines with aging, reducing iron absorption in the elderly.

Effect of the Amount and Form of Iron in Food. Food contains two types of iron—**heme iron** and **nonheme iron**. Heme iron is a part of hemoglobin and myoglobin, so it is found only in animal tissue. Heme iron is much more absorbable than nonheme iron. Although meat, fish, and poultry contain various amounts of heme iron and nonheme iron, the mix averages about 50 percent heme iron and 50 percent nonheme iron.[9] In contrast, plant-based and iron-fortified foods contain only nonheme iron. (See **Figure 12.7.**) Vegetarian diets, by definition, contain little to no heme iron.

Heme iron is two to three times more absorbable than nonheme iron. Depending on the body's iron stores, heme iron absorption ranges from 15 to 35 percent of the amount ingested.[10] As the amount of iron ingested increases, the proportion absorbed decreases.

Dietary Factors That Enhance Iron Absorption. Heme iron absorption is relatively independent of meal composition. On the other hand, meal composition strongly influences nonheme iron absorption. **Table 12.2** lists factors that inhibit or enhance absorption of iron. The two most important dietary factors that boost absorption of nonheme iron are organic acids, especially vitamin C (ascorbic acid), and meat, including fish and poultry. Organic acids maintain the iron in a soluble, bioavailable form as the stomach contents enter the duodenum. To exert this effect, ascorbic acid must be present in the same meal as the nonheme iron. Other organic acids (e.g., citric, malic, and tartaric acids) appear to have effects comparable to those of ascorbic acid. It is unclear exactly how meat enhances absorption of nonheme iron, but the presence of meat, fish, or poultry increases absorption efficiency. In fact, one study found

MEAT

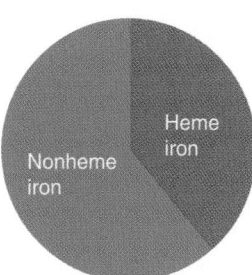

Beef, chicken, and fish contain about 40% heme and 60% nonheme iron. Eggs and dairy products contain no hemoglobin or myoglobin, so they contain only nonheme iron.

LEGUMES AND VEGETABLES

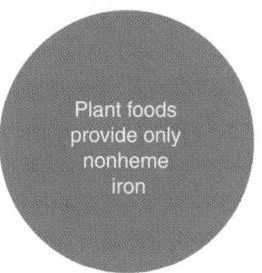

Beans, fortified cereals, soybeans, and green leafy vegetables are sources of nonheme iron.

AVERAGE DAILY DIET

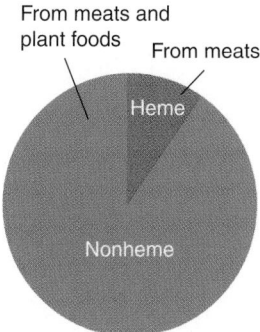

Table 12.2 **Factors That Affect Iron Absorption**

Inhibitors	Enhancers
Fiber and phytate	Vitamin C (ascorbic acid)
Calcium and phosphorus (milk/dairy)	Factor in meat, poultry, and fish
Tannins, found in tea	HCl secreted in the stomach
Polyphenols	Citric, malic, and tartaric acid
Oxalate	

Figure 12.7 **Sources of heme and nonheme iron.** Heme iron is found only in meats. Nonheme iron is found in both plant and animal foods. Eggs and dairy products contain small amounts of nonheme iron only.

polyphenols Organic compounds that include an unsaturated ring containing more than one −OH group as part of their chemical structures; may produce bitterness in coffee and tea.

that nonheme iron absorption in nonvegetarians was more than double that in lacto-ovo-vegetarians.[11] Despite this difference in absorption, this same study did not find evidence of iron deficiency in the vegetarians.[12]

Dietary Factors That Inhibit Iron Absorption. The most significant inhibitors of iron absorption are phytic acid (phytate), which is found in whole grains, and **polyphenols**, which are found in tea, coffee, other beverages, and many plants. (See **Figure 12.8.**) Even though minute amounts of these substances can reduce iron absorption, eating foods rich in vitamin C at the same meal counteracts this effect. The benefits of eating whole grains, which are nutrient dense and rich in fiber, outweigh the negative impact on iron absorption. Rather than cut back on whole grains, include small amounts of meat and/or generous amounts of vitamin C–rich fruits and vegetables with meals to improve iron absorption.

Other inhibitors of nonheme iron absorption include soy, calcium, zinc, oxalates, and fiber. The long-term significance of these inhibitory factors on iron status is unclear. Because many women take calcium supplements to prevent osteoporosis, calcium's inhibition of iron absorption has come under scrutiny. One study found that six months of calcium supplementation (1,200 milligrams per day) reduces short-term iron absorption, yet leaves overall iron status unaffected.[13] To be safe, some experts recommend taking calcium supplements alone at bedtime rather than with meals.[14]

Zinc competes with iron for absorption. When they are taken together, large amounts of either mineral can inhibit the absorption of the other. Deficiency of both nutrients is common, so some developing countries promote enrichment of foods with balanced amounts of both iron and zinc.

Iron Transport and Storage

Transferrin delivers iron from the intestines to the tissues and redistributes iron from storage sites to various body compartments. Individual cells take up the iron transported on transferrin via **transferrin receptors** on the cell

Figure 12.8 **Iron absorption from foods.** Phytates, polyphenols, and fiber inhibit iron absorption, so the bioavailability of iron from plant foods is much lower than that from animal foods. **Source:** Figure by Laurie Grace. From Scrimshaw NS. Iron deficiency. *Scientific American.* October 1991:48. Reprinted by permission of Laurie Grace.

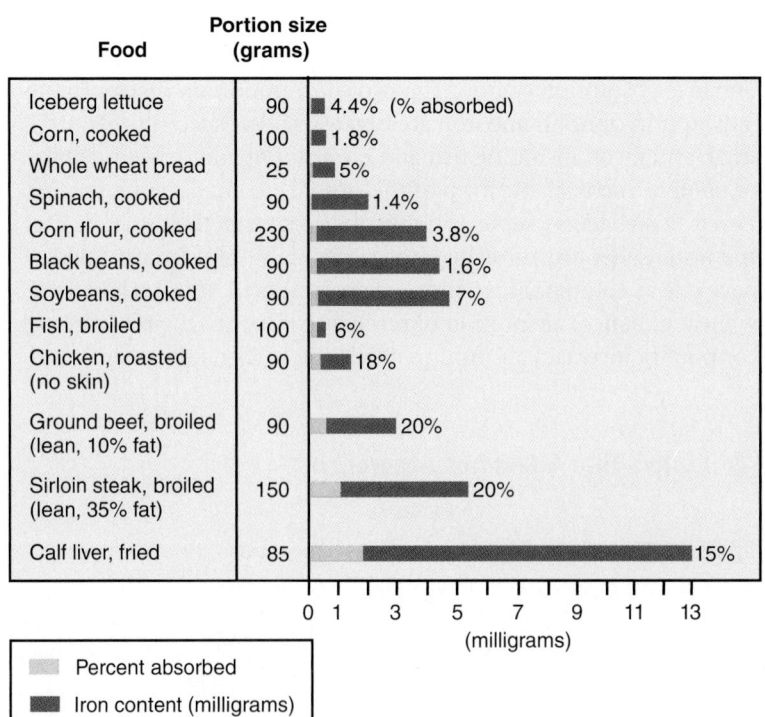

membranes.[15] The number of transferrin receptors varies with the cell's need for iron; tissues with the highest iron need (e.g., bone marrow, liver, and placenta) have the highest concentration of transferrin receptors. (See **Figure 12.9**.)

The body stores surplus iron either as part of the soluble protein complex ferritin or as the insoluble protein complex **hemosiderin**.[16] The liver, bone marrow, spleen, and skeletal muscle harbor most of the body's ferritin and hemosiderin, and small amounts of ferritin circulate in the bloodstream. In healthy people, ferritin contains most of the stored iron.[17] When long-term negative iron balance depletes iron stores, iron deficiency begins.

Iron Turnover and Loss

The body tightly regulates its iron content to ensure adequate stores while protecting against toxicity. It recycles iron, and adjusts absorption and excretion as needed.

Red blood cell formation and destruction are responsible for most iron turnover. In adult men, for example, the breakdown of older red blood cells supplies approximately 95 percent of the iron required to produce new red blood cells. Dietary sources supply only 5 percent. In contrast, this balance is 70/30 in infants, whose growth needs tend to outstrip the recycled supply.

Adults lose about 1 milligram of iron daily in feces and sloughed-off mucosal and skin cells. Women of childbearing age require additional iron

transferrin receptors Specialized receptors on the cell membrane that bind transferrin.

hemosiderin An insoluble form of storage iron.

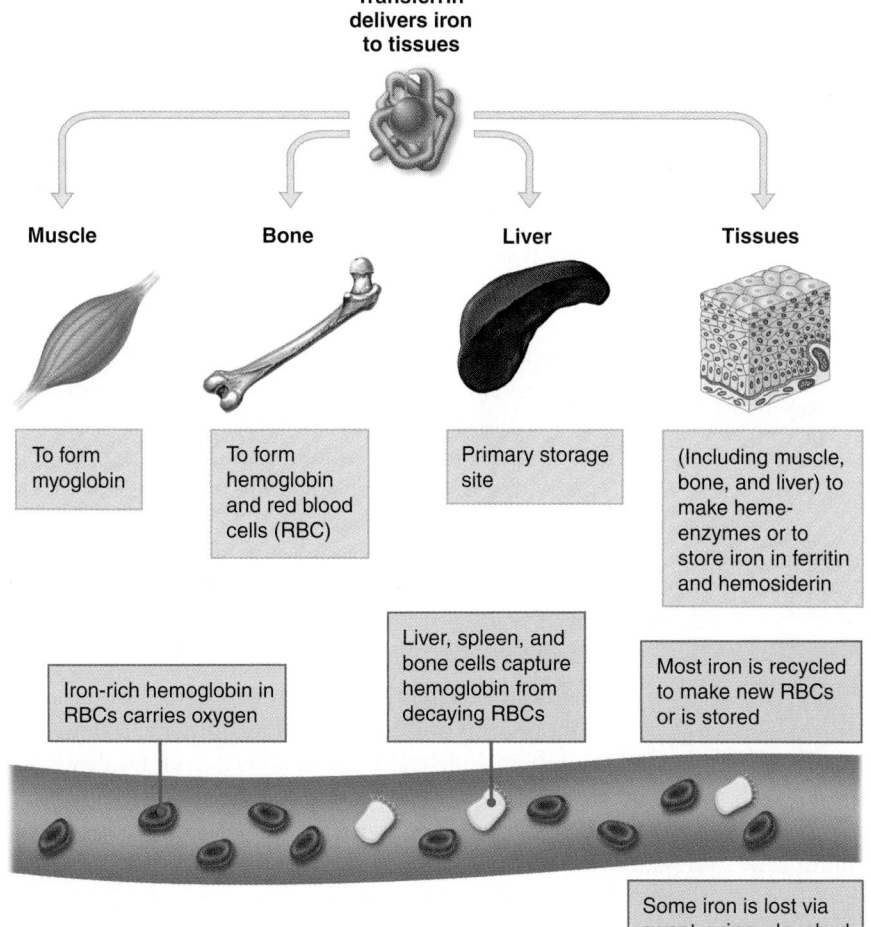

Figure 12.9 **Iron in the body.** Transferrin transports iron to tissues for the synthesis of heme or storage in ferritin and hemosiderin.

(an average of 0.3 to 0.5 mg of iron absorbed daily) to compensate for blood loss during menstruation. Pregnancy increases iron needs markedly to support growth of the fetus and expansion of the maternal blood supply. During pregnancy, a woman requires an absorption of an average of 4 milligrams of additional iron daily over the 280 days of gestation. Blood loss with childbirth depletes iron; thus, women with repeated pregnancies close together are likely to have poor iron status and need extra iron.

All people lose tiny amounts of iron daily in normal gastrointestinal blood loss, but gastrointestinal problems can cause significant iron loss. Peptic ulcer, inflammatory bowel disease, and bowel cancer can cause gastrointestinal bleeding. Hookworm infections, although uncommon in the United States, also are associated with gastrointestinal blood loss and iron depletion.[18]

Dietary Recommendations for Iron

Scientists base recommendations for iron intake on the replacement of daily iron losses and the bioavailability of dietary iron. The primary routes of loss are bleeding, gastrointestinal losses (mainly exfoliation of the intestinal mucosa), sloughing of skin, and sweat. The RDA for iron is based on average losses of 1 milligram per day for adult men and 1.4 milligrams per day for premenopausal women, combined with an absorption percentage of 18 percent from a mixed diet. The RDAs for adults are 8 milligrams per day for men and postmenopausal women and 18 milligrams per day for women of childbearing age.

Dietary intakes of most men actually exceed their RDA, whereas women's intakes are well below the RDA for most age ranges, according to the Third National Health and Nutrition Examination Survey (NHANES III). Researchers attribute the women's lower intake to lower energy intake, since women consume on average 1,800 kilocalories per day and the American diet contains about 6 milligrams iron per 1,000 kilocalories.[19] The average premenopausal woman therefore consumes less than 11 milligrams of iron daily, substantially below the recommended 18 milligrams.

The iron needs of infants are a special concern. During the final weeks of pregnancy, babies ideally store enough iron in the liver, bone marrow, spleen, and hemoglobin-rich blood to see them through their first six months of life. However, if the mother's iron nutrition is poor or the baby is born early, the baby's iron stores are smaller and do not last. To help ensure that babies have adequate iron, pregnant women are urged to meet the RDA of 27 milligrams per day. Infant baby cereal and many infant formulas are fortified with iron.

Sources of Iron

Beef is an excellent dietary source of iron, in terms of both amount and bioavailability. Other excellent sources include clams, oysters, and liver. Poultry, fish, pork, lamb, tofu, and legumes are also good sources. Whole-grain and enriched-grain products contain less bioavailable iron than meat but are significant sources of iron because they constitute a major part of our diets. Fortified cereals also make an important contribution to iron intake in the United States. Dairy products are low in iron. **Figure 12.10** shows the iron content of some foods.

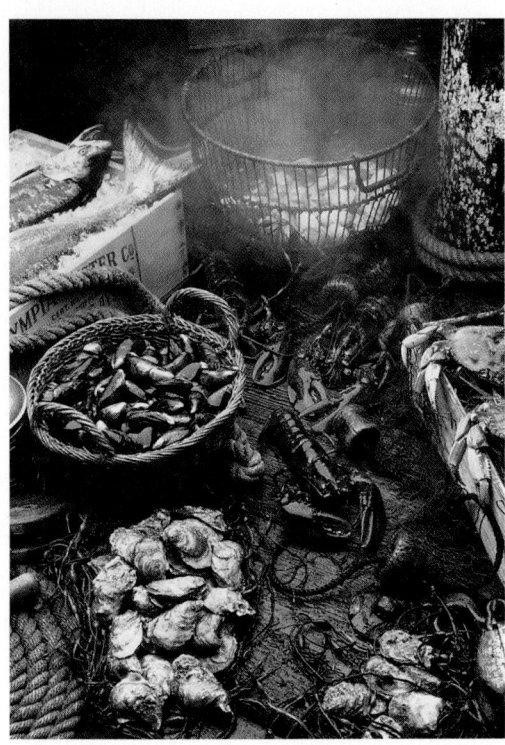

IRON

Daily Value = 18 mg

	Exceptionally good source		
High: 20% DV or more	Clams, cooked	85 g (3 oz)	23.8 mg
	Cheerios cereal	30 g (1 cup)	10.3 mg
	Oysters, cooked	85 g (3 oz)	10.2 mg
	Corn flakes cereal	30 g (~1 cup)	8.7 mg
	Beef liver, cooked	85 g (3 oz)	5.6 mg
	Soybeans, cooked	90 g (~1/2 cup)	4.6 mg
	All Bran cereal	30 g (~1/2 cup)	4.5 mg
Good: 10–19% DV	Lentils, cooked	90 g (~1/2 cup)	3.0 mg
	Steak, porterhouse, cooked	85 g (3 oz)	2.8 mg
	Shrimp, cooked	85 g (3 oz)	2.6 mg
	Spinach, raw	90 g (~3 cups)	2.3 mg
	Tofu, calcium processed	85 g (~1/3 cup)	2.3 mg
	Lima beans, cooked	90 g (~1/2 cup)	2.2 mg
	Turkey, dark meat, cooked	85 g (3 oz)	2.0 mg
	Spaghetti, enriched, cooked	140 g (~1 cup)	1.9 mg

Figure 12.10 **Food sources of iron.** Iron is found in red meats, certain seafoods, vegetables, and legumes, and is added to enriched grains and breakfast cereals.
Source: U.S. Department of Agriculture, Agricultural Research Service. USDA National Nutrient Database for Standard Reference, Release 18. 2005. http://www.ars.usda.gov/nutrientdata.

A varied diet (adequate in calories, rich in fruits and vegetables, and with small amounts of lean animal flesh) generally provides adequate iron. Vegetarians who consume no animal tissue can maximize iron bioavailability from other sources by consuming vitamin C–rich fruits and vegetables with every meal.

Iron Deficiency and Measurement of Iron Status

Iron deficiency is the most common nutritional deficiency worldwide. Although significantly more prevalent in developing countries than in the rest of the world, it is still a public health concern in the United States. Infants and toddlers, adolescent girls, women of childbearing age, and pregnant women are particularly vulnerable.

Iron deficiency is most prevalent in 6- to 24-month-old children, who are in a period of rapid brain growth and development of cognitive and motor skills. Iron stores from fetal development have been depleted, and a major source of energy in the young child's diet is milk, a poor source of iron. If iron stores are not replaced before the child passes critical developmental milestones, developmental deficits from iron deficiency may be irreversible.

Studies of infants and children show a link between iron deficiency and delays in behavioral and cognitive development, but we do not yet understand how iron affects the brain.[20] Research in this area is complicated by the difficulty of separating the roles of iron deficiency and other environmental factors (e.g., generalized malnutrition, poverty, and low parental education) that also impair psychomotor and mental development.

Progression of Iron Deficiency

Iron deficiency progresses through three distinct stages, shown in **Table 12.3**. The third stage is iron-deficiency anemia, a severe form of iron deficiency that is defined by low hemoglobin levels.

Depletion of iron stores is the first stage of iron deficiency, which causes no physiological impairments. Because serum ferritin is proportional to the body's total iron stores, a test of serum ferritin is a good way to assess iron deficiency.

Depletion of functional and transport iron is the second stage of iron deficiency—the stage between iron depletion and actual anemia. The newest and most sensitive measure of this intermediate stage is the serum level of transferrin receptors (TfRs). As the body's iron status falls, TfR levels increase in proportion to the iron deficit. Other blood values used to detect this stage are **transferrin saturation** and **protoporphyrin** levels. Transferrin saturation is a measure of the residual binding capacity for iron, which increases when a lack of iron does not saturate transferrin. Protoporphyrin and iron combine to make heme, the iron-containing portion of hemoglobin. When the supply of iron is inadequate for heme synthesis, blood levels of protoporphyrin rise.

Quick Bites

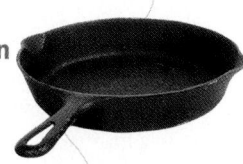

Grandma's Cast-Iron Skillet Helped Her Avoid Iron Deficiency

Iron deficiency is the most common form of malnutrition in the United States. However, this is a relatively recent phenomenon. Americans used to cook using cast-iron pots and pans. A study showed that using these utensils to cook acidic foods like spaghetti sauce and apple butter increases the iron content of such foods by a factor of 30- to 100-fold. Our preference for stainless steel, aluminum, and enamelware does not allow us this fortification.

Table 12.3 Stages of Iron Deficiency

Stage	Biochemical Sign	Functional Implications
Depletion of iron stores	Decreased ferritin	None
Depletion of functional iron	Decreased transferrin saturation Increased erythrocyte protoporphyrin	Decreased physical performance
Iron-deficiency anemia	Decreased hemoglobin Decreased hematocrit Decreased red cell size	Cognitive impairment, poor growth, decreased performance, and decreased exercise tolerance

hematocrit Percentage volume occupied by packed red blood cells in a centrifuged sample of whole blood.

iron overload Toxicity from excess iron.

Normal cells

Decrease in iron stores

↓

Decrease in iron transport

↓   Development of iron deficiency

Fall in hemoglobin synthesis

↓

Anemia

Anemic cells

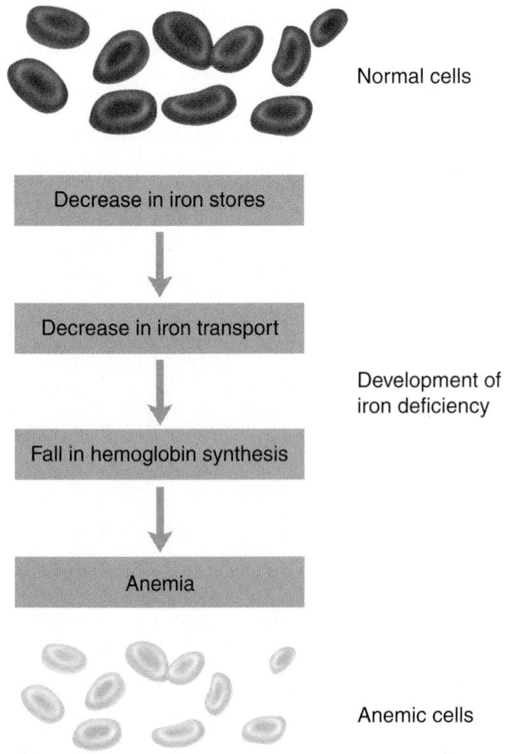

Figure 12.11 **Normal and anemic red blood cells.** Iron deficiency can progress to iron-deficiency anemia, a severe form of iron deficiency that is accompanied by low hemoglobin levels.

Because second-stage iron depletion impairs the function of iron-requiring enzymes needed for aerobic energy production, an iron-depleted person may be unable to work at full capacity. Animal research shows a decreased exercise capacity among iron-deficient animals without anemia. Research in young women with iron deficiency but without anemia shows a similar decrease in their physical performance.[21] More human studies are required to determine whether iron depletion affects other physiological processes.

The third and most severe stage of iron deficiency is anemia—a disease characterized by insufficient and/or defective red blood cells. A lack of iron inhibits production of normal red blood cells, while normal cell turnover continues to deplete the red blood cell population. Red blood cell production falters, producing red blood cells that are pale and smaller than normal. Hemoglobin and **hematocrit** (concentration of red blood cells in the blood) levels also are low. This type of anemia, known for its small, pale red blood cells, is called microcytic hypochromic anemia. Inadequate vitamin B_6 also can cause microcytic hypochromic anemia. Another type of anemia, megaloblastic anemia, is known for its abnormally large, immature red blood cells and is caused by inadequate folate or vitamin B_{12}. (See Chapter 10, "Water-Soluble Vitamins," for more details.) **Figure 12.11** shows normal and anemic blood cells.

The symptoms of microcytic hypochromic anemia vary according to its severity and the speed of its development. They include fatigue, pallor, breathlessness with exertion, decreased tolerance of cold, behavioral changes, deficits in immune function, cognitive impairment, decreased work performance, and impaired growth. In children, iron deficiency is associated with apathy, short attention span, irritability, and reduced ability to learn.[22]

Iron Toxicity

The Tolerable Upper Intake Level (UL) for iron is based on the level that causes gastrointestinal distress. For adults, the UL for iron is 45 milligrams per day.

Iron Poisoning in Children

Accidental iron overdose is a leading cause of poisoning deaths in children younger than 6 years in the United States.[23] The iron products involved range from nonprescription daily multivitamin/mineral supplements for children to high-potency prescription iron supplements for pregnant women. Parents who are cautious about keeping other medications out of reach often do not realize that over-the-counter iron tablets and iron-containing multivitamin/mineral supplements can be toxic to children. Even a few pills can cause the death of a small child. Symptoms of iron intoxication include nausea, vomiting, diarrhea, rapid heartbeat, dizziness, and confusion. Death can occur within hours of ingestion. If iron poisoning is suspected, the child should receive immediate emergency medical care.

Hereditary Hemochromatosis

Hereditary hemochromatosis, a form of chronic **iron overload**, was once thought to be rare but now is known to be quite common. A genetic defect causes excessive iron absorption. Over the years, iron can build up in many parts of the body, leading to severe organ damage and even death. Diabetes, heart disease, cirrhosis, liver cancer, and arthritis can all be consequences of hemochromatosis.

Serious complications of hemochromatosis are five to ten times more common in men than women, primarily because of women's blood loss associated with menstruation and pregnancy. Treatment of hemochromatosis includes minimizing iron intake and frequent phlebotomy (removal of blood) to withdraw some of the iron that blood carries in cells. With early diagnosis and treatment, a person with hemochromatosis can avoid organ damage and other complications and have a normal life span.

Iron overload is highly prevalent in some African communities. Researchers originally thought the custom of consuming beer brewed in steel drums was entirely responsible. These beverages have a large amount of highly bioavailable iron, and alcohol enhances the absorption of iron. However, researchers have found strong evidence for a gene, distinct from the hemochromatosis gene in Caucasians, that may predispose individuals to this disorder.[24]

Key Concepts: *Iron is essential for life but highly toxic in excess. Iron is a key component of the oxygen transporters hemoglobin and myoglobin, and of many enzymes involved in energy metabolism. Heme iron is absorbed more efficiently than nonheme iron. The body carefully regulates iron absorption; iron can be bound to transferrin for transport, or stored as ferritin or hemosiderin. The best dietary source of iron is red meat. Iron deficiency develops gradually, with anemia being the most severe manifestation of deficiency. Iron poisoning is potentially deadly, especially for young children. Hereditary hemochromatosis is a common genetic disease that causes iron overload.*

Zinc

It's hard to believe that a nutrient so important to health could go unnoticed until as recently as 40 years ago, but that is the case with zinc (Zn). Some people may think of zinc only in connection with the "zinc oxide" cream used topically as a sunscreen or with zinc lozenges promoted as a treatment for colds; few consumers realize that dietary zinc is absolutely essential for health.

Scientists first recognized human zinc deficiency in 1961.[25] They found severe zinc deficiencies in young, severely growth-retarded, Iranian men. In addition to suffering from dwarfism, these men were anemic and extremely lethargic and had **hypogonadism** (poorly developed genitals), and some couldn't see well in the dark. Their diets consisted mainly of wheat bread and was almost devoid of animal protein. These men also were known to eat clay (**geophagia**). Scientists hypothesized that the high phytate content of their diet, along with the geophagia, impaired absorption of both zinc and iron. Six years later, a study in Egypt confirmed zinc's role; zinc supplementation improved growth and genital development.[26]

Functions of Zinc

The body contains a small amount of zinc—between 1.5 and 2.5 grams, or about the same amount of zinc as is in a **galvanized** nail, which has a thin layer of zinc to protect it from corrosion. Zinc is a component of every living cell. Zinc is best known for its participation in enzyme structure and function, but it also supports many other diverse biological activities through a role in controlling gene regulation. **Figure 12.12** illustrates the functions of zinc in the body.

Zinc and Enzymes

Zinc is critical to the proper function of more than 80 enzymes and other **metalloproteins**, which are proteins that have a mineral as an essential part of their structures.[27] It is essential for their structural integrity and function, regulation of their activities, and their ability to catalyze reactions. In the cytoplasm, zinc and copper are key components of superoxide dismutase,

hypogonadism Decreased functional activity of the gonads (ovaries or testes) with retardation of growth and sexual development.

geophagia Ingestion of clay or dirt.

galvanized Iron or steel with a thin layer of zinc plated onto it to protect against corrosion.

metalloproteins Proteins with a mineral element as an essential part of their structure.

Quick Bites

Bizarre Behavior or Nutritional Deficiency?

In all cultures, races, and geographic regions, certain people have strange cravings for nonfood items. These cravings include ice (pagophagia), clay and dirt (geophagia), cornstarch (amylophagia), stone (lithophagia), paper, toilet tissue, soap, and foam. Pica, the compulsive consumption of nonfood items, often is associated with either iron or zinc deficiency, but it may also be the result of cultural beliefs or a response to family stresses. Whatever the cause, the behavior is not benign. It can injure teeth as well as cause constipation, intestinal obstruction or perforation, lead poisoning, pregnancy complications, poor growth in children, and mineral deficiencies.

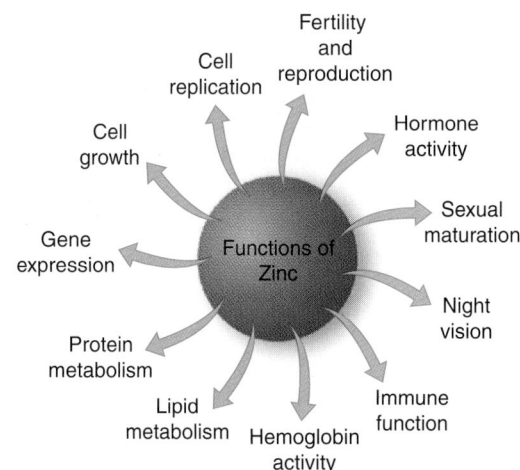

Figure 12.12 **Functions of zinc in the body.** Because zinc is involved in so many different functions, it is fortunate that overt zinc deficiency is rare.

an enzyme that speeds antioxidant reactions and helps protect cells from free radical damage.

Zinc's Role in Nucleic Acid Metabolism

Zinc also is inextricably linked to gene expression. In severe zinc deficiency, cells fail to replicate. This may be why zinc is so important for normal growth of children and sexual maturation of adolescents. Furthermore, certain tissues with high turnover rates, such as cells lining the GI tract, skin cells, immune cells, and blood cells, are particularly vulnerable to a zinc deficiency. As a result, zinc-deficient people often have diarrhea, dermatitis, and depressed immunity.

Zinc and the Immune System

Zinc is vital to a vigorous immune response and is essential to the proper development and maintenance of the immune system. Without zinc, your body could not fight off invading viruses, bacteria, and fungi. Even mild deficiency may increase the risk of infection.

Zinc and Vision

Zinc-deficient people may show signs of night blindness or other classic signs of vitamin A deficiency. Zinc is a key component of the enzyme that activates vitamin A in the retina. Thus, a lack of zinc interferes with vitamin A activity in the eye.

Zinc and Gene Regulation

Zinc enables certain small proteins to fold and form a stable "zinc-finger" structure. This structure interacts with a region of DNA. Without zinc, that area of a gene won't function.[28] This function of zinc may explain how it influences the immune system. Discovery and characterization of zinc-finger protein families is an active area of nutrition research.

Other Zinc Functions

Zinc is essential for a number of other diverse biological functions:

- *Hormonal.* Zinc interacts with a number of hormones, including insulin.
- *Growth and reproduction.* Zinc plays an important role in pregnancy outcome, fetal development, and bone health.
- *Hemoglobin activity.* Zinc increases the affinity of hemoglobin for oxygen and indirectly influences hemoglobin synthesis.
- *Taste.* Some studies show that zinc participates in taste perception and appetite regulation.
- *Cell death.* Zinc can induce as well as inhibit the process of apoptosis, also known as programmed cell death.[29]

Regulation of Zinc in the Body

Zinc Absorption

The body absorbs small amounts of zinc more effectively than large doses, and absorption ranges between 10 and 35 percent—a range similar to heme iron absorption. The degree of zinc absorption depends on the person's zinc status and zinc needs, the zinc content of the meal, and the presence of competing minerals. People with zinc deficiency absorb zinc more thoroughly than those with optimal zinc status. Absorption increases during times of increased need, such as growth spurts, pregnancy, and lactation. On the other hand, certain dietary factors such as phytate and fiber can impair absorption of zinc. **Figure 12.13** shows the zinc absorption process.

metallothionein An abundant, nonenzymatic, zinc-containing protein.

Dietary Factors That Inhibit Zinc Absorption

Because of phytate and fiber, the body absorbs zinc poorly from whole grains—less than 15 percent on average.[30] Phytate can bind zinc in insoluble complexes, thus inhibiting zinc's absorption. Dietary fiber may also reduce zinc absorption, but to a lesser extent than phytate. Calcium in a meal does not appear to affect zinc absorption, but supplemental calcium taken with meals high in phytate may increase phytate's ability to bind zinc and may decrease zinc's bioavailability.[31] However, American diets typically do not contain enough phytate and fiber to depress zinc absorption significantly. Exceptions are vegetarian diets that are high in phytate and fiber.[32]

The negative effect of high-dose nonheme iron supplementation (such as during pregnancy) on zinc absorption is well documented.[33] On the other hand, your body absorbs heme iron (from meat) differently, so heme iron has no effect on zinc absorption. Also, iron inhibits zinc absorption only when there is a high iron-to-zinc ratio.[34] Eating iron-fortified foods is unlikely to inhibit zinc absorption.

Zinc Transport and Distribution

Zinc circulates in the bloodstream loosely bound to albumin and more tightly bound to another protein, alpha$_2$-macroglobulin. Zinc travels to the liver and to the tissues where it is most needed. Muscle and bone contain 90 percent of the body's zinc; the remainder is divided primarily among the liver, kidney, pancreas, brain, skin, and prostate. **Figure 12.14** shows zinc in the body.

Zinc Homeostasis and Excretion

The body has no long-term storehouse of zinc to draw upon when dietary zinc is low. Despite the lack of zinc storage, the body balances zinc absorption and excretion, thus maintaining zinc homeostasis even when confronted with varying needs and dietary conditions.

Intestinal cells act as temporary buffers that help regulate zinc absorption. The protein **metallothionein** binds zinc in the intestinal mucosal cells and impedes its movement into the bloodstream. When zinc intake is high, the body makes more metallothionein to retain more zinc in the intestinal cells. Intestinal cells and other cells produce zinc transporter proteins, which help to maintain body homeostasis.[35]

During digestion, the pancreas secretes as much as 4.0 milligrams of zinc per day in the pancreatic juice. When the body needs zinc, intestinal cells reabsorb most of this secreted zinc. Otherwise, the body excretes it in the feces along with unabsorbed dietary zinc and sloughed, zinc-containing intestinal cells. The body also excretes zinc in minor amounts via urine, sweat, skin, hair, semen, and menstrual fluids.

Key

● Zinc

● Nonheme iron

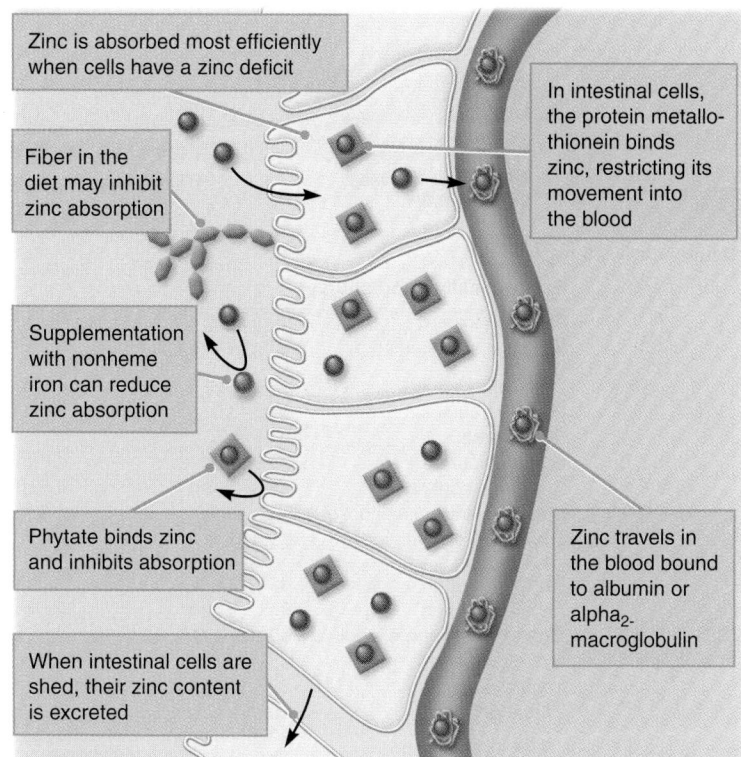

Zinc is absorbed most efficiently when cells have a zinc deficit

Fiber in the diet may inhibit zinc absorption

Supplementation with nonheme iron can reduce zinc absorption

Phytate binds zinc and inhibits absorption

When intestinal cells are shed, their zinc content is excreted

In intestinal cells, the protein metallothionein binds zinc, restricting its movement into the blood

Zinc travels in the blood bound to albumin or alpha$_2$-macroglobulin

Figure 12.13 **Zinc absorption.** Intestinal cells act as temporary buffers that help regulate zinc absorption.

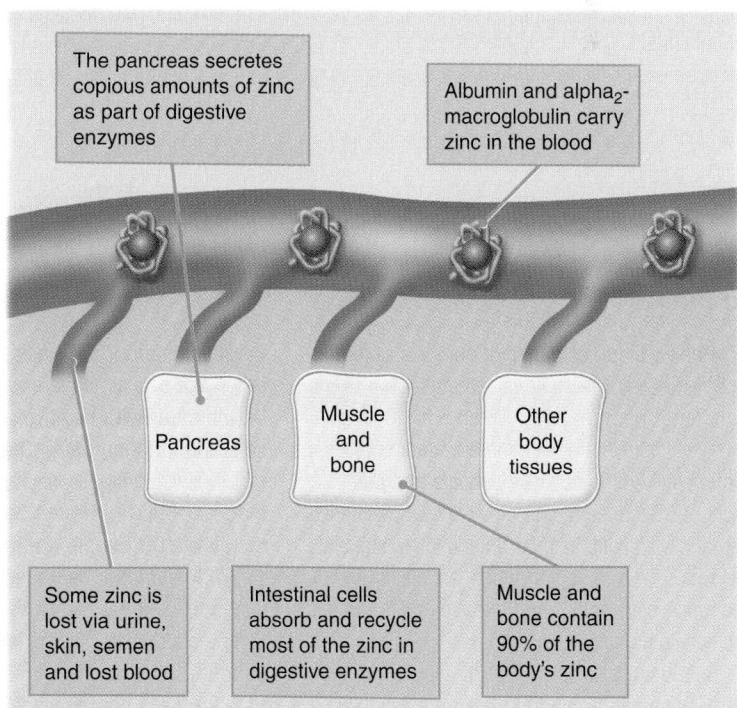

The pancreas secretes copious amounts of zinc as part of digestive enzymes

Albumin and alpha$_2$-macroglobulin carry zinc in the blood

Pancreas

Muscle and bone

Other body tissues

Some zinc is lost via urine, skin, semen and lost blood

Intestinal cells absorb and recycle most of the zinc in digestive enzymes

Muscle and bone contain 90% of the body's zinc

Figure 12.14 **Zinc in the body.** Zinc is a component of every living cell and helps stabilize cell membranes. More than 80 enzymes contain zinc.

Dietary Recommendations for Zinc

The RDA for adult males is 11 milligrams per day, and for females it is 8 milligrams per day. Experts recommend increasing zinc intake to 11 milligrams per day during pregnancy to provide for the growing fetus, and to 12 milligrams per day during lactation.

Average zinc intake in the United States is generally below the RDA.[36] These dietary data raise the important question of whether marginal zinc deficiency is common or the RDA is set too high. Since RDA levels are set higher than the assumed average requirement, average population intakes that are lower than the RDA may not be of concern.

Sources of Zinc

Zinc usually is abundant in foods that are good sources of protein, especially red meat, seafood, oysters, and clams. Dark meat is a richer source than white meat, and unrefined whole grains have more zinc than processed grains. However, the bioavailability of zinc is just as important as the amount present. Although wheat-bran bread has a relatively high amount of zinc (2.4 milligrams), much of it is unavailable due to poor absorption (7 percent).[37] The bioavailability of zinc is highest from red meats, liver, eggs, and seafood. Fruits and vegetables generally are poor sources of dietary zinc.

In the United States, 44 percent of dietary zinc comes from meat, poultry, and seafood, 19 percent from dairy sources, and 17 percent from grains.[38] Adequate zinc intake is of special concern for vegetarians because they do not eat many of the foods that are the best sources of this mineral. **Figure 12.15** shows the zinc content of some foods.

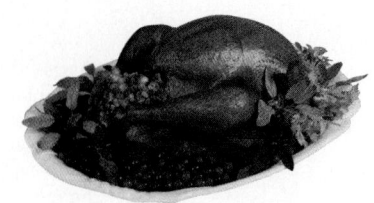

ZINC

Daily Value = 15 mg

Exceptionally good sources

Oysters, cooked	85 g (3 oz)	154 mg
Wheat-bran flakes cereal	30 g (~3/4 cup)	15.8 mg
Crab, Alaska King, cooked	85 g (3 oz)	6.5 mg
Ground beef, extra lean, cooked	85 g (3 oz)	5.5 mg
Cheerios cereal	30 g (~1 cup)	4.6 mg
Beef liver, cooked	85 g (3 oz)	4.5 mg
Steak, porterhouse, cooked	85 g (3 oz)	4.3 mg
Turkey, dark meat, cooked	85 g (3 oz)	3.8 mg
Ham, extra lean, cooked	85 g (3 oz)	2.8 mg
Lobster, cooked	85 g (3 oz)	2.5 mg
Chicken, dark meat, cooked	85 g (3 oz)	2.4 mg
Clams, cooked	85 g (3 oz)	2.3 mg
Yogurt, plain, nonfat	225 g (1 8-oz container)	2.2 mg
Wheat germ	15 g (1/4 cup)	1.8 mg
All Bran cereal	30 g (~1/2 cup)	1.5 mg
Refried beans, canned	130 g (~1/2 cup)	1.5 mg

High: 20% DV or more

Good: 10–19% DV

Figure 12.15 **Food sources of zinc.** Meats, organ meats, and seafoods are the best sources of zinc.
Source: U.S. Department of Agriculture, Agricultural Research Service. USDA National Nutrient Database for Standard Reference, Release 18. 2005. http://www.ars.usda.gov /nutrientdata.

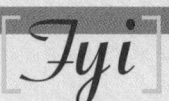 **Zinc and the Common Cold**

FOR YOUR INFORMATION

The common cold, one of our most common illnesses, affects American adults two to four times per year and children 6 to 10 times per year.[1] Colds are even more frequent in young children in day care settings and preschools. Because of missed work and decreased productivity, colds can be an economic stressor as well as a physical nuisance. A cure for the common cold would be of great benefit, and scientists have long pursued this goal.

Because of zinc's role in immune function, 11 placebo-controlled studies between 1984 and 1998 investigated the effect of zinc lozenges on the common cold. Roughly half of

the studies produced positive results and the other half had negative findings.

One study with positive results gained considerable attention from the press. As a result, zinc lozenges are on nearly every pharmacy shelf in the United States. This study recruited 100 people during the winter of 1994. Researchers enrolled subjects within 24 hours of the onset of their common cold symptoms. Every 2 hours while awake, half the subjects took placebo lozenges and half took lozenges containing 13 milligrams of zinc, an average of six lozenges per day. They could take acetaminophen, but they were

asked to refrain from taking other cold medicines or antibiotics during the trial. In the zinc group, colds resolved in an average of 4 days. In comparison, cold symptoms in the placebo group persisted for 7 days.[2]

Though scientists have suggested several hypotheses, the mechanism for the effect is unclear. Zinc deficiency is known to impair immune function, but could all these people have been zinc deficient? This is doubtful. Some speculate that zinc may inhibit viral replication.

During the trial, many of the experimental subjects experienced side effects, including

Zinc Deficiency

Zinc deficiency is most prevalent in populations that subsist on cereal proteins, which have poorly available zinc.[39] Diarrhea and chronic infections such as pneumonia can cause excessive zinc excretion. These diseases are commonplace in developing countries, where zinc deficiency may be widespread. In some of these areas, zinc supplementation has decreased the incidence of acute lower respiratory infection, diarrhea, and attacks of malaria in children.

As **Table 12.4** shows, the primary culprits in marginal zinc deficiency are increased needs, poor intake, poor absorption, and excessive losses. During pregnancy, zinc deficiency may contribute to complications and low birth weight.[40] Zinc-deficient preschool-aged children and patients on **hemodialysis** may have a poor appetite and a diminished sense of taste.[41] Malabsorption syndromes such as cystic fibrosis and **Crohn's disease**

hemodialysis Technique for removing waste products by filtering blood, usually performed on patients with kidney failure.

Crohn's disease A disease that causes inflammation and ulceration along sections of the intestinal tract.

Table 12.4 **Risk Factors for Zinc Deficiency**

Dietary Deficiency	Protein-energy malnutrition Poor food choices	Vegan diets IV feeding without zinc
Increased Requirements	Burn patients Growth spurts	Pregnancy and lactation Chronic infection
Malabsorption	Acrodermatitis enteropathica Celiac disease, Crohn's disease Cystic fibrosis	Geophagia or pica High-phytate diets Chronic iron supplementation
Increased Losses	Sickle cell disease Diabetes Renal disease	Burns and surgery Chronic diarrhea

nausea, bad taste, and sore mouths. In addition to the mild side effects and the cost of the lozenges, such high doses of zinc could have harmful effects. Long-term use of high doses of zinc induces copper deficiency. On average, those in the experimental group took close to 480 milligrams of zinc during the week of their cold. If children have eight colds per year and take nearly 500 milligrams of zinc per cold, could that be enough to induce widespread copper deficiency?

The same research group studied 249 randomly selected children in a double-blind, placebo-controlled trial. The experimental group took zinc gluconate lozenges at the first sign of cold symptoms. Depending on age, each child received 50 to 60 milligrams of zinc per day. There was no difference between groups in the time for all cold symptoms to resolve—a median of 9 days. Although the researchers noted several limitations of their study, they concluded that we still need additional studies to determine what role, if any, zinc has in treatment of the common cold.[3]

Because only half of the studies produced positive effects and excess zinc intake can cause deficiencies of other minerals, we should think twice before routinely giving children (and ourselves) zinc lozenges every time a cold strikes.

1 National Institute of Allergy and Infectious Diseases. Common cold. http://www3.niaid.nih.gov/healthscience /healthtopics/colds. Accessed 12/31/06.

2 Mossad SB, Macknin ML, Medendorp SV, Mason P. Zinc gluconate lozenges for treating the common cold: a randomized, double-blind placebo-controlled study. *Ann Intern Med.* 1996;125:81–88.

3 Macknin ML, Piedmonte M, Calendine C, et al. Zinc gluconate lozenges for treating the common cold in children: a randomized controlled trial. *JAMA.* 1998;279:1962–1967.

Table 12.5 Effects of Zinc Deficiency

Severe Deficiency	Moderate Deficiency
Hypogonadism	Delayed sexual maturation
Cessation of growth	
Patchy loss of hair	Growth retardation
Skin lesions and rashes	Pregnancy complications
Impaired taste (hypogeusia)	
	Acne
Loss of appetite/anorexia	Increased infections
Diarrhea	
Decreased thyroid hormone synthesis	
Night blindness	
Recurrent infections	

acrodermatitis enteropathica A genetic disorder that results in a deficiency in the absorption of zinc.

Wilson's disease Genetic disorder of increased copper absorption, which leads to toxic levels in the liver and heart.

Keshan disease Selenium-deficiency disease that impairs the structure and function of the heart.

impair zinc absorption. Symptoms of moderate to severe zinc deficiency include poor growth, impaired immune response, and other conditions that may include impaired taste acuity. **Table 12.5** lists these and other characteristics of moderate and severe zinc deficiency.

Although severe zinc deficiency is uncommon, it can be caused by **acrodermatitis enteropathica**, a rare genetic disorder that impairs zinc absorption and produces skin problems and infections. In the past, long-term intravenous feeding severely depleted zinc in patients who could not eat normally. Today, trace minerals are added to intravenous solutions.

Zinc Toxicity

Because the body efficiently rids itself of excess zinc, toxicity from high dietary zinc intake is rare. Yet there have been isolated accounts of acute zinc toxicity in people who consumed large amounts of acidic foods or beverages that had been stored in galvanized containers. High doses of zinc may cause acute gastrointestinal distress, nausea, vomiting, and cramping.

Chronic intake of moderately elevated amounts of zinc is a more common cause of zinc toxicity. Usually, excessive zinc supplementation is at fault. In elderly patients, intakes of 100 to 150 milligrams of zinc per day for several weeks decreased immune function.[42] Doses as low as 50 milligrams per day typically cause vomiting.[43] Excess zinc intake also adversely affects blood lipids by elevating LDL and depressing HDL levels.[44] The UL for zinc is set at 40 milligrams per day.

Chronic high intakes of zinc relative to copper can inhibit copper absorption and with time may induce a copper deficiency. Doctors use the interaction of zinc and copper to treat patients with **Wilson's disease**, a genetic disorder of hyperabsorption and accumulation of copper in such patients. Daily doses of between 100 and 150 milligrams zinc effectively inhibit the harmful accumulation of copper in the liver.[45]

Key Concepts: *Zinc is important for normal growth and development, immune function, and the function of many enzymes. Zinc homeostasis is maintained by regulating intestinal absorption. Iron, zinc, and copper all compete for absorption, but problems don't usually occur if these minerals are coming from balanced dietary rather than supplemental sources. The best food sources for zinc are beef, oysters, crab, legumes, and unrefined whole grains. Zinc deficiency is most prevalent in populations that subsist on cereal protein.*

Selenium

The story of selenium (Se) is a recent one and becomes more complex as scientists explore its role at the molecular level. Historically, because animals grazing on selenium-rich soils suffered selenium poisoning, scientists focused on its toxicity. This changed in 1957, when researchers first demonstrated selenium's nutritional benefits in vitamin E–deficient animals. But not until 1979 did evidence emerge that selenium is essential for humans. Chinese scientists reported an association between low selenium status and **Keshan disease**, a heart disorder that strikes children in the Keshan province of China. The Chinese scientists demonstrated that selenium supplements could prevent the disease. Although selenium deficiency does not cause the disease, it predisposes a child to heart damage after a particular type of viral infection. When selenium intake is adequate, the virus apparently does not cause Keshan disease.

Functions of Selenium

Although scientists have identified nearly 50 selenium-containing proteins, two amino acid derivatives—**selenomethionine**, a methionine derivative, and **selenocysteine**, a cysteine derivative—contain most of the body's selenium. Selenomethionine is a selenium "storage compartment," and selenocysteine is selenium's biologically active form. As selenocysteine, selenium is a component of enzymes involved in antioxidant protection and thyroid hormone metabolism.

Selenium is best known as a component of glutathione peroxidases, a family of antioxidant enzymes. The discovery of these enzymes resolved a puzzling overlap in the functions of selenium and vitamin E. Both nutrients play a role in preventing lipid peroxidation and membrane damage. Glutathione peroxidases promote the breakdown of fatty acids that have undergone peroxidation, thus eliminating highly reactive free radicals. (See **Figure 12.16a**.) This reduction in free radicals spares vitamin E, making it available to stop other chain reactions of free radicals. (See **Figure 12.16b**.) Since glutathione peroxidases require selenium, dietary selenium indirectly spares vitamin E.

In recent years, scientists have identified selenium as a component of enzymes involved in the metabolism of iodine and thyroid hormone. Iodine deficiency alone causes **hypothyroidism**, and a combined deficiency of selenium and iodine increases the severity of the disease. There also is some evidence that a combined deficiency of both minerals during pregnancy is involved in some forms of **cretinism** in newborns.

selenomethionine A selenium-containing amino acid derived from methionine that is the storage form of selenium.

selenocysteine A selenium-containing amino acid that is the biologically active form of selenium.

hypothyroidism The result of a lowered level of circulating thyroid hormone, with slowing of mental and physical functions.

cretinism A congenital condition often caused by severe iodine deficiency during gestation, which is characterized by arrested physical and mental development.

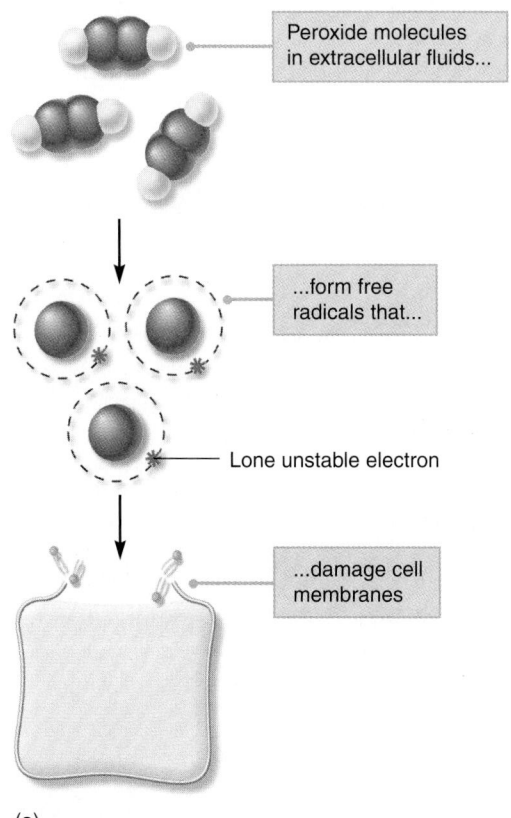

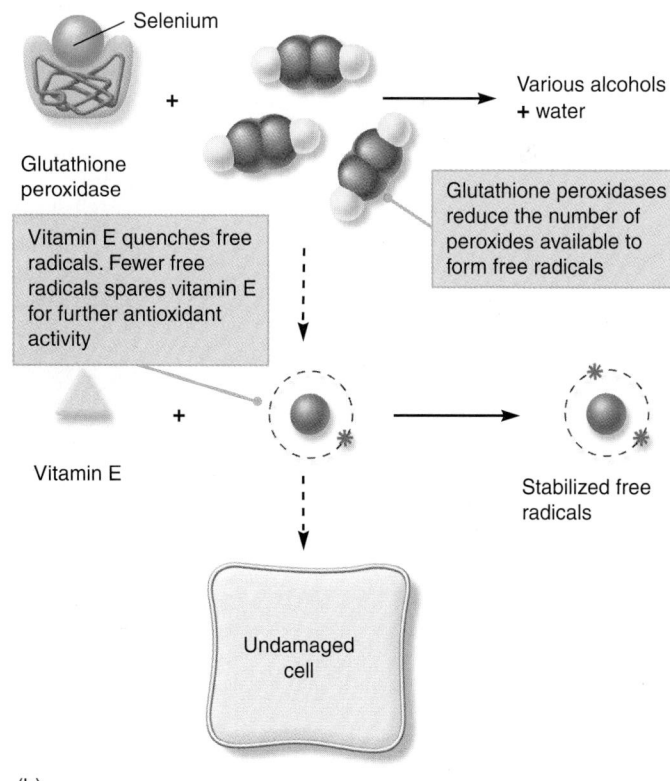

(a) (b)

Figure 12.16 **Free radicals.** (a) Peroxides form free radicals that damage cell membranes and have been implicated in heart disease. (b) Selenium and vitamin E help combat free radicals. Since glutathione peroxidases require selenium, dietary selenium indirectly spares vitamin E.

Selenium is important in the immune system and its response to infections. Research also tentatively links low selenium status to increased cancer risk;[46] however, because small increases in selenium intake can be toxic, selenium supplements are not recommended for cancer prevention. Much more research and large-scale trials are needed to clarify selenium's relationship to cancer.

Regulation of Selenium in the Body

Selenomethionine and selenocysteine are the principal dietary forms of selenium. The body efficiently absorbs these selenoamino acids, with estimates ranging from 50 to 90 percent.[47] The presence of vitamins A, C, and E and reduced glutathione enhance selenium absorption, but phytates and heavy metals such as mercury interfere with its bioavailability.

The selenium regulatory process maintains a low concentration of highly reactive free selenocysteine, and achieves homeostasis through excretion of excess mineral. The major routes of selenium excretion are the urine and the feces. When intake is excessive, the skin and lungs serve as additional excretory routes.

Selenium status, like the status of many trace minerals, is difficult to evaluate. There are no sensitive tests that can readily distinguish between adequate and suboptimal levels of selenium.

Dietary Recommendations for Selenium

Selenium is one of the "youngest" nutrients for which an RDA exists. The first RDA for selenium was established in 1989. The RDA was based on data from Chinese scientists who conducted repletion experiments in selenium-depleted subjects living in areas where Keshan disease was endemic. The RDA for selenium was revised in 2000. For both men and women, the selenium RDA is 55 micrograms per day.[48]

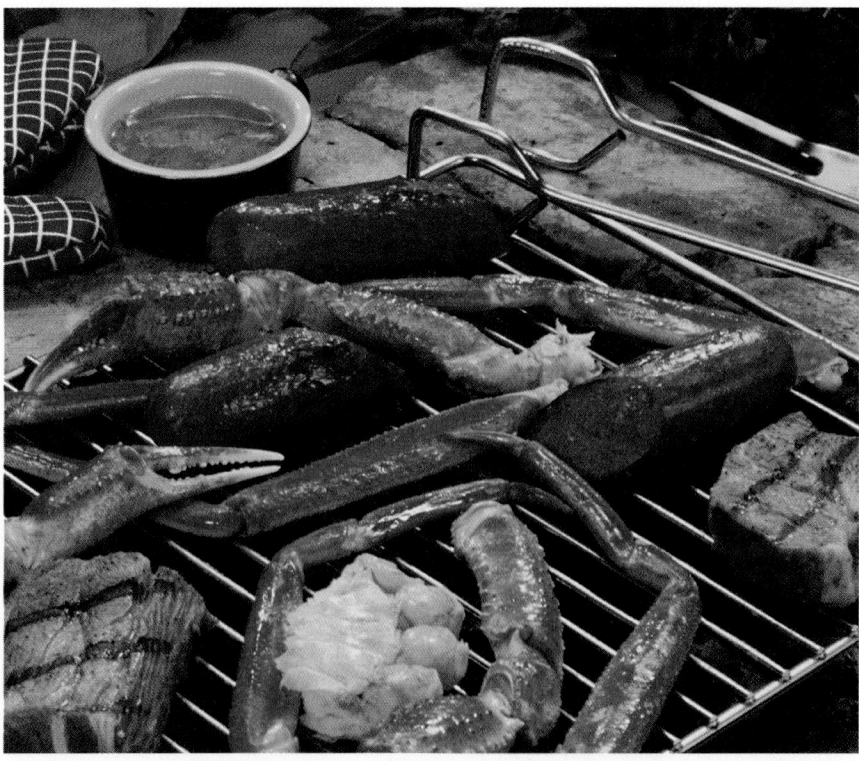

Sources of Selenium

Because animals accumulate selenium in their tissues, the selenium content of food from animal sources generally is more consistent than the selenium content of plants. Organ meats and seafood are consistently good selenium sources. Other meats contain somewhat lower amounts of the mineral. The typical American diet provides adequate selenium. **Figure 12.17** shows some food sources of selenium.

Selenium Deficiency

Selenium deficiency predisposes a person to Keshan disease. Until recently, this disease was a major public health problem in China's Keshan province. Doctors have found selenium deficiency in people who receive long-term **total parenteral nutrition (TPN).** Although after several years of TPN these patients may suffer heart problems and muscle weakness, no specific visible symptoms have been defined for selenium deficiency.

Selenium Toxicity

Chronic consumption of excess selenium can cause brittle hair and nails, and their eventual loss. Although typical dietary intakes are unlikely to exceed safe amounts, selenium supplements can cause problems. Overenthusiastic media reports of research on selenium and cancer, coupled with easy access to selenium supplements, may cause some people to consume unhealthful quantities. The UL is set at 400 micrograms per day for adults.[49]

Key Concepts: *Selenium is best known for its role as an essential component of the antioxidant enzymes glutathione peroxidases. Selenium interacts with vitamin E in antioxidant systems and with iodine in thyroid hormone metabolism. It also is important for good immune function. Good dietary sources for selenium are organ meats and seafood. A deficiency of selenium may predispose a child to Keshan disease, a rare heart disease caused by a virus. New research also links marginal selenium status to cancer risk.*

total parenteral nutrition (TPN) Feeding a person by giving all essential nutrients intravenously.

SELENIUM

Daily Value = 70 μg

High: 20% DV or more

Oysters, cooked	85 g (3 oz)	60.9 μg
Tuna, canned	55 g (2 oz)	44.2 μg
Pork, loin, cooked, lean only	85 g (~3 oz)	40.9 μg
Spaghetti, cooked	140 g (~1 cup)	37.0 μg
Lobster, cooked	85 g (3 oz)	36.3 μg
Shrimp, cooked	85 g (3 oz)	33.7 μg
Beef liver, cooked	85 g (3 oz)	30.7 μg
White bread, enriched	50 g (2 slices)	19.9 μg
Whole-wheat bread	50 g (2 slices)	18.3 μg
Egg, hard cooked	50 g (1 large)	15.4 μg

Good: 10–19% DV

Rice, brown, cooked	140 g (~3/4 cup)	13.7 μg
Oatmeal, cooked	1 cup	11.9 μg
Cheese, cottage	110 g (~1/2 cup)	11.2 μg
Rice, white, enriched, cooked	140 g (~3/4 cup)	10.5 μg
Cheerios cereal	30 g (1 cup)	10.4 μg
Grits, corn, enriched, cooked	1 cup	7.5 μg

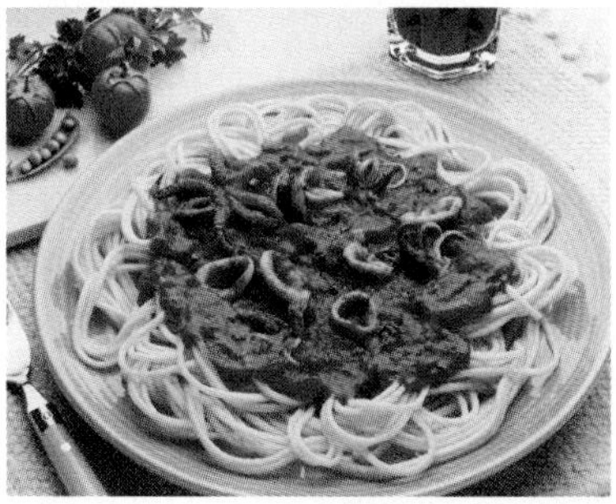

Figure 12.17 **Food sources of selenium.** Selenium is found mainly in meats, organ meats, seafood, and grains.
Source: U.S. Department of Agriculture, Agricultural Research Service. USDA National Nutrient Database for Standard Reference, Release 18. 2005. http://www.ars.usda.gov/nutrientdata.

goiter A chronic enlargement of the thyroid gland, visible as a swelling at the front of the neck; usually associated with iodine deficiency.

triiodothyronine (T3) An iodine-containing thyroid hormone with several times the biologic activity of thyroxine (T4).

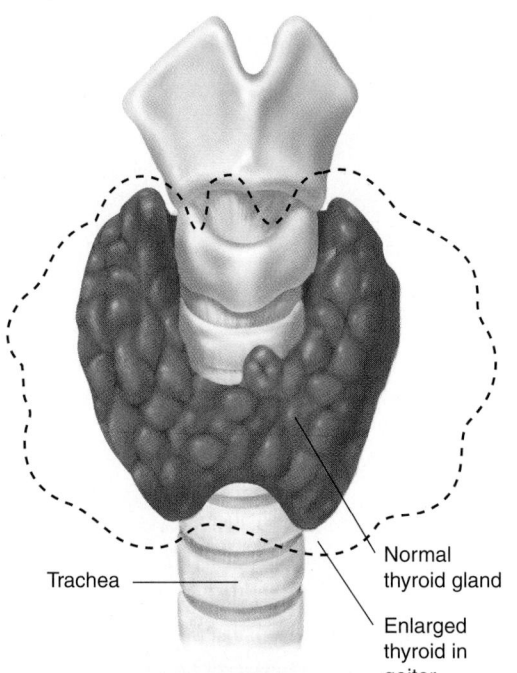

Trachea

Normal thyroid gland

Enlarged thyroid in goiter

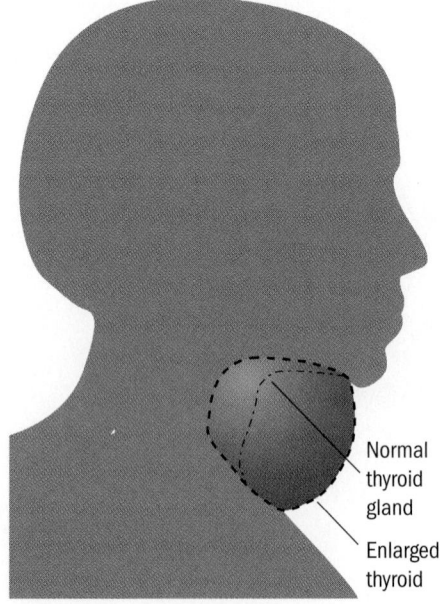

Normal thyroid gland

Enlarged thyroid

Figure 12.18 **Enlargement of the thyroid gland in goiter.** Iodine deficiency results in goiter. Use of iodized salt dramatically reduces goiter rates. This finding led to the widespread fortification of table salt with iodine.

Iodine

Ancient Chinese writings first recorded descriptions of what we now know to be the iodine-deficiency diseases cretinism and **goiter** (see **Figure 12.18**). Cretins were described as feeble-minded dwarfs with puffy facial features and a stumbling gait. In the Middle Ages, European paintings commonly depicted cretins as angels or demons.[50] As late as the early 1900s, goiter was common in certain parts of the United States, particularly the upper Midwest. In 1922 scientists demonstrated that the use of iodized salt by 50,000 school children dramatically reduced goiter rates. These findings led to the widespread fortification of table salt with iodine (I). Although iodine deficiency remains a problem in many parts of the world, the World Health Organization plans to eradicate iodine-deficiency disorders within the next decade through the use of iodized salt programs.[51]

Functions of Iodine

Iodine is an essential component of the two thyroid hormones: **triiodothyronine (T3)** and **thyroxine (T4)**. Thyroid hormones control the regulation of body temperature, basal metabolic rate, reproduction, and growth. Although the thyroid hormones released by the thyroid gland are about 93 percent thyroxine and only 7 percent triiodothyronine, triiodothyronine is about four times more potent than thyroxine.[52] Within a few days of secretion, the body converts most of the thyroxine to the more active triiodothyronine.

Iodine Absorption and Metabolism

Much of the iodine in foods is in the form of iodide (the reduced form) and iodates. The intestine absorbs nearly all of it, from 95 to 100 percent. The entire body contains between 15 and 20 milligrams, 70 to 80 percent of which resides in the thyroid gland. Each day the thyroid gland "traps" between 60 and 120 micrograms of iodide for eventual incorporation into the thyroid hormones. Enzymes oxidize the iodide, and then other enzymes bind it to **thyroglobulin**, the storage form of thyroid hormones.

Thyroid stimulating hormone (TSH) signals the thyroid gland to cleave T3 and T4 from thyroglobulin and release them into the bloodstream. In various body organs, three different enzymes convert most of the T4 to T3. Research reveals that all three of these converting enzymes are selenium dependent. Therefore, a deficiency in selenium may lead to inefficient use of iodine in thyroid hormones.

The kidneys excrete most excess iodine in urine, but some is lost in sweat, especially in hot, humid climates.

Dietary Recommendations for Iodine

To replace losses and prevent deficiency of iodine, the thyroid gland needs at least 60 micrograms daily. Because iodine absorption is very efficient, intakes of 75 micrograms per day should be sufficient for adults. To provide a margin of safety, however, the RDA is set at 150 micrograms per day for both men and women.

Sources of Iodine

Because the ocean is the best source of iodine, the best food sources are seafoods. Saltwater fish have higher concentrations of iodine than fresh water fish. The dairy industry adds iodide to cattle feed and uses sanitizing

Think About It

solutions that contain iodine. These measures add substantial amounts of iodine to milk and dairy products. Natural iodine levels in plants reflect soil levels. For many people, iodized salt used in cooking and at the table is their primary source of iodine. In the United States, iodized salt contains an average of 76 micrograms of iodine per gram of salt.

Excluding iodized salt, the average U.S. diet contains between 230 and 400 micrograms of iodine per day. After salt, dairy products supply most of our dietary iodine, followed by 10 to 15 percent from meat, fish, and poultry and 5 to 15 percent from grains and cereals. Salt added during cooking and at the table contributes 35 to 70 micrograms of iodide to the average adult's daily diet. **Figure 12.19** shows the iodine content of some foods.

Iodine Deficiency

As early as 1830, iodine deficiency was linked to the presence of goiter. We now understand that a deficiency of iodine inhibits the synthesis of thyroid hormones. As the body senses the lack of thyroid hormones, it produces more and more TSH. TSH causes the thyroid gland to grow, eventually resulting in a goiter. Goiter in children has been linked to depressed IQ[53] in addition to the usual symptoms of hypothyroidism—cold intolerance, weight gain, sluggishness, and a decreased body temperature.

Severe iodine deficiency during early pregnancy causes cretinism. Most cretins have stunted growth and are deaf, mute, and mentally retarded. A selenium deficiency may be partly responsible for a form of cretinism commonly seen in Africa.

Raw cabbage, turnips, rutabagas, and cassava contain compounds known as **goitrogens**, which are compounds that block the body's absorption and use of iodine. Consuming large amounts of these foods in their raw form can cause problems; cooking inactivates the goitrogens. Iodine-deficiency disorders are common in developing countries where iodine consumption is low and raw cassava and similar vegetables are a major part of the diet.

Iodine Toxicity

Because high amounts of iodine inhibit synthesis of thyroid hormones and stimulate growth of the thyroid gland, iodine toxicity also can cause goiter. Overzealous supplementation is the most common cause of iodine toxicity. A successful program of iodine fortification must be balanced against the risk of iodine-induced hyperthyroidism, especially in areas of severe iodine deficiency. The UL for iodine is 1,100 micrograms per day.

Key Concepts: *Iodine is an essential component of thyroid hormones. Iodine deficiency causes overstimulation of the thyroid gland and eventual goiter. The best food source of iodine is seafood. Many people around the world are still at risk for iodine deficiency, but iodization of salt is a powerful preventive measure.*

IODINE

Daily Value = 150 μg

High: 20% DV or more	Cod, cooked	85 g (3 oz)	99 μg
	Corn grits, enriched, cooked	1 cup	68 μg
	Milk, 2% milkfat	240 ml (1 cup)	56 μg
	Milk, nonfat	240 ml (1 cup)	51 μg
	White bread	50 g (~2 slices)	46 μg
	Tortilla, flour	55 g	41 μg
	Beef liver, cooked	85 g (3 oz)	36 μg
	Navy beans, cooked	90 g (~1/2 cup)	35 μg
	Shrimp, cooked	85 g (3 oz)	35 μg
	Potato, baked	110 g (1 small)	34 μg
	Turkey breast, cooked	85 g (3 oz)	34 μg
	Whole-wheat bread	50 g (~2 slices)	32 μg
Good: 10–19% DV	Egg, cooked	50 g (1 large)	24 μg
	Oatmeal, cooked	1 cup	16 μg

Figure 12.19 **Food sources of iodine.** Few foods are rich in iodine; it is found mainly in milk, seafood, and some grain products.
Source: Pennington JAT. *Bowes and Church's Food Values of Portions Commonly Used.* 17th ed. Philadelphia, PA: Lippincott-Raven Publishers, 1998.

Quick Bites

Iodine or Iodide: What's in a Name?

Iodine (I_2) is a bluish-black solid that gives off a purple vapor, which gives the element its name. Iodine stems from the Greek word *iôdêdes*, meaning "violet-colored."

Iodide (I^-) is the colorless negative ion of iodine. Iodine circulates in the body bound either to protein or as free iodide ions. Sodium iodide and potassium iodide are iodide salts commonly used in medicines.

thyroxine (T4) An iodine-containing hormone secreted by the thyroid gland to regulate the rate of cell metabolism; known chemically as tetraiodothyronine.

thyroglobulin The storage form of thyroid hormone in the thyroid gland.

thyroid-stimulating hormone (TSH) Secreted from the pituitary gland at the base of the brain, a hormone that regulates synthesis of thyroid hormones.

goitrogens Compounds that can induce goiter.

Menkes' syndrome A genetic disorder that results in copper deficiency.

ceruloplasmin A copper-dependent enzyme responsible for the oxidation of ferrous ion (Fe^{2+}) to ferric ion (Fe^{3+}), enabling iron to bind to transferrin. Also known as ferroxidase I.

Copper

Researchers first recognized the essential nature of copper (Cu) for experimental animals in 1928, but not until the 1960s did evidence emerge that copper deficiency occurs in humans. Cloning of the genes for two genetic disorders of copper metabolism—Wilson's disease (copper toxicity) and **Menkes' syndrome** (copper deficiency)—has fueled interest in copper and led to exciting new discoveries about its metabolism and physiological role. Although simple dietary copper deficiency is not a significant public health concern, excessive supplementation with other trace minerals can cause a secondary copper deficiency.

Functions of Copper

Copper-containing enzymes have many functions, including acting as an antioxidant, participating in the electron transport chain, and aiding the biosynthesis of the pigment melanin and the connective tissue proteins collagen and elastin. Perhaps the most important function of copper is as a component of **ceruloplasmin**, the enzyme that catalyzes the oxidation of ferrous (Fe^{2+}) to ferric (Fe^{3+}) iron for incorporation into transferrin. The absence of ceruloplasmin leads to accumulation of iron in the liver, similar to what is seen in iron overload or hemochromatosis. Copper is an important component of the superoxide dismutases, enzymes involved in antioxidant reactions. Copper also plays a role in various other activities, including the myelinization of the nervous tissue, immune function, and cardiovascular function.

Copper Absorption, Use, and Metabolism

Depending on the amount of copper in the meal and other dietary factors, the intestine absorbs approximately 50 percent of dietary copper. Amino acids, particularly histidine, enhance copper absorption. On the other hand, a number of minerals, most notably iron and zinc, may interfere with copper absorption. Because high-dose iron supplementation is more common than zinc supplementation, the iron–copper interaction is of greater concern. Dietary phytates do not appear to inhibit copper absorption. Because copper is best absorbed in an acidic environment, antacids can reduce copper absorption.

Albumin transports copper from the intestinal cells to the liver, where about two-thirds is incorporated into ceruloplasmin. The average healthy adult body contains approximately 100 milligrams of copper at any time, mainly distributed among the liver, brain, blood, and bone marrow. The body stores relatively little copper, and excretes nearly all excess copper in feces and a minor amount in the urine. Copper excreted in the feces includes unabsorbed dietary copper, copper released in bile, and copper in cells sloughed from the intestinal wall.

Dietary Recommendations and Food Sources for Copper

There is no single reliable index of copper status. Balance studies have been previously used to estimate copper needs. However, balance studies in humans are problematic, so a combination of plasma, serum, and blood cell measures were used to develop the copper RDA.[54] The RDA for both men and women is 900 micrograms per day.

Copper is widely distributed in foods. The richest food sources include organ meats (e.g., liver), shellfish, nuts and seeds, legumes, peanut butter, and chocolate. (See **Figure 12.20**.) Although information about the copper

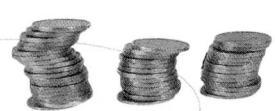

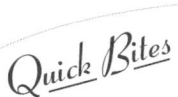

Quick Bites

A Penny for Your …

How do the amounts of zinc and copper in a U.S. penny compare to the amounts in your body? Today's penny is mostly zinc (2.4 grams), covered with some copper plating (62.5 mg). A penny's zinc is in the upper range of the body's zinc content, but the amount of copper falls short. It takes the copper in about $1\frac{1}{2}$ pennies to equal the amount of copper in your body.

content of foods is incomplete, dietary surveys in the United States suggest that adults consume an average of about 1,000 to 1,600 micrograms of copper per day.[55]

Copper Deficiency

Overt copper deficiency is relatively rare in humans. Copper deficiency occurs most commonly in preterm infants. These babies have low copper stores at birth and a rapid growth rate, which elevates needs. Because cow's milk has little copper and it is poorly bioavailable, infants who are inappropriately fed unmodified cow's milk are more likely to develop a deficiency than breastfed infants. Doctors have also observed copper deficiency, albeit less frequently than zinc deficiency, in people with malabsorption syndromes.[56]

Copper deficiency most commonly causes anemia, decreased numbers of white blood cells, and bone abnormalities. In copper-deficiency anemia, low ceruloplasmin activity causes defective iron mobilization. Copper-deficient young children often suffer bone abnormalities. Probably caused by poor synthesis of connective tissue, these abnormalities mimic the changes observed in scurvy. In experimental settings, copper deficiency causes elevated blood cholesterol, impaired glucose tolerance, and heart-related abnormalities. Some scientists suggest that copper deficiency during pregnancy may cause numerous gross structural and biochemical birth defects.[57]

Menkes' syndrome is an extremely rare (~ 1 in 100,000 live births) genetic copper disorder in which there is a failure to absorb copper into the bloodstream and therefore a lack of functional copper-containing proteins such as ceruloplasmin. Serum copper and ceruloplasmin levels are low, but copper accumulates in the intestinal mucosal cells and in the muscle, spleen, and kidney.[58] Menkes' syndrome causes neurological degeneration, peculiar kinky hair, abnormal connective tissue development, osteoporosis,

Quick Bites

Egg Whites? Please Stand Up!

Although cooking food in a copper pot is inadvisable, copper mixing bowls can be a plus. Meringues made in ceramic or steel bowls tend to be snowy white and drier than those made in copper bowls. Making meringue in a copper bowl leads to a creamier, yellowish foam that is harder to overbeat into a lumpy liquid. The copper bowl contributes copper ions to conalbumin, a metal-binding egg protein, thus stabilizing the whipped egg whites.

COPPER

Daily Value = 2 mg

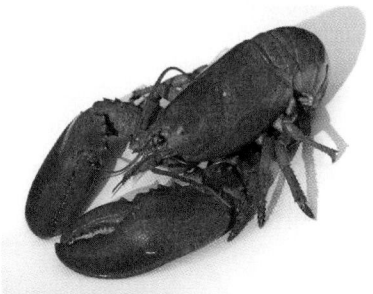

Exceptionally good sources		
Beef liver, cooked	85 g (3 oz)	12.1 mg
Oysters, cooked	85 g (3 oz)	6.4 mg

High: 20% DV or more

Lobster, cooked	85 g (3 oz)	1.6 mg
Crab, Alaska King, cooked	85 g (3 oz)	1.0 mg
Cashews	30 g (~1 oz)	0.6 mg
Clams, cooked	85 g (3 oz)	0.6 mg
Sunflower seeds	30 g (~1 oz)	0.5 mg
Hazelnuts	30 g (~1 oz)	0.5 mg
Mushrooms, cooked	85 g (~1/2 cup)	0.4 mg
Navy beans, cooked	90 g (~1/2 cup)	0.4 mg
Soy milk	240 ml (1 cup)	0.4 mg

Good: 10–19% DV

Tofu, calcium processed	85 g (~1/3 cup)	0.3 mg
Baked beans, canned	130 g (~1/2 cup)	0.3 mg
Peanuts	30 g (1 oz)	0.3 mg
Refried beans, canned	130 g (~1/2 cup)	0.2 mg
Cocoa, dry powder	1 Tbsp	0.2 mg

Figure 12.20 **Food sources of copper.** Copper is found in a limited variety of foods. The best sources are seafood, legumes, and nuts.

Source: U.S. Department of Agriculture, Agricultural Research Service. USDA National Nutrient Database for Standard Reference, Release 18. 2005. http://www.ars.usda.gov/nutrientdata.

chelation therapy Use of a chelator (e.g., EDTA) to bind metal ions to remove them from the body.

Quick Bites

Cooking in Copper

Because the copper imparted a bright green color to cooked green vegetables, cooking vegetables in uncoated copper pans was once encouraged. This practice often led to decreased liver and brain function. The Swedish military recognized copper toxicity and banned copper cooking utensils in 1753.

Quick Bites

Highway Harvest

Oil companies often add a type of manganese to modern gasoline as an antiknock compound to increase the octane rating for high-compression engines. It is now evident that plants along highways accumulate manganese from passing cars.

and poor growth. Although this syndrome is usually fatal in infancy or early childhood, copper-histidine treatment within the first few days of life may prevent irreversible damage.[59]

Copper Toxicity

Compared to other trace elements, copper is relatively nontoxic. The UL for copper is 10,000 micrograms per day. Wilson's disease is a rare (1 in 200,000) genetic copper toxicity disorder that impairs copper excretion in bile, causing toxic accumulation in the liver, brain, kidney, and eye. As copper accumulates in red blood cells, it causes anemia. People with Wilson's disease frequently appear healthy until adolescence or early adulthood. Without treatment, they develop serious liver and neurological problems. Copper toxicity may be treated either by **chelation therapy** to bind and remove copper or with zinc supplementation to decrease copper absorption. Lifelong treatment can prevent many complications of Wilson's disease.

Key Concepts: *The most important function of copper is as a component of ceruloplasmin, the enzyme that catalyzes the oxidation of iron for transport in transferrin. Food sources for copper include organ meats, shellfish, nuts and seeds, legumes, peanut butter, chocolate, and dried fruits. Copper deficiency is relatively rare in humans. Usual copper intakes fall below the current safe and adequate level.*

Manganese

Recognized for centuries, manganese (Mn) derives its name from a Greek term for magic. Although its many functions are not magical, they are unique. Manganese is essential not only in biological systems but also in iron and steel production. It has many industrial uses in such diverse products as dry-cell batteries, glass, ceramics, paints, varnishes, inks, dyes, and fertilizers. Industrial exposure, rather than excessive intake, is the more frequent cause of manganese toxicity.

Functions of Manganese

The body contains between 10 and 20 milligrams of manganese, which is concentrated primarily in the bone, liver, pancreas, and brain. Despite this limited quantity, manganese is a key component of several enzymes:

- *Mn-superoxide dismutase,* located in the mitochondria of cells, is an antioxidant that prevents tissue damage due to lipid oxidation.
- *Arginase* helps form urea in the urea cycle.
- *Pyruvate carboxylase* helps convert pyruvate to oxaloacetate.

Manganese also activates numerous enzymes involved in the formation of cartilage in bone and skin.

Manganese Absorption, Use, and Homeostasis

Absorption of manganese is poor, only 1 to 15 percent. This low absorption rate may protect against toxicity. Some research suggests that high levels of iron, calcium, and phosphorus may inhibit absorption. Fiber and phytate also may limit manganese absorption, but to a lesser degree than they affect the absorption of most other trace minerals. Following absorption, transferrin binds manganese and transports it in the bloodstream.

Excretion, rather than absorption, regulates the body's manganese. Bile is the main excretory route. Should the intestine absorb excess manganese, the body may quickly dump this excess back into the intestine as part of bile. There is no storage form of manganese. As with zinc, there does not appear to be a reliable indicator of manganese status in adults.

Dietary Recommendations and Food Sources for Manganese

The AI for manganese is 2.3 milligrams per day for men and 1.8 milligrams per day for women. Before 2001, manganese recommendations were higher: 2.0 to 5.0 milligrams per day. These recommendations were questioned, however, because they were close to the toxic levels suggested by the Environmental Protection Agency: more than 10 milligrams manganese per day from food or more than 4.2 milligrams from water.[60]

Tea, nuts, cereals, and some fruits are the best food sources of manganese. Some estimates suggest that coffee or tea supplies as much as 20 to 30 percent of our daily manganese intake. Meat, dairy products, poultry, fish, and refined foods are poor sources; they contain little manganese. **Figure 12.21** shows the manganese content of some foods.

Manganese Deficiency

Although people who consume normal varied diets do not appear to be at risk for manganese deficiency, certain disorders may cause suboptimal status. Studies report low manganese or altered manganese metabolism in some patients with nontrauma epilepsy, phenylketonuria (PKU),[61] **amyotrophic lateral sclerosis (ALS)**,[62] and **multiple sclerosis**. In animal studies, manganese deficiency has dramatic effects—impaired growth, skeletal abnormalities, a staggering gait, and impaired fat and carbohydrate metabolism.

amyotrophic lateral sclerosis (ALS) A syndrome marked by muscular weakness and atrophy due to a degeneration of motor neurons of the spinal cord.

multiple sclerosis A progressive disease that destroys the myelin sheath surrounding nerve fibers of the brain and spinal cord.

MANGANESE

Daily Value = 2 mg

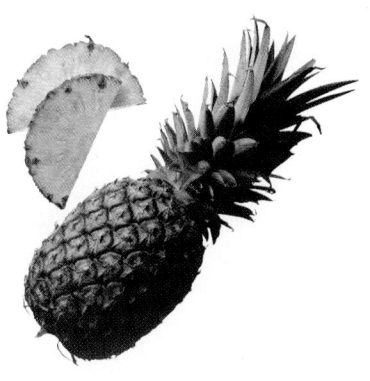

Exceptionally good sources

Pineapple, fresh	140 g (~1 cup)	2.2 mg
Wheat germ	15 g (1/4 cup)	2.0 mg
Hazelnuts	30 g (~1 oz)	1.9 mg
Wheat-bran flakes cereal	30 g (3/4 cup)	1.6 mg
Oatmeal, cooked	1 cup	1.3 mg
Rice, brown, cooked	140 g (~3/4 cup)	1.3 mg
Whole-wheat bread	50 g (2 slices)	1.2 mg
Lima beans, cooked	90 g (~1/2 cup)	1.1 mg
Blackberries, fresh	140 g (~1 cup)	0.9 mg
Spinach, cooked	85 g (~1/2 cup)	0.8 mg
Soybeans, cooked	90 g (~1/2 cup)	0.5 mg
Tea, brewed	240 ml (1 cup)	0.5 mg
Sweet potato, cooked	110 g (1 small)	0.5 mg
Okra, cooked	85 g (~1/2 cup)	0.3 mg
Turnip greens, cooked	85 g (~1/2 cup)	0.3 mg
Beets, cooked	85 g (~1/2 cup)	0.3 mg
Broccoli, cooked	85 g (~1/2 cup)	0.2 mg
Cocoa, dry powder	1 Tbsp	0.2 mg

High: 20% DV or more

Good: 10–19% DV

Figure 12.21 **Food sources of manganese.** Manganese is found mainly in plant foods such as grains, legumes, vegetables, and some fruits.
Source: U.S. Department of Agriculture, Agricultural Research Service. USDA National Nutrient Database for Standard Reference, Release 18. 2005. http://www.ars.usda.gov/nutrientdata.

mineralization The addition of minerals, such as calcium and phosphorus, to bones and teeth.

fluorosis Mottled discoloration and pitting of tooth enamel caused by prolonged ingestion of excessive fluoride.

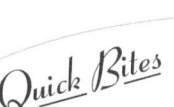

Quick Bites

Accidental Discovery

*I*n the early 1900s people noticed that inhabitants of towns with naturally high levels of fluoride in their water had healthier teeth. To test the correlation between fluoride and tooth decay, in 1945 four cities in the United States and one in Canada took part in a controlled study of water fluoridation. The results were impressive, establishing that fluoride helps to prevent tooth decay.

Manganese Toxicity

Manganese toxicity is a greater threat than manganese deficiency. Foundry workers exposed to airborne manganese dust have experienced severe manganese toxicity. Their symptoms included irritability, hallucinations, and severe lack of coordination. Lower doses of airborne manganese can impair memory and cause impaired motor coordination similar to that experienced in Parkinson's disease. The UL for manganese is 11 milligrams per day.

Key Concepts: *Manganese is important to the functioning of several enzymes in the human body. Our usual intake of manganese falls within the currently recommended intake range. Food sources for manganese are tea, coffee, cereals, and some fruits. Toxicity is more a threat than deficiency is, primarily to people who are exposed industrially to high levels of manganese dust.*

Fluoride

Fluoride (F), the ionized form of fluorine, has the unique ability to prevent dental caries. Although people first observed this beneficial effect in the early 1800s, scientific proof did not emerge until the time of World War II. In 1945 many U.S. water suppliers began voluntarily fluoridating water to improve the dental health of children. Now that use of fluoridated toothpaste and mouthwash is widespread, some experts are raising concerns about potential harm from excessive fluoride intake.

Functions of Fluoride

Bones and teeth contain nearly 99 percent of the body's fluoride. Fluoride supports the **mineralization** of bones and teeth by promoting the deposition of calcium and phosphorus.

Fluoride's cavity-prevention activity is an effect localized in the mouth. Bacteria in the mouth cause dental caries, an infectious disease. When a person eats food, especially carbohydrate foods, these oral bacteria multiply and produce organic acids that eat away tooth enamel, especially beneath plaque. When food leaves the mouth, remineralization begins. If remineralization does not keep pace with demineralization, your teeth become pitted with dental caries. Fluoride decreases the demineralization of tooth enamel and accelerates the subsequent remineralization process. It also inhibits bacterial activity in dental plaques. These cavity-fighting actions can help make your next trip to the dentist a pleasant one.

Regular ingestion of fluoride is especially important during the eruption of new teeth in children. When administered topically, fluoride's support of tooth enamel remineralization can benefit people of all ages.

Fluoride Absorption and Excretion

Your body absorbs almost all the fluoride in water and other liquid beverages. The bioavailability of fluoride in food ranges between 50 and 80 percent. After absorption, the body distributes fluoride in "hard" tissues, mainly the bones and teeth. Excess fluoride is excreted mainly in the urine.

Dietary Recommendations for Fluoride

The AI for fluoride is 4 milligrams per day for adult men, and 3 milligrams per day for women. As of 1995, the American Dental Association and American Academy of Pediatrics no longer recommend fluoride supplementation from birth, and suggest it only for children whose drinking water supplies less than 0.6 milligram per liter. The AI for fluoride for infants is 0.01 milligram per day for ages 0 to 5 months and 0.5 milligram per day for ages 6 to 11 months.

Sources of Fluoride

Water is the main source of fluoride, whether the fluoride is naturally present or added. Artificially fluoridated water contains 0.7 to 1.2 milligrams per liter. Fluoride naturally present in drinking water may vary from less than 0.1 milligram to more than 10 milligrams per liter. The Environmental Protection Agency's regulations require public drinking water systems to remove excess fluoride so that it does not exceed 4.0 milligrams per liter. Almost two-thirds of the U.S. population receive optimally fluoridated water;[63] most other developed countries do not fluoridate their water.

The balance between the positive effects of just enough fluoride and the negative effects of too much fluoride has become the subject of debate. Some scientists argue that artificial fluoridation is an outdated practice. Fluoridation was instituted 50 years ago, when it served as the exclusive source of fluoride for children. Now, however, there are other fluoride sources, including ready-to-feed infant formulas, fluoride supplements, mouthwash, toothpaste, and some beverages. The combination of all of these sources may put children at increased risk for excessive fluoride intake and **fluorosis**.

Because there are so many sources of fluoride, it is difficult to determine the current effectiveness of artificial fluoridation of the water supply. Some opponents argue that artificial fluoridation is inappropriate and "equal to mass medication of the population."[64] However, the dramatic decline in dental carries since fluoridation was initiated is undeniable. To retain the benefits yet avoid overconsumption, the American Dental Association recommends the fluoridation of all water supplies and regulation of other fluoride sources.

Fluoride Deficiency, Toxicity, and Pharmacological Applications

Low fluoride intake increases the risk for dental caries and may hamper the integrity of bone. Adequate fluoride intake in childhood can decrease the incidence of tooth decay by 30 to 60 percent. During tooth development, prolonged excessive fluoride intake can cause fluorosis. (See **Figure 12.22**.) In mild fluorosis, white specks form on the teeth. Severe fluorosis can cause permanent brownish stains and weakened teeth. Consumption of water naturally high in fluoride is the main cause of fluorosis, but children who chronically swallow large amounts of fluoridated toothpaste are also at risk. The UL for fluoride is 10 milligrams per day.

Hemodialysis patients who have been given too much fluoride can suffer acute fluoride toxicity with symptoms that include headaches, nausea, and abnormal heart rhythms. Other observed effects of fluorosis include hip fractures, chronic gastritis, and weak, stiff joints.

Researchers have studied fluoride for the treatment of osteoporosis in postmenopausal women. A daily dose of 75 milligrams of sodium fluoride increased spinal bone density, but it also increased the number of nonspine fractures.[65] Subsequent studies using lower amounts of fluoride (25 mg/day) combined with supplemental calcium reduced the risk of fracture. Fluoride is not an approved treatment for osteoporosis.

Think
About It
4

American Dietetic Association

The Impact of Fluoride on Health

The American Dietetic Association reaffirms that fluoride is an important element for all mineralized tissues in the body. Appropriate fluoride exposure and usage is beneficial to bone and tooth integrity and, as such, has an important, positive impact on health throughout life.

J Am Diet Assoc. 2005;105:1620–1628.
Reprinted with permission.

Quick Bites

Conspiracy Theory

Although the U.S. Public Health Service and the World Health Organization officially endorsed the fluoridation of water in the 1950s, some groups continue to oppose the practice. Objectors claim that water fluoridation violates civil rights, that fluoride is a "nerve poison," and that fluoride is unwanted compulsory medication that can have dangerous side effects. Some groups even claim that fluoridation is a component of a conspiracy for national destruction. So far, objectors have been unable to substantiate their claims and the courts have upheld the constitutionality of fluoridation.

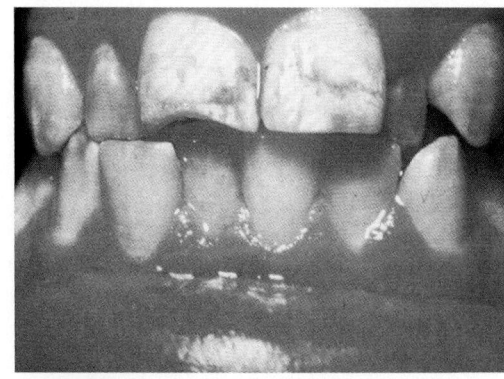

Figure 12.22 **Tooth mottling in fluorosis.** During tooth development, prolonged excessive fluoride intake can cause fluorosis, which discolors and damages teeth.

Key Concepts: *Bones and teeth contain 99 percent of body fluoride. Fluoride supports remineralization, and its major function is the prevention of dental caries. Fluoride is unique in that the main dietary source is water, not food. The majority of our nation's municipal water supplies are artificially fluoridated. Excess fluoride can cause fluorosis. Mild fluorosis with mottling of the teeth is primarily a cosmetic problem; severe fluorosis can weaken teeth.*

Chromium

Chromium (Cr) plays an important but poorly understood role in moving glucose into cells, and in lipid metabolism. Although researchers established chromium's essential role in glucose tolerance during the late 1950s and early 1960s, the development of reliable analytical methods took another 20 years. As with many trace minerals, low levels in biological tissues and the potential for sample contamination make chromium assessment particularly challenging.[66]

Functions of Chromium

Chromium enhances the effects of insulin and is important for proper metabolism of carbohydrates and lipids. It also may play a role in metabolism of nucleic acids and in immune function and growth. Athletes are especially interested in chromium because of its purported effects on body composition.

Chromium Absorption, Transport, and Excretion

Little is known about chromium absorption. Uptake of the inorganic form is thought to be low (about 1 to 2 percent); absorption of organic chromium (a combination of chromium and an organic acid such as chromium picolinate) may be higher (10 to 25 percent). Absorption increases with need and decreases with higher amounts in the diet. Other substances can influence chromium absorption. For example, vitamin C and aspirin increase chromium absorption, and antacids decrease it.[67]

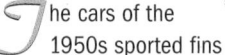

Quick Bites

Chrome-Plated Cars

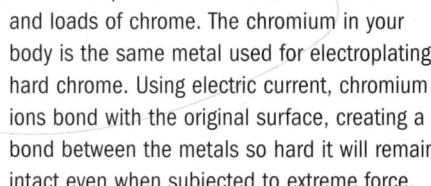

The cars of the 1950s sported fins and loads of chrome. The chromium in your body is the same metal used for electroplating hard chrome. Using electric current, chromium ions bond with the original surface, creating a bond between the metals so hard it will remain intact even when subjected to extreme force.

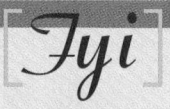

[*Fyi*] Chromium, Exercise, and Body Composition

FOR YOUR INFORMATION

Because chromium supplements are purported to increase lean body mass (LBM) and decrease body fat during resistance training, they have generated a great deal of popular interest. Yet study results are contradictory and chromium's influence on body composition is controversial. The USDA's Human Nutrition Research Center in Beltsville, Maryland, reviewed numerous studies of chromium and body composition.[1] Although several of the studies show that chromium supplementation positively affects gains achieved with resistance training, a number of other experiments show no effect.[2]

What are the issues raised by these studies and how are we to understand the contradictory results? After researchers reported the initial positive results, the press and supplement advertisers overstated the benefits of chromium supplementation, thereby creating unrealistic expectations for improvement in muscle mass. Supplement makers marketed chromium picolinate, the form used in most studies, as the healthy alternative to anabolic steroids, and inappropriately extended the research findings to suggest that chromium would be effective as a weight-loss product.[3] Although one study did show a decrease in percentage of body fat in a

group of sedentary subjects, 20 *years* of studies show that chromium has no significant effect as a weight-loss agent.[4] In 1996 the Federal Trade Commission (FTC) ordered the maker of chromium picolinate to stop making unsubstantiated claims of weight loss and health benefits.

Differences in experimental design explain many of these inconsistent results. In some studies the dosage may have been too low and the time period may have been too short to show any effect. One of the limitations of any chromium study is the inability to assess the initial status of the subjects.

Transferrin and **albumin** transport chromium in the bloodstream. The body contains approximately 4 to 6 milligrams of chromium, mostly in the liver, spleen, and bone; the remainder is widely dispersed at very low concentrations. The body excretes excess chromium in the urine.

Chromium levels in hair, sweat, and serum decrease with age, but study results raise the question as to whether the decline is normal or an effect of the Western diet on chromium levels.[68] Some researchers speculate that the age-related decline in chromium may contribute to the high incidence of insulin resistance and type 2 diabetes in Western countries.

Dietary Recommendations and Food Sources for Chromium

For adults aged 19 to 50 years, the AI for chromium is 35 micrograms per day for men and 25 micrograms per day for women. The AI for older adults is 5 micrograms less. More data on actual requirements for chromium and the chromium content of foods are needed for more specific dietary recommendations.

The chromium content of foods varies widely. Good sources include brewer's yeast, processed meats, whole grains, green beans, broccoli, and spices. Cooking acidic foods in stainless steel containers leaches some chromium into the food.

Chromium Deficiency

The difficulty of assessing chromium status makes it hard to determine the effects of deficiency. Nevertheless, studies in animals and humans point to the following signs of chromium deficiency: decreased insulin-mediated glucose uptake by cells, decreased insulin sensitivity, elevated blood glucose and insulin, and blood lipid abnormalities. Doctors have observed more severe signs, such as brain and nerve disorders, in patients who subsist on total parenteral nutrition that has inadequate chromium.[69]

albumin A protein that circulates in the blood and functions in the transport of many minerals and some drugs.

There is no evidence that chromium supplements provide a "quick fix" for athletes, and long-term chromium intake probably has a minimal effect on body composition and body weight. Although the risk of toxicity from supplemental chromium alone is low, chromium can interact with iron and zinc, which raises concern about adverse effects. As is the case with many trace minerals, only further investigation will clarify the role of chromium in human health.

Studies have raised safety issues about chromium picolinate supplements. This organic form of chromium is very stable, and cells may acquire it intact. Within cells it can interact with peroxide to form the potentially DNA-damaging hydroxyl radical.[5] Researchers have found that chromium picolinate can cause chromosomal abnormalities in Chinese hamster ovary cells.[6] In addition, absorption rates of chromium picolinate in humans may be high enough to allow tissue levels similar to those shown to produce DNA damage.[7] Numerous health groups advise consumers to avoid chromium picolinate supplements.

The best advice for achieving a healthy, fit body? A varied diet, and regular exercise—not reliance on supplements.

1 Anderson RA. Effects of chromium on body composition and weight loss. *Nutr Rev.* 1998;56:266–270.

2 Evans GW. The effect of chromium picolinate on insulin controlled parameters in humans. *Int J Biosoc Med Res.* 1989;11:163–180.

3 Haymes EM, Clarkson PM. Minerals and trace minerals. In: Berning JR, Steen SN, eds. *Nutrition for Sport and Exercise.* 2nd ed. Sudbury, MA: Jones and Bartlett, 1998:95–98.

4 Anderson RA. Op. cit.

5 Speetjens JK, Collins RA, Vincent JB, Woski SA. The nutritional supplement chromium(III) tris(picolinate) cleaves DNA. *Chem Res Toxicol.* 1999;12:483–487.

6 Stearns DM, Wise JP, Patierno SR, Wetterhahn KE. Chromium(III) picolinate produces chromosome damage in Chinese hamster ovary cells. *FASEB J.* 1995;9:1643–1848.

7 Stearns DM, Belbruno JJ, Wetterhahn KE. A prediction of chromium(III) accumulation in humans from chromium dietary supplements. *FASEB J.* 1995;9:1650–1657.

Chromium Toxicity

The only known cases of chromium toxicity occurred in people exposed to airborne chromium compounds in industrial settings. Because inorganic chromium is so poorly absorbed, extremely high oral intakes would be necessary to attain toxic levels. Numerous experiments show 200 micrograms of inorganic chromium to be a safe dose for supplementation. Studies of chromium picolinate supplements show DNA damage in animal cells and have raised safety concerns about this supplemental form (see the FYI feature "Chromium, Exercise, and Body Composition"). To date, no UL has been set for chromium.

Key Concepts: *The primary function of chromium in the body is to potentiate the effects of insulin. Sources of chromium include mushrooms, dark chocolate, prunes, nuts, asparagus, whole grains, wine, brewer's yeast, and some beers. Reliable assessment of chromium status is difficult.*

Molybdenum

Molybdenum (Mo) is essential to both plants and animals. In humans, molybdenum functions as a cofactor for several enzymes that induce oxidation.

Molybdenum Absorption, Use, and Metabolism

The intestine absorbs molybdenum efficiently—some studies suggest up to 80 to 90 percent of the amount consumed. However, the body excretes it rapidly in urine and in bile. Fiber and phytate have no effect on its absorption. Dietary copper is the only significant inhibitor of molybdenum absorption. The body contains about 2 milligrams of molybdenum, 90 percent of which is located in the liver.

Dietary Recommendations and Food Sources for Molybdenum

For adults, the molybdenum RDA is 45 micrograms per day. Although data are limited, typical intakes in the United States exceed the RDA. Peas, beans, and some breakfast cereals are the richest food sources for molybdenum. Organ meats such as liver and kidney also are fairly rich sources, but other meats tend to be poor sources.

Molybdenum Deficiency and Toxicity

Molybdenum deficiency does not occur in people who eat a normal diet. People on total parenteral nutrition who do not receive molybdenum can suffer weakness, mental confusion, and night blindness. People with a rare congenital disorder have deficient amounts of sulfite oxidase, a molybdenum-dependent enzyme. These people suffer from neurological problems similar to those of severe molybdenum deficiency.

Scientists first recognized the interaction between dietary copper and molybdenum in sheep and cattle that grazed on grass grown on soil either very poor or very rich in molybdenum. If the soil content was low in molybdenum, the animals suffered copper toxicity; if the soil was rich, they were deficient in copper. Doctors exploit this interaction when they use a form of molybdenum to treat patients with Wilson's disease. Despite the possible interaction with copper, molybdenum salts are considered relatively nontoxic. The UL for molybdenum is 2,000 micrograms per day.

Quick Bites

Molybdenum Takes a Stand Against the Elements

Molybdenum is a silvery-gray metal that is not found free in nature. It has properties similar to tungsten and is used as an alloy to strengthen and protect metal from corrosion.

Key Concepts: *Several important enzymes require molybdenum. Good food sources include peas, beans, and some breakfast cereals. Healthy people with normal diets do not suffer molybdenum deficiency. High intakes of molybdenum may inhibit absorption of copper.*

Other Trace Elements and Ultratrace Elements

The body contains minuscule amounts of "ultratrace" minerals and may require less than 1 milligram per day of each one. At least 18 minerals could be considered ultratrace: aluminum, arsenic, boron, bromide, cadmium, chromium, fluoride, germanium, iodine, lead, lithium, molybdenum, nickel, rubidium, selenium, silicon, tin, and vanadium.[70] Dietary recommendations are fairly clear and there is substantial research on five of these minerals: iodine, fluoride, manganese, molybdenum, and selenium (all discussed previously). The functions of the remaining minerals are less clear. Although new evidence and media coverage have focused on arsenic, boron, nickel, silicon, and vanadium, data do not exist for the establishment of AIs or RDAs for these minerals. ULs have been set for boron, nickel, and vanadium. (See **Table 12.6.**)

Arsenic

Although arsenic (As) has been an infamous poison for centuries, inorganic arsenic may actually be an essential ultratrace element.[71] As a colorless, tasteless toxin, arsenic trioxide can be fatal in a dose as low as 2 milligrams. On the other hand, arsenic-deprived laboratory animals have poor growth and abnormal reproduction. Arsenic may also participate in methionine metabolism. Estimates of dietary intake of arsenic range from 15 micrograms per day for children to 60 micrograms per day for adult males.[72] The most concentrated food sources are oysters, mussels, and fish. In a typical diet, meat and fish supply about 30 percent of dietary arsenic, cereals and breads supply 20 percent, and starchy vegetables provide 15 percent. A UL has not been established for arsenic. Given arsenic's highly poisonous nature, much more careful research is required to establish recommended intake and UL levels.

Boron

Boron (B) appears to play an important role in bone metabolism, probably in conjunction with other nutrients such as calcium, magnesium, and vitamin D. Boron deficiency depresses growth and is worsened by a vitamin D deficiency. Conversely, boron supplementation lessens the bone abnormalities observed in vitamin D deficiency.

Fruits, nuts, vegetables, and legumes are the main sources of boron. The body absorbs close to 90 percent of the amount consumed and then promptly excretes most of it in the urine. The usual dietary intake of boron is between 1 and 2 milligrams per day.[73] Based on average consumption as well as supplementation studies, scientists estimate that the daily boron requirement is 1 milligram per day. Chronic boron toxicity symptoms include poor appetite, nausea, weight loss, and decreased sexual activity, seminal volume, and sperm count.[74] More research is needed to set safe lower limits for dietary intake. The UL for boron is 20 milligrams per day.

Nickel

Nickel (Ni) is widely distributed throughout the body in very low concentrations that add up to a total body content of approximately 10 milligrams. Most of the research on nickel has been conducted in animals; by extrapolation, scientists assume nickel is essential in humans.

Table 12.6	Tolerable Upper Intake Levels (UL) for Ultratrace Elements	
Arsenic		No UL set
Boron		20 mg/day
Nickel		1 mg/day
Silicon		No UL set
Vanadium		1.8 mg/day

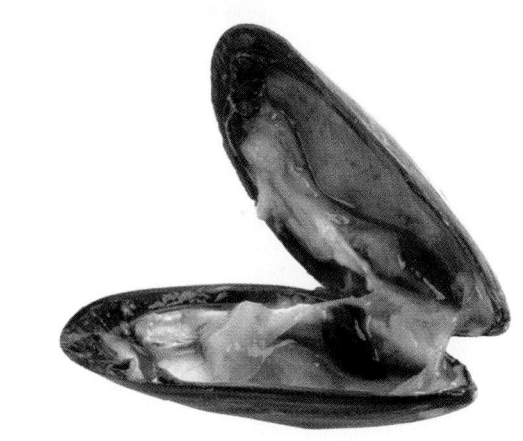

A few nickel-containing enzymes have been identified, and nickel can activate or inhibit a number of enzymes that usually contain other elements. Nickel alters the properties of cell membranes and affects oxidation-reduction systems in cells. Nickel also may function in vitamin B_{12} and folate metabolism.[75]

Nuts, legumes, grains, and vegetables are the best sources of nickel. Depending on the amount of plant foods consumed, dietary intake of nickel varies widely. An acceptable dietary intake of 100 to 300 micrograms per day has been proposed.[76] There is no known nickel deficiency in humans. Toxicity has occurred only in workers exposed to nickel dust or nickel carbonyl in industrial settings. The UL for nickel is 1 milligram per day.

Silicon

Silicon (Si) is the most common element in the earth's crust. The human body contains roughly 1.5 grams of silicon—less than the amount of magnesium, but about the same as iron and zinc. Connective tissues such as the aorta, trachea, tendon, bone, and skin contain much of the body's silicon. From animal studies, scientists hypothesize that silicon helps strengthen collagen and elastin. Experimental diets lacking silicon caused poor growth and skeletal abnormalities in baby chickens. However, there are no known symptoms of silicon deficiency in humans. Studies suggest silicon may help prevent atherosclerosis in the elderly. This element is relatively nontoxic when ingested orally, and no UL has been set for it. However, breathing airborne silicon particles may cause **silicosis**, a type of silicon toxicity.

silicosis A disease that results from excess silicon exposure.

Unrefined grains, cereals, vegetables, and fruits supply most of our dietary silicon. Animal foods are poor sources. Determining a dietary recommendation is difficult because of the lack of human studies showing signs of deficiency. A balance study conducted in the late 1970s suggests that adequate intake is between 21 and 46 milligrams per day.[77] The Total Diet Study conducted in the United States reported silicon intake between 19 and 40 milligrams per day.

Vanadium

In the body, vanadium (V) can exist in a form that is structurally similar to phosphate. Interestingly, in the late 1970s it was noted that *in vitro* vanadium inhibits ATP synthase, an enzyme required for ATP production. Presumably, vanadium replaces phosphate and blocks the reaction. In rats with experimentally induced diabetes, vanadium has also been shown to mimic insulin. However, a precise function for vanadium in humans has not been found, and given the tiny amounts that we consume, deficiencies have not been observed. The UL for vanadium is 1.8 milligrams per day.

Key Concepts: *Ultratrace minerals are elements with very low estimated requirements. Although specific biochemical functions have not been defined for the minerals arsenic, boron, nickel, silicon, and vanadium, they are thought to be essential for humans.*

Label [to] **Table**

If you looked at a list of minerals, could you pick out the trace minerals? Let's see how well you do! Look at the accompanying Nutrition Facts label from a breakfast cereal and guess how many trace minerals are listed.

You should be able to spot three trace minerals on the label: iron, zinc, and copper. Looking at the "ingredients" and "vitamins and minerals" lists, you can see that the iron and zinc were added but the copper appears to come naturally from the cereal. Why do you think these trace minerals are added to this cereal? Many people (especially children) eat marginal amounts of iron and zinc. The best sources of these minerals are meats, liver, and shellfish. Most children don't eat much shellfish or liver, so adding the minerals to cereals, which they do eat, is an easy way to make sure they get 45 percent and 25 percent of Daily Values for iron and zinc, respectively.

The last mineral you see listed is copper. There is 2% of the Daily Value for copper in one serving of this cereal. That's 0.04 milligram (2% of 2 mg).

Nutrition Facts

Serving Size: 1 cup (30g)
Servings Per Container about 9

Amount Per Serving	Cheerios	with ½ cup skim milk
Calories	110	150
Calories from Fat	15	20

	Cheerios % Daily Value**	with ½ cup skim milk
Total Fat 2g*	3%	3%
Saturated Fat 0g	0%	3%
Trans Fat 0g		
Polyunsaturated Fat 0.5g		
Monounsaturated Fat 0.5g		
Cholesterol 0mg	0%	1%
Sodium 280mg	12%	15%
Total Carbohydrate 22g	7%	9%
Dietary Fiber 3g	11%	11%
Soluble Fiber 1g	11%	11%
Sugars 1g	11%	11%
Other carbohydrates 1g		
Protein 3g		
Vitamin A	10%	15%
Vitamin C	10%	10%
Calcium	4%	20%
Iron	45%	45%
Vitamin D	10%	25%
Thiamin	25%	30%
Riboflavin	25%	35%
Niacin	25%	25%
Vitamin B₆	25%	25%
Folic Acid	50%	50%
Vitamin B₁₂	25%	35%
Phosphorus	10%	25%
Magnesium	8%	10%
Zinc	25%	30%
Copper	2%	2%

*Amount in Cereal. A serving of cereal plus skim milk provides 2g total fat (0.5g saturated fat, 1g monosaturated fat). less than 5mg cholesterol, 350mg sodium, 300mg potassium, 28g total carbohydrate (7g sugars) and 7g protein.

**Percent Daily Values are based on a 2,000 calorie diet. Your daily values may be higher or lower depending on your calorie needs:

	Calories:	2,000	2,500
Total Fat	Less Than	65g	80g
Sat Fat	Less Than	20g	25g
Cholesterol	Less Than	300mg	300mg
Sodium	Less Than	2,400mg	2,400mg
Potassium		3,500mg	3,500mg
Total Carbohydrate		300g	375g
Dietary Fiber	25g	30g	

INGREDIENTS: WHOLE GRAIN OATS (INCLUDES THE OAT BRAN), MODIFIED FOOD STARCH, SUGAR, SALT, OAT FIBER, TRISODIUM PHOSPHATE, CALCIUM CARBONATE, VITAMIN E (MIXED TOCOPHEROLS) ADDED TO PRESERVE FRESHNESS.

VITAMINS AND MINERALS: IRON AND ZINC (MINERAL NUTRIENTS), VITAMIN C (SODIUM ASCORBATE), A B VITAMIN (NIACINAMIDE), VITAMIN B₆ (PYRIDOXINE HYDROCHLORIDE), VITAMIN B₂ (RIBOFLAVIN), VITAMIN B₁ (THIAMIN MONONITRATE), VITAMIN A (PALMITATE), A B VITAMIN (FOLIC ACID), VITAMIN B₁₂, VITAMIN D.

LEARNING *Portfolio* c h a p t e r   1 2

Key Terms

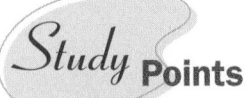

	page		page
acrodermatitis enteropathica	512	Keshan disease	512
albumin	525	Menkes' syndrome	518
amyotrophic lateral sclerosis (ALS)	521	metalloproteins	507
		metallothionein	508
ceruloplasmin	518	mineralization	522
chelation therapy	520	multiple sclerosis	521
cretinism	513	myelinization	499
Crohn's disease	511	myoglobin	498
cytochromes	499	nonheme iron	500
ferric iron (Fe³⁺)	498	polyphenols	502
ferritin	500	protoporphyrin	505
ferrous iron (Fe²⁺)	498	selenocysteine	513
fluorosis	522	selenomethionine	513
galvanized	507	silicosis	528
geophagia	507	thyroglobulin	517
goiter	516	thyroid-stimulating hormone (TSH)	517
goitrogens	517		
hematocrit	506	thyroxine (T4)	517
heme	498	total parenteral nutrition (TPN)	515
heme iron	500		
hemodialysis	511	transferrin	500
hemosiderin	503	transferrin receptors	503
hypogonadism	507	transferrin saturation	505
hypothyroidism	513	triiodothyronine (T3)	516
iron overload	506	Wilson's disease	512

Study Points

➤ Trace elements are minerals that the body needs in small amounts. They are involved in a variety of structural and regulatory functions and are found in both animal and plant foods.

➤ Iron functions in oxygen transport as part of hemoglobin and myoglobin. It is also an enzyme cofactor, important for immune function, and involved in normal brain function.

➤ Iron balance is regulated through absorption; absorption increases when body status is low, and decreases when stores are normal. Meat, vitamin C, and stomach acid tend to increase nonheme iron absorption. Phytate, phenolic compounds, and high doses of other minerals tend to decrease iron absorption.

➤ Recommendations for iron intake consider the amount needed to replace daily losses and the bioavailability of iron from a typical mixed diet. Due to regular iron losses via menstrual bleeding, women of childbearing age need more iron than adult men do.

➤ The best sources of iron are meats. Enriched and whole grains are significant sources in the American diet.

➤ Iron deficiency is the most common nutritional deficiency worldwide. The most severe stage of deficiency, following reduction of iron stores and transport iron, results in anemia.

➤ Iron toxicity can result from acute ingestion of high doses or from chronic excessive iron absorption. Accidental iron overdose is a leading cause of poisoning deaths of children younger than age 6 in the United States.

➤ Zinc is a cofactor for numerous enzymes and is crucial for normal growth, development, and immune function. It is found in protein-rich foods, particularly red meats.

➤ Zinc deficiency results in poor growth, impaired taste, delayed wound healing, and impaired immune response.

➤ Selenium functions as part of the glutathione peroxidases, important antioxidant enzymes. Good sources of selenium are organ meats and seafood. Deficiency of selenium appears to be rare, but has been described in an area of China called the Keshan region.

- ➤ Iodine is necessary for the formation of thyroid hormones, which regulate metabolic rate and body temperature. Much of the iodide in the American diet comes from iodized salt. Iodine deficiency results in goiter. If severe deficiency occurs during pregnancy, the child may be born with cretinism.

- ➤ Copper functions in many enzyme systems, including those involved with antioxidant mechanisms, iron utilization, and immune function. The richest food sources of copper include organ meats, shellfish, nuts and seeds, peanut butter, and chocolate.

- ➤ Copper deficiency results in anemia, decreased numbers of white blood cells, and bone abnormalities.

- ➤ Manganese functions in conjunction with several enzyme systems. The best food sources include tea, coffee, nuts, cereals, and some fruits. Manganese deficiency and toxicity are uncommon; toxicity is usually associated with exposure through manganese mines.

- ➤ Fluoride promotes mineralization of bones and teeth and protects the teeth from caries. Water is a major source of fluoride, due to either naturally high content or added fluoride. Fluorosis is the result of excessive fluoride intake and results in mottling of the teeth.

- ➤ Chromium functions in the normal use of insulin to promote glucose use. Rich sources of chromium are mushrooms, dark chocolate, prunes, nuts, asparagus, whole grains, wine, brewer's yeast, and some beers. Chromium deficiency in humans is difficult to assess, and toxicity of inorganic chromium is unlikely.

- ➤ Although the body contains only about 2 milligrams of molybdenum, it is an important enzyme cofactor. Good food sources are peas, beans, and some breakfast cereals. Molybdenum deficiency and toxicity are both rare.

- ➤ Ultratrace minerals are those required in extremely small amounts; the specific function of many of these nutrients is unknown. Some ultratrace minerals are arsenic, boron, nickel, silicon, and vanadium.

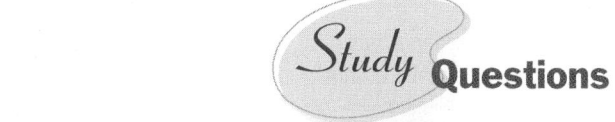

Study Questions

1. In what two ways do trace minerals differ from major minerals?

2. Name two ways that minerals differ from most vitamins.

3. List five factors that can affect a mineral's bioavailability.

4. Explain the differences between "heme" and "nonheme" iron. Which is absorbed better?

5. List the three stages of iron deficiency and the effects of each.

6. What are some of the main functions of zinc?

7. Describe the common causes of zinc deficiency.

8. What are the main functions of selenium?

9. Iodine is a component of which hormones? What are the functions of these hormones? How is selenium linked to these hormones?

10. What are goitrogens and how are they related to goiter?

11. Define Wilson's disease and Menkes' syndrome.

12. What are the functions of manganese in the body?

13. How does fluoride prevent dental caries?

14. Which foods contain chromium, and why is chromium important?

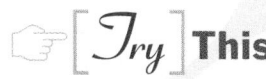

A Simple Check on Your Zinc

Reported in the *Lancet* in the early 1980s, this simple test can provide a rough signal of your zinc status. Buy some zinc sulfate at a health food store. Dissolve it in distilled water to make a 0.1 percent zinc sulfate solution. Refrain from eating, drinking, and smoking for at least an hour before the test. Then swish a teaspoon of the solution around your mouth for 10 seconds. If it tastes unpleasant or metallic, your level of zinc is probably adequate. However, if the solution tastes like water, you may be consuming less zinc than you need.

What About Bobbie?

Let's take a look at Bobbie's intake of the trace minerals iron, zinc, and selenium. Refer to Chapter 1 to review Bobbie's complete food record. Bobbie's intakes of iron, zinc, and selenium exceeded the Recommended Dietary Allowances for her age. This reflects the fact that Bobbie's calorie intake is high enough to satisfy her needs and she selected a wide variety of foods. Below you'll see the foods she ate that contributed the most to her trace mineral intake.

Iron

Bobbie's intake	*20 mg*
Bobbie's RDA	*18 mg*

Most of Bobbie's iron came from enriched grains and red meat. Here are her top four iron sources and the amount each provided:

Spaghetti pasta	*2.9 mg iron*
Bagel	*2.7 mg*
Meatballs	*2.3 mg*
Pizza	*1.5 mg*

Zinc

Bobbie's intake	*14 mg*
Bobbie's RDA	*8 mg*

Bobbie's best source of zinc is red meat—the meatballs she had on her spaghetti. Here are her top four zinc sources and the amount each provided:

Meatballs	*4.9 mg zinc*
Pizza (cheese)	*2.2 mg*
Spaghetti pasta	*1.1 mg*
Bagel	*0.8 mg*

Selenium

Bobbie's intake	*126 μg*
Bobbie's RDA	*55 μg*

Bobbie's best sources of selenium are grain products and meats. Here are her top four selenium sources and the amount each provided:

Spaghetti	*44 μg selenium*
Bagel	*22 μg*
Meatballs	*18 μg*
Turkey	*18 μg*

References

1 Bothwell TH. Overview and mechanisms of iron regulation. *Nutr Rev.* 1995;53(9):237–245.

2 Walter T, Olivares M, Pizarro F, Munoz C. Iron, anemia and infection. *Nutr Rev.* 1997;55(4):111–124.

3 Kretchmer N, Beard JL, Carlson S. The role of nutrition in the development of normal cognition. *Am J Clin Nutr.* 1996; 63:997S–1001S.

4 De Andraca I, Castillo M, Walter T. Psychomotor development and behavior in iron-deficient anemic infants. *Nutr Rev.* 1997; 55(4):125–132.

5 Centers for Disease Control and Prevention (CDC). Recommendations to report and control iron deficiency in the United States. *MMWR.* 1998;7(RR–3).

6 Bothwell TH. Op. cit.

7 Beard JL, Dawson BS, Pinero DJ. Iron metabolism: a comprehensive review. *Nutr Rev.* 1996;54(10):295–317.

8 Bothwell TH. Op. cit.

9 Otten JJ, Hellwig JP, Meyers JD, eds. *Dietary Reference Intakes: The Essential Guide to Nutrient Requirements.* Washington, DC: National Academies Press; 2006.

10 Groff JL, Gropper SS. *Advanced Nutrition and Human Metabolism.* 3rd ed. Belmont, CA: Wadsworth, 2000.

11 Hunt JR, Roughead ZK. Nonheme-iron absorption, fecal ferritin excretion, and blood indexes of iron status in women consuming controlled lactoovovegetarian diets for 8 wk. *Am J Clin Nutr.* 1999;69:944–952.

12 Ibid.

13 Minihane AM, Fairweather-Tait SJ. Effect of calcium supplementation on daily nonheme-iron absorption and long-term iron status. *Am J Clin Nutr.* 1998;68:96–102.

14 Hallberg L. Does calcium interfere with iron absorption? *Am J Clin Nutr.* 1998;68:3–4.

15 Baynes, RD. Refining the assessment of body iron status. *Am J Clin Nutr.* 1996;64:793–794.

16 Bothwell TH. Op. cit.

17 CDC. Op. cit.

18 Stoltzfus RJ, Chwaya HM, Tielsch JM, et al. Epidemiology of iron deficiency anemia in Zanzibari schoolchildren: the importance of hookworms. *Am J Clin Nutr.* 1997;65:153–159.

19 McDowell MA, Briefel RR, Alaimo K, et al. *Energy and Macronutrient Intakes of Persons Ages 2 Months and Older in the United States. Third National Health and Nutrition Examination Survey, Phase I, 1988–1991.* Huntsville, MD: National Center for Health Statistics, 1994. NCH publication 255.

20 Pollitt E. Iron deficiency and educational deficiency. *Nutr Rev.* 1997;55(4):133–140.

21 Zhu YI, Haas JD. Iron depletion without anemia and physical performance in young women. *Am J Clin Nutr.* 1997; 66:334–341.

22 Institute of Medicine, Food and Nutrition Board. *Dietary Reference Intakes for Vitamin A, Vitamin K, Arsenic, Boron, Chromium, Copper, Iodine, Iron, Manganese, Molybdenum, Nickel, Silicon, Vanadium, and Zinc.* Washington, DC: National Academy Press, 2001.

23 Preventing iron poisoning in children. *FDA Backgrounder.* January 15, 1997.

24 Gordeuk V, Mukiibi J, Hasstedt SJ, et al. Iron overload in Africa: interaction between a gene and dietary iron content. *N Engl J Med.* 1992;326(12):95–100.

25 Prasad AS, Helstead JA, Nadami M. Syndrome of iron deficiency anemia, hepatosplenomegaly, hypogonadism, dwarfism and geophagia. *Am J Med.* 1961;31:532–546.

26 Sandstead HH, Prasad AS, Schubert AR, et al. Human zinc deficiency endocrine manifestations and response to treatment. *Am J Clin Nutr.* 1967;20;422–442.

27 Stein JH. *Internal Medicine.* 4th ed. St. Louis: Mosby-Year Book, 1994.

28 King JC, Cousins RJ. Zinc. In: Shils ME, Shike M, Ross AC, Cabellero B, Cousins RJ, eds. *Modern Nutrition in Health and Disease.* 10th ed. Philadelphia: Lippincott, Williams, & Wilkins, 2006:271–285.

29 Ibid.

30 Sandstrom B. Absorption of zinc from soy protein meals in humans. *J Nutr.* 1987;117:321–327.

31 Yan L, Prentice A, Dibba B, et al. Effect of long-term calcium supplementation on indices of iron, zinc, and magnesium status in lactating Gambian women. *Br J Nutr.* 1996;76(6):821–831.

32 Gibson RS. Content and bioavailability of trace elements in vegetarian diets. *Am J Clin Nutr.* 1994;59(suppl):1223–1232.

33 Krebs NF. Overview of zinc absorption and excretion in the human gastrointestinal tract. *J Nutr.* 2000;130:1374S–1377S.

34 Lonnerdal B. Dietary factors influencing zinc absorption. *J Nutr.* 2000;130:1378S–1383S.

35 King JC, Cousins RJ. Op. cit.

36 Briefel RR, Bialostosky K, Kennedy-Stephenson J, et al. Zinc intake of the U.S. population: findings from the Third National Health and Nutrition Examination Survey, 1988–1994. *J Nutr.* 2000;130:1367S–1373S.

37 Navert B, Sandstrom B, Cederblad A. Reduction of the phytate content of bran by leavening in bread and its effect on absorption of zinc in man. *Br J Nutr.* 1985;53:47–53.

38 Gerrior SA, Zizza C. *Nutrient Content of the U.S. Food Supply, 1909–1990.* Washington, DC: US Department of Agriculture, 1994. Home Economics Research Report, No. 52.

39 Prasad AS. Zinc: an overview. *Nutrition.* 1995;11:93.

40 Tamura T, Goldenberg RL. Zinc nutriture and pregnancy outcome. *Nutr Res.* 1996.

41 Heyneman CA. Zinc deficiency and taste disorders. *Ann Pharmacother.* 1996;30:186–187.

42 Bogden JD, Oleske JM, Lavenhar MA, et al. Effects of one year of supplementation with zinc and other micronutrients on cellular immunity in the elderly. *J Am Coll Nutr.* 1990;9:214–225.

43 King JC, Cousins RJ. Op. cit.

44 Institute of Medicine. 2001. Op cit.

45 Hoogenraad T, Van den Hamer C, van Hattum J. Effective treatment of Wilson's disease with oral zinc sulphate: two case reports. *Br Med J.* 1984;289:273–276.

46 Institute of Medicine, Food and Nutrition Board. *Dietary Reference Intakes for Vitamin C, Vitamin E, Selenium, and Beta-Carotene, and Other Carotenoids.* Washington, DC: National Academy Press, 2000.

47 Ibid.

48 Ibid.

49 Ibid.

50 Hetzel BS. *The Story of Iodine Deficiency: An International Challenge in Nutrition.* Oxford, England: Oxford University Press, 1989.

51 World Health Organization sets out to eliminate iodine deficiency disorder. WHO press release; May 25, 1999.

52 Guyton, AC, Hall, JE. *Medical Textbook of Physiology.* 10th ed. Philadelphia: WB Saunders, 2000.

53 Bautista A. Effects of oral iodized salt on intelligence, thyroid status, and somatic growth in school-aged children from an area with endemic goiter. *Am J Clin Nutr.* 1982;35:127–134.

54 Institute of Medicine. 2001. Op. cit.

55 Klevay LM, Buchet JP, Bunker VW, et al. Copper in the Western diet. In: Anke M, Meissner D, Mills CF, eds. *Trace Elements in Man and Animals.* Gersdorf, Germany: Verlag Media Touristik, 1993:207–210.

56 Williams DM. Copper deficiency in humans. *Semin Hematol.* 1983;20:118–128.

57 Keen CL, Uriu-Hare JY, Hawk SN, et al. Effect of copper deficiency on prenatal development and pregnancy outcome. *Am J Clin Nutr.* 1998;67(suppl):1003S–1011S.

58 Turnland JR. Copper. In: Shils ME, Shike M, Ross AC, Cabellero B, Cousins RJ, eds. *Modern Nutrition in Health and Disease.* 10th ed. Philadelphia: Lippincott, Williams, & Wilkins, 2006: 286–299.

59 Kaler SG. Diagnosis and therapy of Menkes' syndrome, a genetic form of copper deficiency. *Am J Clin Nutr.* 1998; 67(suppl):1029S–1034S.

60 Greger JL. Dietary standards for manganese: overlap between nutritional and toxicological studies. *J Nutr.* 1998;128: 368S–371S.

61 Keen CL, Zidenberg-Cherr S. Manganese. In: Ziegler E, Filer L, eds. *Present Knowledge in Nutrition.* 7th ed. Washington, DC: International Life Sciences Institute, 1996:334–343.

62 Kapaki E, Zournas C, Kanias G, et al. Essential trace element alterations in amyotrophic lateral sclerosis. *J Neurol Sci.* 1997; 147(2):171–175.

63 Centers for Disease Control and Prevention. Populations receiving optimally fluoridated public drinking water—United States, 2000. *MMWR.* 2002;51(7):144–147.

64 Simko LC. Water fluoridation: time to reexamine the issue. *Pediatr Nurs.* 1997;23(2):155–159.

65 Riggs BL, Hodgson SF, O'Fallon WM, et al. Effect of fluoride treatment on the fracture rate in women with osteoporosis. *N Engl J Med.* 1990;322:802–809.

66 Mertz W. Confirmation: chromium levels in serum, hair, and sweat decline with age. *Nutr Rev.* 1997;55(10):373–375.

67 Nielson FH. Should you take a chromium supplement? *Healthline.* December 1995.

68 Davis S, McLaren HJ, Hunnisett A, Howard M. Age-related decreases in chromium levels in 51,665 hair, sweat, and serum samples from 40,872 patients: implications for the prevention of cardiovascular disease and type II diabetes mellitus. *Metabolism.* 1997;46:469–473.

69 Anderson RA. Effects of chromium on body composition and weight loss. *Nutr Rev.* 1998;56(9):266–270.

70 Nielsen FH. How should dietary guidance be given for mineral elements with beneficial actions or suspected of being essential? *J Nutr.* 1996;126:2377–2385S.

71 Eckhert CD. Other trace elements. In: Shils ME, Shike M, Ross AC, Cabellero B, Cousins RJ, eds. *Modern Nutrition in Health and Disease.* 10th ed. Philadelphia: Lippincott, Williams, & Wilkins, 2006:338–350.

72 Dabeka RW, McKenzie AD, Lacroix GM, et al. Survey of arsenic in total diet food composites and estimation of the dietary intake of arsenic by Canadian adults and children. *J AOAC Int.* 1993;76(1):14–25.

73 Anderson D, Cunningham W, Lindstrom T. Concentrations and intakes of H, B, S, K, Na, Cl, and NaCl in foods. *J Food Comp Anal.* 1994;7:59–82.

74 Eckhert CD. Op cit.

75 Uthus EO, Poellot RA. Dietary folate affects the response of rats to nickel deprivation. *Biol Trace Elem Res.* 1996;52:23–35.

76 Uthus EO, Seaborn CD. Deliberations and evaluations of the approaches, endpoints, and paradigms for dietary recommendations of the other trace elements. *J Nutr.* 1996;126:2452S–2459S.

77 Kelsay JL, Behall KM, Prather E. Effect of fiber from fruits and vegetables on metabolic responses in human subjects. II: Calcium, magnesium, iron, and silicon balances. *Am J Clin Nutr.* 1979;32:1876–1880.

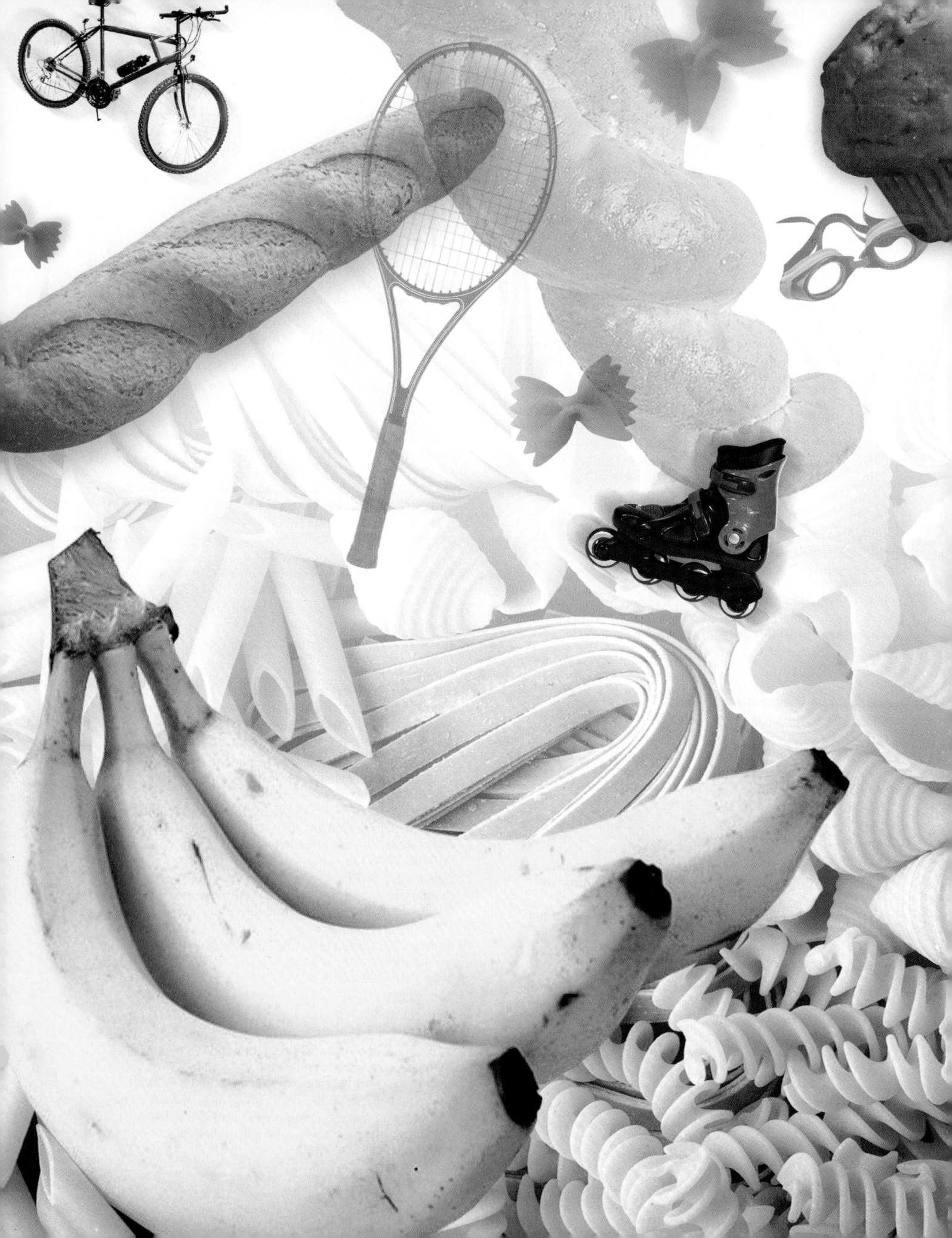

Chapter 13

Sports Nutrition

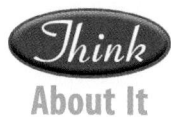

Think About It

1 How much importance do you place on being physically active?

2 How often do you suffer from muscle fatigue? What do you think causes it?

3 How often do you think about food choices when you're planning a physical activity?

4 What kind of protein do you emphasize in your diet?

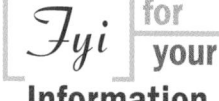

Fyi for your Information

This chapter's FYI boxes include practical information on the following topics:

• Lactate Is Not a Metabolic Dead End

• To Zone or Not to Zone? That Is the Question

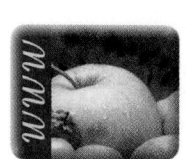

The Web site for this book offers many useful tools and is a great source for additional nutrition information for both students and instructors. For information on sports nutrition, visit the site at **nutrition.jbpub.com.** You'll find exercises that explore the following topics:

• Effective Training

• Sports Nutrition from a Sports Drink Company

• Scan SCAN

Key to Illustrations

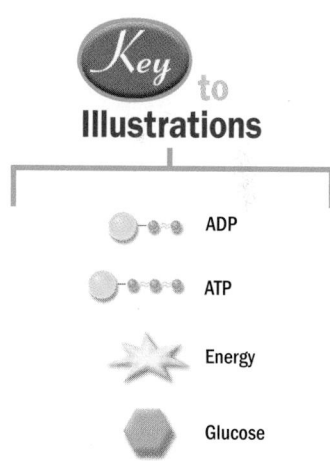

ADP

ATP

Energy

Glucose

What About Bobbie?

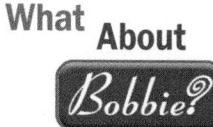

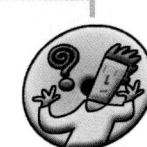

Track the choices Bobbie is making with Nutritionist Pro or EatRight Analysis software.

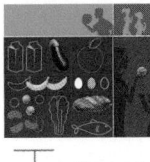

Today is the big 10,000-meter race. You've trained for months. Fans in the crowd shade their eyes as they watch you and your competitors walk onto the track. "Ready," shouts the starter. "Get set." You toe the starting line and adrenaline courses through your blood vessels, increasing your heart rate, diverting blood to your muscles, and mobilizing energy stores in your liver, muscles, and fat. "Go!" Within a fraction of a second, a torrent of calcium flows into your muscle cells, causing your muscles to contract and launch you away from the starting line.

How will you perform in this race? Will your breakfast help or hinder your performance? Will what you ate yesterday and the day before affect your stamina? Does it matter what you eat after you finish the race? Read on for the answers to these questions and learn about the links between nutrition and sports performance.

Nutrition and Physical Performance

Just how physically active do you need to be? (See **Figure 13.1**.) Both the National Institutes of Health (NIH) and Health Canada have found that even small to moderate amounts of physical activity can produce substantial health benefits. Physically active people have a lower risk of developing many chronic diseases, such as coronary heart disease, diabetes, hypertension, osteoporosis, and obesity. Active people also experience an increased sense of well-being and are much better equipped to cope with stress. Health Canada recommends choosing a variety of activities from three types of exercise: endurance, flexibility, and strength. (See **Figure 13.2**.) See Appendix D for *Canada's Physical Activity Guide to Healthy Active Living.*

The American College of Sports Medicine (ACSM) notes an important distinction between physical activity as it relates to health and exercise for physical fitness.[1] According to the ACSM, the level of physical activity that may reduce the risk of various chronic diseases may not be enough—in quantity or quality—to improve physical fitness. According to the Food and Nutrition Board, a minimum of 30 minutes of moderate-intensity physical activity on most days of the week will result in some health benefits. However, 60 minutes of daily physical activity is needed to prevent weight gain and fully achieve health benefits.[2]

What is physical fitness? Measures of fitness may include such factors as strength, endurance, flexibility, and breathing capacity. The ACSM defines physical fitness as "the ability to perform moderate to vigorous levels of physical activity without undue fatigue and the capability of maintaining this level of activity throughout life."[3] In other words, it is more than being able to run a long distance or lift a lot of weight at the gym. Being fit is not defined only by what kind of activity you do, how long you do it, or at what level of intensity. Although these are important measures of fitness, they only address single areas. Overall fitness is made up of five main components:

1. *Cardiorespiratory fitness:* The ability of the body's circulatory and respiratory systems to supply fuel during sustained physical activity.

2. *Muscular strength:* The ability of the muscle to exert force during an activity.

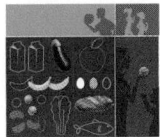

Dietary Guidelines for Americans, 2005

key recommendations

- Engage in regular physical activity and reduce sedentary activities to promote health, psychological well-being, and a healthy body weight.
  - To reduce the risk of chronic disease in adulthood: Engage in at least 30 minutes of moderate-intensity physical activity, above usual activity, at work or home on most days of the week.
  - For most people, greater health benefits can be obtained by engaging in physical activity of more vigorous intensity or longer duration.
  - To help manage body weight and prevent gradual, unhealthy body weight gain in adulthood: Engage in approximately 60 minutes of moderate- to vigorous-intensity activity on most days of the week while not exceeding caloric intake requirements.
  - To sustain weight loss in adulthood: Participate in at least 60 to 90 minutes of daily moderate-intensity physical activity while not exceeding caloric intake requirements. Some people may need to consult with a health care provider before participating in this level of activity.
- Achieve physical fitness by including cardiovascular conditioning, stretching exercises for flexibility, and resistance exercises or calisthenics for muscle strength and endurance.

Key Recommendations for Specific Population Groups

- *Children and adolescents.* Engage in at least 60 minutes of physical activity on most, preferably all, days of the week.
- *Pregnant women.* In the absence of medical or obstetric complications, incorporate 30 minutes or more of moderate-intensity physical activity on most, if not all, days of the week. Avoid activities with a high risk of falling or abdominal trauma.
- *Breastfeeding women.* Be aware that neither acute nor regular exercise adversely affects the mother's ability to successfully breastfeed.
- *Older adults.* Participate in regular physical activity to reduce functional declines associated with aging and to achieve the other benefits of physical activity identified for all adults.

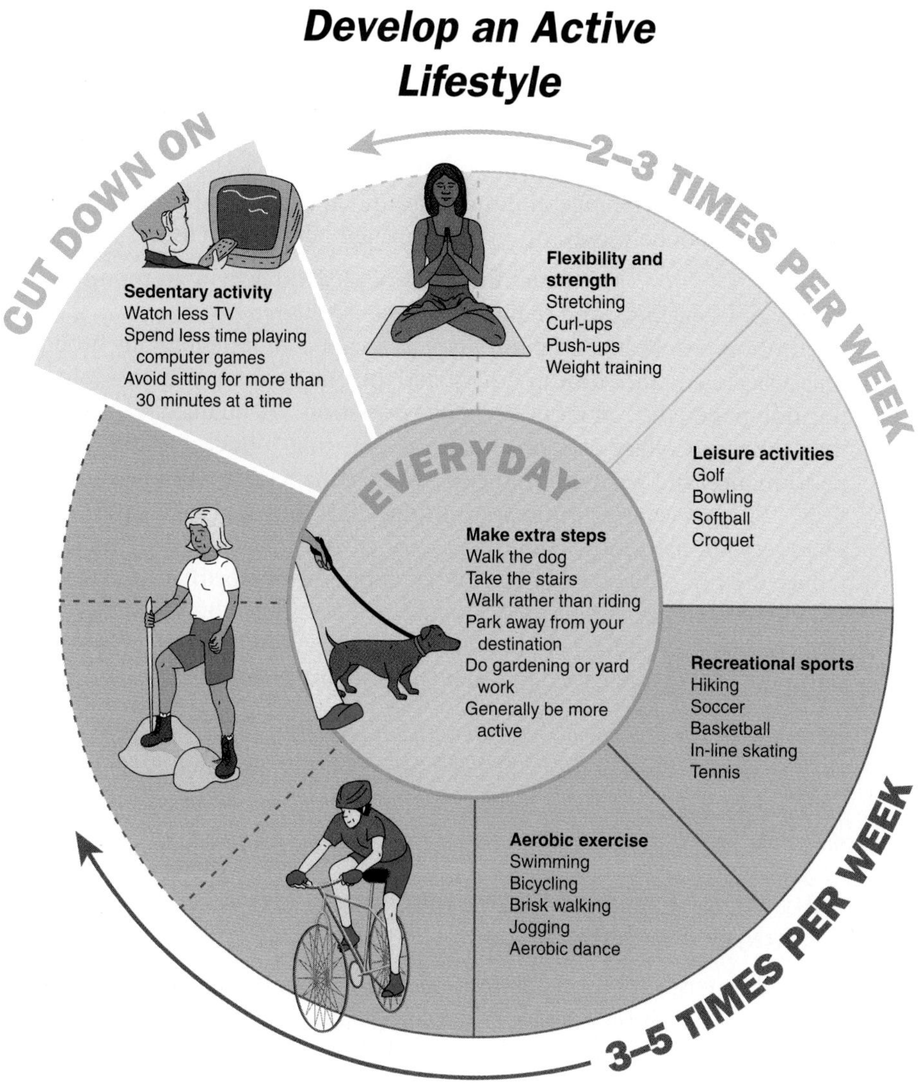

Develop an Active Lifestyle

CUT DOWN ON

2–3 TIMES PER WEEK

Sedentary activity
Watch less TV
Spend less time playing
computer games
Avoid sitting for more than
30 minutes at a time

Flexibility and strength
Stretching
Curl-ups
Push-ups
Weight training

Leisure activities
Golf
Bowling
Softball
Croquet

EVERYDAY

Make extra steps
Walk the dog
Take the stairs
Walk rather than riding
Park away from your
destination
Do gardening or yard
work
Generally be more
active

Recreational sports
Hiking
Soccer
Basketball
In-line skating
Tennis

Aerobic exercise
Swimming
Bicycling
Brisk walking
Jogging
Aerobic dance

3–5 TIMES PER WEEK

Figure 13.1 **Be active.** Perhaps the most important aspect of increasing physical activity is to have fun.

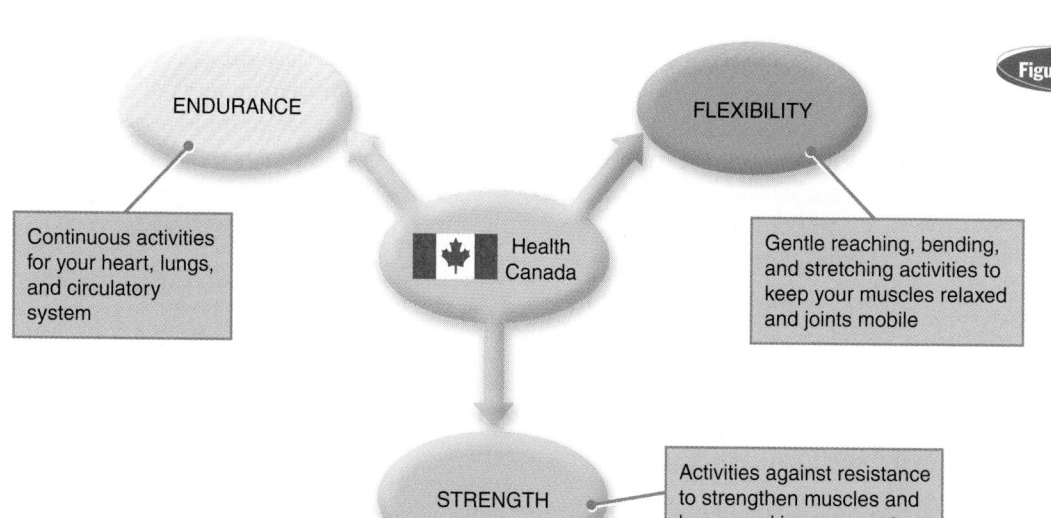

ENDURANCE

FLEXIBILITY

Health Canada

Continuous activities for your heart, lungs, and circulatory system

Gentle reaching, bending, and stretching activities to keep your muscles relaxed and joints mobile

STRENGTH

Activities against resistance to strengthen muscles and bones and improve posture

Figure 13.2 **Variety is the spice of life.** Health Canada recommends that you do a variety of activities from each group—endurance, flexibility, and strength—to receive the most health benefits.
Source: Adapted from *Canada's Physical Activity Guide to Healthy Active Living.*

Table 13.1 Guidelines for Physical Activity: Health and Fitness

Guidelines for Promoting Health

Frequency: daily activity
Intensity: any level of intensity
Duration: accumulation of a minimum of 30 minutes of total daily activity
Mode: any activity

Guidelines for Achieving and Maintaining Physical Fitness

Frequency: 3 to 5 days per week
Intensity: 50 to 90 percent of maximum heart rate
Duration: 20 to 60 minutes of continuous or intermittent aerobic activity (minimum of 10-minute bouts accumulated during the day)
Mode: activity using large muscle groups maintained continuously in a rhythmic and aerobic manner
Resistance training: 2 to 3 days per week to enhance strength and muscular endurance, and maintain fat-free mass
Flexibility training: minimum of 2 days per week, incorporated into overall fitness program to develop and maintain range of motion

Sources: American College of Sports Medicine. Position stand: the recommended quantity and quality of exercise for developing and maintaining cardiorespiratory and muscular fitness and flexibility in healthy adults. *Med Sci Sports Exerc.* 1998;30:975–991; and American College of Sports Medicine. Position Stand: progression models in resistance training for healthy adults. *Med Sci Sports Exerc.* 2002;34:364–380.

skeletal muscles Muscles composed of bundles of parallel, striated muscle fibers under voluntary control. Also called voluntary muscle or striated muscle.

muscle fibers Individual muscle cells.

slow-twitch (ST) fibers Muscle fibers that develop tension more slowly and to a lesser extent than fast-twitch muscle fibers. ST fibers have high oxidative capacities and are slower to fatigue than fast-twitch fibers.

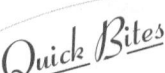

Quick Bites

Pound for Pound?

*W*omen's muscles have smaller muscle fiber cross sections and less muscle mass than men. For a given amount of muscle, however, there is no difference in strength between men and women.

3. *Muscular endurance:* The ability of the muscle to continue to perform without fatigue.

4. *Body composition:* The relative amounts of fat and lean body mass. Body composition is an important component to consider for health and managing your weight.

5. *Flexibility:* The range of motion around a joint. Good flexibility in the joints can help prevent injuries through all stages of life.

Table 13.1 shows guidelines for levels of physical activity to promote health and to achieve and maintain fitness.

Nutrition has taken its rightful place as a vital component of any program that seeks to enhance health, fitness, and athletic performance. In a joint position paper, the American Dietetic Association, Dietitians of Canada, and the American College of Sports Medicine state that "physical activity, athletic performance, and recovery from exercise are enhanced by optimal nutrition."[4] But just what is "optimal nutrition?" Is it the same for a child who plays recreational softball and for a senior citizen who takes daily walks to reduce the risk of type 2 diabetes? What about the competitive athlete who strives to maximize athletic performance and uses nutrition to gain a competitive edge? To understand the relationship between physical activity and nutrition, you first need to appreciate how we use energy during exercise.

Key Concepts: *Exercise provides numerous health benefits, including reduced risk of chronic disease. Physical fitness includes strength, endurance, and flexibility. For optimal physical performance, nutrition is an essential part of all athletic training programs.*

Muscles, Energy Systems, and Physical Performance

Physical activity and sports performance rely on energy production. Just as a race car depends on a high-performance engine and energy-dense fuel to win in record time, our muscles process fuel in the form of chemical energy to produce power for physical performance.

Muscles and Muscle Fibers

Your body contains hundreds of muscles that help control a myriad of functions, from regulating blood pressure to climbing stairs. **Skeletal muscles** are bundles of parallel, striated fibers attached to your skeleton. (See **Figure 13.3.**) These muscles are responsible for your physical movement and are under your conscious control. If you decide to bend your arm, for example, you consciously contract your biceps. Your body contains more than 600 skeletal muscles and uses 9 of them just to control your thumb!

Individual muscle cells are called **muscle fibers**. Skeletal muscle has two primary types:

- **Slow-twitch (ST) fibers**
- **Fast-twitch (FT) fibers**

They derive their names from the difference in their speed of action. One type of fast-twitch fiber can contract 10 times faster than slow-twitch fibers.[5]

Slow-Twitch Fibers

To power their activity, slow-twitch fibers efficiently produce energy by breaking down carbohydrate and fat via aerobic pathways—metabolic reactions that require oxygen. As long as the aerobic pathways are active, ST fibers can produce energy to sustain their movement. With a sufficient supply of oxygen, ST fibers can maintain muscular activity for a prolonged time. This ability is known as **aerobic endurance**.

Because ST fibers have high aerobic endurance, your body predominantly relies on them during low-intensity endurance events, such as a marathon, and during everyday activities, such as walking.

Fast-Twitch Fibers

Compared with ST fibers, fast-twitch fibers have poor aerobic endurance. They are optimized to perform anaerobically (when the oxygen supply is limited). FT fibers can efficiently produce energy for their use via metabolic pathways that do not require oxygen. Bundles of FT fibers exert considerably more force than bundles of ST fibers; due to their limited endurance, however, FT fibers tire quickly.

The body recruits both ST and FT fibers during shorter, higher-intensity endurance events, such as the mile run or the 400-meter swim. During highly explosive events such as the 100-meter dash and the 50-meter sprint swim, the body still recruits both types, but FT fibers contribute most of the muscle power generated.

Fiber Type and the Athlete

Genes determine the relative proportion of muscle fiber types in athletes. Although distance runners who have a high percentage of ST fibers are well suited for endurance events, they will not succeed as elite sprinters. Conversely, sprinters who have predominantly FT fibers are better equipped for explosive events, but they will not become competitive marathon runners. (See **Figure 13.4**.)

Key Concepts: *A muscle cell is called a muscle fiber. The two main types of skeletal muscle fibers are slow-twitch and fast-twitch fibers. Slow-twitch fibers generate fuel through aerobic pathways, whereas fast-twitch fibers produce energy using anaerobic pathways. Fast-twitch fibers can exert more force but have limited endurance.*

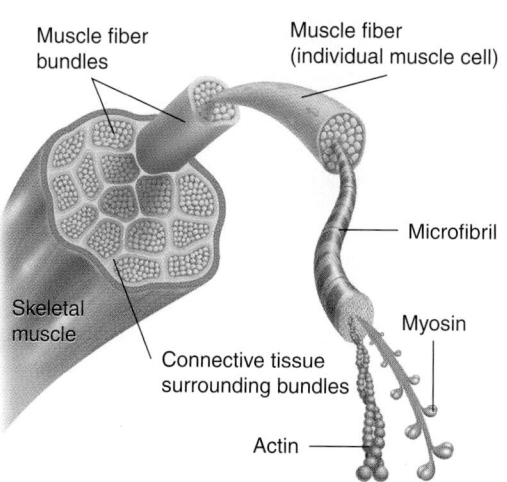

Figure 13.3 **Basic structure of skeletal muscle.**
A muscle fiber is an individual muscle cell that usually extends the entire length of the muscle. Each muscle fiber contains hundreds to thousands of microfibrils. Each microfibril contains thousands of actin and myosin filaments, large protein molecules responsible for muscle contractions.

Labels: Muscle fiber bundles; Muscle fiber (individual muscle cell); Microfibril; Myosin; Actin; Connective tissue surrounding bundles; Skeletal muscle

---

Quick Bites

Fast-Twitch Fish

A large percentage (40 to 60 percent) of a fish's body weight is muscle tissue. Although it spends much of its life slowly cruising, a fish must be able to execute occasional quick bursts of high speed to escape predators or catch a meal. Thus, fish muscle is composed of approximately 75 to 90 percent fast-twitch fibers and fish flesh often is white. The slow-twitch fibers generally are concentrated just under the skin or near fins that are used during slow or high speeds. This arrangement is possible only because fish are buoyant. Land animals could not survive dragging around a large mass of muscle that they used only occasionally in extreme situations.

fast-twitch (FT) fibers Muscle fibers that can develop high tension rapidly. These fibers can fatigue quickly, but are well suited to explosive movements in sprinting, jumping, and weight lifting.

aerobic endurance The ability of skeletal muscle to obtain a sufficient supply of oxygen from the heart and lungs to maintain muscular activity for a prolonged time.

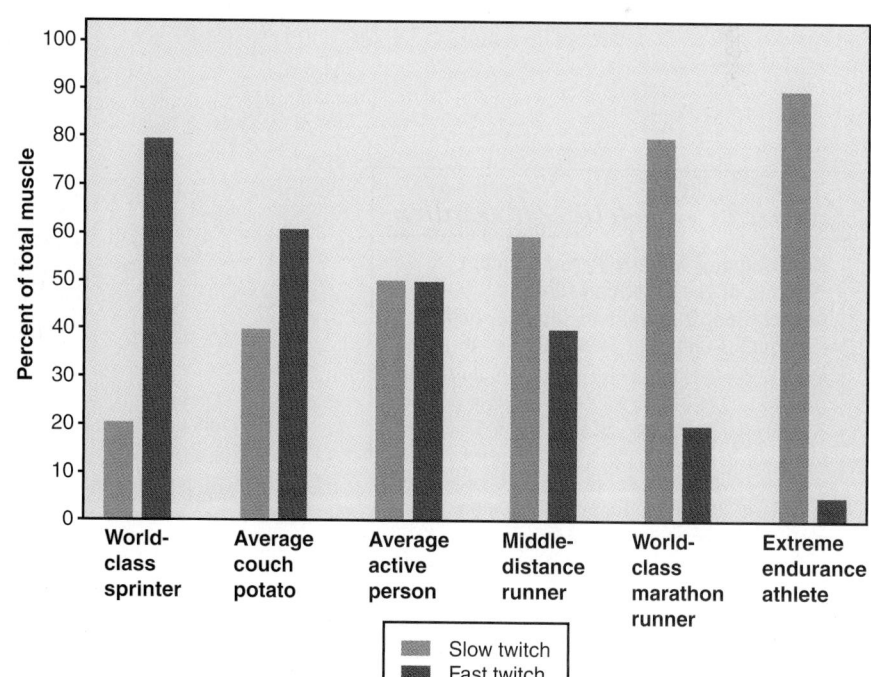

Figure 13.4 **What's your mix of muscle fibers?** If you are best at events requiring explosive movements, you may have a greater percentage of fast-twitch muscle fibers. If endurance events are your specialty, you may have more slow-twitch fibers.
Source: Adapted from Andersen JL, Scherling P, Saltin B. *Muscle, genes and athletic performance. Scientific American.* 2000;283(3):49.

creatine phosphate An energy-rich compound that supplies energy and a phosphate group for the formation of ATP. Also called phosphocreatine.

phosphocreatine See *creatine phosphate*.

ATP-CP energy system A simple and immediate anaerobic energy system that maintains ATP levels. Creatine phosphate is broken down, releasing energy and a phosphate group, which is used to form ATP.

lactic acid energy system Anaerobic energy system; using glycolysis, it rapidly produces energy (ATP) and lactate. Also called anaerobic glycolysis.

ATP-CP Energy System

Let's return to your race. As you launch yourself from the starting line, it takes less than a second for your contracting muscles to burn their entire reserve of adenosine triphosphate (ATP), the immediate energy source for cells. Luckily, your body has a small reservoir of **creatine phosphate** (also called **phosphocreatine**) that your muscles can convert quickly to ATP. (See **Figure 13.5.**) The body stores four to six times more creatine phosphate than ATP.[6] Together, your available ATP and creatine phosphate, the **ATP-CP energy system**, can power an all-out effort for only 3 to 15 seconds.[7] To continue the race, you must enlist carbohydrate stored as glycogen in your muscles and liver. Your cells rapidly disassemble glycogen to glucose, from which they can extract ATP.

Lactic Acid Energy System

For the next minute or two, the acceleration stage, your body uses the simplest and speediest chemical pathways to produce ATP from glucose: the **lactic acid energy system**. (See **Figure 13.6.**) Like the ATP-CP energy system, these pathways are anaerobic—they do not require oxygen. The raw material, glucose, is much more plentiful than creatine phosphate, but its breakdown also produces a by-product: lactate (lactic acid). Although new research shows that cells can extract some energy from lactic acid aerobically,[8] most lactic acid accumulates in cells, making them more acidic. A rise in acidity impairs the breakdown of glucose and inhibits calcium binding. Without calcium, muscles cannot contract. For years, coaches and athletes have blamed lactic acid for muscle fatigue. But it's the change in pH, rather than the lactic acid substance itself, that is the primary culprit.[9]

To continue running beyond the first few minutes, your body employs a sophisticated, oxygen-based system to process lactic acid and squeeze out much more ATP from glucose.

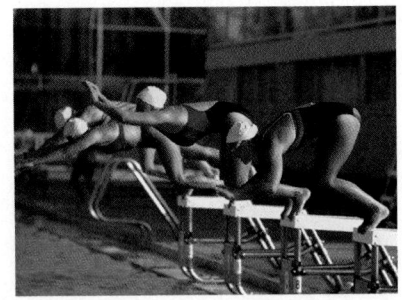

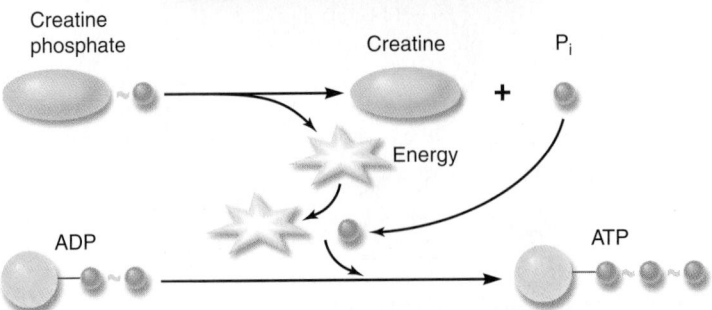

Creatine phosphate   Creatine   P$_i$

Energy

ADP   ATP

Figure 13.5 **ATP-CP energy system.** To maintain relatively constant ATP levels during an initial explosive burst of high-intensity activity, your body uses its ATP–CP energy system to generate ATP from creatine phosphate.

Fyi Lactate Is Not a Metabolic Dead End

FOR YOUR INFORMATION

Today's race is 200 meters, and you are in the lead. The crowd roars with excitement and your coach screams hoarsely as your feet slam over and over on the hard gray cinder track. Other runners are close behind, and you can feel them breathing and pounding at your heels. Air whistles in and out of your wheezing lungs as you doggedly push to stay ahead. Your muscles are screaming, but they carry you across the finish line. A winner!

As you slump in exhaustion, you wonder how your limp muscles carried you through to the end. Each leg seemed to weigh a thousand pounds. As your muscles tire, lactate levels rise and the pH in your muscle cells drops. Scientists, coaches, and athletes have long believed that lactate was a useless, even toxic, dead-end substance. Research proves otherwise. It is the overall acidification of the muscle tissue, rather than a buildup of lactate, that primarily causes muscle fatigue. Also, lactate is now recognized as a fuel in its own right. In addition to acting as a metabolic shunt, lactate is a useful fuel produced and consumed under all conditions of oxygen availability, while exercising or at rest.

Without the energy supplied by the lactic acid energy system, you would never have crossed the finish line. While your body anaerobically burned muscle glycogen, it produced large amounts of lactate. Where does this lactate come from, and how does your body handle it?

Cori Cycle

During vigorous exercise, your contracting muscle cells quickly extract small amounts of ATP from glucose. This simple pathway, called glycolysis, splits glucose into pyruvate molecules faster than the oxygen energy system can accept them for further processing. Cells divert excess pyruvate to lactate to help alleviate the backup.

Lactate accumulates rapidly in muscle cells, which receive a boost of energy by burning some lactate with oxygen—a strategy that yields far more energy than glycolysis alone.[1] Most lactate diffuses through muscle cell membranes into the bloodstream. The liver picks up the circulating lactate and converts it

back to pyruvate. Using energy-demanding reactions, the liver transforms pyruvate to glucose. Glucose enters the bloodstream and travels back to the skeletal muscle cells, where it reenters energy-producing pathways.

This recurring circular pathway is called the Cori cycle. When pyruvate is backed up in muscle cells, the Cori cycle buys time with a detour through the liver. When oxygen becomes readily available, the oxygen energy system becomes the main pathway.

Lactate Shuttle

The pathways of the Cori cycle are an important, but incomplete, part of the lactate picture. The use of the Cori cycle as a holding pattern led to the mistaken belief that lactate was simply a metabolic dead end. Recent studies describe a more extensive role for this long-maligned substance.

Researchers now recognize lactate as an important means of distributing carbohydrate energy sources after a meal and during sustained physical exercise. Lactate's advantage is its ability to move rapidly between cells. It is a small molecule and, unlike glucose, does not need insulin to cross a cell membrane.

Under resting conditions of plentiful carbohydrate and oxygen, diverse tissues such as

skeletal muscle, liver, and skin produce lactate.[2] In these conditions, the supply of raw materials, rather than limited oxygen, drives the formation of lactate.

According to the lactate shuttle hypothesis, lactate formed in muscle cells becomes an energy source at other sites, either adjacent or remote. Skeletal muscle, once thought simply to produce lactate, also directly uses lactate as a fuel. At times, skeletal muscle actually removes more lactate than it produces. The heart muscle is fully aerobic, but it both produces and consumes lactate. Studies suggest that during exercise lactate is the major fuel for the heart and the preferred fuel for certain muscle fibers.[3]

The next time you complain about sore, tired muscles, don't blame lactate. Instead, think about the daily usefulness of lactate and how this little-respected substance helped power you to the finish.

1 Hashimoto T, Hussien R, Brooks GA. Colocalization of MCT1, CD147, and LDH in mitochondrial inner membrane of L6 muscle cells: evidence of a mitochondrial lactate oxidation complex. *Am J Physiol Endocrinol Metab.* 2006;290(6):E1237–E1244.

2 Brooks GA. Mammalian fuel utilization during sustained exercise. *Comp Biochem Physiol.* 1998;120:89–107.

3 Myers J, Ashley E. Dangerous curves: a perspective on exercise, lactate, and the anaerobic threshold. *Chest.* 1997;111:787–795.

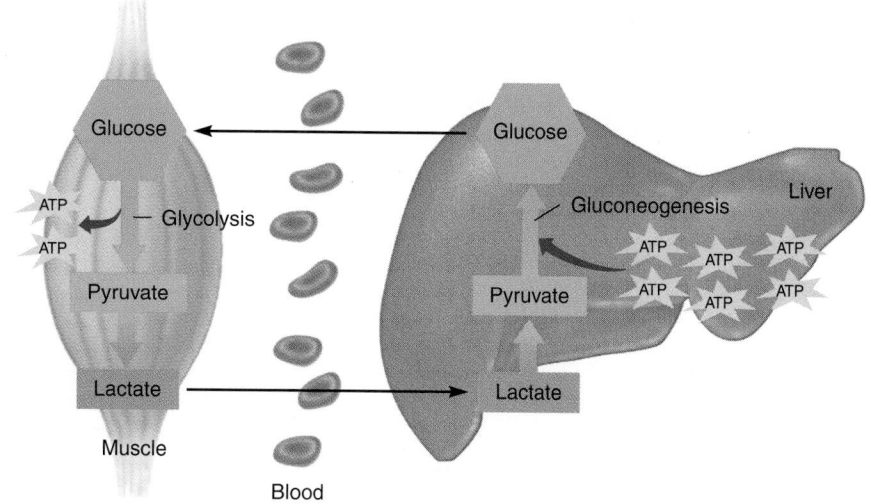

The Cori cycle. The Cori cycle shifts some of the metabolic burden of contracting muscle to the liver. Lactate formed in contracting muscle travels to the liver, which uses it to form glucose. This glucose returns to the muscle to fuel further contractions.

Oxygen Energy System

For the endurance stage, cells can use lengthy, complex chemical pathways in their mitochondria—small units within cells that function as power-generating plants—to convert food and oxygen to ATP. (See **Figure 13.7**.) These reactions are aerobic—they require abundant oxygen. In contracting muscle, blood vessels dilate and deliver a 20-fold increase in oxygen-rich blood to muscle cells,[10] a sufficient supply for mitochondria to produce

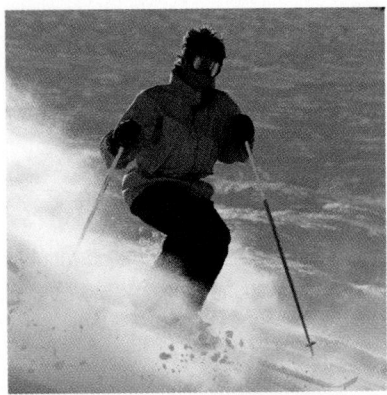

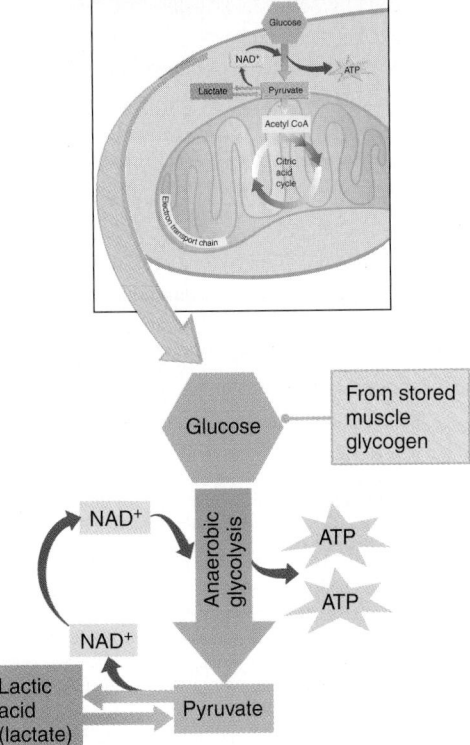

Figure 13.6 **Lactic acid energy system.** During short events requiring power and speed, the lactic acid energy system supplies much of the energy. Because the lactic acid system does not require oxygen, these events are anaerobic activities.

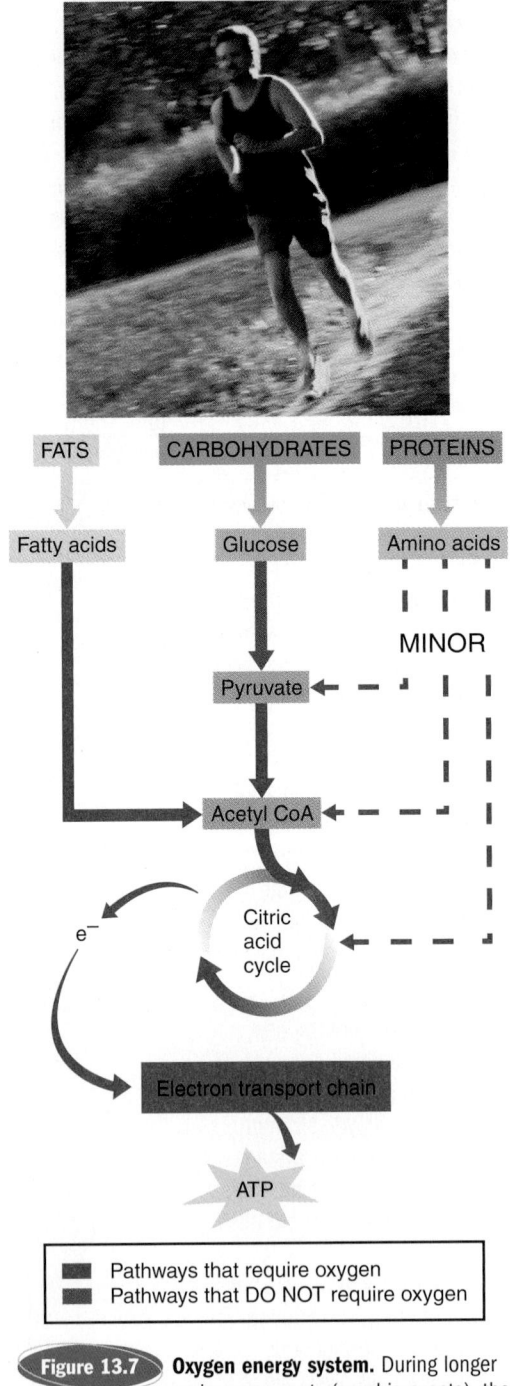

Figure 13.7 **Oxygen energy system.** During longer endurance events (aerobic events), the oxygen energy system supplies most of the energy. This energy system requires oxygen and primarily relies on carbohydrate and fat as fuels.

ATP. In contrast to the two anaerobic systems (ATP-CP system and lactic acid system), the **oxygen energy system** can produce a tremendous amount of ATP. Another advantage is that the oxygen energy system can extract energy from fat as well as glucose. But since the required oxygen must travel a long distance—from the lungs to blood to muscle cells to mitochondria—the oxygen energy system produces ATP at a much slower rate than the anaerobic systems do.

Teamwork in Energy Production

The anaerobic and aerobic energy systems work together to fuel athletic performance. (See **Figure 13.8**.) Although all three energy systems are always active, one system may be the primary fuel source for a particular activity or exercise intensity. As the first 2 minutes of your race elapse, the oxygen energy system is supplying about half of your muscles' energy needs. (See **Figure 13.9**.) By the time you pass the 30-minute mark, this aerobic system is supplying 95 percent; and at two hours or more, the oxygen energy system is supplying 98 percent of your muscles' energy needs.[11]

As long as ATP production by the mitochondria meets energy needs, you are exercising aerobically; highly trained athletes can sustain such exercise for hours. If the exercise rate exceeds your body's ability to supply oxygen to your muscles, you are exercising anaerobically, rapidly depleting your creatine phosphate and glycogen reserves. Once these are exhausted, if available oxygen cannot support the oxygen energy system, performance plummets.

Carbohydrate stores are limited. A 68-kilogram (150-pound) man with 10 to 20 percent body fat, for example, has carbohydrate stores of 1,800 to 2,000 kilocalories in muscle glycogen, liver glycogen, and blood glucose. Compare this to the energy he stores in fat. His fat tissue holds roughly 63,000 to 120,000 kilocalories.[12] Although the body can burn protein for

oxygen energy system A complex energy system that requires oxygen. To release ATP, it completes the breakdown of carbohydrate and fatty acids via the citric acid cycle and electron transport chain.

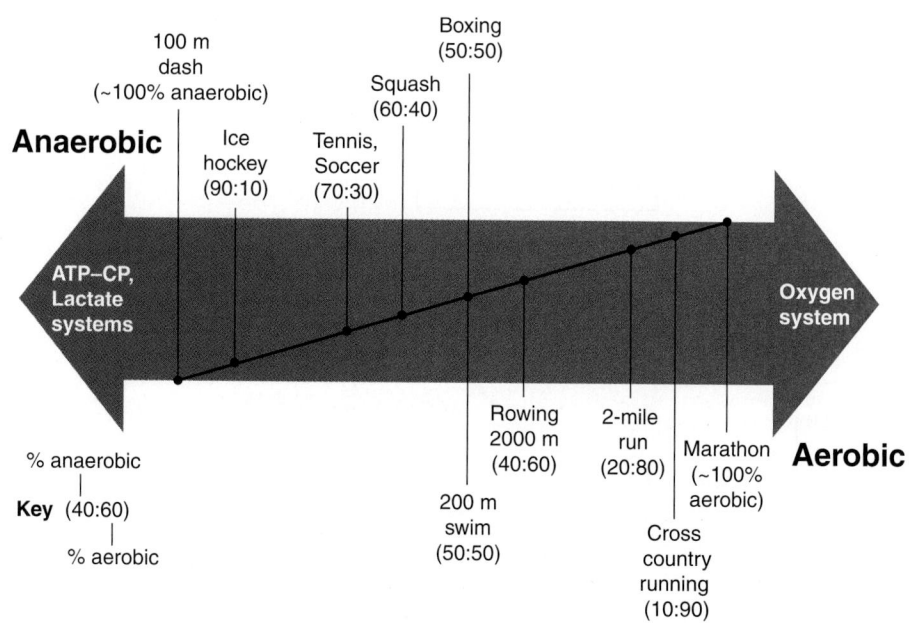

Figure 13.8 **The anaerobic–aerobic continuum.** Most activities use ATP from both anaerobic and aerobic energy systems. However, the 100-meter dash is considered completely anaerobic, and the marathon is considered completely aerobic.

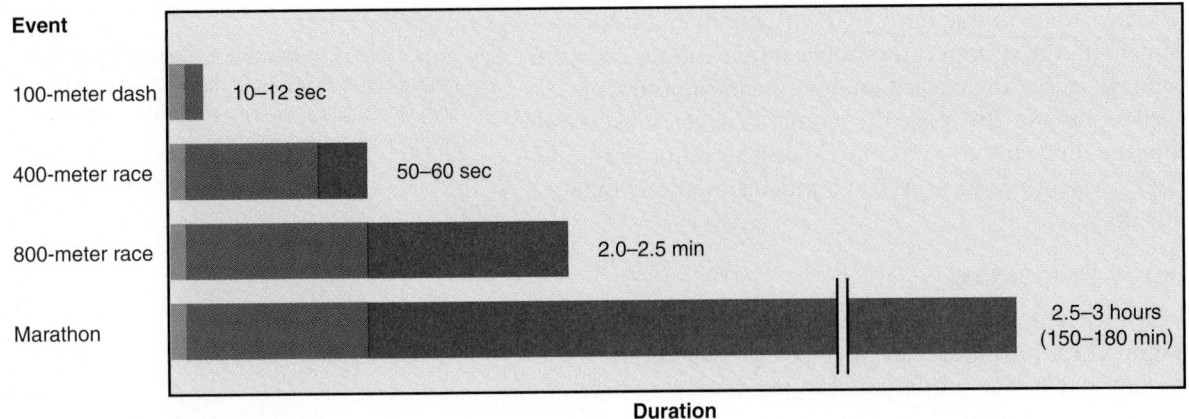

Event

100-meter dash | 10–12 sec

400-meter race | 50–60 sec

800-meter race | 2.0–2.5 min

Marathon | 2.5–3 hours (150–180 min)

Duration

- ☐ ATP–CP energy system
- ☐ Lactic acid energy system
- ☐ Oxygen energy system

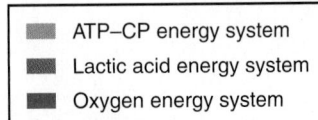 **Sports events and energy systems.** Short-term, explosive events rely upon the ATP-CP and lactic acid energy systems. For longer events, your body turns to the oxygen energy system. During endurance events, your body uses this system to burn fat as well as glucose.

energy, in well-fed people protein probably provides no more than 5 percent of the energy expended in exercise.[13]

Glycogen Depletion

At the beginning of the race, your body rapidly uses muscle glycogen. But as the race grinds on, the rate of glycogen use markedly slows. During the first 1.5 hours, glycogen stores drop steadily to about one-third their starting levels. About 3 hours into the run, as glycogen stores become almost entirely depleted, you may "hit the wall." Your muscles become weak and heavy, your legs shake, and you become confused. Marathon runners commonly experience a sudden onset of exhaustive fatigue around the 18- to 20-mile mark. Drinking fluids that contain glucose can partially compensate for glycogen depletion and soften its effects. Dehydration can cause an even faster onset of fatigue, so drinking plenty of fluids is essential during endurance events.

As exercise intensity increases, glycogen depletion accelerates. Sprinting, for example, uses muscle glycogen 35 to 40 times faster than walking.[14] **Figure 13.10** illustrates how the sensation of fatigue relates to the depletion of muscle glycogen.

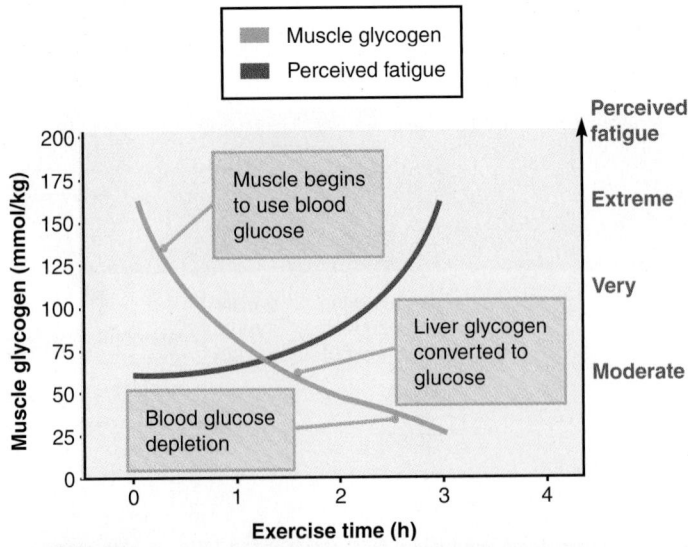

Figure 13.10 **Glycogen depletion and the sensation of fatigue.** As muscle glycogen levels decline, fatigue and eventually exhaustion set in.

Endurance Training

In untrained people, endurance training can increase endurance by as much as 500 percent.[15] To increase endurance, training enhances aerobic capacity by increasing the number of mitochondria and improving the body's ability to deliver oxygen to them. This decreases the reliance on anaerobic energy systems, extending the availability of glycogen reserves and delaying fatigue.

Key Concepts: *Muscle cells use three different energy systems to produce ATP: the ATP-CP energy system, the lactic acid energy system, and the oxygen energy system. The ATP-CP and lactic acid energy systems rely on carbohydrate and do not require oxygen. The oxygen energy system requires oxygen and relies on carbohydrates and fats. During the early minutes of high-intensity exercise, the anaerobic systems are the predominant source of ATP. During lower-intensity endurance events, the third system supplies ATP, although at a much slower rate. Dehydration and depletion of glycogen stores are major factors in fatigue. Training increases the efficiency of oxygen delivery to muscle and increases the number of muscle mitochondria available for aerobic metabolism.*

Optimal Nutrition for Athletic Performance

The optimal diet for most physically active people—from the college student who plays intramural basketball to the 50-year-old woman who enjoys walking during her lunch break—includes a variety of nutrient-dense foods. (See Chapter 2, "Nutrition Guidelines and Assessment.") Food choices should be high in carbohydrate (more than 60 percent of calories), low in fat (less than 30 percent of calories), and moderate in protein. When energy needs are met by eating a variety of foods from each of the MyPyramid food groups, micronutrient (vitamins and minerals) needs are met as well.

Optimal nutrition is an essential part of every athlete's training program and can make a difference when winning is measured in fractions of seconds or inches. General recommendations for competitive athletes include the following:[16]

- Consume adequate energy (calories) and nutrients to support health and performance.

- Maintain appropriate sports-specific ranges for percent body fat and fat-free body mass.

- Promote optimal recovery from training.

- Maintain hydration status.

The underlying foundations of a training diet are similar to the basic principles incorporated in the *Dietary Guidelines for Americans* and Canada's *Guidelines for Healthy Eating*. The primary differences are increased fluid needs to cover an athlete's sweat losses and increased energy needs to fuel physical activity. Studies indicate that athletes often are confused about nutrition and may not follow the dietary recommendations for peak sports performance.[17] Let's take a closer look at the nutritional needs of athletes.

Energy Intake and Exercise

Adequate energy intake is the first nutrition priority for athletes. Meeting energy needs is critical for athletic performance and for maintaining and/or increasing lean body mass. Sports nutritionists recommend eating small, frequent meals to maintain energy metabolism, improve nutrient intake, achieve desired body composition, support a training schedule, and reduce injuries.[18]

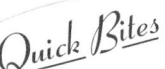

Quick Bites

Use It or Lose It!

The benefits of training begin to disappear after only two weeks of inactivity. Muscular endurance (the ability of a muscle to avoid fatigue) declines, and activities of certain oxidative enzymes drop by as much as 40 percent. By the fourth week, muscle glycogen levels also may drop by 40 percent. Flexibility is quickly lost, and inactivity can substantially decondition the heart muscle and cardiovascular system.

American Heart Association

Physical Activity

Physical inactivity is a major risk factor for developing coronary artery disease. Even moderately intense physical activity such as brisk walking is beneficial when done regularly for a total of 30 minutes or longer on most days.

Reproduced with permission. www.americanheart.org. © 2006, American Heart Association, Inc.

World-class athletes who train strenuously three to four hours each day can almost double their energy needs. The energy demand can be so high that some athletes have trouble consuming enough calories.[19] In contrast, athletes who compete in sports where they are judged by build and in sports with weight classifications often restrict energy intake to avoid weight gain. Energy intakes that are too low can lead to a loss of muscle mass, menstrual dysfunction, lower bone density, and increased risk of fatigue, injury, and illness.[20]

Carbohydrate and Exercise

Guidelines for athletes recommend high carbohydrate intakes during training.[21] A high-carbohydrate diet helps increase glycogen stores and extend endurance. (See **Figure 13.11**.) For endurance athletes, research studies suggest that carbohydrate should supply a minimum of 60 percent of total calories.[22] A high-carbohydrate diet also may prevent mental as well as physical fatigue and is important for stop-and-go sports such as basketball, football, and soccer.[23]

For all athletes, dietary carbohydrates should come mainly from complex carbohydrates, which provide many of the B vitamins necessary for energy metabolism along with iron (if enriched) and fiber (if whole grain). Although added sugars should be minimized, some athletes may need to include more simple sugars to meet energy requirements.

Carbohydrate Loading

Just as you might "top off" the gas tank in a car before a long trip, athletes can fill their glycogen stores prior to training or competition. In a process called **carbohydrate loading**, or **glycogen loading**, athletes manipulate their carbohydrate intake and exercise regimen to maximize muscle glycogen stores. (See **Figure 13.12**.)

Current recommendations for carbohydrate loading include an intake of 60 to 70 percent of total calories from carbohydrate, along with a decrease in exercise intensity and duration prior to competition.[24] **Table 13.2** is a training plan for endurance athletes that includes carbohydrate loading and exercise for the week before an event. The glycogen content of exercised muscles more than doubles in athletes who follow these recommendations, and this extends the duration of higher-

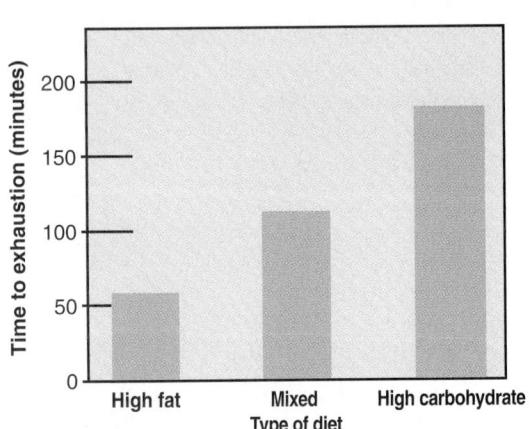

Figure 13.11 **Diet composition and endurance.** Athletes can exercise longer when eating a high-carbohydrate diet.

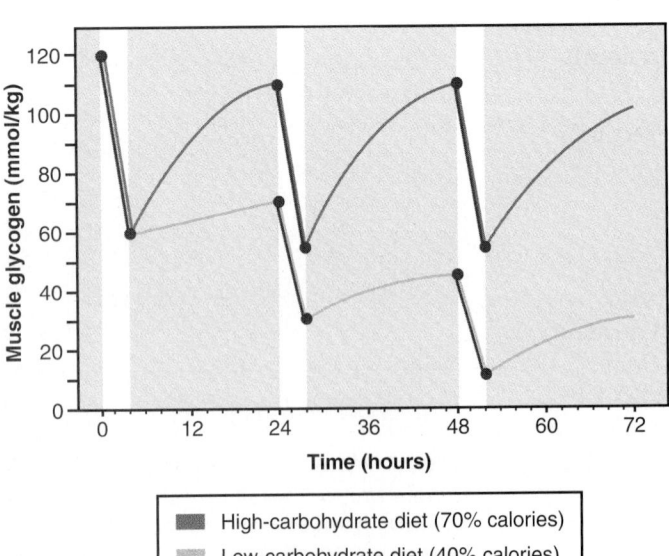

Figure 13.12 **Diet composition, training, and muscle glycogen.** A high-carbohydrate diet replenishes glycogen stores better than a low-carbohydrate diet.
Source: Adapted from Costill DL, Miller JM. Nutrition for endurance sport: carbohydrate and fluid balance. *Int J Sport Nutr.* 1980;1:2–14.

Table 13.2 **Carbohydrate Loading for Endurance Athletes**

Number of Days Before Event	Exercise Duration (mi at 70% of VO$_{2max}$)	Training Diet (g carbohydrate/kg body weight)
6	90	5
5	40	5
4	40	5
3	20	10
2	20	10
1	Rest day	10
Race	Competition	Precompetition food and fluid

Source: Adapted from Coleman EJ. Carbohydrate and exercise. In: Dunford M. *Sports Nutrition.* 4th ed. Chicago: The American Dietetic Association, 2006;14–32. Used with permission.

intensity activity. For example, distance runners who carbohydrate-load may be able to keep a faster pace for a longer time and finish a race sooner.[25]

Even though "extra" glycogen prior to competition sounds like a perfect plan, there is a downside to carbohydrate loading. For each gram of glycogen stored in muscle tissue, the body also stores about 3 grams of water. Many athletes who carbohydrate-load complain about this weight gain and subsequent sluggishness. Some opt to train and compete without carbohydrate loading because, for them, the risk of physical discomfort outweighs the benefit of a greater carbohydrate store.

If you participate in an aerobic activity for fewer than 60 to 90 consecutive minutes, carbohydrate loading probably will provide no benefit. Instead, experts recommend that you taper your training program a few days before competition and eat a diet that provides 70 percent of its calories from carbohydrate for one or two days before the event.[26]

Carbohydrate Intake Before Exercise

Eating carbohydrate two to four hours before morning exercise helps replenish glycogen stores and improve endurance. Because many athletes have problems with GI distress, the carbohydrate and caloric content of the meal should be smaller when eaten closer to a workout. Although some athletes can tolerate solid foods, others prefer liquids to avoid GI distress. Because protein and fat take longer to digest and absorb, preexercise meals should contain no more than 10 to 15 percent of total calories as protein and less than 20 percent of calories from fat. **Table 13.3** offers guidelines for the timing of meals before an event.

Many athletes are confused about whether to eat less than an hour before exercise. To decrease hunger, delay fatigue, and improve performance, athletes who cannot fully refuel several hours prior to a workout must rely on "last minute" carbohydrate intake. Although early research suggested that

carbohydrate loading Changes in dietary carbohydrate intake and exercise regimen before competition to maximize glycogen stores in the muscles. It is appropriate for endurance events lasting 60 to 90 consecutive minutes or longer. Also known as glycogen loading.

glycogen loading See *carbohydrate loading.*

Table 13.3 **Timing Meals Before Events**

Time: 8 A.M. event, such as a road race or swim meet
Meals: Eat a high-carbohydrate dinner and drink extra water the day before. The morning of the event, about 6:00 or 6:30, have a light 200- to 400-calorie meal (depending on your tolerance), such as yogurt and a banana, or one or two energy bars, and extra water. Eat familiar foods. If you want a bigger meal, you might want to get up and eat by 5:00 or 6:00.

Time: 10 A.M. event, such as a bike race or soccer game
Meals: Eat a high-carbohydrate meal and drink extra water the day before. The morning of the event, eat a familiar breakfast by 7:00, to allow 3 hours for the food to digest. This meal will prevent the fatigue that results from low blood sugar. If your body cannot handle any breakfast, eat a late snack before going to bed the night before. This will boost liver glycogen stores and prevent low blood sugar the next morning.

Time: 2 P.M. event, such as a football or lacrosse game
Meals: An afternoon game allows time for you to have either a big, high-carbohydrate breakfast and a light lunch, or a substantial brunch by 10:00, allowing 4 hours for digestion. As always, eat a high-carbohydrate dinner the night before, and drink extra fluids the day before and up to noontime.

Time: 8 P.M. event, such as a basketball game
Meals: A hefty, high-carbohydrate breakfast and lunch will be thoroughly digested by evening. Plan for dinner, as tolerated, by 5:00 or have a lighter meal between 6:00 and 7:00. Drink extra fluids all day.

Time: All-day event, such as a 100-mile bike ride or triathlon training
Meals: Two days before, cut back on your exercise; the day before, take a rest day to allow your muscles the chance to replace depleted glycogen stores. Eat carbohydrate-rich meals at breakfast, lunch, and dinner. Drink extra fluids. The day of the event, eat breakfast according to your tolerance—whatever you usually have before exercising.

Throughout the day, plan to snack at least every 1.5 to 2 hours on wholesome carbohydrates (such as energy bars, dried fruit, or sports drinks) to maintain a normal blood sugar. At lunchtime, eat a carbohydrate meal, but in general, try to distribute your calories evenly throughout the day. Drink fluids before you get thirsty; you should need to urinate at least three times throughout the day.

Source: Reprinted by permission from Nancy Clark. *Nancy Clark's Sports Nutrition Guidebook.* 3rd ed. Champaign, IL: Human Kinetics, 2003:101.

consuming carbohydrate within one hour before activity could cause low blood glucose and early fatigue, later studies report improved performance or no effect.[27]

Preexercise Meals and the Glycemic Index

As you may recall from Chapter 4, "Carbohydrates," individual foods have different effects on blood glucose levels independent of carbohydrate content. The glycemic index of foods is a measure of this effect and has attracted recent interest in relation to the diets of athletes. Current studies have produced mixed results, so it remains unclear whether the glycemic index of carbohydrate in preexercise meals affects performance.[28]

Carbohydrate Intake During Exercise

During exercise, athletes can maintain their carbohydrate supply to exercising muscle by consuming beverages with low to moderate amounts of simple carbohydrate.[29] When an event lasts at least one hour, drinking fluids with 4 to 8 percent carbohydrate, the amount in sports drinks, enables athletes to exercise longer and sprint harder at the finish. (See the Nutrition Science in Action feature "Fourth-Quarter Performance.") Although sports drinks also are suitable during events lasting less than one hour, plain water is adequate for maintaining hydration during these shorter events.[30] Consuming carbohydrate before and during an event improves performance more than either strategy alone.

Carbohydrate Intake Following Exercise

It can take 24 to 48 hours after an event to replenish glycogen stores, and the timing and type of carbohydrates are important factors in the refueling process. Athletes who delay the consumption of carbohydrates for more than four hours after exercising synthesize glycogen only half as fast as athletes who consume carbohydrates during the first two hours after exercising.[31] Some research shows that the first 15 minutes are critical.[32]

The best way to replenish glycogen stores after intense exercise is to consume 1 to 1.5 grams of carbohydrate per kilogram of body weight within 30 minutes after a workout, followed by an additional 1 to 1.5 grams per kilogram two hours later.[33] A 70-kilogram (154-pound) athlete who exercises vigorously for 90 minutes or more, for example, would consume 70 to 100 grams of carbohydrate immediately after exercise, followed by another 70 to 100 grams two hours later. Consuming high-glycemic-index foods enhances glycogen synthesis.[34] Among simple sugars, glucose and sucrose appear equally effective in replenishing glycogen, but fructose alone is not as effective.[35]

Carbohydrate intake after exercise also benefits protein metabolism. Several researchers have shown that these levels of carbohydrates taken immediately or one hour after resistance exercise decrease protein breakdown and enhance protein retention.[36]

Key Concepts: *Energy intake is the most important element of the athlete's diet, and the major source of energy should be carbohydrates. Foods rich in complex carbohydrates, which also can provide fiber, iron, and B vitamins, are best. A high-carbohydrate diet prior to competition helps to maximize glycogen stores and endurance. Carbohydrate loading is a process of adjusting carbohydrate intake and training intensity to maximize glycogen stores just before an event. Consuming carbohydrates soon after exercise enhances the rebuilding of glycogen stores.*

NUTRITION SCIENCE IN ACTION
Fourth-Quarter Performance

Background: Consuming drinks containing carbohydrates during prolonged endurance exercise previously has been demonstrated to improve athletes' exercise outcomes, including endurance and speed, as well as measures of mood. Much less is known about the effects of carbohydrate feedings during intermittent high-intensity exercise, such as playing competitive basketball and soccer.

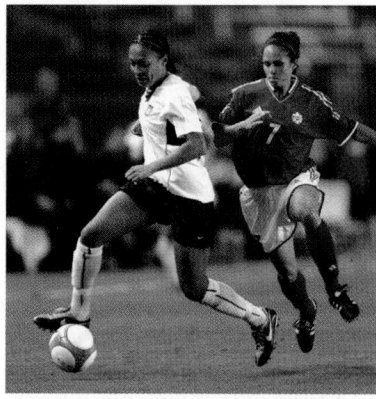

Hypothesis: Carbohydrate feedings during intermittent high-intensity exercise will result in faster sprint times.

Experimental Plan: Twenty active men (N = 10) and women (N = 10) who participate in intermittent high-intensity team sports performed two experimental trials during which they were fed either a carbohydrate solution (CHO) or a flavored placebo (PBO). Experimental trials consisted of four 15-minute quarters of shuttle running with variable intensities ranging from walking to running to maximal sprinting and performing 40 jumps at a target hanging at 80 percent of their maximum vertical jump height. The first and third quarters were followed by 5-minute breaks, and the second quarter by a 20-minute halftime break.

Results: The hypothesis is confirmed. Compared with the placebo, CHO feedings during exercise resulted in faster 20-meter sprint times, especially during the fourth quarter.

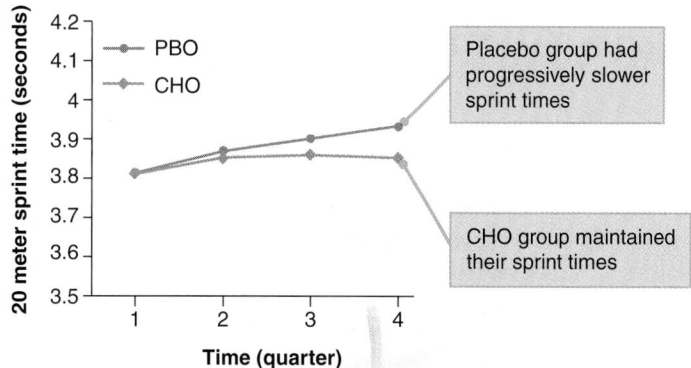

Conclusion and Discussion: These results combined with other measures collected during this experiment show that compared to the placebo, CHO feedings during intermittent high-intensity exercise improved sprinting and jumping performance, speed and agility, and overall mood late in exercise. The results suggest that CHO feedings during team sporting events, such as basketball, can contribute to athletes' ability to perform their best. Future studies of CHO feedings on exercise and cognitive function will be an important contribution to the sports nutrition literature.

Source: Based on Winnick JJ, Davis JM, Welsh RS, et al. Carbohydrate feedings during team sport exercise preserve physical and CNS function. *Med Sci Sports Exerc.* 2005;37(2):306–315.

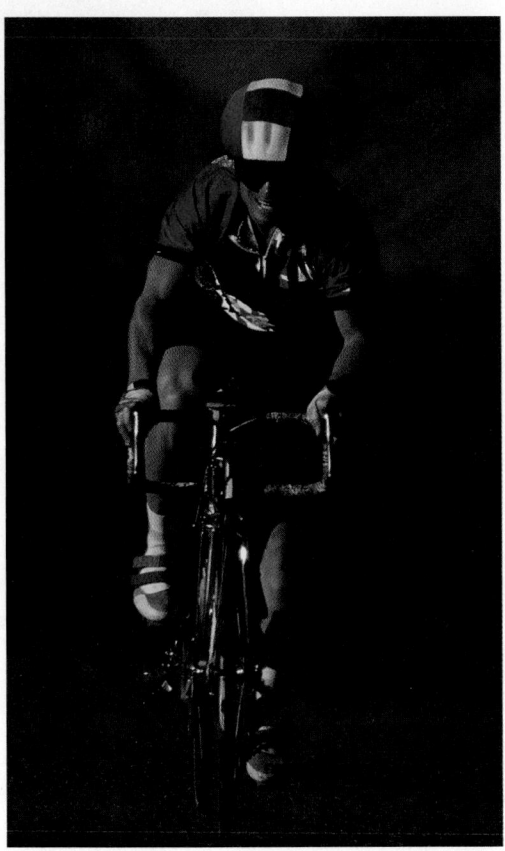

Optimal nutrition is an important part of athletic training.

Dietary Fat and Exercise

During exercise, carbohydrates and fats are the two main fuel sources. Endurance (aerobic) training increases the capacity of your oxygen energy system, enhancing your body's ability to use fat as a fuel. Exercise intensity also affects fuel use. During low- to moderate-intensity exercise, fatty acids are the major fuel source. During high-intensity exercise, the predominant energy source is glucose.

This does not mean that endurance athletes should consume diets high in fat. High-fat diets usually are lower in carbohydrate, thus limiting muscles' ability to replenish glycogen stores. High-fat diets often are high in calories, saturated fat, and cholesterol; your body also digests fat more slowly than carbohydrate.

Fat Intake and the Athlete

Fat intake should not be overly restricted. There is no performance benefit in consuming a diet with less than 15 percent of energy from fat.[37] Extreme fat restriction limits food choices, especially sources of protein, iron, zinc, and essential fatty acids. In addition, athletes with high caloric needs (greater than 5,000 kilocalories per day) may find it difficult to eat enough food without consuming more than 20 to 35 percent of their calories from fat, the range recommended for the general population. Sports nutritionists recommend that any extra fat calories come from monounsaturated and polyunsaturated sources.

Protein and Exercise

Historically, many athletes have believed they could become stronger by eating muscle from animals. Many bodybuilders and weightlifters still believe a meal of steak and eggs is their most important source of calories.[38]

$\mathcal{Fyi}$ To Zone or Not to Zone? That Is the Question

FOR YOUR INFORMATION

Barry Sears, creator of Eicotec bars and author of *Enter the Zone* and *Mastering the Zone*, puts forth the theory that insulin response to high-carbohydrate diets reduces performance by interfering with free fatty acid mobilization and lowering blood glucose. He further asserts that the insulin response facilitates the conversion of carbohydrate to fat and increases adipose tissue stores. The Zone diet books recommend a carbohydrate-restricted diet of exactly 40 percent carbohydrate, 30 percent protein, and 30 percent fat.

The Zone diet proponents assert that high insulin levels increase the production of "bad" eicosanoids. Eicosanoids are hormonelike compounds that help regulate inflammation, the tendency for blood to clot, and the immune system. The protein content of the Zone diet supposedly increases glucagon levels, which in turn support the production of "good" eicosanoids by counteracting the effects of insulin.

The scientific basis of the theory underlying the Zone diet has many faults. There is no evidence that insulin increases the amount of "bad" eicosanoids or that glucagon makes "good" eicosanoids.[1] A high-carbohydrate diet does elicit an insulin response because insulin is needed for the transport of glucose (energy) into the cells. With insulin-mediated glucose uptake, the synthesis of liver and muscle glycogen leads to a decrease in blood glucose. The body preferentially uses carbohydrates for energy and does not readily convert excess carbohydrate to fat. (See the FYI "Do Carbohydrates Turn into Fat?" in Chapter 7, "Metabolism.") During exercise, the release of catecholamines such as epinephrine and norepinephrine drives an increase in blood glucose and a decrease in insulin. Catecholamines also prompt the adipose tissue to release fatty acids into the bloodstream.

Consuming carbohydrate 30 to 60 minutes before exercise is associated with increased

Current research, however, suggests athletes require only slightly higher protein intakes than sedentary people.[39]

Enter the Zone, a popular book with an unscientific premise, recommends a diet of 40 percent carbohydrate, 30 percent fat, and 30 percent protein. With its popularity, athletes' interest in optimal protein intake surged. Athletes—from endurance runners to football players to weekend warriors—are asking the question "Do I need to eat more protein and less carbohydrate for optimal performance?"[40] (See the FYI feature "To Zone or Not To Zone? That Is the Question.")

Protein Recommendations for Athletes

The adult Recommended Dietary Allowance (RDA) for protein is 0.8 gram of protein per kilogram of body weight per day,[41] and people who regularly engage in low-intensity exercise do not need additional protein.[42]

Although the Food and Nutrition Board did not recommend a specific RDA for endurance or strength athletes, studies suggest that endurance athletes involved in heavy training require 1.2 to 1.4 grams of protein per kilogram of body weight per day.[43] Endurance athletes who are training for extreme events, such as the Tour de France, need up to 2 grams per kilogram.[44]

Strength athletes consuming 1.4 grams of protein per kilogram of body weight per day synthesize more body protein than athletes consuming 0.9 grams. Increased protein synthesis during training is an indicator of muscle growth. However, when protein intake was increased to 2.4 grams per kilogram, protein synthesis did not increase further.[45] After adjusting for higher levels of protein oxidation with higher intakes, researchers recommend that strength athletes consume 1.6 to 1.7 grams of protein per kilogram per day.[46] A 91-kilogram (200-pound) strength athlete who wants to build muscle mass would consume about 150 grams of protein. **Table 13.4** shows the protein requirements of various levels of physical activity.

Table 13.4 **Protein Requirements of Sedentary and Active People**

Activity Level	Protein Requirements (g protein/kg body weight)
Sedentary	0.8
Strength athlete	1.6–1.7
Endurance athlete	1.2–1.4
Maximum usable amount for adults	2.0

Source: Adapted from Snyder AC, Naik J. Protein requirements of athletes. In: Berning JR, Steen SN, eds. *Nutrition for Sport and Exercise.* 2nd ed. Sudbury, MA: Jones and Bartlett Publishers, 1998.

insulin and lowered blood glucose. However, those responses are temporary and do not adversely affect performance. In fact, a high-carbohydrate meal one hour before exercise can improve endurance by supplying the exercising muscles with glucose and sparing the loss of glycogen.

Carbohydrates—not fatty acids—are used preferentially for energy during exercise. Muscle glycogen is the body's predominant energy source for most sports. Because it takes longer for fat to become available to muscles as fuel in the form of free fatty acids, the duration of most athletes' workouts is not sufficient to burn significant amounts of fat.

Rather, it is the calorie deficit resulting from the exercise session and negative energy balance during the day that promotes fat loss. When athletes restrict carbohydrate intake, they compromise the amount of carbohydrate stored in their muscles, which is needed to facilitate exercise performance. The Zone diet is a low-energy diet and does not increase the body's ability to burn fat.

It is not realistic to think that a diet composed of 30 percent protein would always contain only 30 percent fat. If you use meats to meet these protein recommendations, it is not difficult to exceed the fat recommendations. And, with a restriction of carbohydrate

foods, a vegetarian-based protein intake is largely ruled out.[2] There are some individuals for whom a high-carbohydrate diet is not recommended. But athletic individuals are not among them.

1 Coleman EJ. Carbohydrate and exercise. In: Dunford M. *Sports Nutrition.* 4th ed. Chicago: The American Dietetic Association, 2006;14–32.

2 Coleman E. Debunking the "Eicotec" myth. *Sports Med Dig.* 1993;15:6–7.

Protein Intake and the Athlete

Athletes don't need protein powders or amino acid supplements to meet the protein demands of athletic performance.[47] Their best protein sources are high-quality protein foods, including legumes, low-fat dairy products, egg whites, lean beef and pork, chicken, turkey, and fish. (See Chapter 6, "Proteins and Amino Acids" for more on protein sources.)

Vegetarian athletes can achieve adequate protein intake and meet their energy needs by eating a variety of protein-rich foods from plant sources, such as grains, nuts, beans, and seeds. Because plant proteins are less digestible than animal foods, the total amount of protein consumed may need to be somewhat higher.

Protein Intake After Exercise

Protein combined with carbohydrate in a postexercise meal increases glycogen synthesis more than carbohydrate alone[48] and also stimulates more protein synthesis.[49] Researchers suggest athletes consume 4 grams of protein for every 10 grams of carbohydrate (grams protein = 40 percent grams carbohydrate).[50] For example, using postexercise recommendations of 1.5 grams of carbohydrate per kilogram of body weight, a 55-kilogram female athlete would need 82.5 grams of carbohydrate (55 g × 1.5 = 82.5 g) and 33 grams protein (82.5 g × 0.40 = 33 g). How does this translate to food? A small bagel, 2 ounces of string cheese, and 8 ounces of low-fat yogurt would be a portable snack to enjoy after a hard workout (provides 86 grams of carbohydrate and 33 grams of protein).

Dangers of High-Protein Intake

diuresis The formation and secretion of urine.

Excessive protein intake from food or supplements enhances **diuresis** (loss of body water) as the body attempts to excrete excess nitrogen through the urine. This increases the risk for dehydration and may contribute to mineral losses. High-protein diets often are high in saturated and total fat and may contribute to obesity, osteoporosis, heart disease, and certain types of cancer. (See Chapter 6, "Proteins and Amino Acids.")

High intakes of single–amino acid supplements may impair absorption of other amino acids. Further, the amount of amino acids contained in supplements is very small compared with the amount in food. For example, one pill may contain 500 milligrams of an amino acid, but 1 ounce of meat, poultry, or fish provides more than 7,000 milligrams of essential and nonessential amino acids! And the cost of supplements is higher.

Key Concepts: *Although fat is an important fuel for exercise, a high-fat diet is not necessary. General recommendations that fat not exceed 20 to 35 percent of total energy intake are appropriate for athletes. Dietary protein is a source of energy and also a source of amino acids for body protein synthesis. The protein requirements of athletes are slightly higher than those of sedentary adults, but still within the normal range of protein consumption. High-protein diets are neither recommended nor necessary. Low-fat dairy products, egg whites, lean beef and pork, chicken, turkey, fish, and legumes are good sources of protein.*

Vitamins, Minerals, and Athletic Performance

Many reactions that support exercise and physical activity require vitamins and minerals. They help extract energy from nutrients, transport oxygen, and repair tissues. Researchers have long debated whether physically active people have greater vitamin and mineral needs than sedentary people.

B Vitamins

Because B vitamins are essential for energy metabolism (see Chapter 10, "Water-Soluble Vitamins"), wouldn't athletes, with their high energy needs, require more B vitamins? There is no need to run to the supplement counter. B vitamins are needed for chemical reactions that release energy. But if athletes consume adequate calories and ample complex carbohydrates, fruits, and vegetables, they eat plenty of B vitamins. However, if athletes consume too few calories or eat mostly refined sugars in lieu of complex carbohydrates, they can compromise their B vitamin intake.

Vegan athletes whose diets do not include fortified foods, such as some soy products and ready-to-eat cereals, may have a problem with vitamin B_{12} intake. They should consult a medical advisor or registered dietitian to determine if they need B_{12} supplements.

Calcium

Calcium is essential for normal muscle function and strong bones. Adequate calcium intake coupled with regular exercise slows the deterioration of the skeleton with age and can reduce the risk of osteoporosis.

Inadequate calcium may increase the risk of stress fractures in athletes. This is of particular concern for the amenorrheic athlete (discussed in the "Female Athlete Triad" section later in this chapter). Athletes should strive to meet the Adequate Intake (AI) level for calcium from a variety of low-fat dairy products and other calcium-rich foods. This is especially true for teens whose calcium needs (1,300 mg/day) are higher than those of adults (1,000 mg/day)

Iron

Iron is vital to oxygen delivery and energy production. As an essential part of hemoglobin and myoglobin, iron helps deliver oxygen to active muscle cells. It is also a key component of several enzymes vital to the production of ATP by the oxygen energy system. (For more details about iron's functional roles, see Chapter 12, "Trace Minerals.")

Because of menstrual losses and lower dietary iron intakes, female athletes have a greater risk of iron deficiency than male athletes. In endurance athletes, the impact of running can cause mechanical trauma to capillaries in the feet and increase the breakdown of red blood cells. The increased breakdown may contribute to low iron status.[51] Some studies suggest that athletes involved in heavy training may need 30 to 70 percent more iron than a nonathlete.[52]

Endurance training also increases the volume of plasma in the blood without initially changing the amount of hemoglobin. This dilutes the hemoglobin, even though training typically maintains or increases the amount of total hemoglobin. This condition, called **sports anemia**, is a false anemia for most athletes and can be remedied with a few days of rest.

Although many elite athletes, especially endurance athletes, have mild iron deficiency, few are anemic.[53] Although anemia can seriously impair a person's capacity to perform activities, mild iron deficiency has little effect on performance.[54]

Other Trace Minerals

Strenuous exercise taxes the body's reserves of copper (essential for red blood cell synthesis) and zinc (vital to the work of many enzymes involved in energy production). During endurance events, increased fluid loss

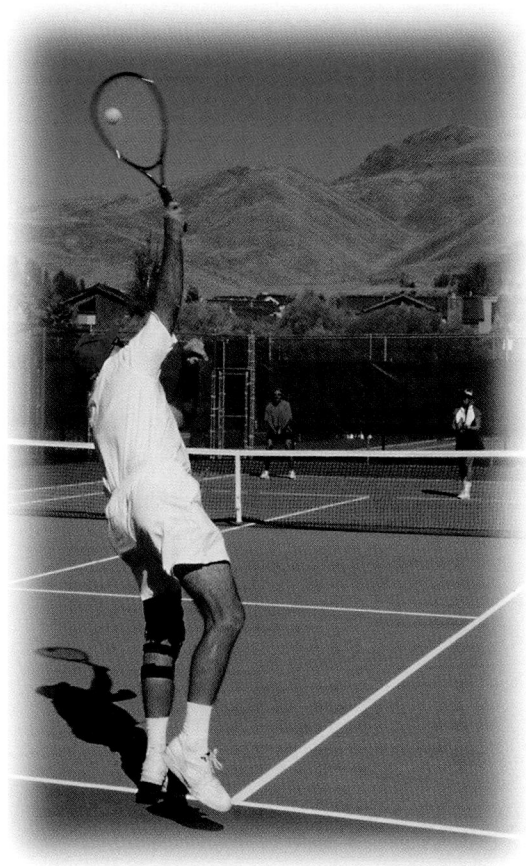

sports anemia A lowered concentration of hemoglobin in the blood due to dilution. The increased plasma volume that dilutes the hemoglobin is a normal consequence of aerobic training.

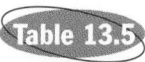

Table 13.5 **A Sample Training Diet**

Athlete performs prolonged daily training
Body weight = 70 kilograms
Energy intake = 3,400 kilocalories

Macronutrients

Carbohydrate	Protein	Fat
535 g	128 g	83 g
63% kcal	15% kcal	22% kcal
7.5 g/kg body weight*	1.8 g/kg body weight**	

Breakfast

8 oz orange juice
2 C Cheerios cereal
8 oz 1% milk
1 large bran muffin

Lunch

2 slices whole-wheat
    bread
2 oz turkey
2 slices tomato
Lettuce leaf
2 tsp mayonnaise
1 med apple
12 oz cranberry juice

Preexercise

8 oz Gatorade
1 cereal bar

Postexercise

1 bagel
2 oz string cheese
16 oz apple juice

Dinner

3 oz chicken breast
1 lg baked potato with
    2 Tbsp low-fat
    sour cream
2 whole-wheat dinner rolls
1 tsp margarine
1 C cooked broccoli
1 C salad greens with
    2 Tbsp Italian salad
    dressing
8 oz 1% milk
1 C low-fat frozen yogurt

* Recommended carbohydrate intake goals for prolonged
   daily training

** Recommended protein intake goals up to 2 g/kg
    body weight for extreme training loads

Quick Bites

Sweating a World Record

When Alberto Salazar ran the Olympic marathon in 1984, he went down in the record books for sweat production. He lost 12 pounds during the 26.2-mile race, despite drinking about 2 liters. His sweat rate was approximately 3.7 liters per hour.

increases mineral losses—zinc in urine and relatively high amounts of both zinc and copper in sweat.

Although these losses may cause marginal deficiencies, supplementation is not necessarily recommended. High-dose supplements of iron, copper, or zinc can interfere with the normal absorption of these and other minerals, so an excess of one can cause a deficiency of the others. **Table 13.5** is an example of a training diet that would meet an athlete's needs for vitamins and minerals through food, which is preferable to taking supplements.

Key Concepts: *Vitamins and minerals are important components of athletes' diets. B vitamins are necessary for normal energy metabolism. Adequate calcium intake can help protect against stress fractures and, coupled with exercise, delays the onset of osteoporosis. Iron is needed to carry oxygen. Strenuous exercise can tax the body's reserves of both copper and zinc.*

Fluid Needs During Exercise

Exercise generates heat, and heavy exercise can increase heat production 15- to 20-fold. The increase in body heat triggers sweating, and sweat cools your body as it evaporates on your skin (see **Figure 13.13**). The body of a well-trained athlete begins to cool itself soon after exercise begins. Even

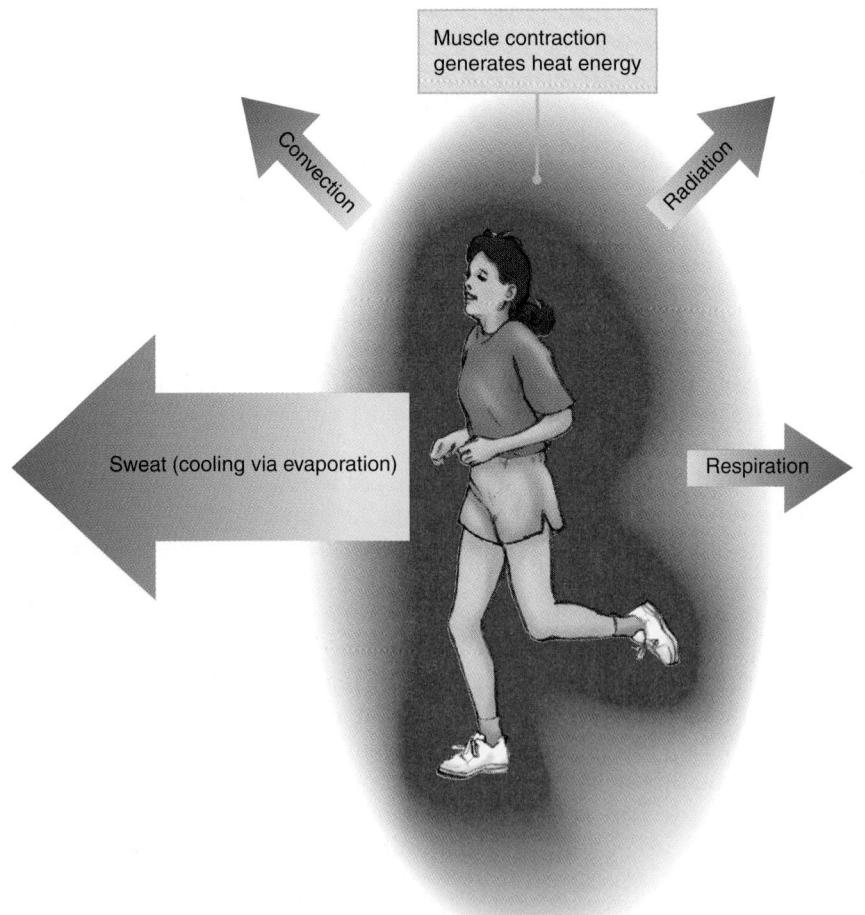

Figure 13.13 **Dissipation of heat during exercise.** During exercise, radiation, convection, and respiration are responsible for some heat loss, but evaporation of sweat dissipates more than 80 percent of the heat generated by increased physical activity.

before core body temperature rises, the athlete's body starts to produce sweat. Sweat rate is affected by environmental temperature (extreme heat or extreme cold), humidity (higher humidity increases the rate of sweat production but reduces efficiency of evaporation), type of clothing, fitness level, and initial fluid balance. During exercise in hot weather, sweat losses of endurance athletes can easily exceed 1 liter per hour.[55]

To keep the body from overheating, blood must flow to the skin, where evaporating sweat can dissipate heat. During exercise, the cooling demand for blood flow to the skin may compete with the cardiovascular demand for blood to deliver fuel to working muscles. Dehydration stresses both systems, making each less efficient. Without fluid replacement during heavy exercise, athletes can become dehydrated quickly, and a water deficit of 1 to 2 percent of body weight degrades athletic performance.[56] Signs of dehydration include the following:

- Elevated heart rate at a given exercise intensity
- Increased rate of **perceived exertion** during activity
- Decreased performance
- Lethargy
- Concentrated urine
- Infrequent urination
- Loss of appetite

Drinking fluid during exercise helps offset fluid loss, minimize cardiovascular changes, reduce perception of effort, and maintain a supply of fuel to working muscles. When possible, athletes should drink fluid at rates that most closely match their sweating rates.[57] Because exercise inhibits the body's thirst signal, you probably won't take in enough fluid if you wait until you are thirsty to replenish your losses. Active people must train themselves to consume adequate amounts of fluid before, during, and after exercise. **Table 13.6** shows how much fluid a person should drink at various levels of physical activity.

Hydration: Drink More!

Athletes should be well hydrated before starting physical activity. The day before an event, the athlete should drink generous amounts of fluid. In the final two to three hours before exercise, the ACSM recommends drinking 400 to 600 milliliters (2 to 3 cups) of fluid.[58] Because even partial dehydration can compromise performance, athletes should maintain fluid balance during the event. After beginning exercise, drinking 150 to 350 milliliters (6 to 12 ounces) every 15 to 20 minutes helps facilitate optimal hydration. Most athletes are unable to replace all lost fluid, so they are somewhat dehydrated when the event ends. To make up for sweat losses and cover obligatory urine production, athletes may need to consume an amount of fluid equal to 1.5 times the body weight lost during the exercise session.

Athletes may choose water, sports drinks, or other beverages to meet fluid needs. During activities that last less than 60 continuous minutes, water can replace fluid lost in sweat and help offset the rise in core temperature. During exercise that lasts longer than 60 continuous minutes, muscle and liver glycogen stores become depleted. Consuming fluids that contain carbohydrate and sodium can delay fatigue (see **Figure 13.14**), enhance palatability of fluids, and promote fluid retention.[59]

Optimal sports drinks provide energy (from glucose, glucose polymers, or sucrose) and electrolytes in a **palatable** solution that promotes rapid

perceived exertion The subjective experience of how difficult an effort is.

palatable Pleasant tasting.

Table 13.6 **Typical Fluid Needs**

Activity Level	Environment	Fluid Requirements (liters per day)
Sedentary	Cool	2–3
Active	Cool	3–6
Sedentary	Warm	3–5
Active	Warm	5–10+

Note that fluid requirements include fluid from all sources—liquids, food, and metabolic water. See Chapter 10, "Water and Major Minerals," for more information.

Source: Murray R. Drink more! Advice from a world class expert. *ACSM's Health and Fitness Journal.* 1997;1:19–23, 50.

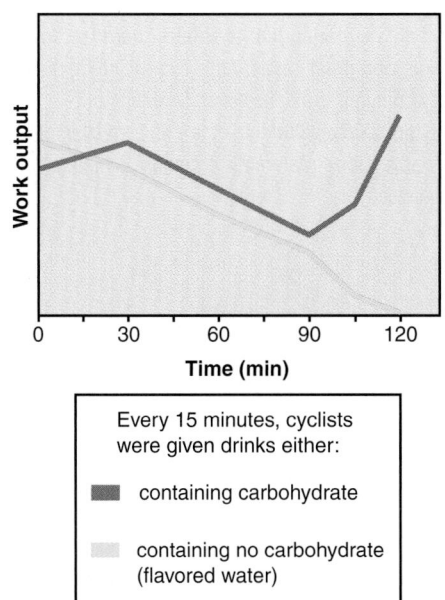

Every 15 minutes, cyclists were given drinks either:

■ containing carbohydrate

▨ containing no carbohydrate (flavored water)

Figure 13.14 **Sports drinks and performance.** Consuming carbohydrate drinks dramatically increases power output after 90 minutes.

absorption (less than 10 percent carbohydrate concentration). (See **Table 13.7**.) The palatability of beverages containing electrolytes and 4 to 8 percent carbohydrate may increase the voluntary intake of fluid.[60] Beverages such as fruit juices and soft drinks are concentrated sources of carbohydrates (more than 10 percent) and may slow gastric emptying. In juices and many soft drinks, the main carbohydrate is fructose, which is associated with slower stomach emptying and abdominal cramps. Carbonated soft drinks may decrease the volume of fluid consumed and delay stomach emptying.

Athletes should avoid beverages that contain alcohol. Alcohol is a diuretic and does not allow complete rehydration. Some athletes use alcohol for psychological benefits—calming nerves, improving self-confidence, and reducing anxiety, pain, and muscle tremor. This misguided effort fails to recognize alcohol's negative influence on physical performance. Alcohol slows reaction time, impairs coordination, and upsets balance. Its diuretic action contributes to dehydration and may impair regulation of body temperature.

For endurance events that last longer than four to five hours (or shorter events in high heat and humidity), athletes who do not replace electrolytes put themselves at risk for abnormally low levels of blood sodium. This life-threatening condition is associated with an excessive loss of electrolytes in sweat and with the excessive consumption of fluid, such as plain water, that does not replace electrolytes. See **Table 13.8** for a summary of the American College of Sports Medicine's position on the amount and type of fluid to consume before, during, and after activity.

Nutrition Needs of Youth in Sport

Young athletes (younger than 19 years) should place a higher priority on nutritional needs for growth and development than on athletic performance.[61] Studies indicate that diets in young athletes are often marginal or

Table 13.7 **Desirable Composition of Sports Beverages**

Characteristic	Comment
Fuel/Calories	Contains a source of carbohydrate: glucose, maltodextrin, sucrose, high-fructose corn syrup. Goal intake is 30–60 g/hr (2–4 cups of a 6 percent carbohydrate drink per hour).
Electrolytes	Enhances fluid uptake and palatability. Contains sodium, potassium, chloride, and phosphorus to replace sweat electrolyte loss in activity longer than four hours. Not an issue in exercise of shorter duration.
Rapid absorption	Carbohydrate concentration less than 10 percent. Carbohydrate concentration over 10 percent can slow gastric emptying. Fructose should not be main or sole form of carbohydrate.
Palatability	Flavor may be biggest key to amount consumed. Taste changes can occur during exercise. Carbonation may decrease amount of fluid consumed.

Source: Shi X, Gisolfi CV. Fluid and carbohydrate replacement during intermittent exercise. *Sports Med.* 1998;25:157–172. Reprinted by permission of Wolters Kluwer Health.

inadequate in energy intake.[62] The consequences of chronic low energy intake include the following:[63]

- Short stature and delayed puberty
- Nutrient deficiencies and dehydration
- Menstrual irregularities
- Poor bone health
- Increased incidence of injuries
- Increased risk of developing eating disorders

Parents and youth need to understand the energy and nutrient demands of growth and training, and many need help in planning meals and snacks to meet those needs. Many sport activities for this age group take place after school, and some schools serve lunch as early as 10:45 A.M. To provide energy for the activity and nutrients for recovery, young people should have meals and snacks before and after exercise. Easily portable snacks include fruit, pretzels, dry cereal, cereal bars, yogurt, sports drinks, sandwiches, and milk. Young athletes must drink adequate fluids during the day as well as at practice and competition. This is especially important because youths have a high tolerance for exercising in heat, which puts them at increased risk for heat exhaustion and heat stroke.

Key Concepts: Exercise of any type increases fluid losses through sweat. Evaporation of sweat from the skin allows the body to cool itself. Fluid losses must be replaced to avoid dehydration. Athletes need to drink plenty of fluid before, during, and after exercise. Fluid choices depend on the duration of activity and the preferences of the athlete. Optimal sports drinks provide energy and electrolytes in a solution that promotes rapid absorption.

Quick Bites

Climbing with Age

Aging does not seem to impair a healthy person's ability to perform activities at a high altitude. On the other hand, aging reduces our ability to sweat; and so as we age, our ability to regulate body temperature declines, thus reducing our ability to exercise safely in hot environments.

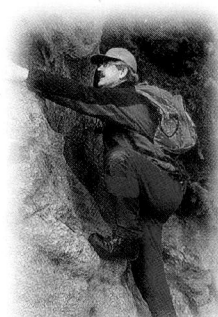

Table 13.8 American College of Sports Medicine Position on Fluid Replacement

Before Activity or Competition

- Drink adequate fluids during the 24 hours before an event, especially during the meal before exercise, to promote proper hydration before exercise or competition.
- Drink about 500 milliliters (~17 ounces) of fluid about two hours before exercise to promote adequate hydration and allow time for excretion of excess ingested water.

During Activity or Competition

- Start drinking early and at regular intervals to consume fluids at a rate sufficient to replace all the water lost through sweating or consume the maximal amount that can be tolerated.
- Fluids should be cooler than ambient temperature and flavored to enhance palatability and promote fluid replacement.

During Competition That Lasts More Than One Hour

- To maintain blood glucose concentration and delay the onset of fatigue, the fluid replacement should contain 4 to 8 percent carbohydrate. Electrolytes (primarily salt) are added to make the solution taste better and reduce the risk of low blood levels of sodium. About 0.5 to 0.7 grams of sodium per liter of water replaces sodium lost by sweating.

Following Activity or Competition

- Complete restoration of the extracellular fluid compartment cannot be sustained without replacement of lost sodium.
- For each pound of body weight lost, consume at least 2 cups of fluid.
- Thirst sensation is *not* an adequate gauge of dehydration, and postexercise consumption stimulates obligatory urine losses. Research shows that drinking an amount of liquid that is 125 to 150 percent of fluid loss is usually enough to promote complete rehydration.

Source: Adapted from Convertino VA, Armstrong LE, Coyle EF, et al. American College of Sports Medicine position stand. Exercise and fluid replacement. *Med Sci Sports Exerc.* 1996;28:i–vii. Reprinted by permission of Lippincott, Williams & Wilkins.

Nutrition Supplements and Ergogenic Aids

The pressure to win contributes to athletes' search for a competitive edge. More than 75 percent of recreational and elite athletes use nutritional supplements and **ergogenic aids** with the expectation of improved performance.[64] Nutrition supplements and ergogenic aids include products that

- Provide calories (e.g., liquid supplements and energy bars)
- Provide vitamins and minerals (including multivitamin supplements)
- Contribute to performance during exercise and enhance recovery after exercise (e.g., sports drinks and carbohydrate supplements)
- Are believed to stimulate and maintain muscle growth (e.g., purified amino acids)[65]
- Contain micronutrients, herbal, and/or cellular components that are promoted as ergogenic aids to enhance performance (e.g., caffeine, chromium picolinate, creatine, and pyruvate)[66]

Most nutrient supplements are unnecessary for athletes who select a variety of foods and meet their energy needs. However, iron and calcium supplements may be recommended for female athletes if their diets are low in these nutrients. Liquid supplements and sports bars that contain carbohydrates, proteins, and fats can provide an easy way to increase energy intake. Sports drinks, gels, and recovery drinks also can contribute to needed fluids and carbohydrates before, during, and after exercise. **Table 13.9** shows the nutrient content of some popular sports bars.

Dietary supplements marketed as performance enhancers are another matter. Herbals, glandulars, enzymes, hormones, and other compounds aimed at athletes carry many attractive claims. Although some products have been well researched, most lack vigorous clinical trials to evaluate efficacy, apply to only one sex (usually males), or are relevant to only one sport (e.g., weight lifting).

Amino Acids

Researchers have studied the use of individual amino acids to enhance performance and have not found clear benefits. Some have proposed that branched-chain amino acids may provide energy and delay central nervous system fatigue, thus improving performance. Studies in humans, however, have shown inconsistent results. Because safety and effectiveness have not been established, they are not recommended.

"Andro" and DHEA

The adrenal gland synthesizes the testosterone precursors **androstenedione ("andro")** and **dehydroepiandrosterone (DHEA)**. Manufacturers claim that supplements of andro and DHEA increase testosterone levels and

ergogenic aids Substances that can enhance athletic performance.

androstenedione ("andro") A steroid precursor secreted by the testes, ovaries, and adrenal cortex.

dehydroepiandrosterone (DHEA) A steroid that is the precursor to androstenedione. DHEA is secreted primarily by the adrenal gland, but also by the testes.

Quick Bites

Office of Dietary Supplements

The mission of the Office of Dietary Supplements is to strengthen knowledge and understanding of dietary supplements by evaluating scientific information, stimulating and supporting research, disseminating research results, and educating the public to foster an enhanced quality of life and health. Visit its Web site at http://dietary-supplements.info.nih.gov/.

Table 13.9 **Nutrient Content of Sports Bars**

Bar	Calories	Carbohydrate (%)	Protein (%)	Fat (%)
Power Bar	225	75	17	8
X-Trainer	220	73	18	9
Tiger Sport	230	70	19	11
Ultra Fuel	490	82	12	6
GatorBar	220	87	5	8
PR Bar	190	40	30	30
Gatorade Energy Bar	260	72	11	17

enhance muscle building—acting as a kind of "natural" steroid. Studies of DHEA have found increases in androgen levels (including testosterone) in women and elderly men with low serum DHA, but not in younger men.[67] Two studies of androstenedione supplementation in men had mixed results. Low doses of andro (100 milligrams per day) did not raise serum testosterone levels, whereas 300 milligrams per day did.[68] In the one of these studies that looked at response to strength training, andro was not effective in improving strength or muscle gains.[69] In both studies, andro use caused estrogen levels to rise, a potentially serious side effect. For DHEA, there is no consistent evidence to support proponents' claims that DHEA supplements improve energy, strength, and immunity.[70]

No long-term studies have tested the safety of androstenedione or DHEA.[71] Despite the success reported anecdotally by a few high-profile athletes, hormone precursors are not recommended because they have many potentially negative effects. In fact, the International Olympic Committee (IOC), National Football League, **NCAA**, and U.S. Tennis Association ban the use of androstenedione.

Little is known about the side effects of these steroidal supplements, but if large quantities of these compounds substantially increase testosterone levels in the body, they also are likely to produce the same side effects as **anabolic steroids**. Anabolic steroid abuse has been associated with a wide range of adverse side effects, ranging from some that are physically unattractive (e.g., acne and breast development in men) to others that are life threatening (e.g., heart attacks and liver cancer). Most are reversible if the abuser stops taking the drugs, but some are permanent.

Caffeine

Caffeine is a natural stimulant. Research suggests that caffeine may affect athletic performance by facilitating signals between the nervous system and the muscles as well as decreasing an athlete's perceived effort during exercise. Caffeine may also increase the body's ability to break down fat for energy. In one well-controlled study, subjects who ingested a high caffeine load one hour before exercise used less muscle glycogen and increased their endurance.[72]

How practical is this regimen? The dose used in the study just described was 9 milligrams of caffeine per kilogram of body weight, which would be 630 milligrams of caffeine for a 70-kilogram person. Considering that one soda has about 30 milligrams of caffeine and one cup of regular coffee about 150 milligrams, that's quite a lot of caffeine! In fact, it's enough to be concerned about stomach discomfort and increasing the concentration of caffeine in the urine above amounts allowed by the IOC—not to mention the fact that caffeine is a mild diuretic, and enhancing urine production is probably not the best course of action right before competition! Lower levels of caffeine intake (e.g., 5–6 mg/kg) also have ergogenic effects and will not cause urine output in excess of IOC limits.[73]

Carnitine

Carnitine, a natural compound in foods, is synthesized in the liver and kidneys from the amino acids lysine and methionine. Carnitine helps transport long-chain fatty acids into the mitochondria, where they are broken down. The appeal to athletes is the idea that supplemental carnitine could help move long-chain fatty acids into the mitochondria faster so they will be metabolized more quickly, thus increasing the use of fat as an energy source. Twenty years of research, however, finds no consistent evidence that carnitine supplements can improve exercise or physical performance in healthy people.[74]

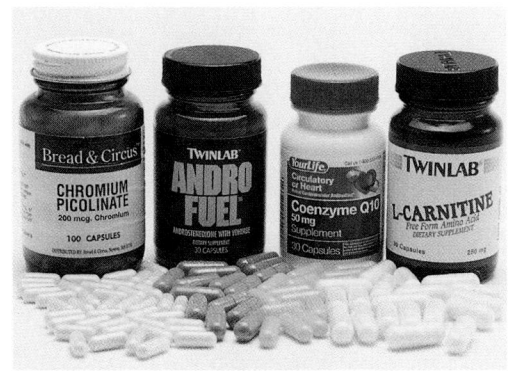

NCAA National Collegiate Athletic Association.
anabolic steroids Several compounds derived from testosterone or prepared synthetically. They promote body growth and masculinization, and oppose the effects of estrogen.

Quick Bites

Placebo Power!

Athletes involved in a heavy weight-lifting program volunteered to participate in a study where they would take what they thought were anabolic steroids. The results were dramatic—during four weeks of treatment these experienced weight lifters had a nearly 7.5-fold increase in the rate of their strength gain. However, they were taking a placebo—an inactive substance identical in appearance to the genuine drug. Because there was no pharmacological effect, gains were solely due to their belief in the treatment.

Chromium

The trace mineral chromium is vital to the movement of glucose into cells. Because of the link between chromium, glucose use, and insulin, chromium has become a popular supplement (typically in the form of chromium picolinate) for both weight loss and athletic performance. The theory is that by enhancing insulin action, chromium increases amino acid uptake, which then increases protein synthesis and promotes a gain in muscle mass. Although the developers of the chromium picolinate supplements had promising results in several studies, a review of 24 studies found no significant reduction in body fat or increase in lean muscle mass.[75] Given these results and the potential risks from chromium picolinate supplementation (see Chapter 12, "Trace Minerals"), this supplement cannot be recommended.

Coenzyme Q_{10} (Ubiquinone)

In the mitochondria of muscle cells, **coenzyme Q_{10} (CoQ_{10})** actively helps transfer electrons in the electron transport chain. CoQ_{10} also may function as an antioxidant and spare vitamin E. In both athletes and sedentary people, supplementation with approximately 100 milligrams per day of CoQ_{10} has shown variable effects on aerobic performance. Early studies that showed positive results had poor study designs (no control group). Studies using control groups show no improvement in exercise performance or reduction in oxidative stress induced by exercise.[76]

Colostrum

If it's good enough for babies, why not athletes? This may be the rationale for the popularity of colostrum supplements. Colostrum is the first milk produced by a new mother. Rich in nutrients, immunoglobulins, and insulin-like growth factors (IGFs), colostrum gets a baby off to a good start and is responsible for jump-starting the enhanced immunity seen in breast-fed infants. The report that may have started the ergogenic supplement craze was published in 1997 and suggested that athletes supplemented with bovine colostrum showed increased levels of IGF-1.[77] IGF-1 is an anabolic hormone that is banned by the IOC as a supplement. But if athletes could increase their IGF levels through colostrum supplementation, it could be a legal route to enhanced performance.

Unfortunately, subsequent studies have not consistently shown increased IGF-1 levels following colostrum supplementation, suggesting errors in the 1997 study.[78] Changes in body composition or performance measures have also not been consistently shown in controlled studies.[79]

Creatine

Creatine, a nitrogenous compound in meats and fish, is synthesized by the liver, pancreas, and kidney. Muscles store creatine mainly as creatine phosphate, which functions as part of the ATP-CP energy system. Creatine has become a popular supplement based on the theory that increasing muscle creatine would prolong short-term energy availability and thus improve performance in short-term, high-intensity activities (such as weight lifting).[80]

Several well-controlled studies have shown improvements in muscle strength when creatine supplementation was added to a strength training regimen.[81] Creatine supplements also may improve the explosive power needed for sprints.[82] But creatine supplements appear to have no benefit for aerobic training. The main side effect seems to be immediate weight gain attributable to water retention.

coenzyme Q_{10} (CoQ_{10}) A compound abundant in cells and vital to the production of ATP in the electron transport chain. Also called ubiquinone.

creatine An important nitrogenous compound found in meats and fish, and synthesized in the body from amino acids (glycine, arginine, and methionine).

Increases in muscle mass are probably a response to the increased stress that an athlete can put on muscle tissue by maximal exercise bursts—the supplement without weight training will have no effect. Also, the ability to store more CP may vary widely among people, so supplements may not be effective for everyone.

With the increasing popularity of creatine supplementation came questions about its long-term safety. Anecdotal reports of muscle cramps, muscle strains, kidney dysfunction, and GI distress have raised concerns. However, college football players who have used creatine for as long as five years have not shown any negative health effects, including no detrimental effects on liver or kidney function.[83] In another study of college football players, creatine supplementation during training did not increase the risk of muscle cramping or injury.[84]

Ephedrine

Ephedrine was a popular ergogenic supplement until its sale in the United States was prohibited by the Food and Drug Administration (FDA) in February 2004.[85] In 2006, this ban was upheld by a federal court. Despite being banned by the NFL, NCAA, and IOC, athletes continue to use ephedrine, either as a weight-loss aid or to gain a performance edge. Ephedrine stimulates the central nervous system and is an effective bronchodilator. In addition, it raises both heart rate and blood pressure. Athletes hoped its stimulatory effects would improve performance, suppress appetite, and promote weight loss. Some studies support these purported benefits, especially when ephedrine is combined with caffeine.[86]

Ephedrine became one of the most controversial supplements on the market. Found in many products as either the herbal ma huang (ephedra) or the synthetic ephedrine, serious side effects and even deaths have been attributed to this supplement. When the 2003 heatstroke-related death of Major League Baseball pitcher Steve Bechler was linked to ephedra use, sports organizations and other groups began to pay more attention. A government-sponsored review of safety and efficacy concluded that the use of ephedrine or the use of ephedra-containing dietary supplements or ephedrine plus caffeine is associated with two to three times the risk of nausea, vomiting, psychiatric symptoms such as anxiety and change in mood, autonomic hyperactivity, and palpitations.[87] Studies such as this led to the FDA's conclusion that ephedrine posed an unreasonable risk of illness or injury.

Ginseng

For thousands of years, Chinese people have used the root of the ginseng plant to treat and prevent numerous disorders. Modern-day use of **ginseng** continues because many people believe it combats a wide range of stressors.[88] Because some reports suggest it improves athletic performance by increasing stamina and aerobic capacity, ginseng also has become popular among athletes.[89]

There is no known mechanism to explain how ginseng might work as an ergogenic aid, and controlled studies do not support ginseng use to improve exercise performance or reduce fatigue. Because the studies that have shown an ergogenic benefit were poorly designed, many researchers question these results.[90] In a European study, for example, elite athletes experienced improved physical work capacity and physiological response after nine weeks of supplementation with 200 milligrams per day of *Panax ginseng*.[91] An American laboratory repeated this study using 200 or 400 milligrams per day of the same

Quick Bites

The Burn to the Finish

The pain a runner feels when approaching the finish line and immediately after the event is called acute muscle soreness. The culprits include a buildup of metabolic by-products, and tissue edema caused by fluid seeping from the bloodstream into surrounding tissues. The pain and soreness usually disappear within minutes or hours.

ginseng A collective term that describes several species of plants of the genus *Panax*.

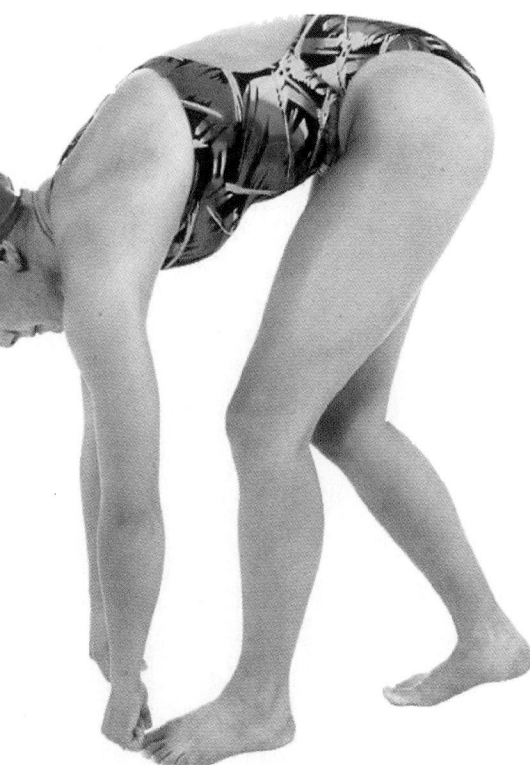

Panax ginseng, but found no effect on heart rate recovery, oxygen use, or aerobic ability.[92] Although testimonials continue to drive ginseng supplementation, further research on this popular herb is needed to evaluate its effectiveness as an ergogenic aid.

soda loading Consumption of bicarbonate (baking soda) to raise blood pH. The intent is to increase the capacity to buffer acids, thus delaying fatigue. Also known as bicarbonate loading.

Glutamine

Glutamine, the nonessential amino acid, is a popular supplement for strength athletes. Glutamine can be classified as a conditionally indispensable amino acid because in situations of severe catabolic stress (e.g., trauma or surgery), endogenous production cannot keep up with the body's use.[93] Proponents of glutamine supplements suggest that intense weight training produces similar catabolic effects on muscle protein and therefore would increase glutamine requirements. However, supplementation studies have not supported an ergogenic effect of glutamine supplementation.[94] Recently, attention has shifted to investigation of a potential immune-enhancing effect of glutamine supplementation in athletes, with some promising results.[95]

Medium-Chain Triglyceride Oil

Medium-chain triglycerides (MCT) are produced from plant oils, primarily coconut oil, and contain saturated fatty acids of medium length (6 to 10 carbons). As with carbohydrate, the body quickly absorbs MCT oil into the blood, where it can become an immediate energy source. One study shows that consumption of carbohydrate combined with MCT may improve cycling performance during endurance events that last more than two hours.[96] The majority of research, however, does not support MCT supplementation as an ergogenic aid.[97] A downside of MCT supplementation is that its taste may be unacceptable, and it may contribute to gastrointestinal distress.

Pyruvate

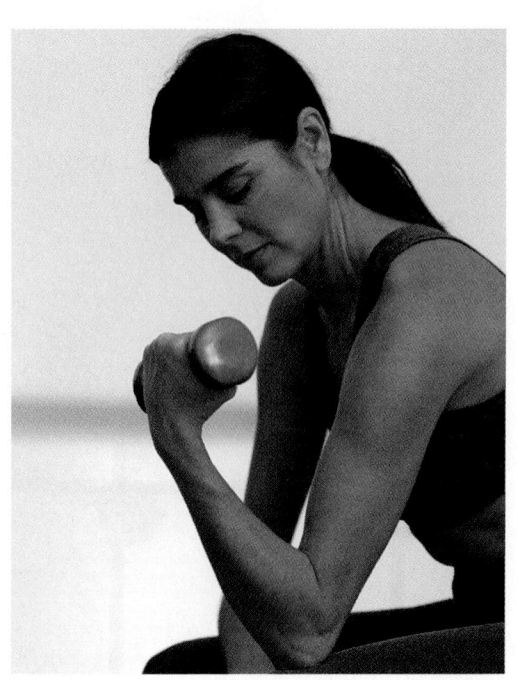

Carbohydrate breakdown produces pyruvate and dihydroxyacetone. In animal studies, pyruvate as a dietary supplement or as a partial replacement for dietary carbohydrate enhanced aerobic endurance capacity.[98] The mechanism of action is unclear, but an increased blood glucose concentration, which would spare muscle glycogen, appears to be responsible for the improvements seen after pyruvate-dihydroxyacetone supplementation. These studies looked only at the aerobic endurance of untrained subjects. A study of trained athletes found that pyruvate administered for five weeks had no beneficial effect on anaerobic exercise performance.[99] Pyruvate supplementation has been associated with GI distress. To support the claim that pyruvate enhances endurance, much more research is needed.[100]

Ribose

Ribose is another supplement that athletes have been talking about. Ribose is a five-carbon monosaccharide that makes up part of the adenosine portion of ATP, and is a key component of DNA and RNA. It has been suggested that ribose supplementation accelerates the synthesis of muscle ATP, which would allow for more intensive training and larger gains. Studies to date do not seem to support these claims.[101]

Sodium Bicarbonate

Some athletes consume sodium bicarbonate (baking soda) in the belief that it will help neutralize the buildup of lactic acid in muscles. Whether **soda loading** actually produces an ergogenic effect is controversial. No improvement in performance has been seen in short-term exercise lasting 30 to 100 seconds.[102] However, comparative studies that evaluate events lasting from 2 to 10 minutes, where lactic acid buildup is most likely, have shown some positive results related to interval training performance.[103]

Bicarbonate loading can produce negative effects. Athletes who follow this regimen report side effects such as intestinal discomfort, stomach distress, nausea, cramping, diarrhea, and water retention. Although bicarbonate loading is not banned, it does have serious health-related consequences. Bicarbonate loading increases blood alkalinity and influences blood pressure. Anyone with high blood pressure (hypertension) should not bicarbonate-load.

Key Concepts: *Numerous dietary supplements, such as caffeine, chromium, CoQ$_{10}$, and ginseng, are marketed for performance-enhancing effects. However, few have been subjected to rigorous clinical trials or long-term safety evaluation. Athletes should consult a physician before adding dietary supplements to their training regimen.*

Weight and Body Composition

Pete, a bodybuilder, wants to bulk up by gaining 15 pounds of muscle and not fat. Sarah, on the other hand, wants to compete as a lightweight rower and needs to lose 7 pounds. Whereas some athletes struggle to lose weight, others find it nearly impossible to gain weight and muscle mass. Whether intentionally gaining or losing weight, weight change should be accomplished slowly—during the off-season or at the beginning of the season before competition starts.

Body composition and body weight are just two of many factors that affect exercise performance. Body composition can affect strength, agility, and appearance. Body weight can influence speed, endurance, and power. Because body fat adds weight without adding strength, many sports emphasize low body fat percentages. Yet, by themselves, body composition and body weight do not accurately predict athletic performance.[104]

Weight Gain: Build Muscle, Lose Fat

Weight gain is influenced by genetics, stage of adolescent development, sex, body mass, diet, training program, prior resistance training, motivation, and use of supplements and anabolic steroids, among other factors. Complex interactions among these factors make it difficult to predict an athlete's ability to meet a weight goal. However, experience tells us the following:

- Untrained male athletes can gain approximately 3 to 4 pounds of lean body mass per month in the early stages of a rigorous resistance-training program.[105] Because of their smaller muscle mass and lean tissue, young women can achieve only 50 to 75 percent of the gains seen in male counterparts, but with the same relative gain in strength.

- Approximately 20 percent of the increase in lean body mass occurs in the first year of resistance training, tapering to 1 to 3 percent in subsequent years. Scientists believe that the rate declines as muscle mass approaches the maximum potential amount determined by genetics.

- Some male athletes of high school age have difficulty gaining muscle mass. These athletes may be in the early stages of the adolescent growth spurt and may lack sufficient levels of the male hormones to stimulate muscle development.

Quick Bites

What's the Best "Fat-Burning" Exercise?

It's a common misconception that low-intensity exercise is superior for "fat burning." Aerobic activities do use a greater percentage of fat as fuel, but it is the total amount of calories expended during exercise that supports increased mobilization of fat in response to a caloric deficit. In terms of actual energy expenditure, higher-intensity exercise requires more calories for a given time period than exercise at a lower intensity. Thus, to lose body fat, the fuel (source of calories) is not as important as the amount of energy expended.

Nutrition plays an important role in increasing lean body mass. Athletes must consume enough calories, along with adequate carbohydrate and protein, to gain the desired muscle mass.[106]

Key Concepts: *Athletes often seek to improve their power and strength by increasing muscle mass. Weight gain as muscle requires increased dietary calories, primarily as carbohydrate, combined with strength training.*

Weight Loss: The Panacea for Optimal Performance?

As the pressure to win increases, many coaches and athletes come to believe that weight loss and lower body fat composition will provide that competitive edge. Athletes strive for lower body weight and lower body fat for three reasons: (1) to improve appearance, especially in aesthetic sports (diving, figure skating, gymnastics); (2) to enhance performance where lower body weight may increase speed (race walking, running, pole vaulting, jumping, cross-country skiing); or (3) to qualify in a lower weight category (wrestling, boxing, and rowing).[107] **Figure 13.15** illustrates the key factors in a successful weight-loss program.

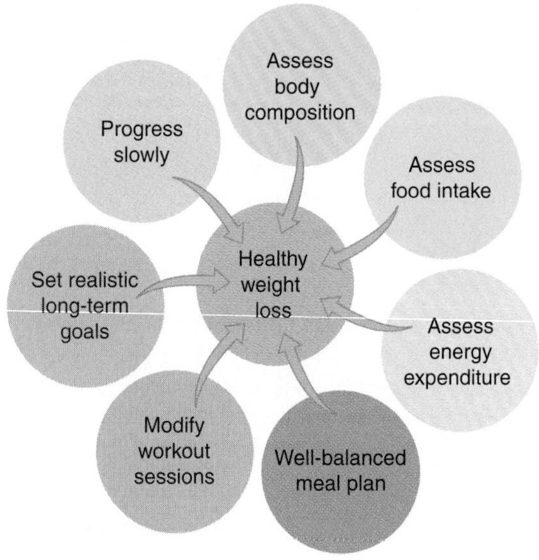

As healthy young adults, men average 15 percent body fat, and women average 25 percent.[108] Although these averages provide starting points, recommendations for individual athletes must account for genetic background, age, sex, sport, health, and weight history. Male athletes should not go below 5 to 7 percent body fat. For female athletes, current research data suggest a minimum 13 to 17 percent body fat to maintain normal menstrual function, which in turn is important for maintaining bone health.[109]

Keeping accurate food and training records provides information on energy intake and expenditure. The best way for athletes to sustain a safe and sensible loss of body fat is to reduce calorie intake moderately and modify the training program. A combination of resistance training and aerobic activity is best for weight loss because it helps maintain or even increase lean body mass while simultaneously decreasing fat mass.

Beware of "fad" weight-loss methods such as ketogenic diets, high-protein diets, and semistarvation diets. These practices can compromise energy reserves, body composition, and psychological well-being, leading to decreased performance and increased health risks. Athletes often are alert to the latest supplements to hit the market. Many claim to accelerate the burning of body fat and augment weight loss. In reality, studies show that most "fat burners" are ineffective or associated with only very modest weight loss in obese subjects.[110]

Key Concepts: *Before embarking on a weight-loss program, athletes should carefully evaluate their goals and set a realistic plan for weight loss and maintenance. Safe weight-loss practices include modest changes in food intake accompanied by gradual increases in aerobic activity.*

Weight Loss: Negative Consequences for the Competitive Athlete?

Changing body size and shape can have detrimental effects. An unrealistic perception of optimal body weight and a belief that weight loss is necessary for improved performance can contribute to unhealthy weight-loss practices.[111] Athletes risk medical problems when dieting goes awry.

Making Weight

Wrestlers, weight lifters, boxers, jockeys, rowers, and coxswains face competitive pressures to "make weight" to compete or to be certified in a lower weight classification. Such athletes often resort to the **pathogenic** weight-control

Figure 13.15 **Keys to successful weight loss.** Just as athletes focus on proper training techniques to avoid injury and improve performance, they should focus on proper weight-loss strategies to lose weight and maintain health.

pathogenic Capable of causing disease.

cardiac output The amount of blood expelled by the heart.

hyperthermia A much higher than normal body temperature.

female athlete triad A syndrome in young female athletes that involves disordered eating, amenorrhea, and lowered bone density.

amenorrhea [A-men-or-Ee-a] Absence or abnormal stoppage of menses in a female; commonly indicated by the absence of three to six consecutive menstrual cycles.

behaviors summarized in **Table 13.10**. Repeated cycles of rapid weight loss and subsequent regain increase the risk of disordered eating, fatigue, psychological distress (anger, anxiety, depression), dehydration, and sudden death.

Studies show that wrestlers, in attempts to gain a competitive advantage, will try to reduce weight a few days before or on the day of competition.[112] Athletes can achieve weight loss of up to 22 pounds (10 kilograms) of body water in one day by fasting, restricting fluids, using diuretics, sitting in a sauna, and exercising in a hot environment using rubber suits. A fluid loss of only 1 to 2 percent of initial body weight (3 pounds for a 150-pound individual) can decrease athletic performance by elevating heart rate and lowering **cardiac output**. Moderate to severe dehydration (more than 3 to 5 percent of body weight) can be dangerous because of increased core body temperature, electrolyte imbalances, and cardiac and kidney changes. These conditions may result in heat illness, including heat cramps, heat exhaustion, or heatstroke.

Rapid weight loss can have serious health consequences. During one month in 1998, three previously healthy collegiate wrestlers died trying to make weight.[113] These athletes had not only dropped significant weight pre-season—more than 20 pounds (9 kilograms)—but also lost between 3.5 to 9 pounds (1.6 to 4 kilograms) in the one to nine hours before their deaths. The wrestlers restricted food and fluid intake. To maximize sweat losses, they wore vapor-impermeable suits under cotton warm-up suits and exercised vigorously in hot environments. Dehydration and **hyperthermia** (elevated body temperature) led to their demise.

Since 1998, the NCAA has revised the guidelines for monitoring weight-loss practices and weigh-in procedures. (See **Figure 13.16**.) This includes educating coaches and athletic trainers about healthy weight-control strategies and limiting the amount of preseason and precompetition weight loss.[114]

Female Athlete Triad

Although the majority of female athletes benefit from increased physical activity, there are those who go too far and risk developing a trio of medical problems. (See "Spotlight on Eating Disorders.") In 1991 the American College of Sports Medicine coined the term **female athlete triad** to describe the interaction of disordered eating, **amenorrhea**, and premature osteoporosis.[115] Female athletes who compete in endurance sports such as long-distance running, aesthetic sports such as gymnastics, antigravitational sports such as indoor rock climbing, and sports with weight classifications such as karate are at the greatest risk.[116]

Disordered Eating

Female athletes who compete in either endurance events, such as long-distance running, or in sports where appearance is important (e.g., gymnastics, figure skating, diving) are at higher risk for disordered eating behaviors. In some cases, disordered eating can progress to an eating disorder. Anorexia nervosa appears to be no more prevalent among female athletes than among nonathletes. On the other hand, the prevalence of bulimia nervosa or subclinical eating disorders is higher in athletes.[117] For more on disordered eating and eating disorders, see the "Spotlight on Eating Disorders."

Amenorrhea

In the general population, 2 to 5 percent of women have amenorrhea. However, the prevalence is much higher in athletes.[118] Research indicates that amenorrhea in athletic women is related to the combined effects of

Table 13.10 **Pathogenic Weight-Loss Practices**

Behavior	Consequence
Fasting	Loss of lean body mass and decreased metabolic rate
Diet pills	Medical side effects and weight regained when discontinued
Fat-free diets	Deficient in macronutrients and micronutrients; difficult to maintain
Diuretics	Dehydration and electrolyte imbalance; no fat loss
Laxatives	Dehydration; no fat loss; may be addicting
Sweating	Dehydration; heat injury; no fat loss
Excessive exercise	Risk of injury and overtraining; no fat loss
Enemas	Dehydration and GI problems; no fat loss
Fluid restriction	Dehydration; heat injury
Self-induced vomiting	Dehydration; acid–base and electrolyte imbalances; esophageal tears and GI bleeding; erosion of dental enamel and swollen parotid glands

Source: Adapted from Otis CL. Too slim, amenorrheic, fracture-prone: the female athlete triad. *ACSM's Health and Fitness*. 1998;2:2–25. Reprinted by permission of Lippincott Williams & Wilkins.

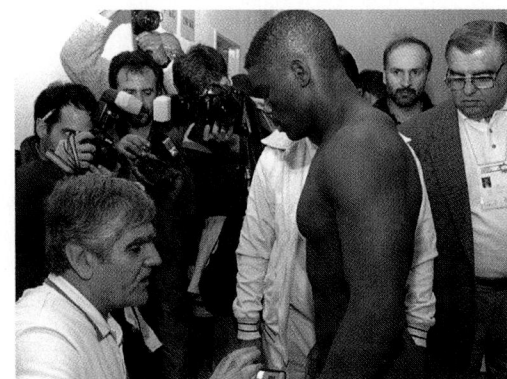

Figure 13.16 **Weighing in.** The NCAA discourages athletes from reducing their weight through intentional dehydration, a dangerous and potentially deadly practice.

increased physical activity, weight loss, low body fat levels, and insufficient energy intake.

Premature Osteoporosis

Health consequences of amenorrhea include premature osteoporosis. Research shows that amenorrheic athletes experience rapid loss of bone mineral density in the spine, which can spread to other parts of the skeleton if amenorrhea continues for a long time.

Treatment involves replacing estrogen, which is low in amenorrheic females. Oral contraceptives are the most common method of estrogen replacement and can also serve as a reliable form of birth control. Calcium supplementation is also recommended. Although bone mineralization may never return to normal in amenorrheic athletes, studies indicate that reducing the intensity of training, improving dietary intake, and increasing body weight can help restore menstruation and increase bone density.[119]

Breaking the Triad

Female athletes at risk are perfectionists, driven to excel in a given sport, who believe that a specific athletic body image is required to excel as an athlete. Some reports estimate that as many as 60 percent of female athletes in aesthetic sports (dance, skating, diving, gymnastics) and weight-dependent sports (rowing, martial arts, horse racing) may be at risk.[120]

Screening, referral, and education are keys to preventing the female athlete triad. Prevention and treatment are most successful when they are multidisciplinary efforts—carried out by a team of medical, athletic,

Quick Bites

Ouch! But I Felt Fine Yesterday. . .

After a bout of heavy exercise, a person may not feel muscle soreness for a day or two. We do not fully understand this painful phenomenon, which is called delayed-onset muscle soreness. Activities that lengthen muscles seem to be the primary cause. The muscles suffer damage with micro-tears in their structure. This leads to an inflammatory response, causing localized muscle pain, swelling, and tenderness.

Table 13.11 **Combating Disordered Eating in Athletes**

De-emphasize body weight. Do not view the athlete's weight as the primary contributor to, or detractor from, athletic performance. Research indicates that athletes can achieve appropriate weight and fitness when the focus is on physical conditioning and strength development as well as the cognitive and emotional aspects of performance.

Eliminate group weigh-ins. Often viewed as a way to motivate the team, the practice of group weigh-ins can be destructive to people who are struggling with their body image and disordered eating. If there is a legitimate reason for weighing an athlete, explain the reason and weigh the athlete privately.

Treat each athlete individually. Many athletes have an unrealistic perception of what an ideal body weight is, especially in sports for which leanness is considered important. Additionally, athletes may strive for weight and body composition that may be realistic in only a few genetically endowed people. It is important to understand that genetic and biological processes, rather than one's willpower to control food intake, affect a person's weight.

Facilitate healthy weight management. Be sensitive to issues related to weight control and dieting. Because many athletes have limited knowledge of sports nutrition, they resort to pathogenic weight-loss practices. Athletes can benefit from nutrition counseling by a sports nutritionist or a registered dietitian who has experience in working with athletes and disordered eating.

Source: Thompson RA, Sherman RT. Reducing the risk of eating disorders in athletics. *Eating Disorders: Journal of Treatment and Prevention.* 1993;1:65–78. Reproduced by permission of Taylor & Francis Group, LLC, www.taylorandfrancis.com.

nutrition, and mental health experts. Proactive sports education includes reducing the emphasis on body weight, eliminating group weigh-ins, treating each athlete individually, and facilitating healthy weight management. (See **Table 13.11**.)

Key Concepts: Pathogenic weight-control practices increase risk of dehydration and compromise performance; they may have long-term serious consequences for athletes. The female athlete triad—disordered eating, amenorrhea, and premature osteoporosis—results from excessive weight loss. Often weight loss is driven by unrealistic ideas of appropriate body weight and shape for competition. Education of coaches and athletes is essential to prevent the female athlete triad.

Label [to] **Table**

Sports drinks are often recommended instead of plain water for those who engage in vigorous physical activity. Their proponents claim that they quickly replenish the body's supply of nutrients, particularly electrolytes. Let's take a look at the Nutrition Facts panel from a popular sports drink, Gatorade.

First, look closely at the serving size—it's not the whole container. This is worth noting because many people might drink the whole container and assume they were getting 50 calories. Not true! The whole container has 200 calories (50 × 4 servings). It's always a good idea to look at the serving size when you are studying a nutrition label.

So what makes this sports drink different from plain (and inexpensive) water? This one has added carbohydrate, sodium, and potassium. Replacing carbohydrate during long workouts prevents complete depletion of glycogen stores. Most sports drinks have between 5 and 8 percent simple sugar. Higher amounts would limit water absorption, and replacement of water is more critical than replacement of glucose.

Sodium and potassium are added to sports drinks to improve taste and help replace electrolytes that are lost during exercise. Gatorade contains 110 milligrams of sodium and 30 milligrams of potassium. For many athletes, and certainly for recreational exercisers, water really is the best fluid replacer. Although both sodium and potassium are lost in sweat, water is lost in greater quantities. Sports drinks have been shown to benefit only athletes who are strenuously exercising for longer than an hour. With prolonged exercise and sweat losses, large losses of electrolytes can make a person dizzy and weak, and may even lead to heat exhaustion or heatstroke.

The next time you head out for a bike ride, consider how long you'll be gone and how strenuous your ride will be, and then consider whether you'll need a sports drink. Also consider your personal taste—if a flavored sports drink will encourage you to replace fluids more than plain water will, that may be an important advantage. Just don't forget to read the label!

Nutrition Facts	
Serving Size 8 fl oz (240mL)	
Servings Per Container 4	
Amount Per Serving	
Calories 50	
	% Daily Value*
Total Fat 0g	0%
Trans Fat 0g	
Sodium 110mg	5%
Potassium 30mg	1%
Total Carbohydrate 14g	5%
Sugars 14g	
Protein 0g	

Not a significant source of Calories from Fat, Saturated Fat, Trans Fat, Cholesterol, Dietary Fiber, Vitamin A, Vitamin C, Calcium, Iron.

* Percent Daily Values are based on a 2,000 calorie diet.

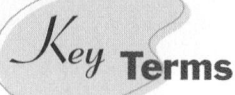
LEARNING *Portfolio*   c h a p t e r   1 3

Key Terms

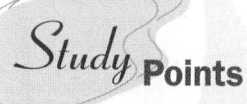
Study Points

➤ Exercise promotes health and reduces risk of chronic diseases.

➤ The ACSM defines physical fitness as "the ability to perform moderate to vigorous levels of physical activity without undue fatigue and the capability of maintaining this level of activity throughout life."

➤ The muscular system contains three types of muscles: smooth, cardiac, and skeletal. There are two types of muscle fibers: slow-twitch (ST) and fast-twitch (FT). ST fibers have high aerobic endurance; FT fibers are optimized to perform anaerobically. Your body depends predominantly on ST fibers for low-intensity events and FT fibers for highly explosive events.

➤ The body uses three systems to produce energy for physical activity: (1) the ATP-CP energy system (anaerobic), (2) the lactic acid energy system (anaerobic), and (3) the oxygen energy system (aerobic).

➤ Anaerobic and aerobic metabolism work together to fuel all types of exercise. During the early minutes of high-intensity exercise, the ATP-CP energy system and the lactic acid energy system provide most of the energy. Endurance activities are fueled primarily by the metabolism of glucose and fatty acids in the oxygen energy system.

➤ Training improves use of fat as a fuel by enhancing oxygen delivery and increasing the number of mitochondria in muscle.

➤ Carbohydrates should be the major source of energy in the athlete's diet and should come from complex carbohydrates, which can provide fiber, iron, and B vitamins. Athletes need carbohydrates so that muscle glycogen stores and blood glucose concentrations will be adequate for training and competitive events. Likewise, carbohydrates are necessary to replenish glycogen stores after intense exercise.

➤ Carbohydrate loading is a process of reducing activity while increasing carbohydrate intake to maximize glycogen stores.

➤ Fat is a major fuel source for exercise, but high fat intake is neither required nor recommended.

➤ Protein needs of athletes are higher than for sedentary individuals, but generally athletes who consume adequate amounts of energy get enough protein. High-protein foods include low-fat dairy products, egg whites, lean beef and pork, chicken, turkey, fish, and legumes.

➤ Other nutrients important to the athlete's diet include B vitamins, iron, zinc, and calcium.

➤ Water is the most essential nutrient and is easily lost from the body with heavy sweating. Replacing fluid with water or sports drinks is important to prevent dehydration. Optimal sports drinks provide energy and electrolytes in a palatable solution that is rapidly absorbed.

➤ Athletes who are still growing have even higher energy and nutrient needs to support both physical activity and normal growth.

➤ Many dietary supplements are promoted as ergogenic aids—substances that enhance performance. Few well-controlled studies on their efficacy and safety have been done, however.

➤ Many athletes strive to either gain or lose weight so as to improve performance. In both cases, realistic goals and gradual changes are necessary for long-term success. Gains in muscle mass require increased calorie intake and weight training. Successful weight loss requires modest reductions in energy intake and increases in aerobic activity.

➤ Weight-control efforts that involve fasting, excessive sweating, purging, diuretics, or laxatives are detrimental to health.

➤ Disordered eating accompanied by amenorrhea and premature osteoporosis is known as the female athlete triad.

Study Questions

1. What are muscle fibers and what are the two major types?

2. List the two anaerobic and one aerobic energy systems that your body uses to generate energy during exercise. When is each active during exercise?

3. What are the general recommendations for an athlete (compared with a nonathlete) in terms of the percentage of calories from carbohydrates, proteins, and fats?

4. What is carbohydrate loading?

5. How do protein recommendations for athletes vary from those for nonathletes?

6. Name three minerals that are of concern for athletes because they may not consume enough.

7. What is sports anemia and why does it happen? How does it compare with other anemias?

8. Define the term *ergogenic aid*. Is there a clear, research-based answer to whether ergogenic supplements work?

9. What is the nutritional strategy for athletes who want to gain muscle mass?

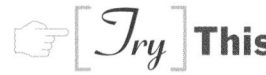 **This**

The Popularity of Ergogenic Aids

Take a trip to a health food store to see just how popular (and expensive!) ergogenic aids are. Try to locate each of the supplements listed in this chapter. Are they all available? What are their prices? Ask a salesperson what he or she knows about each of them. Do his or her answers match what you read in the text?

Commit to Get Fit

Do you meet the American College of Sports Medicine's (ACSM) definition of fitness? Answer the questions below with a yes or no.

1. Do you exercise consistently three to five days per week?
2. When you exercise, does it include 20 to 60 minutes (20 minutes for intense activity and 60 minutes for less intense activity) of continuous aerobic activity?
3. Does your type of exercise use large muscle groups? Can you maintain it? Is it rhythmical and aerobic?
4. Does part of your activity include strength training of a moderate intensity (a minimum of one set of 8 to 12 repetitions of 8 to 10 exercises) at least two days per week?

If you answered no to any of these questions, you are not following the ACSM's suggestions to develop and maintain cardiorespiratory and muscular fitness. Choose a question to which you answered no and set a specific goal to include that factor in your exercise routine.

What About Bobbie?

Imagine that Bobbie is training to compete in a marathon at the end of the semester. She has been exercising consistently and increasing her endurance and mileage times. She hasn't spent much time focusing on her diet, though, and wants to know what changes she could make to improve her nutrition and, therefore, performance. Assume that her current diet meets her calorie needs. How would you compare Bobbie's diet to the guidelines you read about in this chapter?

Macronutrient Contributions

Start with her overall contribution of carbohydrates, proteins, and fats. Compare Bobbie's macronutrient intake to the general sports nutrition recommendations.

	Bobbie's	Recommendations
Carbohydrates	51%	60 to 70%
Proteins	17%	~ 15%
Fats	34%	~ 20%

As you can see, Bobbie's diet is higher in fat and lower in carbohydrates than is recommended for an athlete. If she were to reduce her intake of cream cheese, mayonnaise, cookies, and salad dressing and increase her fruits, vegetables, and whole grains, her diet would come closer to the recommendations for sports nutrition.

Protein

Now let's calculate her protein need based on the athlete's guideline and see if she's consuming enough to maintain lean muscle mass and recover well from exercise.

The protein recommendation for an athlete is approximately 1.2 to 1.4 grams per kilogram of body weight. Bobbie weighs 155 pounds, so her recommended intake is as follows:

155 lb ÷ 2.2 kg per lb = 70.45 kg

70.45 kg × 1.3 g/kg = 91.6 g protein

Bobbie's protein intake was 96 grams, which makes her protein intake a near perfect match for her needs.

Minerals

Look at the two primary minerals that might be inadequate in diets of athletes, especially female athletes. Below is a comparison of Bobbie's calcium and iron intake and her daily recommendations.

	Bobbie's	Recommendations
Calcium	710 mg	1,000 mg
Iron	20 mg	8 mg

As you can see, Bobbie did a very good job of consuming iron, but she is short of her calcium need. If she were to replace the diet soda she had at lunch with 1 cup of nonfat or 1% milk, her intake of calcium would rise to just about 1,000 milligrams. Or she could change her afternoon snack of chips and salsa to a cup of yogurt to accomplish the same thing.

Hydration

Check out Bobbie's intake of fluids in Chapter 1. Although her overall fluid intake is consistent with the AI, how many ounces of plain water did she consume? That's right, she had only 16 ounces! Bobbie is making the same mistake that many athletes do—she's not drinking enough water. Poor hydration status will probably affect her performance adversely. Bobbie's biggest change should be to increase her fluid intake. She'd be smart to drink at least 12 to 16 ounces of water at all of her meals and snacks. This way she'll stay hydrated and be able to perform at an optimal level!

References

1 American College of Sports Medicine (ACSM). Position stand: the recommended quantity and quality of exercise for developing and maintaining cardiorespiratory and muscular fitness and flexibility in healthy adults. *Med Sci Sports Exerc.* 1998; 30:975–991.

2 Institute of Medicine, Food and Nutrition Board. *Dietary Reference Intakes for Energy, Carbohydrate, Fiber, Fat, Fatty Acids, Cholesterol, Protein, and Amino Acids.* Washington, DC: National Academy Press, 2005.

3 ACSM. Op. cit.

4 Position of the American Dietetic Association, Dietitians of Canada, and the American College of Sports Medicine: nutrition and athletic performance. *J Am Diet Assoc.* 2000; 100:1543–1556.

5 Andersen JL, Scherling P, Saltin B. Muscle, genes and athletic performance, *Scientific American.* 2000;283(3):48–55.

6 Connolly-Schoonen J, Holbrook L. Physiology of anaerobic and aerobic exercise. In: Dunford M, ed. *Sports Nutrition.* 4th ed. Chicago: American Dietetic Association, 2006;3–13.

7 Wilmore JH, Costill DL. *Physiology of Sport and Exercise.* 3rd ed. Champaign, IL: Human Kinetics, 2004.

8 Hashimoto T, Hussien R, Brooks GA. Colocalization of MCT1, CD147, and LDH in mitochondrial inner membrane of L6 muscle cells: evidence of a mitochondrial lactate oxidation complex. *Am J Physiol Endocrinol Metab.* 2006; 290(6):E1237–E1244.

9 Brooks GA, Fahey TD, White T. *Exercise Physiology.* Mountain View, CA: Mayfield, 1996:705.

10 Brown GC. Speed limits. *The Sciences.* 2000;40(5):32–37.

11 McArdle WD, Katch FI, Katch VL. *Essentials of Exercise Physiology.* 3rd ed. Baltimore, MD: Lippincott Williams & Wilkins, 2005.

12 Ibid.

13 Position of the American Dietetic Association, Dietitians of Canada, and the American College of Sports Medicine: nutrition and athletic performance. Op. cit.

14 Wilmore JH, Costill DL. Op. cit.

15 Brown GC. *The Energy of Life.* New York: Simon & Schuster, 1999.

16 Berning JR, Steen SN. *Nutrition for Sport and Exercise.* 2nd ed. Sudbury, MA: Jones and Bartlett Publishers, 1998.

17 Hawley J, Dennis SC, Lindsay FH, Noakes TD. Nutritional practices of athletes: are they sub-optimal? *J Sports Sci.* 1995; 13(suppl):S75–S87.

18 Benardot D, Thompson WR. Energy from food for physical activity: enough and on time. *ACSM's Health & Fitness.* 1999; 3:14–18.

19 Vinci DM. Effective nutrition support programs for college athletes. *Int J Sports Nutr.* 1998;8:308–320.

20 Position of the American Dietetic Association, Dietitians of Canada, and the American College of Sports Medicine: nutrition and athletic performance. Op. cit.

21 Burke LM, Cox GR, Culmmings NK, Desbrow B. Guidelines for daily carbohydrate intake: do athletes achieve them? *Sports Med.* 2001;31:267–299.

22 Coleman EJ. Carbohydrate and exercise. In: Rosenbloom CA, ed. *Sports Nutrition.* 3rd ed. Chicago: American Dietetic Association, 2000.

23 Shattuck D. Sports nutritionists fuel the competitive edge. *J Am Diet Assoc.* 2001;101:517–518.

24 Coleman EJ. Op. cit.

25 Ibid.

26 Walberg-Rankin J. Dietary carbohydrate as an ergogenic aid for prolonged and brief competitions in sport. *Int J Sport Nutr.* 1995;5:513–528.

27 Position of the American Dietetic Association, Dietitians of Canada, and the American College of Sports Medicine: nutrition and athletic performance. Op. cit.

28 Ibid.

29 Walton P, Rhodes EC. Glycemic index and optimal performance. *Sports Med.* 1997;23:164–172.

30 Position of the American Dietetic Association, Dietitians of Canada, and the American College of Sports Medicine: nutrition and athletic performance. Op. cit.

31 Ivy JL, Lee MC, Broznick JT, Reed MJ. Muscle glycogen storage after different amounts of carbohydrate ingestion. *J Appl Physiol.* 1988;65:2018–2023.

32 Coleman EJ. Carbohydrate and exercise. In: Dunford M, ed. *Sports Nutrition.* 4th ed. Chicago: American Dietetic Association, 2006;14–32.

33 Coleman EJ. Op. cit.

34 Hawley J, Burke L. *Peak Performance: Training and Nutritional Strategies for Sport.* Leonards, Australia: Allen & Unwin, 1998.

35 Position of the American Dietetic Association, Dietitians of Canada, and the American College of Sports Medicine: nutrition and athletic performance. Op. cit.

36 Roy B, Tarnopolosky M, MacDougall J, et al. Effect of glucose supplement timing on protein metabolism after resistance training. *J Appl Physiol.* 1997;82:1882–1888.

37 Ibid.

38 Kleiner SM, Bazzarre TL, Ainsworth BE. Nutritional status of nationally ranked elite bodybuilders. *Int J Sport Nutr.* 1994; 4:54-69.

39 Lemon PWR. Effects of exercise on dietary protein requirements. *Int J Sports Nutr.* 1998;8:426–447.

40 Clark N, Rosenbloom, C. To zone or not to zone: people respond to The Zone diet plan. *Scan's Pulse.* 1997;16:5–7.

41 Institute of Medicine, Food and Nutrition Board. Op. cit.

42 Gibala MJ, Howarth KR. Protein and exercise. In: Dunford M, ed. *Sports Nutrition.* 4th ed. Chicago: American Dietetic Association, 2006;33–49.

43 Lemon PW. Dietary protein requirements in athletes. *J Nutr Biochem.* 1997;8:52.

44 Hawley J, Burke L. Op. cit.

45 Tarnopolosky MA, Atkinson SA, MacDougall JD, et al. Evaluation of protein requirements for trained strength athletes. *J Appl Physiol.* 1992;73:1986.

46 Lemon PW. Op. cit.

47 Hargreaves MH, Snow R. Amino acids and endurance exercise. *Int J Sport Nutr Exerc Metab.* 2001;11:133–145.

48 Storlie J. Op. cit.; and Tipton KD, Wolfe RR. Exercise, protein metabolism, and muscle growth. *Int J Sport Nutr Exerc Metab.* 2001;11:109–132.

49 Miller SL, Tipton KD, Chinkes DL, Wolf SE, Wolfe RR. Independent and combined effects of amino acids and glucose after resistance exercise. *Med Sci Sports Exerc.* 2003; 35(3):449–455.

50 Storlie J. From fork to muscle. *Training and Conditioning.* 1998;8:26, 28–29, 32–33.

51 Clarkson PM, Haymes EM. Exercise and mineral status of athletes: calcium, magnesium, phosphorus, and iron. *Med Sci Sports Exerc.* 1995;27:831–843.

52 Institute of Medicine, Food and Nutrition Board. *Dietary Reference Intakes for Vitamin A, Vitamin K, Arsenic, Boron, Chromium, Copper, Iodine, Iron, Manganese, Molybdenum, Nickel, Silicon, Vanadium, and Zinc.* Washington, DC: National Academy Press, 2001.

53 Fogelholm M. Indicators of vitamin and mineral status in athletes' blood: a review. *Int J Sport Nutr.* 1995;5:267–284.

54 Zhu YI, Haas JD. Iron depletion without anemia and physical performance in young women. *Am J Clin Nutr.* 1997; 66:334–341.

55 Institute of Medicine, Food and Nutrition Board. *Dietary Reference Intakes for Water, Potassium, Sodium, Chloride, and Sulfate.* Washington, DC: National Academy Press, 2004.

56 Ibid.

57 Coyle EF. Fluid and fuel intake during exercise. *J Sports Sci.* 2004;22(1):39–55.

58 Convertino VA, Armstrong LE, Coyle EF, et al. American College of Sports Medicine position stand: exercise and fluid replacement. *Med Sci Sports Exerc.* 1996;28:i–vii.

59 Ibid.

60 Burke LM. Nutritional needs for exercise in heat. *Comp Biochem Physiol A Mol Integr Physiol.* 2001;128:735–748.

61 American Academy of Pediatrics Committee on Sports Medicine and Fitness. Promotion of healthy weight-control practices in young athletes. *Pediatrics.* 2005;116(6):1557–1564.

62 Thompson JL. Energy balance in young athletes. *Int J Sports Nutr.* 1998;8:160–174.

63 Ibid.

64 Ahrendt DM. Ergogenic aids: counseling the athlete. *Am Fam Physician.* 2001;63:913–922.

65 Dunford M, Smith M. Dietary supplements and ergogenic aids. In: Dunford M, ed. *Sports Nutrition.* 4th ed. Chicago: American Dietetic Association, 2006;116–141.

66 Ibid.

67 Clarkson PM, Rawson ES. Nutritional supplements to increase muscle mass. *Crit Rev Food Sci Nutr.* 1999;39:317–328; Kreider RB. Dietary supplements and the promotion of muscle growth with resistance exercise. *Sports Med.* 1999;27:97–110; and Villareal DT, Holloszy JO, Kohrt WM. Effects of DHEA replacement on bone mineral density and body composition in elderly women and men. *Clin Endocrinol.* 2000;53(5):561–568.

68 King DS, Sharp RL, Vukovich MD, et al. Effect of oral androstenedione on serum testosterone and adaptations to resistance training in young men. *JAMA.* 1999;281:2020–2028; and Leder BZ, Longcope C, Catlin DH, et al. Oral androstenedione administration and serum testosterone concentrations in young men. *JAMA.* 2000;283:779–782.

69 King DS, Sharp RL, Vukovich MD, et al. Op. cit.

70 National Institute on Aging. Pills, patches, and shots: can hormones prevent aging? http://www.niapublications.org/tipsheets/pills.asp. Accessed 7/31/06.

71 Sarubin Fragakis A. *The Health Professional's Guide to Popular Dietary Supplements.* 2nd ed. Chicago: American Dietetic Association, 2003.

72 Spriet L. Caffeine and performance. *Int J Sport Nutr.* 1995; 5(suppl):S84–S99.

73 Bell DG, McLellan TM. Exercise endurance 1, 3, and 6 h after caffeine ingestion in caffeine users and nonusers. *J Appl Physiol.* 2002;93(4):1227–1234; and Cox GR, Desbrow B, Montgomery PG, et al. Effect of different protocols of caffeine intake on metabolism and endurance performance. *J Appl Physiol.* 2002;93(3):990–999.

74 Brass EP. Carnitine and sports medicine: use or abuse? *Ann N Y Acad Sci* 2004;1033:67–78.

75 Vincent JB. The potential value and toxicity of chromium picolinate as a nutritional supplement, weight loss agent and muscle development agent. *Sports Med.* 2003;33:213–230.

76 Sarubin Fragakis A. Op. cit.

77 Mero A, Miikkulainen H, Riski J, et al. Effects of bovine colostrum supplementation on serum IGF-I, IgG, hormone, and saliva IgA during training. *J Appl Physiol.* 1997;84(4): 1144–1151.

78 Kuipers H, van Breda E, Verlaan G, Smeets R. Effects of bovine colostrum supplementation on serum insulin-like growth factor-I levels. *Nutrition.* 2002;18(7–8):566–567.

79 Brinkworth GD, Buckley JD, Bourdon PC, Gulbin JP, David A. Oral bovine colostrum supplementation enhances buffer capacity but not rowing performance in elite female rowers. *Int J Sport Nutr Exerc Metab.* 2002;12(3):349–365; and Hofman Z, Smeets R, Verlaan G, Lugt R, Verstappen PA. The effect of bovine colostrum supplementation on exercise performance in elite field hockey players. *Int J Sport Nutr Exerc Metab.* 2002;12(4):461–469.

80 Toler SM. Creatine is an ergogen for anaerobic exercise. *Nutr Rev.* 1997;55:21–25.

81 Engelhardt M, Neumann G, Berbalk A, Reuter I. Creatine supplementation in endurance sports. *Med Sci Sports Exerc.* 1998; 30:1123.

82 Skare OC, Skalberg AR. Creatine supplementation improves sprint performance in male sprinters. *Scand J Med Sci Sports.* 2001;11:96–102.

83 Kreider RB, Melton C, Rasmussen CJ, et al. Long-term creatine supplementation does not significantly affect clinical markers of health in athletes. *Mol Cell Biochem.* 2003;244(1–2):95–104; and Mayhew DL, Mayhew JL, Ware JS. Effects of long-term creatine supplementation on liver and kidney functions in American college football players. *Int J Sport Nutr Exerc Metab.* 2003;12(4):453–460.

84 Greenwood M, Kreider RB, Melton C, et al. Creatine supplementation during college football training does not increase the incidence of cramping or injury. *Mol Cell Biochem.* 2003; 244(1–2):83–88.

85 US Food and Drug Administration. FDA issues regulation prohibiting sale of dietary supplements containing ephedrine alkaloids and reiterates its advice that consumers stop using these products. *FDA News.* February 6, 2004. http://www.cfsan .fda.gov/~lrd/fpephed6.html. Accessed 1/6/07.

86 Bell DG, McLellan TM, Sabiston CM. Effect of ingesting caffeine and ephedrine on 10-km run performance. *Med Sci Sports Exerc.* 2002;34(2):344–349; Jacobs I, Pasternak H, Bell DG. Effects of ephedrine, caffeine, and their combination on muscular endurance. *Med Sci Sports Exerc.* 2003;35(6):987–994; and Shekelle PG, Hardy ML, Morton SG, et al. Efficacy and safety of ephedra and ephedrine for weight loss and athletic performance: a meta-analysis. *JAMA.* 2003;289(12):1537–1545.

87 Shekelle PG, Hardy ML, Morton SG, et al. Op. cit.

88 Williams MH. *The Ergogenics Edge: Pushing the Limits of Sports Performance.* Champaign, IL: Human Kinetics, 1998.

89 Engles HJ, Wirth JC. No ergogenic effects of ginseng (*Panax ginseng* C.A. Meyer) during graded maximal aerobic exercise. *J Am Diet Assoc.* 1997:1110–1115.

90 Sarubin Fragakis A. Op. cit.

91 Engles HJ, Wirth JC. Op. cit.

92 Ibid.

93 Institute of Medicine, Food and Nutrition Board. 2002. Op. cit.

94 Antonio J, Sanders MS, Kalman D, Woodgate D, Street C. The effects of high-dose glutamine ingestion on weightlifting performance. *J Strength Cond Res.* 2002;16(1):157–160; Haub MD, Potteiger JA, Nau KL, Webster MJ, Zebas CJ. Acute L-glutamine ingestion does not improve maximal effort exercise. *J Sports Med Phys Fitness.* 1998;38(3):240–244.

95 Castell L. Glutamine supplementation in vitro and in vivo, in exercise and in immunodepression. *Sports Med.* 2003; 33(5):323–345; and Krieger JW, Blank SE. Chronic glutamine supplementation influences nasal SigA but not salivary SigA during short-term overreaching run training. *Med Sci Sports Exerc.* 2003;35:S381.

96 Van Zyl CG, Lambert EV, Hawley JA, et. al. Effects of medium-chain triglyceride ingestion on fuel metabolism and cycling performance. *J Appl Physiol.* 1996;80:2217–2225.

97 Dunford M, Smith M. Op. cit.

98 Ivy JL. Effect of pyruvate and dihydroxyacetone on metabolism and aerobic endurance capacity. *Med Sci Sports Exerc.* 1998; 6:837.

99 Stone MH, Sanborn K, Smith LL, et. al. Effects of in-season (5 weeks) creatine and pyruvate supplementation on anaerobic performance and body composition in American football players. *Int J Sport Nutr.* 1999;9:146–165.

100 Sarubin Fragakis A. Op. cit.

101 Kreider RB, Melton C, Greenwood M, et al. Effects of oral D-ribose supplementation on anaerobic capacity and selected metabolic markers in healthy males. *Int J Sport Nutr Exerc Metab.* 2003;13(1):87–96; and Berardi JM, Ziegenfuss TN. Effects of ribose supplementation on repeated sprint performance in men. *J Strength Cond Res.* 2003;17(1):47–52.

102 Horswill CA. Effects of bicarbonate, citrate, and phosphate loading on performance. *Int J Sport Nutr.* 1995;5(suppl): S111–S119.

103 Ibid.

104 Houtkooper LB. Body composition. In: Manore MM, Thompson JL. *Sport Nutrition for Health and Performance.* Champaign, IL: Human Kinetics, 2000:199–219.

105 Rozenek R, Ward P, Long S, Garhammer J. Effects of high-calorie supplements on body composition and muscular strength following resistance training. *J Sports Med Phys Fitness.* 2002;42(3):340–347.

106 Storlie J. From fork to muscle. Op. cit.

107 McArdle WD, Katch FI, Katch VL. Op. cit.

108 Ibid.

109 Ibid.

110 Clarkson PM. The skinny on weight loss supplements and drugs. *ACSM's Health & Fitness.* 1998;2:18–26, 55.

111 Thompson JL. Op. cit.

112 Metz G. The NCAA weighs in. *Training and Conditioning.* 1998;8:16–17, 19, 21–23.

113 Centers for Disease Control and Prevention. Rapid weight loss in wrestlers results in death. *MMWR.* 1998;47(6): 105–108.

114 Metz G. Op. cit.

115 Otis CL, Drinkwater B, Johnson M, et al. American College of Sports Medicine. Position stand: the female athlete triad. *Med Sci Sports Exerc.* 1997;29:i–ix.

116 Torstveit MK, Sundgot-Borgen J. The female athlete triad: are elite athletes at increased risk? *Med Sci Sports Exerc.* 2005; 37:184–193.

117 Sundgot-Borgen J. Risk and trigger factors for the developing of eating disorders in female elite athletes. *Med Sci Sports Exerc.* 1994;4:414–419.

118 Smith AD. The female athlete triad: causes, diagnosis, and treatment. *Physician Sportsmed.* 1996;24:67–70, 75–76, 86.

119 Dueck CA, Manore MM, Matt KS. Role of energy balance in athletic menstrual dysfunction. *Int J Sport Nutr.* 1996; 6:165–190

120 Otis CL, Drinkwater B, Johnson M, et al. Op. cit.

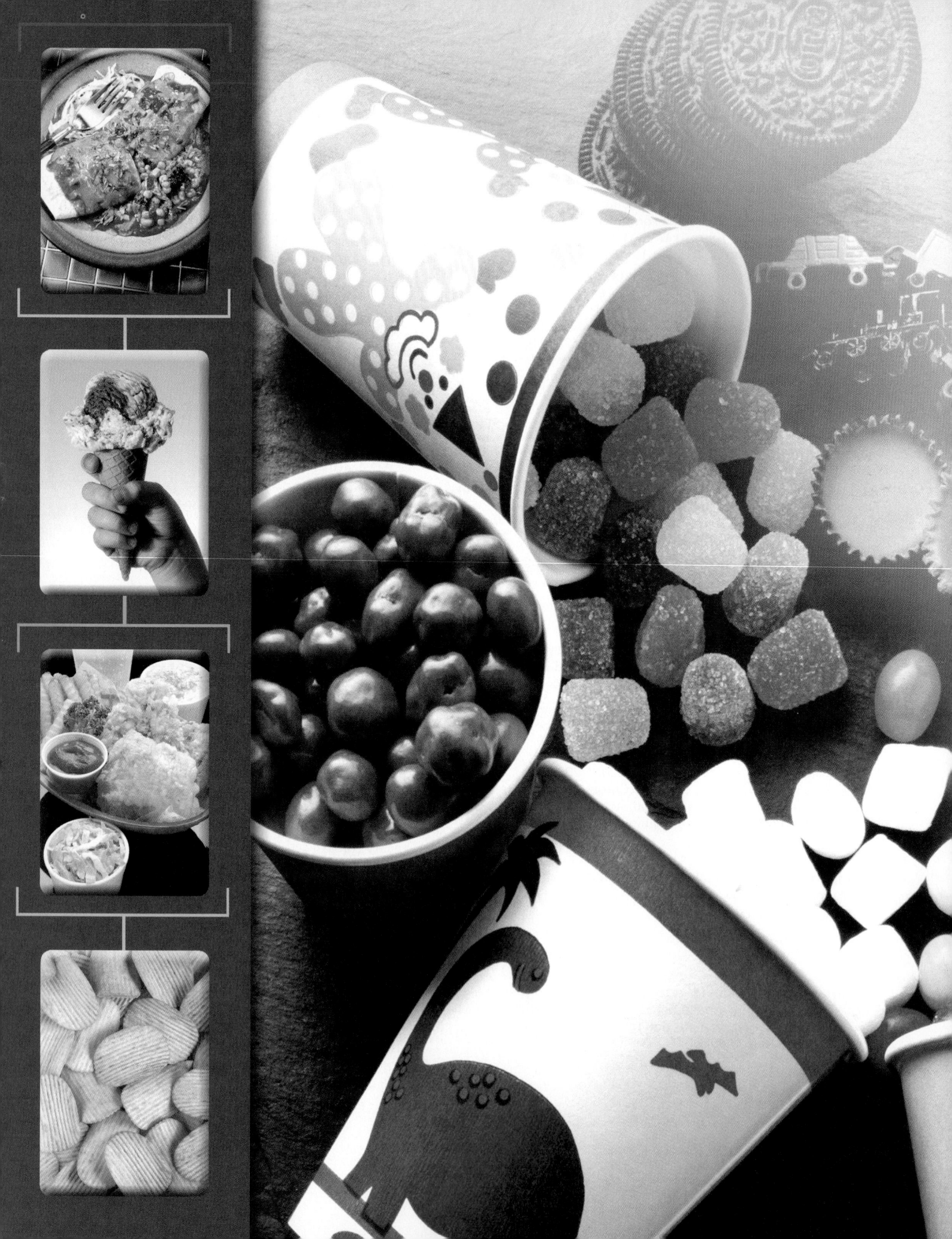

Spotlight on

Eating Disorders

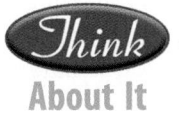 **Think About It**

1. What's your view of the ideal female body?
2. When should you be concerned that you—or someone you know—is dieting obsessively?
3. Given the right situation, what foods are you likely to binge on?
4. How many magazines do you read that promote dieting or encourage thinness?

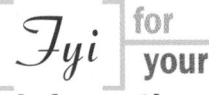 *Fyi* **for your Information**

This chapter's FYI box includes practical information on the following topic:
- Diary of an Eating Disorder

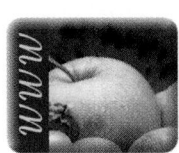 The Web site for this book offers many useful tools and is a great source for additional nutrition information for both students and instructors. For information on eating disorders, visit the site at **nutrition.jbpub.com**. You'll find exercises that explore the following topics:
- Age and Eating Disorders
- Body Image
- The Genetics of Eating Disorders

What About 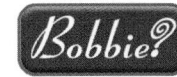 *Bobbie?*

Track the choices Bobbie is making with Nutritionist Pro or EatRight Analysis software.

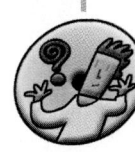

eating disorders A spectrum of abnormal eating patterns that eventually may endanger a person's health or increase the risk for other diseases. Generally, psychological factors play a key role.

disordered eating An abnormal change in eating pattern related to an illness, a stressful event, or a desire to improve one's health or appearance. If it persists it may lead to an eating disorder.

anorexia nervosa [an-or-EX-ee-uh ner-VOH-sah] An eating disorder marked by prolonged decrease of appetite and refusal to eat, leading to self-starvation and excessive weight loss. It results in part from a distorted body image and intense fear of becoming fat, often linked to social pressures.

body image A person's mental concept of his or her physical appearance, constructed from many different influences.

binge-eating disorder An eating disorder marked by repeated episodes of binge eating and a feeling of loss of control. The diagnosis is based on a person's having an average of at least two binge-eating episodes per week for six months.

compulsive overeating See *binge-eating disorder*.

bulimia nervosa [bull-EEM-ee-uh] An eating disorder marked by consumption of large amounts of food at one time (binge eating) followed by a behavior such as self-induced vomiting, use of laxatives, excessive exercise, fasting, or other practices to avoid weight gain.

A gaunt, hollow-cheeked college freshman confides to her roommate that she feels chubby. After an enormous lunch, a secretary works her way through a bag of cookies and polishes off a box of chocolates. A swimming champion who obsesses over every calorie becomes concerned that she hasn't had a period in two months. Disordered eating? Very likely! Eating disorder? Possibly!

Eating disorders and **disordered eating** are not the same. An eating disorder such as anorexia nervosa or bulimia nervosa is an illness that can seriously interfere with daily activities. Disordered eating is usually a temporary or mild change in eating patterns. Although it can occur after an illness or stressful event, it often is related to a dietary change intended to improve one's health or appearance. Unless disordered eating persists, it rarely requires professional intervention. Disordered eating, however, can lead to an eating disorder.

For most of us, eating is a pleasure. For people with an eating disorder, however, food is a source of continual stress and anxiety. (See **Figure SED.1**.) Eating disorders require professional intervention. They include a spectrum of emotional illnesses ranging from self-imposed starvation to chronic binge eating. These illnesses stem from severe distortions of the eating process and produce physical consequences that are often life threatening.[1]

Most of us have eaten to the point of discomfort on particular occasions. (Thanksgiving dinner comes to mind.) And many of us have cut out desserts at one time or another, hoping to fit into a special outfit or to make weight for an athletic event or job interview. But stuffing yourself at a holiday meal or going on an *occasional* diet does not constitute an eating disorder. According to the *Manual of Clinical Dietetics,* a defining characteristic of an eating disorder is a persistent inability to eat in moderation.[2]

The Eating Disorder Continuum

The 1994 edition of the American Psychiatric Association's *Diagnostic and Statistical Manual of Mental Disorders* (DSM-IV) divides eating disorders into three categories, with small but significant areas of overlap. These categories form a continuum, with self-starvation at one end and compulsive overeating at the other. (See **Figure SED.2**.) **Anorexia nervosa** occurs at the self-starvation end of the continuum. Anorexia is a self-imposed starvation syndrome that is triggered by a severely distorted **body image**. People with anorexia are at war with their bodies. Even when they are dangerously

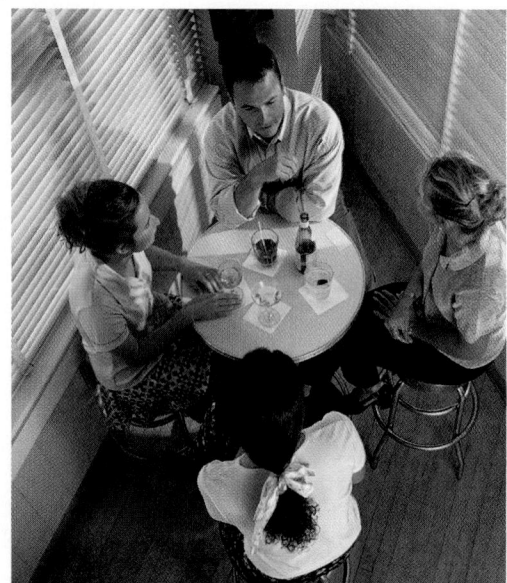

Figure SED.1 **Can you spot the person with the eating disorder?** Some people with eating disorders have normal body weights and are difficult to spot.

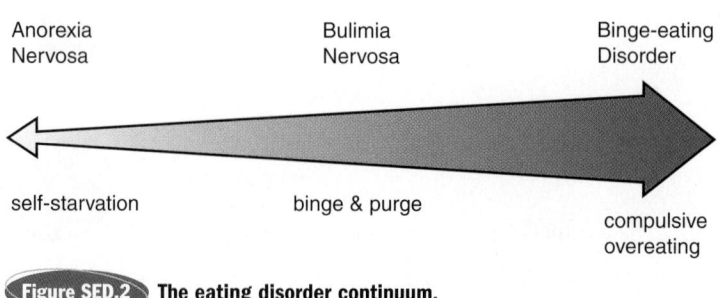

Anorexia Nervosa Bulimia Nervosa Binge-eating Disorder

self-starvation binge & purge compulsive overeating

Figure SED.2 **The eating disorder continuum.**

underweight, people with anorexia typically see themselves as fat. Severely restricting food intake is another symptom of anorexia nervosa. It may also involve purging (self-induced vomiting) and exercising excessively. Anorexia is most prevalent among adolescent females.

At the opposite end of the continuum is **binge-eating disorder**, formerly known as **compulsive overeating**. People with this disorder chronically consume massive quantities of food. Sufferers are typically obese; however, not all obese people binge eat. Diagnosis of binge-eating disorder is based on a person having an average of two binge-eating episodes per week for six months. Such episodes often are triggered by emotions such as frustration, anger, depression, and anxiety.[3]

In the middle of the continuum is **bulimia nervosa**. Like those with binge-eating disorder, people with bulimia nervosa compulsively gorge themselves. Like those with anorexia, people with bulimia desperately want to be thin and resort to purging to reach this goal. After gorging, people with bulimia often become disgusted with themselves and feel terrified of getting fat. To compensate, they make themselves vomit, use laxatives, exercise excessively, and take other actions to avoid gaining weight.

It is important to realize that few people who suffer from eating disorders are purely anorexic, bulimic, or binge eaters. Many swing from one disordered eating pattern to another, alternately starving and gorging themselves. People may suffer from binge-eating disorder at one point in their lives, and anorexia or bulimia at another.[4] **Table SED.1** shows the diagnostic criteria for these eating disorders.

History of a Modern Malady

Contrary to public perception, eating disorders are not New Age diseases. In fact, the first formal report of anorexia nervosa appeared in the medical literature in the 1870s.[5] Informal reports of a "condition of a nervous consumption" were written as early as 1689.[6] Some nutritional anthropologists argue that eating disorders can be traced to even more ancient times. During the Middle Ages, for instance, early Christian ascetics, who led lives of contemplation and rigorous self-denial, shunned worldly pleasures, including food, to show obedience and become closer to God. These people alternated periods of semistarvation with frequent fasts. Was this anorexia disguised as religious devotion? Some scholars think so.[7]

Early Greeks and Romans, in contrast, exhibited exaggerated bingeing and purging behavior at banquets that lasted for days. Guests gorged to the point of physical pain, and then tickled their throats with feathers to induce vomiting. Once their stomachs were empty, they returned to the table. Rather than finding this behavior repulsive or shameful, the ancient Romans glorified it. They even built areas known as vomitoriums into their banquet halls.[8]

Some scholars contend these ancient Romans had bulimia. Others disagree, arguing that the Roman men ate for pleasure in the company of others and purged only so they could rejoin the feast. In contrast, modern bulimia sufferers are usually females who gorge and purge in isolation—and in hopes of achieving an unrealistic cultural standard of beauty. Furthermore, today's bulimia sufferers invariably feel shame, low self-esteem, and even self-hate connected with their eating habits.

Although eating disorders are not an exclusively modern malady, it's clear that eating disorders have become increasingly common in the past few decades. A British model named Twiggy, nicknamed for her sticklike

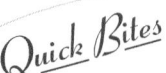

Quick Bites

Scary Statistics

About 5 million Americans have anorexia nervosa, bulimia nervosa, or binge-eating disorder. Researchers estimate that 15 percent of young women have disordered eating attitudes and behaviors. Every year an estimated 1,000 people die from anorexia nervosa.

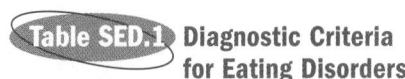

Table SED.1 **Diagnostic Criteria for Eating Disorders**

Anorexia nervosa

- Body weight < 85% of expected weight (or BMI ≤ 17.5 kg/m²)
- Intense fear of weight gain
- Inaccurate perception of own body size, weight, or shape
- Amenorrhea (in females after menarche)

Bulimia nervosa

- Recurrent binge eating (at least two times per week for three months)
- Recurrent purging, excessive exercise, or fasting (at least two times per week for three months)
- Excessive concern about body weight or shape
- Absence of anorexia nervosa

Binge-eating disorder

- Recurrent binge eating (at least two times per week for six months)
- Marked distress with at least three of the following:
  - Eating very rapidly
  - Eating until uncomfortably full
  - Eating when not hungry
  - Eating alone
  - Feeling disgusted or guilty after a binge
- No recurrent purging, no excessive exercising, and no fasting
- Absence of anorexia nervosa

Source: Becker AE, Grinspoon SK, Klibanski A, Herzog DB. Eating disorders. *N Engl J Med.* 1999;340(14): 1092–1098. Copyright © 1999. Massachusetts Medical Society. All rights reserved. Adapted with permission.

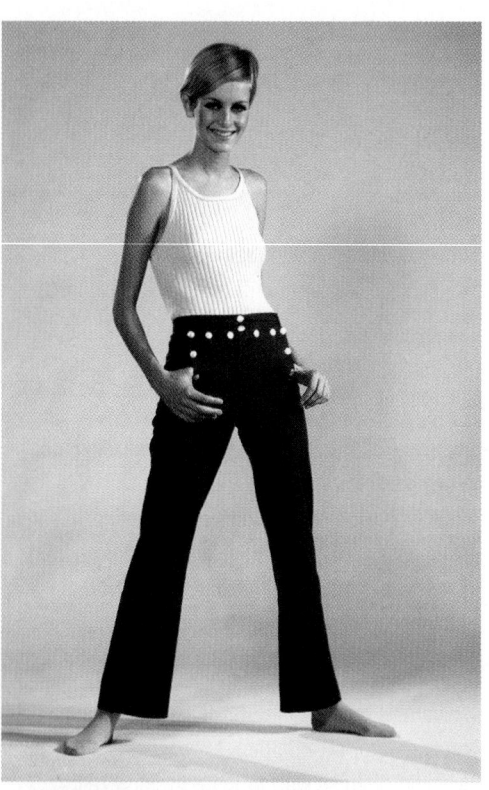

Figure SED.3 **Eye of the beholder.** In the 1960s, Twiggy became the new role model for young women who wanted to be thin and glamorous.

appearance, ushered in the epidemic in the early 1960s. Fashion magazine stories reported that she subsisted on water, lettuce, and a single daily serving of steak and that she had learned to suppress her hunger pangs. Rather than condemn these clearly dangerous eating habits, the magazines held Twiggy up as a model of self-control for girls and young women. (See **Figure SED.3**.)

Our national denial regarding the dangers of semistarvation ended abruptly and dramatically in 1983 with the highly publicized death of 32-year-old pop singer Karen Carpenter from complications of anorexia. Widespread media coverage of her death highlighted the lethal potential of eating disorders and made the terms *anorexia* and *bulimia* household words. Soon, other stars of film, TV, sports, and the fashion world revealed that they too suffered from eating disorders and described the physical, emotional, and social damage these diseases caused in their own lives. But, ironically, increased visibility and knowledge have not stemmed the tide of eating disorders. To the contrary, the prevalence of eating disorders and disordered eating continues to increase.[9]

Key Concepts: *Eating disorders, which are unhealthy conditions known to exist from ancient times, have become alarmingly common in industrialized countries, particularly the United States. Eating disorders range from the self-starvation of anorexia nervosa to the compulsive overeating of binge-eating disorder.*

No Simple Causes

Certain people appear to have a predisposition to eating disorders that may be rooted in psychological, biological, or cultural causes. A person who suffers from depression or **obsessive-compulsive disorder**, for example, may have an increased risk of developing an eating disorder. The vulnerability also may be biological. Indeed, there is evidence that genetic factors may create an increased risk for eating disorders. Another important factor in the development of eating disorders is society's emphasis on extreme thinness. It is clear that eating disorders are complex problems, with multiple causes. Social, psychological, and biological factors all play roles.

Eating disorders can develop when people, especially women, feel social pressure to achieve an unrealistic standard of thinness. Modern Western culture would have women weigh less than what is considered healthy. This means that most women cannot attain what society considers the "ideal" female form without significant food deprivation. These pressures affect even very young girls, starting with their first Barbie doll and her unnatural shape (see **Figure SED.4**), if not before.[10]

Psychological factors are important as well. These encompass everything from peer relationships to relationships with parents. Studies have shown that adolescent girls who were teased about their weight by peers had a more negative image of their bodies and lower self-esteem regardless of a girl's actual weight.[11] Findings were similar for adolescent boys and for teens of varied racial and ethnic backgrounds. Studies also have linked more severe forms of emotional trauma to disordered eating. For example, researchers at Texas A&M University detected symptoms of **post-traumatic stress disorder (PTSD)** in more than half of the anorexia and bulimia patients they studied.[12] PTSD occurs in people who have endured a significant trauma, such as child abuse or rape. Eating disorders also may be associated with dysfunctional family relationships. Some psychologists believe that people with anorexia and bulimia are trying to fulfill unrealistic

Think About It
1

parental expectations of perfection, in part by succumbing to societal pressure to be very thin.

In recent years, scientists have made major advances in understanding the biological foundation of eating disorders, and studies link abnormal levels of neurotransmitters, especially serotonin, to eating disorders.[13] Researchers, for example, have shown that bulimia patients experience spontaneous improvement in eating habits when they take antidepressant medication that increases brain levels of serotonin.[14] Many antiobesity drugs also affect serotonin levels.[15]

Neurotransmitters are just one focus of research into the biology of eating disorders. Another line of investigation focuses on genes. Recently, researchers have confirmed that eating disorders run in families. In addition, eating disorders occur most frequently in families with a history of obsessive-compulsive disorders, anxiety disorders, and depression.[16] Both depression and obsessive-compulsive behavior have been linked to atypical levels of serotonin and norepinephrine in the brain.[17]

It's likely that many genes are involved in the development of eating disorders. Two recently discovered genes are involved in the synthesis and release of the hormones leptin and **orexins** (named after the Greek word *orexis*, meaning "appetite").[18] The leptin gene regulates the body's production of leptin, a hormone that causes rapid weight loss in genetically obese mice. (Unfortunately, leptin has not stimulated the same reaction in humans.) The orexin gene regulates production of two appetite-stimulating hormones, orexin A and orexin B. In experiments, rodents injected with either hormone increased their food consumption 8- to 10-fold.[19]

The discoveries of the leptin and orexin genes significantly advance our understanding of brain chemistry and eating disorders and may eventually lead to new classes of more effective drugs. Drugs that mimic orexins, for example, might help patients with anorexia or other wasting syndromes by increasing their appetites. Conversely, drugs that block orexins might help patients struggling with obesity and binge eating. Or a leptinlike drug may eventually be used to stimulate weight loss. At the very least, discovery of these genes supports the idea that biological factors probably contribute to the development of eating disorders in vulnerable people.

Key Concepts: *The precise causes of eating disorders remain obscure. Researchers have debated whether eating disorders are primarily psychological or genetic in origin. The current view is that eating disorders are a result of the complex interaction of social, biological, and psychological factors. In other words, eating disorders occur in biologically susceptible individuals exposed to particular types of environmental stimuli.*

Anorexia Nervosa

Until the 1960s, few doctors ever saw a case of anorexia nervosa in their own practices, although they learned about the condition in medical school. By the mid-1970s, however, physicians were reporting many cases of anorexia, particularly among young women. Today this serious disorder occurs in an estimated 1 in 200 women, usually starting in adolescence. More than 90 percent of the cases occur in women, and the death rate from anorexia nervosa is about 10 times the death rate of women without anorexia.[20]

The term *anorexia nervosa*, which translates to "nervous loss of appetite," is misleading. People diagnosed with anorexia don't lose their appetite

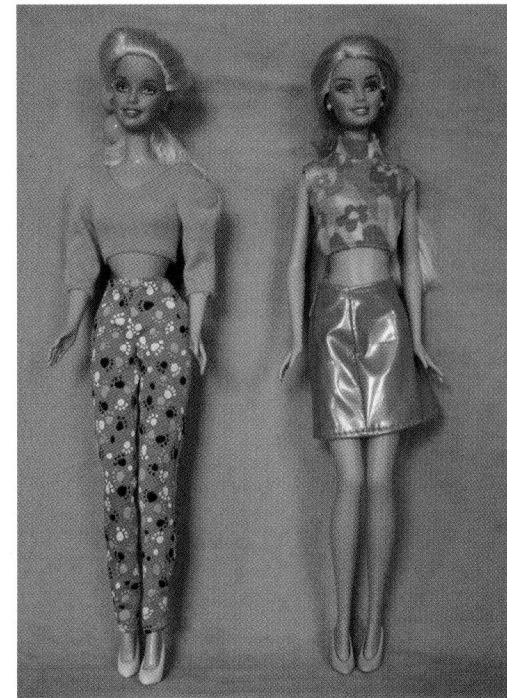

Figure SED.4 **Thin is in.** In 1998, Mattel overhauled Barbie's look for the millennium, giving her slimmer hips, a wider waist, and smaller breasts. Barbie's periodic overhauls are meant to fit the fashion of the times. Does the new Barbie (right) represent a realistic role model for today's young girls?

Quick Bites

Magazine Manipulations

When researchers studied fifth- through twelfth-grade girls in a working-class suburb in the Northeast, nearly 50 percent reported that they wanted to lose weight because of pictures in magazines. Frequent readers of fashion magazines were two to three times more likely to be influenced to diet or exercise to lose weight. Seventy percent of the girls reported that magazine pictures influenced their conception of the perfect body.

obsessive-compulsive disorder A disorder in which a person attempts to relieve anxiety by ritualistic behavior and continuous repetition of certain acts.

post-traumatic stress disorder (PTSD) An anxiety disorder characterized by an emotional response to a traumatic event or situation involving severe external stress.

orexins A class of hormones in the brain that may affect food consumption.

emetics Agents that induce vomiting.

enemas Infusions of fluid into the rectum, usually for cleansing or other therapeutic purposes.

diuretics [dye-u-RET-iks] Drugs or other substances that promote the formation and release of urine. Diuretics are given to reduce body fluid volume in treating such disorders as high blood pressure, congestive heart disease, and edema. Both alcohol and caffeine act as diuretics.

laxatives Substances that promote evacuation of the bowel by increasing the bulk of the feces, lubricating the intestinal wall, or softening the stool.

except in the final stages of the disorder. Instead, they are obsessed with food. But their obsession with thinness is even greater. The German term for the disorder, *pubertätsmagersucht,* or "mania for leanness," more accurately reflects the nature of the disease. The hallmark of anorexia nervosa is dramatic loss of weight, usually to less than 85 percent of the expected weight for height, or a body mass index (BMI) of less than or equal to 17.5 kg/m². (See **Figure SED.5**.)

Anorexia is more prevalent in industrialized societies that share an abundance of food and an attitude that equates beauty, particularly feminine beauty, with thinness. Nine of 10 anorexia sufferers are female—probably because Western society emphasizes thinness more for women than for men.[21] Studies show that the peak age of onset is between 15 and 19 years old.[22] In the past, the typical anorexia sufferer was an upper-class Caucasian female adolescent. Unfortunately, during the past decade anorexia has become more of an equal-opportunity disorder. Physicians have reported cases of the disorder in young women from all social and ethnic backgrounds; it is especially prevalent in women who participate in activities that emphasize leanness, including modeling, ballet, and gymnastics. In addition, anorexia has increased significantly among African American women.[23]

Causes of Anorexia Nervosa

On the surface, anorexia nervosa usually seems to result from a weight-loss program gone awry. A high school freshman may go on a diet after her boyfriend or gymnastics coach tells her she is too heavy An eighth-grader may want to lose weight to be more popular at a new school. The diet may start out just fine, but it never stops.

Beneath the surface, psychological issues are typically at work. Because most cases of anorexia begin around the age of puberty, some psychologists theorize that anorexic behavior is an attempt to prevent or delay sexual maturation. By retaining a child's body, a young girl may hope to avoid the

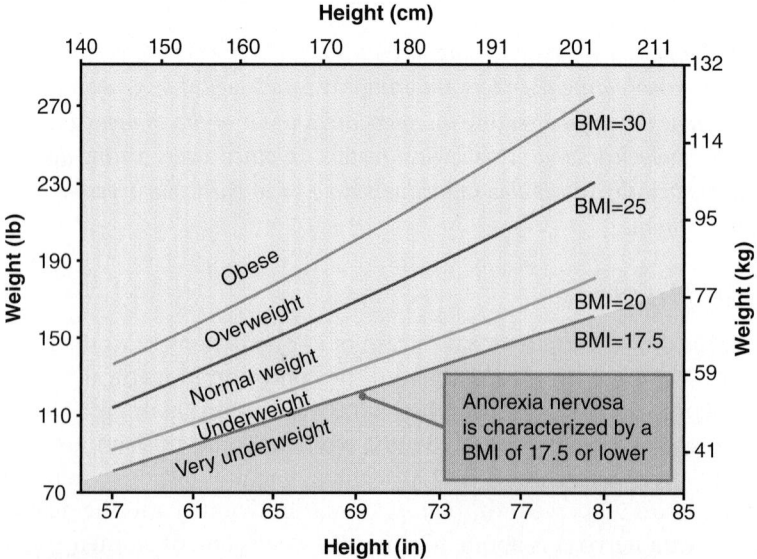

Figure SED.5 **BMI and underweight.** When managing eating disorders, BMI can help guide decisions about nutrition, medications, and psychotherapy.

pressures of the teen years and the responsibilities of adulthood. In addition, psychologists report that anorexia sufferers tend to be rigid, perfectionistic, all-or-nothing thinkers. Sufferers tend to lack a sense of independence and control over their own destiny. They may attempt to compensate for this through acts of intense self-discipline. Parents may facilitate this syndrome by being overly protective or rigid or by holding a child to excessively high standards of achievement.[24]

Warning Signs

Parents and friends of people with anorexia often miss early signs of the disease. It can be easy to mistake a loved one's obsession with dieting, avoidance of particular foods, or rigorous exercise schedule for a reasonable desire to lose weight.[25] When asked about a child who has been diagnosed with anorexia, most parents will describe a "wonderful" daughter—one who has always been cooperative, obedient, an exceptional student, and unusually neat and organized. When she started to diet, she did so with the same zeal and dedication she exhibited in other areas of her life.[26]

Initially, someone with anorexia has a feeling of power. Sufferers enjoy a feeling of control as they learn to deny their hunger and limit their food intake. Early warning signs include obsessively counting calories; developing lists of "safe" foods and foods to avoid; cutting foods, even peas, into small pieces; and spending a great deal of time rearranging food on a plate. To suppress hunger, a person with anorexia may drink up to 30 cups of water or diet soda a day. Anorexia sufferers also may channel their obsessions with food into the preparation of elaborate meals for others without eating any of the food themselves.[27] **Table SED.2** lists the warning signs of anorexia.

As the disease progresses, anorexia sufferers become increasingly disillusioned, withdrawn, and hostile. Success always seems beyond their grasp. No matter how thin they are, they see themselves as overweight. (See **Figure SED.6**.) When they eat more than they think they should, they may induce vomiting or use **emetics**, **enemas**, **diuretics**, or **laxatives**. They may also exercise relentlessly. Eventually, their efforts to avoid obesity take over their lives. They start to avoid social situations that may expose their behaviors and so withdraw more and more from friends and family. Groggy and irritable from food deprivation and sleep disturbances, people with advanced anorexia spend so little time on their schoolwork or jobs that their performance deteriorates. Yet when confronted with their obsessive dieting or deteriorating behavior, they will deny that anything is unusual.[28]

Treatment

Just as there is no one cause for anorexia nervosa, there is no single way to cure it. In fact, most experts doubt that patients with anorexia can ever be cured. Research suggests that with intensive therapy, most patients can achieve normal weight. However, they may struggle all their lives with a moderate to severe preoccupation with food and body weight, poor social relationships, and depression. The earlier a patient begins treatment, the better the prognosis.

The course of anorexia varies greatly. In rare instances, a sufferer recovers spontaneously without treatment. More typically, a patient recovers only after a variety of treatments or enters a cyclical pattern of weight gain and relapse. From 30 to 50 percent of anorexia patients also have

Think About It 2

Table SED.2 Warning Signs of Anorexia

Anorexia nervosa is a disorder in which preoccupation with dieting and thinness leads to excessive weight loss. The person with anorexia may not acknowledge that weight loss or restricted eating is a problem. Family and friends can help by recognizing that the following are warning signs:

- Loss of a significant amount of weight
- Continuing to diet (although thin)
- Feeling fat, even after losing weight
- Fear of weight gain
- Cessation of monthly menstrual periods
- Preoccupation with food, calories, nutrition, and/or cooking
- Preferring to eat in isolation
- Exercising compulsively
- Bingeing and purging

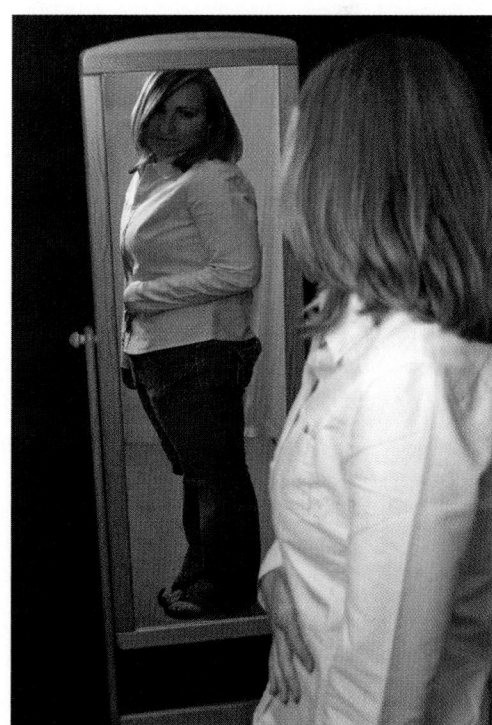

Figure SED.6 Distorted body image.

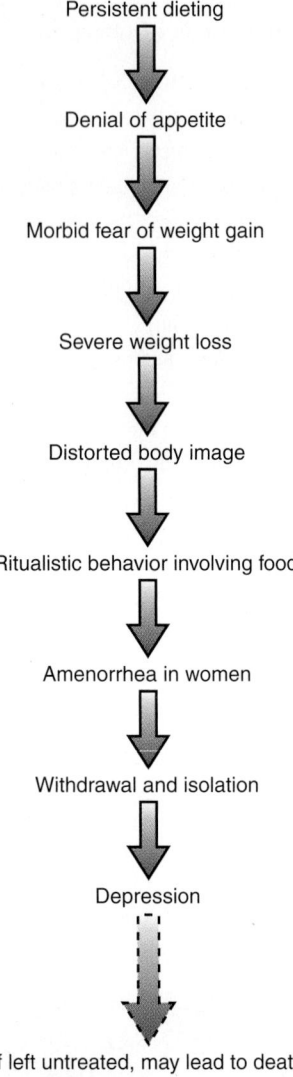

Persistent dieting

Denial of appetite

Morbid fear of weight gain

Severe weight loss

Distorted body image

Ritualistic behavior involving food

Amenorrhea in women

Withdrawal and isolation

Depression

If left untreated, may lead to death

Figure SED.7 The progression of anorexia.

symptoms of bulimia, which can complicate diagnosis and treatment.[29] Tragically, in 6 to 18 percent of cases, the disease proves fatal. (See **Figure SED.7**.) Patients who have other emotional disorders, such as major depression or substance abuse, are the most likely to die from complications of the disease. Potentially fatal complications of anorexia include starvation and suicide.[30]

As with many other behavioral disorders, people with anorexia usually deny the danger of their situation. Thus family and friends must intervene to get sufferers to treatment—often by getting together and supportively confronting the person with evidence that something is seriously wrong. This common technique helps people accept the need for at least an initial medical screening. The complex and multifaceted nature of anorexia requires a team of experienced health care professionals, including physicians, clinical dietitians, and psychotherapists, so that both the physical and psychological aspects of the disorder can be addressed. One of the best places to find an experienced team of therapists is at an eating disorder clinic associated with a major medical facility.[31]

The first goal of treatment is to stabilize the patient's physical condition. The second is to convert the patient, who is typically reluctant, into a willing participant in the treatment plan. A combination of hospitalization, psychotherapy, and pharmacotherapy is often necessary.

Restoring the patient's nutritional status is of prime importance. Otherwise, dehydration, starvation, and electrolyte imbalances can lead to serious health problems and even death. (See **Table SED.3**.) The American Dietetic Association recommends hospitalization if a person's weight drops below 75 percent of the standard weight considered healthy for height. The American Psychiatric Association considers hospitalization essential for a person who has lost more than 20 percent of body weight over a three-month period or weighs 85 percent or less of the standard weight. (See **Table SED.4**.) Once the patient's physical condition has stabilized and

Table SED.3 Side Effects of Excessive Weight Loss in Anorexia Nervosa

Emaciation

- Loss of fat stores and muscle mass
- Reduced thyroid metabolism
- Cold intolerance
- Difficulty maintaining core body temperature

Hematological

- Leukopenia (abnormal decrease of white blood cells)
- Iron-deficiency anemia

Other

- Growth of lanugo (fine, baby-like hairs) over the trunk
- Osteopenia (mineral depletion in bone)
- Premature osteoporosis

Neuropsychiatric

- Abnormal taste sensation
- Depression
- Impaired thought process

Cardiac

- Loss of cardiac muscle, resulting in a smaller heart
- Abnormal heart rhythm
- Increased risk of sudden death

Gastrointestinal

- Delayed gastric emptying
- Bloating
- Constipation
- Abdominal pain

some physical symptoms of starvation have disappeared, psychotherapy can begin in earnest. Many therapists use a cognitive behavioral approach to help the patient challenge irrational beliefs and establish healthy attitudes and behaviors for gaining and maintaining weight.

The early phases of weight gain are fraught with challenges for both patient and clinician. Patients must gain a certain amount of weight to prevent death or permanent damage, while the psychotherapeutic portion of their treatment is still in the very early phases. At first, the patient is encouraged to simply eat enough food to minimize or stop weight loss. Next, the patient is started on a very slow process of weight gain, all the while receiving intensive psychotherapy. The first sign of weight gain can precipitate a crisis. Phobia of obesity may return with renewed vengeance. Many patients refuse to eat. Others resist treatment in covert ways. If not restricted to bed and closely supervised, they may try to burn off calories through relentless exercise or by purging. To avoid detection, they adopt a series of behaviors to conceal their lack of weight gain. These include wearing concealing clothes or "bulking up" before weigh-ins by filling their pockets with coins or drinking large amounts of water or diet soda.[32]

Psychologists use a variety of psychotherapeutic techniques to help the patient deal with underlying emotional issues, such as depression. Treatment programs generally use a combination of behavioral therapy, individual psychotherapy, patient education, family education, and family therapy. Frequently, therapists find family conflicts are at the heart of the eating disorder. Ongoing therapy for the patient and family is key to successful recovery. As the patient's symptoms resolve, she or he must find new ways to relate to and communicate with family members. Family members must remain open and willing to change their behavior toward the person with the eating disorder.

Dietitians work closely with the psychotherapist to help patients develop a realistic view of food and to reshape their food selection and eating behaviors. Although no pharmaceutical agent has been developed specifically to treat anorexia, some antidepressants have proved useful.

Most patients with anorexia nervosa require continued intervention after discharge from the hospital or treatment program. Support groups for people with eating disorders and their families can be an important link in the recovery process. Support groups also can be a useful technique for easing a resistant patient into treatment. With expert help and ongoing therapy, patients with anorexia can develop new mechanisms for coping with life's stresses, eventually replacing their disordered relationship with food with new, healthier interpersonal relationships.

Key Concepts: The hallmark symptoms of anorexia nervosa are a mania for thinness and self-imposed starvation. Sufferers manifest a body weight as much as 15 percent below normal, a severely distorted body image, withdrawal from family and friends, and various physical and psychological changes related to starvation.

Bulimia Nervosa

Although the behavior we now call bulimia was practiced in Greek and Roman times, it has only been recognized as a psychiatric illness for about 20 years. Gerald Russell, a British psychiatrist, first coined the term *bulimia nervosa* in 1979 to describe a syndrome of bingeing and purging in young Caucasian females. The average patient with bulimia is an unmarried Caucasian female in her twenties or thirties with a normal or near-normal

Table SED.4 When Hospitalization Is Needed

Suggested criteria for hospitalization for individuals with anorexia nervosa include:

- Weight loss of greater than 20 percent over three months
- Severe metabolic disturbance
- Severe depression or suicide risk
- Severe bingeing and purging
- Failure to maintain outpatient weight contract
- Psychosis
- Family crisis

Source: American Psychiatric Association. *Diagnostic and Statistical Manual of Mental Disorders.* 4th ed. Text revision. Washington, DC: American Psychiatric Association, 2000. Reprinted with permission.

American Dietetic Association

Nutrition Intervention in the Treatment of Anorexia Nervosa, Bulimia Nervosa, and Other Eating Disorders

It is the position of the American Dietetic Association (ADA) that nutrition intervention, including nutritional counseling, by a registered dietitian is an essential component of the team treatment of patients with anorexia nervosa, bulimia nervosa, and other eating disorders during assessment and treatment across the continuum of care.

J Am Diet Assoc. 2006;106:2073–2082. Reprinted with permission.

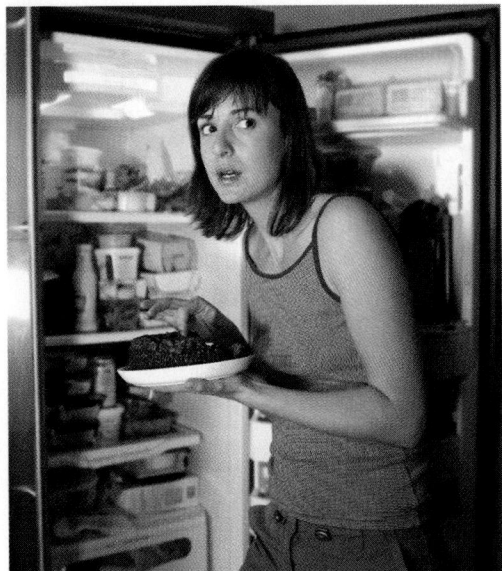

Figure SED.8 The typical person suffering from bulimia is an unmarried Caucasian woman in her twenties or thirties.

Quick Bites

I'm So Hungry I Could Eat an Ox!

The term *bulimia* is derived from the Greek word *bous*, meaning "ox," and *limos*, meaning "hunger."

body weight. (See **Figure SED.8**.) Patients with bulimia are more likely to be sexually active than are those with anorexia and often are involved in destructive relationships with members of the opposite sex. Almost anyone can be affected, however.

The relationships among dieting, bingeing severity, and alcohol use were studied in a sample of women in their first year of college. A positive relationship was found between dieting and bingeing severity and the frequency, intensity, and negative consequences of alcohol use in young women.[33]

People with bulimia nervosa tend to feel very disorganized. They report suffering from depression and low self-esteem. Many were sexually abused as children. Food was often a source of comfort, and eating gradually evolved into a tool for dealing with every unpleasant event, from boredom to major life crises.

It is estimated that between 1 percent and 3 percent of American adolescent and young adult females have bulimia. But bulimia, particularly in its milder forms, often goes undetected. This is because individuals with bulimia are very secretive about their behaviors, typically limiting their binge-and-purge episodes to the middle of the night or times when they are assured of privacy. Also, unlike patients with anorexia or binge-eating disorder, whose body weights may hint at their underlying psychiatric disorder, the body weight of a patient with bulimia is usually average or only slightly above average. Several studies have found that as many as 40 percent of college-aged women occasionally binge and purge—often enough to raise concern but too infrequently for an official diagnosis of bulimia.[34] **Table SED.5** lists the warning signs of bulimia.

Causes of Bulimia

Bulimia seems to occur most often in people who have an intense desire to nurture themselves with food but who are also strongly influenced by our societal obsession with thinness. One description of people with bulimia characterizes them as being obsessed with food but repulsed by fat. In con-

---

[*Fyi*] Diary of an Eating Disorder

FOR YOUR INFORMATION

Every time I leave one of my sessions I feel better. We talk about stuff; I feel, express, and even cry. Today was the third time since I left her office to come home and throw up. I think things are getting better despite the fact that my mind focuses 80 percent of the time on food during the 55 minutes. But it's like the kitchen is a refuge for my mind. I always know it will be there, waiting to embrace me when I get home.

Alone is how I hope to find it. I have been thinking of what I will sink my teeth into first. Usually I go for the fat-free chocolate

cake, then to the frozen yogurt (which makes it all come up much smoother). I don't think this is normal, though I am not really concerned. I feel like a million-pound weight has been swept away by the effortless flush of the toilet. The hardest thing is to look in the mirror after I have thrown up. Sometimes I wipe my face before I look. Other times I leave the spit, bile, and food on my mouth and hands. I just stand there holding my hands up, with my shoulders slumped over. I produce this expression of absolute helplessness—then I laugh.

I guess I am amazed by the act I've just committed. I can't explain why, I can't believe that it is really me doing this. Why would I do something like throw up? I really have no reason to torture myself. Bulimia was always *them*—I can't possibly be like that. I throw up, but I am not a bulimic. I sure as hell don't have an eating disorder.

I am totally for this whole counseling thing because I feel sad a lot and I want to feel better. But I can't leave there and not feel that I have to get this crap out. All this stuff that we talk about.

Table SED.5 Warning Signs of Bulimia

Bulimia nervosa involves frequent episodes of binge eating, almost always followed by purging and intense feelings of guilt or shame. The sufferer feels out of control and recognizes that the behavior is not normal. The signs that a person may have bulimia include:

- Bingeing, or eating uncontrollably
- Compensating for binges by strict dieting, fasting, vigorous exercise, vomiting, or abusing laxatives or diuretics in an attempt to lose weight
- Using the bathroom frequently after meals
- Preoccupation with body weight
- Depression or mood swings
- Irregular menstrual periods
- Dental problems, swollen cheeks or glands, heartburn, or bloating
- Personal or family problems with drugs or alcohol

trast to people with anorexia, people with bulimia focus more on food than on thinness.

Psychologists who have treated patients with bulimia have found that they typically did not receive sufficient nurturing during their formative years. Whereas families of anorexic patients tend to have a lot of rigidly defined roles and rules, families of bulimic patients tend to lack structure. Roles may be loosely defined. Parents are often described as distant and judgmental. Significant family conflict usually exists. Patients often feel that their families failed to provide an adequate sense of security and protection.

Obsessed by Thoughts of Food

A person with bulimia chronically **binges** and **purges**. To meet the official *DSM-IV* definition of the disorder, bingeing and purging must occur at least twice a week for at least three months. Purging may be accompanied or

binge Consumption of a very large amount of food in a brief time (e.g., 2 hours) accompanied by a loss of control over how much and what is eaten.

purge Emptying of the GI tract by self-induced vomiting and/or misuse of laxatives, diuretics, or enemas.

Today, Dr. Tant asked me when this all began. My first thought was, "Oh this throwing up thing? I can't remember." But I do recall one time when my ex-boyfriend Matt and I had gone to a really nice dinner. My recollection of the evening was that it was perfect. I remember thinking about how this food was really fattening, though, and how it would make me fat if I kept it down. I didn't know or have the willpower to just not eat it. Over and over I tortured and berated myself about the effects this dinner would have on my body. I couldn't bear it. This dinner was no longer one meal; it was going to ruin my body and make me fat. I couldn't stand that food being inside me another moment. Looking back I can't imagine how I could have thrown up right there on the side of the road. It was like I had no couth. I told Matt to pull over, and I just stuck my hand down my throat. Rationalizing the act while engaging in it, I then jumped back in the truck to carry on with the night. We never discussed my vile act other than Matt saying, "I can't believe you just did that."

"I know," I responded, "but it just was making me feel so sick. I mean, my stomach was really nauseous [sic]." Basically I don't know when I began this war with myself, but I know it caused me to fear myself. The rest is a blur—its beginning, its incentive. I heard Dr. Tant's question. I just didn't have the answer.

Chelsea Browning Smith

Source: Smith C. *Diary of an Eating Disorder.* Dallas, TX: Taylor Publishing Company, 1998. Reprinted by permission of Taylor Publishing, an imprint of Rowman & Littlefield Publishing Group.

Figure SED.9 The binge-and-purge cycle of bulimia.

replaced by fasting, excessive exercise, or other behaviors that compensate for the binge episode. Between binges, people with bulimia typically restrict their dietary intake to a limited number of low-calorie foods they consider "safe." This dietary control is an illusion, however. The average bulimic sufferer is obsessed by thoughts of food and spends a great deal of time both planning the next binge and trying to resist the urge to binge.[35] **Figure SED.9** illustrates the binge-and-purge pattern of bulimia.

Just what triggers a binge is not clear. People with bulimia tend to be all-or-nothing thinkers. If they eat a single piece of food from their forbidden list, such as a cookie, they feel driven to consume the entire box. Some researchers believe that hunger caused by very restrictive dieting, combined with a buildup of everyday stresses, overwhelms the person's resolve and precipitates a binge.

During a binge, individuals with bulimia typically consume massive quantities of highly palatable "forbidden" foods such as pastry, ice cream, and candy. This gorging takes place over a relatively short time span—say, an hour or two. Binges may contain up to 10,000 kilocalories. Afterward, feeling physically ill from overindulgence, sufferers use a variety of purging techniques, such as self-induced vomiting or excessive quantities of laxatives, to rid themselves of the food. Or they may follow a binge with a period of very strict fasting and heightened exercise.

Purging leads to a variety of physical symptoms. Over time, the gastric acid in vomit burns the lining of the pharynx, esophagus, and mouth, erodes tooth enamel, and may even result in loss of teeth. Repeated vomiting also can enlarge the salivary glands and erode the lining of the stomach and esophagus.

Excessive self-induced vomiting and diarrhea can upset the body's delicate biochemical balance through loss of electrolytes and body water. Among other dangers, changes in electrolyte balance can trigger an irregular heartbeat and precipitate a life-threatening medical crisis. For example, Terri Schiavo, the focus of intense media attention in 2005, suffered from bulimia and collapsed when her potassium levels dipped frighteningly low. Her heart stopped, which likely caused decreased blood flow to her brain, leading to brain damage.

Excessive use of emetics (drugs to induce vomiting) and laxatives carries its own risks. Repeated use of emetics is toxic to the liver and kidneys, and abuse of laxatives can damage the lining of the large intestine. **Figure SED.10** shows the side effects of bulimic purging.

Treatment

Little research has been done on the long-term course of bulimia. It appears, however, that bulimia is easier to treat than anorexia, perhaps because bulimic patients tend to recognize that their behavior is abnormal. Following treatment, more than half of patients report an improvement in their binge-eating and coping behaviors. About 30 percent of patients eventually become symptom-free. The rest, however, struggle with the disorder to some degree throughout their lives. To reduce the risk of relapse, therapists encourage patients to stay involved in support groups after completing formal therapy.

Cognitive behavior therapy is key to helping patients reshape their attitudes about food and identify situations that trigger bingeing. The therapist's goal is to help patients let go of their need to categorize foods as safe or dangerous, good or bad. Patients must learn techniques for dealing with stress and uncomfortable or painful memories and feelings. Depression, which typically accompanies this disorder, must be treated as well. Many patients with bulimia also require treatment for substance abuse. A patient

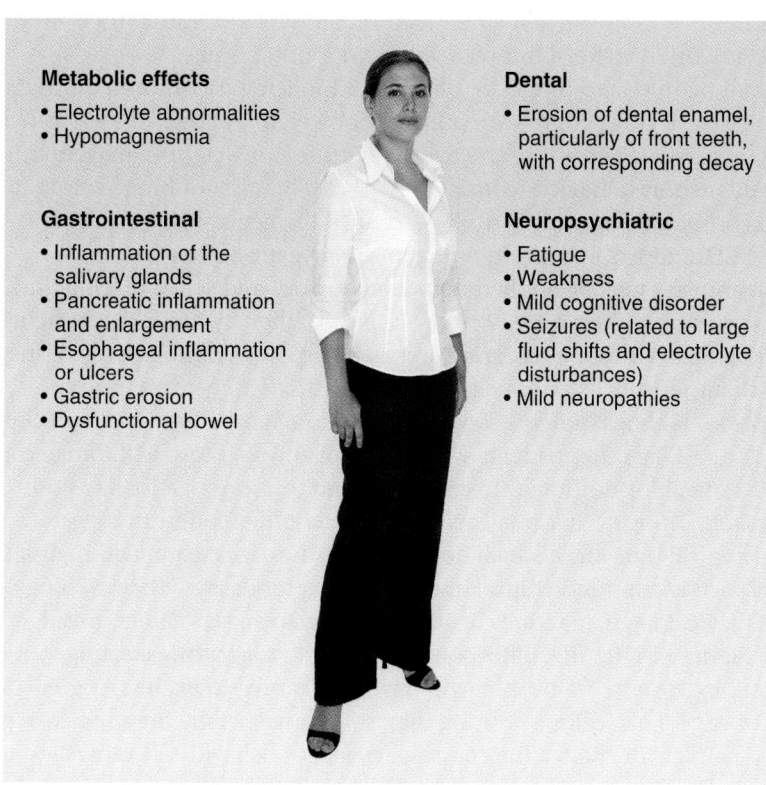

Metabolic effects
- Electrolyte abnormalities
- Hypomagnesmia

Gastrointestinal
- Inflammation of the salivary glands
- Pancreatic inflammation and enlargement
- Esophageal inflammation or ulcers
- Gastric erosion
- Dysfunctional bowel

Dental
- Erosion of dental enamel, particularly of front teeth, with corresponding decay

Neuropsychiatric
- Fatigue
- Weakness
- Mild cognitive disorder
- Seizures (related to large fluid shifts and electrolyte disturbances)
- Mild neuropathies

Figure SED.10 Bulimia and side effects of purging.

is hospitalized only when severely depressed or when purging is so frequent that physical damage has occurred or is imminent.

Medication can be an effective adjunct to psychotherapy. Serotonin-enhancing antidepressants have been used successfully to treat bulimia.

Key Concepts: *Key symptoms of bulimia nervosa are binge-eating episodes at least twice a week for three months, followed by behaviors that compensate for the binges, such as severe dieting, purging, or a combination of dieting and purging. The body weights of people with bulimia are typically close to or slightly above that considered healthy for their heights.*

Binge-Eating Disorder

Overeating has been reported in the medical literature since scribes first put stylus to tablet. Over the generations, societies, including our own, have considered obesity a sign of good health, wealth, and even fertility. But modern Western society is not among these. Binge eating is the most common eating disorder in industrialized nations. It occurs only in societies where people have access to an abundant supply of food. Its precise causes are unclear. However, the condition seems to be related to an intense desire to nurture oneself with food or to reduce stress by eating.[36] In 1994 the American Psychiatric Association recognized binge-eating disorder as an emotional illness.

Stress and Conflict Often Trigger Binge Eating

A person with binge-eating disorder consumes excessive quantities of food in a relatively short period of time at least twice a week. Unlike the bulimia sufferer, however, the person with binge-eating disorder does not attempt to compensate by purging or other means. In some instances, binge eaters adopt a grazing pattern. "Grazers" eat constantly for extended periods of time, eventually consuming an exceptionally large quantity of food. This

Quick Bites

When Plumpness Was Valued

In centuries past, extra pounds displayed one's wealth and prosperity. The wealthy could afford abundant food and didn't perform physical labor.

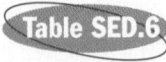 **Table SED.6** **Warning Signs of Binge-Eating Disorder**

Binge eaters, like bulimia sufferers, experience periods of uncontrolled eating that they usually keep secret. Binge eaters often are depressed and sometimes have other psychological problems. Signs that a person may have a binge-eating disorder include:

- Episodes of binge eating
- Eating when not physically hungry
- Frequent dieting
- Feeling unable to stop eating voluntarily
- Awareness that eating patterns are abnormal
- Weight fluctuations
- Depressed mood
- Attribution of social and professional successes and failures to weight

Figure SED.11 Feelings of loneliness, depression, anxiety, or stress can trigger a binge-eating episode.

pattern of overindulgence may be seen in people who restrict their food intake at work or school but seek solace in food at home.

Not all people who binge are obese. But bingeing is common among the severely obese and people with a history of weight cycling. In the United States, at least 30 percent of the people enrolled in weight-management programs report behaviors consistent with a diagnosis of binge-eating disorder, compared with only 3 to 5 percent of the general population.[37] **Table SED.6** describes warning signs of binge-eating disorder.

Many binge eaters begin dieting in grade school and start bingeing during adolescence or in their early twenties. Typically, they try numerous weight-loss programs without long-term success. Binge eaters exhibit many of the same characteristics as bulimic patients. More than 50 percent have clinical depression. Feelings of depression, loneliness, anxiety, or stress can precipitate a binge. Like other patients with eating disorders, those with binge-eating disorder are all-or-nothing thinkers. They tend to categorize foods as safe or dangerous. Eating even a small serving of a forbidden food can trigger a binge. Typical binge foods include sweets, pastries, ice cream, and high-fat snacks such as nuts and chips. However, if junk foods aren't handy, binge eaters may eat large quantities of starchy foods, such as potatoes, bread, and pasta. **Figure SED.11** illustrates some factors that trigger binge eating.

Most binge eaters are people who have not learned to express or even acknowledge their feelings. During therapy sessions, many binge eaters report feeling helpless to change the course of events or behaviors of others around them. Rather than acknowledge their feelings, they swallow them—aided by large quantities of food. They become addicted to the behavior itself because it is the only way they can get relief from stress. (See **Figure SED.12**.)

Binge eating often is a learned response to stress or conflict, passed down from one generation to the next. Parents may use food rather than affection and discussion to shape their children's behavior. Food is used for celebration and consolation, for reward and punishment. Children growing up in such environments learn to eat in response to emotions rather than hunger. As adults, they turn to food to satisfy all their emotional needs.

Treatment

Little is known about the course and prognosis of binge-eating disorder. However, people who become obese as a result of this disorder are at risk of developing weight-related health problems, including type 2 diabetes, hypertension, degenerative joint disease, heart disease, and even certain cancers.

People who have binge-eating disorder are rarely able to control the condition themselves. They usually require therapy to help them identify their long-buried emotions and learn techniques for giving voice to their feelings. Therapists experienced in treating this disorder discourage patients from trying to lose weight initially. Any attempts to restrict food intake can backfire by creating anxiety and provoking a binge. The major focus of therapy is to help patients identify their emotions and separate true biological hunger from emotional hunger. Once significant progress is made in these areas, the patient is better equipped psychologically to address weight issues.

Long-term support is key to keeping binge eaters from relapsing. Self-help groups such as Overeaters Anonymous are one source of support. These groups are organized according to the 12-step philosophy of Alcoholics Anonymous. In addition, many hospitals in large urban areas have support groups led by trained therapists. Hospitals and clinics that provide medically supervised fasting programs such as Optifast often supply this type of service as well. (See Chapter 8, "Energy Balance, Body Composition, and Weight Management," for further information on this type of weight-control program.)

Many patients with binge-eating disorder benefit from antidepressant medications. These drugs reduce the urge to binge, most likely by altering the brain's serotonin level. Various weight-management medications are now in development. These also may curb the urge to binge.

Key Concepts: *Binge-eating disorder is the most common eating disorder seen in people of all ages and backgrounds. Like people with bulimia, those with binge-eating disorder consume significantly more food than is typically eaten in a given period of time. Unlike bulimia, those with binge-eating disorder do not purge or fast. Not all binge eaters are obese, although many obese people binge.*

Body Dysmorphic Disorder

People with **body dysmorphic disorder (BDD)** are preoccupied with an imagined or slight defect in appearance, worrying, for example, that their skin is scarred, that they are balding, or that their nose is too big. Patients may engage in long rituals of grooming, repeatedly combing hair, applying makeup, or picking at their skin. The condition's severity varies. Whereas some people can manage it, for others the preoccupation causes significant distress and impairment: They may have few friends, avoid dating, miss school or work, and feel very self-conscious in social situations.

Many patients with BDD have coexisting conditions, such as obsessive-compulsive disorder, major depression, delusions, or social phobia. Approximately 2 to 7 percent of patients who undergo plastic surgery have BDD and are generally unhappy with the results.

BDD affects 1 to 2 percent of the general population; however, BDD frequently goes undiagnosed. Patients are ashamed of their problem and fail to report it to their physicians. Even though it is a serious and distressing condition, it is easily trivialized. In addition, even many health professionals are unaware that BDD is a psychiatric disorder that often responds to psychiatric treatment. Many people seek treatment from dermatologists, plastic surgeons, and other physicians, but these professionals often are ignorant of this disorder and thus are unhelpful.

Psychiatric treatment, including medication and cognitive behavior therapy, can effectively decrease symptoms and suffering. The therapist helps the person with BDD resist compulsive BDD behaviors (for example, mirror checking), face avoided situations (for example, social situations), and develop a more realistic view of his or her appearance. Medications, including selective serotonin reuptake inhibitors (SSRIs), can relieve obsession and decrease distress and depression.[38]

Key Concepts: *Body dysmorphic disorder is often seen with coexisting conditions such as obsessive-compulsive disorder, major depression, delusions, or social phobia. Patients with BDD magnify slight defects and are preoccupied with their appearance.*

Night-Eating Syndrome

When a person grazes through the evening, finds herself plotting midnight refrigerator raids, and wakes at night to eat, she may have **night-eating syndrome (NES)**. A person with this disorder

- Eats more than half of daily calories during and after the evening meal

- Wakes up at least once a night to eat, especially high-carbohydrate snacks

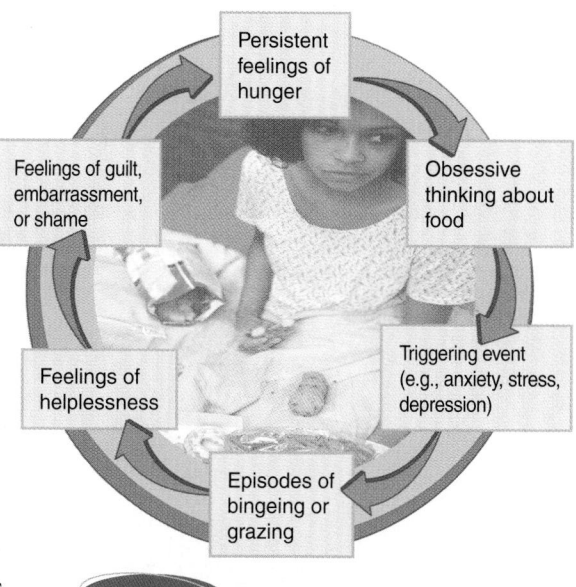

Figure SED.12 **The vicious cycle of binge eating.** Binge-eating disorder is the most common eating disorder.

body dysmorphic disorder (BDD) An eating disorder in which a distressing and impairing preoccupation with an imagined or slight defect in appearance is the primary symptom.

night-eating syndrome (NES) An eating disorder in which a habitual pattern of interrupting sleep to eat is the primary symptom.

- Feels tense, anxious, worried, or guilty while eating
- Lacks appetite for breakfast and postpones it for hours
- Persists in this behavior for at least three months

Night-eating syndrome is a fairly uncommon eating disorder in the general population—perhaps only 1 to 2 percent of adults in the general population have this problem—but it affects up to a quarter of obese people. Although underlying causes are not fully understood, the disorder may result from a combination of biological, genetic, and emotional factors. Researchers have noted several hormonal imbalances among NES sufferers: Levels of both melatonin (a sleep-inducing hormone) and leptin (an appetite-suppressing hormone) were significantly reduced from normal levels. Cortisol—the so-called stress hormone that kicks in when we feel tense—appears higher at night in night eaters, perhaps arousing them to wake and head for the kitchen. Stress, depression, and anxiety commonly affect mood among those with the condition.

Night-eating syndrome involves a disturbed food intake circadian rhythm, which may be out of sync by as much as four to five hours with a person's normal sleep rhythm. It is possibly the first clinical disorder to manifest differing circadian rhythms of two biological systems.

The heavy preference for carbohydrates, which trigger the brain to produce "feel-good" neurochemicals, suggests that night eating may be an attempt to self-medicate mood problems. A dietitian can help develop meal plans that distribute intake more evenly throughout the day so that a person is not as vulnerable to caloric loading in the evening. Stress-reduction programs, including psychological therapy, can be helpful.

Key Concepts: *Night-eating syndrome, though uncommon, affects up to a quarter of obese people. People with NES interrupt normal sleep to eat and often feel stressed, anxious, and depressed. They typically have hormonal imbalances. Psychotherapy and stress reduction therapy can be helpful.*

Males: An Overlooked Population

As many as a million boys and men in the United States struggle with eating disorders.[39] Yet males with eating disorders have been "ignored, neglected or dismissed because of statistical infrequency of the disease, combined with the pervasive myth that eating disorders are a female disease," according to Arnold E. Andersen, former director of the Eating and Weight Disorders Clinic at Johns Hopkins University and scientific editor of the book *Males with Eating Disorders.*[40]

Women who develop eating disorders may feel fat, but they typically are near average weight. In contrast, most men who develop these diseases are overweight. Many were seriously teased about their weight as children. Whereas women are concerned primarily with weight, men are concerned with shape and muscle definition. Indeed, men often develop disordered eating habits while trying to improve their athletic performance. Finally, more men than women diet to prevent medical consequences associated with being overweight.

Why do fewer males than females develop full-blown eating disorders? Anderson contends that there is a "dose-response" relationship between the amount of sociocultural pressure to be thin and the probability of developing an eating disorder. Consider that articles and advertisements that promote dieting usually are targeted at young women rather than young men. When men are exposed to activities that require leanness, such as wrestling, swimming, running, and horse racing, they exhibit a substantial increase in anorexic behavior. It seems clear that cultural conditioning, not sex, contributes to the incidence of eating disorders.[41]

Furthermore, the degree of thinness held up as desirable for women is 15 percent below a healthy body weight, whereas the degree of thinness held up as desirable for men is well within the healthy limits of normal weight. Thus, women are more likely than men to alter their eating habits to achieve the desired appearance.

An Unrecognized Disorder

Like women, most men develop eating disorders during adolescence. But males can develop eating disorders during preadolescence and young adulthood as well. The diagnostic criteria for anorexia and bulimia in men and women are similar. But doctors are so conditioned to viewing eating disorders as a female phenomenon that they often miss eating disorders in males. Likewise, the patient, his family, and friends may not recognize disordered eating patterns. (See **Table SED.7**.) Because our culture accepts overeating among men more readily than in females, binge eating in particular may go unrecognized in men. In addition, anorexia may elude diagnosis in men more often than in women because malnourished men don't experience definitive symptoms, such as a woman's loss of menstrual periods, that can alert professionals and others to the problem. Men also tend to view an eating disorder as a "woman's disease," so they often are hesitant to seek medical attention.[42]

Quick Bites

When Men Starve

During World War II, researchers at the University of Minnesota conducted a starvation study on 36 male volunteers, all conscientious objectors. Their typical food intake was cut in half and they lost about 25 percent of their body weight. Researchers noted significant psychological changes as well. The subjects began obsessing about food, collecting recipes and cookbooks, and hoarding food-related objects. They became apathetic, chronically exhausted, and lost all interest in sex. Most were afraid to leave the experimental conditions for fear of losing control in the outside world.

Table SED.7 Signs of an Undisclosed Eating Disorder

People with eating disorders usually exhibit several of the following signs.

Physical

- Arrested growth
- Marked change or frequent fluctuations in weight
- Inability to gain weight
- Fatigue
- Constipation or diarrhea
- Susceptibility to fractures
- Delayed menarche
- Calcium or phosphorus imbalances, abnormal blood pH, or high serum amylase levels

Behavioral

- Change in eating habits
- Difficulty in social settings
- Reluctance to be weighed
- Depression
- Social withdrawal
- Repeated absence from school or work
- Deceptive or secretive behavior
- Stealing (e.g., to obtain food)
- Substance abuse
- Excessive exercise

Source: Becker AE, Grinspoon SK, Klibanski A, Herzog DB. Eating disorders. *N Engl J Med.* 1999;340(14):1092–1098. Copyright © 1999. Massachusetts Medical Society. All rights reserved. Reprinted with permission.

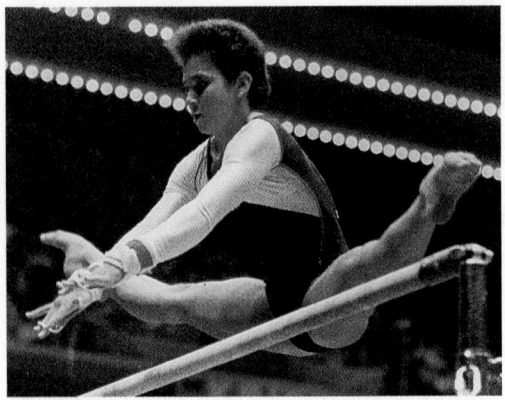

Christy Henrich, a top Olympic gymnast, weighed less than 60 pounds when she died in 1994 at age 22 of multiple organ failure, a complication resulting from anorexia and bulimia.

anorexia athletica Eating disorder associated with competitive participation in athletic activity.

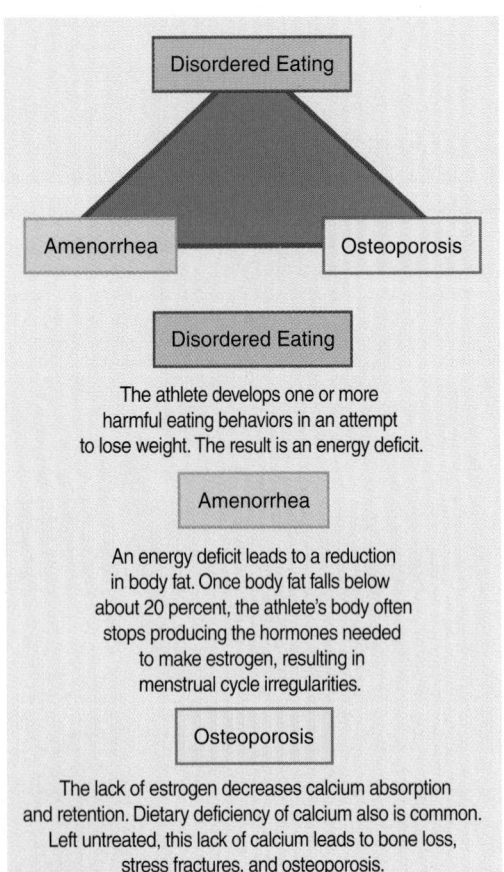

Figure SED.13 **Female athlete triad.** Disordered eating that results in excessive weight loss can lead to amenorrhea, which in turn leads to osteoporosis.

Key Concepts: Men also suffer from eating disorders, although at rates much lower than those of women. Like women, men typically develop eating disorders during adolescence and young adulthood but are more often overweight and striving for a particular body shape and muscularity. Although the diagnostic criteria are the same, with the exception of amenorrhea, eating disorders in men are often undiagnosed due to societal conditioning that views eating disorders as "female" diseases.

Anorexia Athletica

Participation in competitive athletics seems to be a common link in the development of eating disorders among males and females, regardless of their social or ethnic backgrounds. Sports-related eating disorders are known as **anorexia athletica**.[43] Although studies have not found higher rates of disordered eating in athletes as compared with nonathletes, those athletes who compete in lean sports are at higher risk.[44] Lean sports—those that emphasize leanness or body image—include distance running and swimming, gymnastics, dance, and diving. Athletes who have anorexia athletica seek to attain an unrealistic body size that they consider desirable for purposes of competition. In many cases, athletes with mild eating disorders are able to disguise their disease as attention to fitness. People who seem to be addicted to their exercise routine are at greater risk of developing eating disorders.[45]

Coaches and trainers play a significant role in the development of eating disorders among athletes.[46] The attitude that leanness equals performance, exemplified by sayings such as "get down to your fighting weight," still prevails.

The Female Athlete Triad

Female athletes who fall prey to the "thin-at-any-cost" philosophy are at risk of developing a condition known as the female athlete triad. (See **Figure SED.13.**) This syndrome is characterized by disordered eating, amenorrhea (absence of menstruation), and abnormally low bone density.[47] This triad occurs especially in young women involved in sports that involve appearance (e.g., gymnastics) and endurance (e.g., long-distance running). Once body fat falls below 20 percent, women's estrogen can drop significantly. As a result, women's bodies enter a menopause-like state years ahead of time. Their periods become irregular or cease altogether. Bone loss accelerates, just as it would after natural menopause. Many female athletes who suffer from this triad have the bone density of women in their fifties and sixties. Weakened bones are more likely to fracture during exercise or daily activities. Stress fractures can be a red flag for female athlete triad. Because much of this bone loss is irreversible, women who suffer from the female athlete triad are at increased risk of developing osteoporosis.[48]

To help combat this alarming trend, the American College of Sports Medicine and the National Collegiate Athletic Association (NCAA) have established an eating disorders awareness campaign aimed at coaches and trainers. The NCAA also has a three-part video series, *Nutrition and Eating Disorders*, to acquaint coaches and trainers with the causes and effects of eating disorders as well as the steps to take when they suspect an athlete has an eating disorder.

Key Concepts: Athletics can be a gateway to eating disorders. Female athletes who develop restrictive eating habits are at risk for developing a more severe syndrome known as the female athlete triad. Disordered eating, amenorrhea, and abnor-

mally low bone density characterize this syndrome. If not corrected, the female athlete triad can hinder athletic performance and set the stage for lifelong health problems.

Vegetarianism and Eating Disorders

Some researchers have found a strong correlation between vegetarianism and eating disorders in teenagers. A study conducted in Minnesota schools found that 81 percent of students who classified themselves as vegetarians were female. Compared with nonvegetarian peers, these self-described vegetarians were twice as likely to participate in frequent diets, four times as likely to report intentional vomiting, and eight times as likely to report laxative use.[49] Some people with eating disorders try to disguise a change in eating habits by adopting a strict vegetarian diet.[50]

Smoking and Eating Disorders

British medical researcher Arthur Crisp described a new variation on eating disorders in 1998. His previous studies showed that smoking was more common among teens with eating disorders than in the general teenage population. His later research indicates that despite ample knowledge of the health risks of smoking, girls of average or slightly above average weight are taking up smoking in record numbers to curb their appetites. Though not frankly anorexic or bulimic, many young subjects report that they periodically combine smoking with self-induced vomiting to enhance weight-control efforts.[51] This combined behavior is of particular interest and concern to researchers.

Baryophobia

Baryophobia, a disorder characterized by fear of fat, was virtually unheard of until the late 1970s, when pediatricians began reporting a surprising number of young patients from affluent backgrounds whose growth appeared to be stunted because of poor nutrition. In some instances, the stunting occurs when a child secretly starts to diet in order to fit in better with his or her trimmer classmates. More often, however, the child's parents are at the root of the problem. Many well-intentioned parents underfeed their children in an attempt to "protect" them from inheriting their family's tendency toward obesity, heart disease, or diabetes. But the low-fat, high-carbohydrate diet beneficial to many adults may supply too few calories to meet the energy demands of active, growing children. In such instances, the entire family needs nutritional counseling to help them understand what constitutes a healthful diet and realistic body weight for a growing child.[52]

baryophobia [barry-oh-FO-bee-ah] An uncommon eating disorder that stunts growth in children and young adults as a result of underfeeding.

Infantile Anorexia

Unwitting parents can even create disordered eating in infants, perhaps setting the stage for eating disorders later in life.[53] Childhood nutrition specialist Ellyn Satter has analyzed videotapes of infant feedings. Satter examined whether parents responded to—or ignored—their babies' nonverbal eating readiness cues. She concluded that many parents fail to recognize their babies' body language: They feed their babies too rapidly or too slowly, they offer foods the baby doesn't care for, or they persist in trying to feed a clearly full baby who is turning away from food. These well-meaning parents may inadvertently teach their babies to ignore hunger and satiety (fullness) cues and, instead, to eat in response to outside influences.[54]

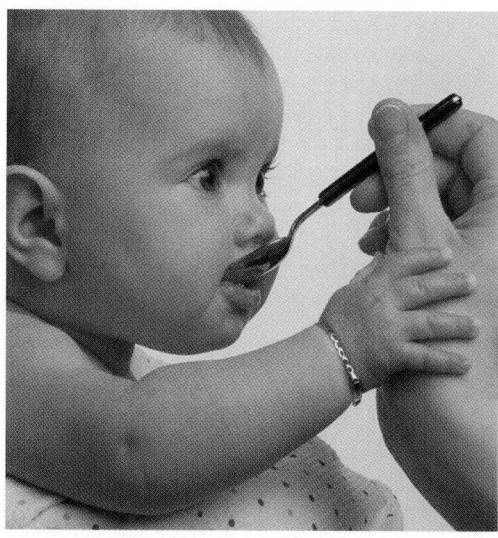

infantile anorexia Severe feeding difficulties that begin with the introduction of solid foods to infants. Symptoms include persistent food refusal for more than one month, malnutrition, parental concern about the child's poor food intake, and significant caregiver–infant conflict during feeding.

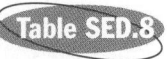 **Table SED.8** **Preventing Eating Disorders**

To join the effort to prevent eating disorders, follow these tips:

- Celebrate the diversity of human body shapes and sizes.

- Present accurate information about nutrition, weight management, and health.

- Discourage restrictive eating practices, including skipping meals.

- Encourage people to eat in response to hunger, not emotions.

- Reinforce messages about good eating and activity patterns at school and at home.

- Carefully phrase comments about a person's weight, body, or fitness level.

- Teach children and young people how to constructively express negative emotions.

- Encourage parents, teachers, coaches, and other professionals who work with children to do likewise.

- Encourage people of all ages to focus on personal qualities rather than physical appearance, of themselves and others.

- Find and promote images of fit people of all sizes and shapes.

Reports of a new disorder called **infantile anorexia** lend support to Satter's observations.[55] A team of child psychiatrists at the Children's National Medical Center in Washington, DC, described this disorder, in which severe feeding difficulties begin as an infant is introduced to solid foods.[56] Symptoms include persistent food refusal for more than a month, malnutrition, parental concern about the child's poor food intake, and significant caregiver-infant conflict during feeding. The disorder typically starts or worsens during the transition from nursing to spoon-feeding and self-feeding, between ages 6 months and 3 years.

Babies with infantile anorexia should not be confused with picky eaters. Picky eaters may initially refuse all foods but allow themselves to be coaxed into eating. Picky eaters have strong food likes and dislikes but are not malnourished. And the relationship between the picky eaters and their parents or caregivers lacks the element of frustration and conflict seen in infantile anorexia.

Infantile anorexia has many serious consequences. Malnutrition can impair the developing brain and adds special stress to the parent-infant relationship. Furthermore, early conflict around meals may herald a life-long unhealthy relationship with food.

Key Concepts: *Researchers are continuously recognizing associations between eating disorders and behaviors such as vegetarianism and smoking. Even babies and young children may suffer from disordered eating patterns.*

Combating Eating Disorders

Eating disorders are extremely difficult to treat, although advances in neurochemistry and scientific understanding of the mind-body connection may provide new avenues of treatment. Most experts agree that emphasis should be placed on preventing eating disorders.

The NIH believes that health care professionals should lead the eating disorder prevention effort by learning to promote self-esteem in their patients and teaching patients that people can be healthy at every size. Ideally, this approach would have a ripple effect: Patients would transmit these beliefs to others. A variety of public information campaigns aimed at parents and people who work with children and adolescents have evolved over the past decade to help promote eating disorder awareness. One of the most prominent examples is the Body Size Acceptance campaign coordinated through the University of California, Berkeley, under the direction of Joanne Ikeda. (See **Table SED.8.**)

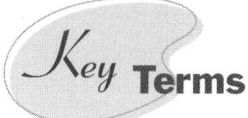

LEARNING *Portfolio*

Key Terms

Study Points

➤ An eating disorder is a complex emotional illness, the primary symptom of which is significantly altered eating habits. Eating disorders occur in biologically susceptible people exposed to particular types of environmental stimuli.

➤ Although eating disorders existed even in ancient times, they have become alarmingly common in industrialized countries.

➤ Eating disorders involve highly restrictive eating patterns (seen in anorexia nervosa), a combination of compulsive overeating and purging (seen in bulimia nervosa), or unrestricted binge eating.

➤ Eating disorders are common in people who participate in body-conscious activities such as dance, wrestling, gymnastics, and bodybuilding.

➤ From 1 to 5 percent of people with eating disorders are male.

➤ Anorexia nervosa is an obsession for thinness manifested in self-imposed starvation.

➤ The typical person with anorexia nervosa is a young Caucasian woman from an upper-class, achievement-oriented family.

➤ Victims of anorexia nervosa have a body weight at least 15 percent below normal, a distorted body image, and physical and psychological symptoms related to starvation.

➤ The body weight of people with bulimia nervosa is close to or even slightly above that considered healthy for their height.

➤ Key symptoms of bulimia nervosa are binge-eating episodes occurring at least twice a week for three months, followed by severe dieting, purging, or a combination of dieting and purging.

➤ Binge-eating disorder is the most common eating disorder.

➤ Like those with bulimia, people with binge-eating disorder consume more food than is typically eaten in a given period of time.

➤ People with body dysmorphic disorder (BDD) are preoccupied with an imagined or slight defect in appearance.

➤ In night-eating syndrome, the food intake rhythm may be out of sync with a person's normal sleep rhythm by as much as four to five hours.

➤ Many competitive athletes, both male and female, have disordered eating behaviors.

➤ Disordered eating, amenorrhea, and abnormally low bone density characterize the female athlete triad.

➤ The best treatment for eating disorders is prevention. Once an eating disorder has become entrenched, intensive and prolonged treatment is typically required. Many people require lifelong support to maintain healthful eating and lifestyle habits.

Study Questions

1. **What three factors play a role in most, if not all, eating disorders?**

2. **What are the warning signs of anorexia nervosa?**

3. **What is the usual treatment for people with anorexia nervosa, and what do most experts say about their potential for recovery?**

4. **What is the typical profile of a person with bulimia nervosa?**

5. **Describe an eating binge and all the behaviors that constitute purging.**

6. **List some common traits of people with binge-eating disorder.**

7. **What are the three components of the female athlete triad?**

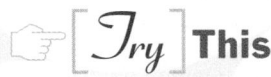 **This**

Is There Any Help Out There?

How much help is available in your community for people with eating disorders? Scan the telephone directory (Yellow Pages) for eating disorder clinics, programs, and centers. Call them to inquire about their services. Do they have a psychologist, medical doctor, dietitian, nurse, and/or social worker on staff? Is it an inpatient or outpatient program? What is their philosophy of therapy? What is their success rate? What are their payment plans?

What About Bobbie?

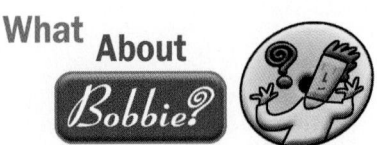

Bobbie's friend Janet has been struggling with anorexia nervosa for some time. Bobbie recently expressed concern again and asked Janet about her eating habits. Janet told Bobbie she eats the following foods in a typical day:

"Breakfast"
1 head of iceberg lettuce, with salt and pepper but no dressing
(If she wakes up really hungry, she'll have another with vinegar on it.)

"Snack"
6 to 8 white mushrooms

"Lunch"
3 or 4 dill pickles

"Dinner"
1 12-ounce can artichoke hearts (rinsed)

Fluids include mineral water, diet cola, and/or caffeinated tea.

Let's compare this intake with Bobbie's (see Chapter 1 to review Bobbie's one-day diet). First, Janet's daily intake is just under 300 kilocalories compared with Bobbie's 2,440. Not only is Janet at risk due to her lack of calories, but her intake of protein is approximately 0 grams. Her body has already used any glycogen it had as reserve fuel. In addition, at 5 feet 3 inches and 98 pounds, she has very little reserve fat tissue for future energy needs. Without intake of dietary protein, her organ and muscle tissues have become prime targets for degradation. Even though Janet takes a multivitamin and a mineral supplement, if she doesn't seek help soon, she may suffer the typical symptoms and effects of starvation and malnutrition.

References

1 American Dietetic Association. Position of the American Dietetic Association: nutrition intervention in the treatment of anorexia nervosa, bulimia nervosa, and eating disorders not otherwise specified (EDNOS). *J Am Diet Assoc.* 2003; 103(6):748–765.

2 American Dietetic Association. *Manual of Clinical Dietetics.* 6th ed. Chicago: American Dietetic Association, 2000.

3 Crowther JH, Sanftner J, Bonifazi DZ, Sheperd KL. The role of daily hassles in binge eating. *Int J Eat Disord.* 2001; 29:449–454.

4 Johnson JG, Cohen P, Kasen S, Brook JS. Eating disorders during adolescence and the risk for physical and mental disorders during early adulthood. *Arch Gen Psych.* 2002;59:545–552.

5 Pearce JM. Richard Morton: origins of anorexia nervosa. *Eur Neurol.* 2004;52:191–192.

6 Ibid.

7 Suraf M. Holy anorexia and anorexia nervosa: society and the concept of disease. *Pharo.* 1998;61(4):2–4.

8 Reid TR. The world according to Rome. *National Geographic.* 1997;8:54–83.

9 U.S. Department of Health and Human Services. *Eating Disorders.* http://www.4woman.gov/owh/pub/factsheets /eatingdisorders.pdf. Accessed 11/12/06.

10 Neumark-Sztainer D, Story M, Hannan PJ, Perry CL, Irving LM. Weight-related concerns and behaviors among overweight and nonoverweight adolescents: implications for preventing weight-related disorders. *Arch Pediatr Adolesc Med.* 2002; 156:171–178.

11 Eisenberg ME, Neumark-Sztainer D, Story M. Associations of weight-based teasing and emotional well-being among adolescents. *Arch Pediatr Adolesc Med.* 2003;157:733–738.

12 Gleaves DH. Scope and significance of posttraumatic symptomatology among women hospitalized for an eating disorder. *Int J Eat Disord.* 1998;2:147–156.

13 Kaye WH, Frank GK, Bailer UF, Henry SE. Neurobiology of anorexia nervosa: clinical implications of alterations in the function of serotonin and other neuronal systems. *Int J Eat Disord.* 2005;37:S15–S19.

14 Mayer LE, Walsh BT. The use of selective serotonin reuptake inhibitors in eating disorders. *J Clin Psychiatry.* 1998;59(suppl 15):28–34.

15 Kaye W, Gendall K, Strober M. Serotonin neuronal function and selective serotonin reuptake inhibitor treatment in anorexia and bulimia nervosa. *Biol Psychiatry.* 1998;44:825–838.

16 Lilenfeld LR, Kaye WH, Greeno CG, et al. A controlled family study of anorexia nervosa and bulimia nervosa: psychiatric disorders in first-degree relatives and effects of proband comorbidity. *Arch Gen Psychiatry.* 1998;55:603–610.

17 Aragona M, Vella G. Psychopathological considerations on the relationship between bulimia and obsessive-compulsive disorder. *Psychopathology.* 1998;31:197–205.

18 Shirasaka T, Takasaki M, Kannan H. Cardiovascular effects of leptin and orexins. *Am J Physiol Regul Integr Comp Physiol.* 2003;284(3):R639–R651.

19 Sakurai T, Amemiya A, Ishii M, et al. Orexins and orexin receptors: a family of hypothalamic neuropeptides and G protein-coupled receptors that regulate feeding behavior. *Cell.* 1998; 92:573–585.

20 American Medical Association. JAMA patient page: anorexia nervosa. *JAMA.* 2006;295(22):2684.

21 American Psychiatric Association. *Diagnostic and Statistical Manual of Mental Disorders.* 4th ed. Text revision. Washington, DC: American Psychiatric Association, 2000.

22 Bulik CM, Reba L, Siega-Riz AM. Anorexia nervosa: definition, epidemiology, and cycle of risk. *Int J Eat Disord.* 2005; 37:S2–S9.

23 Sim LA, Sadowski CM, Whiteside SP, Wells LA. Family-based therapy for adolescents with anorexia nervosa. *Mayo Clin Proc.* 2004;79:1305–1308.

24 Keel PK, Dorer DJ, Eddy KT, et al. Predictors of mortality in eating disorders. *Arch Gen Psych.* 2003;60:179–183.

25 Ibid.

26 Neumark-Sztainer D, Story M, Hannan PJ, et al. Op. cit.

27 Keel PK, Dorer DJ, Eddy KT, et al. Op. cit.

28 American Dietetic Association. 2003. Op. cit.

29 National Institutes of Health. National Center for Health Statistics. www.nih.gov. Accessed 7/31/06.

30 American Psychiatric Association. Op. cit.

31 Brownell K, Fairburn M. *Eating Disorders and Obesity: A Comprehensive Handbook.* 2nd ed. New York: Guilford Press, 2002.

32 Keel PK, Dorer DJ, Eddy KT, et al. Op. cit.

33 Krahn DD, Kurth CL, Gomberg E, Drewnowski A. Pathological dieting and alcohol use in college women—a continuum of behaviors. *Eat Behav.* 2005;6(1):43–52.

34 Keel PK, Dorer DJ, Eddy KT, et al. Op. cit.

35 French SA, Leffert N, Story M, et al. Adolescent binge/purge and weight loss behaviors: associations with developmental assets. *J Adolesc Health.* 2001;28:211–221.

36 American Psychiatric Association. Op. cit.

37 Ibid.

38 Veale D. Body dysmorphic disorder. *Postgrad Med J.* 2004; 80:67–71.

39 Andersen AE, Cohn L, Holbrook T. *Making Weight: Men's Conflicts with Food, Weight, Shape, and Appearance.* Carlsbad, CA: Gurze Books, 2000.

40 Andersen AE. *Males with Eating Disorders.* New York: Brunner Mazel, 1990.

41 Strober M, Freeman R, Lampert C, et al. Males with anorexia nervosa: a controlled study of eating disorders in first-degree relatives. *Int J Eat Disord.* 2001;29:263–269.

42 Andersen AE, Cohn L, Holbrook T. Op. cit.

43 Sudi K, Öttl K, Payerl D, et al. Anorexia athletica. *Nutrition.* 2004;20:657–661.

44 Reinking MF, Alexander LE. Prevalence of disordered-eating behaviors in undergraduate females collegiate athletes and nonathletes. *J Athl Train.* 2005;40:47–51.

45 Benyo R. *The Exercise Fix.* Berkeley, CA: Leisure Press, 1991.

46 American Academy of Pediatrics Committee on Sports Medicine and Fitness. Promotion of healthy weight-control practices in young athletes [published errata in *Pediatrics* 2006;117(4):1467]. *Pediatrics* 2005;116(6):1557–1564.

47 Otis CI, Drinkwater B, Johnson M, et al. American College of Sports Medicine position stand. The female athlete triad. *Med Sci Sports Exerc.* 1997;29:i–ix.

48 Ruud JS, Woolsy MN, Dorfman L. Eating disorders in athletes. In: Rosenbloom CA, ed. *Sports Nutrition,* 3rd ed. Chicago: American Dietetic Association, 2000.

49 Perry CL, McGuire MT, Neumark-Sztainer D, Story M. Characteristics of vegetarian adolescents in a multiethnic urban population. *J Adolesc Health.* 2001;29(6):406–416.

50 Klopp SA, Heiss CJ, Smith HS. Self-reported vegetarianism may be a marker for college women at risk for disordered eating. *J Am Diet Assoc.* 2003;103:745–747.

51 Crisp AH, Halek C, Sedgewick P, et al. Smoking and pursuit of thinness in schoolgirls in London and Ottawa. *Postgrad Med J.* 1998;74:473–479.

52 Ganley T, Sherman C. Exercise and children's health. *Physician Sportsmed.* 2000;28(2):85–93.

53 Ibid.

54 Satter E. *Child of Mine.* Denver, CO: Bull Publishing, 2000.

55 Satter E. The feeding relationship: implications for dietitians. Paper presented at: annual meeting of the American Dietetic Association; October 1992; Washington, DC.

56 Chatoor I. Feeding disorders in infants and toddlers: diagnosis and treatment. *Child Adolesc Psychiatr Clin North Am.* 2002; 11:163–183.

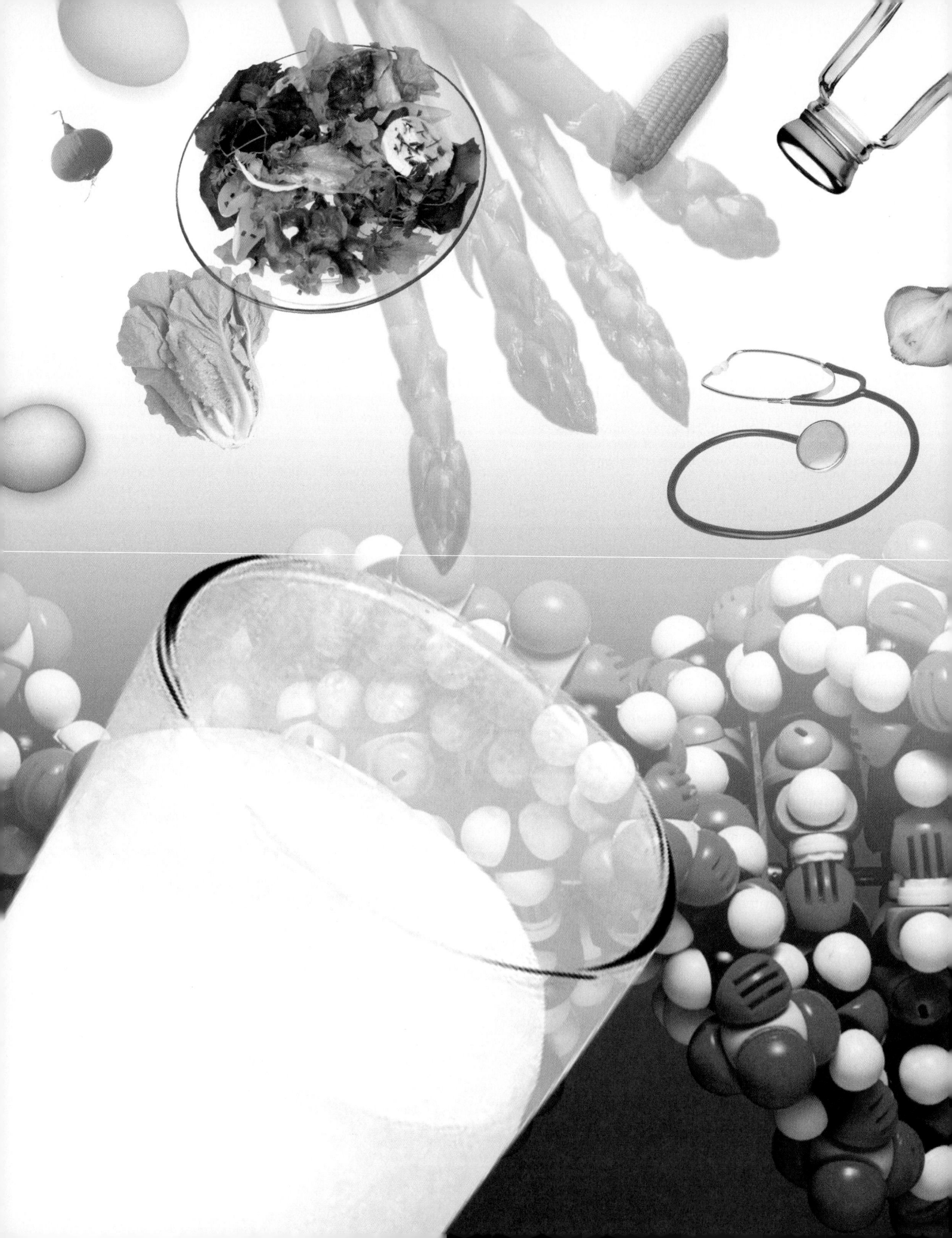

Chapter 14

Diet and Health

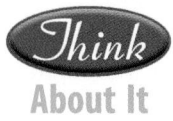

Think **About It**

1 Is there a history of heart disease in your family?

2 Do you know your blood pressure?

3 How often do you salt your food before tasting it?

4 How often do you worry about your personal risk of cancer?

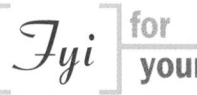

Fyi **for your Information**

This chapter's FYI boxes include practical information on the following topics:

• Overweight and Obesity: Health Consequences

• The Pima Indians

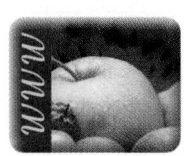

The Web site for this book offers many useful tools and is a great source for additional nutrition information for both students and instructors. Visit the site at **nutrition.jbpub.com** for information on fat-soluble vitamins. You'll find exercises that explore the following topics:

• Heart Attack: Warning Signs and Lifesaving Actions

• Understanding Cancer

• Educating People with Diabetes

What About 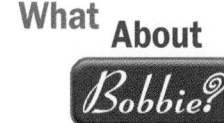 *Bobbie?*

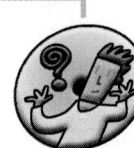

Track the choices Bobbie is making with Nutritionist Pro or EatRight Analysis software.

*W*hat caused Joel Smith to have a heart attack at age 48? Not his age. Few men suffer heart attacks before age 50. What about his cholesterol? Possibly. Joel inherited the tendency to have high levels of both LDL cholesterol and homocysteine. Could his diet have been a contributing factor? Over his lifetime, Joe has enjoyed plenty of hearty meals with lots of meat, gravy, pie, and ice cream. He never developed the habit of eating many fruits or vegetables.

Joel was an athlete in high school, wasn't he? Just prior to his heart attack, Joel was playing a spirited game of basketball with his kids. Yet despite his enjoyment of sports, he limited his physical activity to an occasional weekend basketball game. Some time before his heart attack, Joel developed a respiratory infection from bacteria called *Chlamydia pneumoniae* (thought by some experts to be a cause of arterial damage and atherosclerosis).

All of these factors, including the unaccustomed vigorous activity, contributed to Joel's heart attack. It is difficult to separate out the relative importance of each factor, but taken collectively they culminated in a potentially fatal event. With some changes in his lifestyle, Joel might have avoided his heart attack. Eating more fruits and vegetables and limiting intake of fat would have helped, as would shooting hoops on a more regular basis or taking a brisk, 60-minute walk each day. You cannot change the inherited tendency to develop a disease, but you almost always can reduce your risk by modifying your lifestyle.

Nutrition and Chronic Disease

What does it mean to be healthy? The World Health Organization (WHO) defines health as "a state of complete physical, mental, and social well-being and not merely the absence of disease or infirmity."[1] Although most of us focus on the last part of that definition, "the absence of disease or infirmity," the first part is equally important. As you have learned, nutrition is an important part of physical, mental, and social well-being. It also is important for preventing disease.

Disease can be defined as "an impairment of the normal state of a living animal or one of its parts" and can arise from environmental factors or specific infectious agents (e.g., bacteria or viruses).[2] Diseases may be acute (short-lived illnesses that arise and resolve quickly) or they may be chronic (diseases with a slow onset and long duration). Although nutrition can affect the susceptibility to acute diseases, and certainly contaminated food is a source of acute disease, our food choices are more likely to affect our risk for developing chronic diseases such as heart disease or cancer. In its report *Diet, Nutrition and the Prevention of Chronic Diseases*, the WHO states that "the diets people eat, in all their cultural variety, define to a large extent people's health, growth, and development."[3] Other lifestyle factors, such as smoking and exercise, as well as genetic factors, may also determine who gets sick and who remains healthy.

Healthy People 2010

In 2000, the U.S. Department of Health and Human Services published *Healthy People 2010*, a comprehensive set of disease prevention and health promotion objectives for the nation.[4] The Healthy People 2010 initiative includes two overarching goals: (1) increase the quality and years of healthy life and (2) eliminate health disparities. These two goals are supported by specific objectives in 28 focus areas (see **Figure 14.1**). "Nutrition and Overweight" is one of the focus areas; its objectives include increasing intake of fruits, vegetables, and whole grains while decreasing intake of fat, saturated fat, and sodium. These ideas probably sound familiar; they are the same concepts found in the *Dietary Guidelines for Americans*.

Obesity and Chronic Disease

Once considered merely an aesthetic issue, obesity is now widely recognized as a major public health problem. It is a risk factor for the major chronic diseases of public health significance in the United States and Canada: coronary heart disease, cancer, diabetes, hypertension, and metabolic syndrome. Good health habits and proper weight management are

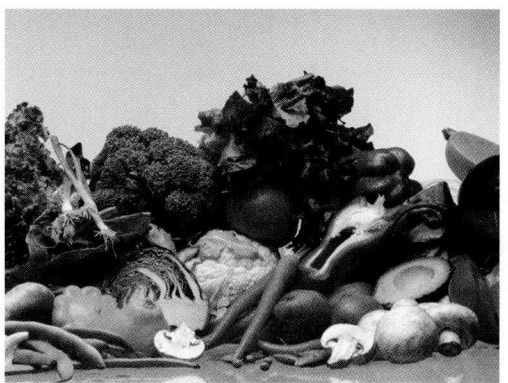

American Dietetic Association

The Role of Dietetics Professionals in Health Promotion and Disease Prevention

It is the position of the American Dietetic Association that primary prevention is the most effective, affordable course of action for preventing and reducing risk for chronic disease. Registered dietitians and dietetic technicians, registered, are leaders in delivering preventive services in both clinical and community settings, including advocating for funding and inclusion of these services in programs and policy initiatives at local, state, and federal levels. In addition, registered dietitians are leaders in facilitating and participating in research in chronic disease prevention and health promotion.

J Am Diet Assoc. 2006;106:1875–1884.
Reprinted with permission.

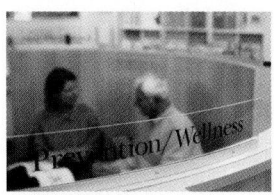

- Access to Quality Health Services
- Arthritis, Osteoporosis, and Chronic Back Conditions
- Cancer
- Chronic Kidney Disease
- Disability and Secondary Conditions
- Educational and Community-Based Programs
- Environmental Health
- Family Planning
- Food Safety
- Health Communication
- Heart Disease and Stroke
- HIV
- Immunization and Infectious Diseases
- Injury and Violence Prevention
- Maternal, Infant, and Child Health
- Medical Product Safety
- Mental Health and Mental Disorders

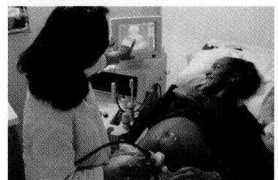
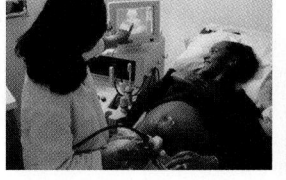
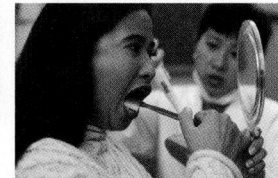

- Nutrition and Overweight
- Occupational Health and Safety
- Oral Health
- Physical Activity and Fitness
- Public Health Infrastructure
- Respiratory Diseases
- Sexually Transmitted Diseases
- Substance Abuse
- Tobacco Use
- Vision and Hearing

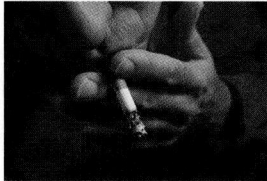
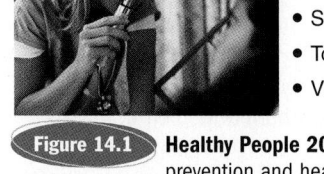

Figure 14.1 **Healthy People 2010.** Healthy People 2010 is a comprehensive set of disease prevention and health promotion objectives for the United States to achieve over the first decade of the new century. Specific objectives in each of these 28 focus areas support the overarching objectives of increasing quality and years of healthy life, and eliminating health disparities. For more on Healthy People 2010, visit http://www.healthypeople.gov.

key components of a healthy lifestyle that avoids or at least delays the onset of these diseases. Often, weight loss or, at a minimum, no further weight gain can improve health outcomes dramatically.

As you learned in Chapter 8, "Energy Balance, Body Composition, and Weight Management," overweight and obesity are defined in terms of body mass index (BMI) values. Ideally, measuring body fatness would be a better indicator of chronic disease risk, because it is excess body fatness rather than excess body weight that is linked to increased risks. Waist circumference, for example, can be a valuable screening tool for identifying excess abdominal fatness. Public health objectives, such as those in Healthy People 2010, emphasize the need for healthful eating behaviors, beginning in childhood, that allow for the achievement and maintenance of a healthy weight.

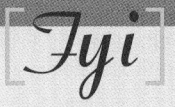

Overweight and Obesity: Health Consequences

FOR YOUR INFORMATION

Health problems resulting from overweight and obesity could reverse many of the health gains achieved in the United States in recent decades. Overweight and obesity may soon cause as much preventable disease and death as cigarette smoking. The primary concern of overweight and obesity is one of health, not appearance.

Potential consequences of overweight and obesity are summarized here. In many cases, a small amount of weight loss can reverse chronic disease risks. (See Chapter 8, "Energy Balance, Body Composition, and Weight Management.")

Premature Death
- An estimated 300,000 deaths per year may be attributable to obesity.
- The risk of death rises with increasing weight.
- Even moderate weight excess (10 to 20 pounds for a person of average height) increases the risk of death, particularly among adults aged 30 to 64 years.
- Individuals who are obese (BMI > 30 kg/m²) have a 50 to 100 percent increased risk of premature death from all causes, compared with individuals with a healthy weight.

Heart Disease
- The incidence of heart disease (heart attack, congestive heart failure, sudden

cardiac death, angina or chest pain, and abnormal heart rhythm) is increased in persons who are overweight or obese (BMI > 25 kg/m²).
- High blood pressure is twice as common in adults who are obese than in those who are at a healthy weight.
- Obesity is associated with elevated triglycerides (blood fat) and decreased HDL cholesterol ("good cholesterol").

Diabetes
- A weight gain of 11 to 18 pounds increases a person's risk of developing type 2 diabetes to twice that of individuals who have not gained weight.
- Over 80 percent of people with diabetes are overweight or obese.

Cancer
- Overweight and obesity are associated with an increased risk for some types of cancer, including endometrial (cancer of the lining of the uterus), colon, gall bladder, prostate, kidney, and post-menopausal breast cancer.
- Women who gain more than 20 pounds from age 18 to midlife double their risk of postmenopausal breast cancer compared with women whose weight remains stable.

Breathing Problems
- Sleep apnea (interrupted breathing while sleeping) is more common in obese persons.
- Obesity is associated with a higher prevalence of asthma.

Arthritis
- For every 2-pound increase in weight, the risk of developing arthritis is increased by 9 to 13 percent.
- Symptoms of arthritis can improve with weight loss.

Reproductive Complications
- Obesity in premenopausal women is associated with irregular menstrual cycles and infertility.
- Complications of pregnancy
  - Obesity during pregnancy is associated with increased risk of death in both the baby and the mother and increases the risk of maternal high blood pressure by 10 times.
  - In addition to many other complications, women who are obese during pregnancy are more likely to have gestational diabetes and problems with labor and delivery.
  - Infants born to women who are obese during pregnancy are more likely to be high birth weight, and

Physical Inactivity and Chronic Disease

A sedentary lifestyle is also a significant risk factor for chronic disease. Physically active people generally outlive those who are inactive, and inactivity is almost as significant a risk factor for heart disease as high blood pressure, smoking, or high blood cholesterol! Physical activity also plays a significant role in long-term weight management. Including at least 30 minutes per day of moderate physical activity such as brisk walking or cycling will help reduce chronic disease risk; weight-management efforts are enhanced by higher amounts of exercise—at least 60 minutes per day. See Chapter 13, "Sports Nutrition," for more on physical activity recommendations.

therefore the need for cesarean section delivery increases as well as the infant's risk of low blood sugar (which can be associated with brain damage and seizures).

- Obesity during pregnancy is associated with an increased risk of birth defects, particularly neural tube defects such as spina bifida.

Additional Health Consequences

- Overweight and obesity are associated with increased risks of gallbladder disease, incontinence, and depression as well as increased surgical risk.
- Obesity can affect the quality of life through limited mobility and decreased physical endurance as well as through social, academic, and job discrimination.

Children and Adolescents

- Risk factors for heart disease, such as high cholesterol and high blood pressure, occur with increased frequency in overweight children and adolescents compared with those with a healthy weight.
- Type 2 diabetes, previously considered an adult disease, has increased dramatically in children and adolescents. Overweight is closely linked to type 2 diabetes.

- Overweight adolescents have a 70 percent chance of becoming overweight or obese adults. This increases to 80 percent if one or more parent is overweight or obese.
- The most immediate consequence of overweight, as perceived by children themselves, is social discrimination.

Benefits of Weight Loss

- Weight loss as modest as 5 to 15 percent of total body weight in a person who is overweight or obese reduces the risk factors for some diseases, particularly heart disease.
- Weight loss can result in lower blood pressure, lower blood sugar, and improved cholesterol levels.
- A person with a BMI above the healthy weight range may benefit from weight loss, especially if he or she has other health risk factors, such as high blood pressure, high cholesterol, smoking, diabetes, a sedentary lifestyle, and a personal and/or family history of heart disease.

People tend to think of overweight and obesity as strictly a personal matter, but there is much that local communities can and should do to address these problems and improve the health of the population in general.

Actions for Communities

- Ensure daily, quality physical education in all school grades.
- Build physical activity into regular routines and playtime for children and their families.
- Create more opportunities for physical activity at worksites.
- Make community facilities available and accessible for physical activity for all people, including the elderly.
- Promote healthier food choices, including at least five servings of fruits and vegetables each day, and reasonable portion sizes at home, in schools, at worksites, and in communities.
- Ensure that schools provide healthful foods and beverages on school campuses and at school events.

Source: US Department of Health and Human Services. *The Surgeon General's Call to Action to Prevent and Decrease Overweight and Obesity.* 2001. http://www.surgeongeneral.gov/topics/obesity. Accessed 8/7/06.

genes Sections of DNA that contain hereditary information. Most genes contain information for making proteins.

Human Genome Project An effort coordinated by the Department of Energy and the National Institutes of Health to map the genes in human DNA.

nucleotides Subunits of DNA or RNA consisting of a nitrogenous base (adenine, guanine, thymine, or cytosine in DNA; adenine, guanine, uracil, or cytosine in RNA), a phosphate molecule, and a sugar molecule (deoxyribose in DNA and ribose in RNA). Thousands of nucleotides are linked to form a DNA or RNA molecule.

base pair Two nitrogenous bases (adenine and thymine or guanine and cytosine), held together by weak bonds, that form a "rung" of the "DNA ladder." The bonds between base pairs hold the DNA molecule together in the shape of a double helix.

complementary sequence Nucleic acid base sequence that can form a double-stranded structure with another DNA fragment by following base-pairing rules (A pairs with T, and C pairs with G). The complementary sequence to GTAC, for example, is CATG.

genetic code The instructions in a gene that tell the cell how to make a specific protein. A, T, G, and C are the "letters" of the DNA code; they stand for the chemicals adenine, thymine, guanine, and cytosine, respectively, which make up the nucleotide bases of DNA. Each gene's code combines the four chemicals in various ways to spell out three-letter "words" that specify which amino acid is needed at every step in making a protein.

mutation A permanent structural alteration in DNA. In most cases, DNA changes either have no effect or cause harm. Occasionally, a mutation can improve an organism's chance of surviving and passing the beneficial change on to its descendants. Certain mutations may lead to cancer or other diseases.

gene expression The process by which proteins are made from the instructions encoded in DNA.

Quick Bites

Biological Blueprint

Nearly all of the 100 trillion cells in the human body contain a copy of the entire human genome, the complete set of genetic instructions necessary to build a human being.

Genetics and Disease

In the last several years, knowledge regarding the relationship between our genetic makeup and disease has exploded. We now recognize that nearly all diseases have some genetic component. Most human illnesses occur because of the interaction of many genetic, environmental, nutritional, and lifestyle factors. (See **Figure 14.2.**) As the number one killer in the United States and Canada, cardiovascular disease is a good example of how genetic influences affect the development of disease.[5] Family history of heart disease is an important risk factor for developing the disease.

Although a few relatively rare cancers have a primarily genetic basis and affect many members of a given family, most cancers seem to be caused by a variety of factors. A study of nearly 45,000 twins showed that environmental factors contribute more to the development of most common cancers than genetic factors, but genetics still exerts a major effect on whether we get cancer. By comparing cancer rates in identical twins (who share all the same **genes**) with fraternal twins (who, on average, share half their genes), the researchers could estimate the contribution of genetics in developing cancer. Inherited genetic factors contributed between 27 and 42 percent of the causation of colon and rectal cancers, breast cancer, and prostate cancer.[6]

Understanding how our genes influence our risk for disease has been a major goal of the **Human Genome Project**, an international effort spearheaded by the U.S. National Institutes of Health (NIH). The Human Genome Project is providing scientists with clues to the genetic variations that are responsible for common illnesses. Understanding the genetics of diseases will allow researchers to develop more effective medications and may lead to routine gene-based treatments.[7]

The Workings of DNA and Genes

Our genetic instructions are carried by deoxyribonucleic acid (DNA), a molecule that can be visualized as an immensely long, corkscrew-shaped ladder—a double helix. (See **Figure 14.3.**) DNA is made of subunits called **nucleotides**. Each nucleotide contains one sugar molecule (deoxyribose—a five-carbon sugar), one phosphate molecule, and one base. The sugar and phosphate molecules make up the "side rails" of a DNA molecule, and the bases form the "rungs." That is, the base in each nucleotide of one "side rail" joins with a base in a nucleotide on the opposite "side rail." DNA has only four bases—adenine (A), thymine (T), guanine (G), and cytosine (C)—and each base is picky about its partner. To form a **base pair**, A always joins with T, and G always joins with C. Thus, the sequence of bases on one side of the ladder (for example, AGCGT) determines the **complementary sequence** on the other side (TCGCA). Using this "genetic alphabet," an enormous number of messages can be written.

Genes are sequences of DNA that carry the **genetic code** for making proteins. The genetic code combines the four "letters" of the genetic alphabet in various ways to spell out three-letter "words" that specify which amino acid is needed at each step in making a protein. Errors in the code may be harmless, or they may lead to serious disease. For example, people with sickle cell anemia have a mistake (called a **mutation**) in their genetic code for the amino acids making up the protein beta-globin. Beta-globin is part of the oxygen-carrying protein hemoglobin found in red blood cells. This section of sickle cell anemia patients' genetic code contains the sequence GTG (the code for valine) instead of GAG (the code for glutamate), so their cells manufacture beta-globin proteins with the wrong amino acid. Hemoglobin containing this faulty protein cannot carry a full load of oxygen and causes red blood cells to form a sickle shape.

Diet influences **gene expression**—the making of proteins. Components in the diet can enhance or inhibit gene expression, thereby increasing or decreasing protein synthesis. Folate status, for example, influences the genetic instructions for the production of an enzyme called MTHFR (methylenetetrahydrofolate reductase). This enzyme works in folate metabolism to convert homocysteine to methionine. People with a particular DNA mutation have reduced enzyme activity and, as a result, higher homocysteine levels. When their folate status is low, their risk for heart disease is significantly elevated.[8] Scientists are also studying how folate status and this genetic mutation may influence cancer risk.

Nutritional genomics, which focuses on the influences of food components on gene expression, is in its infancy. (See the Chapter 1 FYI feature "Are Nutrigenomics in Your Future?") As we learn more about the genetic causes of disease and the lifestyle factors that influence them, we will be able to better screen individuals for disease susceptibility, and then target appropriate lifestyle interventions to reduce their risk.[9]

Key Concepts: *Diseases can be acute or chronic. Nutrition and other lifestyle factors such as obesity and physical inactivity have a major influence on the risk of developing chronic diseases. Our genetic makeup also influences disease risk. Genes are segments of DNA that contain the code for making proteins. Gene expression can be modified by diet. Understanding how our genes can influence the course of a disease may influence future population screening and produce targeted interventions to reduce disease risk.*

Chronic diseases	Dietary risk factors						Nondietary risk factors					
	High-fat diet	Excessive alcohol intake	Low complex carbohydrate/fiber	Low vitamin and/or mineral intake	High sugar intake	High intake of salty or pickled foods	Genetics	Age	Sedentary lifestyle	Smoking and tobacco use	Stress	Environmental contaminants
Cancers	?*	X	X	X		X	X	X	X	X		X
Hypertension	X	X		X		in salt sensitive people	X	X	X	X	X	
Diabetes (type 2)	X		X				X	X	X			
Osteoporosis		X		X			X	X	X	X		
Atherosclerosis	X		X				X	X	X	X	X	
Obesity	X	X	X		X		X		X			
Stroke	X		X				X	X	X	X	X	
Diverticulosis	X		X	X				X	X			
Dental and oral diseases				X	X		X			X		

* The Nurses' Health Study, a large prospective study, found no evidence linking higher total fat intake with increased risk of breast cancer. These results call into question theories that link dietary fat to other cancers.

Figure 14.2 **Risk factors for chronic diseases.** Diet, lifestyle choices, and genetics interact to shape a person's risk profile.

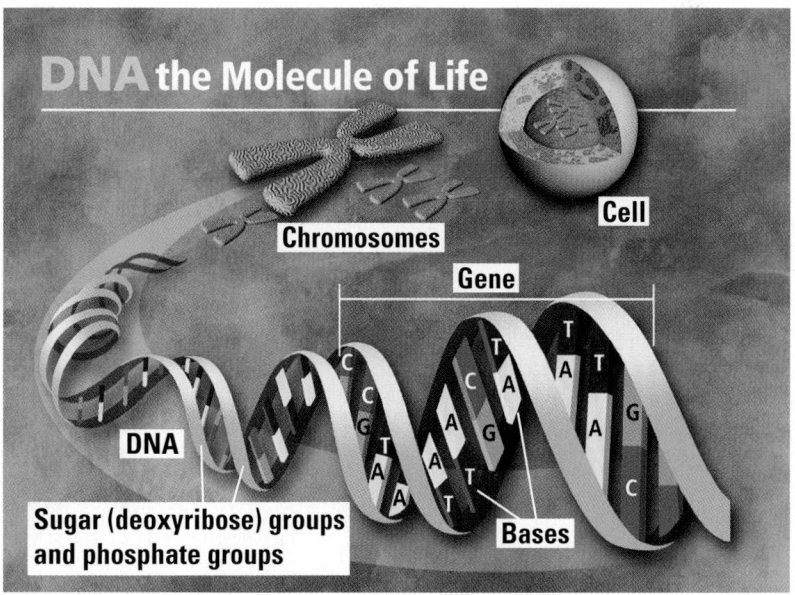

Figure 14.3 **Structure of DNA.** All the instructions needed to direct cellular activities are contained within the chemical DNA (deoxyribonucleic acid). The DNA sequence is the particular side-by-side arrangement of bases along the DNA strand (e.g., ATTCCGGA). This order spells out the exact instructions required to build proteins and create a unique person. **Source:** US Department of Energy Human Genome Program, http://www.ornl.gov/hgmis

cardiovascular disease (CVD) Any abnormal condition characterized by dysfunction of the heart and blood vessels. CVD includes atherosclerosis (especially coronary heart disease, which can lead to heart attacks), cerebrovascular disease (e.g., stroke), and hypertension (high blood pressure).

coronary heart disease (CHD) A type of heart disease caused by narrowing of the coronary arteries that feed the heart, which needs a constant supply of oxygen and nutrients carried by the blood in the coronary arteries. When the coronary arteries become narrowed or clogged by fat and cholesterol deposits and cannot supply enough blood to the heart, CHD results.

Cardiovascular Disease

Cardiovascular disease (CVD) is the leading cause of death in the United States and Canada, claiming one life every 37 seconds. Nearly half of all Americans alive today will die from CVD. Although we typically think of CVD as primarily affecting men and older adults, heart attack is the number one killer of American women, and 45 percent of heart attacks occur in people younger than 65.[10] But not all the news is bad. In the past 50 years, lifestyle changes and medical advances have led to significant progress in the fight against CVD.

Much of the incidence of CVD is attributable to the so-called American way of life. Too many Americans eat a high-fat diet, are overweight and sedentary, smoke cigarettes, manage stress ineffectively, have uncontrolled high blood pressure or high blood cholesterol levels, and do not know the signs of CVD. Of course, not all the risk factors for CVD are controllable—some people have an inherited tendency toward high blood pressure. But many factors can be changed, treated, or modified, so you have the power to significantly reduce your risk.

The Cardiovascular System and Cardiovascular Disease

The cardiovascular system consists of the heart and blood vessels (veins, arteries, and capillaries). (See **Figure 14.4**.) Together, they pump and circulate blood throughout the body. A person weighing 150 pounds has about 5 quarts of blood, which circulates about once every minute.

When we talk about diet and heart disease, we are usually referring to **coronary heart disease (CHD)**. CHD is caused by atherosclerosis and, when serious, may result in angina pectoris (chest pain) or myocardial infarction (heart attack). Atherosclerosis of the cerebral arteries leading to the brain can cause a stroke.

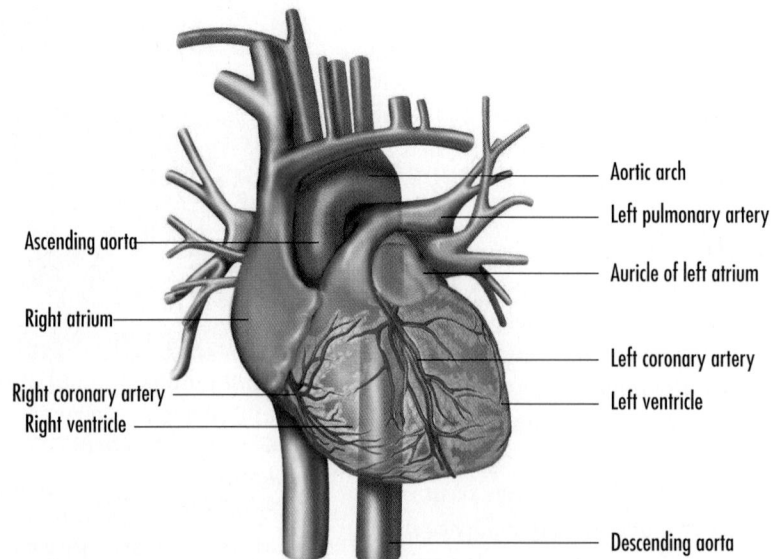

Ascending aorta

Right atrium

Right coronary artery
Right ventricle

Aortic arch
Left pulmonary artery
Auricle of left atrium
Left coronary artery
Left ventricle

Descending aorta

Figure 14.4 **The heart and major arteries.** Oxygenated blood is pumped through the arteries (red) and oxygen-depleted blood is returned to the heart via the veins (blue).

What Is Atherosclerosis?

Atherosclerosis is a slow, progressive hardening and narrowing of the arteries. (See **Figure 14.5.**) It is one type of arteriosclerosis, which literally means "hardening of the arteries." In atherosclerosis, arteries become narrowed by deposits of fat, cholesterol, and other substances. As these deposits, called **plaque**, accumulate along the artery walls, the arteries lose their elasticity and their ability to expand and contract, thereby restricting blood flow. Once narrowed in this way, an artery is vulnerable to plaque rupture and blockage by blood clots.

Plaque buildup begins when excess lipid particles collect beneath the cells that line an artery, called **endothelial cells** or the **endothelium**. High cholesterol, high blood pressure, smoking, and diabetes can all damage the endothelium and initiate atherosclerosis. Certain viral and bacterial infections also may damage blood vessels.[11]

Platelets, components of one of the body's protective mechanisms, collect at the damaged area and form a cap of cells, thereby isolating the plaque within the artery wall. The narrowed artery is vulnerable to blockage by clots that can form if the cap breaks and the fatty core of the plaque combines again with platelets and other clot-producing factors in the blood. If the heart, brain, or other organs are deprived of blood, and the vital oxygen that blood carries, the effects of atherosclerosis can be deadly.

Cholesterol and Atherosclerosis

In the early 1960s researchers identified high blood cholesterol, or **hypercholesterolemia**, along with smoking and high blood pressure, as principal risk factors for coronary heart disease. They understood that a high-fat, high-cholesterol diet tends to raise blood cholesterol, and high blood cholesterol levels promote atherosclerosis. Atherosclerosis leads to artery disease and often causes heart attacks or strokes.

Total cholesterol levels do not tell the entire story. The levels of LDL and HDL cholesterol predict a person's risk for developing atherosclerosis more accurately than the individual's total cholesterol levels. High LDL cholesterol is a greater risk than high total cholesterol, with some kinds of LDL being more dangerous than others. For example, high levels of **lipoprotein a [Lp(a)]**, a low-density lipoprotein, seem especially harmful. High levels

Quick Bites

Who Discovered Atherosclerosis?

Leonardo da Vinci offered the first detailed analysis of diseased blood vessels and was also the first to attribute this pathology to diet.

American Heart Association

Cardiovascular Disease Risk Reduction

- Balance calorie intake and physical activity to achieve or maintain a healthy body weight.
- Consume a diet rich in vegetables and fruits.
- Choose whole-grain, high-fiber foods.
- Consume fish, especially oily fish, at least twice a week.
- Limit your intake of saturated fat to <7% of energy, trans fat to <1% of energy, and cholesterol to <300 mg per day by
  —choosing lean meats and vegetable alternatives;
  —selecting fat-free (skim), 1%-fat, and low-fat dairy products; and
  —minimizing intake of partially hydrogenated fats.
- Minimize your intake of beverages and foods with added sugars.
- Choose and prepare foods with little or no salt.
- If you consume alcohol, do so in moderation.
- When you eat food that is prepared outside of the home, follow the AHA Diet and Lifestyle Recommendations.

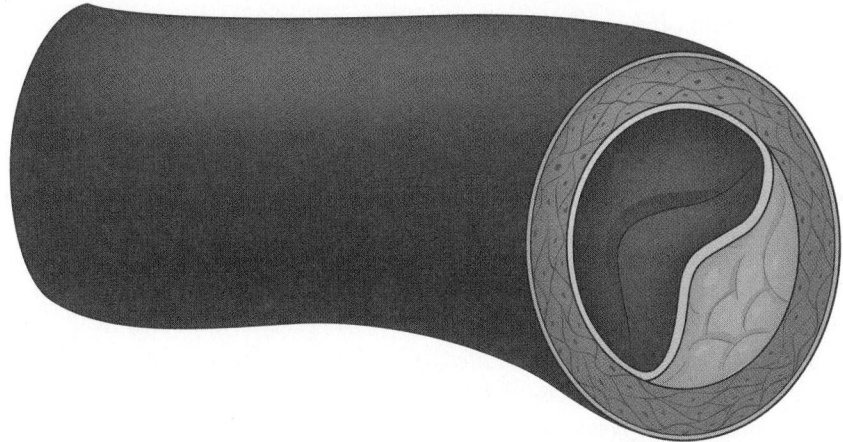

Figure 14.5 **Development of atherosclerosis.** Atherosclerotic plaque is formed by a buildup of fatty material in the wall of an artery. An artery narrowed by plaque is vulnerable to blockage by a blood clot, causing a heart attack or stroke.

C-reactive protein (CRP) A protein released by the body in response to acute injury, infection, or other inflammatory stimuli. CRP is associated with future cardiovascular events.

risk factors Anything that increases a person's chance of developing a disease, including substances, agents, genetic alterations, traits, habits, or conditions.

Quick Bites

How Do Cholesterol-Lowering Medications Work?

One class of cholesterol-lowering medications, the bile acid sequestrants, works by combining bile acid and cholesterol in the intestine to form compounds that the body cannot absorb. Because this cholesterol is then lost in feces, cholesterol must be taken from the blood to make more bile, thus lowering the blood cholesterol level. Another popular type of medication, the statins, interferes with cholesterol synthesis in the liver.

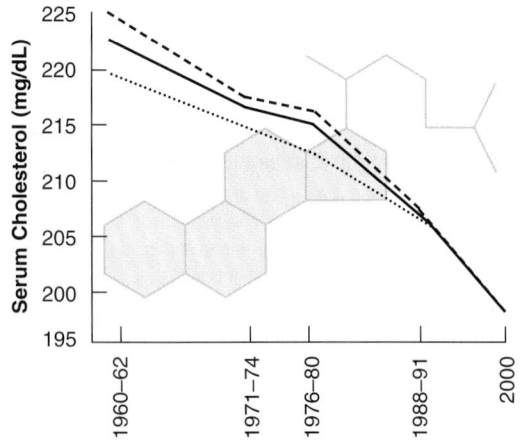

Key

.... men

- - - - - women

———— total

Figure 14.6 **Trends in age-adjusted mean serum cholesterol.** Since the 1960s, mean serum cholesterol levels have steadily declined, along with a decline in death rates from coronary heart disease.

of Lp(a) prevent the normal breakup of blood clots that cause heart attack or stroke. Although Lp(a) is associated with heart attack, it remains unclear whether and how it is influenced by diet.[12] Low HDL cholesterol levels increase the risk of a future cardiovascular event, as do high levels of triglycerides and other blood lipids.[13] See Chapter 5, "Lipids," for more on cholesterol and lipoproteins.

Deaths from coronary heart disease have fallen dramatically, by more than 50 percent over the past 30 years. That drop seems to be correlated with the 28 percent drop in hypercholesterolemia from 1976 to 1994 (see **Figure 14.6**), which in turn parallels a reduced consumption of cholesterol and a lower percentage of calories from fat.[14]

But has eating less fat and cholesterol made us more heart healthy? Or do falling death rates simply reflect better treatment of heart attacks and existing heart disease? Although the weight of the evidence supports the effectiveness of preventive efforts, including diet, several studies suggest that treatment, rather than prevention, has been the more important factor in reducing deaths from heart disease.[15] And, since most heart attacks occur in people with average to moderately high blood cholesterol levels, researchers are exploring other factors, such as infections, that may produce these heart attacks.[16]

Inflammation and Atherosclerosis

The idea that chronic infection can lead to unsuspected disease is not new. Bacterial infection, for example, is known to cause stomach ulcers. In fact, antibiotic therapy is the currently favored treatment for ulcers. Infection caused by bacteria or viruses is suspected to be a factor in heart disease as well. Laboratory evidence and autopsy studies suggest that the inflammatory process resulting from infection may play a role in heart disease, possibly explaining why aspirin, an anti-inflammatory medication, has proved effective in reducing the risk of a heart attack. Clinical trials currently are testing this idea.

C-reactive protein (CRP), a protein released in response to acute injury, infection, or other inflammatory stimuli, may offer a new assessment tool for CVD risk.[17] Independent of other risk factors, researchers found that men with elevated levels of CRP have a threefold increase in their risk of heart attack and a twofold increase in their risk of stroke.[18] These results were confirmed in a study of women.[19] Another report, based on an eight-year follow-up of more than 14,000 initially healthy women, found that elevated levels of CRP help in predicting future cardiovascular events, such as heart attack.[20]

Scientists hypothesize that inflammation (indicated by an elevated CRP level) makes the cap over a plaque more likely to rupture. Elevated CRP levels have been associated with smoking and obesity, and lower CRP levels are found in people who are physically active.

Key Concepts: *Cardiovascular disease is the leading cause of death in the United States and Canada. Much of the prevalence of CVD can be attributed to unhealthy aspects of the American lifestyle, such as smoking, overeating, lack of exercise, high cholesterol levels, and uncontrolled blood pressure. An infection caused by bacteria or viruses may also lead to heart disease. The body releases C-reactive protein (CRP) in response to acute injury, infection, or other inflammatory stimuli; CRP levels may be predictive of heart disease risk.*

Risk Factors for Atherosclerosis

Risk factors are conditions or behaviors that increase your likelihood of developing a disease. When you have more than one risk factor for atherosclerosis, for example, your chance of having a heart attack or stroke greatly multiplies. Fortunately, most of the heart disease risk factors are largely within your control. Risk factors for atherosclerosis that are under your control include

- High blood pressure
- High blood cholesterol
- Cigarette smoking
- Diabetes
- Overweight
- Physical inactivity

Risk factors beyond your control include

- Age (45 or older for men; 55 or older for women)
- Family history of early heart disease (having a mother or sister who has been diagnosed with heart disease before age 65, or a father or brother diagnosed before age 55)

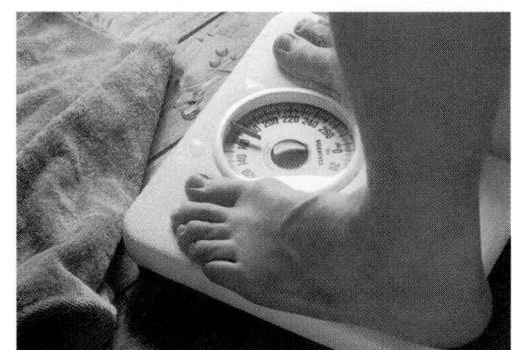

Table 14.1 shows not only factors associated with increased risk of cardiovascular disease, but also factors that may decrease risk. Focusing on risk reduction factors is an important public health strategy for reducing the burden of atherosclerosis in the United States and Canada.

Dietary and Lifestyle Factors for Reducing Atherosclerosis Risk

In June 2006, the American Heart Association (AHA) released new diet and lifestyle recommendations for reducing cardiovascular disease risk.[21] The 2006 AHA Diet and Lifestyle Recommendations are part of a comprehensive

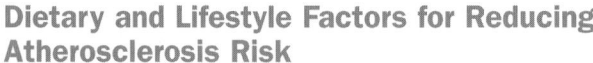

Table 14.1 Strength of Evidence Regarding Lifestyle Factors and Risk of Cardiovascular Disease

	Decreased Risk	No Relationship	Increased Risk
Convincing	Regular exercise	Vitamin E supplements	Myristic and palmitic acid (saturated fatty acids)
	Linoleic acid		*Trans* fatty acids
	Fish and fish oils (EPA, DHA)		High sodium intake
	Vegetables and fruits		Overweight
	Potassium		High alcohol intake (for stroke)
	Low to moderate alcohol intake (for CHD)		Smoking
Probable	α-linolenic acid	Stearic acid	Dietary cholesterol
	Oleic acid		Unfiltered boiled coffee
	Nonstarch polysaccharides (fiber)		
	Whole-grain cereals		
	Nuts (unsalted)		
	Plant sterols/stanols		
	Folate		

Source: Diet, nutrition and the prevention of chronic diseases: a report of a joint WHO/FAO expert consultation. WHO Technical Report Series 916. Geneva, Switzerland, 2003.

plan to reduce the incidence of atherosclerosis and are appropriate for anyone over the age of 2. Major diet and lifestyle goals are (1) consuming an overall healthy diet, (2) aiming for a healthy body weight (defined as a BMI of 18.5 to 24.9 kg/m²), (3) aiming for a desirable lipid profile as defined by the National Cholesterol Education Program (NCEP) of the National Heart, Lung, and Blood Institute (NHLBI) (see **Table 14.2**), (4) aiming for a normal blood pressure, (5) aiming for a normal blood glucose level, (6) being physically active, and (7) avoiding use of and exposure to tobacco products. The specific AHA recommendations along with other diet and lifestyle factors related to cardiovascular disease risk reduction are summarized in the following subsections.

Balance Calorie Intake and Physical Activity to Achieve or Maintain a Healthy Body Weight

Obesity is an independent risk factor for cardiovascular disease, and weight gain during the teen years and in adulthood is associated with increased risk of heart disease.[22] To avoid weight gain, calorie intake needs to match calorie output. Awareness of the calorie content of foods and beverages and control of portion sizes are major steps toward calorie control.

Physical activity helps reduce cardiovascular disease risk in a dose-response fashion.[23] Current recommendations suggest engaging in a minimum of 30 minutes of moderate-intensity activity on most days of the week; more activity would reduce heart disease risk further. In a study of postmenopausal women, brisk walking and more vigorous exercise (e.g., aerobics, tennis) were equally beneficial in reducing cardiovascular events.[24]

Consume a Diet Rich in Fruits and Vegetables

Fruits and vegetables are rich in nutrients and fiber and also low in calories. Eating more fruits and vegetables helps meet nutrient intake requirements without overindulging in calories. In addition, diets that emphasize fruits and vegetables have consistently been shown to lower cardiovascular disease risk factors. (See the Nutrition Science in Action feature "Coronary Heart Disease.") A variety of vegetables and fruits, with an emphasis on whole,

Table 14.2 Adult Blood Cholesterol and Triglyceride Levels

Total Cholesterol		LDL Cholesterol	
Desirable	< 200	Optimal	< 100
Borderline high	200–239	Near or above optimal	100–129
High	≥ 240	Borderline high	130–159
		High	160–189
		Very high	≥ 190
Triglyceride		**HDL Cholesterol**	
Normal	< 150	Low	< 40
Borderline high	150–199	High	≥ 60
High	200–499		
Very high	≥ 500		

Note: All units are mg/dL.

Sources: National Cholesterol Education Program. *Third Report of the Expert Panel on Detection, Evaluation, and Treatment of High Blood Cholesterol in Adults (Adult Treatment Panel III), Final Report.* Washington, DC: US Department of Health and Human Services, 2003. NIH publication 02-5215.

NUTRITION SCIENCE IN ACTION

Coronary Heart Disease

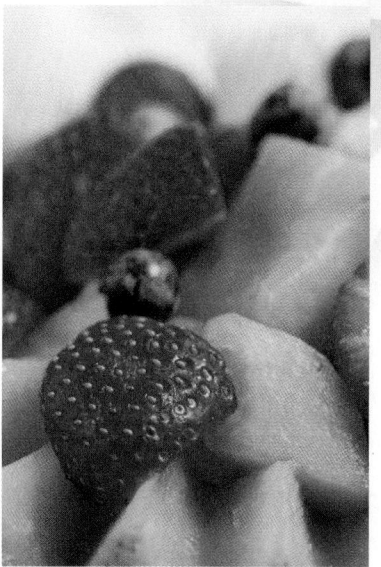

Background: A number of studies have shown that components of fruits and vegetables may reduce the risk of coronary heart disease (CHD). Few studies, however, have examined the relationship between fruit and vegetable consumption and the risk for CHD.

Hypothesis: People with high intakes of fruits and vegetables will have a lower risk of CHD events (heart attacks) than people with low intakes.

Experimental Plan: Using food-frequency questionnaires, follow participants in the Nurses' Health Study and the Health Professionals' Follow-up Study for 14 years. Select men and women free of diagnosed cardiovascular disease, cancer, and diabetes. Control for standard CHD risk factors and compare the lowest and highest intake of fruit and vegetables with the incidence of CHD events.

Results: The hypothesis is confirmed. After controlling for other risk factors, people in the highest fruit and vegetable intake group (top 20 percent, who averaged 9 to 10 servings per day) had significantly fewer CHD events compared with those in the lowest fruit and vegetable intake group (lowest 20 percent, who averaged fewer than 3 servings per day).

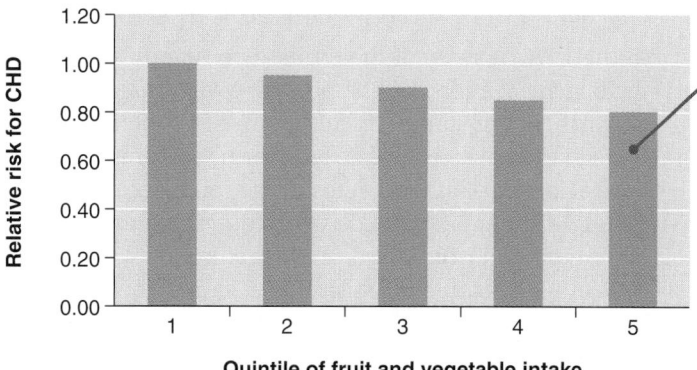

As fruit and vegetable consumption increased, risk for CHD was reduced

Conclusion and Discussion: People with high intakes of fruits and vegetables were older, smoked less, and generally had healthier living habits than those with low intakes. Although the lower incidence of heart attacks in the high-intake group is partially explained by health factors other than diet, it also was associated independently with high fruit and vegetable intake. This study suggests that consumption of fruits and vegetables, particularly green leafy vegetables and vitamin C–rich fruits and vegetables, reduces the risk of CHD. Future studies might look at the effects of taking certain supplements to enhance the effects of consuming green leafy vegetables and vitamin C–rich fruits.

Source: Based on Joshipura KJ, Hu FB, Manson JE, Stampfer MJ, et al. The effect of fruit and vegetable intake on risk for coronary heart disease. *Ann Intern Med.* 2001;134(12):1106–1114.

unprocessed sources, is recommended. Preparation methods that do not add calories, saturated or *trans* fat, sugar, and salt are also recommended.

Brightly colored vegetables and fruits are not only nutrient-rich, but also are good sources of phytochemicals, including antioxidants. In the blood, oxygen free radicals can attack and oxidize low-density lipoproteins; as these oxidized LDL are deposited in blood vessel walls, the process of building up plaque begins.[25] Although some studies suggest that consumption of a diet high in vitamin E and other antioxidants may inhibit oxidation and subsequent atherosclerosis,[26] recent trials using supplements of vitamin E alone or a combination of vitamin E, vitamin C, and beta-carotene have not supported a beneficial effect on CVD outcomes, at least in high-risk individuals.[27] Even so, diets rich in fruits and vegetables—sources of these vitamins and other antioxidant compounds—are recommended.

Choose Whole-Grain, High-Fiber Foods

Diets that emphasize whole grains and other foods rich in fiber have been linked to improved overall diet quality and reduced cardiovascular disease risk.[28] As described in Chapter 4, "Carbohydrates," certain types of fiber can bind to bile acids in the gastrointestinal tract, so these bile acids are excreted in the feces rather than recycled and reused. Additional bile acids must then be made from cholesterol, lowering the total amount in the body. In the large intestine, intestinal bacteria partially digest fiber and then produce short-chain fatty acids, which are linked to reduced cholesterol synthesis.[29] The Adequate Intake (AI) level for fiber (14 grams per 1,000 kilocalories) is based on the amount of fiber that has been shown to reduce CVD risk.[30] The American Heart Association and the *Dietary Guidelines for Americans* recommend that at least half of grain intake come from whole grains.

Consume Fish, Especially Oily Fish, at Least Twice a Week

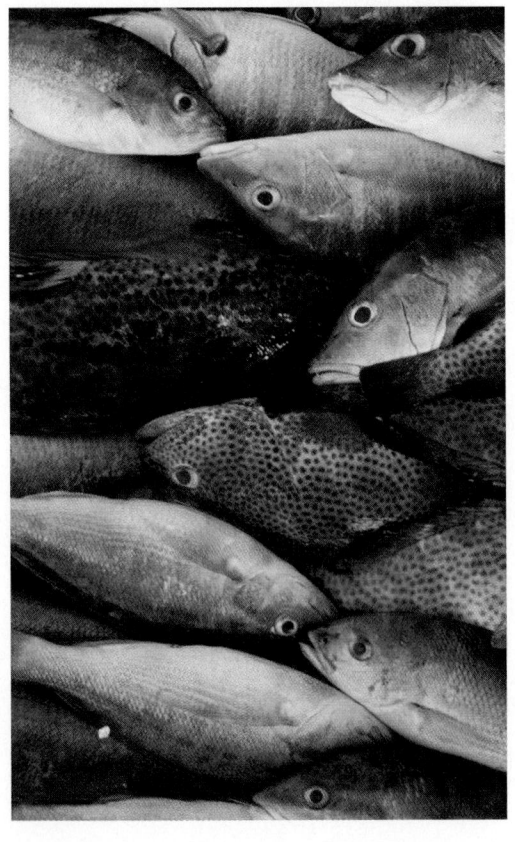

In the 1970s a study of the Inuits (Greenland Eskimos) focused attention on the beneficial effects of EPA and DHA, the *omega*-3 fatty acids in fish fats.[31] Researchers were puzzled: This group of people had a high intake of fat, saturated fat, and cholesterol from marine mammals and fish, yet they showed little evidence of atherosclerosis. The Inuits were compared to the Danes, among whom atherosclerosis was common and whose diet was similarly high in fat, but from meats and dairy products. It became clear that the high EPA and DHA content of fish in the Inuit diet protects against heart disease by discouraging blood cells from clotting and from sticking to artery walls, and by reducing inflammation. Studies of other groups have since shown similar results. The Japanese, for example, with their generous fish intake, have low rates of atherosclerosis. Many other studies point in the same direction; some show that as few as two or three servings of fish weekly can be protective. Not only does fish provide EPA and DHA, but it can also displace other foods higher in saturated and *trans* fatty acids from the diet.

Other studies continue to support the idea that consuming *omega*-3s from fish and fish oils protects against heart disease and its many complications.[32] The Nurses' Health Study shows that higher consumption of fish or *omega*-3 fatty acids also reduces the risk of stroke caused by blood clots.[33] Scientists are also investigating whether *omega*-3s may help some chronic inflammatory conditions such as rheumatoid arthritis,[34] asthma,[35] and psoriasis, although research in these areas has yielded mixed results.[36] All in all, there are certainly enough positive results to encourage further study and recommend regular consumption of cold-water fish (e.g., salmon, cod) for EPA and DHA, as well as plant foods with *alpha*-linolenic acid.[37]

Limit Your Intake of Saturated and Trans Fat and Cholesterol

Saturated and *trans* fatty acids raise total and LDL cholesterol and should be minimized in a heart-healthy diet. Saturated fatty acids raise LDL cholesterol more than *trans* fatty acids do, but saturated fatty acids also raise HDL cholesterol.[38] The American Heart Association recommends limiting saturated fat intake to less than 7 percent of total calories, and *trans* fat intake to less than 1 percent (the 2005 *Dietary Guidelines* recommend keeping *trans* fat intake "as low as possible"). This is a significant reduction from the typical U.S. consumption of 11.2 percent of calories from saturated fat and 2.7 percent of calories from *trans* fat.[39] Replacing saturated fats with monounsaturated or *omega*-6 polyunsaturated fatty acids lowers both total and LDL cholesterol. Research also shows that consuming monounsaturated fats, such as olive oil, lowers total and LDL cholesterol without lowering HDL.[40]

This positive effect of olive oil may explain why Greeks, Turks, Italians, and others around the Mediterranean who eat a diet high in fat still have low rates of heart disease. Their overall diet pattern seems to model AHA recommendations—ample fresh fruits, vegetables, pasta, and whole grains; small amounts of meat and poultry; and generous use of olive oil. Favorable results from both epidemiological and intervention studies have made the Mediterranean diet popular.[41]

Does the total amount of fat consumed make a difference? The AHA supports recommendations of the Institute of Medicine (the DRI values) and the NCEP for a total fat intake of 25 to 35 percent of energy intake. When researchers compared replacement of saturated fat calories with either protein or monounsaturated fat, they found that a high-protein diet (25 percent of calories from protein, 48 percent from carbohydrate, and 27 percent from fat) reduced blood pressure and lowered LDL cholesterol, but also lowered HDL cholesterol.[42] The higher-fat diet (37 percent of calories from fat, 48 percent from carbohydrate, and 15 percent from protein) resulted in lower blood pressure, no change in LDL cholesterol, and increased HDL cholesterol. In this diet, 21 percent of the calories came from monounsaturated fat, mostly olive and canola oils.

What about cholesterol intake? Some evidence links cholesterol intake to blood cholesterol levels, and because cholesterol is not essential in the diet, it should be limited. When people reduce their saturated fat intake by limiting fat from dairy products and meats, cholesterol intake usually goes down. The AHA recommends limiting cholesterol intake to less than 300 milligrams per day.

Minimize Your Intake of Beverages and Foods with Added Sugars

As discussed in Chapter 4, "Carbohydrates," added sugar intake in the United States has risen dramatically in the last 20 years. Reducing consumption of added sugars helps to improve the nutrient quality of the diet and also reduces calorie intake. Paying attention to sources of added sugars will help individuals achieve weight goals.

Choose and Prepare Foods with Little or No Salt

Hypertension is one of the major risk factors for cardiovascular disease, and generally, blood pressure rises as salt intake rises. Further discussion of salt, sodium, other minerals, and blood pressure follows in the section "Hypertension" later in this chapter. The AHA suggests that reducing sodium intake to 2,300 milligrams per day or less is an achievable goal.

If You Consume Alcohol, Do So in Moderation

Numerous studies associate moderate alcohol consumption with a substantial decrease in heart disease risk.[43] Although the positive effects of alcohol are generally associated with wine, and particularly red wine consumption, the benefits are found with other forms of alcohol.[44] However, alcohol is addictive, and high intake can have adverse effects on the body. So, the AHA recommends limiting alcohol intake to no more than one drink per day for women and two drinks per day for men, ideally with meals.

The positive effects of alcohol on heart disease risk provide at least a partial explanation for the "French Paradox," the fact that the French eat rich cheeses and fatty meats, yet still have low rates of heart disease. They also have relatively high intakes of fruits, vegetables, and red wine—all rich sources of antioxidant phytochemicals.[45] Antioxidants and moderate alcohol consumption may offset some of the adverse effects of poor food choices and perhaps protect against heart disease.

When You Eat Food That Is Prepared Outside of the Home, Follow the AHA 2006 Diet and Lifestyle Recommendations

More and more of our meals are either eaten away from home or brought home as takeout food. All too often, our choices away from home are high in saturated and *trans* fat, cholesterol, added sugars, and sodium and low in fiber, fruits, and vegetables. Also, portion sizes at restaurants are typically more than those recommended by MyPyramid. Consumers need to make wise choices both at home and away from home. Splitting entrée portions with a companion, choosing steamed vegetables instead of a loaded baked potato, or substituting a salad with low-fat dressing for french fries will help individuals follow the AHA guidelines. For more tips for heart-healthy choices when dining out, see **Table 14.3**.

Other Dietary Factors

B Vitamins. Folate and vitamins B_6 and B_{12} are involved in pathways that convert one amino acid, homocysteine, to another amino acid, methionine. As noted earlier, high levels of homocysteine may contribute to heart disease by promoting atherosclerosis, excessive blood clotting, or blood vessel rigidity. Folate and vitamins B_6 and B_{12} can help reduce destructive levels of homocysteine. Scientists believe that consumption of a diet rich in these vitamins helps prevent blood vessel damage from homocysteine.[46] For more information, see the FYI feature "The B Vitamins and Heart Disease" in Chapter 10, "Water-Soluble Vitamins."

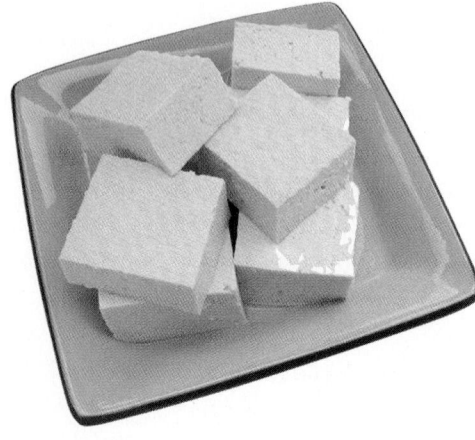

Soy. Soy-based foods, such as soy milks, soy burgers, tofu, and tempeh, have become popular items in grocery stores. In October 1999, the U.S. Food and Drug Administration (FDA) approved labeling for foods containing soy protein as protective against coronary heart disease. Since then, many well controlled studies on soy protein substantially added to our scientific knowledge base. The American Heart Association Nutrition Committee reevaluated the evidence on soy protein and found that the direct cardiovascular health benefit of soy protein is minimal at best.[47]

Other components in soybeans may provide favorable effects. Because many soy products have high content of polyunsaturated fats, fiber, vitamins, and minerals and low content of saturated fat, using these foods to replace foods high in animal protein, fat, and cholesterol may confer benefits to cardiovascular health.

Soy also contains isoflavones, a group of compounds often referred to as phytoestrogens because of their hormonelike effects. Phytoestrogens are

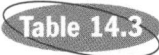 **Table 14.3** Tips for Dining Out

Are you able to stick to your low-saturated-fat, low-cholesterol diet when eating out? If not, you will be able to if you follow these tips:

- Choose restaurants that have low-saturated-fat, low-cholesterol menu choices. Don't be afraid to make special requests—it's your right as a paying customer.
- Control serving sizes by asking for a side-dish or appetizer-size serving, sharing a dish with a companion, or taking some home.
- Ask that gravy, butter, rich sauces, and salad dressing be served on the side. That way, you can control the amount of saturated fat and cholesterol that you eat.
- Ask to substitute a salad or baked potato for chips, fries, coleslaw, or other extras—or just ask that the extras be left off your plate.
- When ordering pizza, order vegetable toppings such as green pepper, onions, and mushrooms instead of meat or extra cheese. To make your pizza even lower in saturated fat and cholesterol, order it with half the cheese or no cheese.
- At fast food restaurants, go for salads, grilled (not fried or breaded) skinless chicken sandwiches, regular-sized hamburgers, or roast beef sandwiches. Go easy on the regular salad dressings and fatty sauces. Limit your consumption of jumbo or deluxe burgers, sandwiches, french fries, and other foods.

Reading the Menu

- Choose low-saturated-fat, low-cholesterol cooking methods. Look for terms such as the following: steamed, in its own juice (au jus), garden fresh, broiled, baked, roasted, poached, tomato juice, dry boiled (in wine or lemon juice), and lightly sautéed or lightly stir-fried.
- Be aware of dishes that are high in saturated fat and cholesterol. Watch out for terms such as the following: butter sauce, fried, crispy, creamed, in cream or cheese sauce, au gratin, au fromage, escalloped, parmesan, hollandaise, bernaise, marinated (in oil), stewed, basted, sautéed, stir-fried, casserole, hash, prime, pot pie, pastry crust.

Source: National Heart Lung and Blood Institute. Dining out on the TLC diet. http://www.nhlbi.nih.gov/chd/Tipsheets/diningout.htm. Accessed 8/28/06.

also found in lignins from flax seed, whole grains, and some fruits. Although phytoestrogens do not appear to have any effect on blood lipids,[48] isoflavones may help improve endothelial function.[49]

Putting It All Together

Healthy People 2010 objectives target reducing deaths from heart disease and stroke as well as reducing the number of adults with high blood cholesterol levels. To accomplish these goals, dietitians recommend lowering total fat intake, lowering saturated and *trans* fat intake, maintaining a healthy body weight, and exercising on a regular basis. Eating fruits, vegetables, legumes, and grains that contain fiber helps lower cholesterol levels too. These foods contain antioxidants and B vitamins, such as B_6 and folate, that may also reduce the risk of heart disease. Substituting fish or soy foods for high-fat meats and cheeses can be beneficial as well.

Key Concepts: To reduce your risk of heart disease, get regular exercise, control your weight, and don't smoke. Dietary changes you can make to reduce your heart disease risk include eating less fat, saturated and trans fat, and cholesterol while increasing intake of fruits, vegetables, and whole grains. Look for sources of omega-3 fatty acids and fiber in your food choices.

Hypertension

Persistent high blood pressure (**hypertension**) often is called a "silent killer" because it usually has no specific symptoms or early warning signs. You can be hypertensive for years without realizing it. During those years, untreated hypertension may cause damage to vital organs, particularly the heart, the brain, the kidneys, and the eyes. It increases the risk of heart attack, congestive heart failure, stroke, and kidney failure. The good news is that hypertension can be treated and controlled. Hypertension affects

hypertension When resting blood pressure persistently exceeds 140 mm Hg systolic or 90 mm Hg diastolic.

nearly one-fourth of American adults and more than two-thirds of people older than 65.[50]

What Is Blood Pressure?

Blood pressure is the force exerted by the blood on the walls of the blood vessels, especially the arteries. This force is created by the pumping action of the heart. Every time the heart contracts, or beats (systole), blood pressure increases. When the heart relaxes between beats (diastole), the pressure decreases. Blood pressure can fluctuate considerably, depending on various factors. When you are excited, afraid, or exercising, for example, your heart pumps more blood into your arteries and your blood pressure rises. Blood pressure rises and falls during the day. When it stays elevated over time, it's called hypertension.

Blood pressure is measured using a **sphygmomanometer** (blood pressure cuff) (see **Figure 14.7**), and is expressed as two numbers. The **systolic** pressure is the higher number and represents pressure during the heart's contraction. The **diastolic** pressure is the lower number, measured during the heart's resting phase. Normal blood pressure is defined as a systolic pressure less than 120 mm Hg (millimeters mercury) and a diastolic pressure less than 80 mm Hg.

What Is Hypertension?

The Joint National Committee on Prevention, Detection, Evaluation, and Treatment of High Blood Pressure (JNC) released new classifications for hypertension in 2003.[51] (See **Table 14.4**.) The JNC 7 report added a new category of "prehypertension," recognizing that individuals with blood pressure between 130/80 and 139/89 mm Hg are twice as likely to develop hypertension as those with lower values.

Persistent high blood pressure of unknown cause (90 percent of cases) is called **essential hypertension**. Essential hypertension most likely has many causes, including diet, obesity, alcohol abuse, lack of exercise, physical and emotional stress, and psychological and genetic factors. When the condition results from another problem, such as a kidney defect, it is called **secondary hypertension**. In secondary hypertension, blood pressure usually returns to normal when the underlying defect is corrected.

Renin and Hypertension

The enzyme renin is associated with some cases of essential hypertension. This enzyme promotes the formation of angiotensin proteins, which cause the arteries to constrict. Some people with essential hypertension have higher than normal levels of renin in their blood. People with high renin levels have an increased incidence of heart attacks, strokes, and kidney failure.

Other people with essential hypertension have lower than normal levels of renin in their blood. Their hypertension may be caused primarily by increased blood volume. This condition could result either from decreased sodium excretion by the kidneys or from increased secretion of aldosterone, a hormone that causes the kidneys to retain sodium and water.

Stress and Hypertension

Stress may contribute to sustained high blood pressure. When stressors, either internal or external, activate the sympathetic nervous system, heart rate increases, arteries constrict, and the blood exerts greater force on the artery walls. Chronic stress has been implicated in heart disease.

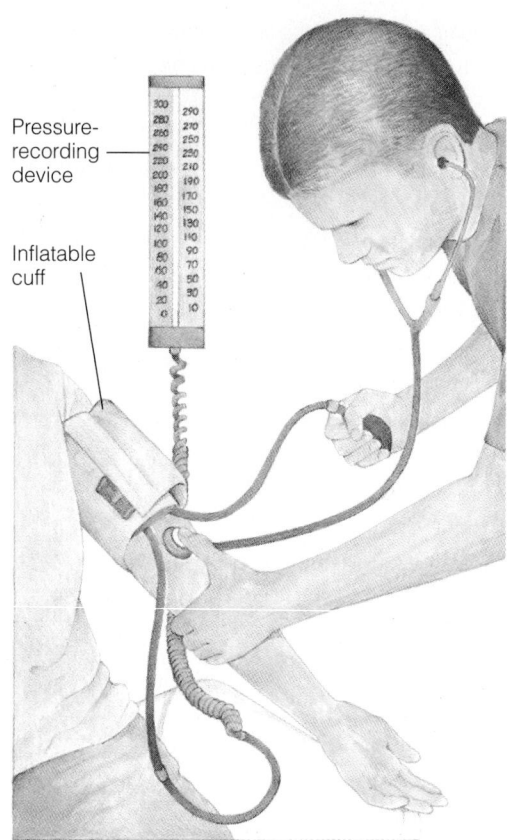

(a)

(b)

Figure 14.7 **Blood pressure reading. (a)** A sphygmomanometer (blood pressure cuff) is used to determine blood pressure. **(b)** As shown, the blood pressure rises and falls with each contraction of the heart.
① When the pressure in the cuff exceeds the arterial peak pressure, blood flow stops. No sound is heard.
② As cuff pressure is gradually released, a sound can be heard as pressure in the cuff falls below the peak arterial pressure. At this point, called systolic pressure, blood begins flowing through the artery again.
③ As cuff pressure continues to drop, the sound stops when the cuff pressure is equal to the lowest pressure in the artery. At this point, called the diastolic pressure, the artery is fully open.

Table 14.4 **Blood Pressure Classifications for Adults**[a]

Category	Systolic (mm Hg)[b]		Diastolic (mm Hg)[b]
Normal	Less than 120	and	Less than 80
Prehypertension	120–139	or	80–89
Stage 1 Hypertension	140–159	or	90–99
Stage 2 Hypertension	160 or higher	or	100 or higher

[a] For adults 18 and older who are not on medicine for high blood pressure and do not have a short-term serious illness.

[b] Millimeters of mercury

Source: Chobanian AV, Bakris GL, Black HR, et al. The Seventh Report of the Joint National Committee on Prevention, Detection, Evaluation, and Treatment of High Blood Pressure: the JNC 7 report. *JAMA.* 2003;289(19):2560–2572.

Risk Factors for Hypertension

Even though the cause for most cases of hypertension is unknown, several factors clearly contribute to hypertension. As with heart disease risk, some hypertension risk factors are controllable and others are uncontrollable. Risk factors for hypertension under your control include the following:

- *Obesity.* People with a BMI of 30 kg/m² or higher are more likely to develop high blood pressure.

- *Eating too much salt.* High sodium intake increases blood pressure in some people.

- *Lack of physical activity.* A sedentary lifestyle is associated with overweight and increased blood pressure.

- *Drinking too much alcohol.* Heavy and regular use of alcohol increases blood pressure.

Risk factors for hypertension that are beyond your control include the following:

- *Race.* African Americans develop high blood pressure more often, at earlier ages, and with more severity than Caucasians.[52]

- *Age.* Blood pressure risk rises with age; people with normal blood pressure at age 55 have a 90 percent lifetime risk of developing hypertension.[53]

- *Heredity.* Family history of hypertension is a strong predictive factor.

Dietary and Lifestyle Factors for Reducing Hypertension

The National High Blood Pressure Education Program (NHBPEP) has updated its recommendations for preventing hypertension.[54] These recommendations are very similar to the AHA recommendations for reducing heart disease risk:

- Maintain normal body weight for adults (BMI 18.5–24.9 kg/m²).

- Reduce dietary sodium intake to no more than 6,000 milligrams of sodium chloride or 2,400 milligrams of sodium per day.

- Engage in regular aerobic physical activity, such as brisk walking, at least 30 minutes per day most days of the week.

blood pressure The pressure of blood against the walls of a blood vessel or heart chamber. Unless there is reference to another location, such as the pulmonary artery or one of the heart chambers, this term refers to the pressure in the systemic arteries, as measured, for example, in the forearm.

sphygmomanometer [sfig-mo-ma-NOM-eh-ter] An instrument for measuring blood pressure and especially arterial blood pressure.

systolic Pertaining to a heart contraction. Systolic blood pressure is measured during a heart contraction, a time period known as systole.

diastolic Pertaining to the time between heart contractions, a period known as diastole. Diastolic blood pressure is measured at the point of maximum cardiac relaxation.

essential hypertension Hypertension for which no specific cause can be identified. Ninety to 95 percent of people with hypertension have essential hypertension.

secondary hypertension Hypertension caused by an underlying condition such as a kidney disorder. Once the underlying condition is treated, the blood pressure usually returns to normal.

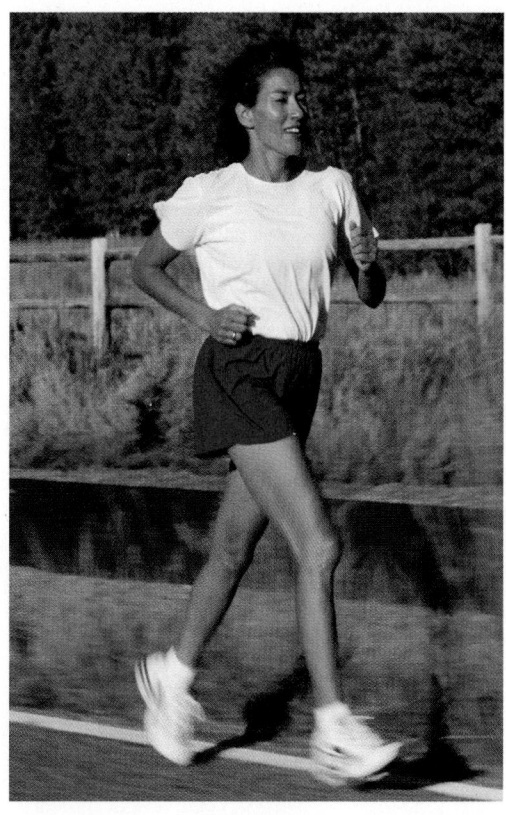

- Limit alcohol consumption to no more than 1 ounce of ethanol per day for most men and no more than 0.5 ounce for most women.

- Maintain adequate intake of dietary potassium (more than 3,500 milligrams per day).

- Consume a diet rich in fruits and vegetables, low-fat dairy products, and foods with a reduced content of saturated and total fat (DASH eating plan).

Sodium

Excessive sodium can hold excessive fluid in the body, at least temporarily. These excesses can be burdensome on the kidneys, heart, and blood vessels. The consensus among heart disease experts is that too much sodium, ingested routinely over the years, plays a role in the underlying causes of hypertension in genetically predisposed or "salt-sensitive" people. The more salt they eat, the higher their blood pressure.

Population studies appear to bear this conclusion out. Rates of hypertension are higher in countries with high sodium intakes. On the other hand, primitive people, whose diets contain very little sodium, seldom have hypertension. Their blood pressure does not rise with age if they continue to eat their traditional diet. If they adopt a "modern" (higher-sodium) diet, however, their blood pressure tends to rise, and they are more likely to become hypertensive.[55]

Other Dietary Factors

Sodium is not the only dietary factor associated with hypertension. Excess weight tends to raise blood pressure; regular exercise and weight loss help to reduce blood pressure. Reducing consumption of alcohol also tends to reduce blood pressure and improves the effectiveness of antihypertensive medications. Eating a diet rich in calcium, magnesium, and potassium reduces blood pressure as well.[56] The mechanism by which these minerals act on hypertension may in part reflect their interrelationship with sodium metabolism.

The DASH Diet

The **DASH (Dietary Approaches to Stop Hypertension)** study, a multicenter NHLBI-sponsored trial, tested the effects of different dietary patterns on blood pressure. After a control period, the 459 subjects in this study received one of three diets for an eight-week period:[57]

1. *Control diet:* Macronutrient and fiber content equal to U.S. average; 4 servings of fruits and vegetables per day; 0.5 serving of dairy products per day; potassium, magnesium, and calcium levels close to the 25th percentile of U.S. consumption.

2. *Fruit and vegetable diet:* 8.5 servings of fruits and vegetables per day; potassium and magnesium levels at the 75th percentile of U.S. consumption; other nutrients similar to control diet.

3. *Combination diet:* 10 servings of fruits and vegetables per day; 2.7 servings of low-fat dairy products per day; less fat, saturated fat, and cholesterol than control diet; potassium, magnesium, and calcium levels at the 75th percentile of U.S. consumption.

The sodium content of the diets averaged about 3,000 milligrams per day. The study excluded subjects who were taking antihypertensive medications, unless their physicians had given them permission to discontinue their medication for the course of the study.[58]

Think
About It
3

Both the fruit and vegetable diet and the combination diet significantly lowered the systolic and diastolic blood pressure in all subjects and in subgroups analyzed by sex, ethnicity, and hypertensive/normotensive status. For hypertensive individuals, the DASH combination diet lowered blood pressure as much as antihypertensive drugs. Widespread adoption of the DASH combination diet could lead to a downward shift in the incidence and severity of the disease. Because recent data indicate a slight rise in the incidence of stroke, kidney disease, and heart failure and a leveling of the heart disease death rate among U.S. adults, the NHLBI recommends that all Americans—not just those with hypertension—follow the DASH combination diet.[59] **Table 14.5** shows sample meals from the three DASH diets used in the study.

Results from a follow-up study, the DASH-Sodium trial, support both the DASH-style dietary changes and lower sodium intake. This study used different levels of daily sodium restriction (3,300 mg, 2,400 mg, and 1,500 mg) and two diet plans (a "typical" American diet and the DASH diet). Approximately 41 percent of the participants had hypertension. Reducing sodium intake lowered blood pressure for participants in both dietary treatment arms, but the DASH diet in combination with sodium restriction was more effective than the low-sodium control diet alone.[60]

To help keep blood pressure at healthy levels, the DASH eating plan is rich in potassium. A potassium-rich diet may help to reduce elevated or high

DASH (Dietary Approaches to Stop Hypertension) An eating plan low in total fat, saturated fat, and cholesterol, and rich in fruits, vegetables, and low-fat dairy products that has been shown to reduce elevated blood pressure.

Table 14.5 Sample Menus from the DASH Study

Meal	Control Diet	Fruit and Vegetable Diet	DASH Combination Diet
Breakfast	Apple juice Sugar-frosted flakes White toast Butter Jelly Whole milk	Orange juice Oat bran muffin Raisins Dried apricots Butter	Orange juice Granola bar Fat-free yogurt 1% low-fat milk Banana
Lunch	Ham-and-chicken sandwich on white bread, with lettuce, pickles, mustard, and mayonnaise Fruit cocktail	Ham-and-Swiss cheese sandwich on whole-wheat bread Banana	Smoked turkey sandwich on whole-wheat bread with lettuce and mayonnaise Fresh orange
Dinner	Spiced cod Scallion rice Carrots Butter French rolls	Spiced cod Scallion rice Lima beans Butter Dinner rolls Melon balls	Spiced cod Scallion rice Spinach Margarine Dinner rolls Melon balls 1% low-fat milk
Snack	Graham crackers Vanilla frosting Tropical fruit punch	Peanuts	Peanuts Dried apricots Melon balls

Source: Karanja NM, Obarzanek E, Lin P-H, et al. Descriptive characteristics of the dietary patterns used in the Dietary Approaches to Stop Hypertension trial. *J Am Diet Assoc.* 1999; 99(suppl 8):S19–S27.

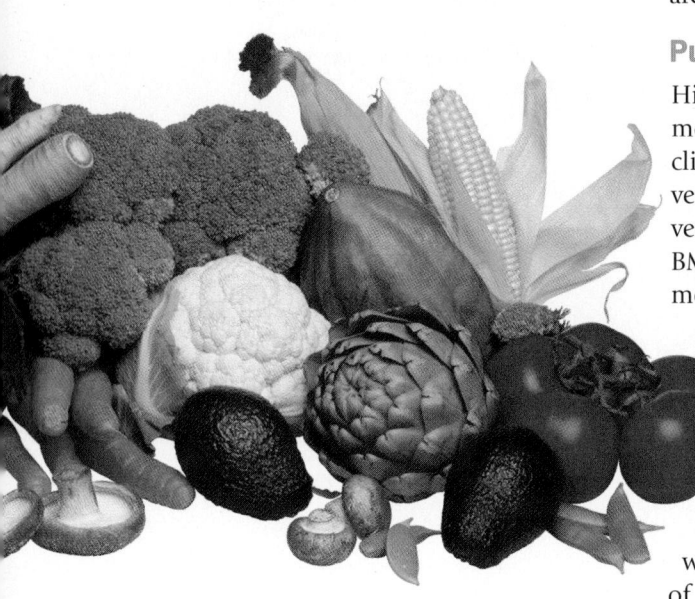

blood pressure, but be sure to get your potassium from food sources, not from supplements. Many fruits and vegetables, some milk products, and fish are rich sources of potassium. (See Chapter 11, "Water and Major Minerals.")

Putting It All Together

High blood pressure can be controlled and even prevented by making modifications in diet and lifestyle as described previously. The PREMIER clinical trial was designed to assess the effects of behavioral lifestyle interventions on blood pressure over a six-month period.[61] The behavioral interventions included weight loss of at least 15 pounds for individuals with a BMI greater than or equal to 25 kg/m^2, at least 180 minutes per week of moderate-intensity physical activity, and restricted intake of sodium (2,400 mg/day or less) and alcohol (1 ounce or less for men and 0.5 ounce or less for women). One study group received general advice on factors that affect blood pressure, while two other groups received regular group and individual counseling. One of the groups receiving behavioral counseling was also instructed on the DASH diet.

Weight loss occurred in all three groups, but only the behavioral intervention groups showed improvements in fitness. Blood pressure was significantly reduced in the groups making lifestyle changes. Control of existing hypertension was most successful in the group following the DASH diet.[62]

These results support the advice of the NHBPEP described earlier and provide a mechanism by which to achieve the Healthy People 2010 objective of reducing the proportion of adults with hypertension. Blood pressure can be unhealthy even if it stays only slightly above the optimal level of less than 120/80 mm Hg. The higher blood pressure rises above normal, the greater the health risk. Recognition and control of high blood pressure is essential for avoiding damage to vital organs. Taking your blood pressure on a regular basis is the key to detecting this silent killer.

Key Concepts: Hypertension is a risk factor for atherosclerosis, kidney disease, and stroke. Blood pressure tends to rise with age, and rates of hypertension are higher among African Americans. Sodium intake affects blood pressure, especially in those individuals who are salt sensitive. Low intake of potassium, calcium, and possibly magnesium also may contribute to the development of hypertension. Eating a diet replete with fresh foods and avoiding processed foods will not only improve the balance of minerals in our diet but may also reduce risk of disease.

Cancer

Cancer is the second leading cause of death in the United States and Canada.[63] In fact, one in every four deaths in these nations is attributable to cancer. Reducing both the number of new cancer cases and the death rates from cancer are key objectives of Healthy People 2010. Cancer comprises a group of more than 100 diseases that involve the uncontrolled division of the body's cells. Although it can develop in virtually any of the body's tissues, and each type of cancer has its unique features, the basic processes that produce cancer are quite similar in all forms of the disease. To understand cancer, it is helpful to know what happens when normal cells become cancerous.

What Is Cancer?

The body consists of many types of cells. Normally, cells grow and divide to produce more cells only when the body needs them. This orderly process helps keep the body healthy. Sometimes, however, cells keep dividing when new cells are not needed. These extra cells form a mass of **tissue**, called a growth or **tumor**.

Tumors can be **benign** or **malignant**. Benign tumors are not cancer. They can often be removed and, in most cases, they do not regrow. Cells from benign tumors do not spread to other parts of the body. Most important, benign tumors rarely pose a threat to life. In contrast, malignant tumors are cancer. Cells in these tumors are abnormal and divide without control or order. As a result, they can invade and damage nearby tissues and organs. Also, cancer cells can break away from a malignant tumor and enter the bloodstream or the lymphatic system. In this way, cancer can spread from the original cancer site to form new tumors in other organs. The spread of cancer is called **metastasis**.

Most cancers are named for the organ or type of cell in which they begin. Cancer that begins in the lung is lung cancer, for example, and cancer that begins in skin cells known as **melanocytes** is called **melanoma**. **Leukemia** and **lymphoma** are cancers that arise in blood-forming cells. The abnormal blood cells circulate in the bloodstream and lymphatic system. They may also invade (infiltrate) body organs and form tumors.

Cancer develops in a multistage process that can take many years. There are typically three phases of development.

1. *Initiation* occurs when something alters a cell's genetic structure and prepares it to act abnormally during later stages.

2. *Promotion*, a reversible stage, occurs when a chemical or other factor encourages initiated cells to become active.

3. *Progression* occurs when promoted cells multiply and perhaps invade surrounding healthy tissue.

When cancer spreads (metastasizes), cancer cells are often found in nearby or regional **lymph nodes** (sometimes called lymph glands). If the cancer has reached these nodes, it means that cancer cells may have spread to other organs, such as the liver, bones, or brain. (See **Figure 14.8**.) When cancer spreads from its original location to another part of the body, the new tumor has the same kind of abnormal cells and the same name as the primary tumor. If lung cancer spreads to the brain, for example, the cancer cells in the brain are actually lung cancer cells. The disease is called metastatic lung cancer (it is not brain cancer).

Risk Factors for Cancer

The more we can learn about what causes cancer, the more likely we are to find ways to prevent it. Although doctors can seldom explain why one person gets cancer and another does not, they know that cancer is not caused by an injury, such as a bump or bruise. Also, although being infected with certain viruses may increase the risk of some types of cancer, cancer is not contagious; no one can "catch" cancer from another person.

Cancer usually develops over time. It results from a complex mix of factors related to lifestyle, heredity, and environment. Researchers have identified a number of factors that increase a person's chance of developing cancer. Many types of cancer are related to the use of tobacco, items that people eat and drink, exposure to ultraviolet (UV) radiation from the sun, and exposure to cancer-causing agents (**carcinogens**) in the environment and the workplace. Some people are more sensitive than others to factors that cause cancer.

Think About It
4

cancer A term for diseases in which abnormal cells divide without control. Cancer cells can invade nearby tissues and can spread through the bloodstream and lymphatic system to other parts of the body.

tissue [TISH-yoo] A group or layer of cells that are alike and that work together to perform a specific function.

tumor [TOO-mer] An abnormal mass of tissue that results from excessive cell division. Tumors perform no useful body function. They may be benign (not cancerous) or malignant (cancerous).

benign [beh-NINE] Not cancerous; does not invade nearby tissue or spread to other parts of the body.

malignant [ma-LIG-nant] Cancerous; a growth with a tendency to invade and destroy nearby tissue and spread to other parts of the body.

metastasis [meh-TAS-ta-sis] The spread of cancer from one part of the body to another. Tumors formed from cells that have spread are called "secondary tumors" and contain cells that are like those in the original (primary) tumor. The plural is *metastases*.

melanocytes [mel-AN-o-sites] Cells in the skin that produce and contain the pigment called melanin.

melanoma A form of skin cancer that arises in melanocytes, the cells that produce pigment. Melanoma usually begins in a mole.

leukemia [loo-KEE-mee-a] Cancer of blood-forming tissue.

lymphoma [lim-FO-ma] Cancer that arises in cells of the lymphatic system.

lymph nodes [limf nodes] Rounded masses of lymphatic tissue that are surrounded by a capsule of connective tissue. Lymph nodes filter lymph (lymphatic fluid), and they store lymphocytes (white blood cells). They are located along lymphatic vessels. Also called lymph glands.

carcinogens [kar-SIN-o-jins] Any substances that cause cancer.

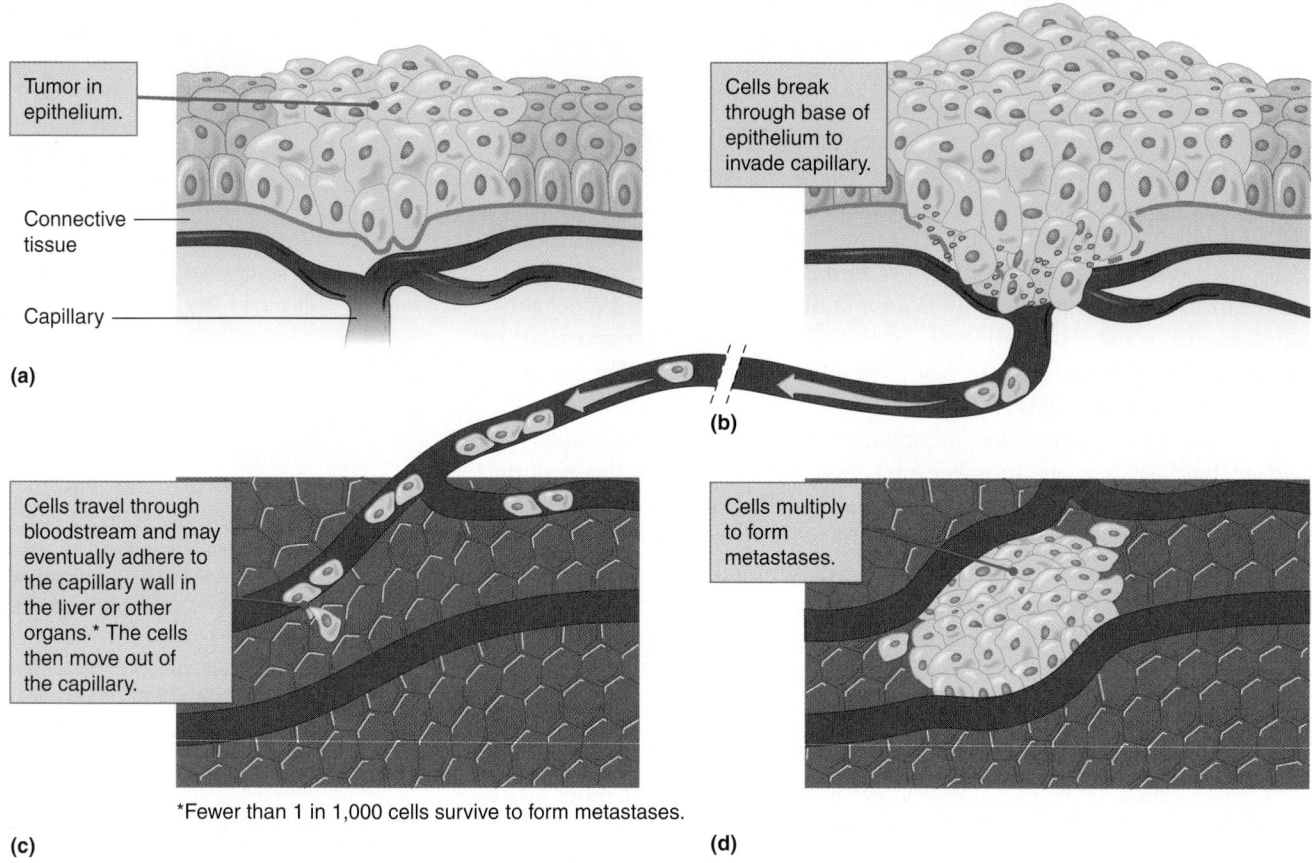

Tumor in epithelium.

Connective tissue

Capillary

(a)

Cells break through base of epithelium to invade capillary.

(b)

Cells travel through bloodstream and may eventually adhere to the capillary wall in the liver or other organs.* The cells then move out of the capillary.

Cells multiply to form metastases.

*Fewer than 1 in 1,000 cells survive to form metastases.

(c)

(d)

Figure 14.8 **How cancer cells multiply and spread.** Cancer cells can break away from a malignant tumor, enter the bloodstream or the lymphatic system, and travel to new sites to form new tumors in other organs.

Nevertheless, most people who develop cancer have none of the known risk factors. And most people who do have risk factors do not develop the disease. Researchers have learned that cancer is caused by changes (called mutations or alterations) in genes that control normal cell growth and cell death. Most cancer-causing gene changes are generated by factors in a person's lifestyle or the environment. However, some alterations that may lead to cancer are inherited; that is, they are passed from parent to child. Having such an inherited gene alteration increases the risk of cancer, but it does not mean that the person is certain to develop cancer.

The Diet–Cancer Link

Although evidence suggests that between 20 and 30 percent of cancers are due to poor food choices and physical inactivity, the role played by nutrition and diet in cancer development is complex.[64] Some dietary factors may act as promoters; many others may have protective roles, blocking the cellular changes in one of the developmental stages. **Table 14.6** summarizes the evidence regarding diet–cancer links.

Food choices interact with other lifestyle factors and also with genetics to affect cancer risk.[65] As the field of nutritional genomics evolves, it will enhance our ability to target dietary interventions for cancer prevention and treatment.[66] Until that time, general dietary guidelines from the American Cancer Society can be used.

Dietary and Lifestyle Factors for Reducing Cancer Risk

In 2002, the American Cancer Society released its *Nutrition and Physical Activity Guidelines for Cancer Prevention.*[67] These guidelines emphasize physical activity and weight control and also suggest how communities can provide opportunities for Americans to be physically active. Note that the four major recommendations are similar to the guidelines for reducing the risk of heart disease.

1. Eat a variety of healthful foods, with an emphasis on plant sources.

   - Eat five or more servings of a variety of vegetables and fruits each day.

   - Choose whole grains in preference to processed (refined) grains and sugars.

   - Limit consumption of red meats, especially processed meats and those high in fat.

   - Choose foods that help you maintain a healthful weight.

2. Adopt a physically active lifestyle.

   - *For adults:* At least 30 minutes of moderate activity per day for five or more days of the week. Note that current DRIs recommend more physical activity—60 minutes per day.[68]

   - *For children and adolescents:* At least 60 minutes per day of moderate to vigorous activity at least five days a week.

3. Maintain a healthful weight throughout life.

   - Balance caloric intake with physical activity.

   - Lose weight if you are currently overweight or obese.

4. If you drink alcoholic beverages, limit consumption.

   - Limit intake to no more than two drinks per day for men and one drink per day for women. Regular consumption of even a few drinks per week has been associated with an increased risk of breast cancer in women.

 **Table 14.6** **Strength of Evidence Linking Diet and Physical Activity to Cancer Risk at Various Sites**

Evidence	Decreased Risk	Increased Risk
Convincing	Physical activity (colon)	Overweight/obesity (esophagus, colorectum, breast, endometrium, kidney)
		Alcohol (oral cavity, pharynx, larynx, esophagus, liver, breast)
		Aflatoxin (liver)
		Chinese-style salted fish (nasopharynx)
Probable	Fruits and vegetables (oral cavity, esophagus, stomach, colorectal)	Preserved meat (colorectal)
	Physical activity (breast)	Salt-preserved foods and salt (stomach)
		Very hot (thermally) drinks and food (oral cavity, pharynx, esophagus)

Source: Diet, nutrition and the prevention of chronic diseases: a report of a joint WHO/FAO expert consultation. WHO Technical Report Series 916. Geneva, Switzerland, 2003.

aflatoxin A toxin produced by a mold that grows on crops, such as peanuts, tree nuts, corn, wheat, and oil seeds (like cottonseed).

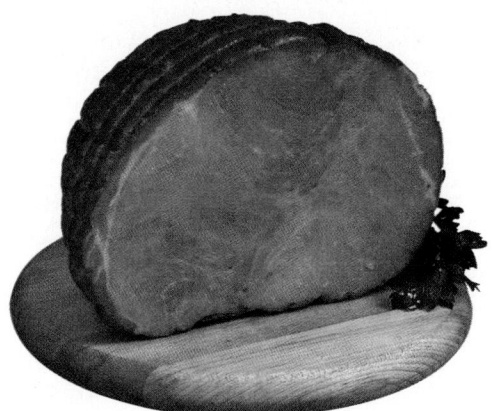

The WHO report *Diet, Nutrition and the Prevention of Chronic Diseases* supports these recommendations and adds four others: (1) reduce consumption of Chinese-style fermented salted fish, salt-preserved foods, and salt; (2) minimize exposure to **aflatoxin** in foods; (3) reduce consumption of preserved meat (e.g., sausages, salami, bacon, ham); and (4) avoid consuming foods or drinks when they are at a scalding hot temperature.[69]

Fat

High-fat diets have been associated with an increase in the risk of cancers of the colon and rectum, prostate, and endometrium. The association between high-fat diets and breast cancer appears to be much weaker. The Nurses' Health Study followed more than 121,000 women for 14 years and found no evidence that higher total fat intake was associated with an increased risk of breast cancer.[70] These results call into question theories that link dietary fat with other cancers. Others, however, have questioned the dietary assessment methodology of the Nurses' Health Study, suggesting that the food frequency questionnaires used may not be a sensitive enough measure of fat intake.[71]

High intake of red meat (beef, pork, lamb) and processed meat (bacon, sausage, hot dogs, lunch meat) is associated with some types of colorectal cancer; long-term consumption of poultry and fish is associated with reduced risk.[72] High intake of red meat, total fat, and animal fat has been linked to prostate cancer.[73] Overall, calorie intake (and the resulting obesity from excess calories) may be a more important factor than fat intake.[74]

Vegetables and Fruits

Evidence that vegetable and fruit consumption reduces cancer risk has led to attempts to isolate specific nutrients and to administer these in pharmacological doses to high-risk populations. Most of these attempts have failed to prevent cancer and, in some cases, have produced adverse effects. Notable examples include the three randomized trials of beta-carotene for the prevention of lung cancer, undertaken because many observational epidemiological studies showed that people eating foods high in beta-carotene have a lower risk of lung cancer. Two of the clinical trials showed that smokers taking high-dose beta-carotene supplements developed lung cancer at higher rates than those taking a placebo,[75] while a third study showed no effect.[76] These findings support the idea that beta-carotene may be only a proxy for other single nutrients or combinations of nutrients found in whole foods and that taking a single nutrient in large amounts may be harmful.

It remains unclear which components of vegetables and fruits are most protective against cancer. Vegetables and fruits are complex foods, with each containing more than 100 potentially beneficial substances, including vitamins, minerals, and fiber. Specific phytochemicals, such as carotenoids, flavonoids, terpenes, sterols, indoles, and phenols, show benefit against certain cancers in experimental studies. (For more on phytochemicals, see the "Spotlight on Complementary and Alternative Nutrition.") In addition to having antioxidant effects, nutrients and other phytochemicals may inhibit multiplication of cancer cells, alter enzymes, inhibit the conversion of chemicals into toxins, and alter hormone metabolism. Until more is known about specific food components, however, the best advice is to eat five or more servings of a variety of vegetables and fruits in their various forms: fresh, frozen, canned, dried, and juiced.

Despite recommendations from numerous health agencies to eat at least five servings of vegetables and fruits each day, intake of these foods remains low among both adults and children.[77] In 1991, concern about low intake levels prompted a nationwide initiative—the National 5 a Day for Better

Health program—to help ensure that vegetables and fruits are available and accessible to all population groups and to increase vegetable and fruit consumption to five to nine servings per day.[78]

Whole Grains and Legumes

Whole grains are an important source of many vitamins and minerals, such as folate, vitamin E, and selenium, all of which have been associated with lower risk of colon cancer.[79] Whole grains are higher in fiber, certain vitamins, and minerals than are processed (refined) flour products. Although evidence for the association between fiber and cancer risk is inconclusive,[80] consumption of high-fiber foods is still recommended. Because the benefits that grain-based foods impart may derive from their other nutrients and phytochemicals, as well as from fiber, it is best to obtain fiber from whole grains—and vegetables and fruits—rather than from fiber supplements.

Beans and other legumes are excellent sources of many vitamins and minerals, protein, and fiber. Legumes are especially rich in nutrients and phytochemicals that may protect against cancer[81] and can be a useful low-fat, high-protein alternative to meat.

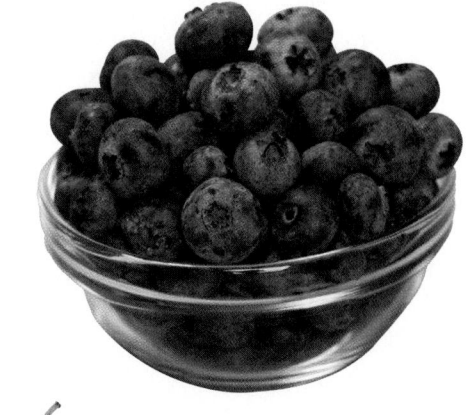

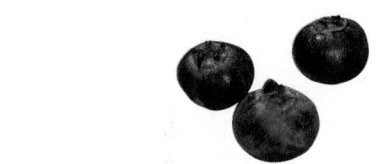

Putting It All Together

Some cancer risk factors can be avoided. Others, such as inherited factors, are unavoidable, but it may be helpful to be aware of them. People can help protect themselves by avoiding known risk factors whenever possible. They can also talk with their doctors about regular checkups and the value of cancer screening tests (see **Figure 14.9**). Reducing both the number of new cancer cases and the death rates from cancer are key objectives of Healthy People 2010.

To reduce your cancer risk, eat a moderately low-fat diet and increase your consumption of fruits, vegetables, and whole grains. Maintain a healthy weight, exercise regularly, don't smoke, and don't use alcohol excessively. If these recommendations are beginning to sound like a broken record, you're right—the same lifestyle changes that reduce risk of atherosclerosis and hypertension can reduce risk of cancer.

Key Concepts: *Cancer develops when something alters cellular DNA so that cells divide and multiply uncontrollably. Both genetic factors and environmental factors, including diet, influence cancer risk. Although the evidence linking dietary fats with cancer is contradictory, many other dietary factors play key roles in reducing risk. Strategies for reducing cancer risk include eating more fruits, vegetables, and whole grains; increasing physical activity; maintaining a healthy weight; and limiting alcohol consumption.*

Diabetes Mellitus

Almost everyone knows someone who has diabetes. An estimated 17 million people—6.2 percent of the population—in the United States have diabetes mellitus. Although an estimated 11.1 million have been diagnosed, unfortunately 5.9 million people (or one-third) do not realize that they have this serious, lifelong condition.

What Is Diabetes?

Diabetes is a disorder of carbohydrate metabolism—the way our bodies use digested carbohydrates for growth and energy. Recall from Chapter 4, "Carbohydrates," that carbohydrates in food are digested and absorbed, and

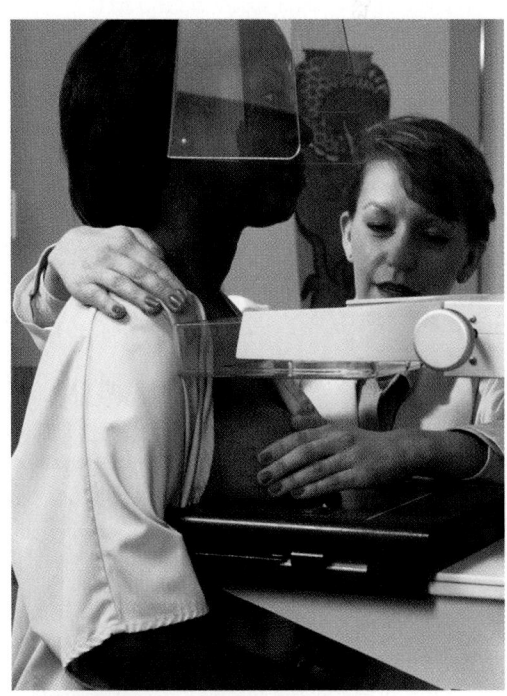

Figure 14.9 **Cancer screening tests.** Mammograms can detect breast cancer at an early stage and improve chances for successful treatment.

end up as glucose in the blood. Glucose is a major source of fuel for the body. After digestion, glucose passes into the bloodstream and into cells, where it is used for growth and energy. For glucose to get into most types of cells, insulin must be present. Insulin is a hormone produced by the pancreas.

When we eat carbohydrates, the pancreas should automatically produce the right amount of insulin to move glucose from blood into our cells. In people with diabetes, however, the pancreas either produces little or no insulin, or the cells do not respond appropriately to the insulin that is produced. As a result, glucose builds up in the blood, causing **hyperglycemia**—an abnormally high blood glucose level that is the hallmark of diabetes mellitus.

Because the overly abundant blood glucose is unable to enter starving cells and fuel their needs, diabetes often is called a disease of "starvation in the midst of plenty." In an ironic twist of fate, these starving cells signal the liver to make more glucose, worsening the hyperglycemia. The kidneys are taxed beyond their capacities to reabsorb glucose, and the excess spills into the urine, where it can be detected by urine glucose tests. Thus, even though the blood contains large amounts of glucose, the body loses access to its main source of fuel.

Unable to use glucose, cells turn to other energy sources—fat and protein. But these options can lead to other problems. Excessive use of fat as an energy source, without available glucose in the cell, causes ketosis and acidosis, dangerously high acidity levels in the blood. Use of muscle proteins causes muscle wasting and weakness. Abnormalities in fat and protein metabolism often accompany hyperglycemia.[82]

Over time, abnormally high blood glucose concentrations cause damage. Excess glucose in the blood reacts with and damages body proteins and tissues, especially in the eyes, kidneys, nerves, and blood vessels. Complications of diabetes can contribute to degenerative conditions such as peripheral vascular disease (disease of blood vessels that supply the feet and legs), deterioration of the eye and eventual blindness, kidney disease, and progressive nerve damage. Diabetes is responsible for 50 percent of all amputations of the lower extremities and 25 percent of all kidney failure in adults.[83] Diabetes is also the leading cause of blindness in adults.[84] People with diabetes are four times more likely to develop premature heart disease than people without diabetes. In the United States and Canada, diabetes is one of the leading contributors to death and disability.

Diagnosis of Diabetes Mellitus

A diagnosis of diabetes mellitus is usually made by measuring plasma glucose concentration either after an overnight fast, as part of an oral glucose tolerance test (OGTT) (see **Figure 14.10**), or any time of the day if a patient presents with symptoms of diabetes. The classic symptoms of diabetes mellitus are polyuria (excessive urination), polydipsia (excessive thirst), and unexplained weight loss, sometimes with polyphagia (excessive eating). The diagnostic criteria for diabetes mellitus are shown in **Table 14.7**.

Three major types of diabetes exist:

1. *Type 1 diabetes*. Type 1 diabetes usually is diagnosed in children and young adults and was previously known as insulin-dependent diabetes (IDDM) or juvenile diabetes. In type 1 diabetes, the body fails to produce insulin, the hormone that "unlocks" cells, allowing glucose to enter and fuel them. Roughly 5 to 10 percent of Americans who are diagnosed with diabetes have type 1 diabetes.

hyperglycemia [HIGH-per-gly-SEE-me-uh] Abnormally high concentration of glucose in the blood.

type 1 diabetes Diabetes that occurs when the body's immune system attacks beta cells in the pancreas, causing them to lose their ability to make insulin.

type 2 diabetes Diabetes that occurs when target cells (e.g., fat and muscle cells) lose the ability to respond normally to insulin.

pre-diabetes Blood glucose levels higher than normal but not high enough to warrant a diagnosis of diabetes.

insulin resistance State in which enough insulin is produced but cells do not respond to the action of insulin. Also called insulin insensitivity.

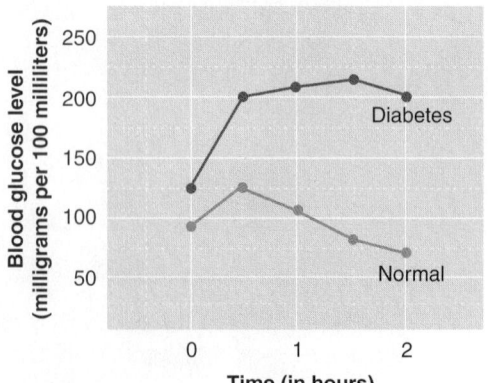

Figure 14.10 **Glucose tolerance test.** A glucose tolerance test measures the level of glucose in the blood following consumption of a standard dose of glucose. Glucose tolerance tests are used to diagnose diabetes.

2. *Type 2 diabetes.* In type 2 diabetes, either the body does not produce enough insulin or cells ignore the insulin. Type 2 diabetes was previously known as non-insulin-dependent diabetes (NIDDM) or adult-onset diabetes. Approximately 90 to 95 percent (16 million) of all Americans with diabetes mellitus have type 2 diabetes.

   • *Pre-diabetes.* Pre-diabetes is a condition in which a person's blood glucose levels are higher than normal but not high enough to warrant a diagnosis of type 2 diabetes. At least 16 million Americans have pre-diabetes, in addition to the 17 million with diabetes.

3. *Gestational diabetes.* Gestational diabetes occurs in a pregnant woman who has never had diabetes, but who develops hyperglycemia during pregnancy. It affects approximately 4 percent of all pregnant women—about 135,000 cases in the United States each year.

Type 1 Diabetes Mellitus

Type 1 diabetes usually occurs in people younger than 30 and often develops suddenly. People with type 1 diabetes lack insulin, usually because an autoimmune response has destroyed insulin-producing cells of the pancreas. Symptoms include excessive thirst, frequent urination, rapid weight loss, and blurred vision.[85] When blood glucose levels rise, glucose spills into the urine, taking water with it and causing frequent urination and increased thirst. Although blood glucose levels are high, the lack of insulin prevents glucose from entering cells to be burned for energy. The result is weight loss and feelings of hunger.

People with type 1 diabetes require lifelong, daily insulin injections balanced with a healthful diet and regular exercise to maintain blood glucose levels in the normal range. Because exercise lowers blood glucose levels, individuals must consider the timing of exercise in addition to food intake and insulin injections to avoid lowering blood glucose levels excessively.

Type 2 Diabetes Mellitus

When type 2 diabetes is diagnosed, the pancreas usually is producing enough insulin, but, for unknown reasons, the body cannot use the insulin efficiently, a condition called **insulin resistance**. After several years, insulin production decreases. The result is the same as for type 1 diabetes—glucose builds up in the blood and the body cannot use its main source of fuel efficiently. Type 2 diabetes is often part of a metabolic syndrome that includes obesity, elevated blood pressure, and high levels of blood triglycerides. (See the "Metabolic Syndrome" section later in this chapter.)

In contrast to the sudden onset of type 1 diabetes, the symptoms of type 2 diabetes develop gradually, and some people may not show symptoms for many years. Symptoms of type 2 diabetes may eventually include fatigue or nausea, frequent urination, unusual thirst, weight loss, blurred vision, frequent infections, and slow healing of wounds or sores.

Pre-diabetes

Before people develop type 2 diabetes, they almost always have pre-diabetes—impaired glucose tolerance that results in a blood glucose level that is higher than normal yet not high enough to be diagnosed as diabetes. Recent research has shown that some long-term damage to the body, especially to the heart and circulatory system, may already be occurring during the pre-diabetes stage.

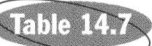

Table 14.7 Diagnostic Criteria for Diabetes Mellitus

Symptoms of diabetes plus casual plasma glucose concentration ≥ 200 mg/dL (11.1 mmol/L)

or

Fasting plasma glucose ≥ 126 mg/dL (7.0 mmol/L)

or

Two-hour postload glucose ≥ 200 mg/dL (11.1 mmol/L) during an oral glucose tolerance test

Source: American Diabetes Association. Diagnosis and Classification of Diabetes Mellitus. *Diabetes Care.* 2007;30(suppl 1): S42–S47. Reprinted by permission.

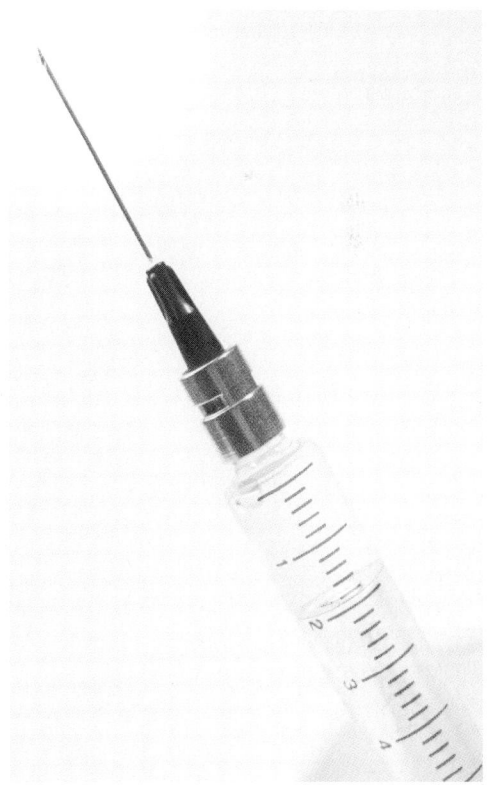

gestational diabetes A condition that results in high blood glucose levels during pregnancy.

People who have pre-diabetes are at increased risk for developing both type 2 diabetes and heart disease. Unless they take steps to prevent or delay diabetes, such as dietary changes, moderate weight loss, and regular exercise, many will develop type 2 diabetes within 10 years.

Gestational Diabetes Mellitus

Pregnant women who have never had diabetes before but who develop impaired glucose tolerance during pregnancy are said to have **gestational diabetes**. Although the cause of gestational diabetes remains unknown, researchers have uncovered certain clues. The placenta produces hormones that help the baby develop. Unfortunately, these hormones also block the action of the mother's insulin in her body. This insulin resistance makes it difficult for the mother's body to use insulin and can triple the amount of insulin needed to get sufficient glucose into her cells.

Gestational diabetes usually goes away after pregnancy. Once a woman has had gestational diabetes, however, her chances are 2 in 3 that it will return in future pregnancies. In a few women, pregnancy reveals preexisting type 1 or type 2 diabetes. These women will need to continue diabetes treatment after pregnancy.

Many women who had gestational diabetes will develop type 2 diabetes later in life. Both forms of diabetes involve insulin resistance. Gestational diabetes occurs more often in African Americans, Native Americans, Hispanic Americans, and people with a family history of diabetes.

Key Concepts: *An estimated 17 million people in the United States have diabetes mellitus, a leading cause of death and disability. Unfortunately, 5.9 million of these people (or one-third) are unaware that they have the disease. Three major types of diabetes have been identified: type 1, type 2, and gestational diabetes. Type 1, the most severe form, requires a daily regimen of insulin, careful diet control, and physical activity. In type 2 diabetes, the treatment focuses on diet and weight loss. Gestational diabetes occurs during pregnancy but usually goes away after delivery.*

Risk Factors for Diabetes

Anyone with a family history of diabetes has an increased risk. (See **Table 14.8.**) In most cases of type 1 diabetes, people must inherit risk factors from both parents, and whites have the highest rate of this disease.[86] Yet genes do not tell the complete story. When one identical twin has type 1 diabetes, for example, the other twin gets the disease at most only half the time.[87] Possible environmental triggers include exposure to cold weather and certain viruses or other infectious agents that activate the immune system. Early diet also may play a role. For example, type 1 diabetes is less common in people who were breastfed and began eating solid food at older ages.[88]

A family history of type 2 diabetes is one of the strongest risk factors for getting the disease.[89] Type 2 diabetes occurs most frequently in Native Americans, Hispanic Americans, and African Americans. But this increased risk seems to matter only in people who follow a Western lifestyle—a lifestyle characterized by too much fat; too little fruits, vegetables, and fiber; and too little exercise. In contrast, people who live in areas that have not become Westernized tend not to get type 2 diabetes, no matter how high their genetic risk.[90]

The risk of developing type 2 diabetes increases progressively as body fat increases, especially around the midsection. The dramatic surge in obesity rates in the United States is a major reason that the incidence of type 2 dia-

 **Table 14.8** Risk Factors for Type 1 and Type 2 Diabetes Mellitus

Risk Factors for Type 1 Diabetes

- First-degree relative (parent, sibling) with type 1 diabetes

Risk Factors for Type 2 Diabetes

- Age ≥ 45 years
- Overweight (BMI ≥ 25 kg/m^2)
- First-degree relative with diabetes
- Sedentary lifestyle
- Ethnicity: African American, Latino, Native American, Asian American, Pacific Islander
- Previously identified pre-diabetes
- History of gestational diabetes
- Hypertension (≥ 140/90 mm Hg)
- HDL cholesterol level ≤ 35 mg/dL and/or triglyceride level ≥ 250 mg/dL
- History of vascular disease

Source: American Diabetes Association. Position statement: prevention of type 1 diabetes mellitus. *Diabetes Care.* 2003;26(suppl 1):S140; and Position statement: the prevention or delay of type 2 diabetes. *Diabetes Care.* 2003;26(suppl 1):S62–S69.

betes has tripled since 1970.[91] Compared to a normal-weight person, an obese person can have 40 times the risk of type 2 diabetes.[92] Most, but not all, people diagnosed with type 2 diabetes are obese at the time of their diagnosis. Unfortunately, as more children and adolescents become overweight, type 2 diabetes is becoming more common in young people. Contrary to popular opinion, high sugar or high carbohydrate intake does not by itself cause diabetes as long as it does not contribute to excess energy intake and obesity.

Do other dietary factors make a difference? The Nurses' Health Study suggests that total, saturated, and monounsaturated fat intakes are not associated with risk of type 2 diabetes in women, but that *trans* fatty acids increase risk and polyunsaturated fatty acids reduce risk.[93] Other studies have shown that high saturated fat intake is associated with higher risk of impaired glucose tolerance and higher fasting glucose and insulin levels.[94] Numerous studies have shown a protective effect of increased consumption of nonstarch polysaccharides (fiber).[95] **Table 14.9** summarizes the evidence linking lifestyle factors and type 2 diabetes risk.

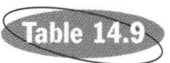 **Table 14.9** Strength of Evidence Related to Lifestyle and Type 2 Diabetes Risk

Evidence	Decreased Risk	Increased Risk
Convincing	Voluntary weight loss in overweight/obese people	Overweight and obesity
	Physical activity	Abdominal obesity
		Physical inactivity
		Maternal diabetes
Probable	Nonstarch polysaccharides	Saturated fats
		Intrauterine growth retardation

Source: Diet, nutrition and the prevention of chronic diseases: a report of a joint WHO/FAO expert consultation. WHO Technical Report Series 916. Geneva, Switzerland, 2003.

Dietary and Lifestyle Factors for Reducing Diabetes Risk

The best measures for preventing pre-diabetes and obesity-related type 2 diabetes are a healthful diet and regular exercise. Reducing excess body fat will improve glucose tolerance and reduce related risk factors for heart disease. Regular exercise will improve carbohydrate and lipid metabolism and increase insulin sensitivity. (See **Figure 14.11**.) In addition, exercise improves blood flow to the extremities, bringing blood pressure down to normal levels and reducing risk of heart disease.

Fyi The Pima Indians

FOR YOUR INFORMATION

The Pima Indians of Arizona, along with teams of scientists and doctors from the National Institutes of Health, have been responsible for unraveling some of the complex interactions between genetics, lifestyle, and disease. Thirty years ago, Pima volunteers and scientists began to work together to try to understand why the Pimas have extremely high rates of obesity as well as the highest known rate of type 2 diabetes of any community in the world. Half of all adult Pima Indians have diabetes, and 95 percent of those with diabetes are obese. Complications of diabetes such as kidney disease are extremely common in the Pima community.[1]

The ravages of diabetes were not always a problem for the Pimas. Hundreds of years ago they developed a sophisticated irrigation system that allowed them to cultivate such crops as wheat, beans, squash, and cotton. Hard physical work and a low-fat, high-fiber diet were the norm. Obesity and diabetes were essentially nonexistent. The Pimas lived this traditional lifestyle until the late nineteenth century, when American farmers living upstream diverted their water supply. Their way of life was seriously disrupted, resulting in poverty and severe malnutrition. The U.S. government gave the Pimas lard, sugar, and flour to help them survive. Although life improved for the Pimas as the economy rebounded after World War II, the increasing prosperity was accompanied by high-fat and sugary foods, more leisure time, and less physical work, resulting in an epidemic of obesity and diabetes.

Modern Pima Indians are not much different from most Americans in their diet and exercise habits, but they have much higher rates of obesity and diabetes. Scientists have postulated that they have inherited "thrifty genes" that allow them to retain fat more easily than most people. This genetic trait helped the ancestors of modern Pima Indians survive the hard times when food was not plentiful. During times of plenty, the "thrifty genes" allowed them to store extra fat so that they would not starve when famine struck. Unfortunately, the genetic traits that once helped them survive became a liability in modern times, when high-fat/high-calorie foods are readily available and the need for physical work is greatly diminished. In the 1890s, the traditional Pima Indian diet consisted of only about 15 percent fat; today, it is nearly 40 percent fat. Genetically, this is a recipe for disaster.

Although the specific genes for the inheritance of type 2 diabetes have not yet been located, several genes that play a role in insulin resistance (a major factor in the development of type 2 diabetes) have been found to be much more common in Pima Indians than in the general U.S. population. Pima Indians with diabetes develop kidney failure more often and at a younger age than non–Native Americans with diabetes. Ongoing research seeks to identify the genetic reasons for the high rate of kidney disease among Pima families.[2]

Further evidence for the effects of diet and exercise on health is seen when the Arizona Pimas are compared with a genetically similar population in Mexico. The Pimas who currently live in Arizona migrated there from the Sierra Madre mountains of Mexico hundreds of years ago. A Pima community still exists in a remote part of those mountains. These Mexican Pimas live much as their ancestors did, farming mostly by hand and eating a traditional diet that is very low in fat and high in fiber. Although the people in this region are genetically similar to the Arizona Pimas, obesity and diabetes are rarely seen among them.[3]

The challenge for the Arizona Pimas is to incorporate some of the healthy practices of their ancestors into their modern way of life. This is really the same challenge faced by most of us in the twenty-first century. Until the last 100 years, most humans had to engage in heavy physical work on a daily basis to survive. Our bodies simply were not designed to handle the amount of high-fat, high-calorie foods that most Americans eat, especially when sedentary pursuits occupy the bulk of our time.

1 National Institute of Diabetes and Digestive and Kidney Diseases. The Pima Indians: pathfinders for health. www.niddk.nih.gov/health/diabetes/pima/obesity/obesity.htm. Accessed 8/7/06.

2 National Diabetes Information Clearinghouse. American Indians, Alaska natives, and diabetes. http://www.niddk.nih.gov/health/diabetes/pubs/amindian/amindian.htm. Accessed 8/7/06.

3 National Institute of Diabetes and Digestive and Kidney Diseases. Op. cit.

The Diabetes Prevention Program study of more than 3,000 people, 45 percent of whom were minorities, found that people who received intensive lifestyle intervention were able to reduce their risk of developing type 2 diabetes by 58 percent. The lifestyle interventions included walking or other moderate physical exercise for about 30 minutes per day and weight reduction of 5 to 7 percent.[96]

Management of Diabetes

Before the discovery of insulin in 1921, everyone with type 1 diabetes died within a few years after diagnosis. Although insulin therapy is not a cure, its discovery represented the first major breakthrough in diabetes treatment.

Today, healthy eating, physical activity, and insulin delivery via injection (see **Figure 14.12**) or an insulin pump are the basic therapies for type 1 diabetes. The amount of insulin must be balanced with food intake and daily activities. Blood glucose concentrations must be closely monitored.

Healthy eating, physical activity, and blood glucose testing are the basic management tools for type 2 diabetes, and weight loss often restores normal glucose metabolism.[97] Exercise increases the sensitivity of body cells to insulin, so the body needs less insulin to let glucose into cells. If diet and exercise fail to maintain blood glucose levels in the normal range, people with type 2 diabetes sometimes need medications to either increase insulin production or improve glucose uptake by cells. In some cases, insulin is needed to normalize blood glucose levels.

Nutrition

Although people with diabetes have the same nutritional needs as anyone else, good diabetes control requires that they monitor their food intake carefully. By eating well-balanced meals in the correct amounts, people can keep their blood glucose levels as close to normal (non-diabetes level) as possible. The Exchange Lists for Meal Planning (see Appendix B) help people with diabetes plan their diets.

Specific meal plans should be based on an individual's usual food intake. People with type 1 diabetes should eat at about the same time each day and should try to be consistent regarding the types of food they choose. Keeping calories and carbohydrate intake consistent helps to prevent blood glucose levels from becoming too high or too low. People with type 2 diabetes should consume a diet that is well balanced and low in fat.

Having diabetes once meant a lifetime of meals that lacked the most pleasant aspect of taste: sweetness. Current recommendations suggest a diet with carbohydrates from fruits, vegetables, whole grains, legumes, and low-fat milk that is low in saturated and *trans* fat.[98] Although in the past dietary treatment of diabetes eliminated simple sugars from the diet, current recommendations allow individuals with diabetes to include moderate amounts of simple sugars in their diet as long as sugar intake does not contribute to excess energy intake and obesity.[99]

Putting It All Together

Researchers continue to search for the cause or causes of diabetes and ways to prevent and cure it. Some genetic markers for type 1 diabetes have been identified, and it is now possible to screen relatives of people with type 1 diabetes to see whether they are at increased risk of developing the disease. In the future, it may be possible to administer insulin through inhalers, a pill, or a patch. Devices also are being developed that can monitor blood glucose levels without having to prick a finger to get a blood sample.

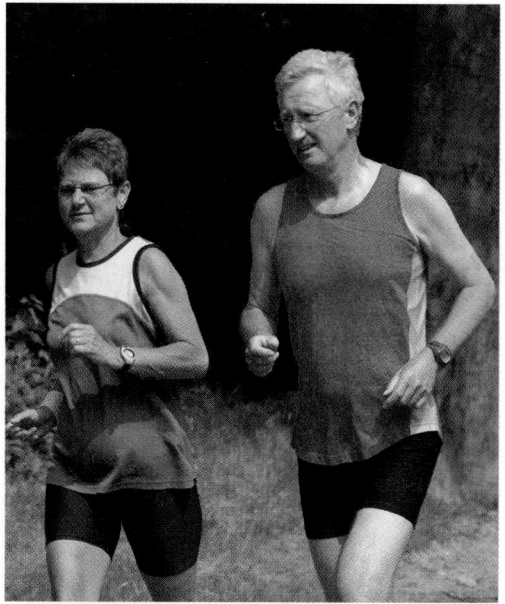

Figure 14.11 **Exercise and diabetes.** Regular physical activity improves glucose tolerance and helps reduce the risk of developing type 2 diabetes later in life.

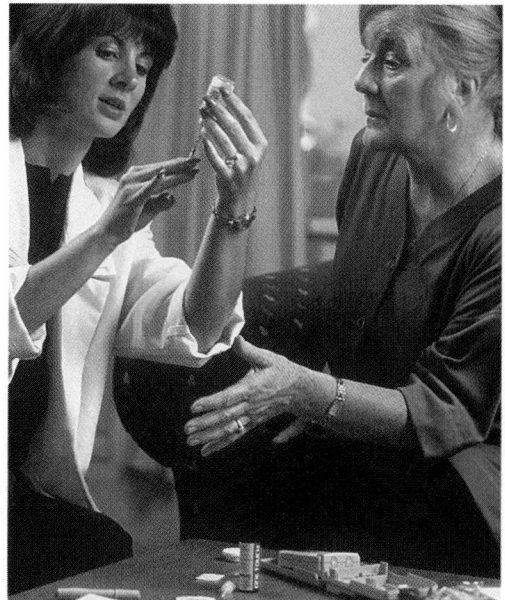

Figure 14.12 **Insulin injections.** In type 1 diabetes and some cases of type 2 diabetes, people need daily insulin injections to normalize blood glucose levels.

metabolic syndrome A cluster of at least three of the following risk factors for heart disease: hypertriglyceridemia (high blood triglycerides), low HDL cholesterol, hyperglycemia (high blood glucose), hypertension (high blood pressure), and excess abdominal fat.

For now, the challenge is to slow the rate at which diabetes incidence is increasing. Healthy People 2010 objectives include a reduction in incidence of diabetes along with the economic burden it presents. Results from the Diabetes Prevention Program show that relatively modest changes in weight and exercise can be enough to reduce diabetes incidence. We turn, once again, to advice encouraging healthful eating (consumption of more fruits, vegetables, and fiber), regular physical activity, and lifelong weight management.

Key Concepts: *Family history is a risk factor for both type 1 and type 2 diabetes. For type 2 diabetes, additional risk factors include increasing age, overweight, sedentary lifestyle, and ethnicity. Risk reduction can be achieved through healthy eating, modest weight loss, and increases in physical activity.*

Metabolic Syndrome

One in five adults in the United States has **metabolic syndrome**, and the prevalence will continue to grow because of the tendency toward a sedentary lifestyle, according to the Centers for Disease Control and Prevention.[100] By 2010, as many as 50 to 75 million Americans may exhibit the syndrome.[101] Metabolic syndrome is a cluster of at least three of the following signs:[102]

- *Excess abdominal fat:* For most men, a 40-inch waist or greater; for women, a waist of 35 inches or greater
- *High blood glucose:* At least 110 mg/dL after fasting
- *High serum triglycerides:* At least 150 mg/dL
- *Low HDL cholesterol:* Less than 40 mg/dL for men; less than 50 mg/dL for women
- *Elevated blood pressure:* 130 mm Hg or above systolic or 85 mm Hg or above diastolic

Taken individually, these risk factors may not look particularly serious. When you put them together, however, the problems rise substantially. Individuals with metabolic syndrome are at increased risk for both cardiovascular disease and type 2 diabetes.[103] More study is needed to understand the relationship between the risk factors embodied in metabolic syndrome, but researchers have identified people with metabolic syndrome as having the greatest risk of death from heart attack.

Although some scientists think that metabolic syndrome is genetically based, it is unlikely that metabolic syndrome results from a single cause. The primary underlying risk factors appear to be insulin resistance and abdominal obesity. For many people, poor diet and lack of physical activity combined with a genetic predisposition lead to the development of the syndrome. The high prevalence of metabolic syndrome underscores an urgent need to develop comprehensive efforts directed at controlling the obesity epidemic and improving physical activity levels.

People with metabolic syndrome should work with their doctors to

- Monitor blood glucose, lipoproteins, and blood pressure
- Achieve and maintain a healthy body weight and increase physical activity—both are time-tested methods of improving insulin sensitivity, blood pressure, and lipoprotein levels
- Treat diabetes and hyperlipidemia according to established guidelines

- Choose drug therapy for hypertension with care—different medications have different effects on insulin sensitivity

Key Concepts: *Metabolic syndrome, associated with an increased risk of death from heart attack, is a cluster including at least three of the following signs: abdominal fat, elevated blood glucose, elevated triglycerides and HDL cholesterol, and elevated blood pressure. A poor diet and sedentary lifestyle combined with a genetic predisposition are thought to be the underlying causes.*

Osteoporosis

Osteoporosis is a major public health problem, affecting more than 10 million Americans over the age of 50, with another 34 million people at risk.[104] Without a concerted effort to reduce risk, it is estimated that by the year 2020 half of all Americans over 50 will either have osteoporosis or be at high risk. Although 80 percent of those with osteoporosis are women, by age 75 one-third of all men have osteoporosis. However, women are most at risk for bone fractures related to osteoporosis. Experts estimate that 40 percent of U.S. white women aged 50 or older will experience a spine, hip, or wrist fracture.[105] Although we often associate osteoporosis with being elderly, the stage for its emergence is actually set much earlier in life, much like other chronic diseases. Fortunately, diet and lifestyle changes can help to delay the onset of osteoporosis and may prevent related fractures.

What Is Osteoporosis?

Osteoporosis means "porous bone." It's a good description because bone mass or density declines and bone quality deteriorates, leaving the bones fragile and vulnerable to fracture. The hip, spine, and wrist bones are especially vulnerable. Often called a "silent disease," osteoporosis develops over several years without outward symptoms. Eventually bone loss makes bones so weak that they break with a mild strain, bump, or a fall. In fact, in some cases, the break may occur first and cause the fall!

Bone strength depends on two main features: bone density and bone quality. Bone density is determined by peak bone mass and amount of bone loss. Bone quality refers to architecture, turnover, damage accumulation (e.g., microfractures), and mineralization. Currently, no accurate measure of overall bone strength exists. Bone mineral density (BMD) is frequently used as a proxy measure and accounts for approximately 70 percent of bone strength.

Low bone mineral density is an important predictor of future bone fractures. Other predictors include a history of falls, low physical function such as slow gait speed and decreased leg muscle strength, impaired cognition, impaired vision, and the presence of environmental hazards (e.g., throw rugs). Some risks for fracture, such as age, low BMI, and low levels of physical activity, probably increase the rate of fractures through decreased bone density, increased propensity to fall, and inability to absorb impact.

Risk Factors for Osteoporosis

A common misperception is that osteoporosis always results from excessive bone loss. Bone loss commonly occurs as men and women age; however, a person who does not reach optimal (i.e., peak) bone mass during childhood and adolescence may develop osteoporosis without the occurrence of accelerated bone loss. Hence suboptimal bone growth in childhood and

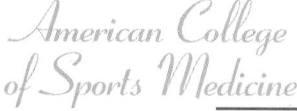

American College of Sports Medicine

Physical Activity and Bone Health

Maintaining a vigorous level of physical activity across the lifespan should be viewed as an essential component of the prescription for achieving and maintaining optimal bone health. The following exercise prescription is recommended to help preserve bone health during adulthood:

- Mode: weight-bearing endurance activities (tennis; stair climbing; jogging, at least intermittently during walking), activities that involve jumping (volleyball, basketball), and resistance exercise (weight lifting)
- Intensity: moderate to high, in terms of bone-loading forces
- Frequency: weight-bearing endurance activities 3–5 times per week; resistance exercise 2–3 times per week
- Duration: 30–60 minutes per day of a combination of weight-bearing endurance activities, activities that involve jumping, and resistance exercise that targets all major muscle groups

Source: Kohrt, WM, Bloomfield, SA, Little, KD, et al. American College of Sports Medicine Stand. Physical activity and bone health. *Med Sci Sports Exerc.* 2004;36:1985–1996. Reprinted with permission.

Table 14.10	Risk Factors for Osteoporosis

Advanced age

Female

Thin and/or small frame

Family history of osteoporosis

Early menopause, whether natural or surgically induced

Low testosterone levels in men

Abnormal absence of menstrual periods (amenorrhea)

Anorexia nervosa or bulimia nervosa

Medical conditions, such as thyroid disease, rheumatoid arthritis, and problems that block intestinal absorption of calcium

Use of certain medications, such as corticosteroids and anticonvulsants

Insufficient dietary calcium

Lack of weight-bearing exercise

Cigarette smoking

Excessive use of alcohol or caffeine

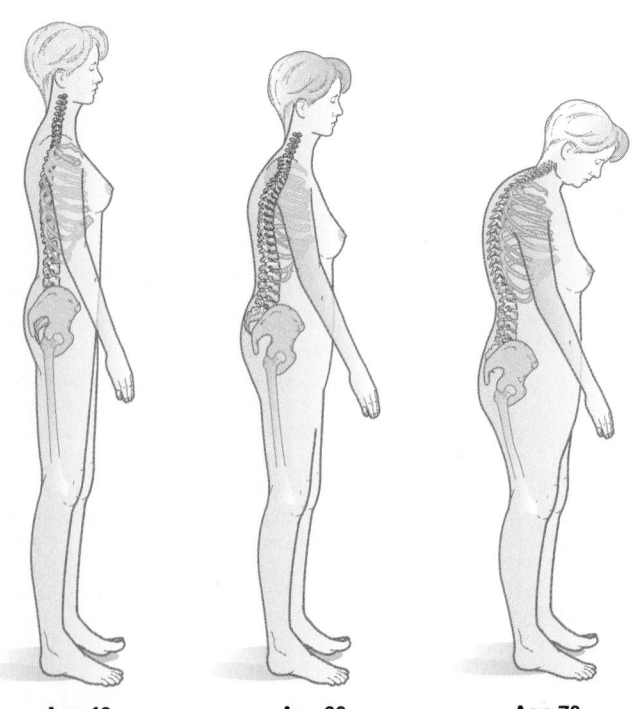

| Age 40 | Age 60 | Age 70 |

Figure 14.13 Progression of dowager's hump.

adolescence is as important as bone loss to the development of osteoporosis. **Table 14.10** lists the risk factors for osteoporosis.

Bone mass typically peaks sometime around age 30. Starting in midlife, bone breakdown exceeds bone formation, and the progressive loss of bone begins. If earlier calcium and vitamin D intakes maximized bone mass, then when bone loss begins you are likely to be a long way from low bone density and fractures.

Because declining estrogen levels accelerate bone loss, postmenopausal women have the highest risk of developing osteoporosis. By age 65, some women have lost half their skeletal mass, and they may show deformities of the upper spine, known as a "dowager's hump." (See **Figures 14.13** and **14.14**.) Women who reach menopause with low bone mass have a greatly increased risk of fractures.

Many medical disorders, such as genetic disorders, endocrine disorders, congestive heart failure, kidney disease, and alcoholism, as well as administration of certain drugs such as steroids, also may lead to osteoporosis and increased fracture risk.

Dietary and Lifestyle Factors for Reducing Osteoporosis Risk

The main factor in reducing risk of osteoporosis and related fractures is maximum peak bone mass. Dietary components such as calcium and vitamin D help to achieve and maintain bone mass. Engaging in physical activity, especially weight-bearing exercise, helps to increase peak bone mass early in life and helps to maintain muscle strength and coordination that will reduce risk for falls later in life.

Calcium

Calcium is important for attaining peak bone mass and for preventing and treating osteoporosis. Adequate calcium intake throughout life helps prevent osteoporosis, and good calcium intake during childhood and adolescence helps maximize peak bone mass. Even in adulthood, adequate calcium slows bone loss, and it reduces fracture rates in postmenopausal women.

Calcium is clearly an important nutrient in bone health, but it's not the only one. Normal mineralization and maintenance of bone also require vitamins D, A, and K; phosphorus, fluoride, and magnesium; and protein.

Vitamin D

You need vitamin D for calcium absorption and bone maintenance. Because aging limits the ability to manufacture active vitamin D, older people should use vitamin D–fortified foods such as milk or consider taking vitamin D supplements. Phytate and oxalate, caffeine, and smoking can reduce calcium absorption or increase excretion rates.

Vitamin D deficiency, which occurs more often in postmenopausal women and older Americans,[106] has been associated with a greater incidence of hip fractures.[107] Because bone loss increases the risk of fractures, vitamin D supplementation may help prevent osteoporotic fractures.[108] It's important to be cautious with vitamin D supplements, because toxicity can quickly develop. For more on vitamin D, see Chapter 9, "Fat-Soluble Vitamins."

Vitamin A

Although vitamin A is essential for normal bone formation, animal, human, and laboratory research findings suggest an association between excessive vitamin A intake and weaker bones.[109] Researchers have also noticed that worldwide, the highest incidence of osteoporosis occurs in northern Europe, a population with a high intake of vitamin A.[110] However, this region has lower levels of sun exposure, which leads to decreased biosynthesis of vitamin D and may be at least partially responsible for these findings.

In the Nurses' Health Study, women who consumed the most vitamin A in foods and supplements (greater than or equal to 3,000 micrograms per day as retinol—more than triple the recommended intake) had a significantly increased risk of experiencing a hip fracture compared with those consuming the least amount (less than 1,250 micrograms per day of retinol).[111] This increased risk was attributed to retinol and not to vitamin A as beta-carotene.

On the other hand, the Centers for Disease Control and Prevention reviewed data from the Third National Health and Nutrition Examination survey (NHANES III), 1988–1994, to determine whether any association existed between bone mineral density and fasting blood levels of retinyl esters, a form of vitamin A.[112] Blood levels of retinyl esters in 5,800 participants were in the normal range, and researchers did not identify any significant associations between bone mineral density and blood levels of retinyl esters.

No evidence indicates an association between beta-carotene intake and increased risk of osteoporosis. Instead, current evidence points to a possible association with vitamin A as retinol only. Because current studies yield conflicting results, additional research is needed to clarify the association between high levels of vitamin A intake and osteoporosis.[113]

Exercise

Regular weight-bearing exercise enhances bone remodeling and strength. Exercise helps maximize bone mass when you're young and will slow bone loss during your later years. To promote bone health and slow the development of osteoporosis, fitness experts make the following suggestions:

- Exercise should be weight-bearing and should put stress on bones. Examples include walking and running.

- For continued improvement, exercise intensity should increase progressively.

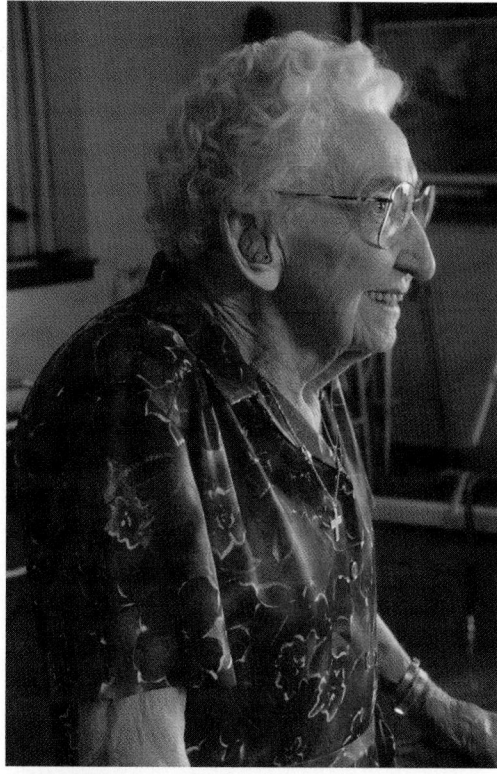

Figure 14.14 **Dowager's hump.** In people with osteoporosis, the bones in the upper spine develop small compression fractures. These bones heal into wedge shapes, and the upper spine assumes a deformed, curved shape known as a "dowager's hump."

Quick Bites

Lost in Space

Knowing that stress on bones maintains their strength, what would you guess happens in the gravity-free environment of outer space? Experience with prolonged space travel has made it clear that extensive bone and mineral loss are one health hazard of living without gravity's constant pull. Interestingly, changes in non-weight-bearing bones were not seen in studies of space travelers. As humans spend longer periods in space, scientists will be challenged to discover how to preserve bone strength without the constant stimulation of gravity on weight-bearing bones.

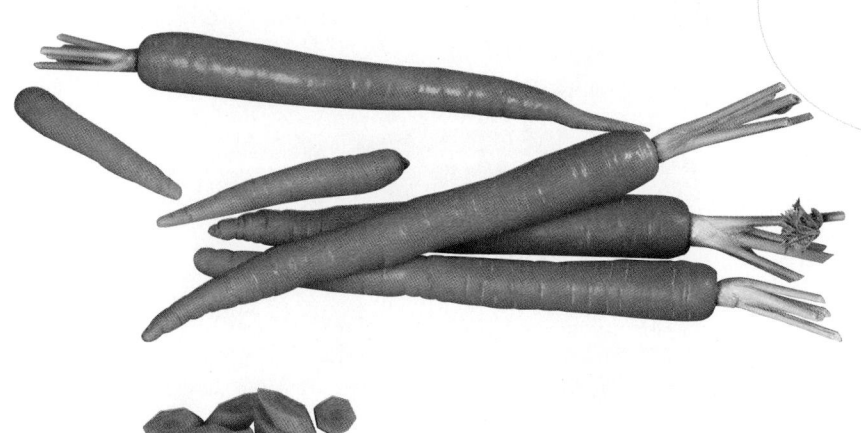

American Dietetic Association

Nutrition and Women's Health

It is the position of the American Dietetic Association (ADA) and Dietitians of Canada (DC) that women have specific nutritional needs and vulnerabilities and, as such, are at unique risk for various nutrition-related diseases and conditions. Therefore, ADA and DC strongly support research, health promotion activities, health services, and advocacy efforts that will enable women to adopt desirable nutrition practices for optimal health.

J Am Diet Assoc. 2004;104:984–1001.
Reprinted with permission.

- People with small total bone mass have the greatest potential for improvement.

- There is a maximum achievable bone density. As this point is approached, greater efforts are needed to achieve smaller gains.

- Discontinuing an exercise program reverses the benefits.

Putting It All Together

Osteoporosis is a debilitating degenerative disease that contributes to poor quality of life in elders. Although bone loss with age is a major contributor to osteoporosis, maximizing peak bone mass early in life can go a long way toward preventing or at least delaying osteoporosis. Reducing the proportion of adults with osteoporosis is one of the Healthy People 2010 objectives.

To improve your bone health, the U.S. Surgeon General suggests the following: Eat foods rich in calcium and vitamin D, be physically active every day, maintain a healthy body weight throughout your life, protect yourself from falls, avoid smoking and limit alcohol intake, and discuss increased risks with your doctor.[114] Postmenopausal women with low bone density may be advised to consider new drugs that prevent or reduce bone loss.[115]

Key Concepts: *Osteoporosis is the progressive loss of bone mass, resulting in fragile bones that break easily. Osteoporosis primarily affects postmenopausal women who have lower estrogen levels and accelerated rates of bone loss. Adequate calcium intake early in life helps maximize peak bone mass and reduces the risk of osteoporosis. Adequate amounts of vitamin D and regular exercise also are important for bone health.*

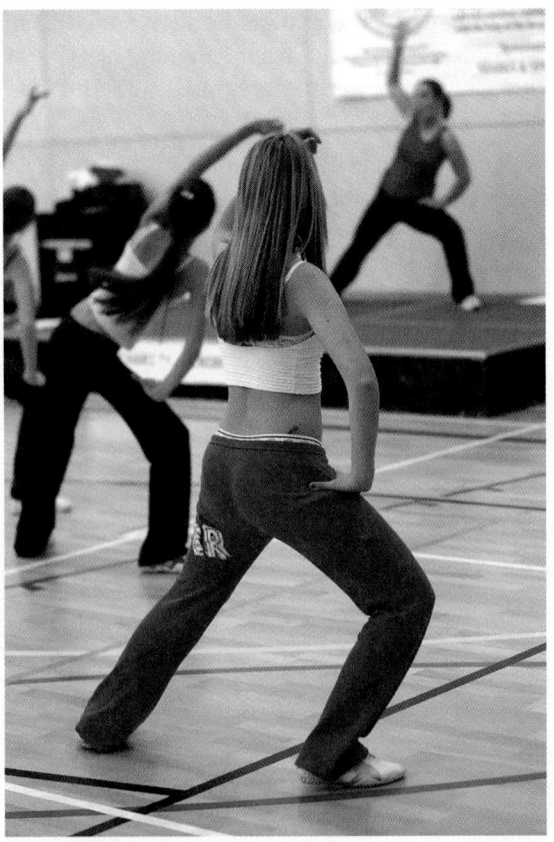

Label [to] **Table**

Sodium is found naturally in many foods, but processed foods account for most of the salt and sodium Americans consume. Processed foods with high amounts of salt include regular canned vegetables and soups, frozen dinners, lunch meats, instant and ready-to-eat cereals, and salty chips and other snacks. You can use food labels to choose products lower in sodium.

Compare Labels

Which of these two items is lower in sodium? To tell, check the Percent Daily Value.

The frozen peas are lower in sodium, with just 5% of the DV per $^1/_2$ cup serving. The canned peas have three times more sodium than the frozen peas: 16% of the DV in one serving.

Sodium also is found in many foods that may surprise you, such as baking soda, soy sauce, and monosodium glutamate (MSG), and sodium is found in some antacids—the range is wide. For more on sodium content of foods, see Chapter 11, "Water and Major Minerals."

Before trying salt substitutes, check with your doctor, especially if you have high blood pressure. Many salt substitutes contain potassium chloride and may be harmful for individuals who have certain medical conditions or who take diuretic medications.

Frozen Peas

Nutrition Facts

Serving Size: 1/2 cup
Servings Per Container: about 3

Amount Per Serving

Calories: 60	**Calories from Fat:** 0

	% Daily Value*
Total Fat 0g	
Saturated Fat 0g	0%
Trans Fat 0g	0%
Cholesterol 0mg	
Sodium 125mg	0%
Total Carbohydrate 11g	5%
Dietary Fiber 6g	4%
Sugars 5g	22%
Protein 5g	

Vitamin A 15%	Vitamin C 30%
Calcium 0%	Iron 6%

*Percent Daily Values are based on a 2,000 calorie diet.

Canned Peas

Nutrition Facts

Serving Size: 1/2 cup
Servings Per Container: about 3

Amount Per Serving

Calories: 60	**Calories from Fat:** 0

	% Daily Value*
	0%
	0%
Total Fat 0g	
Saturated Fat 0g	0%
Trans Fat 0g	16%
Cholesterol 0mg	4%
Sodium 380mg	14%
Total Carbohydrate 12g	
Dietary Fiber 3g	
Sugars 4g	
Protein 4g	

Vitamin A 6%	Vitamin C 10%
Calcium 2%	Iron 8%

*Percent Daily Values are based on a 2,000 calorie diet.

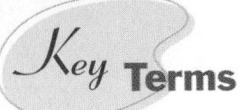

LEARNING *Portfolio* c h a p t e r 1 4

Key Terms

Study Points

> Genetics plays a part in nearly all human diseases.

> Much of the prevalence of cardiovascular disease and cancer can be attributed to smoking, consumption of a high-fat diet, and sedentary lifestyle.

> LDL and HDL cholesterol levels predict heart disease risks more accurately than do total cholesterol levels. Infection and the inflammatory process may play a role in heart disease, and C-reactive protein may offer a new assessment of CVD risk.

> Ways to reduce risk for CVD include stopping smoking, exercising daily, managing weight, controlling blood pressure, and eating a healthful diet. Studies of groups with generous fish intakes show a low incidence of heart disease. Antioxidants and moderate alcohol consumption also may help protect against heart disease.

> Because hypertension usually has no specific symptoms or early warning signs, it is often called a "silent killer."

> Added weight places greater demands on the cardiovascular system, so people who are overweight are at higher risk for hypertension. Rates of hypertension are higher in countries with high sodium intakes.

> The three phases in the development of cancer are initiation, promotion, and progression.

> Evidence shows that generous intake of vegetables and fruits reduces risk of cancer.

> An estimated 17 million people—6.2 percent of the population—in the United States have diabetes mellitus, and one-third of these are unaware of their condition.

> Three major types of diabetes are type 1, type 2, and gestational diabetes.

> The dramatic surge in obesity rates in the United States is a major reason why the incidence of type 2 diabetes has tripled since 1970.

> Dietary recommendations for people with diabetes emphasize consuming diets rich in complex carbohydrates (including fiber) and low in fat.

> Often called a "silent disease," osteoporosis develops over several years without outward symptoms or diagnosis. Osteoporosis affects more than 25 million Americans, making it a major public health problem.

> To promote bone health and slow the development of osteoporosis, fitness experts suggest that exercise should be weight-bearing and should put stress on bones. Examples include walking and running.

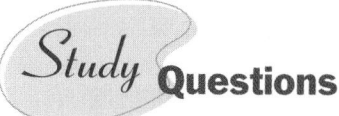

Study Questions

1. In what ways do diet and exercise affect your health?
2. What is the major goal of the Human Genome Project?
3. What are the diet-related guidelines for reducing heart disease risk?
4. How do high levels of homocysteine contribute to heart disease?
5. What are the risk factors for hypertension?
6. How can people with hypertension lower their blood pressure?
7. What is the difference between cancer initiation and cancer promotion?
8. What are the major types of diabetes? Describe the differences between them.
9. What is metabolic syndrome?
10. What vitamin and mineral are most important for maximizing bone mass and reducing risk of osteoporosis?

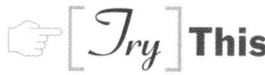

Learn CPR!

The CPR (cardiopulmonary resuscitation) courses given by the American Red Cross, the American Heart Association, your local fire department, and other groups may help you save a life some day. Anyone can take these courses and become qualified to perform CPR. Investigate CPR courses in your community, and sign up to take one.

What's Your Family History?

Look into your family medical history. Is there cardiovascular disease in your family, as indicated by premature deaths from heart attack, stroke, or congestive heart failure? Are there any cases of cancer in your family, and has anyone died of cancer? How about diabetes, hypertension, or osteoporosis? Interview your parents and other relatives and develop a history of chronic disease in your family. These diseases may be risk factors for you. Keep that point in mind as you consider whether you need to make lifestyle changes to stay healthy and avoid chronic disease.

What About Bobbie?

Bobbie recently found out that her mother (age 50) has been diagnosed with hypertension. Her mother's parents both had hypertension, and both died in their early 60s from heart attacks. Bobbie is worried about her mom, but also about her own risk for hypertension and heart disease. After reading about the effectiveness of the DASH diet in lowering blood pressure, she decides to share what she has learned with her mom.

Let's take a look at Bobbie's diet and compare it to the DASH diet. You may want to review her one-day intake in Chapter 1. The National Heart, Lung, and Blood Institute (NHLBI) has information on its Web site describing the DASH Eating Plan (http://www.nhlbi.nih.gov /health/public/heart/hbp/dash/new_dash.pdf).

A key part of the DASH diet is its emphasis on fruits and vegetables. With about three servings of vegetables, but only one serving of fruit, Bobbie is a long way from the DASH diet's 8–10 daily servings of fruits and vegetables! Eating more fruits and vegetables would boost Bobbie's potassium intake, which was low at 2,890 milligrams. Bobbie also is low in dairy products (and calcium). The DASH diet includes 2–3 servings of low-fat or fat-free dairy products, but again Bobbie falls short with a splash of 2% milk in her coffee and cheese on her pizza. The DASH-Sodium study showed that reducing sodium intake, in conjunction with the DASH Eating Plan, reduced blood pressure even further. Bobbie's sodium intake, at 4,820 milligrams, is much higher than the Daily Value of 2,400 milligrams.

To reduce her hypertension risk, Bobbie could snack on fruits and vegetables instead of pizza and chips, include low-fat milk or yogurt on a regular basis, choose fewer canned or processed foods, and exercise regularly. Given her family history, it would be good idea for Bobbie to have her blood pressure checked regularly.

References

1 World Health Organization. WHO definition of health. Preamble to the Constitution of the World Health Organization, 1948. http://www.who.int/about/definition /en/print.html. Accessed 8/7/06.

2 MedlinePlus Medical Dictionary. http://www.nlm.nih.gov /medlineplus/mplusdictionary.html. Accessed 8/7/06.

3 World Health Organization. *Diet, Nutrition and the Prevention of Chronic Diseases: A Report of a Joint WHO/FAO Expert Consultation.* Geneva, Switzerland: World Health Organization, 2003. WHO Technical Report Series 916.

4 US Department of Health and Human Services. *Healthy People 2010.* 2nd ed. With *Understanding and Improving Health and Objectives for Improving Health.* 2 vols. Washington, DC: US Government Printing Office, 2000.

5 DeBusk RM. *Genetics: The Nutrition Connection.* Chicago: American Dietetic Association, 2003.

6 Lichtenstein P, Holm NV, Verkasalo PK, et al. Environmental and heritable factors in the causation of cancer. *N Engl J Med.* 2000;343(2):78–85.

7 Collins FS, McKusick VA. Implications of the Human Genome Project for medical science. *JAMA.* 2001;285(5):540–544.

8 Klerk M, Verhoef P, Clarke R, et al. *MTHFR* 677C→T polymorphism and risk of coronary heart disease: a meta-analysis. *JAMA.* 2002;288(16):2023–2031.

9 Khoury MJ, McCabe LL, McCabe ERB. Population screening in the age of genomic medicine. *N Engl J Med.* 2003; 348(1):50–58.

10 Clinicians Group. *Clinician Reviews.* 2002;12(10):54–60; and Miniño AM, Heron MP, Smith, BL. *Deaths: Preliminary Data for 2004.* Hyattsville, Maryland: National Center for Health Statistics, 2006. National Vital Statistics Reports, Vol. 54, No. 19. http://www.cdc.gov/nchs/data/nvsr/nvsr54/nvsr54_19.pdf. Accessed 8/7/06.

11 Mlot C. Chlamydia linked to atherosclerosis. *Science.* 1996; 272:1422; and Zhou YF, Leon MB, Waclawiw MA, et al. Association between prior cytomegalovirus infection and the risk of restenosis after coronary atherectomy. *N Engl J Med.* 1996;335:624–630.

12 Bostrom AG, Cupples A, Jenner JL. Elevated plasma lipoprotein(a) and coronary heart disease in men aged 55 years and younger: a prospective study. *JAMA.* 1996;276:544–548.

13 Hoeg JM. Evaluating coronary heart disease risk. *JAMA.* 1997;277:1387–1390.

14 National Cholesterol Education Program. *Second Report of the Expert Panel on Detection, Evaluation, and Treatment of High Blood Cholesterol in Adults.* Washington, DC: National Institutes of Health, 1993.

15 Rosamond WD, Chambless LE, Folsom AR, et al. Trends in the incidence of myocardial infarction and in mortality due to coronary heart disease, 1987 to 1994. *N Engl J Med.* 1998;339:861–867.

16 National Heart, Lung, and Blood Institute. Emerging risk factors—science's agenda for the next century. *Heart Memo.* Summer 1998:15.

17 Ridker PM, et al. C-reactive protein levels and outcomes after statin therapy. *N Engl J Med.* 2005;352:20–28.

18 Ridker PM, Cushman M, Stampfer MJ, et al. Inflammation, aspirin, and the risk of cardiovascular disease in apparently healthy men. *N Engl J Med.* 1997;336:973–979.

19 Ridker PM, Hennekens CH, Buring JE, et al. C-reactive protein and other markers of inflammation in the prediction of cardiovascular disease in women. *N Engl J Med.* 2000;342:836–843.

20 Ridker PM, Buring JE, Cook NR, Rifai N. C-reactive protein, the metabolic syndrome, and risk of incident cardiovascular events: an 8-year follow-up of 14,719 initially healthy American women. *Circulation.* 2003;107(3):391–397.

21 Lichtenstein AH, Appel LJ, Brands M et al. Diet and lifestyle recommendations revision 2006: a scientific statement from the American Heart Association Nutrition Committee. *Circulation.* 2006;114:82–96.

22 Sivanandam S, Sinaiko AR, Jacobs DR Jr, et al. Relation of increase in adiposity to increase in left ventricular mass from childhood to young adulthood. *Am J Cardiol.* 2006; 98(3):411–415; and Willett WC, Manson JE, Stampfer MJ, et al. Weight, weight change, and coronary heart disease in women. *JAMA.* 1995;273(6):461–465.

23 World Health Organization. 2003. Op. cit.

24 Manson JE, Greenland P, LaCroix AZ, et al. Walking compared with vigorous exercise for the prevention of cardiovascular events in women. *N Engl J Med.* 2002;347(10):716–725.

25 Witzum JL. The oxidation hypothesis of atherosclerosis. *Lancet.* 1994;344:793–795.

26 Hodis HN, Mack WJ, LaBree L, et al. Serial coronary angiographic evidence that antioxidant vitamin intake reduces progression of coronary artery atherosclerosis. *JAMA.* 1995; 273:1849–1854.

27 Yusuf S, Dagenais G, Pogue J, et al. Vitamin E supplementation and cardiovascular events in high-risk patients. The Heart Outcome Prevention Evaluation Study Investigators. *N Engl J Med.* 2000;342(3):154–160; and Heart Protection Study Collaborative Group. MRC/BHF Heart Protection Study of antioxidant vitamin supplement in 20,536 high-risk individuals: a randomised placebo-controlled trial. *Lancet.* 2002; 360(9326):23–33.

28 Hu FB, Willett WC. Optimal diets for prevention of coronary heart disease. *JAMA.* 2002;288:2569–2578.

29 Anderson JW. Short-chain fatty acids and lipid metabolism. In: Cummings JH, Rombeau JL, Sakata T, eds. *Physiological and Clinical Aspects of Short Chain Fatty Acids.* New York: Cambridge University Press, 1995:509–523.

30 Institute of Medicine, Food and Nutrition Board. *Dietary Reference Intakes for Energy, Carbohydrate, Fiber, Fat, Fatty Acids, Cholesterol, Protein, and Amino Acids.* Washington, DC: National Academy Press, 2005.

31 Bang HO, Dyerberg J. The composition of food consumed by Greenlandic Eskimos. *Acta Med Scand.* 1973;200:69–73.

32 Balk EM, Lichtenstein AH, Chung M, et al. Effects of omega-3 fatty acids on serum markers of cardiovascular disease risk: a systematic review. *Atherosclerosis.* 2006;189:19–30; and Harris WS, Isley WL. Clinical trial evidence for the cardioprotective effects of omega-3 fatty acids. *Curr Atheroscler Rep.* 2001; 3:174–179.

33 Iso H, Rexrode KM, Stampfer MJ, et al. Intake of fish and omega-3 fatty acids and risk of stroke in women. *JAMA.* 2001;285:304–312.

34 Adam O. Anti-inflammatory diet in rheumatic diseases. *Euro J Clin Nutr.* 1995;49:703–717.

35 Lewis RA, Austen K, Soberman RJ. Leukotrienes and other products of the 5-lipoxygenase pathway. *N Engl J Med.* 1990;323;645–655.

36 Soyland E, Funk J, Rajka G, et al. Effect of dietary supplementation with very-long-chain n-3 fatty acids in patients with psoriasis. *N Engl J Med.* 1993;328:1812–1816.

37 Neaton JD, Blackburn H, Jacobs D, et al. Serum cholesterol level and mortality findings for men screened in the Multiple Risk Factor Intervention Trial. Multiple Risk Factor Intervention Trial research group. *Arch Intern Med.* 1992;152:1490–1500; and World Health Organization. 2003. Op. cit.

38 Lichtenstein AH, Ausman LM, Jalbert SM, Schaefer EJ. Effects of different forms of dietary hydrogenated fats on serum lipoprotein cholesterol levels. *N Engl J Med.* 1999;340:1933–1940.

39 Briefel RR, Johnson CL. Secular trends in dietary intake in the United States. *Ann Rev Nutr.* 2004;24:401–431; and Allison DB, Egan SK, Barraj LM, et al. Estimated intakes of trans fatty and other fatty acids in the US population. *J Am Diet Assoc.* 1999;99:166–176.

40 Kris-Etherton PM, Pearson TA, Wan Y, Hargrove RL, Moriarty K, Fishell V, Etherton TD. High-monounsaturated fatty acid diets lower both plasma cholesterol and triacylglycerol concentrations. *Am J Clin Nutr.* 1999;70:1009–1015.

41 Katan MB, Grundy SM, Willett WC. Beyond low fat diets. *N Engl J Med.* 1997;337:563–566; and Kris-Etherton P, Eckel RH, Howard BV, et al. AHA Science Advisory: Lyon Diet Heart Study: Benefits of a Mediterranean-style, National Cholesterol Education Program/American Heart Association Step I dietary pattern on cardiovascular disease. *Circulation.* 2001;103(13):1823–1825.

42 Appel LJ, Sacks FM, Carey VJ, et al. Effects of protein, monounsaturated fat, and carbohydrate intake on blood pressure and serum lipids: results of the OmniHeart randomized trial. *JAMA.* 2005;294:2455–2464.

43 Klatsky AL. Should patients with heart disease drink red wine? *JAMA.* 2001;285:2004–2006; and US Department of Health and Human Services and US Department of Agriculture. *Dietary Guidelines for Americans, 2005.* 6th ed. Washington, DC: US Government Printing Office, 2005.

44 Flesch M, Rosenkranz S, Erdmann E, Bohm M. Alcohol and the risk of myocardial infarction. *Basic Res Cardiol.* 2001;96:128–135.

45 Drewnowski A, Henderson SA, Shore AB. Diet quality and dietary diversity in France: implications for the French paradox. *J Am Diet Assoc.* 1996;96:663–669.

46 Epstein FH. Homocysteine and atherothrombosis. *N Engl J Med.* 1998;338:1042–1060.

47 Sacks FM, Lichtenstein A, Van Horn L, et al. Soy protein, isoflavones, and cardiovascular health: an American Heart Association science advisory for professionals from the nutrition committee. *Circulation.* 2006; 113;1034–1044.

48 Jenkins DJ, Kendall CW, Jackson CJ, et al. Effects of high- and low-isoflavone soyfoods on blood lipids, oxidized LDL, homocysteine, and blood pressure in hyperlipidemic men and women. *Am J Clin Nutr.* 2002;76(2):365–372; and

Lichtenstein AH, Jalbert SM, Adlercreutz H, et al. Lipoprotein response to diets high in soy or animal protein with and without isoflavones in moderately hypercholesterolemic subjects. *Arterioscler Thromb Vasc Biol.* 2002;22(11):1852–1858.

49 Steinberg FM, Guthrie NL, Villablanca AC, Kumar K, Murray MJ. Soy protein with isoflavones has favorable effects on endothelial function that are independent of lipid and antioxidant effects in healthy postmenopausal women. *Am J Clin Nutr.* 2003;78(1):123–130.

50 Chobanian AV, Bakris GL, Black HR, et al. and the National High Blood Pressure Education Program Coordinating Committee. The Seventh Report of the Joint National Committee on Prevention, Detection, Evaluation, and Treatment of High Blood Pressure: the JNC 7 report. *JAMA.* 2003;289(19):2560–2572.

51 Ibid.

52 Zemel MB. Dietary pattern and hypertension: the DASH study. *Nutr Rev.* 1997;55:303–308.

53 Vasan RS, Beiser A, Seshadri S, et al. Residual life-time risk for developing hypertension in middle-aged women and men: the Framingham Heart Study. *JAMA.* 2002;287:1003–1010.

54 Whelton PK, He J, Appel LJ, et al. Primary prevention of hypertension: clinical and public health advisory from the National High Blood Pressure Education Program. *JAMA.* 2002;288(15):1882–1888.

55 Ibid.

56 Kotchen TA, McCarron DA. Dietary electrolytes and blood pressure: a statement for healthcare professionals from the American Heart Association Nutrition Committee. *Circulation.* 1998;6:613–617.

57 Harsha DW, Lin PW, Obarzanek E, et al. Dietary approaches to stop hypertension: a summary of study results. *J Am Diet Assoc.* 1999;99(8 suppl):S35–S39.

58 Vogt TM, Appel LJ, Obarzanek E, et al. Dietary approaches to stop hypertension: rationale, design, and methods. *J Am Diet Assoc.* 1999;99(8 suppl):S12–S18.

59 Recommendations updated for hypertension. *Harvard Health Letter.* 1998;1:6–7.

60 Svetkey LP, Sacks FM, Obarzanek E, et al. The DASH Diet, Sodium Intake and Blood Pressure Trial (DASH-Sodium): rationale and design. DASH-Sodium Collaborative Research Group. *J Am Diet Assoc.* 1999;99:S96–S104; and NHLBI study shows large blood pressure benefit from reduced dietary sodium. NIH news release; May 17, 2000. http://www.nhlbi.nih.gov/new/press/may17-00.htm. Accessed 8/7/06.

61 Svetkey LP, Harsha DW, Vollmer WM, et al. Premier: a clinical trial of comprehensive lifestyle modification for blood pressure control: rational, design and baseline characteristics. *Ann Epidemiol.* 2003;13(6):462–471.

62 PREMIER Collaborative Research Group. Effects of comprehensive lifestyle modification on blood pressure control: main results of the PREMIER clinical trial. *JAMA.* 2003;289(16):2083–2093.

63 National Center for Health Statistics. Leading causes of deaths. http://www.cdc.gov/nchs/fastats/lcod.htm. Accessed 8/7/06; and Statistic Canada. Cancer. http://www.cihr-irsc.gc.ca/e/24937.html. Accessed 1/6/07.

64 Key TJ, Allen NE, Spencer EA, Travis RC. The effect of diet on risk of cancer. *Lancet.* 2002;360(9336):861–868.

65 Lichtenstein P, Holm NV, Verkasalo PK, et al. Op. cit.

66 Kim H. New nutrition, proteomics, and how both can enhance studies in cancer prevention and therapy. *J Nutr.* 2005;135:2715–2718.

67 Byers T, Nestle M, McTiernan A, Doyle C, Currie-Williams A, Gansler T, Thun M, and the American Cancer Society 2001 Nutrition and Physical Activity Guidelines Advisory Committee. American Cancer Society Guidelines on nutrition and physical activity for cancer prevention: Reducing the risk of cancer with healthy food choices and physical activity. *CA Cancer J Clin.* 2002;52:92–119.

68 Institute of Medicine, Food and Nutrition Board. Op. cit.

69 World Health Organization. 2003. Op. cit.

70 Holmes MD, Hunter DJ, Colditz GA, et al. Association of dietary intake of fat and fatty acids with risk of breast cancer. *JAMA.* 1999;281:914–920.

71 Bingham SA, Luben R, Welch A, et al. Are imprecise methods obscuring a relation between fat and breast cancer? *Lancet.* 2003;362:212–214.

72 Giovannucci E. Diet, body weight, and colorectal cancer: a summary of the epidemiologic evidence. *J Women's Health.* 2003;12(2):173–182; and Chao A, Thun MJ, Connell CJ, et al. Meat consumption and risk of colorectal cancer. *JAMA.* 2005;293:172–182.

73 Nelson WG, DeMarzo AM, Isaacs WB. Prostate cancer. *N Engl J Med.* 2003;394(4):366–381.

74 Katan MB, Grundy SM, Willett WC. Op. cit.

75 The Alpha-Tocopherol, Beta Carotene Cancer Prevention Study Group. The effect of vitamin E and beta carotene on the incidence of lung cancer and other cancers in male smokers. *N Engl J Med.* 1994;330:1029–1035; and Omenn G, Goodman G, Thornquist M, et al. Effects of a combination of beta carotene and vitamin A on lung cancer and cardiovascular disease. *N Engl J Med.* 1996;334:1150–1155.

76 Henneken SC, Buring J, Manson J, et al. Lack of effect of long term supplementation with beta-carotene on the incidence of malignant neoplasms and cardiovascular disease. *N Engl J Med.* 1996;334:1145–1149.

77 Life Sciences Research Office, Federation of American Societies for Experimental Biology. *Third Report on Nutrition Monitoring in the United States.* Washington, DC: US Government Printing Office, 1995; Havas S, Heimendinger J, Damron D, et al. 5 A Day for better health: Nine community research projects to increase fruit and vegetable consumption. *Public Health Rep.* 1995;110:68–79.

78 Potter JD, Finnegan JR, Guinard J-X, et al. *5 A Day for Better Health Program Evaluation Report.* Bethesda, MD: National Institutes of Health, National Cancer Institute, 2000. NIH publication 01-4904; and US Department of Health and Human Services. Eat 5 to 9 a day for better health. http://www.5aday.gov/index.html. Accessed 8/28/06.

79 Slavin JL. Mechanisms for the impact of whole grain foods on cancer risk. *J Am Coll Nutr.* 2000;19:3002–3075.

80 Schatzkin A, Lanza E, Corle D, et al. Lack of effect of a low-fat, high-fiber diet on the recurrence of colorectal adenomas. Polyp Prevention Trial Study Group. *N Engl J Med.* 2000;342:1149–1155; and Alberts DS, Martinez, ME, Roe DJ, et al. Lack of effect of a high-fiber cereal supplement on the recurrence of colorectal adenomas. Phoenix Colon Cancer Prevention Physicians' Network. *N Engl J Med.* 2000; 342:1156–1162.

81 Messina M, Erdman JW, eds. Modern applications for an ancient bean: soybeans and the prevention and treatment of chronic disease. *J Nutr.* 1995;125:567–569.

82 O'Brien T, Nguyen TT, Zimmerman BR. Hyperlipidemia and diabetes mellitus. *Mayo Clin Proc.* 1998;73:969–976.

83 Anderson JW, Geil PB. Nutritional management of diabetes mellitus. In: Shils ME, Olson JA, Shike M, eds. *Modern Nutrition in Health and Disease.* 9th ed. Philadelphia: Lippincott Williams & Wilkins, 1999:1259–1286.

84 Ibid.

85 American Diabetes Association. Diagnosis and classification of diabetes mellitus. *Diabetes Care.* 2007;30(suppl 1):S42–S47.

86 American Diabetes Association. Genetics of diabetes. http://www.diabetes.org/genetics.jsp. Accessed 8/7/06.

87 Ibid.

88 Ibid.

89 Ibid.

90 Ibid.

91 Diabetes Prevention Program Research Group. Reduction in the incidence of type 2 diabetes with lifestyle intervention or metformin. *N Engl J Med.* 2002;346:393–403.

92 Pickup JC, Williams G, eds. *Textbook of Diabetes.* 2nd ed. Malden, MA: Blackwell Science, 1997.

93 Salmeron J, Hu FB, Manson JE, et al. Dietary fat intake and risk of type 2 diabetes in women. *Am J Clin Nutr.* 2001; 73:1019–1026.

94 Feskens EJ, Virtanen SM, Rasanen L, et al. Dietary factors determining diabetes and impaired glucose tolerance: a 20-year follow-up of the Finnish and Dutch cohorts of the Seven Countries Study. *Diabetes Care.* 1995;18(8):1104–1112.

95 World Health Organization. 2003. Op cit.

96 Diabetes Prevention Program Research Group. Op. cit.

97 Franz MJ. Managing obesity in patients with comorbidities. *J Am Diet Assoc.* 1998;98(suppl):S39–S43; and Burke JP, Haffner SM, Gaskill SP, et al. Reversion from type 2 diabetes to nondiabetic status. Influence of the 1997 American Diabetes Association criteria. *Diabetes Care.* 1998;21:1266–1270.

98 American Diabetes Association. Nutrition recommendations and interventions for diabetes. A position statement of the American Diabetes Association. *Diabetes Care.* 2007;30(suppl 1):S48–S65.

99 Ibid.

100 Ford ES, Giles WH, Dietz WH. Prevalence of the metabolic syndrome among US adults: findings from the Third National Health and Nutrition Examination Survey. *JAMA*. 2002;287:356–359.

101 Hansen BC. The metabolic syndrome X. *Ann N Y Acad Sci*. 1999;892:1–24.

102 Grundy SM, Cleeman JI, Daniels SR, et al. Diagnosis and management of the metabolic syndrome: an American Heart Association/National Heart, Lung, and Blood Institute Scientific Statement. *Circulation*. 2005;112:2735–2752.

103 Ibid.

104 US Department of Health and Human Services. *Bone Health and Osteoporosis: A Report of the Surgeon General*. Rockville, MD: US Department of Health and Human Services, Office of the Surgeon General, 2004.

105 Ibid.

106 Institute of Medicine, Food and Nutrition Board. *Dietary Reference Intakes: Calcium, Phosphorus, Magnesium, Vitamin D and Fluoride*. Washington, DC: National Academy Press, 1997.

107 Reid IR. The roles of calcium and vitamin D in the prevention of osteoporosis. *Endocrinol Metab Clin North Am*. 1998;27:389–398.

108 Meunier PJ, Delmas PD, Eastell R, et al. Diagnosis and management of osteoporosis in postmenopausal women: clinical guidelines. International Committee for Osteoporosis Clinical Guidelines. *Clin Ther*. 1999;21:1025–1044.

109 Binkley N, Krueger D. Hypervitaminosis A and bone. *Nutr Rev*. 2000;58:138–144.

110 Johansson S, Melhus H. Vitamin A antagonizes calcium response to vitamin D in man. *J Bone Miner Res*. 2001; 16:1899–1905.

111 Feskanich D, Singh V, Willett WC, Colditz GA. Vitamin A intake and hip fractures among postmenopausal women. *JAMA*. 2002;287:47–54.

112 Ballew C, Galuska D, Gillespie C. High serum retinyl esters are not associated with reduced bone mineral density in the Third National Health and Nutrition Examination Survey, 1988–1994. *J Bone Miner Res*. 2001;16:2306–2312.

113 Institute of Medicine, Food and Nutrition Board. *Dietary Reference Intakes for Vitamin A, Vitamin K, Arsenic, Boron, Chromium, Copper, Iodine, Iron, Manganese, Molybdenum, Nickel, Silicon, Vanadium, and Zinc*. Washington, DC: National Academy Press, 2001.

114 US Department of Health and Human Services. 2004. *Op cit.*

115 New SA, Bolton-Smith C, Grubb DA, Reid DM. Nutritional influences on bone mineral density: a cross-sectional study in premenopausal women. *Am J Clin Nutr*. 1997;65(6):1831–1839.

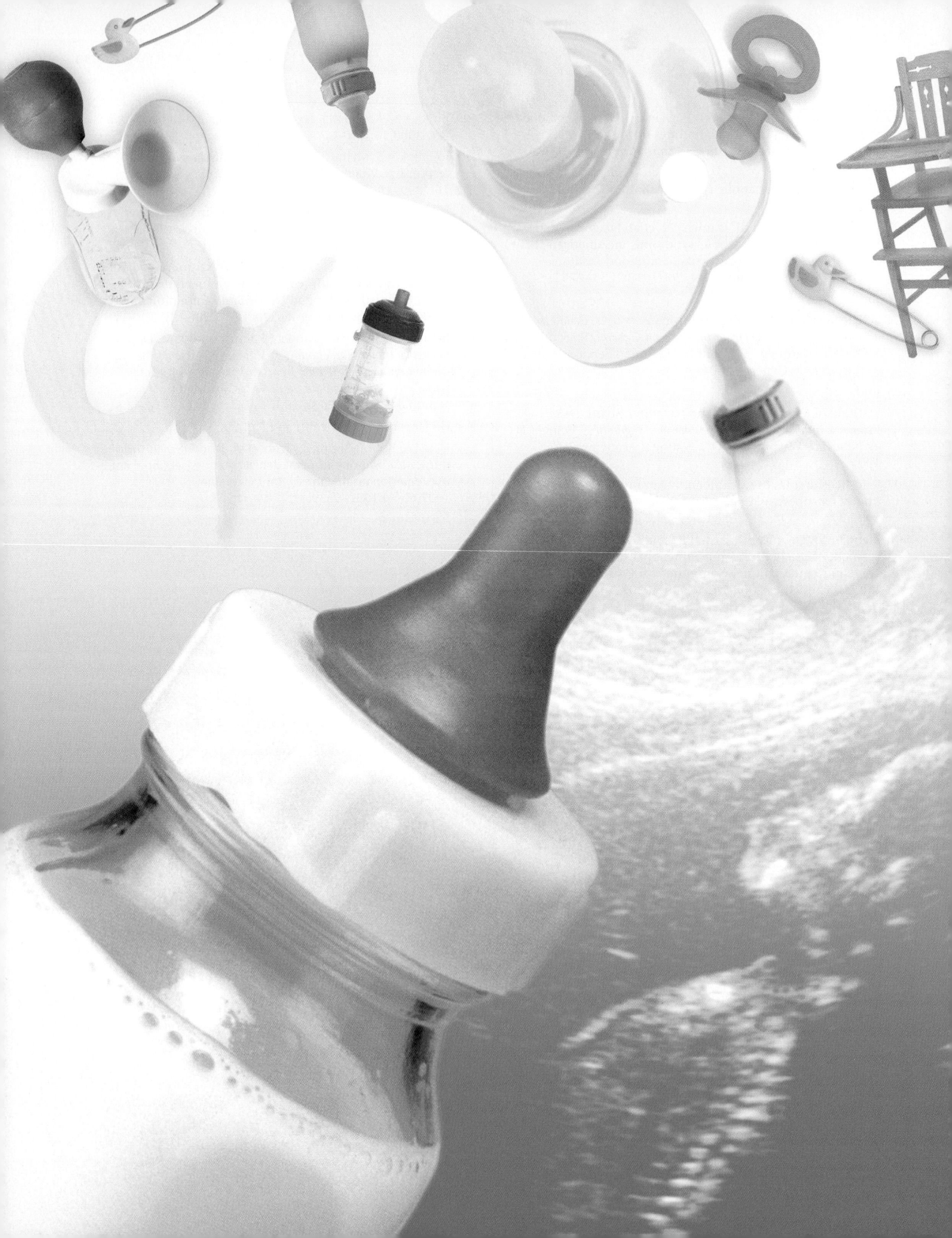

Chapter 15

Life Cycle: Maternal and Infant Nutrition

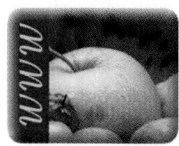
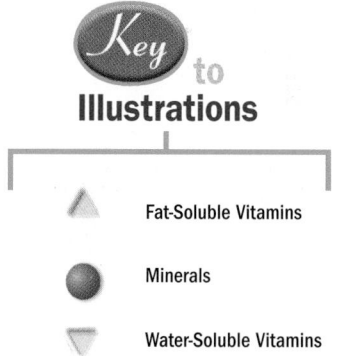
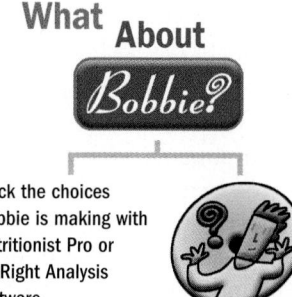

*I*magine waking up tomorrow and finding a newborn baby in the house! Play along for a moment with the idea that it's *your* baby. Would your current eating habits have been sufficient to support the nutritional demands of pregnancy? If not, what changes should you have made and why? What about other aspects of your lifestyle that might need to be modified *before* pregnancy, such as smoking, alcohol use, and exercise? How would you feed a new baby? Breastfeeding poses its own nutritional demands but has many benefits for the infant. If you've never shopped for infant formula or baby food before, you may be surprised at the variety of choices and confused as to which is best. So, although the likelihood of waking up tomorrow and finding a newborn in the house is remote, it's never too early to learn about the nutritional implications of pregnancy, breastfeeding, and infant feeding.

Pregnancy

Pregnancy is a time of tremendous physiological changes, and these changes demand healthful dietary and lifestyle choices. Energy and nutrient needs both increase, but the need for calories increases by a smaller percentage than the need for most vitamins and minerals. As a result, food choices during pregnancy must be nutrient dense.

What about tobacco and alcohol? Research clearly shows that both have damaging effects on a developing fetus; it's essential to abstain from both during pregnancy. Although research about the effects of caffeine is less conclusive, most health care professionals also recommend limiting caffeine intake during pregnancy.

Nutrition Before Conception

Everyone knows a woman needs to eat well once she becomes pregnant. But her nutritional status at the moment of conception is also important. Vitamin status at conception, for example, can mean the difference between a healthy baby and one with a devastating birth defect. In addition, a woman's weight at conception can influence her pregnancy and delivery and the baby's health.

For these reasons, it's important for a woman to get care before she gets pregnant. Many experts recommend extending prenatal care—the routine health care that a woman receives during her pregnancy—to include the preconception period as well. (See **Figure 15.1**.) Although this is certainly a worthy goal, it is important to realize that about half of the pregnancies in the United States are unplanned. Hence, good nutrition for all women of childbearing age is an important public health objective.

Preconception care has three main components: risk assessment, health promotion, and intervention. Nutrition is an important aspect of all three components. (See **Table 15.1**.) Risk assessment includes an evaluation of a prospective mother's vitamin status and weight, as well as her health habits—including use of alcohol, tobacco, and other substances—and her overall medical condition. Health promotion means providing the would-be mother with information about the steps she can take to maximize her chances of a trouble-free pregnancy, an uneventful delivery, and a healthy, full-term baby. The third component of preconception care, intervention, can be as simple as recommending a folic acid supplement or as complex

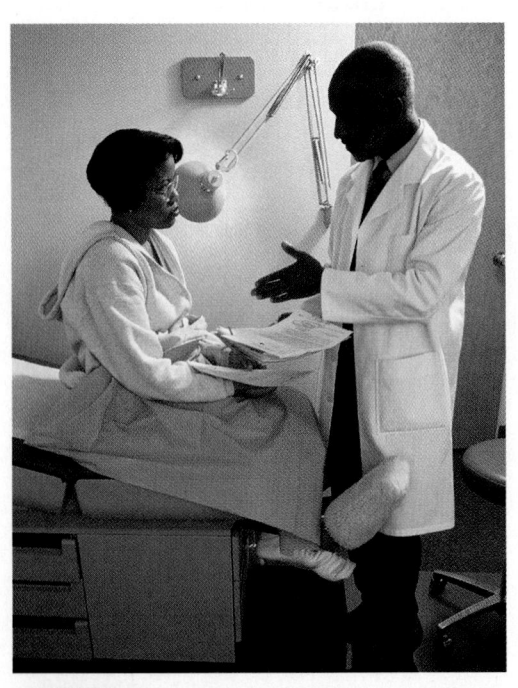

Figure 15.1 **Preconception care.** Planning and care before pregnancy are recommended for all prospective mothers.

as treating an eating disorder or substance abuse. Before conception, the goal is to resolve the nutrition and health issues that could harm a mother or her baby.

Weight

Although everyone should be concerned about maintaining a healthful weight, a woman contemplating pregnancy needs to pay careful attention to her weight. Maternal obesity can complicate pregnancy and delivery and may compromise a baby's health. Being too thin, meanwhile, carries its own risks.

Body mass index (BMI) is an indicator of a prospective mother's weight status. (See Chapter 8, "Energy Balance, Body Composition, and Weight Management" to review how to calculate BMI.) Lean women with a BMI less than 20 kg/m² have increased risks of **preterm delivery** and delivering a **low-birth-weight infant**.[1] At the other end of the spectrum, overweight and obese women have increased risks of several problems, including preterm delivery and stillbirth.[2] In addition, obese women are at higher risk for the following:[3]

- High blood pressure
- **Gestational diabetes** (a form of diabetes that is associated with pregnancy; it often is controlled through diet alone)
- **Preeclampsia** (a condition marked by high blood pressure, fluid retention, and protein in the urine)
- Prolonged labor
- Unplanned cesarean section
- Difficulty initiating and continuing breastfeeding

Of course, the time to lose or gain weight is well before a pregnancy begins. It is not a good idea for pregnant women, even obese pregnant women, to diet. And a thin woman who finds it hard to put on weight under normal circumstances is unlikely to find it any easier when she's pregnant, especially if she experiences **morning sickness**.

Women with eating disorders have special pregnancy-related risks. Ideally, anorexia nervosa or bulimia nervosa is diagnosed and treated well before conception, to give the prospective mother's body plenty of time to

preterm delivery A delivery that occurs before the 37th week of gestation.

low-birth-weight infant A newborn who weighs less than 2,500 grams (5.5 lb) as a result of either premature birth or inadequate growth in utero.

gestational diabetes A condition that results in high glucose levels during pregnancy.

preeclampsia A condition of late pregnancy characterized by hypertension, and proteinuria.

morning sickness A persistent or recurring nausea that often occurs in the morning during early pregnancy.

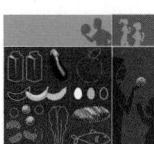

Dietary Guidelines for Americans, 2005
key recommendations

- Consume a variety of nutrient-dense foods and beverages within and among the basic food groups while choosing foods that limit the intake of saturated and *trans* fats, cholesterol, added sugars, salt, and alcohol.
- Meet recommended intakes within energy needs by adopting a balanced eating pattern, such as the USDA Food Guide or the DASH Eating Plan.

Key Recommendations for Specific Population Groups

- *Women of childbearing age who may become pregnant.* Eat foods high in heme iron and/or consume iron-rich plant foods or iron-fortified foods with an enhancer of iron absorption, such as vitamin C–rich foods.
- *Women of childbearing age who may become pregnant and those in the first trimester of pregnancy.* Consume adequate synthetic folic acid daily (from fortified foods or supplements) in addition to food forms of folate from a varied diet.

Table 15.1 **Nutrition-Related Components of Preconception Care**

Risk Assessment

Age, diet, substance use (tobacco, alcohol, illicit drugs)
Existing medical condition(s)
Barriers to prenatal care and primary health care

Health Promotion

Healthful diet and refraining from substance use
Compliance with prenatal care

Interventions

Referral to high-risk pregnancy programs if necessary
Referral for treatment of adverse health behaviors
Nutrition counseling, supplementation, or referral to improve diet as needed

Source: Adapted in part from Jack B, et al. *Perspectives on Prenatal Care.* New York: Elsevier Science, 1990.

trimesters Three equal time periods of pregnancy, each lasting approximately 13 to 14 weeks.

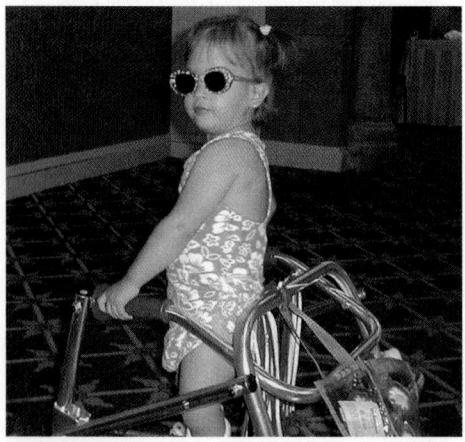

Figure 15.2 **Child with spina bifida.** Spina bifida causes varying degrees of limb paralysis. Some children will be able to walk using leg braces or crutches while others will require a wheelchair.
Source: Photo courtesy of Spina Bifida Association of America, www.sbaa.org.

recover and prepare for the rigors of pregnancy, birth, and breastfeeding. A woman who begins her pregnancy with an active eating disorder may not gain enough weight—or may vomit too much—to sustain a growing fetus. Risks can include premature delivery, a low-birth-weight infant, and even fetal death. Women with pica crave nonfood items, such as dirt or chalk. Eating nonfood substances may interfere with nutrient absorption of food and cause a deficiency. Pica cravings are also of concern because nonfood items may contain toxic or parasitic ingredients.

Vitamins

A good diet goes a long way toward meeting the demands of pregnancy, but even a diet that includes all the food groups may not contain enough of certain nutrients. This is especially true for folic acid, a nutrient needed to prevent neural tube defects, which are birth defects that involve the spinal column.[4] One of the most common neural tube defects is spina bifida, a birth defect in which part of the spinal cord protrudes through the spinal column, causing varying degrees of paralysis and lack of bowel and bladder control. (See **Figure 15.2**.)

The U.S. Public Health Service and the Institute of Medicine of the National Academy of Sciences both recommend that all women of childbearing age consume 400 micrograms of synthetic folic acid each day from fortified foods or supplements to reduce the risk of having an infant affected with a neural tube defect. This recommendation covers *all* women of childbearing age—not just pregnant women—because neural tube development occurs before the sixth week of fetal life. During this period, a woman may not know she is pregnant or may not have made appropriate dietary changes. This recommended intake of folic acid is in addition to folate (the natural form of the vitamin) consumed from other foods. Remember that folic acid is added to all enriched grain products and to many ready-to-eat cereals (see Chapter 10, "Water-Soluble Vitamins"). **Table 15.2** presents the folate content of selected grain products.

The rate of neural tube defects has been declining in recent years, in part as a result of folic acid fortification. In 2004, one of every 5,100 live births in the United States was afflicted with spina bifida. This rate is significantly less than in 1995, when spina bifida occurred every 3,500 live births.[5]

While it's important to get enough folic acid, it is also crucial to avoid getting too much vitamin A (retinol) during pregnancy. Some vitamin A is good for you; too much may be teratogenic. A teratogen is a substance that causes birth defects—literally, the term means "monster-producing." The Institute of Medicine considered this link between excessive retinol intake and birth defects in setting the Tolerable Upper Intake Level (UL) of retinol

Table 15.2 **Folate in Grain Products**

Foods	Folate (μg DFE)
Ready-to-eat cereals (25% DV), 1 C	170
Pasta, enriched, cooked, 1 C	140–160
Rice, enriched, cooked, 1 C	170
Tortilla, flour, enriched, 1 (10" diameter)	140
Bagel, enriched, 2 oz (3" diameter)	70
Bread, white, enriched, 1 slice	25–40

Source: Data compiled from Suitor CW, Bailey LB. Dietary folate equivalents: interpretation and application. *J Am Diet Assoc.* 2000;100:88–94.

for women of childbearing age. The UL is 3,000 micrograms (10,000 IU) of retinol from food and supplements for women over the age of 18. For teens, the UL is 2,800 micrograms (9,300 IU).

Any woman who might become pregnant must avoid using drugs that contain vitamin A or vitamin A analogs; examples are the acne medications isotretinoin (Accutane) and tretinoin (Retin-A). Because these medications are potent teratogens,[6] doctors prescribe such drugs to women of childbearing age only if tests show that a woman is not pregnant, and she practices birth control. In 2006, the Food and Drug Administration (FDA) launched a computer-based risk management program called iPledge designed to ensure that no women taking isotretinoin become pregnant and that no one who is already pregnant be prescribed isotretinoin.[7]

Pregnant women can—and should—eat as much as they like of fruits and vegetables rich in beta-carotene and other carotenoids. These foods pose no risk of birth defects and offer many health benefits.

Substance Use

Many women plan to give up cigarettes, alcohol, or other drugs when they get pregnant. A better plan is to give up these substances well before becoming pregnant. (See **Figure 15.3**.) A woman who uses or abuses tobacco, alcohol, or illicit drugs prior to conception is likely to enter pregnancy with a low BMI and deficient nutritional stores.[8]

Key Concepts: *Ideally, the time to prepare nutritionally for pregnancy is well before conception. A woman who has adequate nutrient stores, particularly of folic acid, and is at a healthy weight can reduce the risk for maternal and fetal complications during pregnancy. In addition to healthful diet selections, avoiding cigarettes, alcohol, and other drugs is important when contemplating pregnancy.*

Physiology of Pregnancy

Pregnancy is an awe-inspiring process of growth and development that affects both mother and fetus. An understanding of the stages of growth and development of the fetus, along with the physiological changes that occur in the mother during pregnancy, will help to explain the nutrient needs of a pregnant woman.

Stages of Human Fetal Growth

How long does pregnancy last? Nine months, right? Well, it depends on when you start counting. When a health care provider gives an expectant mother a due date, it is typically calculated as 40 weeks from the date of the start of her last menstrual period, roughly 10 to 14 days *before* the actual date of conception. This 40-week period is often divided into three **trimesters** of 13 or 14 weeks each; however, this division does not reflect specific stages in fetal development.

Figure 15.4 illustrates the early stages of pregnancy. Following fertilization of the egg (ovum)

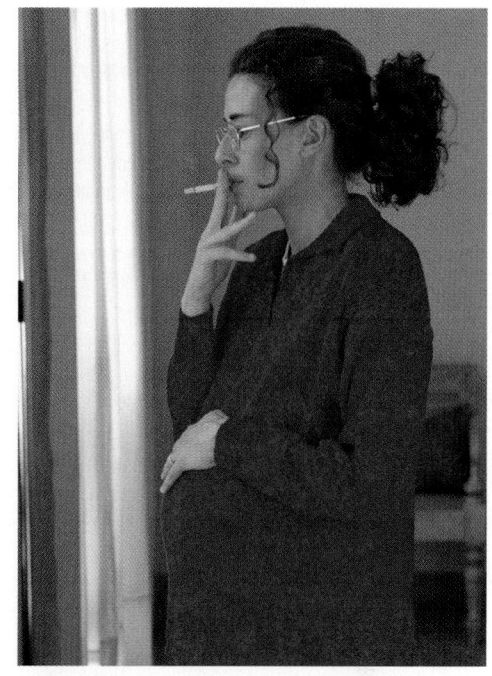

Figure 15.3 **Substance use.** Using tobacco, alcohol, or illicit drugs before and during pregnancy puts the baby at risk. If you use these substances, stop before becoming pregnant.

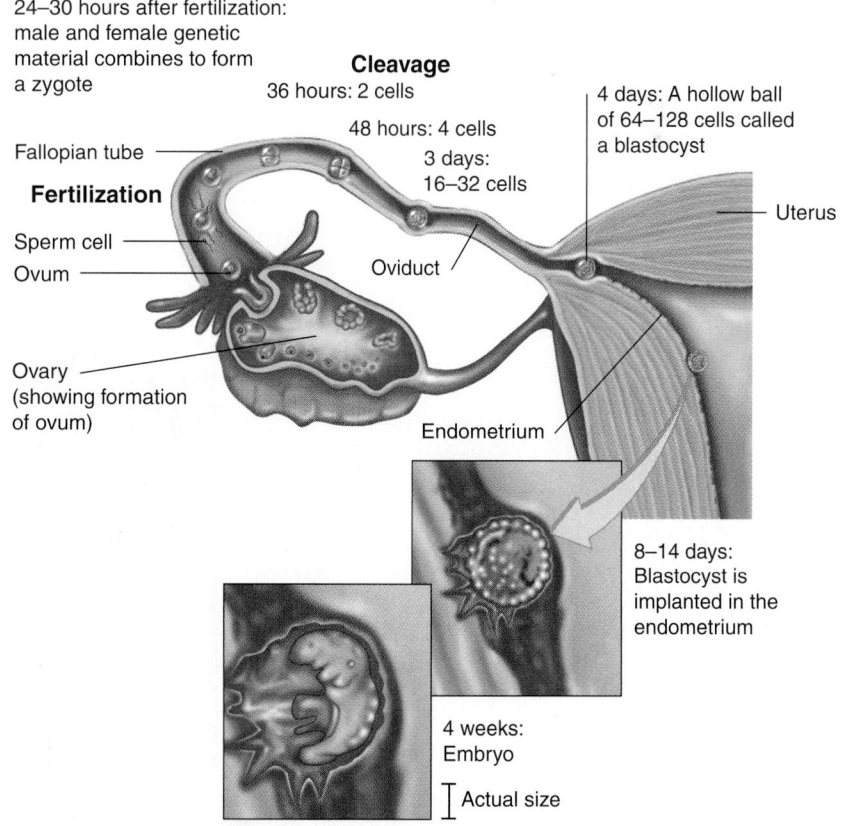

Figure 15.4 **Early stages of pregnancy.** The fertilized egg divides rapidly and begins to differentiate. The inner cells become the fetus, and the outer cells become the placenta.

blastogenic stage The first stage of gestation, during which tissue proliferation by rapid cell division begins.

placenta The organ formed during pregnancy that produces hormones for the maintenance of pregnancy and across which oxygen and nutrients are transferred from mother to infant; it also allows waste materials to be transferred from infant to mother.

embryonic stage The developmental stage between the time of implantation (about two weeks after fertilization) through the seventh or eighth week; the stage of major organ system differentiation and development of main external features.

organogenesis The period when organ systems are developing in a growing fetus.

critical period of development Time during which the environment has the greatest impact on the developing embryo.

comes the **blastogenic stage**—a period of rapid cell division. As these cells divide, they begin to differentiate. The inner cells in this growing mass will form the fetus; the outer layer of cells will become the **placenta**. During this stage, which lasts about two weeks, the fertilized ovum implants itself in the wall of its mother's uterus.

The next period of pregnancy, the **embryonic stage**, extends from the end of the second week through the eighth week after conception. The placenta, a vital organ that serves as a conduit between mother and child, forms on the uterine wall during this stage. Attached to the placenta by the umbilical cord, the embryo now receives its nourishment from its mother, and nearly everything the mother eats, drinks, or smokes reaches the embryo.

The embryonic stage also is a period of **organogenesis**. By the time the embryo is 8 weeks old, all of the main internal organs have formed, along with the major external body structures. (See **Figure 15.5**.) Because nutrient deficiencies or excesses and intake of harmful substances can result in congenital abnormalities (birth defects) or spontaneous abortion (miscarriage), this stage is a **critical period of development**.

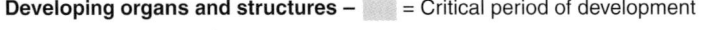

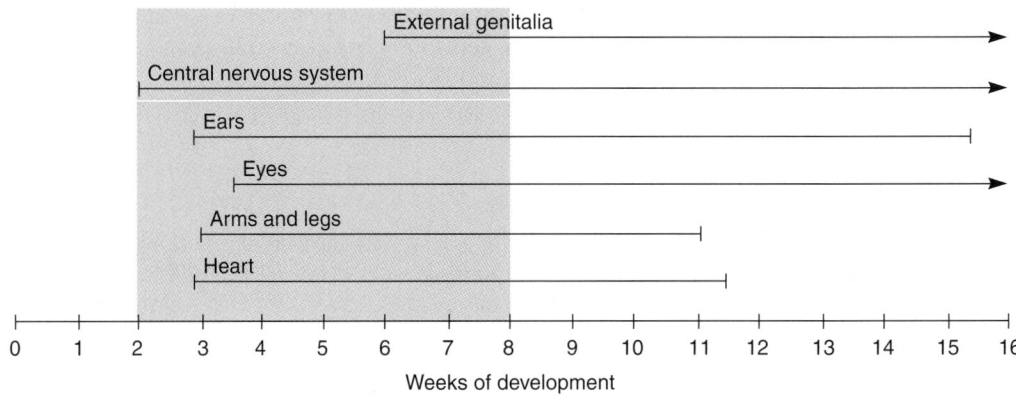

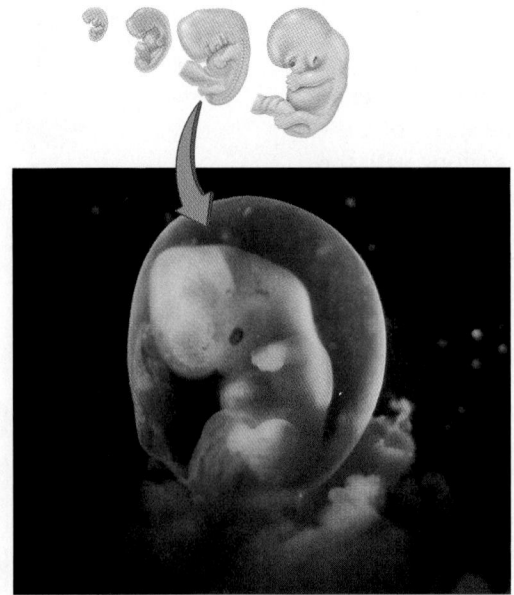

Figure 15.5 **Embryonic development.** During the embryonic stage—week 2 through week 8—all the major organ systems are forming. During this critical period of development, the embryo is highly vulnerable to nutrient deficiencies and toxicities as well as harmful substances like tobacco smoke.

The longest period of pregnancy is the **fetal stage**, the period from the end of the embryonic period until the baby is born. During this time, the fetus is growing rapidly, with dramatic changes in body proportions. From the end of the third month of pregnancy until delivery at full term, fetal weight increases nearly 500-fold. The typical newborn is about 20 inches long and weighs approximately 7 pounds 7 ounces.

Key Concepts: *From conception to full-term baby, the process of fetal development is typically divided into three stages. The blastogenic stage involves rapid cell division of the fertilized ovum and its implantation in the uterine wall. Cells differentiate and organ systems and body structures are formed during the embryonic stage. The fetal stage, the longest stage of pregnancy, is marked by growth in size and change in body proportions.*

Maternal Physiological Changes and Nutrition

While the fertilized ovum is developing from a mass of dividing cells to an embryo and then to a fetus, changes are occurring in the mother's body as well. (See **Figure 15.6**.) These changes occur as the result of various hormones secreted mainly by the placenta.

Growth of Maternal Tissue. Maternal tissues, including the breasts, uterus, and adipose stores, increase in size during pregnancy. Hormones promote growth and changes in the breast tissue to prepare for **lactation**. Fat stores increase to provide energy for late pregnancy and for lactation and are a major component of maternal weight gain.

Maternal Blood Volume. During the course of pregnancy, blood volume expands by nearly 50 percent. Production of red blood cells also increases. Iron, folate, and vitamin B$_{12}$ are all key nutrients in red blood cell production. Hemoglobin and hematocrit values during pregnancy are lower than

fetal stage The period of rapid growth from the end of the embryonic stage until birth.

lactation The process of synthesizing and secreting breast milk.

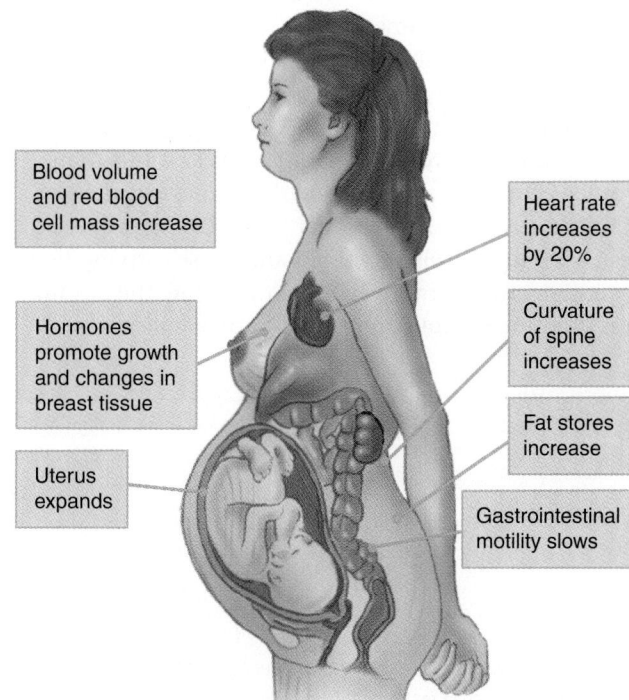

Blood volume and red blood cell mass increase

Hormones promote growth and changes in breast tissue

Uterus expands

Heart rate increases by 20%

Curvature of spine increases

Fat stores increase

Gastrointestinal motility slows

Figure 15.6 **Maternal changes during pregnancy.** Hormones released throughout pregnancy influence the growth of the baby and alter the way the mother's organs function.

amniotic fluid The fluid that surrounds the fetus; contained in the amniotic sac inside the uterus.

when a woman is not pregnant, but this is more often due to the dilution of the blood cells by an increase in plasma volume (also known as hemodilution) than to nutrient deficiency. Even so, regular monitoring of such markers of hematologic status is an important component of prenatal care so that true deficiencies can be identified and treated early.

Gastrointestinal Change. During pregnancy, gastrointestinal motility slows, and food moves more slowly through the intestinal tract. On the plus side, nutrient absorption is increased because nutrients spend more time in the small intestine. On the other hand, slower motility can contribute to nausea, heartburn, constipation, and hemorrhoids.

Key Concepts: *The mother's body is undergoing various changes during pregnancy, guided by changing levels of hormones. Uterine, breast, and adipose tissues grow; blood volume expands; and gastrointestinal motility slows. All of these changes have nutritional and dietary implications for pregnant women.*

Maternal Weight Gain

How much weight should a woman gain during pregnancy? Doctors' recommendations have varied over the years from minimal weight gain to unlimited weight gain to recommendations based on prepregnancy BMI, as shown in **Table 15.3**. For women with a BMI of 19.8 to 26 kg/m², the recommended weight gain is 25 to 35 pounds (12.5–18 kg).[9] For the heaviest women—those with BMIs greater than 29 kg/m² at the start of pregnancy—a weight gain of at least 15 pounds (6 kg) is recommended. When maternal weight gain is within these limits, infants are more likely to be born normal weight and at term. However, weight gain varies widely among women who give birth to healthy, full-term infants.[10]

Twin births account for one of every 34 live births in the United States. Of course, women who carry two, or more, fetuses need to gain more weight, 35 to 45 pounds (16–20.5 kg), than women who carry just one. A higher weight gain is also recommended for women who were underweight prior to pregnancy. When an expectant mother's prepregnancy BMI is less than 19.8 kg/m², the recommended weight gain is 28 to 40 pounds (13–18 kg).

The pattern of weight gain is also important to a healthy pregnancy outcome. During the first trimester, average weight gain is low, less than 5 pounds for most women. Over the second and third trimesters, the suggested weight gain is a little less than 1 pound per week (0.4 kg per week), with more gain suggested for underweight women and those carrying twins, and a lower gain for women who are overweight.[11] Monitoring the amount and rate of weight gain is an important component of prenatal care.

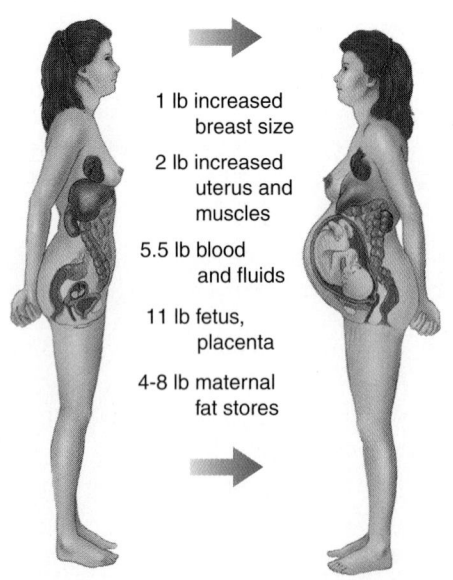

1 lb increased breast size

2 lb increased uterus and muscles

5.5 lb blood and fluids

11 lb fetus, placenta

4-8 lb maternal fat stores

(a) First trimester   (b) Third trimester

Figure 15.7 **Components of maternal weight gain.** During the first trimester, most women gain less than 5 pounds. Over the second and third trimesters, the suggested weight gain is a little less than 1 pound per week.

Table 15.3 **Guidelines for Weight Gain During Pregnancy**

Prepregnancy BMI (kg/m²)	Weight Gain* (lb)	(kg)
Low (< 19.8)	28–40	12.5–18
Normal (19.8–26)	25–35	11.5–16
High (> 26–29)	15–25	7.0–11.5
Obese (> 29)	≥ 15	≥ 6

*Young adolescents should strive for gains at the upper end of the recommended range. Short women (< 157 cm or 62 in.) should strive for gains at the lower end of the range.

Source: Adapted from *Nutrition During Pregnancy.* Reprinted with permission from the National Academies Press. Copyright © 1990, National Academy of Sciences.

The weight gained during pregnancy can be divided into (1) the fetus and associated tissues and fluids and (2) maternal tissue growth. In a typical total weight gain of 27.5 pounds (12.5 kg), the fetus, placenta, and **amniotic fluid** account for nearly 40 percent of that weight. Maternal tissues (i.e., adipose stores, breast and uterine growth, and expanded blood and extracellular fluid volumes) account for the remaining 60 percent. (See **Figure 15.7.**)

Key Concepts: *Weight gained during pregnancy is a combination of fetal and maternal tissues and fluids. Weight gain recommendations are based on BMI prior to pregnancy. Women of normal weight (BMI = 19.8–26 kg/m²) should gain 25 to 35 pounds over the course of pregnancy. Most of this weight gain occurs during the second and third trimesters.*

Energy and Nutrition During Pregnancy

A pregnant woman requires added calories to grow and maintain not just her developing fetus, but also the placenta, increased breast tissue, and fat stores. Growth and development of the fetus also require protein, vitamins, and minerals.

Energy

Resting Energy Expenditure (REE) increases during pregnancy because of the energy expenditure of the fetus and placenta, and the increased workload on the heart and lungs.[12] Energy is also needed to support weight gain, primarily in the second and third trimesters. Researchers have found that actual energy expended by pregnant woman varies widely.[13] Using median energy expenditure as a guide, pregnant women need approximately 340 extra kilocalories per day during the second trimester and an extra 450 kilocalories per day during the third trimester.[14] Weight gain during pregnancy is probably the best indicator of adequate calorie intake.

As mentioned in the discussion of preconception care, women should never diet to lose weight or sharply restrict weight gain during pregnancy. Inadequate energy intake during the first trimester is associated with higher rates of premature delivery, fetal death, and malformations of the infant's central nervous system. During the second and third trimesters, restricting intake results in slowed fetal growth so that the fetus is underdeveloped for his or her age.

Nutrients to Support Pregnancy

Most healthy women who eat a well-balanced diet have no trouble meeting the majority of their nutrient requirements during pregnancy without vitamin and mineral supplements. However, even middle- to upper-income pregnant women have difficulty getting adequate iron from food alone, and intake of magnesium and folate may also be lacking.[15] (See the Nutrition Science in Action feature "Eating for Two.") Essential nutrients can be divided into two broad categories: macronutrients (proteins, fats, and carbohydrates) and micronutrients (vitamins and minerals). **Table 15.4** shows the nutrient recommendations for pregnant women compared with nonpregnant women.

Macronutrients

Macronutrients supply energy and provide the building blocks for protein synthesis. The recommended balance of energy sources does not change during pregnancy. A low-fat, moderate-protein, high-carbohydrate diet is still appropriate.

Table 15.4 **Nutritional Recommendations for Pregnancy**

	Nonpregnant	Pregnant	% increase
Energy (kcal)	2,400	2,740/2,852	14–18
Protein (g)	46	71	54
Vitamin A (μg RAE)	700	770	10
Vitamin D (μg)	5	5	0
Vitamin E (mg)	15	15	0
Vitamin K (μg)	90	90	0
Thiamin (mg)	1.1	1.4	27
Riboflavin (mg)	1.1	1.4	27
Niacin (mg)	14	18	29
Vitamin B_6 (mg)	1.3	1.9	46
Folate (μg)	400	600	50
Vitamin B_{12} (μg)	2.4	2.6	8
Pantothenic acid (mg)	5	6	20
Biotin (μg)	30	30	0
Choline (mg)	425	450	6
Vitamin C (mg)	75	85	13
Calcium (mg)	1,000	1,000	0
Phosphorus (mg)	700	700	0
Magnesium (mg)	310	350	13
Iron (mg)	18	27	50
Zinc (mg)	8	11	38
Selenium (μg)	55	60	9
Iodine (μg)	150	220	47
Fluoride (mg)	3	3	0
Copper (μg)	900	1,000	11
Chromium (μg)	25	30	20
Manganese (mg)	1.8	2	11
Molybdenum (μg)	45	50	11
Sodium (mg)	1,500	1,500	0
Chloride (mg)	2,300	2,300	0
Potassium (mg)	4,700	4,700	0
Water (mL)	2,700	3,000	11

Needs for most nutrients increase during pregnancy. Generally, vitamin and mineral needs increase more than energy needs, which means that food choices should be nutrient-dense. Values for energy are based on Estimated Energy Requirements (EER) for a reference 19-year-old active woman. The first number for pregnancy represents the second trimester; the other number is for the third trimester. Values for protein, vitamins, minerals, and water are RDAs or AIs for ages 19 to 30.

Think About It

1

NUTRITION SCIENCE IN ACTION

Eating for Two

Background: Most studies that have shown less than adequate dietary intakes for vitamins and minerals (especially iron) have focused on low-income (high-risk) pregnant women. Few studies have examined a low-risk population that would be more likely to consume an adequate diet before and during pregnancy. Estimated Average Requirement (EAR) values are the most appropriate comparison standards for assessing the nutrient intakes of groups.

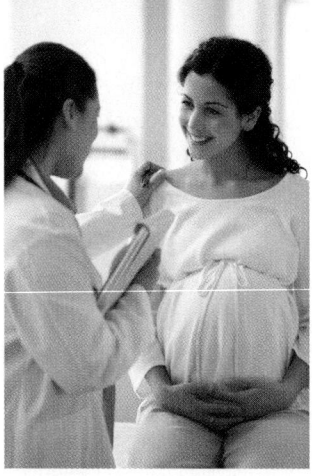

Hypothesis: Diet records will show that study participants will fail to consume adequate amounts of iron from food to meet the EAR for iron during pregnancy.

Experimental Plan: Recruit healthy women in their first trimester, who have household incomes in the middle to upper range. Have subjects complete three-day diet records every month of their pregnancy. Analyze data and compare iron intakes to EAR values.

Results: The hypothesis is confirmed. The median iron intake of the 63 women who participated in the study was significantly less than the EAR.

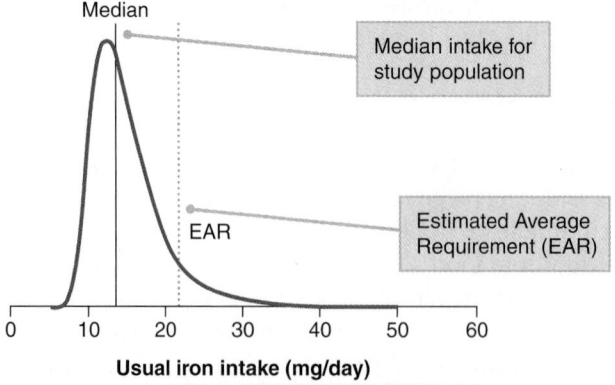

Conclusion and Discussion: Pregnant women do not obtain adequate iron from diet alone, and the results of this study support the current recommendations for iron supplementation during pregnancy. For other nutrients, the mother's diet quality should be evaluated before recommending nutrient supplements. Most pregnant women probably need folic acid supplements to meet the increased requirements of pregnancy. Future studies might test the effects of peer support on healthful diet selection in pregnant women.

Source: Based on Turner RE, Langkamp-Henken B, Littell RC, et al. Comparing nutrient intake from food to the estimated average requirements shows middle- to upper-income pregnant women lack iron and possibly magnesium. *J Am Diet Assoc.* 2003;103(4):461–466.

Protein. Extra protein is needed during pregnancy for the synthesis of new maternal, placental, and fetal tissues. A pregnant woman's RDA for protein is 1.1 grams per kilogram per day (an additional 25 grams per day over nonpregnant needs). This amount of protein is easily supplied in typical American diets consumed by nonpregnant women. Thus many women need not increase their protein intake to reach the levels recommended for pregnancy. Pregnant women who are vegetarians, including vegans, also should be able to meet their protein needs from food sources alone—as long as they select a variety of protein sources and consume enough total calories. (See the FYI feature "Vegetarianism and Pregnancy.")

Fats. Dietary fats provide vital fuel for the mother and for the development of placental tissues. Needs for essential fatty acids during pregnancy are slightly higher than for nonpregnant women.[16] The pregnant woman's body also stores fats to support breastfeeding after childbirth. Very low fat diets (in which fewer than 10 percent of daily calories come from dietary fats) are not recommended for pregnancy. Such diets are unlikely to supply sufficient amounts of essential fatty acids, fat-soluble vitamins, or calories.

Carbohydrates. Carbohydrates provide the main source of extra calories during pregnancy. Food choices should emphasize complex carbohydrates such as whole-grain breads, fortified cereals, rice, and pasta. In addition to supplying vitamins and minerals, these foods can increase fiber intake substantially. A fiber-rich diet is recommended during pregnancy to help prevent constipation and hemorrhoids. The AI for fiber increases from 25 to 28 grams per day during pregnancy.

Key Concepts: *Most healthy women with well-balanced diets meet the majority of their nutrient requirements during pregnancy. The actual increase in energy need varies substantially among women. The adequacy of energy intake can be measured by the amount of weight gained. Weight loss is not advised during pregnancy, even for obese women. As long as energy intake is adequate and a variety of foods are eaten, protein intake should be more than adequate to support prenatal growth and development.*

Micronutrients

A pregnant woman has an increased need for many vitamins and minerals that support growth and development. In addition, her increased energy needs mean she requires higher amounts of nutrients such as the B vitamins thiamin, riboflavin, niacin, and pantothenic acid that are essential for energy metabolism.

Needs for the other B vitamins (except biotin) also increase. Folate and vitamin B_{12} are used in synthesis of DNA and red blood cells, and vitamin B_6 is crucial for metabolism of amino acids. Of these vitamins, folate needs increase the most, from 400 micrograms per day to 600 micrograms per day during pregnancy. Vitamin C needs increase slightly during pregnancy, from 75 to 85 milligrams per day for women aged 19 to 50 years. For the fat-soluble vitamins, the RDA for vitamin A increases slightly during pregnancy, while the recommended intake levels for vitamins D, E, and K are unchanged.

For most minerals, recommended intakes are higher during pregnancy—most dramatically for iron. The RDA for iron increases from 18 milligrams per day to 27 milligrams per day. Iron is necessary to make red blood cells and is important for normal growth and energy metabolism. Iron deficiency and its associated anemia is the most common nutrient deficiency in

Table 15.5 Factors Associated with Increased Risk for Iron Deficiency During Pregnancy

Young age (e.g., 15 to 19 years)
Multiple pregnancies
Diets low in meat and ascorbic acid
Diets high in coffee and tea
Low socioeconomic status
Low level of education
Black or Hispanic ethnicity

Source: Adapted from Puolakka J, Janne O, Pakarinen A, Vihko R. Serum ferritin in the diagnosis of anemia during pregnancy. *Acta Obstet Gynecol Scand.* 1980;95 (suppl):57–63.

pregnancy. **Table 15.5** lists the characteristics of women who are at particularly high risk for iron deficiency.

Because getting 27 milligrams of iron in the daily diet is not easy, experts recommend iron supplementation for the general population of pregnant women.[17] A single-salt iron supplement such as ferrous sulfate is best. A woman can maximize absorption of an iron supplement by eating it on an empty stomach (between meals or at bedtime) and washing it down with liquids other than milk, tea, or coffee, which inhibit absorption.

Key Concepts: *Needs for vitamins and minerals increase during pregnancy, some more than others. Extra vitamins and minerals are needed to support growth and development as well as increased energy use. Recommended intake levels increase most dramatically for folate and iron.*

Food Choices for Pregnant Women

You may be surprised to learn that the recommended diet for a pregnant woman is not much different from that for adults in the general population. Variety is the key to a well-balanced diet. The extra calories needed for

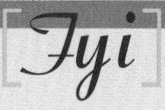

Fyi Vegetarianism and Pregnancy

FOR YOUR INFORMATION

Can pregnant women meet all of their nutritional needs on a vegetarian diet? A fair question. Common vegetarian practices include the avoidance of meat, poultry, and fish (lacto-ovo-vegetarian and lactovegetarian) and the avoidance of all animal foods (vegan). These foods are important sources of iron, zinc, calcium, vitamin B[12], and other nutrients. Although vegetarian diets can provide reasonable quantities of trace elements, animal-derived foods frequently contribute larger amounts that the body absorbs more easily. To meet the demands of pregnancy, supplementation may be in order.

Supplemental iron is generally recommended for all pregnant women. Supplemental vitamin B[12] (2.0 micrograms per day) is also recommended for vegan mothers. If their sun exposure is limited, they also may need daily supplementation of 10 micrograms of vitamin D.[1] Vegetarians with low calcium intake (<600 milligrams per day) should consume a supplement that provides at least 500 milligrams per day. Some vegan foods, such as fortified soy milks, may contain these important nutrients. It is important to check the label to be sure.

The overall nutrient content of a vegetarian diet depends on both the energy content and the variety of the foods consumed. The suggested dietary patterns in Table 1 will meet the average energy levels recommended for pregnant women.

1 Institute of Medicine. *Dietary Reference Intakes for Calcium, Phosphorus, Magnesium, Vitamin D, and Fluoride.* Washington, DC: National Academy Press, 1997.

Table 1 Suggested Servings for Pregnant Vegans

Food Group	2,200 kcal	2,800 kcal
Bread, grains, cereals (50% whole-grain products)	10	12
Legumes, plant proteins	2	3
Vegetables	3	4
Dark-green leafy vegetables	2	2
Fruits	4	6
Nuts, seeds	1	1
Fortified soy drinks* and tofu	3	3
Added fats and oils	4	6
Approximate Composition		
Protein (g)	76	95
% kcal as fat	24	25
% kcal as carbohydrate	62	61

* Milk alternatives fortified with calcium, vitamin D, and vitamin B[12]

Source: Adapted from Haddad EH. Development of a vegetarian food guide. *Am J Clin Nutr.* 1994;59(suppl):1248S–1254S.

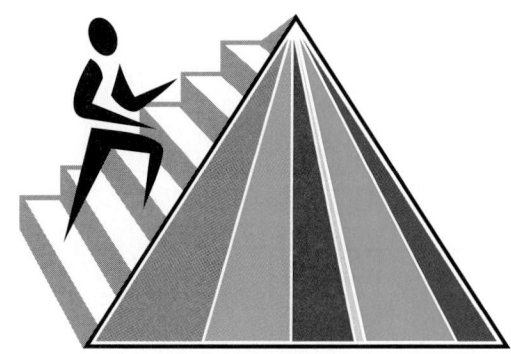

pregnancy are easy to obtain from an additional serving from each of the following food groups: grains, vegetables, fruits, and low-fat milk. Because the increased need for energy is proportionately less than the increased need for most nutrients, nutrient-dense foods are important. There is little room in the diet plan for high-calorie, high-fat, low-nutrient "extras." In a study that assessed dietary intake of pregnant and nonpregnant women using the Healthy Eating Index (HEI), pregnant women generally consumed more servings of fruit and dairy products.[18] However, about 40 percent of the pregnant women did not meet the minimum recommended number of servings from all food groups.

Supplementation

Other than iron and folate, a pregnant woman can get all of the nutrients she needs by making healthful choices using the food intake patterns of MyPyramid. In an ideal world, health care providers would evaluate the dietary intake of all prenatal patients and recommend dietary changes to improve nutrition where needed. In reality, this seldom happens, and pregnant women in the United States and Canada routinely receive prescriptions for prenatal vitamin/mineral supplements. The amount and balance of nutrients in prenatal formulations is appropriate for pregnancy. Because toxic levels can be reached quickly, especially for vitamins A and D, pregnant women should avoid high doses and multiple supplements. In addition, because most herbal preparations have not been evaluated for safety during pregnancy, they are not recommended.

Foods to Avoid

With the exception of alcohol, no foods are completely off limits to pregnant women. If a mother-to-be is experiencing problems with nausea and vomiting, she may want to abstain for a while from foods that aggravate these symptoms. Cultural traditions may dictate changes in diet during pregnancy, but these tend to reflect traditional beliefs and practices rather than health science.

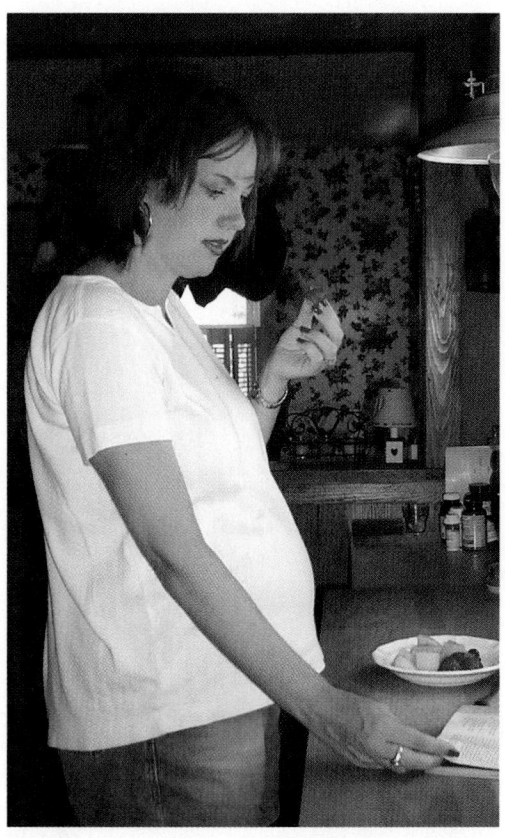

The FDA and the Environmental Protection Agency (EPA) advise women who may become pregnant, pregnant women, lactating mothers, and young children to avoid certain types of fish that are likely to contain significant amounts of mercury, enough to potentially harm a fetus or young child. The FDA and EPA recommend the following for women and young children:[19]

- Avoid eating shark, swordfish, king mackerel, or tilefish because they contain high levels of mercury.
- Eat up to 12 ounces a week of a variety of fish and shellfish that are lower in mercury, such as shrimp, canned light tuna, salmon, pollock, and catfish.
- Check local advisories about the safety of fish caught by family and friends in local lakes, rivers, and coastal areas.

The need to restrict or eliminate caffeine during pregnancy remains controversial. High caffeine intake has been shown to be teratogenic in animal studies and has been linked to low birth weight in humans. Studies suggest that low birth weight with high caffeine consumption occurs only in combination with smoking. Nonetheless, because caffeine sources tend to be low in nutrients, it is prudent to limit caffeine intake during pregnancy.

Key Concepts: *With the exception of iron and folate, a well-balanced, varied diet can easily meet all of a pregnant woman's nutrient needs. Pregnant women should choose nutrient-dense and high-carbohydrate foods in the proportions found in the MyPyramid food system. Although vitamin and mineral supplementation is common during pregnancy, it probably is not needed other than for iron and folate. When supplements are used, they should be designed for pregnant women. Pregnant women should avoid alcohol and moderate their intake of caffeine.*

Substance Use and Pregnancy Outcome

When a pregnant woman eats, she eats for two. When she smokes, drinks, or uses drugs, she does so for two as well. The consequences of these behaviors may be felt for generations.

Tobacco and Alcohol

Smoking during pregnancy increases the risks of miscarrying, delivering a stillborn infant, giving birth prematurely, and delivering a low-birth-weight baby.[20] Women in lower socioeconomic groups have the highest rates of cigarette use before, during, and after pregnancy. Women in the highest socioeconomic groups, meanwhile, are the most likely to quit smoking during pregnancy, but are just as likely as other women to take up the habit again after giving birth.

Fetal alcohol syndrome (FAS) describes a consistent pattern of physical, cognitive, and behavioral problems in infants born to women who use alcohol heavily during pregnancy. Children severely afflicted by the syndrome show marked growth deficiencies before and after birth; physical anomalies such as a small head, certain characteristic facial deformities (see **Figure 15.8**), heart defects, and joint and limb irregularities; mental retardation; and central nervous system disorders. The greater a mother's alcohol use during pregnancy, the more severe the symptoms of FAS tend to be in the child. There is no known safe threshold for alcohol use in pregnancy. The only way to avoid alcohol-related risks to a fetus is to avoid all alcohol during pregnancy.

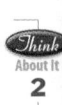

Drugs

A pregnant woman who smokes marijuana increases the risk for miscarriage, premature delivery, and low birth weight. In addition, maternal marijuana use may result in some of the same physical abnormalities seen in infants with FAS. Effects on the fetus vary depending on the mother's diet, frequency of marijuana use, and use of other drugs.

Cocaine use has reached epidemic proportions among women of childbearing age in the United States, with the greatest use among African American and Hispanic women.[21] In addition to addicting the newborn, cocaine use increases risks of stroke, prematurity, fetal growth retardation, miscarriage, and certain birth defects.[22] Some of these problems may stem from nutritional deficiencies in the mother both before and during pregnancy, as well as from concurrent tobacco and alcohol use, which is common among cocaine users. **Figure 15.9** illustrates the possible effects of a woman's drug use while she is pregnant.

Key Concepts: *Smoking, alcohol, and illicit drug use during pregnancy can all have devastating effects on fetal development. Low birth weight, preterm delivery, and birth defects are some of the consequences. Fetal alcohol syndrome is a specific set of physical, mental, and behavioral defects caused by alcohol consumption during pregnancy. A pregnant woman should avoid all these substances.*

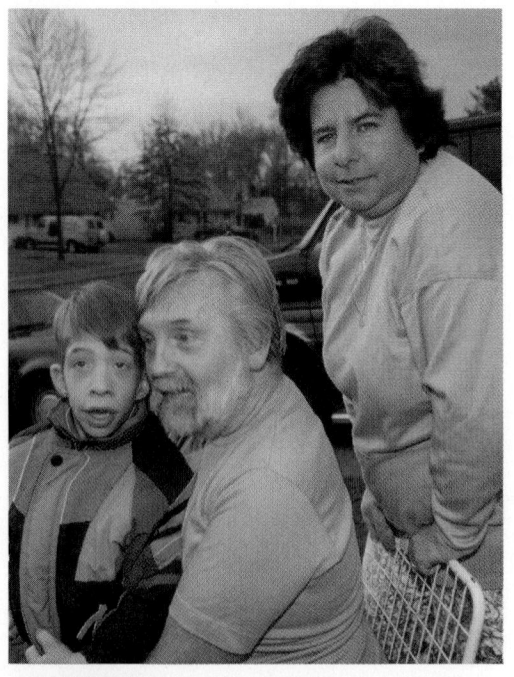

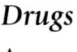 **Figure 15.8** **Fetal alcohol syndrome.** The facial characteristics of a child with fetal alcohol syndrome include a short nose with a flattened bridge, eyelids with extra folds, and a thin upper lip with no groove below the nose.

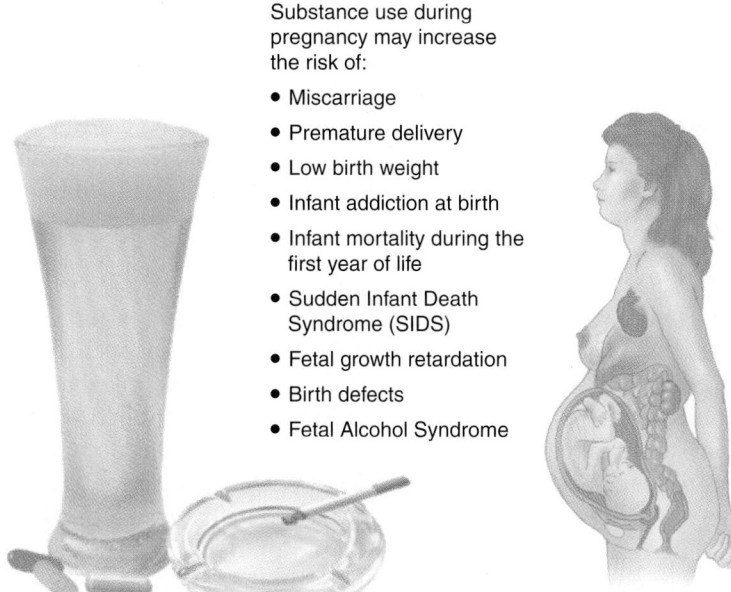

Substance use during pregnancy may increase the risk of:

- Miscarriage
- Premature delivery
- Low birth weight
- Infant addiction at birth
- Infant mortality during the first year of life
- Sudden Infant Death Syndrome (SIDS)
- Fetal growth retardation
- Birth defects
- Fetal Alcohol Syndrome

Figure 15.9 **Substance use affects the developing fetus.** When a pregnant woman smokes, drinks, or uses drugs, so does her growing baby. The consequences of these behaviors may be felt for generations.

Special Situations During Pregnancy

Most women progress through pregnancy with no more than a mild period of morning sickness or problems with constipation or heartburn. However, complications such as abnormal glucose tolerance or elevated blood pressure may affect dietary choices and nutritional status. In addition, some women have unique nutritional needs during pregnancy.

Gastrointestinal Distress

Morning sickness, or nausea associated with pregnancy, is most common early in pregnancy as the mother's body adjusts to changes in hormone levels. Many pregnant women find they experience less morning sickness if they eat dry cereal, toast, or crackers about half an hour before getting out of bed. (See **Figure 15.10**.) Keeping some food in the stomach throughout the day helps too. This means eating smaller, more frequent meals, and drinking liquids between meals instead of with food. Avoiding food aromas that trigger nausea is another useful tactic.

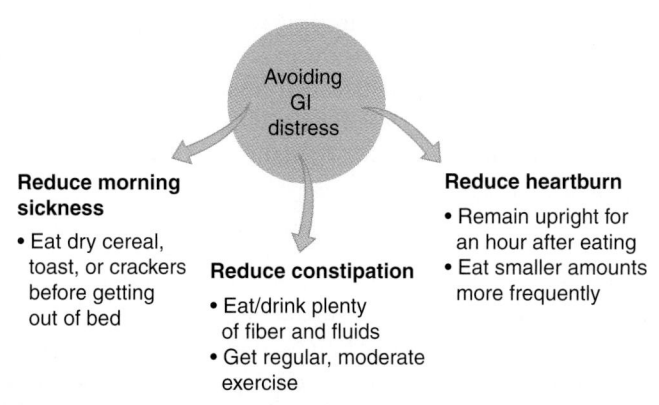

Avoiding GI distress

Reduce morning sickness
- Eat dry cereal, toast, or crackers before getting out of bed

Reduce constipation
- Eat/drink plenty of fiber and fluids
- Get regular, moderate exercise

Reduce heartburn
- Remain upright for an hour after eating
- Eat smaller amounts more frequently

Figure 15.10 **Strategies for avoiding GI distress.** During pregnancy, most women experience GI distress as morning sickness, constipation, or heartburn.

Heartburn and constipation are the result of slowed GI movement. Remaining upright for at least an hour after eating and having smaller, more frequent meals may prevent heartburn. Getting plenty of fiber and fluids in the diet and getting regular mild to moderate exercise can limit constipation. Of course, a pregnant woman should always consult her health care provider before using a prescription drug, over-the-counter medicine, herbal supplement, or home remedy for nausea, vomiting, heartburn, or constipation.

Food Cravings and Aversions

Many pregnant women experience specific food cravings and/or aversions, and we often laugh at stories about unusual combinations such as pickles and ice cream. These changes in food preferences may be linked to taste and metabolic changes, but they rarely are based on a nutrient deficiency or other physiological condition. Most cravings and aversions do not affect the quality of the diet unless food choices become very narrow.

Some pregnant women crave nonfood items such as starch or clay. The term *pica* describes routine consumption of nonfood items such as dirt, clay, laundry starch, ice, or burnt matches. Although this behavior may seem outlandish, in many cases it is a culturally accepted practice that affects significant numbers of pregnant women, especially in rural areas of the southeastern United States.[23] The etiology of pica is unknown, and although research reports have associated pica with mineral deficiencies, it is not clear whether pica is a potential cause or effect.[24] Pica can be harmful if nonfood items crowd nutritious foods out of the diet. In addition, nonfood items may contain toxins, lead, bacteria, and parasites; in the case of laundry starch, a significant number of calories may be consumed without providing any vitamins and minerals.

Hypertension

Measurement of blood pressure is a routine part of prenatal care. When not accompanied by other symptoms, increased blood pressure during pregnancy is usually temporary and carries little risk. However, the combination of hypertension, edema, and proteinuria (protein in the urine) indicates the condition known as preeclampsia. If preeclampsia progresses to **eclampsia**, it can be life-threatening for both mother and baby.

Preeclampsia is more common in women who are pregnant for the first time, adolescents, women older than 35, and women with preexisting diabetes or hypertension. In mild cases, bed rest and close monitoring are the treatments of choice. Sodium restriction and drug therapy are not recommended. Severe cases may require more aggressive treatment. Calcium supplementation may be useful for prevention for women with low calcium intake;[25] however, conclusive links between nutrient intake and development or prevention of preeclampsia have not been found.[26] Early identification of preeclampsia through routine prenatal care is important for good maternal and fetal outcomes.

Diabetes

A woman with diabetes faces special challenges in pregnancy. She has an increased risk of developing preeclampsia and a greater-than-average chance of problems that affect the fetus, including fetal death. However, with early prenatal intervention and careful control of blood glucose levels, these risks can be reduced to the same level as in nondiabetic pregnancies.[27]

eclampsia The occurrence of seizures in a pregnant woman that are unrelated to brain conditions.

Pregnancy may require frequent adjustments of both diet and insulin to keep blood sugar in check. Insulin requirements often decrease during the first half of pregnancy, but increase during the second half. Women who did not need insulin before they became pregnant and were able to control their blood sugar through diet alone may begin to need insulin during their pregnancy.

Gestational Diabetes

Gestational diabetes is a condition in which abnormal glucose tolerance exists only during pregnancy and resolves after delivery. The hormones of pregnancy tend to counteract insulin, and in about 4 percent of pregnancies, this results in a rise in blood glucose. **Table 15.6** lists factors associated with an increased risk of gestational diabetes. Women at high risk should be screened for gestational diabetes through an oral glucose tolerance test as soon as possible. If gestational diabetes is not found at that time, rescreening should be done between the 24th and 28th weeks of pregnancy.[28] Gestational diabetes often can be controlled through diet, although some cases may require insulin therapy.

HIV/AIDS

Women infected with the human immunodeficiency virus (HIV) can potentially pass the virus to their children during pregnancy, delivery, or breastfeeding. Medical treatments used routinely in the United States and other developed countries reduce the risk of transmission during pregnancy and delivery to less than 2 percent.[29] In developing countries where treatments are not available, women with HIV or AIDS are likely to have multiple nutrition problems, including protein-energy malnutrition, vitamin and mineral deficiencies, and inadequate weight gain, all of which pose risks to the fetus.

Adolescence

Despite prevention efforts, adolescent pregnancy rates in the United States are among the highest in the developed world.[30] Pregnant adolescents are nutritionally at risk. Their own needs for growth and development are compromised by the extra demands posed by the growth and development of the fetus. Risks for preeclampsia, anemia, premature birth, low-birth-weight babies, infant mortality, and sexually transmitted diseases are all increased for pregnant adolescents younger than 16.[31]

Even before becoming pregnant, many teenagers do not demonstrate healthful eating patterns. Their diets are likely to be inadequate in total calories, calcium, iron, zinc, riboflavin, folic acid, and vitamins A, D, and B$_6$. Poverty, smoking, and abuse of alcohol and other substances compound the negative effects of adolescent nutritional inadequacies.

Nutrition care for pregnant teens starts with determining daily energy needs. The Institute of Medicine recommends that pregnant adolescents be encouraged to strive for weight gains toward the upper end of the range recommended for adult mothers (see Table 15.3).[32] The need for supplemental vitamins and minerals is also greater in this age group.

Key Concepts: *Numerous factors affect the dietary needs and choices of pregnant women. Routine prenatal care is important to identify unhealthful eating behaviors and potential complications such as preeclampsia and gestational diabetes. Pregnant women with diabetes or AIDS need special dietary intervention. Pregnant teens have especially high nutrient needs to fuel not only fetal growth but also their own adolescent growth.*

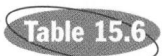 **Table 15.6** **Factors Associated with Risk for Gestational Diabetes**

Being older than 25 years
Obesity, at any age
Family history of diabetes mellitus
Previous poor pregnancy outcome
History of abnormal glucose tolerance
Ethnicity associated with high incidence of diabetes

Lactation

During pregnancy, physiological changes in breast tissue and fat stores prepare the woman's body for the demands of lactation. Preparation for lactation also involves education. Although breastfeeding is one of the most natural functions of a woman's body, knowledge about lactation can make breastfeeding a success for both mother and infant.

Breastfeeding Trends

Public health goals since the late 1970s have been to increase the percentage of infants who are breastfed. The goal of Healthy People 2010 is to increase the proportion of newborns who are initially breastfed to at least 75 percent. Efforts to promote breastfeeding have been successful; more than 70 percent of infants are now breastfed initially,[33] up from a low of around 20 percent in the early 1970s.[34]

However, only about 35 percent of infants are still being breastfed at 6 months of age, a much lower rate than the Healthy People 2010 goal of 50 percent. What are the reasons for this trend? Lack of knowledge about the benefits of breastfeeding for both mother and baby surely plays a role. Societal attitudes regarding the acceptability of breastfeeding also are influential, and vary across cultural and demographic groups. The decline in breastfeeding through the 1950s and 1960s affected the attitudes and knowledge base of today's grandmothers and also the once common practice of seeing women nursing an infant. Most states now have laws protecting a woman's right to breastfeed her child in a public place; many have specific language noting that breastfeeding is not indecent exposure! Parents should make decisions about feeding their infants based on accurate information, so providing information about the mechanics of breastfeeding as well as the benefits for both mother and baby should be an integral part of prenatal care.

Physiology of Lactation

Virtually every woman who wants to breastfeed her newborn can do so.[35] The size or shape of the breast has no impact on the lactation process. **Figure 15.11** shows the anatomy of a normal breast.

Changes During Adolescence and Pregnancy

Although mammary tissue is present in newborns, that tissue does not grow and develop until the onset of puberty. Throughout adolescence, the amount of breast tissue grows and the mammary glands and ducts develop. An adolescent who becomes pregnant shortly after her first period or who has had only irregular periods prior to becoming pregnant may have underdeveloped mammary glands and insufficient breast tissue to support lactation. However, most teen mothers have no difficulty breastfeeding their babies.

During pregnancy, the breast tissue changes so that milk production is possible. Not only does the breast change in size, but the structure of the glands and ducts also becomes more intricate, and secretory cells are formed. The mammary tissue is mature and capable of producing milk by the start of the third trimester.

After Delivery

Although birth triggers a rapid increase in milk production and secretion, full lactation does not begin as soon as the baby is born. One of the best ways to establish lactation is to put the newborn to the breast as soon after

American Dietetic Association

Promoting and Supporting Breastfeeding

It is the position of the American Dietetic Association (ADA) that exclusive breastfeeding provides optimal nutrition and health protection for the first 6 months of life, and breastfeeding with complementary foods for at least 12 months is the ideal feeding pattern for infants. Breastfeeding is also a public health strategy for improving infant and child health survival, improving maternal morbidity, controlling health care costs, and conserving natural resources.

J Am Diet Assoc. 2005;105:810–818.
Reprinted with permission.

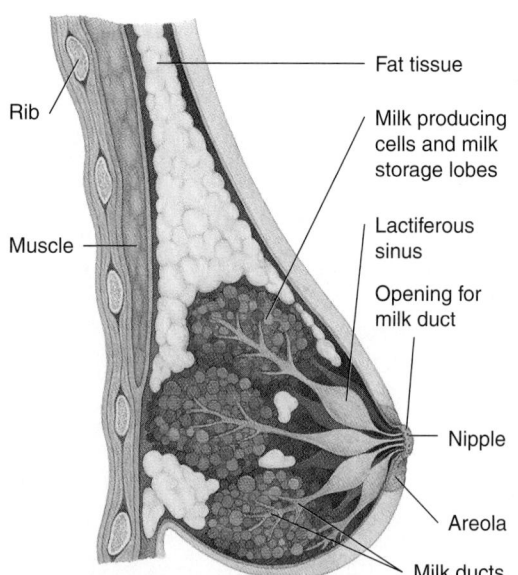

Rib
Muscle

Fat tissue
Milk producing cells and milk storage lobes
Lactiferous sinus
Opening for milk duct
Nipple
Areola
Milk ducts

Figure 15.11 **Anatomy of the breast.** During pregnancy, breasts increase in size and undergo internal development. By the start of the third trimester, breasts are capable of producing milk.

delivery as possible. During the first two or three days after birth, a nursing infant receives **colostrum**, an immature milk that is quite high in protein and immunoglobulins (immunoprotective factors). If the newborn is fed regularly at the breast, lactation will be firmly established within two or three weeks after birth, and mature milk will be produced.

Hormonal Controls

Maturation of breast tissue and the production and release of breast milk are controlled by several hormones. During lactation, the pituitary gland produces two important hormones—**prolactin** and **oxytocin**. (See **Figure 15.12**.) The infant suckling at the breast stimulates the release of prolactin from the pituitary gland. In turn, prolactin stimulates the production of milk in the breast tissue. Giving water or infant formula to the baby reduces the time spent nursing at the breast, and milk production declines.

The second hormone, oxytocin, allows milk to be released from the mammary glands to the nipple and therefore to the hungry infant. It would be inconvenient and messy if milk were released from the breast as soon as it was produced! So, the infant suckling at the breast signals the pituitary gland to release oxytocin, which in turn stimulates the release of milk. This process, often called the **let-down reflex**, may be accompanied by a tingling sensation in the breast that lets the mother know the infant is receiving milk. Let-down can be inhibited by anxiety, stress, and fatigue. It can also be stimulated by thoughts of the baby or hearing the baby cry.

Key Concepts: *Increasing the proportion of infants who are breastfed is an important public health goal. Prenatal care should include information about the physiology of lactation and benefits for mother and baby. Changes in breast tissue that allow lactation culminate at delivery. Breast milk changes in the two or three weeks following the infant's birth. The first milk, colostrum, is high in protein and immune factors. Key hormones that regulate milk production and release are prolactin and oxytocin.*

Nutrition for Breastfeeding Women

To provide adequate nutrition for her baby while protecting her own nutritional status, a breastfeeding mother must choose a varied, healthful, nutrient-dense diet. Her needs for energy and most nutrients are higher or the same as for pregnancy.

colostrum A thick yellow fluid secreted by the breast during pregnancy and the first days after delivery.

prolactin A pituitary hormone that stimulates the production of milk in the breast tissue.

oxytocin A pituitary hormone that stimulates the release of milk from the breast.

let-down reflex The release of milk from the breast tissue in response to the stimulus of the hormone oxytocin. The major stimulus for oxytocin release is the infant suckling at the breast.

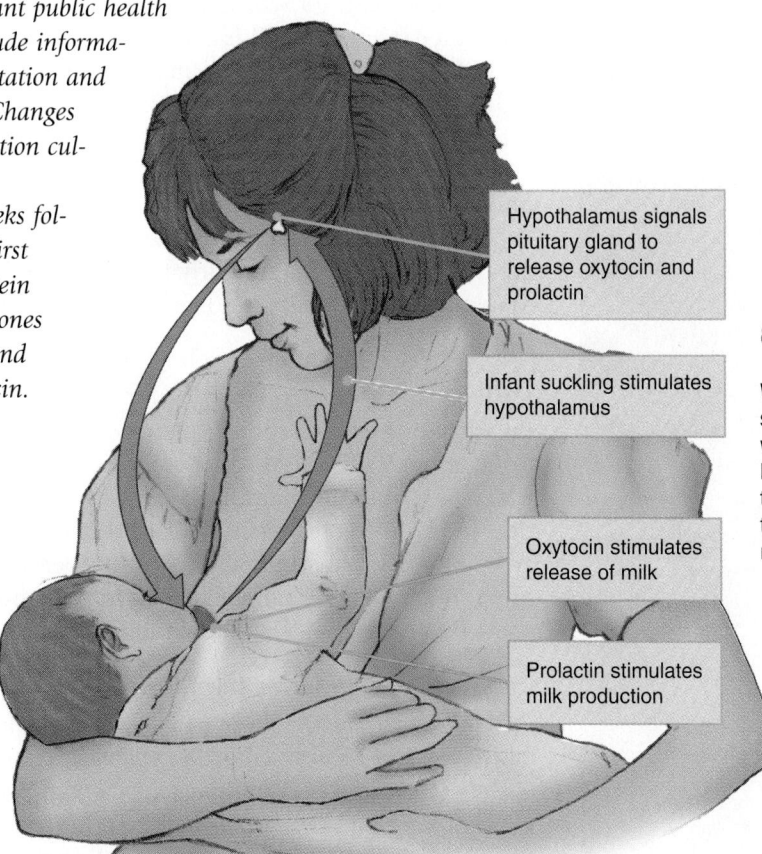

Hypothalamus signals pituitary gland to release oxytocin and prolactin

Infant suckling stimulates hypothalamus

Oxytocin stimulates release of milk

Prolactin stimulates milk production

Figure 15.12 **Hormonal control of lactation.** When an infant nurses, the infant's suckling stimulates the nipple, which sends nerve signals to the hypothalamus. In turn, the hypothalamus signals the pituitary gland to release hormones that stimulate milk production and release.

Energy

The energy needed to support milk production is obtained in part by mobilization of fat stores, with the remaining kilocalories provided by the diet. During the first six months of lactation, the energy cost of milk production is about 500 kilocalories per day.[36] On average, well-nourished breastfeeding women lose weight slowly, about 0.8 kilogram (~1.75 pounds) per month, with weight stabilizing after about six months. Based on this rate of weight loss, which provides about 170 kilocalories per day, a breastfeeding woman needs an extra intake of 330 kilocalories per day during the first six months of lactation and 400 extra kilocalories daily during the second six months.[37] This may be an overestimation of actual needs for many women, especially those who are sedentary. To ensure adequate milk production and avoid nutrient deficiencies, a nursing mother should consume at least 1,800 kilocalories per day.

Protein

Adequate protein intake is also important while nursing. The RDA for protein is the same as during pregnancy: 1.3 grams per kilogram per day or an additional 25 grams over the nonpregnant RDA. Unless calorie intake is very low, lack of dietary protein is uncommon among women in the United States and Canada.

Vitamins and Minerals

Breastfeeding women need higher amounts of most vitamins than during pregnancy. Exceptions include vitamins D, K, and thiamin, for which the recommended intake is the same during lactation and pregnancy, and niacin and folate, for which the RDA is lower during lactation than during pregnancy (although still higher than for women in the general population). When vitamin intake is inadequate, the vitamin content of breast milk can diminish, which puts the infant at risk for deficiency.

For minerals, current RDA and AI values suggest increased needs during lactation (as compared with pregnancy) for all minerals except calcium, phosphorus, magnesium, iron, fluoride, and molybdenum. Iron needs decrease below nonpregnant values because iron losses from menstruation are not present during the early months of exclusive breastfeeding. Maternal intake of minerals has less influence on levels in breast milk than is true for vitamins.

Water

Breastfeeding women require plenty of fluids. A nursing mother should drink about 2 liters (~8 cups) of water per day and at least one cup of water each time she breastfeeds her baby. The AI for total water (beverages plus foods) is 3.8 liters per day. Coffee and other caffeinated beverages are acceptable if limited to one or two cups per day—and if they do not replace other fluids. Because caffeine passes into the breast milk, caffeine can make some breastfed infants wakeful and jittery.

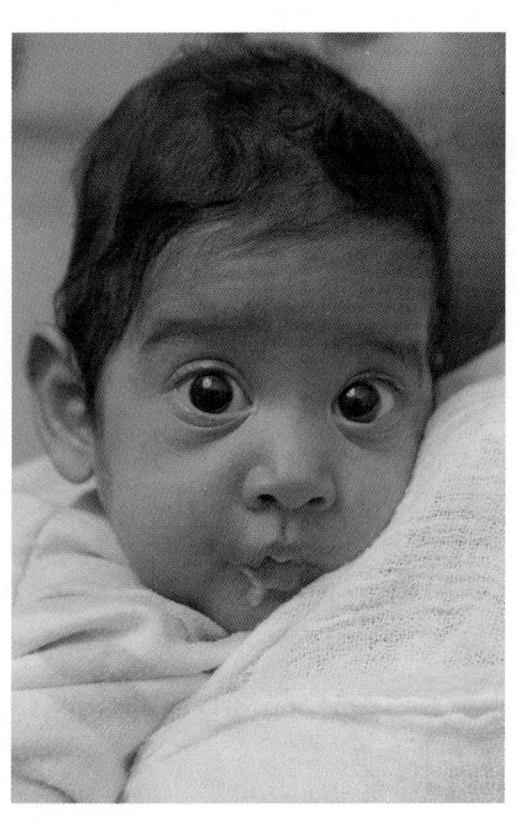

Key Concepts: *Energy and nutrient needs are usually even higher during lactation than during pregnancy. Intake recommendations suggest an additional 330 to 400 kilocalories and 25 extra grams of protein each day above nonpregnant needs. Low vitamin intake affects the nutritional quality of breast milk. Recommended intake levels for minerals are generally higher during lactation than during pregnancy. Fluids are also important for adequate milk production.*

Food Choices

Choosing a variety of foods from MyPyramid is the best way to meet the nutritional demands of lactation. Following the food intake patterns of MyPyramid, diets of 2,200 to 2,800 kilocalories per day can easily meet most nutrient needs.

Nursing mothers should eat plenty of vegetables, the source of many essential micronutrients. Although vegetables in the cabbage family, including broccoli, cauliflower, kale, and Brussels sprouts, have long been considered causes of **colic** symptoms in breastfed infants, these cruciferous vegetables may have an unwarranted bad reputation. Scientific evidence that these vegetables cause distress for infants remains weak. Removal of numerous foods from the diet should be done only under the supervision of a registered dietitian.

Supplementation

In general, breastfeeding women do not need routine vitamin/mineral supplementation. The exceptions are those women who do not follow dietary guidelines and vegan women who avoid all animal products. Vitamin B_{12} is likely to be too low in the milk of nursing vegans, so they should take a B_{12} supplement.[38] For breastfeeding women who do not get regular sun exposure and do not drink milk or other fortified products, a vitamin D supplement may be warranted.[39] For most nursing mothers, though, dietary counseling is the preferred way to address nutrient imbalances.

Practices to Avoid During Lactation

When a nursing mother smokes or uses alcohol or other drugs, these substances wind up in her breast milk. Cigarette smoking can decrease production of breast milk.[40] It is a myth that drinking alcohol enhances the let-down reflex, making it easier to nurse. Rather, alcohol inhibits the milk-ejection reflex so that the baby gets less milk but with a higher concentration of alcohol. Illicit drugs also show up in breast milk and can be transferred to the infant. If a new mother cannot abstain from using these drugs, she should not breastfeed.

Key Concepts: *Food choices during lactation should follow MyPyramid and emphasize nutrient-dense foods. With good choices and adequate calories, a lactating woman may not need vitamin and mineral supplements. During pregnancy and lactation, a woman should avoid smoking, alcohol, and illicit drugs. She should consult a health care professional before taking medications or dietary supplements.*

Benefits of Breastfeeding

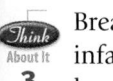

Breast milk is the optimal food for the health, growth, and development of infants.[41] Both mother and infant benefit from breastfeeding; in fact, the larger society benefits through reduced infant illness and health care costs.

Benefits for Infants

Human milk provides optimal nutrition for babies, as you will see in the section "Energy and Nutrient Needs of Infancy" later in this chapter. Breast milk provides more than nutrients, however, and the health-promoting factors in breast milk are difficult, if not impossible, to replicate in infant formula.

Breast milk has been shown to reduce the incidence of respiratory, gastrointestinal, and ear infections; allergies; diarrhea; and bacterial meningitis. Evidence suggests that these effects occur in a dose-response relationship,

colic Periodic inconsolable crying in an otherwise healthy infant that appears to result from abdominal cramping and discomfort.

Table 15.7 Suggested Protective Benefits of Human Milk

Breastfeeding may reduce a baby's risk of these disorders during infancy or later in life:

- Diarrhea and gastrointestinal illness
- Lower respiratory infection
- Otitis media
- Bacterial meningitis
- Allergic diseases
- Childhood asthma
- Childhood leukemia
- Childhood obesity
- Sudden infant death syndrome (SIDS)
- Type 1 diabetes mellitus
- Cardiovascular diseases

Source: American Dietetic Association. Position of the American Dietetic Association: promoting and supporting breastfeeding. *J Am Diet Assoc.* 2005;105:810–818.

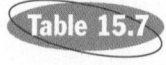
Quick Bites

Breastfeeding and Birth Control

Does breastfeeding prevent pregnancy? No. But under certain conditions, breastfeeding can dramatically reduce the chances of becoming pregnant. During the first six months after giving birth, a woman who has not yet had a period and fully breastfeeds her baby (no other liquids or solids) has less than a 2 percent chance of pregnancy.

galactosemia [gah-LAK-toh-see-mee-ah]
An inherited disorder of galactose metabolism marked by high levels of galactose in the blood and the buildup of toxic substances.

with the best outcomes for infants who are exclusively breastfed for at least six months.[42] Colostrum contains substantial amounts of antibodies, including immunoglobulin A (IgA), the first line of defense against most infectious agents.[43] Breastfeeding also appears to stimulate development of the infant's own immune system.[44]

Breastfeeding promotes a close bond between mother and infant that may be important to normal psychological development.[45] It is important for mothers (and fathers) who bottle-feed to promote the same type of closeness while feeding. A well-designed study examined the relationships between the duration of breastfeeding and adult intelligence. It found that babies who are breastfed longer have higher intelligence scores as adults.[46]

As long as mother and baby are in reasonably close proximity, breast milk is always ready when the baby is ready to eat. There's nothing to prepare, mix, or heat; and for a hungry infant, that's an important advantage! Breast milk is always the perfect temperature and is sterile. In addition, links between breastfeeding and reduced risk of disorders such as type 1 diabetes, cardiovascular disease, childhood obesity, and Crohn's disease have been suggested; these need further study. **Table 15.7** lists some of the possible protective benefits of human milk.

Benefits for Mother

Breastfeeding stimulates uterine contractions, which help the uterus return to its normal size. If the baby is put to the breast immediately after delivery, these same contractions (an effect of oxytocin) also can help control blood loss. Although not an effective method of birth control, exclusive breastfeeding suppresses ovulation in many women.

Breastfeeding is as convenient for mother as it is for baby and is certainly less expensive than formula feeding. Although more comprehensive studies are needed, there is some evidence that breastfeeding will reduce a woman's risk of ovarian cancer, breast cancer, and osteoporosis.[47] If, as expected, a breastfed baby has fewer episodes of infectious illness, this reduces health care costs and reduces employee absence and lost income for working mothers.

Contraindications to Breastfeeding

Nearly all women who want to breastfeed can do so successfully, and breastfeeding is experiencing a resurgence in popularity.[48] There are times, however, when breastfeeding is inappropriate because of infant or maternal disease or drug use. Depending on the specifics of the operation, breast enlargement or reduction surgery may or may not preclude breastfeeding.[49] The main concern is whether milk ducts and major nerves were cut or damaged.

If an infant has **galactosemia**, an inborn error in carbohydrate metabolism, the child cannot metabolize galactose. Unless given a galactose-free diet, the afflicted infant will fail to develop mentally and physically in a normal way. Because the digestion of human milk produces galactose, infants with galactosemia must consume a special lactose-free formula. Infants with phenylketonuria (PKU), however, can be breastfed and receive supplemental low-phenylalanine formula.

In the case of infectious or chronic diseases, individual situations should be discussed with the health care provider. For example, a woman with untreated tuberculosis should not breastfeed because the illness may be transmitted to her child. In the United States and Canada, where safe feeding alternatives exist, women infected with HIV are advised not to breastfeed because HIV can be transmitted to the baby through breast milk.

Some medications pass directly into human milk, and some prescribed medications may preclude breastfeeding. Women taking prescription or over-the-counter medicines or herbal supplements should discuss the effects of these products on breast milk with their health care providers.

Key Concepts: *Health benefits and convenience are key advantages of breastfeeding. For the infant, breastfeeding has been linked to reduced incidence of many infectious diseases as well as other conditions. For a mother, breastfeeding speeds recovery of normal uterine size and may reduce her disease risk. Although breastfeeding is the preferred method of infant feeding, there are times when breastfeeding is contraindicated. These situations should be identified and discussed as part of prenatal care.*

Resources for Pregnant and Lactating Women and Their Children

Many agencies support research and education programs that promote the health of pregnant and breastfeeding women and their children. You may be familiar with the March of Dimes and its efforts to reduce birth defects and prematurity through optimal nutrition during pregnancy. La Leche League is a voluntary health and education organization that offers programs and educational materials to help breastfeeding mothers learn about the benefits and practice of breastfeeding.

The **Special Supplemental Nutrition Program for Women, Infants, and Children (WIC)** is a much-acclaimed program of the Food and Nutrition Service of the U.S. Department of Agriculture (USDA). WIC provides food assistance, nutrition education, and referrals to health care services for low-income pregnant, postpartum, and breastfeeding women, as well as infants and children up to the age of 5. Compared with at-risk women and children who are eligible for WIC but do not participate in the program, WIC participants have significantly fewer problems such as low-birth-weight infants.[50]

WIC services include intensive breastfeeding education and support. Over the first six months of life, breastfed infants enrolled in WIC use about $500 less in WIC and Medicaid services than do formula-fed infants enrolled in WIC, according to a study conducted in Colorado.[51] Continued promotion of breastfeeding by WIC and other public health programs can have both health and economic benefits. Periodically, WIC participants are required to bring their infants into the local WIC office. These visits give WIC staff an opportunity to evaluate the infant's growth and provide the caregiver with additional nutrition education.

Infancy

Infancy is the period of a child's life between birth and 1 year. Because of the rapid growth that occurs during this time, nutritional needs are higher per unit of body weight than at any other time in the life cycle. Despite the critical importance of nutrition at this stage, feeding an infant is a fairly simple process. Human milk provides all of the nutrients an infant needs and is the model for infant formulas. By 4 to 6 months, the infant's physical development and physiological maturation signal readiness for the addition of "solid" foods to the diet.

Human infants need love as much as they need food. Without love and nurturing, a baby can fail to thrive even if she is offered all of the right nutrients. If an infant is not nourished emotionally, nutrition recommendations and requirements become meaningless.[52]

Quick Bites

Breastfeeding to Control Blood Pressure?

Oxytocin, the hormone produced while breastfeeding, can lower the blood pressure of nursing mothers. Research shows that breastfeeding mothers had lower blood pressures after nursing than did bottle-feeding mothers. When asked to discuss stressful events, nursing mothers also showed smaller increases in blood pressure than the bottle-feeders showed. Mothers often claim that they feel relaxed during breastfeeding, which may account for the difference in blood pressure.

Special Supplemental Nutrition Program for Women, Infants, and Children (WIC) A USDA program that provides federal grants to states for supplemental foods, health care referrals, and nutrition education for low-income pregnant, breastfeeding, and non-breastfeeding postpartum women, and to infants and children at nutritional risk.

infancy The period between birth and 12 months of age.

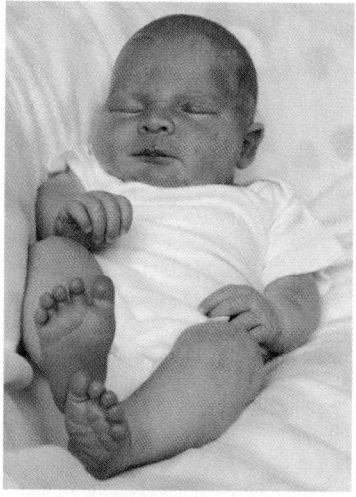

(a)

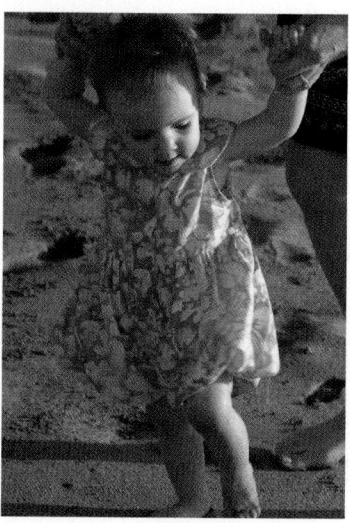

(b)

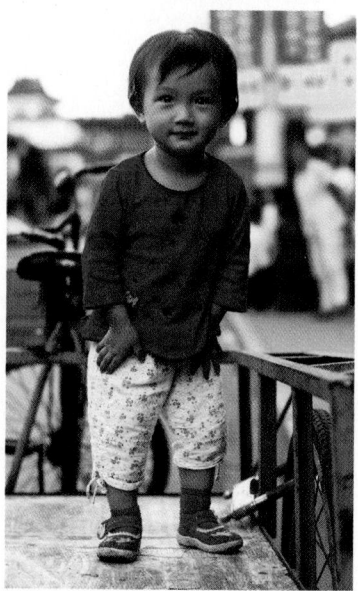

(c)

Figure 15.13 **Different stages of infancy.** (a) Newborn. (b) 4 to 6 months. (c) 12 months.

Infant Growth and Development

Birth weight is the best predictor of the child's health in the first year of life; however, it is important to correlate weight with **gestational age**. The risk profile of an infant who has a low birth weight because of **prematurity** is different from that of a **full-term baby** with a low birth weight.

Immediately after birth, an infant loses about 6 percent of his body weight. This is normal and expected. By 10 to 14 days, the infant should return to his birth weight. Over the next 12 months, his growth will be phenomenal. By the age of 4 to 6 months, a healthy infant will have doubled his birth weight. By his first birthday, the infant will have tripled his birth weight and increased his length by about 50 percent. The infant's body proportions change too, so that by age 1 he is looking less like a baby and more like a **toddler**. (See **Figure 15.13**.)

Length (used instead of height because infants can't stand) and **head circumference** are more sensitive measures than weight for assessing a baby's growth and nutritional status. Weight alone reflects just recent nutritional intake. Head circumference measures brain growth and development. Chronic malnutrition can limit this growth and is reflected in inadequate gains in head size. Regular measurements of head circumference, therefore, can verify proper growth. Head circumference measurements are useful in infants and children up to age 2.

Growth Charts

During routine checkups throughout infancy (and during childhood and adolescence), health care practitioners measure weight, length or height, and head circumference and plot these values on **growth charts**. (See **Figure 15.14**.) Charts for weight-for-age, length- (or height-) for-age, head circumference-for-age, weight-for-length, and BMI-for-age are available for boys and girls, and for two age ranges: birth to 36 months, and 2 to 20 years. (See Appendix I.) Health care practitioners use growth charts to show the growth of an individual baby over time. These charts also allow comparison of one child's growth with that of children in the general population.

Key Concepts: *A typical infant doubles her birth weight by age 4 to 6 months and triples it by 12 months. Infant length increases about 50 percent during the first year. Health care practitioners use growth charts to follow and assess an infant's growth in weight, length, and head circumference.*

Energy and Nutrient Needs of Infancy

How do you suppose scientists determine the nutrient needs of newborns and young infants? Studies with babies as subjects are rare—the logistical and ethical questions are daunting! So how else can we know what babies need? It's simple: We just look at breast milk—the food designed especially

---

gestational age Age of the fetus measured from the first day of the mother's last menstrual period until birth.

prematurity Birth before 37 weeks of gestation.

full-term baby A baby delivered during the normal period of human gestation, between 38 and 41 weeks.

toddler A child between 12 and 36 months of age.

head circumference Measurement of the largest part of the infant's head (just above the eyebrows and ears); used to determine brain growth.

growth charts Charts that plot the weight, length, and head circumference of infants and children as they grow.

for babies. The composition of human milk is the gold standard by which infant nutrient needs are determined. Babies who are not breastfed are given infant formula. In the United States, most infant formulas have a base of modified cow's milk or soy protein. To assure that formula meets all of an infant's nutrient needs, federal regulations require that the formula's composition complies with nutritional standards.

Energy

An infant's energy need is the amount of energy she requires for basal functions such as respiration and metabolism, in addition to growth and activity. An infant's basal energy needs, relative to her size, are about twice that of an adult. The amount of energy an infant needs for activity varies throughout the first year of life, increasing as the child becomes more mobile. (See **Figure 15.15.**) In general, a newborn requires about 100 kilocalories per kilogram of body weight.[53] **Table 15.8** lists the specific equations for calculating infants' estimated energy requirements (EER).

The appropriate balance of energy sources (carbohydrate, fat, and protein) is different for infants than for adults. (See **Figure 15.16.**) The best diet for infants (as modeled by human milk) is high in fat and moderate in carbohydrate. Infants have high calorie needs but can consume only a small amount at any one time. An infant's stomach is quite small; a newborn can consume only about 1 to 2 ounces of liquid at a feeding. Because fat is the most concentrated source of calories, a high-fat diet supplies adequate calories in a smaller volume. A high-fat diet also is necessary for normal brain growth, which continues until about 18 to 24 months of age. **Figure 15.17** shows the primary functions of energy-yielding nutrients in infants, which we discuss in the next sections.

Protein

Protein needs during infancy are higher than at any other time in the life cycle. In fact, protein needs (measured in grams per kilogram of body weight) during the first six months of life are nearly twice as high as an adult's needs. **Table 15.9** lists the protein recommendations for infants.

Nine indispensable amino acids are required in infancy. Deficiency in any of them can retard growth. During times of stress, such as illness, three conditionally indispensable amino acids—cysteine, tyrosine, and taurine—may become indispensable to an infant. In addition, these nutrients may be indispensable for premature infants and for babies who suffer from

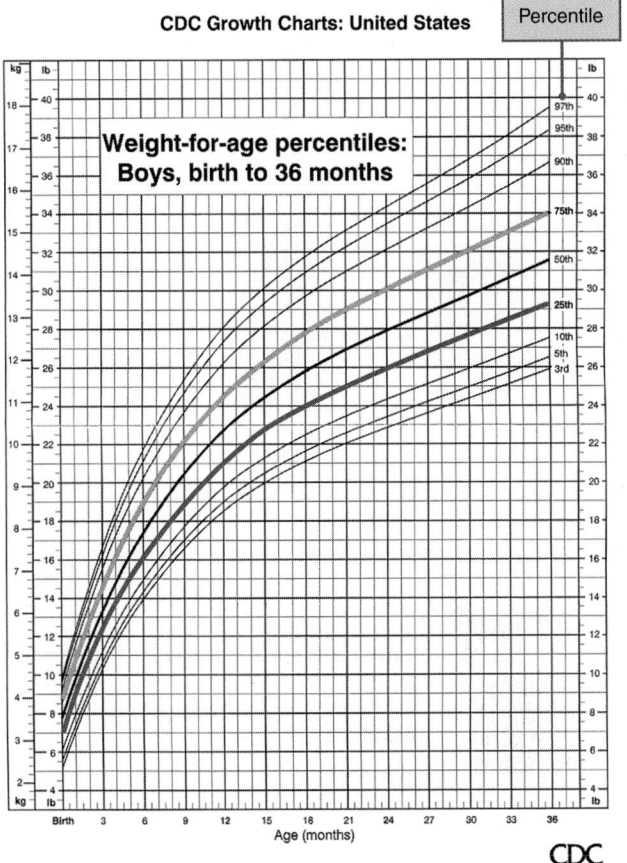

Figure 15.14 **Growth chart.** The CDC (Centers for Disease Control and Prevention) has complete sets of growth charts available on the Internet at www.cdc.gov/growthcharts. See Appendix I for full-scale samples of growth charts for boys and girls aged 2 to 20 years.
Source: Developed by the National Center for Health Statistics in collaboration with the National Center for Chronic Disease Prevention and Health Promotion (2000).

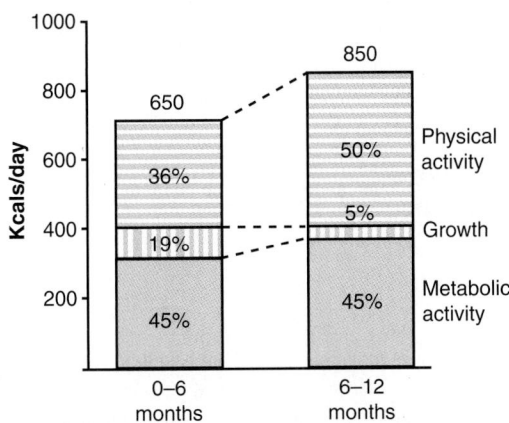

Figure 15.15 **Allocation of energy expenditure.** During the second six months, infants increase their energy expenditure for physical activity.
Source: Adapted from Foman SJ, Bell EF. Energy. In: Foman SJ, ed. *Nutrition of Normal Infants.* St. Louis: Mosby, 1993.

Table 15.8 Estimated Energy Requirement (EER) During Infancy

Age (mo)	EER Equation
0–3	$(89 \times \text{wt [kg]} - 100) + 175$ kcal/day
4–6	$(89 \times \text{wt [kg]} - 100) + 56$ kcal/day
7–12	$(89 \times \text{wt [kg]} - 100) + 22$ kcal/day

Source: Institute of Medicine, Food and Nutrition Board. *Dietary Reference Intakes for Energy, Carbohydrate, Fiber, Fat, Fatty Acids, Cholesterol, Protein, and Amino Acids.* Washington, DC: National Academies Press, 2005. Reprinted with permission from the National Academy of Sciences.

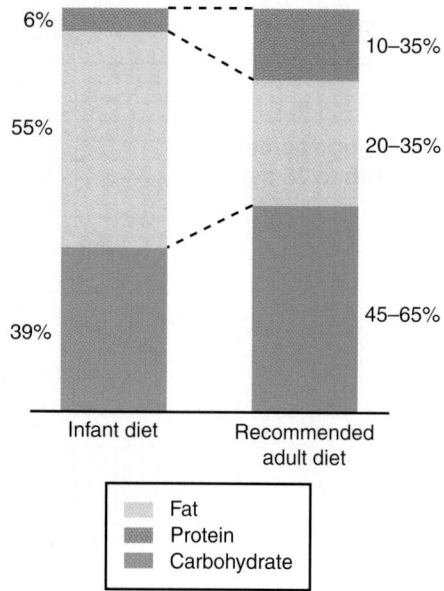

Figure 15.16 **Percentages of energy-yielding nutrients in infant and adult diets.** The best diets for infants are high in fat and moderate in carbohydrate. Infants need a high-fat diet for normal brain growth and to provide adequate calories in a smaller volume.

Protein
Growth

Carbohydrate (lactose)
Energy
Enhances absorption of calcium and phosphorus

Fat
Energy
Nervous system development
Accumulation of fat stores

Figure 15.17 **Primary functions of energy-yielding nutrients for infants.** To support growth, protein needs (per kg body weight) are higher in infancy than in any other life stage.

Table 15.9 **Protein AI or RDA for Infants**

Age (mo)	g/kg	g/d*
0–6	1.52	9
7–12	1.2	11

* The values for grams per day are based on reference weights of infants. Needs of individual infants vary.

Source: Institute of Medicine, Food and Nutrition Board. *Dietary Reference Intakes for Energy, Carbohydrate, Fiber, Fat, Fatty Acids, Cholesterol, Protein, and Amino Acids.* Washington, DC: National Academies Press, 2005. Reprinted with permission from the National Academy of Sciences.

certain **inborn errors of metabolism**. The carnitine and glycine content of human milk suggests that these amino acids are required in higher amounts during infancy as well. Both human milk and infant formula provide complete protein with all the indispensable amino acids.

One of the major differences between human milk and the milk of other mammals (such as cows) is the amount and type of protein that each contains. The main types of proteins in any milk are casein (phosphorus-containing proteins) and whey proteins. Human milk has larger amounts of the whey protein **alpha-lactalbumin**, for example. This protein contains all of the indispensable amino acids infants need, and human babies easily digest and absorb it. Cow's milk, in contrast, contains larger amounts of casein, a large protein that forms hard curds in the infant's stomach. Infants cannot digest or absorb casein easily, and too much may cause intestinal blood loss. The protein content of human milk is lower than that of unmodified cow's milk. This level is appropriate for the **neonate**, whose kidneys and GI tract are still immature. Indeed, excessive protein may disturb an infant's fragile hydration status, which is one reason that regular cow's milk is inappropriate for infants.

Carbohydrate and Fat

Carbohydrates and triglycerides are the major energy sources for infants. This allows protein to be used primarily for growth and not as an energy source. Nearly all of the carbohydrate in human milk and in the infant formulas made from cow's milk is lactose. Infants digest lactose easily and tolerate it well.

Triglycerides are the major energy source in human milk, providing about 50 to 55 percent of the calories. Fats in milk also enhance a baby's sense of fullness between feedings. Experts recommend that infants get at least 30 grams of fat per day.[54] Breast milk is rich in essential fatty acids: the *omega*-6 fatty acid arachidonic acid (ARA) and two long-chain *omega*-3 fatty acids, eicosapentaenoic acid and docosahexaenoic acid. These fatty acids have roles in neurological development, so some researchers have suggested that they should be considered provisionally essential for human infants.[55] The Food and Nutrition Board has set an AI for newborns (0 to 6 months of age) of 4.4 grams per day of linoleic acid and 0.5 gram per day of *alpha*-linolenic acid.[56] Infants also need cholesterol for brain development. Human milk is rich in cholesterol, containing about 20 to 30 milligrams per 100 milliliters.[57]

Water

Because water as a percentage of body weight is higher in babies than adults, infants have higher fluid needs. The AI for water during infancy is 0.7 liter per day in the first six months (assumed to be from human milk) and 0.8 liter per day from 7 months to 1 year of age. Human milk fulfills not only the nutrient needs of the neonate, but also the fluid requirements. Properly prepared formula accomplishes the same task. During the first four to six months, supplemental water is not necessary for healthy infants who are exclusively breastfed or who receive properly mixed formula. This is true even in hot, humid weather.[58] Once solid foods are introduced, a baby's water needs change, and additional water may be required.

Vitamins and Minerals

Human milk provides the amounts of vitamins and minerals that human babies need. Therefore, the micronutrient composition of human milk is the reference point for designing infant formula. As long as an infant is receiving adequate calories from breast milk or infant formula, nearly all vitamin and mineral needs also are being met. Human milk is lower in a few nutrients (e.g., iron and vitamin D), but infants absorb these nutrients more efficiently from breast milk than from formula. This section focuses on a few vitamins and minerals that may be of concern for infants. (See Figure 15.18.)

Vitamin D. Vitamin D is a key nutrient for calcium absorption and mineralization of bone. Human milk is low in vitamin D; however, inadequate vitamin D usually is not a problem because breastfed infants absorb it well and can make enough vitamin D from exposure to sunlight. It may be a concern, though, for infants who are not exposed to sunlight, as well as for those with darkly pigmented skin. These babies make less vitamin D from the same amount of sunlight exposure than do lighter-skinned infants. If a breastfed baby does not get adequate sunlight exposure and if the baby's mother is deficient in vitamin D, the infant's risk is especially high. The American Academy of Pediatrics (AAP) recommends that all breastfed infants receive a daily supplement of 5 micrograms (200 IU) of vitamin D.[59]

Vitamin K. Vitamin K is necessary for the production of prothrombin, a substance needed for blood to clot. Although intestinal bacteria synthesize vitamin K, the gut is sterile at birth. Because babies are born with minimal stores of vitamin K, it is recommended that a single dose of vitamin K be given at birth. Both human milk and infant formula provide adequate vitamin K; as feeding begins, helpful bacteria begin to flourish in the infant's intestinal tract.

Vitamin B$_{12}$. Vitamin B$_{12}$ is essential for cell division and normal folate metabolism. Mothers who include meat, fish, and dairy products in their diets produce milk that is adequate in vitamin B$_{12}$. This may not be true of strict vegetarians, whose diet—and milk—may be deficient in vitamin B$_{12}$. Breastfed infants of vegan mothers may need a vitamin B$_{12}$ supplement.

Iron. Iron is essential for growth and development, and iron-deficiency anemia is the most common nutritional deficiency in the United States. Human milk is not a rich source of iron, but it does not need to be. Approximately 50 percent of the iron in breast milk is absorbed, compared with only 4 percent of the iron in infant formula. If the mother has consumed an iron-rich diet during pregnancy, the fetus builds up large enough iron stores during gestation to meet most of its iron needs for the first few months of life. These stores begin to diminish during the fourth month of life. By the age of 6 months, a breastfed infant needs an additional iron source. Iron-fortified infant cereals can meet this need. For formula-fed babies, iron supplementation is needed from birth. The AAP therefore recommends iron-fortified formula for all formula-fed babies.[60]

Fluoride. Human milk is low in fluoride, a mineral important for dental health. Current research has led the American Dental Association and the AAP to recommend fluoride supplements for breastfed infants after the age of 6 months.[61] If the local water supply has adequate fluoride and the formula is mixed with tap water, formula-fed infants do not need fluoride supplements. If the water used to mix formula has inadequate fluoride, fluoride supplements are indicated. Fluoridation policies and the fluoride content of tap water vary among municipalities.

inborn errors of metabolism Any kind of biological defect (e.g., PKU) that prevents proper metabolism of a specific nutrient.

alpha-lactalbumin Primary protein in human milk.

neonate An infant from birth to 28 days.

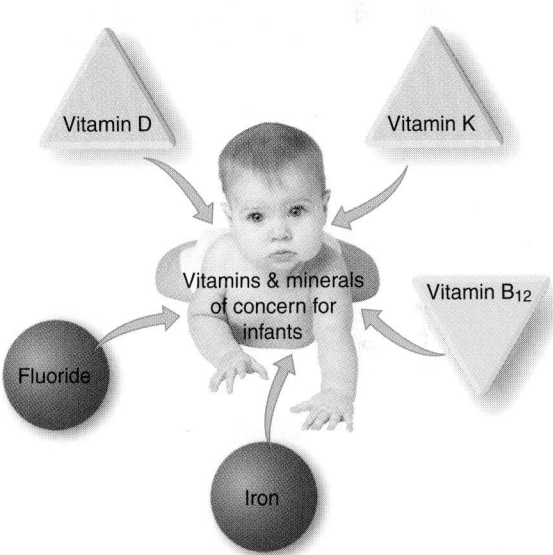

Figure 15.18 **Micronutrients of concern during infancy.** Infants who lack sun exposure can become deficient in vitamin D. A dose of vitamin K usually is given to babies at birth to ensure a sufficient supply. Because vegan mothers can have breast milk deficient in vitamin B$_{12}$, their babies may need a B$_{12}$ supplement. By the age of 6 months, breastfed infants need additional iron. Formula-fed infants should consume iron-fortified formula. Human milk is low in fluoride.

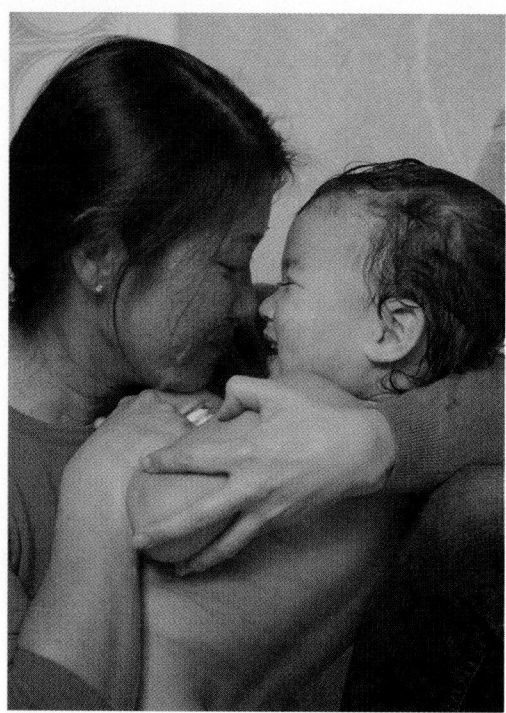

Quick Bites

What's a Biberon?

Many people consider Dr. Nils Rosen von Rosenstein to be the father of pediatrics. In his 1764 textbook, he describes a "biberon," a leather nipple used for artificial infant feeding. He also describes 14 types of infant diarrhea.

Key Concepts: *Energy and nutrient needs for infancy are estimated based on the composition of human milk. Because of their rapid growth and development, infants have high energy and nutrient needs per kilogram of body weight. Caregivers must give special attention to vitamin D, iron, and fluoride to ensure that the infant obtains enough. If breast milk or formula (properly mixed) are meeting energy needs, the fluid needs of the infant also are being met.*

Newborn Breastfeeding

The AAP has identified breastfeeding as the ideal method of feeding to achieve optimal growth and development[62] and recommends that breast-feeding begin as soon after birth as possible and continue at least through the first 12 months of life.[63] Feedings should occur at least every two to three hours, for a total of 8 to 12 feedings per day. Duration of feedings is guided by the infant's behavior and may last from 10 to 15 minutes per breast. Hospitals should provide every opportunity for breastfeeding to begin before the baby goes home. Nurses or **lactation consultants** should be available to offer professional breastfeeding support to new mothers. The AAP recommends that no supplements of formula or water be given to breastfed neonates unless medically indicated.

Alternative Feeding: Infant Formula

Women may decide not to breastfeed or to breastfeed only briefly. Their infants need infant formulas designed to provide adequate nutrition.

Standard Infant Formulas

Standard infant formulas have cow's milk as a base. In making infant formula, manufacturers first remove the milk fat and replace it with vegetable oils. Infant formula is fortified with all essential vitamins and minerals according to guidelines established by the AAP and enforced by the Food and Drug Administration. Infant formulas are available with or without added iron, but because of the decreased bioavailability of iron in infant formulas and the infant's high needs, the AAP recommends using only iron-fortified formulas.

Although formula manufacturers try to mimic the composition of human milk, formula remains an imperfect copy. For example, *alpha*-linolenic acid, an essential *omega*-3 fatty acid, is missing from many formulas. However, several brands of infant formula now contain three fatty acids that are prevalent in human milk: arachidonic acid (ARA), eicosapentaenoic acid (EPA), and docosahexaenoic acid (DHA). Some studies show that supplemental ARA and EPA may benefit infants' visual function and cognitive development.[64] Human milk also contains more cholesterol than infant formulas.

Soy-Based Formulas

Formula-fed infants who develop vomiting, diarrhea, constipation, abdominal pain, or colic are frequently switched to soy-based formulas. In these formulas, soy is the source of protein. To compensate for the inferior digestibility of soy protein, soy formulas contain more protein than formulas based on cow's milk. Soy formulas are lactose free and iron fortified. Corn syrup and sucrose are the carbohydrate sources.

Other Types of Formula

Special formulas are available for infants who are allergic to both cow's milk and soy protein, those who are premature, and those who have rare defects in metabolic pathways. These special formulas often have their protein content modified in either its digestibility or its amino acid composition. Many special formulas contain medium-chain triglycerides as the major fat source. This type of fat is very well digested and absorbed. These special formulas are expensive and often taste bad, but they are essential for many infants.

Formula Preparation

Formulas come in three forms: ready-to-feed, concentrate, and powdered. Although the ready-to-feed version is the most convenient, it is also the most expensive. As the name implies, the formula can be poured directly from the can into a bottle and fed to the baby. Liquid concentrate formula is mixed with an equal amount of water before feeding. Powdered formula also is mixed with water and is the least expensive.

When using infant formulas, principles of food safety must be observed. Infants have immature immune systems and may develop infections from improperly prepared or stored formula. If not fed to the infant immediately, prepared formula should be refrigerated immediately and kept in the refrigerator until needed. If formula is not used within 48 hours, it should be discarded. For at least the first few months, the AAP recommends sterilizing all equipment used for feeding.

Improperly mixed formula is another danger, whether it is a result of ignorance in following instructions or of economics. Some caregivers on limited budgets might purposefully overdilute formula to make it last longer. This deprives the infant of necessary calories and protein and provides too much water. Other caregivers might overconcentrate the formula in the misguided belief that this might encourage faster growth. Overconcentrated formula provides too much protein and too little water and may cause problems with an infant's kidney function and hydration.

Breast Milk or Formula: How Much Is Enough?

It is fairly simple to use DRI values and breast milk or formula composition to estimate an infant's needs based on body weight. For example, a newborn who weighs 7 pounds, 11 ounces (3.5 kg) requires approximately 390 kilocalories and 5 grams of protein each day. This amount is provided by approximately 600 milliliters (~20 oz) of breast milk or infant formula.

It's easy to keep track of how much formula an infant has consumed, but what about the breastfed baby? Although you can't see how much breast milk a nursing infant is consuming, there are other ways to tell that a baby is getting enough to eat. An adequately fed newborn will breastfeed 8 to 12 times, wet at least six diapers, and have at least three loose stools each day in the first week of life. The newborn will also regain its birth weight within the first two weeks. Normal growth, regular elimination patterns, and a satisfied demeanor are the best indicators that a baby is getting enough to eat.

Feeding Technique

Feeding should take place in a loving and warm environment. A breastfeeding mother holds her baby close, at a distance that encourages mother-baby eye contact. (See **Figure 15.19**.) During bottle-feeding, the caregiver needs to hold the baby close and make eye contact. Propping the bottle against a pillow or other object, so that the baby can feed alone, should be avoided.

Babies swallow air while feeding, whether at the breast or with a bottle, and they need to be burped. Babies generally need to be burped after 15 minutes or 2 to 3 ounces of formula. Just as the infant sends signals of readiness for feeding, she also signals fullness. Fullness cues include fussiness, playfulness, sleep, or just turning away. Parents need to learn these cues and respond to them.

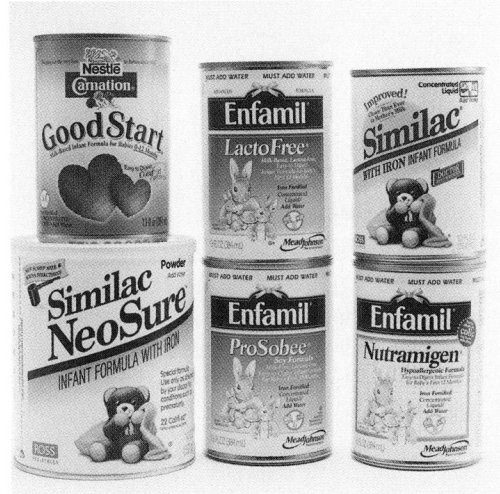

Quick Bites

But the Breast Milk Looks Weak...

Mature breast milk looks similar to nonfat milk—thin, pale, and bluish. Not to worry! This appearance is normal and breast milk always contains the right amount of nutrients for the baby. It is never too weak.

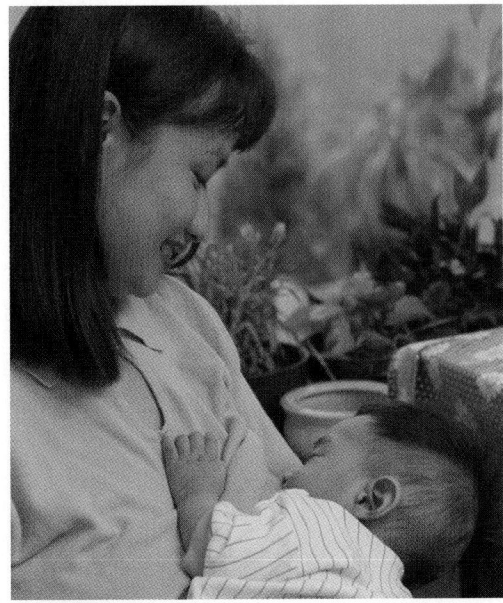

Figure 15.19 **Breastfeeding.** Breastfeeding nurtures an infant emotionally as well as physically. This intensely rewarding time helps to bond a mother and her child.

complementary foods Any foods or liquids other than breast milk or infant formula fed to an infant.

extrusion reflex A young infant's response when a spoon is put in its mouth; the tongue is thrust forward, indicating that the baby is not ready for spoon feeding.

Key Concepts: *Human milk provides all necessary nutrients for growth and development and enhances the immune system of the maturing infant. Infants who are not breastfed receive infant formula, which should be fortified with iron. Careful preparation and storage of the formula ensures proper nutrient composition and food safety. Formula feedings should nourish the baby emotionally as well as nutritionally.*

Introduction of Solid Foods into the Infant's Diet

Based on an infant's physiological needs (e.g., depletion of iron stores) and physical development (e.g., the ability to sit up), solid foods, also called **complementary foods**, are introduced. To say that we are introducing *solid* foods is a bit of a misnomer; we are really referring to pureed and liquefied cereals, fruits, vegetables, and meats that are added to the infant's diet of breast milk or infant formula. According to the American Academy of Pediatrics, complementary foods are not needed in diets of infants fed either breast milk or iron-fortified infant formula before the age of 6 months.[65]

Physiological Indicators of Infant Readiness for Solid Foods

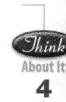

Before a baby reaches 6 months of age, solid food is not necessary for nutrition; in fact, early introduction of supplemental foods can be detrimental. By the age of 6 months, however, an infant is physiologically ready to expand his diet. For example, at this age a baby has increased levels of digestive enzymes, so that foods other than human milk or formula can be digested with ease. In addition, the infant is more able to maintain adequate hydration by the age of 6 months. Before this age, adding cereals or other solid foods to the diet can negatively affect an infant's hydration. It is probably no coincidence that the iron stores acquired in the mother's womb become depleted at the same time the baby is physiologically ready to expand his diet. However, solid food is a supplement to, not a replacement for, human milk or formula at this time.

Developmental Readiness for Solid Foods

If you attempt to spoon-feed a very young infant (e.g., at 3 weeks of age), the infant's tongue will push the spoon and food right back out. This **extrusion reflex** is a sign that the infant is not ready for solid foods. By 6 months of age, the infant will no longer push the food out and is capable of transferring food from the front of the mouth to the back, an ability necessary for swallowing solid foods. Also, the infant can purposefully bring her hand to her mouth, an ability necessary for self-feeding. In addition, if the baby is able to control her head and neck while sitting with minimal support, she is ready to be fed solids.

Start Healthy Feeding Guidelines

The *Start Healthy Feeding Guidelines for Infants and Toddlers* are science-based, practical guidelines for feeding healthy babies for the first two years.[66] The *Dietary Guidelines for Americans* and MyPyramid provide guidance for healthy Americans 2 years old and over. The *Start Healthy Feeding Guidelines* were designed to answer parents' and caregivers' questions, such as "When is my baby ready for complementary foods? What foods should I feed my baby? How do I feed these foods?"[67] The appropriate age for introduction of complementary foods balances physiological and developmental readiness with nutritional requirements for growth and development. **Figure 15.20** summarizes the *Start Healthy Feeding Guidelines*.

Signs of readiness for the introduction of infant cereals and thin, pureed foods include the ability to sit with support and the ability to take food from a spoon and move it forward and backward in the mouth with the

Development Stage	Newborn	Head Up	Supported Sitter	Independent Sitter	Crawler	Beginning to Walk	Independent Toddler
Physical Skills	• Needs head support	• More skillful head control with support emerging	• Sits with help or support • On tummy, pushes up on arms with straight elbows	• Sits independently • Can pick up and hold small object in hand • Leans toward food or spoon	• Learns to crawl • May pull self to stand	• Pulls self to stand • Stands alone • Takes early steps	• Walks well alone • Runs
Eating Skills	• Baby establishes a suck-swallow-breathe pattern during breast or bottle feeding	• Breastfeeds or bottle feeds • Tongue moves forward and back to suck	• May push food out of mouth with tongue, which gradually decreases with age • Moves pureed food forward and backward in mouth with tongue to swallow • Recognizes spoon and holds mouth open as spoon approaches	• Learns to keep thick purees in mouth • Pulls head downward and presses upper lip to draw food from spoon • Tries to rake foods toward self into fist • Can transfer food from one hand to the other • Can drink from a cup held by feeder	• Learns to move tongue from side to side to transfer food around mouth and push food to the side of the mouth so food can be mashed • Begins to use jaw and tongue to mash food • Plays with spoon at mealtime, may bring it to mouth, but does not use it for self-feeding yet • Can feed self finger foods • Holds cup independently • Holds small foods between thumb and first finger	• Feeds self easily with fingers • Can drink from a straw • Can hold cup with two hands and take swallows • More skillful at chewing • Dips spoon in food rather than scooping • Demands to spoon-feed self • Bites through a variety of textures	• Chews and swallows firmer foods skillfully • Learns to use a fork for spearing • Uses spoon with less spilling • Can hold cup in one hand and set it down skillfully
Baby's Hunger & Fullness Cues	• Cries or fusses to show hunger • Gazes at caregiver, opens mouth during feeding indicating desire to continue • Spits out nipple or falls asleep when full • Stops sucking when full	• Cries or fusses to show hunger • Smiles, gazes at caregiver, or coos during feeding to indicate desire to continue • Spits out nipple or falls asleep when full • Stops sucking when full	• Moves head forward to reach spoon when hungry • May swipe the food toward the mouth when hungry • Turns head away from spoon when full • May be distracted or notice surroundings more when full	• Reaches for spoon or food when hungry • Points to food when hungry • Slows down in eating when full • Clenches mouth shut or pushes food away when full	• Reaches for food when hungry • Points to food when hungry • Shows excitement when food is presented when hungry • Pushes food away when full • Slows down in eating when full	• Expresses desire for specific foods with words or sounds • Shakes head to say "no more" when full	• Combines phrases with gestures, such as "want that" and pointing • Can lead parent to refrigerator and point to a desired food or drink • Uses words like "all done" and "get down" • Plays with food or throws food when full
Appropriate Foods & Textures	• Breastmilk or infant formula	• Breastmilk or infant formula	• Breastmilk or infant formula • Infant cereals • Thin pureed foods	• Breastmilk or infant formula • Infant cereals • Thin pureed baby foods • Thicker pureed baby foods • Soft mashed foods without lumps • 100% Juice	• Breastmilk or infant formula • 100% Juice • Infant cereals • Pureed foods • Ground or soft mashed foods with tiny soft noticeable lumps • Foods with soft texture • Crunchy foods that dissolve (such as baby biscuits or crackers) • Increase variety of flavors offered	• Breastmilk or infant formula or whole milk • 100% Juice • Coarsely chopped foods, including foods with noticeable pieces • Foods with soft to moderate texture • Toddler foods • Bite sized pieces of food • Bites through a variety of textures	• Whole milk • 100% Juice • Coarsely chopped foods • Toddler foods • Bite-sized pieces of food • Becomes efficient at eating foods of varying textures and taking controlled bites of soft solids, hard solids, or crunchy foods by 2 years

Figure 15.20 The *Start Healthy Feeding Guidelines.* Summary of physical and eating skills, hunger and fullness cues, and appropriate food textures for children 0 to 24 months of age.

Source: Butte N, Dwyer J, et al. The *Start Healthy Feeding Guidelines for Infants and Toddlers. J Am Diet Assoc.* 2004;104:442–454. Copyright © 2004, with permission from The American Dietetic Association.

tongue. As the infant's body control improves and he can sit independently, he will also develop the ability to pick up and hold objects in his hand. He will be able to take in thicker pureed foods and soft mashed foods without lumps.

Babies who can crawl are also likely to be ready to self-feed finger foods such as baby biscuits or crackers. Babies at this stage can hold small foods between the thumb and first finger, and also hold a cup (preferably one with a cap and spout) independently. A baby is able to participate in the feeding process, and as her dexterity improves, she will be able to pick up small pieces of food. It is important that caregivers monitor the child's eating to make sure the youngster does not choke on food or on nonfood items.

At the end of the first year, when a baby is standing alone and beginning to walk, his diet can expand even further, with bite-size pieces of table foods and a wider variety of textures. Self-feeding with his fingers is much easier, and he desires to self-feed with a spoon as well—a messy but developmentally appropriate thing to do. Most table foods are appropriate for the child at this stage.

There is no scientific evidence to support introduction of complementary foods in any particular order; cultural practices play a large role in determining which foods are introduced first. Introducing a source of iron, such as an iron-fortified infant cereal or pureed meats, is necessary because iron stores developed in pregnancy are declining. No matter what food is introduced first, new foods should be introduced one at a time, at intervals of about one week, to see how well the infant tolerates each food and to be on the lookout for allergic reactions. Throughout the first year, breast milk or infant formula still forms the major portion of the infant's diet. Ideally, however, the child will have been introduced to a variety of foods by his or her first birthday.

Parents and caregivers should take care that complementary foods be soft in texture to avoid the risk of choking. Delaying—until age 1—the introduction of common food allergens, particularly cow's milk, egg whites, and wheat, can prevent food allergies for many infants. In addition to its allergic potential, whole cow's milk provides too much protein and too little iron, is low in essential fatty acids, may impair kidney function and lead to dehydration, and has been linked to development of insulin-dependent diabetes mellitus.[68] In families with a strong history of allergies, introduction of eggs should be delayed until age 2, and peanuts, tree nuts, fish, and shellfish should not be introduced before age 3.

Along with observing the infant's developmental readiness for complementary foods, parents and caregivers need to be alert to an infant's hunger and satiety cues. The suggestions in **Table 15.10** can help new parents establish a healthy feeding relationship with their child.

Various caregivers may be involved in a child's nutrition. In today's society, it is inappropriate to assume that the caregiver is solely the mother, father, grandparent, or even a relative of the child. Many children spend the majority of their feeding time in a child-care setting. Nutrition education and training for child-care workers enhances the likelihood of proper feeding practices in these settings.[69]

Key Concepts: *An infant's physiological needs and developmental readiness usually indicate the appropriate time to introduce solid foods. Semisolid and solid foods should be introduced slowly to check for food intolerances or allergic reactions. The caregiver should choose foods that meet the child's nutritional needs and suit his or her developmental capabilities.*

Table 15.10 **How to Feed Solid Foods**

- Feed your baby when she is hungry and wants to eat, but work toward regular feeding times.
- Put her in her highchair, perhaps propped up with a couple of pillows.
- Have her sit up straight and face you. She'll be able to swallow better and will be less likely to choke.
- Sit right in front of her.
- Hold the spoonful of food about 12 inches away from her face. It may be easier to start out with a long-handled baby spoon.
- Wait for her to pay attention and open her mouth before you try to feed her.
- Feed as slowly or as fast as she wants to eat.
- Let her touch her food.
- Respect her caution. It will take a while for her to get used to the spoon and the flavors of the foods.
- Talk to her, keep her company, but don't be exciting or entertaining.
- Stop feeding as soon as she shows you she is done.

Source: Satter E. *Child of Mine: Feeding with Love and Good Sense.* Boulder, CO: Bull Publishing, 2000.

Feeding Problems During Infancy

Colic

The term *colic* refers to continuous crying and distress in a healthy infant that appears to be due to abdominal cramping and discomfort. Infants with colic usually cry for hours, despite efforts to comfort them. In some cases, a change in formula or a change in the breastfeeding mother's diet provides some relief; however, diet (of either mother or infant) is not considered a cause of colic.[70] Most often, colic goes away on its own, usually by the age of 3 to 4 months.

Early Childhood Caries

Decay in the primary teeth, known as early childhood caries, and sometimes called "baby bottle tooth decay" (see **Figure 15.21**) can result if baby teeth are bathed too long in milk, formula, or juice, which nourish decay-producing bacteria. Other factors, such as inadequate development of tooth enamel, also contribute.[71] The problem is often associated with routinely putting a baby to bed with a bottle, so that the baby's teeth are awash in formula or juice for much or all of the night. Children with early childhood caries are more susceptible to caries in the permanent teeth and the possibility of life-long dental problems.[72]

Iron-Deficiency Anemia: Milk Anemia

Human milk and cow's milk both are low in iron. As discussed earlier, this is usually not a problem—the iron in breast milk is well absorbed, and regular cow's milk is not recommended for babies younger than 1 year. Iron deficiency may develop in older infants who do not eat enough iron-rich foods.

Gastroesophageal Reflux

Gastroesophageal reflux is the regurgitation of the stomach contents into the esophagus after a feeding. This type of spitting up occurs in 3 percent of newborns, usually males, and typically disappears within 12 to 18 months. Concern is warranted if reflux makes a child difficult to feed or results in coughing, choking, or frequent vomiting. Adding cereal to bottle feedings is *not* recommended for a baby who has reflux.

Diarrhea

Stool patterns vary from infant to infant, as well as in the same infant over time. Healthy, thriving breastfed infants may have up to 12 stools per day—or only 1 per week. Formula-fed infants usually have 1 to 7 bowel movements per day. Diarrhea—the frequent passage of loose, watery stools—can rapidly dehydrate an infant. Infants with diarrhea require increased fluids, and caregivers should consult the child's pediatrician for specific advice about how to meet this need.

Failure to Thrive

Full-term infants who experience poor growth in the absence of disease or physical defect suffer from **failure to thrive (FTT)**. (See **Figure 15.22**.) Although this can occur at any age, in infancy it usually occurs in the second half of the first year. Common causes include poverty and a resulting shortage of food, inappropriate foods in an infant's diet, improper formula preparation, or excessive consumption of fruit juice or fruit drinks. (See the FYI feature "Fruit Juices and Drinks.") In addition, well-meaning parents may introduce low-fat or nonfat milk in an attempt to prevent obesity.

gastroesophageal reflux A backflow of stomach contents into the esophagus, accompanied by a burning pain because of the acidity of the gastric juices.

failure to thrive (FTT) Abnormally low gains in length (height) and weight during infancy and childhood; may result from physical problems or poor feeding, but many affected children have no apparent disease or defect.

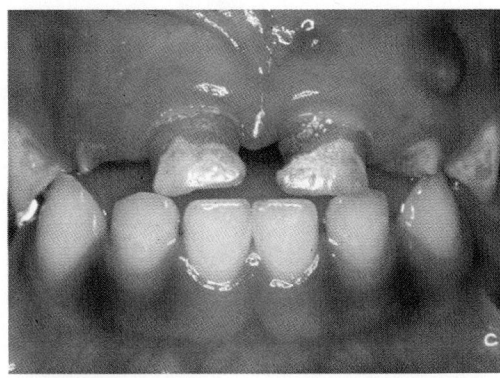

Figure 15.21 **Early childhood caries.** A baby routinely put to bed with a bottle can develop extensive tooth decay.

Quick Bites

Pumping Iron

The use of cow's milk for children younger than 1 year is a common cause of iron deficiency. Cow's milk is low in iron, and drinking cow's milk can cause intestinal bleeding in infants. The amount of iron in breast milk is low, but this iron is highly bioavailable. Breast milk also contains proteins that bind iron, thereby inhibiting the growth of diarrhea-causing bacteria that feed on iron. If formula is used, the AAP recommends that it be iron fortified.

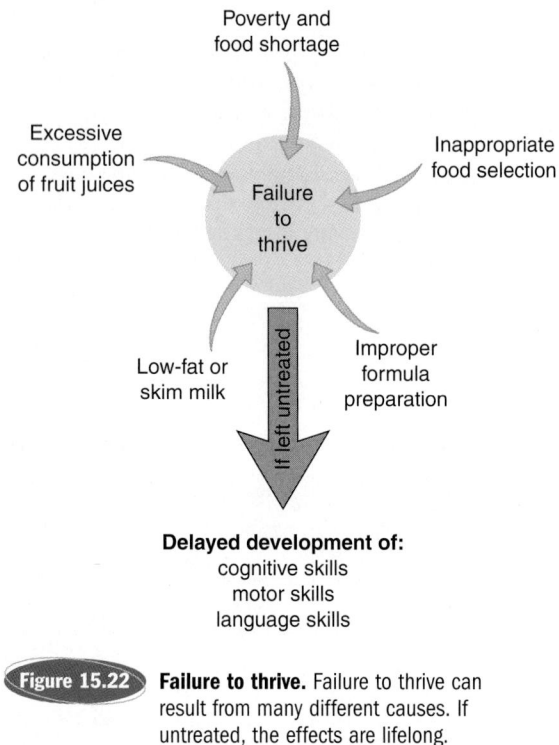

Figure 15.22 **Failure to thrive.** Failure to thrive can result from many different causes. If untreated, the effects are lifelong.

Babies need a high-fat diet to support normal growth and brain development. As stated, regular cow's milk should not be introduced before age 1. Low-fat milks are inappropriate for children younger than 2 years.

Untreated, FTT can delay cognitive, motor, and language development. Studies indicate, however, that intensive intervention can correct FTT and allow resumption of a normal growth pattern. Such intervention includes nutrition education for caregivers, maintenance of food records by the caregiver, frequent weight checks of the infant, and perhaps social service intervention for the family.

Although there is nothing complex about the nutrient needs and food choices appropriate for babies, it is important for caregivers to receive some education about proper feeding. Some of the practices we learn from friends, parents, and other family members, or remember from our own childhood, are inappropriate for babies. Studies show that even people who receive nutrition education in the WIC program introduce solid foods much too early and feed infants sweetened tea, soft drinks, and other inappropriate foods. Newborns don't come with instructions, but caregivers can always turn to a pediatrician or registered dietitian for answers to feeding questions.

Fyi Fruit Juices and Drinks

FOR YOUR INFORMATION

Fruit juices are popular beverages for children aged 6 months to 5 years. Juices do have benefits to the diet. They are refreshing and sweet, accessible and affordable, more healthful than soft drinks, and provide energy, water, and selected minerals and vitamins.[1] A glass of 100 percent fruit juice counts as one fruit serving. If juice is being used as a source of vitamin C, drinking just 3 to 6 fluid ounces per day meets vitamin C intake recommendations.

Fruit juices vary greatly in fiber, pectin, sorbitol, and carbohydrate composition. White grape juice is probably the easiest to digest (it contains similar amounts of glucose and fructose and no sorbitol). Apple and pear juice, while more popular, are less well absorbed due to higher amounts of sorbitol and fructose.[2]

Fruit juice consumption can be a factor in obesity, if excess juice is consumed on top of a well-rounded diet. Paradoxically, fruit juice consumption also can be a factor in failure to thrive. Failure to thrive may result if fruit juices replace other food sources (particularly milk), or if high amounts of sorbitol and fructose cause diarrhea and malabsorption.[3]

The vast array of juice drinks and fruit beverages available in the marketplace makes it difficult for parents to find nutritious choices. At best, these beverages contain added vitamin C and, in some cases, vitamin A and calcium. However, beverages that are less than 100 percent fruit juice are more like soft drinks than fruits and, as such, should be severely limited in the diets of young children.

To keep intake of fruit juices to a healthy level,

- Limit consumption of fruit juice to 12 fluid ounces per day and ideally no more than 3 to 6 fluid ounces per day
- Encourage caregivers to offer fruit rather than juice to children
- Dilute fruit juice with water
- Delay introduction of juices in the diet until the child can drink from a cup, thus avoiding using juice in bottles

1 Lifshitz F. Weaning foods...the role of fruit juice in the diets of infants and children. *J Am Coll Nutr*. 1996;15(suppl): 15–35.

2 Ibid.

3 Nobugrot T, Chasalow F, Lifshitz F. Carbohydrate absorption from one serving of fruit juice in young children: age and carbohydrate composition effects. *J Am Coll Nutr*. 1997;16: 152–158.

Key Concepts: *Feeding-related problems of infancy include colic, early childhood caries, nursing bottle tooth decay, iron-deficiency anemia, gastroesophageal reflux, diarrhea, and failure to thrive. Usually minor adjustments in food choices or feeding techniques solve these problems; however, caregivers may need the guidance of a pediatrician or registered dietitian.*

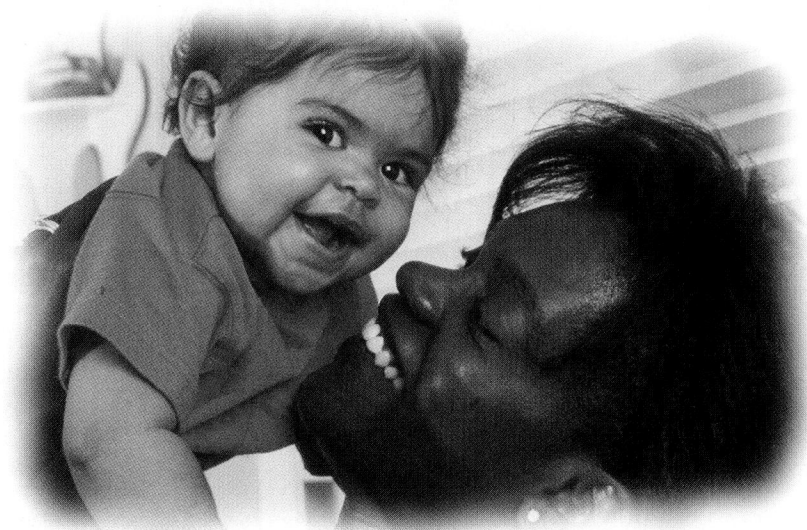

Label [to] **Table**

A pregnant woman requires more nutrients than usual. The RDA for both iron and folate increases by 50 percent during pregnancy. Iron, especially, is difficult to get in this quantity from the diet. Enriched grains and fortified foods, such as cereals, make it easier to obtain these essential nutrients. Let's take a look at the Nutrition Facts label from a popular breakfast cereal.

Take a look at how much folic acid a 1-cup serving of this breakfast cereal contains—50% DV (DV = 400 micrograms). The DV for folate is the same as the RDA for nonpregnant women; for pregnancy, the RDA increases to 600 micrograms. If orange juice accompanies the cereal, another 15% DV (60 µg) is added for a 1-cup serving. So, these two foods provide a substantial amount of the folate that a pregnant woman would need.

Iron also is extremely important for pregnancy because of its role in growth and its importance as blood volume increases during pregnancy. One serving of this breakfast cereal provides almost half of the DV of 18 milligrams (45 percent of 18 milligrams equals 8 milligrams). However, during pregnancy, the RDA for iron is 27 milligrams. So, one serving of this cereal provides nearly one-third of the iron needed each day—a good start. Having orange juice with the cereal will enhance iron absorption.

Nutrition Facts

Serving Size: 1 cup (30g)
Servings Per Container about 9

Amount Per Serving	Cheerios	with ½ cup skim milk
Calories	110	150
Calories from Fat	15	20
	% Daily Value**	
Total Fat 2g	3%	3%
Saturated Fat 0g	0%	3%
Trans Fat 0g		3%
Polyunsaturated Fat 0.5g		
Monounsaturated Fat 0.5g		
Cholesterol 0g	0%	1%
Sodium 280mg	12%	15%
Total Carbohydrate 22g	7%	9%
Dietary Fiber 0g	11%	11%
Sugars 1g		
Protein 3g		
Vitamin A	10%	15%
Vitamin C	10%	10%
Calcium	4%	20%
Iron	45%	45%
Vitamin D	10%	25%
Thiamin	25%	30%
Riboflavin	25%	35%
Niacin	25%	25%
Vitamin B₆	25%	25%
Folic Acid	50%	50%
Vitamin B₁₂	25%	35%
Phosphorus	10%	25%

LEARNING *Portfolio* c h a p t e r 1 5

Key Terms

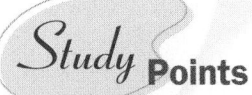

Study Points

➤ Nutritional status before pregnancy is an important part of having a healthy baby. Moreover, it is an integral part of all aspects of preconception care: risk assessment, health promotion, and intervention. Being either overweight or underweight prior to pregnancy increases risk of complications.

➤ Folic acid supplementation before pregnancy has been shown to reduce the risk of neural tube defects such as spina bifida.

➤ Excessive intake of some vitamins (vitamin A, in particular) and use of tobacco, alcohol, and drugs increase the risk of poor pregnancy outcomes; women should discontinue these practices before they become pregnant.

➤ Pregnancy can be divided into three stages: blastogenic, embryonic, and fetal. In the blastogenic stage, the fertilized ovum begins rapid cell division and implants itself in the uterine wall. During the embryonic stage, organ systems and other body structures form. During the fetal stage, the longest period of pregnancy, the fetus grows in size and changes in proportions.

➤ Women who enter pregnancy at a normal BMI should gain 25 to 35 pounds during pregnancy. Underweight women should gain more weight and overweight women less. Energy needs increase by 340 to 450 kilocalories per day for the second and third trimesters.

➤ By using the MyPyramid to plan food intake, pregnant women who consume enough energy should be able to meet all their nutrient needs with the exception of iron and folate. They should get needed extra calories mainly from grains, fruits, and vegetables.

➤ Limiting caffeine intake during pregnancy is recommended. Smoking during pregnancy increases the risk of preterm delivery and low birth weight. Alcohol and drug use can interfere with normal fetal development and should be avoided during pregnancy.

➤ Gastrointestinal distress such as morning sickness, heartburn, and constipation are common during pregnancy and result from the action of various hormones on the GI tract. Although most food cravings or aversions present no problems, excessive consumption of nonfood items, known as pica, interferes with adequate nutrition.

➤ During pregnancy, hormones control the development of breast tissue in preparation for milk production. Colostrum, the first milk, which is rich in protein and antibodies, is produced soon after delivery. By two to three weeks after delivery, lactation is well established, and mature milk is being produced.

➤ The pituitary hormone prolactin stimulates milk production. Oxytocin, another pituitary hormone, stimulates milk release, which is known as the let-down reflex.

➤ Unless they reduce their physical activity, breastfeeding women need about 330 to 400 more kilocalories per day than they did when they were not pregnant. By obtaining adequate energy and using MyPyramid to balance choices, most lactating women can obtain all the nutrients they need from their diet. Cigarettes, alcohol, and illicit drugs should not be used while breastfeeding.

- Mothers benefit from breastfeeding through enhanced physiologic recovery, convenience, and emotional bonding. Contraindications to breastfeeding include infection with HIV or active tuberculosis, and regular use of certain medications.

- Infants receive optimal nutrition from human milk. Breastfeeding can reduce the incidence of infectious diseases, allergies, and other problems during infancy.

- La Leche League, the March of Dimes, and the WIC program for low-income women are among the numerous resources for support and education of pregnant and breastfeeding women.

- Infancy is the fastest growth stage in the life cycle; infants double their birth weight in 4 to 6 months and triple it by 1 year of age. The nutritional status of infants is assessed primarily through measurements of growth.

- Infants' energy needs must be met through a high-fat diet, which provides the maximum calories in minimal volume. Infants' protein and fluid needs are also high.

- Human milk is low in vitamin D; breastfed babies need regular sun exposure or supplemental vitamin D. For breastfed infants, iron-fortified foods need to be introduced by 6 months of age. Formula-fed infants should be given iron-fortified formula.

- Infant formulas usually are based on either cow's milk or soy protein. Unmodified cow's milk is inappropriate for infants throughout the first year of life.

- The FDA regulates the vitamin and mineral composition of infant formulas to ensure adequate infant nutrition. Formula is available in ready-to-feed, liquid concentrate, and powdered forms.

- A nurturing environment is important to the feeding of infants, no matter what the milk source.

- Solid foods are introduced to the infant one at a time, usually beginning with iron-fortified infant cereal. Potential allergens, such as cow's milk, egg whites, and wheat, should be delayed until the baby is at least 12 months old. Developmental markers, such as head and body control and the absence of the extrusion reflex, show readiness for solid foods.

- Colic, although troublesome to infant and caregiver, is not caused by diet. Iron-deficiency anemia is common in infants who lack iron-rich foods. Infants are susceptible to dehydration, especially when diarrhea is prolonged. Failure to thrive describes an infant who is not growing well; intervention may be required to correct feeding practices of caregivers.

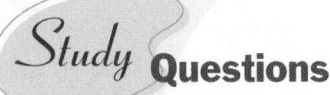

Study Questions

1. Describe the three stages of fetal growth.

2. What are some of the physiological changes that occur to a woman during pregnancy?

3. How do the recommended intake values for calories, protein, folate, and iron change for pregnancy?

4. What contributes to morning sickness, and how can a woman minimize its effects?

5. Is it okay for an infant to experience weight loss immediately after birth? If an infant does lose weight, does it mean he or she is at nutritional risk?

6. What are some of the nutritional benefits of breast milk?

7. How much water does a breastfed or formula-fed infant need each day?

8. Is it necessary to give breastfed infants supplements of vitamins and/or minerals? If so, which ones?

9. Describe the process for introducing solid foods into an infant's diet.

10. List the feeding problems that may occur during infancy.

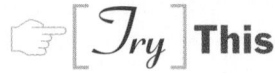

For Just One Week, Can You Eat Like You're Expecting?

The purpose of this exercise is to see if you can follow the nutrition guidelines for pregnancy for just one week. Keep in mind that pregnant women attempt to do this for 38 to 40 weeks! Your goal is to reduce or eliminate caffeine, alcohol, and over-the-counter medications. Make an effort to eat according to MyPyramid each day, selecting the most nutrient-dense choices from each group. You should also take a basic multivitamin/mineral tablet (in place of a woman's prenatal supplement) daily. This will ensure that you consume the amounts of protein, vitamins, and minerals recommended for pregnancy.

Costs of Infant Formula

The purpose of this exercise is to find out how much it might cost to feed an infant. An average 3-month-old baby weighs about 13 pounds (6 kilograms) and would need about 600 kilocalories per day. Using standard infant formula, this baby would need about 30 ounces of formula each day. Now, go to a grocery store and find the infant formulas. If you were to purchase ready-to-feed formula, how much would it cost to feed this baby for one day? What if you were to use concentrated liquid formula? Powdered formula?

What About 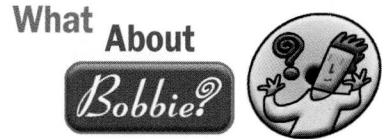 Bobbie?

Let's pretend that Bobbie is pregnant and in her second trimester. She wants to know whether she's meeting her basic nutrient needs by following her usual diet. Refer to Chapter 1 to review her one-day intake. How do you think she's doing? Let's compare Bobbie's intake of nutrients to the recommendations for pregnant women.

Protein

If you remember reviewing Bobbie's diet after reading Chapter 6, "Proteins and Amino Acids," you may recall that it is quite high in protein. Her intake was 96 grams, and her nonpregnancy RDA (based on her weight) was 56 grams. During pregnancy, however, Bobbie needs extra protein to ensure her body can handle the demands of tissue growth. An extra 25 grams per day (for a total of 81 grams) is adequate to meet the needs of pregnancy. Bobbie's intake is higher than this level and could be reduced.

Folate

Bobbie's intake of folate was 650 micrograms, which is consistent with her pregnancy RDA of 600 micrograms. Her intake is mainly from enriched grains. By adding other folate-rich foods to her diet, such as spinach, legumes, and orange juice, she would obtain other vital nutrients. If Bobbie is adhering to proper prenatal care, then she is consuming a prenatal supplement with folic acid as well.

Iron

Bobbie's intake of iron for one day was 20 milligrams. This is substantially lower than her pregnancy RDA of 27 milligrams. This places Bobbie at greater risk for iron deficiency, a common condition in pregnancy. In addition to taking a prenatal supplement that contains iron, Bobbie is advised to continue choosing iron-rich lean red meats such as the beef meatballs for dinner. She would also benefit from adding more dark-green leafy vegetables to her diet, along with a squeeze of lemon (or other source of vitamin C) to increase the absorption of the nonheme iron. With these additions to her diet, Bobbie will lower her chances of having iron deficiency during her pregnancy.

References

1 Cnattingius S, Bergstrom R, Lipworth L, Kramer MS. Prepregnancy weight and the risk of adverse pregnancy outcomes. *N Engl J Med.* 1998;338:147–152.

2 Ibid.

3 Cnattingius S, et al. Op. cit.; and Goldenberg RL, Tamura T. Prepregnancy weight and pregnancy outcome. *JAMA.* 1996; 275:1127–1128.

4 Institute of Medicine, Food and Nutrition Board. *Dietary Reference Intakes for Thiamin, Riboflavin, Niacin, Vitamin B_6, Folate, Vitamin B_{12}, Pantothenic Acid, Biotin, and Choline.* Washington, DC: National Academy Press, 1998.

5 Mathews TJ. Trends in spina bifida and anencephalus in the United States, 1991–2004. Centers for Disease Control and Prevention, National Center for Health Statistics. http://www.cdc.gov/nchs/products/pubs/pubd/hestats/spine_anen.htm. Accessed 1/7/07.

6 Worthington-Roberts B. The role of maternal nutrition in the prevention of birth defects. *J Am Diet Assoc.* 1997;97:S184.

7 US Food and Drug Administration. FDA announces strengthened risk management program to enhance safe use of isotretinoin (Accutane) for treating severe acne. *FDA News.* August 12, 2005. http://www.fda.gov/bbs/topics/NEWS/2005/NEW01218.html. Accessed 8/7/06.

8 Piyathilake CJ, Macaluso M, Hine RJ, et al. Local and systemic effects of cigarette smoking on folate and vitamin B_{12}. *Am J Clin Nutr.* 1994;60:559–566.

9 Institute of Medicine. *Nutrition During Pregnancy.* Washington, DC: National Academy Press, 1990.

10 Ibid.

11 Ibid.

12 Institute of Medicine, Food and Nutrition Board. *Dietary Reference Intakes for Energy, Carbohydrate, Fiber, Fat, Fatty Acids, Cholesterol, Protein, and Amino Acids.* Washington, DC: National Academy Press, 2005.

13 Pitkin RM. Energy in pregnancy. *Am J Clin Nutr.* 1999; 69(4):583.

14 Institute of Medicine, Food and Nutrition Board. 2005. Op. cit.

15 Turner RE, Langkamp-Henken B, Littell RC, Lukowski MJ, Suarez MF. Comparing nutrient intake from food to the estimated average requirements shows middle- to upper-income pregnant women lack iron and possibly magnesium. *J Am Diet Assoc.* 2003;103(4):461–466.

16 Institute of Medicine, Food and Nutrition Board. 2005. Op. cit.

17 Institute of Medicine, Food and Nutrition Board. 1990. Op. cit.

18 Pick ME, Edwards M, Moreau D, Ryan EA. Assessment of diet quality in pregnant women using the Health Eating Index. *J Am Diet Assoc.* 2005;105:240–246.

19 US Department of Health and Human Services and US Environmental Protection Agency. What you need to know about mercury in fish and shellfish. March 2004. http://www.cfsan.fda.gov/~dms/admehg3.html. Accessed 7/18/06.

20 Lowe JB, Balanda KP, Clare G. Evaluation of antenatal smoking cessation programs for pregnant women. *Aust N Z J Pub Health.* 1998;22:55.

21 Pamuk E, Makuc D, Heck K, et al. *Socioeconomic Status and Health Chartbook. Health, United States 1998.* Hyattsville, MD: National Center for Health Statistics, 1998. Updated October 1999.

22 Institute of Medicine, Food and Nutrition Board. 1990. Op. cit.

23 Corbetet RW, Ryan C, Weinrich SP. Pica in pregnancy: does it affect pregnancy outcomes? *Am J Matern Child Nurs.* 2003; 28:183–189.

24 Johnson CD, Koh SH, Shynett B, Koh J, Johnson C. An uncommon dental presentation during pregnancy resulting from multiple eating disorders: pica and bulimia: case report. *Gen Dent.* 2006;54(3):198–200.

25 Roberts JM, Balk JL, Bodnar LM, Belizan JM, Bergl E, Martinez A. Nutrient involvement in preeclampsia. *J Nutr.* 2003; 133:1684S–1692S.

26 Turner RE. Nutrition during pregnancy. In: Shils ME, Ross AC, Shike M, Caballero B, Cousins RJ, eds. *Modern Nutrition in Health and Disease.* 10th ed. Philadelphia: Lippincott Williams & Wilkins, 2006; and Rumbold AR, Crowther CA, Haslam RR, et al. Vitamins C and E and the risks of preeclampsia and perinatal complications. *N Engl J Med.* 2006;354(17):1796–1806.

27 Story M, Alton I. Nutritional guidelines during pregnancy and lactation. In: Wolinsky I, Klimis-Tavantzis D, eds. *Nutritional Concerns of Women.* New York: CRC Press, 1996.

28 American Diabetes Association. Diagnosis and classification of diabetes mellitus. *Diabetes Care.* 2007;30(suppl 1):S42–S47.

29 March of Dimes. HIV and AIDS in pregnancy. November 2002. http://www.marchofdimes.com/professionals/681_1223.asp. Accessed 1/7/07.

30 Centers for Disease Control and Prevention. Assessing adolescent pregnancy. *MMWR.* 1998;47:433.

31 Story M, Alton I. Nutrition issues and adolescent pregnancy. *Nutr Today.* 1995;30:142.

32 Institute of Medicine, Food and Nutrition Board. 1990. Op. cit.

33 Li R, Darling N, Maurice E, Barker L, Grummer-Strawn LM. Breastfeeding rates in the United States by characteristics of the child, mother, or family: the 2002 National Immunization Survey. *Pediatrics.* 2005;155:31–37.

34 Ryan A, Wenjun Z, Acosta A. Breastfeeding continues to increase into the new millennium. *Pediatrics.* 2002;110:1103–1109.

35 Neville MC. Anatomy and physiology of lactation. *Pediatr Clin North Am.* 2001;48:13–34.

36 Institute of Medicine, Food and Nutrition Board. 2005. Op. cit.

37 Ibid.

38 Institute of Medicine, Food and Nutrition Board. 1990. Op. cit.

39 Greer FR. Do breastfed infants need supplemental vitamins? *Pediatr Clin North Am.* 2001;48:415–423.

40 Story M, Alton I. 1996. Op. cit.

41 American Dietetic Association. Position of the American Dietetic Association: promoting and supporting breastfeeding. *J Am Diet Assoc.* 2005;105:810–818.

42 Raisler J, Alexander C, O'Campo P. Breast-feeding and infant illness: a dose-response relationship? *Am J Public Health.* 1999;89:25–30.

43 American Dietetic Association. Op. cit.

44 Hanson LA, Korotkova M, Lundin S, et al. The transfer of immunity from mother to child. *Ann N Y Acad Sci.* 2003; 987:199–206.

45 Worthington-Roberts BS, Williams SR. *Nutrition Through the Life Cycle.* 4th ed. New York: McGraw-Hill, 1999.

46 Mortensen EL, Michaelsen KF, Sanders SA, Reinisch JM. The association between duration of breastfeeding and adult intelligence. *JAMA.* 2002;287:2365–2371.

47 Lawrence A. *A Review of the Medical Benefits and Contraindications to Breastfeeding in the United States.* Arlington, VA: National Center for Education in Maternal and Child Health, 1997. Maternal and Child Health Technical Information Bulletin.

48 Wright AL. The rise of breastfeeding in the United States. *Pediatr Clin North Am.* 2001;48:1–12.

49 Riordan J, Auerbach KG. *Breastfeeding and Human Lactation.* 2nd ed. Sudbury, MA: Jones and Bartlett, 1999.

50 Owen GM. Maternal nutrition. In: Owen AL, Splett PL, Owen GM, eds. *The Art and Science of Delivering Services.* 4th ed. Boston: WCB-McGraw-Hill, 1999:208.

51 Montgomery DL, Splett PL. Economic benefits of breastfeeding infants enrolled in WIC. *J Am Diet Assoc.* 1997; 97:379–386.

52 American Dietetics Association. Why children must play while they eat: an interview with T. Berry Brazelton. *J Am Diet Assoc.* 1993;93:1385–1387.

53 Institute of Medicine, Food and Nutrition Board, Committee on Nutritional Status During Pregnancy and Lactation. *Nutrition During Lactation.* Washington, DC: National Academy Press, 1990.

54 Institute of Medicine, Food and Nutrition Board. 2005. Op. cit.

55 Uauy R, Peirano P, Hoffman D, et al. Role of essential fatty acids in the function of the developing nervous system. *Lipids.* 1996;31:S167–S176.

56 Institute of Medicine, Food and Nutrition Board. 2005. Op. cit.

57 Ibid.

58 Sachdev HP, Krishna J, Puri RK, et al. Water supplementation in exclusively breast-fed infants during summer in the tropics. *Lancet.* 1991;337:929–933.

59 AAP Committee on Fetus and Newborn. *Guidelines for Perinatal Care.* 5th ed. Elk Grove Village, IL: American Academy of Pediatrics, 2002.

60 Ibid.

61 Ibid.

62 American Academy of Pediatrics. Breastfeeding and the use of human milk. *Pediatrics.* 1997;100:1035–1039.

63 Kleinman RE, ed. *Pediatric Nutrition Handbook.* 5th ed. Elk Grove Village, IL: American Academy of Pediatrics, 2004.

64 Auestad N, Scott DT, Janowsky JS, et al. Visual, cognitive, and language assessments at 39 months: a follow-up study of children fed formulas containing long-chain polyunsaturated fatty acids to 1 year of age. *Pediatrics.* 2003;112:177–183; and Thorpe M. Infant formula supplemented with DHA: are there benefits? *J Am Diet Assoc.* 2003;103:551–552.

65 Kleinman RE. Op. cit.

66 Pac S, McMahon K, Ripple M, et al. Development of the Start Healthy Feeding Guidelines for infants and toddlers. *J Am Diet Assoc.* 2004;104:455–467.

67 Butte N, Cobb K, Dwyer J, et al. The Start Healthy Feeding Guidelines for infants and toddlers. *J Am Diet Assoc.* 2004; 104:442–454.

68 American Academy of Pediatrics. Infant feeding practices and their possible relationship to the etiology of diabetes mellitus. *Pediatrics.* 1994;94:752–754.

69 Nahikian-Nelms M. Influential factors of caregiver behavior at mealtime: a study of 24 child care programs. *J Am Diet Assoc.* 1997;97:505–509.

70 Clifford TJ, Campbell K, Speechley KN, Gorodzinsky F. Infant colic: empirical evidence of the absence of an association with source of early infant nutrition. *Arch Pediatr Adolesc Med.* 2002;156:1123–1128.

71 American Academy of Pediatric Dentistry. *Policy on Early Childhood Caries (ECC): Unique Challenges and Treatment Options.* 2003. http://www.aapd.org/media/Policies_Guidelines /P_ECCUniqueChallenges.pdf. Accessed 8/6/06.

72 National Maternal and Child Oral Health Resource Center. *Promoting Awareness, Preventing Pain: Facts on Early Childhood Caries (ECC).* 2nd ed. 2004. http://www.mchoralhealth.org /PDFs/ECCFactSheet.pdf. Accessed 8/6/06.

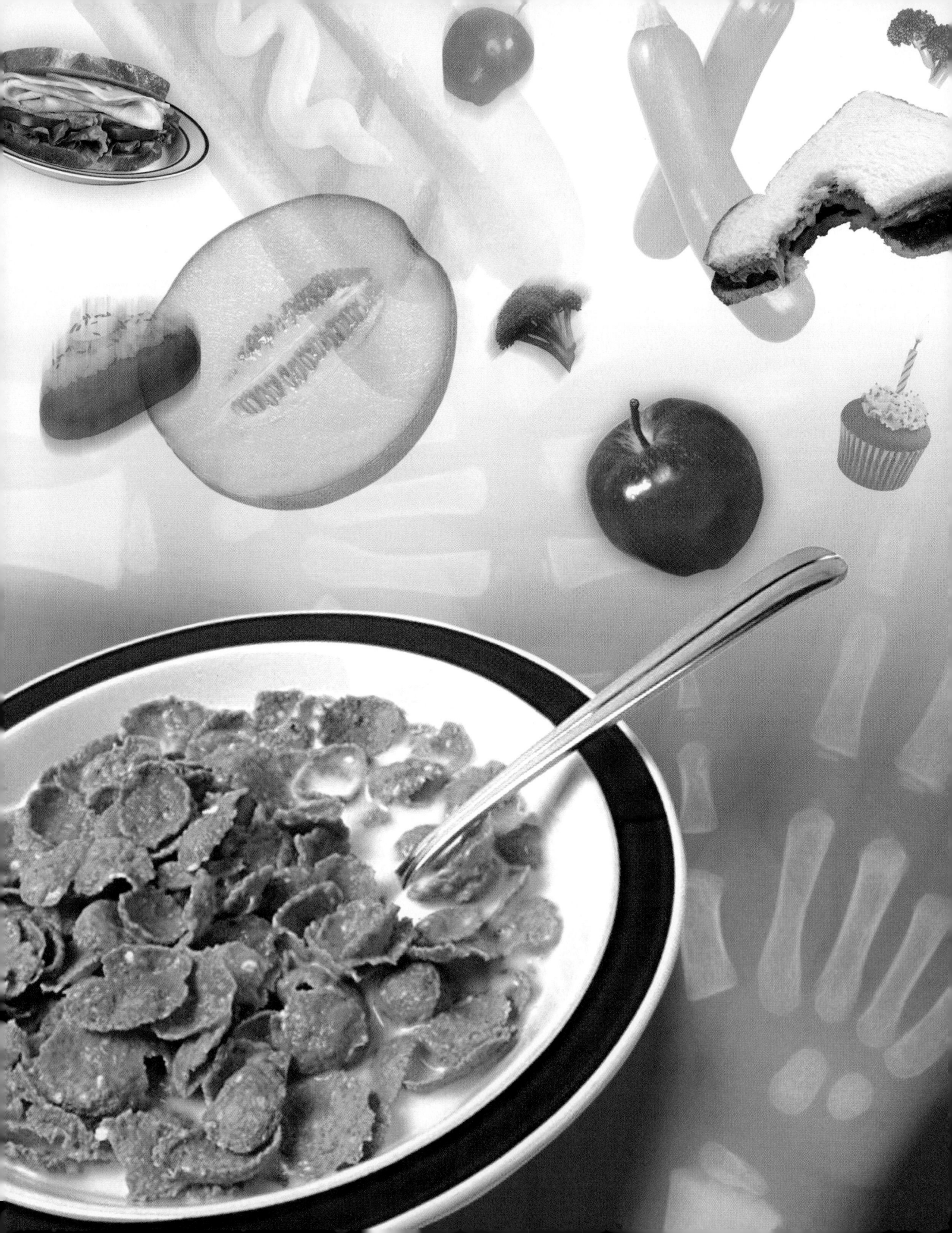

Chapter 16

Life Cycle: From Childhood Through Adulthood

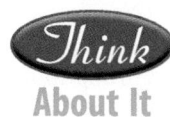

Think About It

1 Were you a "picky" eater as a child? What about now?

2 What's your experience with acne and eating particular foods?

3 What behavior changes would you consider making now that would help you live longer?

4 Your grandfather lives by himself and relies on frozen foods for his nutritional needs. How do you feel about this strategy?

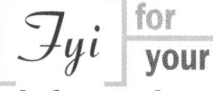

Fyi for your Information

This chapter's FYI boxes include practical information on the following topics:

• Food Hypersensitivities and Allergies

• Overweight in Children and Teens: Whose Problem Is It?

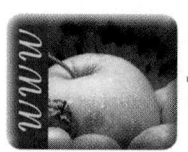

The Web site for this book offers many useful tools and is a great source for additional nutrition information for both students and instructors. For information on nutrition during childhood, adolescence, and adulthood, visit the site at **nutrition.jbpub.com**. You'll find exercises that explore the following topics:

• Got Milk—Allergy?

• Lead

• Childhood Malnutrition

• The Elderly Nutrition Program

• Older Women and B$_{12}$

• Arthritis and Nutrition

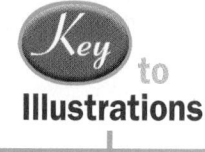

Key to Illustrations

▲ Fat-Soluble Vitamins

● Minerals

▽ Water-Soluble Vitamins

What About 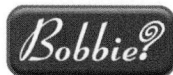 **Bobbie?**

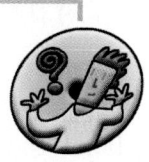

Track the choices Bobbie is making with Nutritionist Pro or EatRight Analysis software.

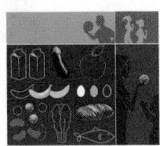

Dietary Guidelines for
Americans, 2005

key recommendations

- Consume a variety of nutrient-dense foods and beverages within and among the basic food groups while choosing foods that limit the intake of saturated and *trans* fats, cholesterol, added sugars, salt, and alcohol.
- Meet recommended intakes within energy needs by adopting a balanced eating pattern, such as the USDA Food Guide or the DASH Eating Plan.

Key Recommendations for Specific Population Groups

- *Children and adolescents.* Consume whole-grain products often; at least half the grains should be whole grains. Children 2 to 8 years should consume 2 cups per day of fat-free or low-fat milk or equivalent milk products. Children 9 years of age and older should consume 3 cups per day of fat-free or low-fat milk or equivalent milk products.

childhood The period of life from age 1 to the onset of puberty.

adolescence The period between onset of puberty and adulthood.

American Dietetic Association

Dietary Guidance for Healthy Children Aged 2 to 11 Years

It is the position of the American Dietetic Association that children ages 2 to 11 years should achieve optimal physical and cognitive development, attain a healthy weight, enjoy food, and reduce the risk of chronic disease through appropriate eating habits and participation in regular physical activity.

J Am Diet Assoc. 2004;104:660–677.
Reprinted with permission.

*I*t's the year 2060. Who are you? Where do you live? What is your life like? How healthy are you? If projections made earlier in the century were accurate, you are part of the largest segment of the population—in 2060 between one-third and one-fourth of Americans are older than 65. Perhaps you have retired recently, or maybe you continue to work in your profession. Think about how technology has changed in your lifetime: New methods of communication have been developed that make e-mail and the Internet seem old-fashioned, so late twentieth century!

Consider how much you have changed over the years. Throughout childhood and adolescence you were growing, sometimes quite rapidly. Whether you fueled that growth with burgers and fries, black beans and rice, chips and soft drinks, or yogurt and salads will have determined a lot about your health status in 2060. Did you continue the eating habits you had in college, and did these allow you to control your weight, blood cholesterol, and blood pressure? Or perhaps in the year 2060 these conditions are no longer of concern. Advances in genetics may have allowed gene therapy to replace diet therapy and medications for chronic diseases.

In the last chapter we explored the nutritional needs of pregnant and breastfeeding women and their babies. Now we will look at how continued growth in childhood and adolescence affects nutritional needs. In addition, we'll see how nutritional needs change as we age, and we'll consider feeding practices, meal planning, and obstacles to healthful eating for each age group.

Childhood

Childhood is the term that refers to the years from age 1 through the beginning of **adolescence**. Growth in childhood, although continuous, occurs at a significantly slower rate than in infancy. During the childhood years, a typical child will gain about 5 pounds and grow 2 to 3 inches each year. Children can be divided into three groups based on their age and development: toddlers (ages 1–3), preschoolers (ages 4–5), and school-aged children (ages 6–10).

Energy and Nutrient Needs During Childhood

Energy and Protein

An average 1-year-old requires about 850 to 1,000 kilocalories per day.[1] This daily energy requirement gradually increases until it almost doubles by around age 10. Estimated Energy Requirements (EER) for children can be calculated based on sex, age, height, weight, and activity level. (See **Table 16.1.**) The added energy cost for growth is only 20 kilocalories per day, much less than the 175 kilocalories per day needed during early infancy. Although total energy requirements increase, the kilocalories needed per kilogram of body weight slowly decrease as children move through childhood. The same is true for protein requirements. (See **Table 16.2.**)

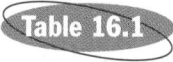

Table 16.1 Estimated Energy Requirement (EER) Equations for Children Age 3 to 8 Years

Males

EER = 88.5 − 61.9 × Age [y] + PA × (26.7 × Weight [kg] + 903 × Height [m]) + 20 kcal/day

Physical activity (PA)

Sedentary = 1.00; Low active = 1.13; Active = 1.26; Very active = 1.42

Females

EER = 135.3 − 30.8 × Age [y] + PA × (10.0 × Weight [kg] + 934 × Height [m]) + 20 kcal/day

Physical Activity (PA)

Sedentary = 1.0; Low active = 1.16; Active = 1.31; Very active = 1.56

Source: Institute of Medicine, Food and Nutrition Board. *Dietary Reference Intakes for Energy, Carbohydrate, Fiber, Fat, Fatty Acids, Cholesterol, Protein, and Amino Acids.* Washington, DC: National Academies Press, 2005. Reprinted with permission from the National Academy of Sciences.

Table 16.2 Protein RDAs for Childhood

Age (y)	Protein (g/kg)	Reference Weight* (kg)	Protein (g/d)
1–3	1.05	12	13
4–8	0.95	20	19

*Reference weights are based on median weights of children in that age group.

Source: Institute of Medicine, Food and Nutrition Board. *Dietary Reference Intakes for Energy, Carbohydrate, Fiber, Fat, Fatty Acids, Cholesterol, Protein, and Amino Acids.* Washington, DC: National Academies Press, 2005. Reprinted with permission from the National Academy of Sciences.

Table 16.3 Iron-Rich Foods and Snacks

Iron-Rich Foods

Ground beef

Poultry

Fish

Legumes

Dark-green vegetables

Enriched breads, cereals, rice, and pasta

Iron-Rich Snacks

Cream of Wheat

Cooked macaroni or pasta

Enriched cereals, either dry or with milk

Tortillas filled with refried beans

Dried apricots

Raisins (for older children)

Bean dip

Chili, mildly seasoned

Peanut butter on enriched bread or graham crackers

Sloppy Joe

Casseroles with meat (many children do not like plain meats)

Vitamins and Minerals

As long as a child cooperates by eating a variety of healthful foods, a well-planned diet should provide most of the nutrients a child needs. One exception is iron. Children ages 4 to 8 years require 10 milligrams of iron per day, but may not get that amount without careful meal planning. High consumption of milk, a poor source of iron, can contribute to inadequate iron intake, and so milk intake during childhood should be limited to 3 to 4 cups per day. This allows room in the diet for high-iron food sources such as lean meats, legumes, fish, poultry, and iron-enriched breads and cereals. (See **Table 16.3**.) Iron deficiency not only affects growth but also can impair the child's mood, attention span, focus, and ability to learn.[2]

A child's diet also may be low in other micronutrients, especially zinc, vitamin D, and vitamin E. (See **Figure 16.1**.) Children often dislike vegetables, or they may be following their parents' low-fat diets, which may be low in zinc and vitamin E.[3]

Vitamin and Mineral Supplements

Many caregivers would rather give a child a vitamin/mineral pill than plan and prepare the meals necessary to ensure an adequate diet. However, the balanced diet a child needs is not much different from the diet an adult needs. In fact, MyPyramid is for anyone age 2 and older (see **Figure 16.2**); children need the same balance of food groups as is recommended for

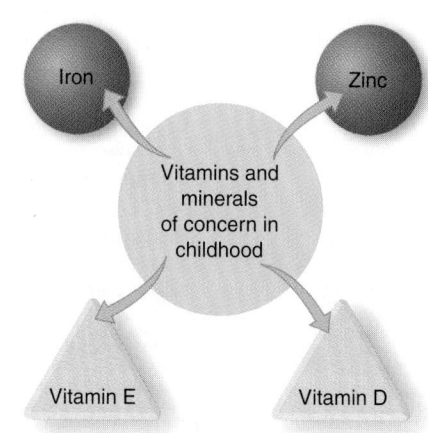

Figure 16.1 **Micronutrients of concern in childhood.** Milk is low in iron, and small children also may have low intakes of zinc, vitamin D, and vitamin E.

adults. Caregivers who understand this may be less tempted to rely on supplements to achieve a balanced diet.

Some children should receive supplements. Among them are children whose diets are restricted for medical reasons, those with chronic diseases, those who are malnourished, and those with food allergies that require them to avoid multiple foods or food groups.[4] (For more on food allergies, see the FYI feature "Food Hypersensitivities and Allergies.") Caregivers need to be reminded that vitamin and mineral supplements for children are dangerous in large doses. Vitamin and mineral preparations must be treated like all medicines and kept safely out of children's reach. Supplements containing iron in doses over 30 milligrams are especially dangerous to children. Accidental consumption of vitamin and mineral or iron supplements should be treated as a poisoning emergency.

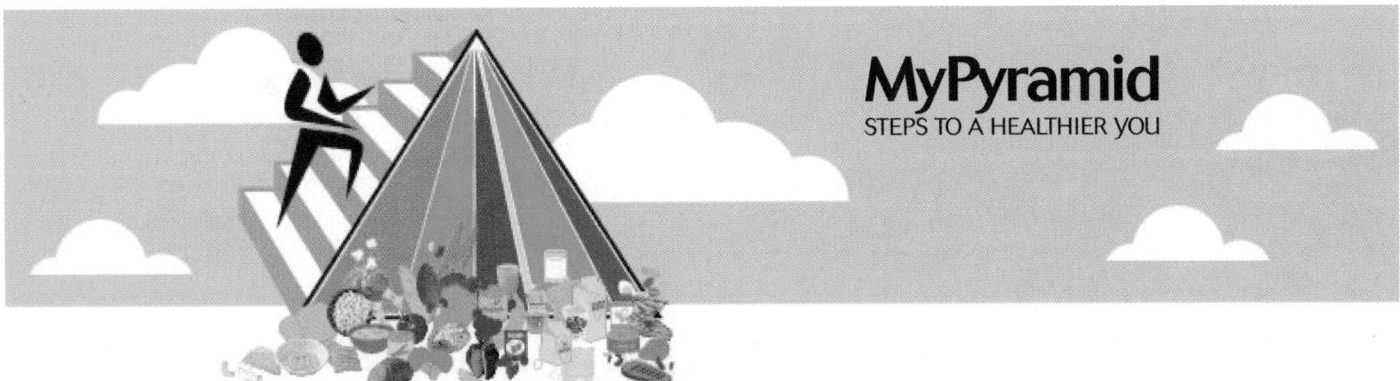

MyPyramid
STEPS TO A HEALTHIER YOU

Based on the information you provided, this is your daily recommended amount from each food group.

GRAINS 6 ounces	VEGETABLES 2 1/2 cups	FRUITS 2 cups	MILK 3 cups	MEAT & BEANS 5 1/2 ounces
Make half your grains whole Aim for at least **3 ounces** of whole grains a day	**Vary your veggies** Aim for these amounts each week: **Dark green veggies** = 3 cups **Orange veggies** = 2 cups **Dry beans & peas** = 3 cups **Starchy veggies** = 3 cups **Other veggies** = 6 1/2 cups	**Focus on fruits** Eat a variety of fruit Go easy on fruit juices	**Get your calcium-rich foods** Go low-fat or fat-free when you choose milk, yogurt, or cheese	**Go lean with protein** Choose low-fat or lean meats and poultry Vary your protein routine—choose more fish, beans, peas, nuts, and seeds

Find your balance between food and physical activity

Be physically active for at least **60 minutes** every day, or most days.

Know your limits on fats, sugars, and sodium

Your allowance for oils is **6 teaspoons a day.**

Limit extras—solid fats and sugars—to **265 calories a day.**

Your results are based on a 2000 calorie pattern.

Name: _____

This calorie level is only an estimate of your needs. Monitor your body weight to see if you need to adjust your calorie intake.

Figure 16.2 **MyPyramid for a young boy.** This MyPyramid reports the recommendations for an 8-year old active boy (engages in physical activity for more than 60 minutes on most days). **Source:** US Department of Agriculture. www.MyPyramid.gov.

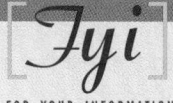 **Food Hypersensitivities and Allergies**

FOR YOUR INFORMATION

Food allergies, or food hypersensitivities, are allergic reactions to food proteins. Allergies are different from food intolerances (such as lactose intolerance), which may involve digestive problems rather than an immune response. Allergies are less likely than intolerances to be transient, and tend to have more serious consequences. Proteins that trigger allergies are known as allergens. The most common food allergens are found in milk, eggs, tree nuts, peanuts, soy, wheat, fish, and shellfish.

Food allergies occur when the immune system mounts a specific reaction to a food protein. Surveys suggest that about 25 percent of people in the general population think they suffer from food allergies. But studies show that only 1 to 2 percent of adults and 6 to 8 percent of children under the age of 3 truly do.[1]

In a true allergic reaction, the immune system responds to an allergen with a cascade of chemical reactions that can cause wheezing, difficulty breathing, and hives, as well as a host of other symptoms. (See **Table 1**.) Food allergy symptoms often affect more than one body system and may change in severity from one reaction to the next.

Anaphylaxis, the most severe allergic reaction, usually takes place within the first hour after eating the offending food. Shock and respiratory failure can rapidly ensue. Anaphylaxis can be fatal, so immediate emergency care is essential.

Allergy symptoms that occur immediately after a food is eaten make detective work easier. If symptoms are slow to evolve, a child may suffer chronic diarrhea and even experience failure to thrive before the problem is identified.

When identification of the food culprit isn't so obvious, an elimination diet can help. All suspected foods are eliminated from the diet and slowly reintroduced, one by one, on a specific schedule. Both intake and reactions are carefully recorded. Prolonged or improper use of such a diet can have severe nutritional consequences. A registered dietitian can help with diet planning to ensure nutritional adequacy.

The double-blind, placebo-controlled food challenge is the gold standard of food allergy testing. Although definitive, it can be dangerous for people prone to anaphylactic reactions. In this test, increasing amounts of a suspected food are given to the patient under the supervision of a physician, who looks for allergy symptoms and signs. This test must be done by trained personnel with emergency equipment handy.

The treatment for food allergy is avoidance of the offending allergen. Each child with a food allergy needs a nutrition assessment that pays attention to the specific nutrients missing as a result of avoiding the offending foods. For example, if a toddler is avoiding milk and milk products due to a cow's milk allergy, the nutrients most at risk would be protein, vitamin D, and calcium. As a child's diet includes more and more foods, careful label reading is the key to identifying allergen-containing foods. As of January 2006, all food labels were required to list in plain English the presence of ingredients that contain protein derived from milk, eggs, fish, crustacean shellfish, tree nuts, peanuts, wheat, or soybeans.[2] These eight foods are responsible for 90 percent of food allergies. Organizations such as the Food Allergy Network provide resource materials for parents and children, including recipes and tips for successful traveling and dining with a child who has food allergies.[3]

Many children naturally outgrow food allergies by the time they are 3 years old. Once outgrown, the food allergy will not return.

1 Simpson HA. Food allergy. *JAMA.* 1997;278:1888–1894.
2 Thompson T, Kane RR, Hager MH. Food Allergen Labeling and Consumer Protection Act of 2004 in effect. *J Am Diet Assoc.* 2006;106:1742–1744.
3 The Food Allergy & Anaphylaxis Network. http://www.foodallergy.org. Accessed 8/2/06.

Table 1 **Symptoms of Food Allergies**

Gastrointestinal Tract	Respiratory Tract
Itching of the lips, mouth, and throat	Runny or stuffed-up nose, sneezing, postnasal discharge
Swelling of the throat	Recurrent croup
Abdominal cramping and distention	Chronic pneumonia
Diarrhea	Middle-ear infections
Colic	
Gastrointestinal bleeding	
Protein-losing enteropathy	*Systemic*
	Anaphylaxis
Skin	Heart rhythm irregularities
	Low blood pressure
Hives	
Swelling	
Eczema, contact dermatitis	

Influences on Childhood Food Habits and Intake

Children develop food preferences at an early age. Toddlers start to exhibit unique feeding practices and styles. For some, this means that one food cannot touch another, or that foods cannot be green, or that *all* foods must be green. All of these "preferences" are merely the toddler's way of exhibiting control over his or her environment while experimenting and exploring. Although it may seem like an eternity to even the most patient caregiver, these food habits are usually temporary. The wise caregiver allows this process to occur naturally, rather than wage food battles that ultimately are always won by the child. Toddlers are ready for most table foods and can eat the same foods as the family, albeit with constant mealtime supervision so they avoid choking. See Appendix J for more about feeding toddlers.

As a child's environment expands, more and more external factors influence the child's diet. It is estimated that children spend more time watching television than doing most other activities. Recognizing the influence that children have on household purchases, advertisers target commercials specifically at children during prime children's viewing hours. Cartoons, for example, feature countless ads for sweetened cereals, fast foods, candy, and other foods high in sugar or fat, none of which are necessary or desirable.[5] When families make television watching a normal part of meal routines, children's diets have fewer fruits and vegetables and more pizzas, snack foods, and sodas than the diets of children in families that separate television viewing and eating.[6]

Social events and parties often promote unhealthful eating habits. No matter what the occasion, the menu for children's parties rarely varies. The staples are pizza, ice cream, soft drinks, and candy. None of these foods alone is a problem, but the fact that these foods are offered at the majority of social gatherings is. Popular snacks and beverages also tend to be too high in sugar and fat. Serving more healthful but still child-friendly snacks, such as those in **Table 16.4**, breaks this tradition.

Key Concepts: *Children grow at a slower rate than they did as infants, but still gain 2 to 3 inches and about 5 pounds per year. They should be able to obtain adequate energy and nutrients from their meals and snacks. Iron-deficiency anemia is the most common nutritional deficiency among American children. Cow's milk is not an adequate source of iron and should be limited to 3 or 4 cups per day to allow for other, high-iron foods. Outside influences, such as television viewing, affect children's preferences for foods with low nutrient density.*

Nutritional Concerns of Childhood

Malnutrition and Hunger in Childhood

Of all of the issues facing children with respect to growth and nutrition, none is so devastating as hunger and subsequent malnutrition. Throughout the world, over half of the deaths of young children can be attributed to undernutrition.[7] Deficiencies in vitamin A, zinc, iron, and protein also result in illness, stunted growth, limited development, and, in the case of vitamin A, possibly permanent blindness.

In the United States, an estimated 3.5 million people will experience homelessness in a given year. Nearly 40 percent of the homeless are children.[8] About 25 percent of children younger than 3 years live in poverty—a higher percentage than in any other age bracket of the population.[9] Children in families with low incomes have a higher prevalence of iron deficiency and poor health status than children in higher-income families.[10] Nearly 12 million children grow up in so-called **food-insecure households** (where

Table 16.4 **Healthy Snacks**

Cereal and milk
Yogurt shake: plain yogurt with fresh fruit
Peanut butter on celery
Popcorn sprinkled with Parmesan cheese
Fresh vegetables and a yogurt dip
Pretzels
Bananas with peanut butter
Graham crackers and peanut butter
Sliced apples with cheese
Bagel and melted cheese
Bran muffins
Pumpkin, banana, or zucchini bread
Mini pizza on English muffin
Homemade pita pocket sandwiches
Yogurt and mini bagel
Fresh fruit
Hot chocolate (made with milk)

calories are adequate, but diet quality has suffered), and more than 2.7 million children experience hunger.[11] Because their bodies need to grow, children are more vulnerable than adults to the effects of malnutrition.

Federal programs such as the Special Supplemental Nutrition Program for Women, Infants, and Children (WIC), **National School Lunch Program, School Breakfast Program,** and **Summer Food Service Program** help to create a safety net for these children. (See **Figure 16.3.**) The WIC program, designed to follow children through their fifth birthday, provides vouchers for milk, eggs, cereal, juice, cheese, and either peanut butter or dried beans. However, participation rates in WIC are less than they could be. Many caregivers either do not understand that WIC is still available after a child is weaned from breast milk or formula or do not have transportation to the WIC site or grocery store.

The National School Lunch and School Breakfast programs offer free or reduced-cost breakfast and lunch at school. Lunches must provide at least one-third of a child's RDA for energy, protein, vitamins A and C, and the minerals iron and calcium; breakfasts must supply one-fourth of the RDA for these nutrients. In addition, school meals must now conform to the *Dietary Guidelines for Americans* and limit total fat calories to 30 percent and saturated fat calories to 10 percent.[12] The Summer Food Service Program was created after the realization that many children who depend on the breakfast and lunch programs during the school year were experiencing hunger during the summer months. For many children, these meals are the major—and, in some cases, only—sources of calories and other nutrients. Those who plan and serve meals have the challenge of balancing popular foods that children will eat with foods that provide good nutrition.

Food and Behavior

Many parents and caregivers mistakenly believe that consuming sugar-laden foods causes **hyperactivity** in children. The myth persists even though a number of carefully controlled studies find no cause-and-effect relationship.[13] The term *hyperactivity* usually is defined as an abnormal increase in activity that is maladaptive and inconsistent with developmental level, but common usage has blurred its meaning. Parents often use this term to describe what they view as unruly behavior in children, particularly in

food-insecure households Households whose members take in enough calories, but have diets of reduced quality that do not meet all daily nutritional requirements.

National School Lunch Program A USDA program that provides nutritious lunches and the opportunity to practice skills learned in classroom nutrition education; enacted in 1946 to provide U.S. children with at least one healthful meal every school day.

School Breakfast Program A USDA program that assists schools in providing a nutritious morning meal to children nationwide.

Summer Food Service Program A USDA program that helps children in lower-income families to continue receiving nutritious meals during long school vacations when they do not have access to school lunch or breakfast.

hyperactivity A maladaptive and abnormal increase in activity that is inconsistent with developmental levels. Includes frequent fidgeting, inappropriate running, excessive talking, and difficulty in engaging in quiet activities.

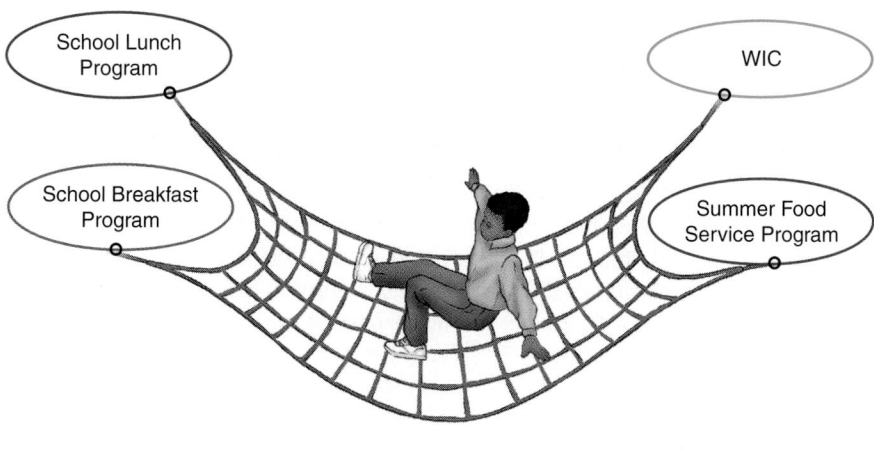

Safety Net for Children

Figure 16.3 **Federal safety net for children.** Children are more vulnerable than adults to the effects of malnutrition. For many children, these federal programs provide the major and, in some cases, the only sources of calories and other nutrients.

social settings such as parties. Many people also believe that certain food additives, including preservatives and colorings, can cause or exacerbate behavioral disorders. However, no studies conclusively link food to behavior. Children typically react to situations surrounding parties (where high-sugar foods are often served) in excitable ways. This is not proof of a cause-and-effect relationship between those foods and those behaviors.

Caffeine products can make children jittery and interfere with their sleep. Because children have small body sizes, the effects of a caffeinated beverage are intensified. Many soft drinks are high in caffeine; examples include Mountain Dew (55 mg per 12-oz can), Surge (51 mg per 12-oz can), and Coca-Cola (36 mg per 12-oz can).

Nutrition and Chronic Disease in Childhood

When is it appropriate to adopt adult dietary guidelines for children? It is well documented that early signs of chronic disease appear in children. Evidence of early plaque development has been seen in the coronary arteries of adolescents and is associated with adult cardiovascular diseases. However, the low-fat, high-fiber diet advocated for adults may jeopardize a very young child's growth. Infants and toddlers younger than 2 years need fat in their diets for growth, organ protection, and central nervous system development. Dietary restrictions at this age are not appropriate.

For children older than 3, however, efforts to lower fat, saturated fat, and cholesterol intake may reduce the risks of chronic disease. The American Heart Association, National Heart, Lung and Blood Institute, and the American Academy of Pediatrics (AAP) all support such efforts.[14] But it's important that parents and caregivers do not misinterpret the recommenda-

---

American Heart Association

Overweight in Children

Overweight children are more likely to be overweight adults. Successfully preventing or treating overweight in childhood may reduce the risk of adult overweight. This may help reduce the risk of heart disease and other diseases.

Reproduced with permission. www.americanheart.org. © 2006, American Heart Association, Inc.

Fyi Overweight in Children and Teens: Whose Problem Is It?

FOR YOUR INFORMATION

The news, whether print or broadcast, is full of stories about the growing problem of overweight in children and adolescents. An epidemic, say some. A sign that all Americans will soon be overweight or obese, say others. What's to be done about it? Will lawsuits against fast food restaurants, snack-food companies, or soft-drink makers help our children's health? Will banning candy and sodas from schools assure healthful food choices? Can we afford to spend more school time on physical education when a school's success is measured by academic test scores?

As with so many public health issues, there are many questions but no easy answers. The prevalence of overweight and its attendant health problems is clearly on the rise among American children. Currently, 11 percent of children ages 2 to 5 years and 15 percent of children age 6 and older are overweight.[1] These values are more than double the rates of overweight in the early 1970s. This rise in prevalence of overweight is accompanied by increased rates of weight-related conditions, including type 2 diabetes. Once considered only an adult disease, rates of type 2 diabetes in children and adolescents have skyrocketed: In 1990, less than 4 percent of children diagnosed with diabetes had type 2; today, that rate is 30 to 50 percent.[2] In addition to posing health risks, overweight in children has many psychosocial and emotional effects, leading some to conclude that obesity is "one of the most stigmatizing and least socially acceptable conditions in childhood."[3]

What's to be done? Most health professionals agree that dieting and significant weight loss are inappropriate for children and teens who are still growing. The Society for Nutrition Education advocates for "health at any size"—an approach that is health centered instead of weight centered, and that focuses on the whole person.[4] This approach promotes lifestyle behavior changes for living actively, eating healthfully, nurturing self-esteem, and respecting cultural and family traditions. This preventive (rather than treatment) approach is gaining acceptance along with the recognition that treatment can lead to other problems, such as eating disorders, nutrient deficiencies, size discrimination, and body hatred.

Promoting healthy lifestyles in children is something with which few can argue, but implementation of programs to promote behavior change can be complicated. Children and teens spend a significant portion of their days at school and with peers,

tions and restrict children's energy intake. During the preschool and school years, gradual changes can bring food choices in line with the *Dietary Guidelines for Americans*.

Many experts feel that before **puberty**, a low-fat diet has no demonstrated benefits for children. Health Canada, the Canadian government's health promotion department, recommends putting a priority on energy intake as well as the intake of nutrients required for proper growth. It recommends against restricting food choices during preschool and childhood. Health Canada recommends gradually adjusting fat intake from 30 to 40 percent of kilocalories for children ages 1 to 3 years down to 25 to 35 percent for ages 4 to 18 years.[15] Caregivers should offer children healthful choices and, as they grow, educate them about proper adult nutrition.

Childhood Overweight

In the United States, overweight in childhood is increasing at an alarming rate. Overweight children run a high risk of becoming obese adults and suffering the ensuing health problems.[16] (See the FYI feature "Overweight in Children and Teens: Whose Problem Is It?") An overweight child is likely to reach maturity earlier than a child of normal weight, but perhaps at the expense of height. Some overweight children already deal with cardiovascular consequences of overweight, such as lipid abnormalities and hypertension, and many overweight children develop type 2 diabetes prior to the teen years. Finally, overweight children experience the psychological trauma associated with overweight in our culture. Factors involved in the development of overweight in childhood include genetics, environment, behavior, and activity levels. (See **Figure 16.4**.)

puberty The period of life during which the secondary sex characteristics develop and the ability to reproduce is attained.

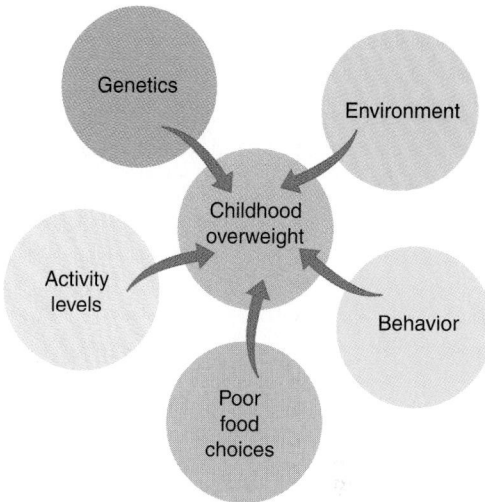

Figure 16.4 **Factors that contribute to childhood overweight.** Childhood overweight is on the rise and predisposes children to health problems when they become adults.

yet they are influenced also by the behaviors and attitudes of parents and other family members. A recent poll by the Harvard Forums on Health found that 65 percent of those surveyed felt that schools should play a major role in helping to fight the obesity problem in the United States, and more than 90 percent supported healthier school lunches, inclusion of healthy eating and exercise topics in health classes, and more physical education in schools.[5] But where will such resources for schools come from? And if changes in schools do occur, how well will parents and the community at large support those programs? It does little good to encourage children to exercise if they lack safe places to play outside or if parents continue to model a couch-potato lifestyle.

Nevertheless, schools and communities are trying. At least 28 states have introduced legislation targeting sales of soft drinks and/or candy in schools, and many school districts have successfully replaced soft drinks with water, 100 percent fruit juice, and milk. Schools are also finding creative ways to promote exercise, turning tired old gymnasiums into fitness centers, using exercycles to power video games, and incorporating exercise principles into the science curriculum. Schools can't buck the overweight trend alone, however, which is why programs must integrate the family and community. For example, a handful of communities are trying out the "Walking School Bus," an effort to promote walking among children who live within a mile of their schools.[6] These and other community-

based initiatives can encourage the small, but sustainable lifestyle changes needed for long-term weight management and reduction of health risks in our nation's youth.

1 Ogden CL, Flegal KM, Carroll MD, Johnson CL. Prevalence and trends in overweight among US children and adolescents, 1999–2000. *JAMA*. 2002;288:1728–1732.

2 IFIC Foundation. The challenge of type 2 diabetes in children. *Food Insight*. January/February, 2003.

3 Schwimmer JB, Burwinkle TM, Varni JW. Health-related quality of life of severely obese children and adolescents. *JAMA*. 2003;289(14):1813–1819.

4 Society for Nutrition Education. Guidelines for childhood obesity prevention programs: promoting healthy weight in children. *J Nutr Educ Behav*. 2003;35(1). http://www.sne .org/Chi_Obesity.pdf. Accessed 8/2/06.

5 The Harvard Forums on Health. *Obesity as a Public Health Issue: A Look at Solutions*. http://www.phsi .harvard.edu/health_reform/poll_results.pdf. Accessed 8/2/06.

6 Walking School Bus. http://www.walkingschoolbus.org. Accessed 8/2/06.

Programs designed to treat childhood overweight generally provide behavior modification, exercise counseling, psychological support or therapy, family counseling, and family meal-planning advice. The goal is not weight loss, but allowing the child's height to catch up with his or her weight. Rather than restrict caloric intake or food choices, the usual strategy is to increase activity and improve food choices.

Lead Toxicity

Lead toxicity can result in slow growth and iron-deficiency anemia and can damage the brain and central nervous system, leading to a host of learning disabilities and behavior problems. Increased blood lead levels are associated with reduced IQ, even at levels less than the CDC/WHO "level of concern" of 10 micrograms per deciliter.[17] Evidence also suggests that lead exposure may delay pubertal development in girls.[18] Lead is present in the plumbing of old homes; old paint; house dust in homes with cracked or peeling lead-based paint; and, in some areas, the soil. Children can ingest lead by drinking contaminated water, eating paint chips, or sucking their fingers after playing in or around lead-contaminated house dust or soil. Lead toxicity occurs more frequently in areas of poverty, where lead contamination is more common and where iron-deficiency anemia is present.

Low intakes of iron, calcium, and zinc tend to result in increased lead absorption. Children with an adequate intake of these micronutrients show less incidence of lead toxicity. Therefore, many of the programs established to reduce the incidence of lead toxicity in children also promote good nutrition, with an emphasis on adequate iron, calcium, and zinc consumption.

Vegetarianism in Childhood

Well-planned lacto-vegetarian, lacto-ovo-vegetarian, and vegan diets satisfy the nutrient needs of children.[19] Vegetarian children have lower intakes of total fat, saturated fat, and cholesterol, and higher intakes of fruits, vegetables, and fiber. Sources of calcium, iron, zinc, vitamin B_{12}, and vitamin D need to be emphasized, especially for children following vegan diets. For a vegan child, legumes and nuts should be substituted for meats, and calcium- and vitamin B_{12}–fortified soy milk should be substituted for cow's milk. At least 20 to 30 minutes of sunlight exposure three times per week should provide enough vitamin D.[20]

Key Concepts: *Hunger and malnutrition affect a significant number of our nation's children. To combat the growing number of hungry children, programs such as WIC, the National School Lunch Program, and the School Breakfast Program are vital. Other concerns common to childhood include overweight, lead toxicity, and chronic disease prevention. Infants and toddlers should not be given low-fat, high-fiber diets; when children reach the age of 3, caregivers should begin to adjust children's diets to follow appropriate dietary guidelines. For vegetarian children, dietary sources of calcium, iron, zinc, vitamin D, and vitamin B_{12} require special attention.*

Adolescence

Adolescents seem to add inches overnight. Many caregivers complain that they cannot keep enough food in the house to satisfy an adolescent's appetite! Adolescence commonly is defined as the time between the onset of puberty and adulthood. This maturation process involves both physical growth and emotional maturation.

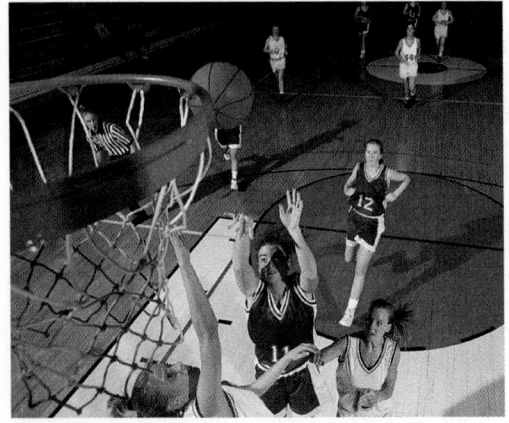

Physical Growth and Development

Hormones drive growth, which varies from child to child. In general, growth spurts begin between ages 10 and 12 for girls and between ages 12 and 14 for boys.[21] This spurt, or period of maximal growth, lasts about 2 years.

Height

The first phase of adolescent growth is linear. On average, boys grow 8 inches and girls grow 6 inches during puberty. This growth is uneven. The hands and feet enlarge first. The calves and forearms lengthen next, followed by expansion of the hips, chest, shoulders, and trunk. As a result, adolescents often appear awkward or clumsy. After the main growth spurt, growth continues for 2 to 3 years, but at a much slower rate.

For girls, peak growth occurs about 1 year before **menarche**, the onset of menstruation. A typical girl has achieved about 95 percent of her adult height by menarche and grows only 2 to 4 inches during the remainder of adolescence. Growth rates are closely related to sexual maturation, reflected in breast development (girls), change of voice (boys), development of sexual organs, and growth of pubic hair. Skeletal growth is completed when the **growth plates**, which separate the ends, or **epiphyses**, from the shafts at the ends of the long bones, close. This is a critical point in development. An adolescent who is malnourished and of small stature at the point of epiphyseal closure may not achieve his or her full potential height.

Weight

The second growth phase of adolescence involves lateral growth. Here, the adolescent "fills out," or gains weight. External factors such as diet and exercise affect weight gain more than linear growth, so weight gain can vary widely among adolescents. However, a typical girl will gain 35 pounds during adolescence; a typical boy will gain 45 pounds. In our weight-sensitive society, adolescents should be prepared for this normal, expected weight gain. Although the bulk of an adolescent's lateral growth occurs after the linear growth spurt, a significant portion of the two growth stages overlap. For girls, for example, peak weight gain usually occurs around the time of menarche.

Body Composition

Before puberty, the body composition of boys and girls does not differ greatly. This changes dramatically during adolescence. Boys experience greater increases in lean body mass, resulting in more obvious muscle definition. Girls accumulate greater stores of body fat, specifically around the hips and buttocks, upper arms, breasts, and upper back. By adulthood, a typical woman's body composition is 23 percent fat; a typical man, in contrast, has 12 percent body fat.

Emotional Maturity: Developmental Tasks

Adolescence is a time not only of great physical growth but also of tremendous emotional growth. This psychological development affects food choices, eating habits, and body image. Many teens become more interested in the healthful aspects of nutrition. Others experiment with unhealthful food choices as an exercise in independence or in an attempt to achieve an idealized body image.

American Heart Association

Fiber and Children's Diets

Children older than 2 years should gradually adopt the American Heart Association Eating Plan. That means saturated fat intake should be 8–10 percent of total calories and dietary cholesterol should be limited to no more than 300 mg daily. Children should also get the majority of calories from complex carbohydrates high in fiber.

A fiber guideline of "age plus 5" has been proposed to set dietary fiber amounts for young children. This means, for example, a 5-year-old should consume 5 + 5 = 10 grams of fiber per day. Once a child's caloric intake approaches that of an adult (1,500 calories or more), 25 total grams should be well tolerated.

Reproduced with permission. www.americanheart.org. © 2006, American Heart Association, Inc.

---

menarche First menstrual period.

growth plates The area of developing tissue near the end of the long bones in children and adolescents.

epiphyses The heads of the long bones that are separated from the shaft of the bone until the bone stops growing.

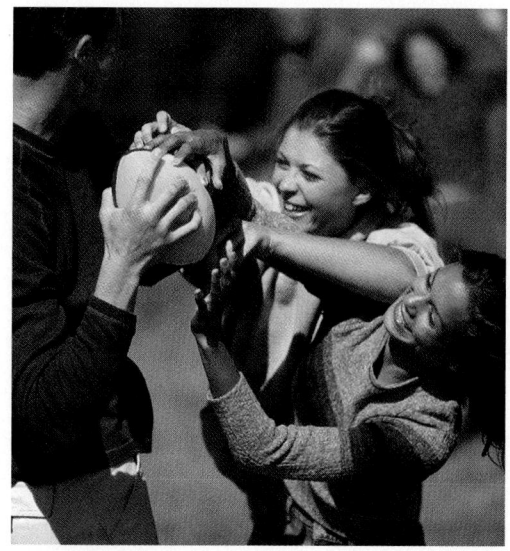

Nutrient Needs of Adolescents

Although growth, not age, should be the ultimate indicator of nutrient needs, Dietary Reference Intakes (DRIs) are established based on age. Separate recommendations for males and females reflect their differences in growth rates and body composition seen during adolescence.

Energy and Protein

Energy needs, as total kilocalories per day, are greater during adolescence than at any other time of life, with the exception of pregnancy and lactation. Equations used to calculate Estimated Energy Requirement (EER) are the same as for children, except for the added energy factor for growth, which is higher for adolescents (see **Table 16.5**). Recommended energy intakes are guidelines only; adjustments often are needed to meet individual requirements.

To support growth, an adolescent's protein needs per unit body weight are higher than an adult's but less than a rapidly growing infant's (see **Table 16.6**). By age 14 to 18, the protein RDA has declined nearly to adult levels (as grams per kilogram body weight), reflecting the end of linear growth for most teens. American teens rarely have a problem with adequate protein intake, but teenage girls risk a lack of protein if they cut calories too drastically in attempts to control weight.

Table 16.5 **Estimated Energy Requirement (EER) Equations for Adolescents Age 9 to 18 Years**

Males

$$EER = 88.5 - 61.9 \times Age\ [y] + PA \times (26.7 \times Weight\ [kg] + 903 \times Height\ [m]) + 25\ kcal/day$$

Physical activity (PA)
Sedentary = 1.00; Low active = 1.13; Active = 1.26; Very active = 1.42

Females

$$EER = 135.3 - 30.8 \times Age\ [y] + PA \times (10.0 \times Weight\ [kg] + 934 \times Height\ [m]) + 25\ kcal/day$$

Physical activity
PA: Sedentary = 1.0; Low active = 1.16; Active = 1.31; Very active = 1.56

Source: Institute of Medicine, Food and Nutrition Board. *Dietary Reference Intakes for Energy, Carbohydrate, Fiber, Fat, Fatty Acids, Cholesterol, Protein, and Amino Acids.* Washington, DC: National Academies Press, 2005. Reprinted with permission from the National Academy of Sciences.

Table 16.6 **Protein RDAs for Adolescence**

Age (y)	Protein (g/kg)	Reference Weight* (kg)	Protein (g/d)
9–13, female and male	0.95	36	34
14–18, female	0.85	54	46
14–18, male	0.85	61	52

*Reference weights are based on median weights for that sex and age group.

Source: Institute of Medicine, Food and Nutrition Board. *Dietary Reference Intakes for Energy, Carbohydrate, Fiber, Fat, Fatty Acids, Cholesterol, Protein, and Amino Acids.* Washington, DC: National Academies Press, 2005. Reprinted with permission from the National Academy of Sciences.

Vitamins and Minerals

Along with increased needs for energy and protein, adolescents have higher vitamin and mineral needs as compared with people at most other life stages. Three nutrients of particular concern for adolescents are vitamin A, calcium, and iron, each of which plays an important role in growth. (See **Figure 16.5**.)

Teens can improve their vitamin A intake by including more fruits and vegetables in their diets. Adequate calcium, essential for bone formation and maximal bone density, can be harder to obtain. Many teens, especially girls, reduce their calcium intake by replacing calcium-rich milk in their diets with soft drinks.[22] During puberty, adolescents gain 15 percent of their full adult height and accumulate half of their ultimate adult bone mass. Adolescents who do not achieve sufficient bone density have a greater risk of developing osteoporosis later in life. The Adequate Intake (AI) for calcium in adolescence is 1,300 milligrams of calcium every day. Dairy products are rich in calcium (about 300 milligrams per cup of milk or yogurt) and convenient to eat; without these or calcium-fortified products, meeting the AI is difficult indeed.

Adolescent boys need added iron to support growth of muscle and lean body mass. Teenage girls need added iron to replace blood lost during menstruation. The recommended intake for boys aged 14 to 18 is 11 milligrams per day; for teen girls, it is 15 milligrams per day. As long as they take in enough calories, both groups should be able to obtain this iron from nutrient-dense foods. During adolescence, however, food selection often is less than optimal. Careful meal planning is required to maximize teenagers' iron consumption.

Influences on Adolescent Food Intake

Teenagers want and need to make their own food choices and purchases and may want to take over preparation of their own food. Although the parent can set a good example, parental influence is much weaker now. Factors that influence an adolescent's food selection and consumption include the desire to be healthy, fitness goals, amount of discretionary income, social practices, and peers. (See **Figure 16.6**.)

Teens have more access to foods than children do. They also usually have their own money and even access to independent transportation. Along with this increased freedom comes greater spending power. Teens enjoy spending money on food and making their own selections. The food industry responds accordingly by marketing directly to teens. The message is enjoyment and pleasure, and advertised products may not be nutritionally adequate.

Teens perceive benefits to eating healthful foods, such as enhanced physical and mental performance, increased energy, and psychological well-being. However, barriers to healthful eating include convenience and personal preference for less healthful alternatives, along with lack of parental or school support and modeling.[23] Teens attending school are faced with more food choices than ever before. In addition to the standard school lunch or breakfast program outlined earlier, most middle schools and high schools have vending machines, snack carts, school stores, or even private vendors supplying foods such as pizza for cafeteria meals.[24] Vending and other food sales can be a major source of revenue for many schools, supporting athletic programs and other after-school activities. Health professionals and others have expressed concern about the presence of low-nutrient-density "competitive" foods (e.g., snacks and soft drinks sold side by side with school lunches),[25] and many states have pursued legislation to

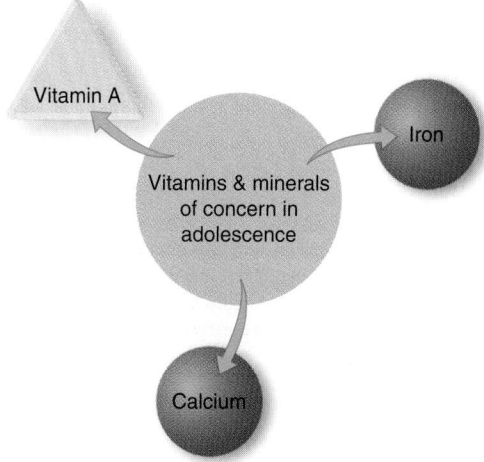

Figure 16.5 **Micronutrients of concern in adolescence.** Vitamin A is important for growth, and calcium is essential for building strong bones. Teen girls especially need adequate iron intake to replace iron lost due to menstruation.

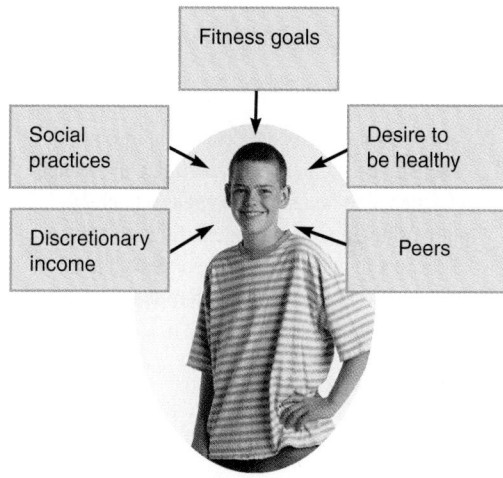

Figure 16.6 **Factors that influence adolescent food choices.** Social, cultural, and psychological factors, especially peer pressure, strongly influence adolescent food choices.

American Dietetic Association

Child and Adolescent Food and Nutrition Programs

It is the position of the American Dietetic Association that all children and adolescents, regardless of age; gender; socioeconomic status; racial, ethnic, or linguistic diversity; or health status, should have access to food and nutrition programs that ensure the availability of a safe and adequate food supply that promotes optimal physical, cognitive, social, and emotional growth and development. Appropriate food and nutrition programs include food assistance and meal programs, nutrition education initiatives, and nutrition screening and assessment followed by appropriate nutrition intervention and anticipatory guidance to promote optimal nutrition status.

J Am Diet Assoc. 2006;106:1467–1475.
Reprinted with permission.

acne An inflammatory skin eruption that usually occurs in or near the sebaceous glands of the face, neck, shoulders, and upper back.

Quick Bites

Early Abusers

These days, youngsters seem to start abusing substances earlier and earlier. Use of alcohol, cigarettes, and inhalants is increasing among fourth-, fifth-, and sixth-graders. By sixth grade, 15 percent of children have tried alcohol and cigarettes. Many children say that peer pressure is their reason for experimentation.

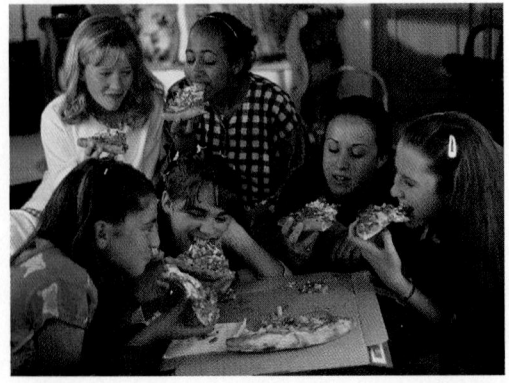

either remove vending machines or change the products available during the school day. A study by the Arizona Department of Education found that replacing sodas, candy, and gum in schools with water, juice, low-fat milk, granola bars, pretzels, fruits, and vegetables resulted in equal or greater revenue for schools.[26]

Key Concepts: *Humans need more calories and nutrients during adolescence than at any other stage of life, with the exception of pregnancy and lactation. Boys grow about 8 inches, gain about 45 pounds, and increase their lean body mass. Girls grow about 6 inches, gain about 35 pounds, and increase their body fat. As at earlier ages, calcium, iron, and vitamin A are often lacking in adolescent diets. Factors that determine food selection and consumption include the desire to be healthy, fitness goals, amount of discretionary income, social practices, and peers.*

Nutrition-Related Concerns for Adolescents

Fitness and Sports

For many adolescents, an interest in fitness becomes the catalyst for learning about nutrition and improving dietary habits. Some teens, unfortunately, become obsessed with their athletic performance, food intake, and body appearance and go to extremes that can jeopardize not only their current athletic performance but also their long-term health. For more information about the nutritional needs of athletes, see Chapter 13, "Sports Nutrition."

Acne

Many teens blame certain foods for their **acne.** Myths surrounding acne and diet abound, but research has not found any correlation between acne and chocolate, greasy foods, soft drinks, nuts, or milk. Nevertheless, differences in acne incidence between westernized and nonwesternized societies are striking, and researchers theorize a connection between diets rich in refined carbohydrates and acne.[27] This theory needs controlled testing before specific recommendations can be made. Effective treatments for acne include topical benzoyl peroxide, low-dose oral antibiotics, and two medications derived from vitamin A—Retin-A and Accutane. Although both of these medications are derivatives of vitamin A, there is no correlation between dietary vitamin A and acne.

Think About It **2**

Eating Disorders

Eating disorders, discussed more thoroughly in the "Spotlight on Eating Disorders," frequently begin during adolescence. Adolescents often become preoccupied with their weight, appearance, and eating habits. Although eating disorders still affect more girls than boys, the prevalence in males is increasing. Thus, eating disorders shouldn't be ignored or dismissed as only a "girl's problem."

Adolescent Overweight

As is the case with younger children, the number of overweight adolescents is climbing. One contributing factor is a decline in physical activity by many teens, particularly girls.[28] Overweight adolescents have an increased risk of developing high blood pressure and abnormal glucose tolerance. They also suffer psychologically from teasing, being ostracized by peers, and from longing to be slimmer. In addition, adolescent overweight sets the stage for adult obesity, with all of its attendant health consequences. (See Chapter 8, "Energy Balance, Body Composition, and Weight Control," for more on overweight and obesity.) Finally, adolescents who engage in unhealthful weight-loss methods are more likely to engage in other risky behaviors, such as tobacco, alcohol, or other drug use, unprotected sex, suicide attempts, and delinquency.[29] **Table 16.7** lists the factors that can put an adolescent at risk for overweight.

Tobacco, Alcohol, and Recreational Drugs

Developmentally, adolescence is a period of experimentation, and many adolescents experiment with illegal substances or drugs. Although survey results from 2005 show a continuing decline in tobacco and drug use, non-medical use of prescription medications continues at a high rate.[30] Nearly one-fourth of high school seniors graduate as smokers, and many young females smoke in an attempt to control appetite and weight. An adolescent who smokes tobacco often has a lower energy intake and subsequently a decreased nutrient intake.

Marijuana has the opposite effect on hunger. Many teens who smoke marijuana will experience "the munchies," a desire to snack and munch—usually on snacks high in calories but with low nutrient density. Smoking marijuana carries the same risks as smoking tobacco. In addition, marijuana sometimes is laced with other drugs, including LSD and amphetamines.

Adolescents who drink alcohol are at greater risk of harming themselves or others through violence and accidental injury.[31] In addition, teens who drink are replacing needed nutrients with empty alcohol calories. Finally, alcohol can interfere with the absorption and metabolism of necessary nutrients. (For more information about nutrition and alcohol, see the "Spotlight on Alcohol," especially the section "Alcoholics and Malnutrition.") Growing adolescents cannot afford to have nutrients replaced or poorly absorbed during growth.

Other drugs, such as cocaine, pose further risks. In using illegal drugs, the adolescent becomes preoccupied with both the acquisition and use of the drug; these activities take priority over food intake or selection. Teens who use drugs are usually underweight and report poor appetites.

Quick Bites

The Dangers of Teenage Smoking

The Centers for Disease Control and Prevention (CDC) estimate that nearly 4 million adolescents smoke regularly. Each day, about 6,000 young people try a cigarette, and more than 3,000 become regular smokers. The CDC predicts that of all young people currently under the age of 18, more than 5 million will die prematurely of a smoking-related disease. New research shows that the earlier a person begins to smoke, the greater the damage.

Table 16.7 **Risk Factors for Overweight in Adolescence**

Risk Factors	Explanations
Social Variables	
Socioeconomic status	Direct relationship for males; inverse relationship for females
Parental obesity	Strong correlation between obesity in parents and over-weight in their children
Race	Higher in white children and African American female adolescents
Family size	Less overweight with larger family size
Television watching	Increased viewing correlates with increasing overweight
Physical Environment	
Region	Greater incidence of overweight in Northeast; urban areas
Seasonal	Higher in winter
Genetic/Metabolic Factors	
Reduced energy expenditure	

Source: Adapted from Bandini LG. Obesity in the adolescent. *Adolesc Med.* 1992;3:459–471.

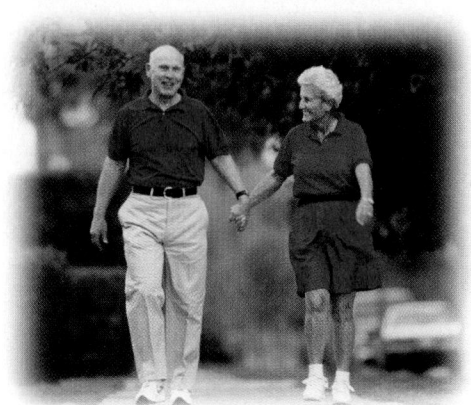

Key Concepts: *Adolescence can be an uncomfortable time for the teen who is concerned with body image, body changes, or athletic activities. Although many teens blame certain foods for their acne, research has not found a definite correlation between acne and diet. Many adolescents are preoccupied with their weight, appearance, and eating habits. Adolescent overweight is on the rise, and eating disorders frequently begin during adolescence. Use of tobacco, alcohol, or recreational drugs can influence nutrient intake and interfere with good nutrition.*

Staying Young While Growing Older

Just when does old age begin? The answer is increasingly elusive as more people remain healthy and active well into their seventies, eighties, and even nineties. Today, older people represent the fastest-growing segment of the U.S. population, and the size of the older population (age 65 or older) is projected to double between 2000 and 2030. (See **Figure 16.7**.) It is estimated that by 2030, nearly one in five Americans will be older than 65. As the baby boomers start turning 85 in 2011, the population aged 85 and older will begin growing the fastest, with a projected increase from 4.2 million in 2000 to nearly 21 million by 2050.[32]

Age-related changes in body composition, sensory abilities, organ systems, and immune function are normal. (See **Figure 16.8**.) We age at different rates, and many age-related declines will have little impact on our day-to-day lives. Other changes affect our nutrient needs and nutrient status (**Table 16.8**), so it becomes especially important to eat nutrient-dense food.

As we get older, many of us fear loss of mental function even more than loss of physical function. Yet, as the years advance, most people maintain cognitive function with only subtle changes. Staying physically and mentally active is a key factor in maintaining function.[33] In most cases, slight changes involving sensory acuity, secondary memory, and information-processing speed do not affect quality of life or lead to progressive or rapid

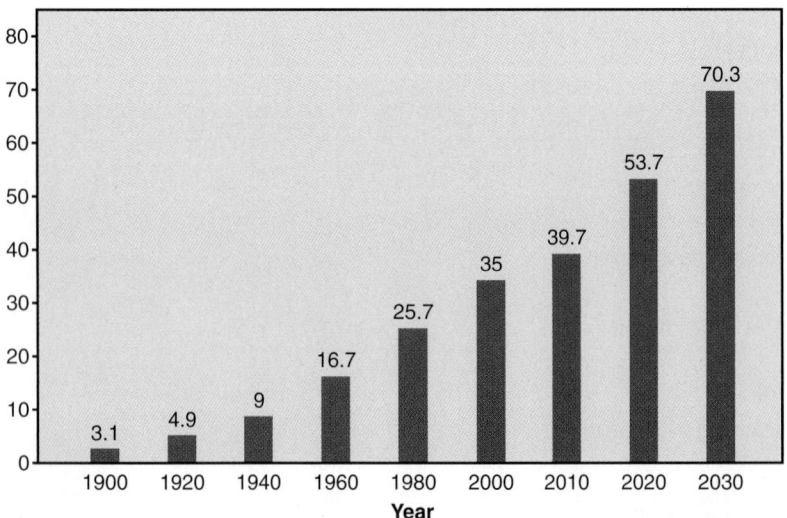

**Number of Persons 65+
1900–2030
(numbers in millions)**

Figure 16.7 **The aging U.S. population.** The number of people over age 65 is growing rapidly.
Source: Administration on Aging, Department of Health and Human Services. A profile of older Americans: 2005. http://www.aoa.gov/PROF/Statistics/profile/2005/profiles2005.asp. Accessed 8/2/06.

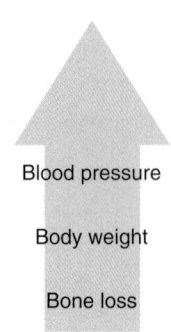

Saliva production
Stomach secretions
Lactase secretion
Gastrointestinal motility
Cardiac output
Blood volume
Kidney function
Liver function
Immune function
Vitamin absorption

Blood pressure
Body weight
Bone loss

Figure 16.8 **Age-related physiological changes.** As we age, most physiological changes emerge gradually.

declines in mental function. On the other hand, when depression or dementia is suspected, professional evaluation becomes necessary. Overmedication or drug interactions, rather than disease, may be responsible for the changes in behavior.

Although it is not possible to stop the aging process, we can control aspects of our lifestyle that contribute to a healthier old age. Many of our choices—food, exercise, smoking, and alcohol—affect not only our risk for chronic disease (see **Figure 16.9**) but also the rate at which we age. Nutrition is a key factor in successful aging, which can be defined as maintaining a lower risk of disease and disease-related disability, high mental and physical function, and active engagement in life.[34]

Weight and Body Composition

People who are overweight when they enter their later years or who gain weight after age 50 have a significantly increased risk of cardiovascular disease.[35] In addition, being overweight often is associated with diabetes, high blood pressure, and some types of cancer.

On the other hand, people who enter their mature years on the lean side—and who remain lean due to a healthy, active lifestyle—increase their chances of enjoying a healthy old age. But thinness alone is not always a health advantage. Obviously, older adults who lose weight due to illness enjoy no health benefits from losing these pounds. Weight loss puts them at increased risk for further illness, including cardiovascular disease and osteoporosis—especially if the original illness also limits activity. And, of course, leanness due to tobacco use or alcoholism increases a person's vulnerability to a decline in health.

Mobility

Muscle mass and strength decline naturally with age. Indeed, physiological functions that affect our mobility begin to decline at the rate of about 1 percent or more per year from about age 30.[36] Our posture begins deteriorating

Think About It 3

Quick Bites

Animal Lifetimes

In general, larger animals live longer than smaller animals, but there are many interesting exceptions. For instance, a mouse, a parakeet, and a bat are approximately the same size, but the mouse has a life span of 2 years, the parakeet 13 years, and the bat up to 50 years!

Quick Bites

Longevity Champions

In the United States, women live an average of five years longer than men do.

Table 16.8 Age-Related Changes and Nutrient Needs

Change in Body Composition or Physiologic Function	Impact on Nutrient Requirement
Decreased muscle mass	Decreased need for energy
Decreased bone density	Increased need for calcium, vitamin D
Decreased immune function	Increased need for vitamin B_6, vitamin E, zinc
Increased gastric pH	Increased need for vitamin B_{12}, folic acid, calcium, iron, zinc
Decreased skin capacity for cholecalciferol synthesis	Increased need for vitamin D
Increased wintertime parathyroid hormone production	Increased need for vitamin D
Decreased calcium bioavailability	Increased need for calcium, vitamin D
Decreased hepatic uptake of retinol	Decreased need for vitamin A
Decreased efficiency in metabolic use of vitamin B_6	Increased need for vitamin B_6
Increased oxidative stress status	Increased need for beta-carotene, vitamin C, vitamin E
Increased levels of homocysteine	Increased need for folate, vitamin B_6, vitamin B_{12}

Source: Blumberg J. Nutritional needs of seniors. *J Am Coll Nutr.* 1997;16(6):517–523.

Chronic diseases	Dietary risk factors						Nondietary risk factors					
	High-fat diet	Excessive alcohol intake	Low complex carbohydrate/fiber	Low vitamin and/or mineral intake	High sugar intake	High intake of salty or pickled foods	Genetics	Age	Sedentary lifestyle	Smoking and tobacco use	Stress	Environmental contaminants
Cancers	?*	X	X	X		X	X	X	X	X		X
Hypertension	X	X		X		in salt sensitive people	X	X	X	X	X	
Diabetes (type 2)	X		X				X	X	X			
Osteoporosis		X		X			X	X	X	X		
Atherosclerosis	X		X	X			X	X	X	X	X	
Obesity	X	X	X		X		X		X			
Stroke	X		X				X	X	X	X	X	
Diverticulosis	X		X	X					X	X		
Dental and oral diseases				X	X		X			X		

* The Nurses' Health Study, a large prospective study, found no evidence linking higher total fat intake with increased risk of breast cancer. These results call into question theories that link dietary fat to other cancers.

Figure 16.9 **Risk factors for disease.** Diet, lifestyle choices, and genetics interact to shape a person's risk profile.

taste threshold The minimum amount of flavor that must be present for a taste to be detected.

in our fifties—a result of bad habits, bone loss, and a decrease in muscle tone. Poor posture can affect lung and cardiovascular function, mobility, and balance. Diseases such as stroke, arthritis, and diabetes become more common and may cause severe physical disability. Medications and nutritional deficiencies may lead to impaired motor function.

Fortunately, exercise can offset much of this decline.[37] Canada, for example, addresses this issue in its *Physical Activity Guide for Older Adults.* (See **Figure 16.10**.) In fact, the benefits of physical activity and strength training may be most profound for those who are aging. Increased self-confidence, better balance and mobility, fewer falls and fractures, enhanced mental acuity, and improved appetite and nutrient intake are but a few of the physical and psychological benefits of exercise during our older years. (See **Figure 16.11**.)

Immunity

In the fifth decade of life, the body's defense mechanisms begin to weaken. The immune system loses some of its ability to fight viruses, bacteria, and other foreign bodies. Elders are more vulnerable to upper respiratory tract infections such as influenza and pneumonia, urinary tract infections, pressure sores, and foodborne illnesses. Physical barriers to infectious agents, foreign bodies, and chemicals weaken as well. These barriers include the

Quick Bites

Losing Water

At birth, 75 percent of the body is composed of water. By the time a person reaches old age, that number has dwindled to 50 percent due to changes in body composition.

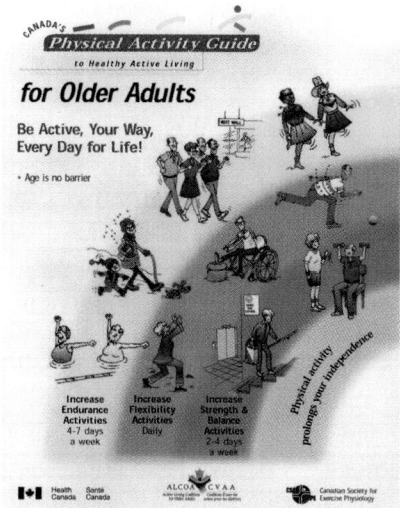
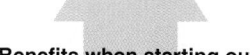

Canada's Physical Activity Guide for Older Adults. The guide explains why physical activity is important, offers tips for increasing physical activity, and recommends levels of activity necessary to good health and improved quality of living. **Source:** *Canada's Physical Activity Guide for Older Adults.* Reproduced with permission from Health Canada. ©Minister of Public Works and Government Services Canada, 2002.

Benefits when starting out:

Meet new people
Feel more relaxed
Sleep better
Have more fun

Benefits from regular physical activity:

Continued independent living
Better physical and mental health
Improved quality of life
More energy
Move with fewer aches and pains
Better posture and balance
Improved self-esteem
Weight maintenance
Stronger muscles and bones
Relaxation and reduced stress

Scientists have proved that being active reduces the risk of:

Heart disease
Falls and injuries
Obesity
High blood pressure
Type 2 diabetes
Osteoporosis
Stroke
Depression
Colon cancer
Premature death

Figure 16.11 **Benefits from increased physical activity.** Physical activity helps adults maintain their health and independence as they age.

skin, the acid environment in the stomach, and swallowing and coughing reflexes.

Inadequate consumption of protein can compromise immunity and health in elders. Because of poor appetite, difficulty chewing, financial constraints, concerns about fat intake, or lactose intolerance, older people may reduce their intake of meat, dairy products, fresh fruits, and vegetables, making it difficult for them to get all the calories and essential nutrients they need. Lack of protein and many of the vitamins and minerals commonly associated with animal foods (i.e., vitamins B_6, B_{12}, and D, calcium, iron, and zinc) can lead to suppressed immunity, decreased muscle mass, slowed wound healing, and osteoporosis.[38] (See **Figure 16.12**.)

Key Concepts: Lifestyle choices, such as diet and exercise, affect how we age. Control of body weight can reduce our risk for many chronic diseases associated with aging. Adequate protein, vitamins, and minerals can protect our immune status. Regular exercise not only enhances our mobility but also reduces disease risk and improves mental health.

Taste and Smell

In older adults, the **taste threshold**—the minimum amount of a flavor that must be present to detect the taste—is more than double that of college-aged adults. Sensitivity to sweet and salty tastes goes first, so older adults often increase their intake of foods high in sugar and sodium—increasing the health problems that stem from overconsumption of these nutrients. Along with taste, our sense of smell diminishes with age, especially in the seventh decade of life and beyond. The idea that older people should be served bland foods is misguided. When food has stronger flavors and

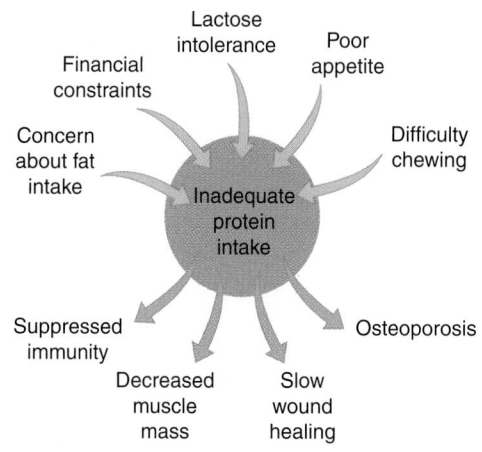

Figure 16.12 **Protein malnutrition in elders.** A combination of several factors can lead to inadequate protein intake that compromises immunity and health.

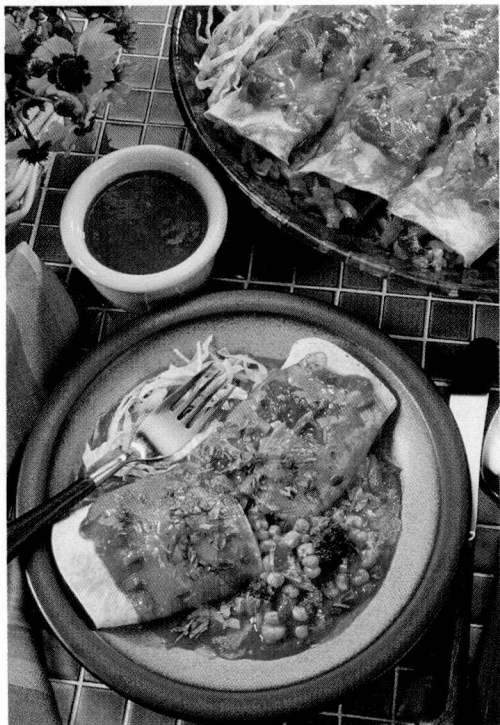

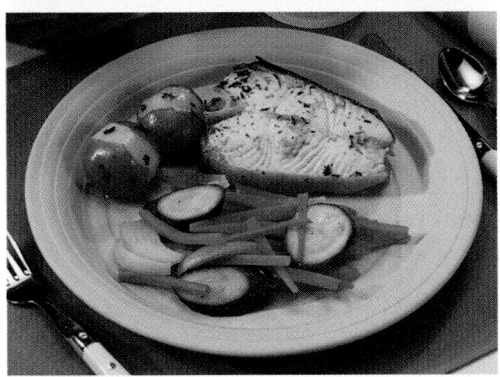

Figure 16.13 **Elders need stronger flavors.** More highly spiced meals rather than bland ones may encourage an elder to eat more.

odors, both healthy and ill elders find it more palatable and eat more, thus increasing their nutrient intake.[39] (See **Figure 16.13**.)

Gastrointestinal Changes

Saliva production tends to decrease as we age, especially in people who take medications for conditions such as congestive heart failure. Lack of saliva affects the preparation of food for digestion and contributes to gum disease—a breach in one of the immune system's first lines of defense against infection.

With age, digestive secretions decline. Most significant are reductions in the stomach secretions of hydrochloric acid and pepsin. These reductions can allow the development of atrophic gastritis—a chronic inflammation of the stomach lining that is common among elders. Atrophic gastritis can affect protein digestion as well as interfere with normal absorption of iron, calcium, vitamin B_{12}, vitamin B_6, and folate.[40] Although reduced lactase production also is associated with aging, a complete intolerance to milk and dairy products is less common than older people often suspect. Most people with reduced lactase production can include some milk, cheese, and yogurt in their diets.

Constipation, gas, and bloating are common complaints of old age. These problems are due to a slowing of gastrointestinal motility with aging, along with decreased physical activity, a diet low in fiber, and low fluid intake. Feelings of fullness may cause older people to eat less. Reduced digestive secretions lower the amount of nutrients elders absorb from the foods they do eat.

Myths and misinformation about the GI effects of various foods, even among the medical community, may steer a person away from nutrient-dense foods such as dairy products, legumes, broccoli, cauliflower, tomatoes, and citrus products. While many elders mistakenly blame these foods for causing problems with gas, others may be sensitive to lactose in dairy products or may have had an adverse reaction to members of the cabbage family or "acid"-containing foods. GI distress also may be caused by factors totally unrelated to the food itself—inappropriate food preparation, lack of adequate fluid, and physical inactivity. Regardless of the cause, once people have an adverse reaction, they may associate it with a recently consumed food and become reluctant to try that food again.

Key Concepts: *The perception of taste declines with age. To detect flavors, older people need food with stronger flavors and odors. This loss of taste may contribute to loss of appetite and poor food intake. Age-related changes in the GI tract reduce nutrient absorption. Decreased motility contributes to constipation.*

Nutrient Needs of the Mature Adult

To live life to its fullest, you need good nutrition. A lifestyle that incorporates the *Dietary Guidelines for Americans,* together with regular physical activity, is essential to a long and productive life. **Figure 16.14** shows MyPyramid for an older adult.

Energy

Our energy requirements decline as we age, mainly because of reduced physical activity and loss of lean body mass. Physical activity can delay some of this loss, thus allowing us to eat more without gaining weight and increasing the likelihood that our diets will be adequate in essential nutrients.

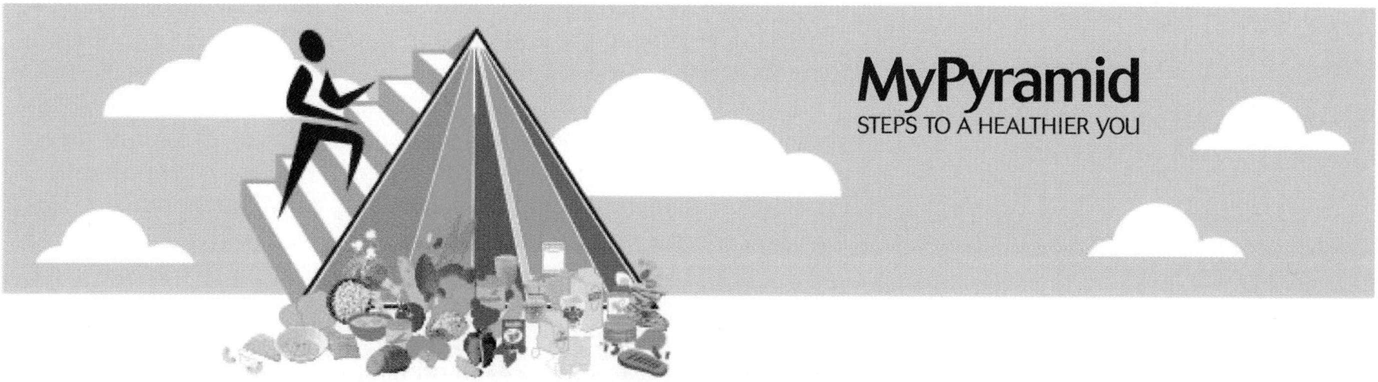

MyPyramid
STEPS TO A HEALTHIER YOU

Based on the information you provided, this is your daily recommended amount from each food group.

GRAINS 5 ounces	VEGETABLES 2 cups	FRUITS 1 1/2 cups	MILK 3 cups	MEAT & BEANS 5 ounces
Make half your grains whole	**Vary your veggies**	**Focus on fruits**	**Get your calcium-rich foods**	**Go lean with protein**
Aim for at least **3 ounces** of whole grains a day	Aim for these amounts **each week:**	Eat a variety of fruit	Go low-fat or fat-free when you choose milk, yogurt, or cheese	Choose low-fat or lean meats and poultry
	Dark green veggies = 2 cups	Go easy on fruit juices		Vary your protein routine— choose more fish, beans, peas, nuts, and seeds
	Orange veggies = 1 1/2 cups			
	Dry beans & peas = 2 1/2 cups			
	Starchy veggies = 2 1/2 cups			
	Other veggies = 5 1/2 cups			

Find your balance between food and physical activity

Be physically active for at least **30 minutes** most days of the week.

Know your limits on fats, sugars, and sodium

Your allowance for oils is **5 teaspoons a day.**

Limit extras–solid fats and sugars–to **130 calories a day.**

Your results are based on a 1600 calorie pattern.

Name: _____

This calorie level is only an estimate of your needs. Monitor your body weight to see if you need to adjust your calorie intake.

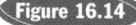 **Figure 16.14** **MyPyramid for an older woman.** This MyPyramid reports the recommendations for an 80-year-old inactive woman (engages in physical activity for less than 30 minutes on most days). **Source:** US Department of Agriculture. www.MyPyramid.gov.

The EER equations are the same for older adults as for younger adults (see Chapter 8, "Energy Balance, Body Composition, and Weight Management"). The decline in total energy expenditure associated with aging is 10 kilocalories per year for men and 7 kilocalories per year for women. In other words, a 60-year-old man who maintains his weight while eating 2,300 kilocalories per day will need only 2,200 kilocalories at age 70. Individual energy needs depend on activity, lean body mass, and the presence of disease; a person who is confined to a bed or chair, for example, usually requires fewer calories than a mobile person.

Protein

Protein needs (as grams per kilogram of body weight) do not change as we age, but may be somewhat harder for us to meet as our overall energy needs decrease and our tastes change. As our caloric needs decrease and our protein needs remain constant, an adequate diet must contain relatively more protein. Although some studies have recommended a protein intake of 1 gram per kilogram of body weight, for healthy older people, the RDA for protein is 0.8 grams per kilogram of body weight, or on average 46 grams per day for women and 56 grams for men. Chronically ill individuals may need more protein to maintain nitrogen balance. Trauma, stress, and infection also may increase protein needs. However, there are risks associated with high protein intake, including dehydration, nitrogen overload, and adverse effects on the kidneys.

Carbohydrate

After infancy, carbohydrates should make up 45 to 65 percent of the calories in the diet. Because foods with primarily simple carbohydrates provide little nutrient value, the best choices are foods with complex carbohydrates.

Fiber, a complex carbohydrate, has many potential benefits, including preventing constipation and diverticulosis, helping to promote a healthy body weight, and reducing risk for diabetes. (See Chapter 4, "Carbohydrates," for more information about fiber.) Because the AI for fiber is based on calorie intake (14 g/1,000 kcal/day) and energy needs decline with age, the AI for fiber is 30 grams per day for men over age 50 and 21 grams per day for women. Fiber also can help to reduce blood cholesterol, making these recommendations especially important for those who are at risk for heart disease. Five or more servings of fruits and vegetables daily, accompanied by whole-grain breads or cereals high in bran, will supply this amount easily. To avoid abdominal discomfort, increase dietary fiber intake gradually. When increasing dietary fiber intake, it is essential to consume adequate fluids—ideally water—to avoid dehydration and constipation.

Fat

Excess dietary fat can lead to obesity, which in turn increases the risk for diabetes, heart disease, and some types of cancer. Younger people should limit their dietary cholesterol and fat, but severe restrictions in elders may be counterproductive. Extreme fat phobia may contribute to nutritional deficiencies among older people who are afraid to drink milk, eat red meat, or even eat poultry or fish. Too few animal products in the diet may contribute to a lack of dietary protein; deficiency of minerals such as calcium, iron, and zinc; and poor vitamin B_{12} intake and absorption.

Healthy people who are at low risk for heart disease should obtain 20 to 35 percent of their daily calories from fat, with no more than 8 to 10 percent of the calories from saturated fat. They should limit their cholesterol intake to 300 milligrams per day. People at increased risk for heart disease should limit saturated fat and cholesterol even more, according to their physicians' advice.

Water

Nutritionists often call water the forgotten nutrient. Water is essential to all body functions, and if intake is inadequate, cellular metabolism becomes difficult, if not impossible. In elders, a decreased thirst response and a reduction in kidney function increase the risk of dehydration.[41] Diuretic medications, alcohol, and caffeine all increase fluid excretion and can contribute to dehydration. Fluid recommendations for elders are the same as for younger adults: 3,700 milliliters per day for men, and 2,700 milliliters per day for women.[42] These fluids are obtained from both beverages and foods.

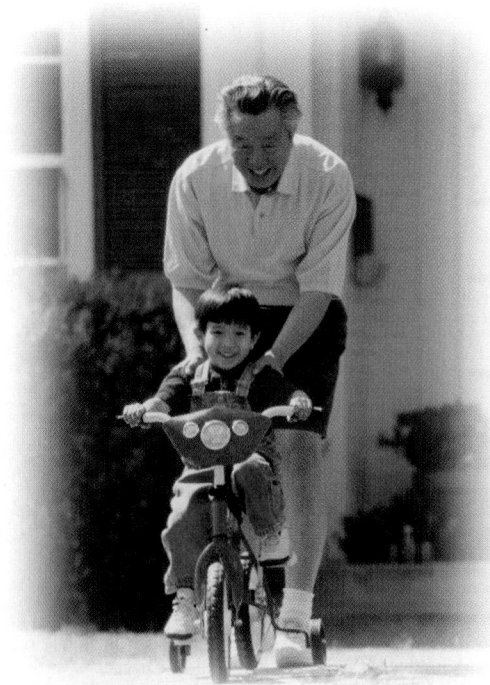

Key Concepts: *Although caloric needs decline with loss of lean tissue and reduced physical activity, protein needs do not change for elders. A high-carbohydrate, moderate-fat diet is still recommended. Water is important; because of their diminished thirst response, older people may not drink enough.*

Vitamins and Minerals

As we age, our micronutrient status changes, especially our needs for vitamin D, vitamin B$_{12}$, and calcium. (See **Figure 16.15**.) In many cases, our vitamin needs remain stable while our energy needs decline. In other cases, age-related declines in absorption, use, or activation of nutrients lead to increased dietary vitamin and mineral needs. Therefore, it is especially important for elders to eat nutrient-dense foods.

Vitamin D

Vitamin D promotes bone health; too little dietary vitamin D can lead to brittle and porous bones that are susceptible to fracture. Elders often have low vitamin D status.[43] Not only are aging tissues less able to take up vitamin D from the blood, but aging skin also is less able to synthesize vitamin D when exposed to sunlight. In addition, many elders spend more time indoors and have reduced exposure to sunlight. When they go outside, many avoid the sun and use sunscreens—a good strategy for skin cancer prevention but one that reduces vitamin D synthesis. Elders with lactose intolerance often avoid dairy products, reducing their vitamin D intake and further compromising vitamin D status. The AI for vitamin D for adults aged 51 though 70 is 10 micrograms per day. For adults 70 and older, the AI is 15 micrograms per day. Younger adults only need 5 micrograms per day.

B Vitamins

The B vitamins deserve special consideration in adults and the aged. Extensive research links inadequate folate, vitamin B$_6$, and vitamin B$_{12}$ to elevated levels of plasma homocysteine, which is associated with an increased risk for cardiovascular disease.[44] High homocysteine levels have also been hypothesized to play a role in dementia.[45] (See Chapter 10, "Water-Soluble Vitamins.")

Vitamin B$_{12}$ deficiency is common in elders, with prevalence varying from 3 to 40 percent.[46] Although most adults consume adequate amounts of dietary vitamin B$_{12}$, from 10 to 30 percent of elders lose their ability to absorb protein-bound vitamin B$_{12}$ from foods. An intake of 2.4 micrograms per day of vitamin B$_{12}$ is recommended for all adults older than 51. Because it is easier to absorb synthetic B$_{12}$ than food-bound B$_{12}$, scientists suggest that adults older than 50 use fortified foods or B$_{12}$-containing supplements to meet their vitamin B$_{12}$ requirements.

Key Concepts: *Vitamin D, folate, vitamin B$_6$, and vitamin B$_{12}$ are key nutrients for elders. Vitamin D status can decline due to reduced intake, synthesis, and activation. Poor folate, B$_{12}$, and B$_6$ status may result in high homocysteine levels, a risk factor for heart disease. Vitamin B$_{12}$ absorption declines with age; B$_{12}$ is more easily absorbed from fortified foods and supplements, so these become important sources for elders.*

Calcium

Maintaining adequate calcium intake reduces the rate of age-related bone loss and the incidence of fractures, especially of the hip.[47] For all adults aged 51 and older, the AI for calcium is 1,200 milligrams per day, 200 milligrams per day higher than the AI for adults 31 to 50 years old.[48]

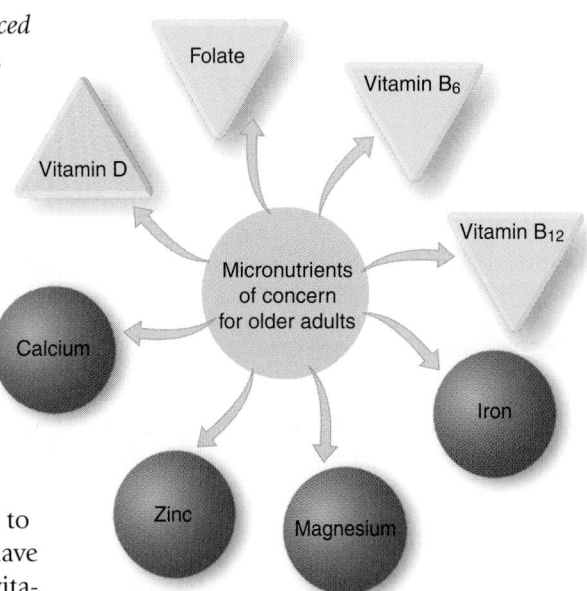

Figure 16.15 **Micronutrients of particular concern for older people.** As we age, our energy needs decline, but our vitamin and mineral needs remain stable. This makes nutrient-dense foods especially important for elders.

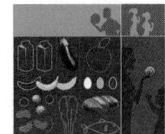

Dietary Guidelines for Americans, 2005
key recommendations

- Consume a variety of nutrient-dense foods and beverages within and among the basic food groups while choosing foods that limit the intake of saturated and *trans* fats, cholesterol, added sugars, salt, and alcohol.
- Meet recommended intakes within energy needs by adopting a balanced eating pattern, such as the USDA Food Guide or the DASH Eating Plan.

Key Recommendations for Specific Population Groups

- *People over age 50.* Consume vitamin B$_{12}$ in its crystalline form (i.e., fortified foods or supplements).
- *Older adults, people with dark skin, and people exposed to insufficient ultraviolet band radiation (i.e., sunlight).* Consume extra vitamin D from vitamin D–fortified foods and/or supplements.

We are less able to absorb calcium as we age, partly because of a loss of vitamin D receptors in the gut. Stomach inflammation also reduces calcium absorption, as does an increase in the consumption of fiber—a practice that doctors recommend for its laxative effects. Because of real or perceived lactose intolerance, many older people have a low intake of dairy foods and therefore of calcium.

Zinc

Although clinical zinc deficiencies are uncommon, older adults frequently have marginal zinc intakes.[49] Stress, especially in hospitalized elders, appears to increase the risk of zinc deficiency and suppress immune function. Studies show that zinc supplementation hastens wound healing, but only in those who are zinc deficient. Because excess zinc may interfere with immune function and the absorption of other minerals and may work to lower HDL cholesterol, people of all ages should avoid excessive and continuous zinc supplementation.

Magnesium

Magnesium plays an essential role in many cellular reactions. Magnesium deficiency has been observed in people with malabsorption syndromes, those with malnutrition or alcoholism, and in elders. However, magnesium deficiency due to inadequate intake is rare. The potential role of increased dietary magnesium in the reduction of high blood pressure, cardiovascular disease, and diabetes is a top research priority.

Iron

Iron remains an important nutrient throughout the life cycle. Following menopause, the RDA for women drops to the same level as for men, 8 milligrams per day. Iron deficiency is a concern for elders who have limited intake of iron from the best sources—red meats, fish, and poultry. Reduced meat consumption may result from taste changes, economics, poor dentition, or a combination of factors.

To Supplement or Not to Supplement

Use of dietary supplements, including vitamins, minerals, and herbal and botanical products, is widespread.[50] Although food is "the best medicine," some elders may feel they need a supplement to meet their nutrient needs. Food is more than the sum of its known nutrients, however, and replacing food with supplements may be a poor trade-off. In addition, some nutrients in large amounts can be toxic; they also can affect the absorption of other nutrients or interfere with the absorption and metabolism of prescription medications.

Excessive use of vitamin supplements by elders may result in **hypervitaminosis**. The need for vitamin A decreases with age, increasing the chances that supplementation may lead to liver dysfunction, bone and joint pain, headaches, and other problems. Also, taking large amounts of vitamin C can increase the likelihood of kidney stones and gastric bleeding. Because we know that many older people use vitamin supplements and that megadoses may have negative effects on health, it is important to inform elders of the Tolerable Upper Intake levels (ULs) for micronutrients. The UL represents a level of intake from a combination of food and dietary supplements that should not be exceeded on a routine basis. (See **Table 16.9**.)

hypervitaminosis High levels of vitamins in the blood, usually as a result of excess supplement intake.

Table 16.9 **UL Values of Vitamins and Minerals for Adults**

Vitamin A (as retinol)	3,000 µg/d
Vitamin C	2,000 mg/d
Vitamin D	50 µg/d
Vitamin E*	1,000 mg/d
Niacin*	35 mg/d
Vitamin B₆	100 mg/d
Folic acid*	1,000 µg/d
Choline	3,500 mg/d
Boron	20 mg/d
Calcium	2,500 mg/d
Chloride	3,600 mg/d
Copper	10,000 µg/d
Fluoride	10 mg/d
Iodine	1,100 µg/d
Iron	45 mg/d
Magnesium*	350 mg/d
Manganese	11 mg/d
Molybdenum	2,000 µg/d
Nickel	1 mg/d
Phosphorus	4,000 mg/d
for >70 yr	3,000 mg/d
Selenium	400 µg/d
Sodium	2,300 mg/d
Vanadium	1.8 mg/d
Zinc	40 mg/d

*From fortified foods and supplements only

Key Concepts: *Important minerals for elders are calcium, zinc, magnesium, and iron. Calcium is important to reduce the risk for osteoporosis. Marginal zinc deficiency has been suspected in many elders and may be the result of reduced intake of red meats. Iron needs decline for women as they go through menopause. Excessive supplementation with certain vitamins or minerals can lead to health problems.*

Nutrition-Related Concerns of Mature Adults

Many factors can interfere with intake or use of nutrients by older adults. Therefore, caretakers, health care practitioners, and seniors themselves must pay attention to nutritional status. To manage acute or chronic nutrition-related conditions, seniors may need to make specific dietary changes.

Drug–Drug and Drug–Nutrient Interactions

Drugs not only affect the way the body uses nutrients but also can alter the activities of other drugs. In turn, foods and nutrients can enhance or interfere with the effects of drugs. (See **Table 16.10**.) Some drugs interfere with appetite; others cause a dry mouth. Because many elders take several medications or are on long-term drug therapy, they may find themselves at increased nutritional risk.

People should view herbal supplements and vitamins or minerals in high doses as drugs, particularly when taken in conjunction with prescription or over-the-counter medications. Although herbal supplements almost certainly interact with other medicines, many interactions are not well documented. In addition to the health and safety issues, supplement therapies can be costly. For more on dietary supplements, see the "Spotlight on Complementary and Alternative Nutrition."

Depression

Many studies report high levels of well-being among elders, especially those who remain independent. Although depression is one of the most common psychological effects of aging, it is most common among institutionalized and low-income people. Researchers believe that depression is related to the loss of receptors for the neurotransmitter serotonin. Loss of these receptors also may cause cognitive difficulties.

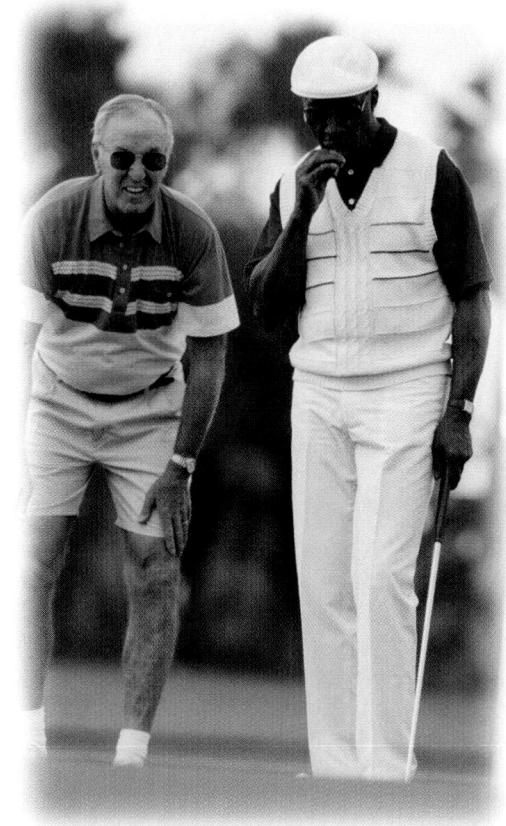

In later life, life transitions and stressful events can become frequent companions that increase the likelihood and severity of depression. Among these stressors are the loss of loved ones, including spouse and friends; physical disability; perceived loss of physical attractiveness; inability to psychologically defend oneself from unpleasant events; inability to care for oneself, which forces one to depend upon

Table 16.10 **Examples of Food–Drug Interactions**

Drug	Food That Interacts	Effect of the Food	What to Do
Analgesic			
Acetaminophen (Tylenol)	Alcohol	Increases risk for liver toxicity	Avoid alcohol.
Antibiotic			
Tetracyclines	Dairy products; iron supplements	Decreases drug absorption	Do not take with milk. Take 1 hr before or 2 hr after food or milk.
Amoxicillin, penicillin	Food	Decreases drug absorption	Take 1 hr before or 2 hr after meals.
Azithromycin (Zithromax), erythromycin	Food	Decreases drug absorption	Take 1 hr before or 2 hr after meals.
Nitrofurantoin (Macrobid)	Food	Decreases GI distress, slows drug absorption	Take with food or milk.
Anticoagulant			
Warfarin (Coumadin)	Foods rich in vitamin K	Decreases drug effectiveness	Limit foods high in vitamin K: liver, broccoli, spinach, kale, cauliflower, and Brussels sprouts.
Antifungal			
Griseofulvin (Fulvicin)	High-fat meal	Increases drug absorption	Take with high-fat meal.
Antihistamine			
Diphenhydramine (Benadryl), chlorphenira-mine (Chlor-Trimeton)	Alcohol	Increases drowsiness	Avoid alcohol.
Antihypertensive			
Felodipine (Plendil), nifedipine	Grapefruit juice	Increases drug absorption	Consult physician or pharmacist before changing diet.
Anti-inflammatory			
Naproxen (Aleve)	Food or milk	Decreases GI irritation	Take with food or milk.
Ibuprofen (Motrin)	Alcohol	Increases risk for liver damage or stomach bleeding	Avoid alcohol.
Diuretic			
Spironolactone (Aldactone)	Food	Decreases GI irritation	Take with food.
Psychotherapeutic (MAO inhibitors)			
Tranylcypromine (Parnate)	Foods high in tyramine: aged cheeses, Chianti wine, pickled herring, brewer's yeast, fava beans	Risk for hypertensive crisis	Avoid foods high in tyramine.

Note: Grapefruit juice contains a compound not found in other citrus juices. This compound increases the absorption of some drugs and can enhance their effects. Talk with your pharmacist or doctor to see if your medicine is affected by grapefruit juice before changing your routine.

Source: Bobroff LB, Lentz A, Turner RE. *Food/Drug and Drug/Nutrient Interactions: What You Should Know About Your Medications.* Gainesville, FL: University of Florida, March 1999. Publication FCS 8092 in a series of the Department of Family, Youth and Community Sciences, Florida Cooperative Extension Service, Institute of Food and Agricultural Sciences.

caregivers and long-term care; social isolation; and, inevitably, the approach of death. In elders, depression often leads to malnutrition and may manifest itself as either anorexia (loss of appetite) or obesity. Anorectic elders lose weight and muscle mass, putting them at risk for chronic conditions such as osteoporosis.

Alcoholism is prevalent among socially isolated or depressed elders. People who consume excessive amounts of alcohol often have diets low in essential nutrients. Over time, excessive alcohol use can cause chronic liver disease, pancreatitis, secondary vitamin and mineral deficiencies, and protein-energy malnutrition.

Anorexia of Aging

Poor food intake can lead to **anorexia of aging**. When older people become ill, anorexia puts them at high risk for developing protein-energy malnutrition.[51] Protein-energy malnutrition, in turn, can contribute to numerous problems, including immune deficiencies, anemia, falls, and cognitive deficits.[52]

It can be difficult to pinpoint treatment strategies for anorexia in older people. However, treating even one aspect of the problem can provide at least temporary improvement. Unfortunately, lifelong inappropriate food habits, social factors, living conditions, and fear of injury may interfere with a person's ability and desire to stay or become healthy.

Key Concepts: Among the problems elders face are lack of appetite and the side effects and interactions of medications they use. Medicines have the potential to interact with food and nutrients in the diet, and a lack of knowledge of these possibilities increases the risk for harmful effects. Although many elders have high levels of well-being, depression is common among institutionalized and low-income seniors.

Arthritis

Arthritis is a general term that describes more than 100 diseases that cause pain and swelling of joints and connective tissue. (See **Figure 16.16**.) Arthritis is a chronic, lifelong affliction that, at its worst, can make

anorexia of aging Loss of appetite and wasting associated with old age.

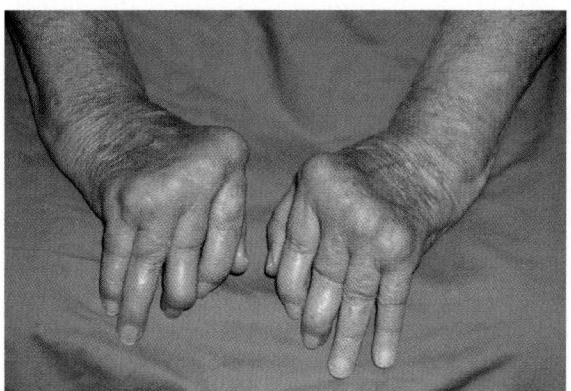

Figure 16.16 **Arthritis.** Degeneration of the finger joints can cause a debilitating lack of function.

Why Elephants Don't Need Dentures

*E*lephants are the only mammals with a built-in tooth replacement system. As they age, elephants go through six sets of teeth, changing about every 10 years. When elephants are around 70 years old, about the maximum life span, the last set of molars wears out.

movement difficult or even impossible. Unfortunately, there is no proven cure for arthritis. At best, appropriate treatment programs reduce symptoms. In terms of nutrition, arthritis pain may impair appetite or make it hard to prepare meals, and some arthritis medications may interfere with nutrient absorption. These factors underscore the importance of a nutrient-dense diet for arthritis sufferers.

Weight management is important in treating arthritis. Excess weight puts undue pressure on the hips and knees. Weight loss by people who are overweight or obese may reduce the risk of developing osteoarthritis, particularly of the knee.[53]

People who have rheumatoid arthritis may benefit from adding foods that are high in unsaturated fatty acids, particularly the *omega*-3 fatty acids in flaxseed and cold-water fish. There is some evidence that these fatty acids may have beneficial effects on the immune system of people with rheumatoid arthritis, thus helping reduce discomfort.[54]

Among the many kinds of arthritis, gout stands out because of the intensity of its pain. The classic attack occurs in someone who goes to bed feeling well and then awakens in the middle of the night with excruciating pain that has been likened to having someone walk on your eyeballs. This often leads to a visit to the emergency room.

Gout is directly linked to an excess of uric acid in the blood. Uric acid, a natural breakdown product of purines (organic compounds) found in all foods and body tissues, is normally dissolved in blood. But excess uric acid can accumulate as microscopic crystals in hand or foot joints, where it leads to painful inflammation, or gouty arthritis. Age-related degenerative osteoarthritis, particularly in the big toe, also enhances the risk of gout.

Certain medications, alcohol, overeating, and an unusual increase in exercise can trigger an attack of gout, but often it strikes without warning. After the attack passes, medications can help control uric acid levels. To reduce the risk of future attacks, people who are overweight should gradually lose weight, cut down on alcohol, and reduce their consumption of foods high in purines, such as organ meats, red meat, shellfish, and beans.

Bowel and Bladder Regulation

As a result of physiological and lifestyle changes, older people are susceptible to problems with their bowels and bladder. Hospitalized or institutionalized elderly patients who require catheters to urinate run an increased risk of **urinary tract infection (UTI)** both during and after the procedure.

urinary tract infection (UTI) An infection of one or more of the structures in the urinary tract; usually caused by bacteria.

Inadequate hydration not only affects the bladder, but also makes constipation more likely. Age-related decreases in intestinal motility and transit time, accompanied by poor food intake, may exacerbate the problem. In addition, lack of physical activity contributes to loss of muscle tone needed for regular elimination.

Chronic constipation is one of the most common health complaints among elders. If they do not have at least one bowel movement per day, many elders wrongly consider themselves constipated and quickly self-prescribe laxatives. However, excessive use of laxatives may cause nutritional deficiencies by decreasing transit time and preventing adequate absorption of nutrients. Decreased transit time also reduces water reabsorption by the GI tract and contributes to dehydration.

Increasing intake of dietary fiber and fluids is one of the most effective treatments for bowel and bladder problems. Elders should gradually switch to—and then maintain—a high-fiber diet. They also should be careful to maintain adequate fluid intake and get regular exercise.

Key Concepts: *Arthritis and changes in bowel and bladder habits are common problems in elders. Weight management is an important component of arthritis treatment. Because of an increased risk of dehydration and constipation, elders should be encouraged to follow a high-fiber diet and consume plenty of fluids.*

Dental Health

The mouth is the gateway to the rest of the gastrointestinal system. Poor oral health impairs the ability to eat and obtain adequate nutrition.[55] Missing teeth or poorly fitting dentures make some elders self-conscious about eating, which leaves them unable to eat comfortably in public. Mouth pain and difficulty swallowing interfere with the process of eating, and tooth loss can alter choices and quality of food. Meats, fresh fruits, and fresh vegetables often are avoided. Oral infections affect the whole body and may increase the risk of other chronic diseases, including heart disease.

Vision Problems

Poor vision and blindness interfere with the ability to buy and prepare food; visually impaired people cannot read food labels, cookbooks, or the settings on stoves or microwave ovens. **Macular degeneration** is a common disease of the eye that gradually leads to loss of vision. It affects about 6 percent of people between the ages of 65 and 74, and about 20 percent of those aged 75 to 85. Research has found that people with a higher intake of green leafy vegetables are less likely to develop this sight-robbing disorder. Foods that contain antioxidants, including carotenoids but not vitamin E, are most strongly associated with a reduced risk.[56] Greens, such as collards and spinach, show the most promise when consumed five or more times per week. By preventing free radical damage, antioxidants in these foods may protect the eye and the blood vessels that supply it. The National Eye Institute's Age-Related Eye Disease Study (AREDS) found that taking a specific high-dose formulation of antioxidants and zinc (beta-carotene, vitamins A, C, and E, copper, and zinc) significantly reduces the risk of advanced age-related macular degeneration and its associated vision loss. Slowing progression of the disease from the intermediate stage to the advanced stage will save the vision of many people.[57]

Osteoporosis

Although osteoporosis affects older adults of both sexes, it is most common in postmenopausal women. Osteoporosis is the deterioration of bone structure until, often without warning, the fragile bone breaks upon the slightest impact.

Nutritional factors, particularly early in life, are thought to play an important role in the development of osteoporosis. While regular weight-bearing exercise helps prevent osteoporosis, inactivity increases osteoporosis risk.

macular degeneration Progressive deterioration of the macula, an area in the center of the retina, that eventually leads to loss of central vision.

Quick Bites

Meno-What?

Most animal species do not go through menopause.

Alzheimer's disease A presenile dementia characterized by accumulation of plaques in certain regions of the brain and degeneration of a certain class of neurons.

Long periods of inactivity, such as may be imposed by complete bed rest or illnesses that limit mobility, can promote the disease. (See Chapter 14, "Diet and Health," for more on osteoporosis, including risk factors.)

Although prevention is the best treatment for osteoporosis, many people enter later life with bad habits—poor nutrition and physical inactivity—that put them at risk. Adopting a diet that is rich in calcium and vitamin D and engaging in regular physical activity, particularly weight-bearing exercises, minimizes osteoporosis risks.

Alzheimer's Disease

Among its other ravages, **Alzheimer's disease** eventually destroys the ability to obtain, prepare, and consume an optimal diet. While genetic factors can affect the risk for Alzheimer's disease, other risk factors include age, head trauma, and possibly exposure to environmental toxins. Although much more research is needed to determine their effects, estrogen and a combination of nonsteroidal anti-inflammatory drugs and antioxidants may offer some protection from the disease.[58]

Most cases of Alzheimer's disease begin after age 70, but it can strike genetically predisposed people at a younger age. During the first stage of the disease, the afflicted person can have difficulty recalling names, frequently lose possessions, and easily become lost. Sensory sensitivity, such as loss of the sense of smell, begins to change gradually and so may not be readily noticed.

As the disease progresses, the person becomes unable to complete simple tasks that require learned motor movement, such as using a can opener. There is an increase in behavior problems, including wandering, aggression, and sleep disorders. These behaviors, if they occur frequently, can affect the person's ability to maintain weight and nutritional status.

The late stages of the disease are marked by inability to communicate, and about one-third of those with Alzheimer's disease develop overactivity that drains the nutritional reserve and increases calorie needs. Eventually, people with Alzheimer's disease become unable to walk and are restricted to a chair or bed. At this time, the caregiver must carefully plan the person's diet to meet psychological and physical needs, paying particular attention to optimum nutrition without excess weight gain.

Key Concepts: *Oral health, vision, and bone health all decline with aging. Tooth loss and oral pain can reduce food intake and nutrient quality. Loss of vision can make food shopping and preparation difficult. Osteoporosis, most common in postmenopausal women, can cause debilitating fractures. Alzheimer's disease eventually destroys the ability to obtain, prepare, and consume an optimal diet. Management of these conditions depends first on their identification by health care professionals.*

Meal Management for Mature Adults

Many elders are at nutritional risk because of economics, social isolation, physical restrictions, inability to shop for or prepare food, and medical conditions. Fortunately, there are a number of ways that older people can remain independent and have access to an adequate diet.

American Dietetic Association

Nutrition Across the Spectrum of Aging

It is the position of the American Dietetic Association that older Americans receive appropriate care; have broadened access to coordinated, comprehensive food and nutrition services; and receive the benefits of ongoing research to identify the most effective food and nutrition programs, interventions, and therapies across the spectrum of aging.

J Am Diet Assoc. 2005;105:616–633.
Reprinted with permission.

Managing Independently

Independent and assisted-living programs allow people to live relatively carefree yet independent lives. Senior-citizen apartment buildings and retirement villages offer a variety of services, including balanced meals. Programs such as **Meals on Wheels** and the **Older Americans Act Nutrition Program** (formerly known as the Elderly Nutrition Program) provide meals to homebound people, as well as to those in congregate (group) settings. Most programs provide meals at least five times per week. The Older Americans Act Nutrition Program is supported primarily with federal funds; volunteer time, in-kind donations, and participant contributions make up the remainder.

An evaluation of the Older Americans Act Nutrition Program showed that program participants had higher nutrient intake levels than nonparticipants and had a higher level of regular social contacts—another important factor in eating well.[59] The **Food Stamp Program** is another option that provides low-income elderly households with the means to purchase food. Unfortunately, because food stamps carry a "welfare" stigma, some elders are reluctant to use them. In addition, many people who need some help buying food cannot meet the eligibility requirements.

Wise Eating for One or Two

Preparing meals that are healthful and tasty is a challenge for those living alone or in small households. As discussed earlier in this chapter, our nutrition needs—with the exception of calories—do not decrease as we age, but our ability to meet them does. Reliance on convenience foods, fast foods, and eating out can adversely affect the nutritional status of elders. Men who live alone are especially likely to eat out or skip meals rather than prepare foods for themselves. For both men and women, physical disability or illness can quash the desire to prepare and eat meals.

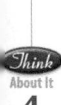

Some simple changes in appliances and food-preparation techniques can help elders overcome common obstacles to food preparation. Those who can't or won't cook can use microwave or toaster ovens and small appliances to prepare simple meals. A meal based on a lower-sodium, low-fat convenience entree can meet nutritional needs if accompanied by vegetables, whole-grain bread, milk, and fruit.

Finding Community Resources

An older person's need for community support typically changes from decade to decade. Sometimes, identifying community resources can be challenging, and financial considerations may further limit access to resources that can assist older people in their own homes. Within local communities, Area Agencies on Aging, Social and Rehabilitation Services, Cooperative Extension Services, churches, and extended-care facilities may have lists of resources and educational programs for elders. **Table 16.11** lists important resources for elders.

Key Concepts: *Older adults who obtain adequate food and nutrient intake while living independently may require assistance from time to time. This assistance may take the form of help with food shopping or preparation or identification of community resources that can stretch the food dollar. Numerous resources exist to assist elders in maintaining a productive, high-quality life.*

Meals on Wheels A voluntary, not-for-profit organization established to provide nutritious meals to homebound people (regardless of age) so they may maintain their independence and quality of life.

Older Americans Act Nutrition Program A federally funded program, formerly known as the Elderly Nutrition Program, that provides older persons with nutritionally sound meals through meals-on-wheels programs or in senior citizen centers and similar congregate settings.

Food Stamp Program A USDA program that helps single people and families with little or no income to buy food.

 **Important Resources for Elders**

Resource Directory for Older People

http://www.aoa.gov/eldfam/How_To_Find/ResourceDirectory/resource_directory.asp
The Resource Directory for Older People is a cooperative effort of the National
Institute on Aging and the Administration on Aging. This directory provides
resources for elders, their caregivers and family members, and those in the
legal and health care professions. Available via the Internet, it provides telephone
numbers (some toll free), names, addresses, and fax numbers for organizations
that work with older adults.

The Eldercare Locator

http://www.eldercare.gov
(800) 677-1116 (toll free)
The National Association of Area Agencies on Aging and the National Association
of State Units on Aging administer the Eldercare Locator, a public service of the
Administration on Aging, U.S. Department of Health and Human Services. The Eldercare
Locator is a nationwide directory-assistance service that helps older persons and their
families identify resources for aging Americans.

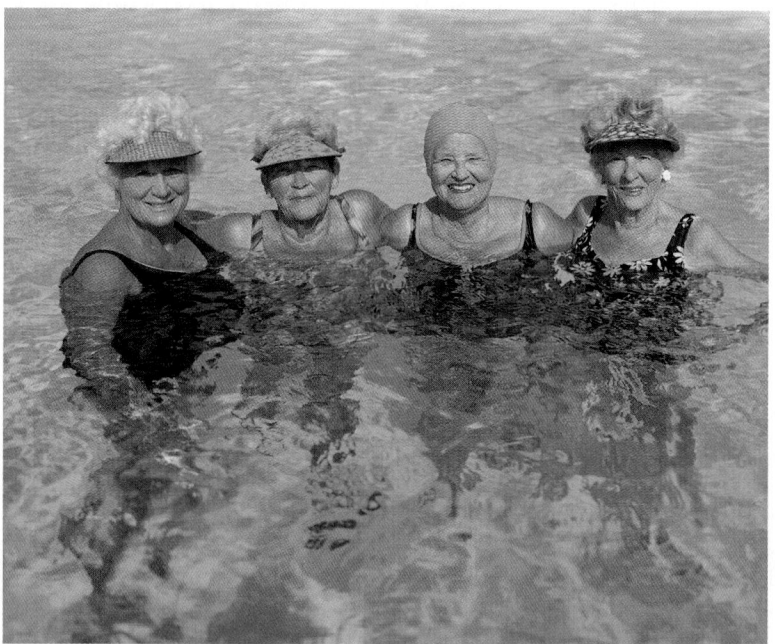

Label [to] **Table**

What is it about fruit snacks that attracts kids? The sweet flavors, bright colors, shapes, and logos of favorite movie or TV characters? Probably all of these. Parents may be attracted by claims for vitamins. So are these nutritious snacks or little more than candy? Let's have a look at the label.

On the positive side, this is a fat-free snack and contains little sodium. However, most of the calories, 56 of 80, come from sugar (14 g $\times$ 4 kcal/g), and the remainder from starch and protein. If you were to see the ingredient list, you would find that the first three ingredients are sugars: corn syrup, sucrose, and fruit juice from concentrate.

The vitamins added to fruit snacks are the only redeeming feature of the product, providing 25% of the DV for vitamins A, C, and E. But is there a better way to get these nutrients? One-half cup of orange juice provides two-thirds of the DV for vitamin C and significant amounts of thiamin, folate, and potassium as well. Just a handful of baby carrots provides more than 100% DV for vitamin A, along with some fiber. Vitamin E is widespread in the food supply—a small amount of salad dressing as a dip for the carrots would add vitamin E.

So, the fruit snacks are not as devoid of nutrients as candy, but are not as nutrient dense as fruits and vegetables. The fruit snacks may have some nutrient value, but they are high in sugar and, like all sugary snacks, should be used sparingly.

Nutrition Facts

Serving Size: 1 pouch (26g/0.9 oz)
Servings Per Container 10

Amount Per Serving

Calories 80

	% Daily Value*
Total Fat 0g	
Sodium 15mg	**0%**
Total Carbohydrate 19g	**1%**
Sugars 14g	**6%**
Protein 1g	

Vitamin A 25%
  (100% as beta carotene)

Vitamin C 25% • Vitamin E 25%

Not a significant source of calories from fat, saturated fat, *trans* fat, cholesterol, dietary fiber, calcium, or iron.

*Percent Daily Values are based on a 2,000 calorie diet. Your daily values may be higher or lower depending on your calorie needs:

		Calories:	2,000	2,500
Total Fat	Less Than		65g	80g
Sat Fat	Less Than		20g	25g
Cholesterol	Less Than		300mg	300mg
Sodium	Less Than		2,400mg	2,400mg
Total Carbohydrate			300g	375g
Dietary Fiber			25g	30g

Calories per gram:
Fat 9 • Carbohydrate 4 • Protein 4

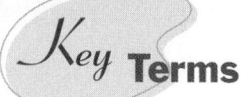

LEARNING *Portfolio* chapter 16

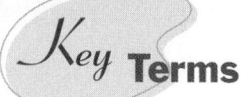

Key Terms

	page		page
acne	700	Meals on Wheels	717
adolescence	688	menarche	697
Alzheimer's disease	716	National School Lunch	
anorexia of aging	713	Program	693
childhood	688	Older Americans Act	
epiphyses	697	Nutrition Program	717
food-insecure households	693	puberty	695
Food Stamp Program	717	School Breakfast Program	693
growth plates	697	Summer Food Service	
hyperactivity	693	Program	693
hypervitaminosis	710	taste threshold	704
macular degeneration	715	urinary tract infection (UTI)	714

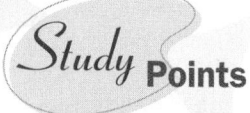

Study Points

➤ For children and adolescents, growth is the key determinant of nutrient needs. If diets are planned carefully, children do not need vitamin/mineral supplementation.

➤ Federally funded nutrition and feeding programs reduce malnutrition and hunger among American children.

➤ Adoption of adult-style diets to reduce risk of chronic disease should begin gradually after the age of 3.

➤ The prevalence of overweight and eating disorders is rising among American children and teens; treatment programs should address food choices and activity levels rather than impose strict calorie limits. Vegetarian diets for children need to be planned carefully to avoid nutrient deficiencies.

➤ Total energy and nutrient needs of adolescents are high to support growth and maturation. Girls need more iron than boys do to compensate for losses after the onset of menstruation. Active teens need more calories and nutrients than sedentary teens; fluid intake is also a priority.

➤ Nutrition and physical activity are two important, controllable components of a healthy life and healthful

aging. Moreover, numerous physiological and psychological aspects of the aging process affect food intake and nutritional status.

➤ Energy needs decline with age, reflecting loss of lean body mass and reduced physical activity. The protein RDA and the recommended balance of carbohydrate and fat calories in the diet are similar for young and older adults. Fluid intake needs special attention due to the reduced thirst response that occurs with age.

➤ Because of reduced intake, synthesis, and activation, vitamin D status declines with age; recommended intake levels are therefore raised. Vitamin B$_{12}$ status may be compromised due to inadequate absorption.

➤ Calcium and zinc intakes are likely to be marginal in the diets of elders. Magnesium and iron remain important.

➤ Dietary supplements, both vitamin/mineral and herbal/botanical, should be used with caution, preferably with professional advice.

➤ Because many elders take multiple medications, they are at risk for drug–nutrient, food–drug, and drug–drug interactions. Anorexia of aging is also a major public health problem.

➤ Arthritis is a prevalent chronic health problem in this age group. Weight management is a key element of arthritis treatment.

➤ Chronic constipation is a common complaint among older adults. Fluids, fiber, and regular exercise can reduce the likelihood of constipation.

➤ Both poor oral and visual health can compromise the ability of elders to consume a nutritionally adequate diet.

➤ Osteoporosis is a major health problem that can be addressed through adequate calcium, vitamin D, regular weight-bearing exercise, and medication if needed.

➤ Adults can maintain independence while aging but may require special assistance to obtain and prepare food. Community resources can help respond to the needs of elders and those of their caretakers and family.

Study **Questions**

1. Which vitamins and minerals are most likely to be deficient in a child's diet?

2. Describe the hunger and malnutrition that occur in U.S. households. What federal programs help to address these problems?

3. Identify several chronic nutrition problems that can affect children. How can these problems be avoided?

4. What are typical nutritional concerns for adolescents?

5. What are some of the consequences of decreased immunity among elders?

6. How does the fact that most older people have less lean body mass affect their need for protein? Compared with a younger adult, does a person older than 65 need more, less, or about the same amount of protein?

7. Why are elders at risk of vitamin D deficiency?

8. Discuss minerals that may need special attention in assessment of an elder's nutrition status.

9. What problems might elders encounter with dietary supplements?

10. List some of the meal/food programs that are available to assist older persons.

11. What is the role of physical activity in osteoporosis prevention? What nutritional factors are important?

☞ [*Try*] **This**

Eat Like a Kid

Children, especially toddlers, tend to be exploratory, and take in the sensory nature of food—the textures, smells, and tastes. In fact, you were probably once this way. The purpose of this exercise is to eat a meal like a kid and gain an appreciation of food's textures and taste. Make some mashed potatoes, macaroni and cheese, buttered peas, or spaghetti (favorite "kid food") and eat it with your fingers. Explore your food and play with it. Try mixing foods. How does this experience make you feel?

Aging Simulation

The purpose of this exercise is to simulate what it can be like to age and experience age-related declines in health. Have you ever thought of how difficult it is to be an older person with health problems and do routine tasks? Invite a few friends over and do the following:

- Put gloves on to simulate the difficulty of losing sensitivity in your hands.
- Use cotton balls in your ears to decrease your hearing ability.
- Apply some petroleum jelly to a pair of glasses or sunglasses to give yourself poor vision.

Now try a simple activity. Make a salad or put a CD in your CD player and listen to it. After completing the activity, switch disabilities with your friends so that everyone has experienced each of the limitations. What is it like to do these everyday activities with your impairment?

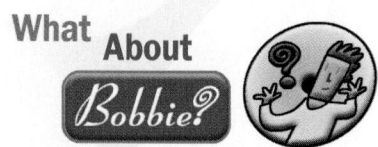

What About Bobbie?

Let's pretend that Bobbie is in her sixties and just read a newspaper article about how older people may have low intakes of vitamins E and B₆, magnesium, calcium, and iron. How do you think her diet compares to the needs of a 65-year-old woman? You may want to review her one-day intake in Chapter 1. Although her calorie intake probably is much higher than that of most women in their sixties, let's look at her intake of these vitamins and minerals.

Bobbie was close to her RDA or AI for vitamin B₆, magnesium, and zinc, but her intake was lower for vitamin E and calcium. This low value for vitamin E likely reflects a lack of complete data for the vitamin E content of foods, since Bobbie's fat intake was ample. As is true of many women in their sixties who don't have an adequate intake of calcium, this increases Bobbie's risk of osteoporosis.

Vitamin E

RDA	15 mg
Bobbie's intake	9 mg

Vitamin B₆

RDA	1.5 mg
Bobbie's intake	2.0 mg

Magnesium

RDA	320 mg
Bobbie's intake	310 mg

Calcium

AI	1,200 mg
Bobbie's intake	745 mg

Zinc

RDA	8 mg
Bobbie's intake	12 mg

References

1 Institute of Medicine, Food and Nutrition Board. *Dietary Reference Intakes for Energy, Carbohydrate, Fiber, Fat, Fatty Acids, Cholesterol, Protein, and Amino Acids.* Washington, DC: National Academy Press, 2005.

2 Kleinman RE, ed. *Pediatric Nutrition Handbook.* 5th ed. Elk Grove Village, IL: American Academy of Pediatrics, 2004.

3 Skinner JD, Carruth BR, Houck KS, et al. Longitudinal study of nutrient and food intakes of infants aged 2 to 24 months. *J Am Diet Assoc.* 1997;97:496–504.

4 Kleinman RE. Op. cit.

5 Kotz K, Story M. Food advertisements during children's Saturday morning television programming: are they consistent with dietary recommendations? *J Am Diet Assoc.* 1994;94:1296–1300.

6 Coon KA, Goldberg J, Rogers BL, Tucker KL. Relationship between use of television during meals and children's food consumption patterns. *Pediatrics.* 2001;107:E7.

7 Caulfield LE, de Onis M, Blossner M, Black RE. Undernutrition as an underlying cause of child deaths associated with diarrhea, pneumonia, malaria, and measles. *Am J Clin Nutr.* 2004;80:193–198.

8 National Coalition for the Homeless. *How Many People Experience Homelessness?* NCH Fact Sheet 2. June 2006. http://www.nationalhomeless.org/publications/facts /How_Many.pdf. Accessed 8/2/06.

9 Zuckerman B, Parker S. Preventive pediatrics: new models of providing needed health services. *Pediatrics.* 1995;95:758–762.

10 Alaimo K, Olson CM, Frongillo EA Jr, Briefel RR. Food insufficiency, family income, and health in US preschool and school-aged children. *Am J Public Health.* 2001;91:781–786.

11 Andrews M, Nord M, Bickel G, Carlson S. *Household Food Security in the United States, 1999.* Alexandria, VA: US Department of Agriculture, Food and Nutrition Service, 2000. Food Assistance and Nutrition Research Report No. 8 (FANRR-8).

12 US Department of Agriculture, Food and Nutrition Service. *National School Lunch Program.* Alexandria, VA: US Department of Agriculture, 2006. http://www.fns.usda.gov/cnd/Lunch /AboutLunch/NSLPFactSheet.pdf. Accessed 8/2/06.

13 Wolraich ML, Lindgren SD, Stumbo PJ, et al. Effects of diets high in sucrose or aspartame on the behavior and cognitive performance of children. *New Engl J Med.* 1994;330:301–307.

14 Gaull G, Giombetti T, Yeaton Woo R. Pediatric dietary lipid guidelines: A policy analysis. *J Am Coll Nutr.* 1995;14:411–418.

15 Health Canada, Office of Nutrition Policy and Promotion. *Nutrition Recommendations for Canadians: Draft Recommendations for Dietary Fat.* May 21, 2004. http://www.hc-sc.gc.ca /hpfb-dgpsa/onpp-bppn/comment_period_rec_on_fat _e.html#fn1. Accessed 11/12/06.

16 Daniels SR, Arnett DK, Eckel RH, et al. Overweight in children and adolescents: pathophysiology, consequences, prevention, and treatment. *Circulation.* 2005;111:1999–2012; and Field AE, Cook NR, Gillman MW. Weight status in childhood as a predictor of becoming overweight or hypertensive in early adulthood. *Obes Res.* 2005;13:163–169.

17 Canfield RL, Henderson CR, Cory-Slechta DA, et al. Intellectual impairment in children with blood lead concentrations below 10 μg per deciliter. *N Engl J Med.* 2003;348(16):1517–1526.

18 Selevan SG, Rice DC, Hogan KA, et al. Blood lead concentration and delayed puberty in girls. *N Engl J Med.* 2003;348(16):1527–1536.

19 Position of the American Dietetic Association and Dietitians of Canada: vegetarian diets. *J Am Diet Assoc.* 2003;103(6):748–765.

20 Kleinman RE. Op. cit.

21 Ibid.

22 Lytle LA. Nutritional issues for adolescents. *J Am Diet Assoc.* 2002;102(3 suppl):S8–S12.

23 O'Dea JA. Why do kids eat healthful food? Perceived benefits of and barriers to healthful eating and physical activity among children and adolescents. *J Am Diet Assoc.* 2003;103(4):497–501.

24 Templeton SB, Arlette MA, Panemangalore M. Competitive foods increase the intake of energy and decrease the intake of certain nutrients by adolescents consuming school lunch. *J Am Diet Assoc.* 2005;105:215–220.

25 Kubik MY, Lytle LA, Story M. Soft drinks, candy, and fast food: what parents and teachers think about the middle school food environment. *J Am Diet Assoc.* 2005;105:233–239.

26 Department of Education, State of Arizona. *Arizona Healthy School Environment Model Policy: Implementation Pilot Study.* February 2005. http://www.asu.edu/educ/epsl/CERU/Articles /CERU-0502-109-OWI.pdf. Accessed 8/2/06.

27 Cordain L, Lindeberg S, Hurtado M, et al. Acne vulgaris: a disease of Western civilization. *Arch Dermatol.* 2002;138(12): 1591–1592.

28 Kimm SYS, Glynn NW, Kriska AM, et al. Decline in physical activity in black girls and white girls during adolescence. *N Engl J Med.* 2002;347(10):709–715.

29 Neumark-Sztainer D, Story M, French SA. Covariations of unhealthy weight loss behaviors and other high-risk behaviors among adolescents. *Arch Pediatr Adolesc Med.* 1996; 150:304–308.

30 Johnston LD, O'Malley PM, Bachman JG, Schulenberg JE. *Monitoring the Future National Results on Adolescent Drug Use: Overview of Key Findings, 2005.* Bethesda, MD: National Institute on Drug Abuse, 2006. NIH publication 06-5882. http://monitoringthefuture.org/pubs/monographs /overview2005.pdf. Accessed 8/2/06.

31 Wechsler H, Lee JE, Kuo M, Lee H. College binge drinking in the 1990s: a continuing problem. *J Am Coll Health.* March 2000;48P:199–210.

32 Federal Interagency Forum on Aging-Related Statistics. *Older Americans 2004: Key Indicators of Well-Being.* Washington, DC: US Government Printing Office, 2004. http://www.agingstats .gov/chartbook2004/default.htm. Accessed 8/2/06.

33 Verghese J, Lipton RB, Katz MJ, et al. Leisure activities and the risk of dementia in the elderly. *N Engl J Med.* 2003; 348:2508–2516.

34 Kuczmarski MF, Weddle DO, for the American Dietetic Association. Position paper of the American Dietetic Association: nutrition across the spectrum of aging. *J Am Diet Assoc.* 2005;105:616–633.

35 Harris TB, Savage PJ, Grethe ST, et al. Carrying the burden of cardiovascular risk in old age: association of weight and weight change with prevalent cardiovascular disease, risk factors, and health statistics in the Cardiovascular Health Study. *Am J Clin Nutr.* 1997;66:837–844.

36 Worthington-Roberts BS, Williams SR. *Nutrition Throughout the Life Cycle.* 3rd ed. St. Louis: Mosby-Year Book, 1996.

37 Chin A, Paw MJ, DeJong N, et al. Physical exercise and/or enriched foods for functional improvement in frail, independently living elderly: a randomized controlled trial. *Arch Phys Med Rehabil.* 2001;82:811–817.

38 Lesourd BM. Nutrition and immunity in the elderly: modification of immune responses with nutritional treatments. *Am J Clin Nutr.* 1997;66(suppl):478S–484S.

39 Schiffman SS. Intensification of sensory properties of foods for the elderly. *J Nutr.* April 2000;130(suppl):927S–930S; and Mathey MF, Siebelink E, de Graaf C, Van Staveren WA. Flavor enhancement of food improves dietary intake and nutritional status of elderly nursing home residents. *J Gerontol A Biol Sci Med Sci.* 2001;56:M200–M205.

40 Worthington-Roberts BS, Williams SR. Op. cit.

41 Institute of Medicine, Food and Nutrition Board. *Dietary Reference Intakes for Water, Potassium, Sodium, Chloride, and Sulfate.* Washington, DC: National Academy Press, 2004.

42 Ibid.

43 Hanley DA, Davison KS. Vitamin D insufficiency in North America. *J Nutr.* 2005;135:332–387.

44 Blumberg J. Nutritional needs of seniors. *J Am Coll Nutr.* 1997;16:517–523; and Fairfield KM, Fletcher RH. Vitamins for chronic disease prevention in adults: scientific review. *JAMA.* 2002;287:3116–3126.

45 Seshadri S, Beiser A, Selhub J, et al. Plasma homocysteine as a risk factor for dementia and Alzheimer's disease. *N Engl J Med.* 2002;346:476–483.

46 Vitamin B_{12} deficiency: recognizing subtle symptoms in older adults. *Geriatrics.* 2003;58(3):30–38.

47 Blumberg J. Op. cit.

48 Institute of Medicine, Food and Nutrition Board. *Dietary Reference Intakes for Calcium, Phosphorus, Magnesium, Vitamin D, and Fluoride.* Washington DC: National Academy Press. 1997.

49 Blumberg J. Op. cit.

50 Wold RS, Lopez ST, Yau CL, et al. Increasing trends in elderly persons' use of nonvitamin, nonmineral dietary supplements and concurrent use of medications. *J Am Diet Assoc.* 2005;105:54–63.

51 Morley JE. Anorexia, body composition, and ageing. *Curr Opin Clin Nutr Metab Care.* 2001;4:9–13.

52 Morley JE. Anorexia of aging: physiologic and pathologic. *Am J Clin Nutr.* 1997;66:760–773.

53 National Institute of Arthritis and Musculoskeletal and Skin Diseases. *Handout on Health: Osteoarthritis.* July 2002; revised May 2006. http://www.niams.nih.gov/hi/topics/arthritis /oahandout.htm. Accessed 8/2/06.

54 James MJ, Cleland LG. Dietary n-3 fatty acids and therapy for rheumatoid arthritis. *Semin Arthritis Rheum.* 1997;27:84–97.

55 Sheiham A, Steele JG, Marcenes W, et al. The relationship among dental status, nutrient intake, and nutritional status in older people. *J Dent Res.* 2001;80:408–413.

56 Stringham JM, Hammond BR Jr. Dietary lutein and zeaxanthin: possible effects on visual function. *Nutr Rev.* 2005; 63:59–64.

57 National Eye Institute. The AREDS formulation and age-related macular degeneration. http://www.nei.nih.gov /amd/summary.asp. Accessed 8/2/06.

58 Cyr M, Calon F, Morissette M, et al. Drugs with estrogen-like potency and brain activity: potential therapeutic application for the CNS. *Curr Pharm Des.* 2000;6:1287–1312; Prasad KN, Hovland AR, Cole WC, et al. Multiple antioxidants in the prevention and treatment of Alzheimer disease: analysis of biologic rationale. *Clin Neuropharmacol.* 2000;23:2–13; and Engelhart MJ, Geerlings MI, Ruitenberg A, et al. Dietary intake of antioxidants and risk of Alzheimer disease. *JAMA.* 2002;287:3223–3229.

59 Millen BE, Ohls JC, Ponza M, McCool AC. The Elderly Nutrition Program: an effective national framework for preventive nutrition interventions. *J Am Diet Assoc.* 2002; 102:234–240.

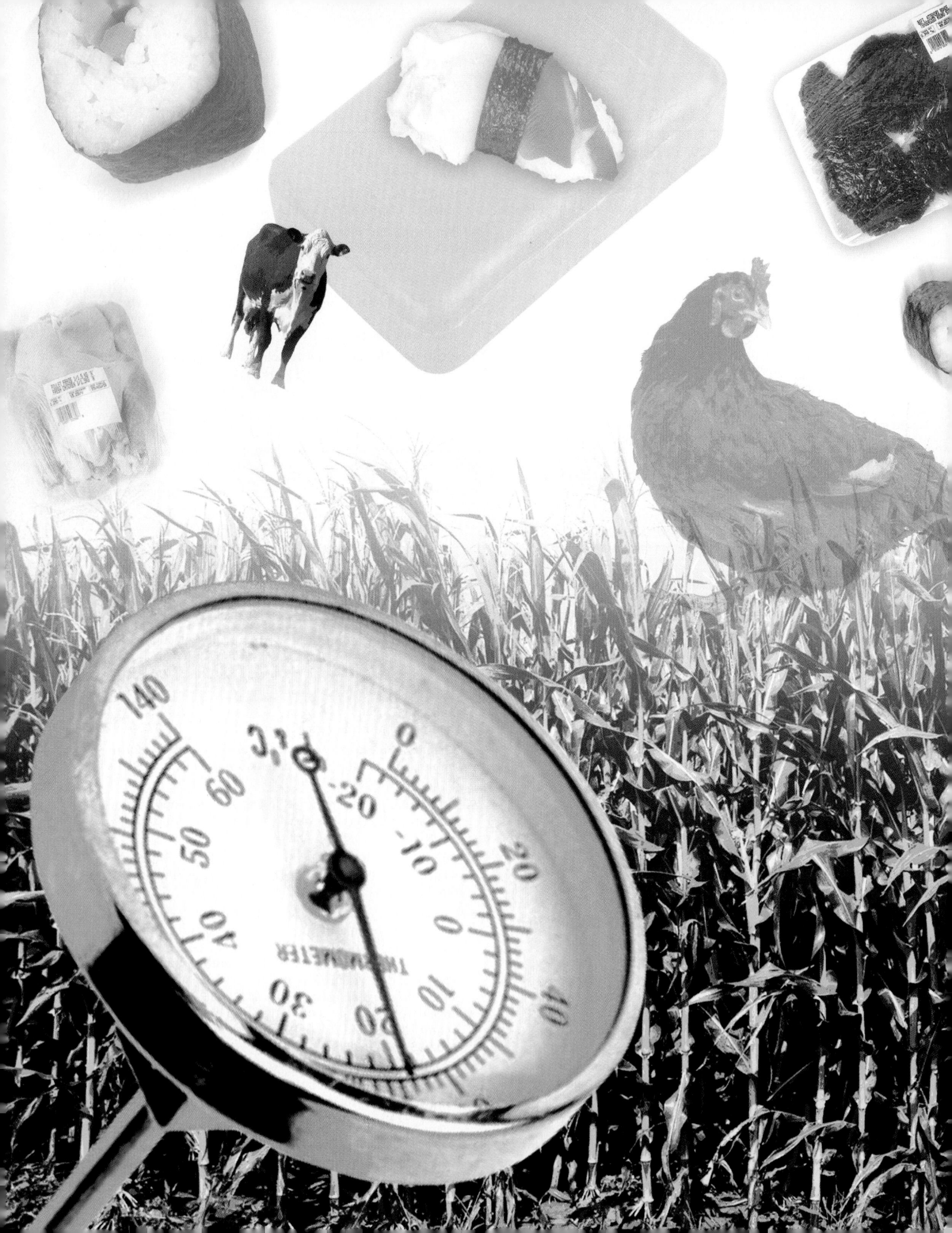

Chapter 17

Food Safety and Technology

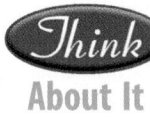

Think About It

1 Do you worry about getting sick from the food you eat?
2 To what extent do you rely on organically grown food to avoid pesticides?
3 What food safety measures, such as thawing meat in the refrigerator, do you practice at home?
4 Would genetically modified rice be welcome at your dinner table?

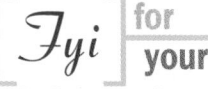

Fyi for your Information

This chapter's FYI boxes include practical information on the following topics:

• Seafood Safety

• At War with Bioterrorism

• Safe Food Practices

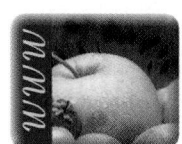

The Web site for this book offers many useful tools and is a great source for additional nutrition information for both students and instructors. For information on food safety and technology, visit the site at **nutrition.jbpub.com**. You'll find exercises that explore the following topics:

• The HACCP Approach to Food Safety

• Genetically Modified Food

• Irradiated Food

• What's Swimming with Your Seafood?

foodborne illness A sickness caused by food contaminated with microorganisms, chemicals, or other substances hazardous to human health.

The newspaper headline screams "Poorly Cooked Hamburger Meat Proves Fatal." You read further and discover that a child's death has been traced to bacteria thriving in undercooked hamburger meat. Additionally, several adults have become ill from the same source. Your search for more information reveals another outbreak that leads to the recall of 19 million pounds of ground beef. This worries you. You hate well-done meat. You especially like your hamburgers blood red and your steaks rare. "Well," you ponder, "maybe I'll move my preferences up a notch to pink hamburgers and medium-rare steaks." Have you made the right choice? Or should you investigate this issue further?

Although once confined mainly to cookbooks and textbooks, today food safety advice shows up in many places—the popular press, the classroom, even the *Dietary Guidelines for Americans*. What has prompted such enthusiasm? Recent headlines tell part of the story. Microbial contamination of such foods as hamburger, apple juice, eggs, raw sprouts, and spinach has seriously sickened thousands and killed many, especially those most susceptible: young children, people with compromised immune systems, and seniors.

Consumers are voicing their concerns about other food safety issues as well, including fears about excessive pesticide residues in plant foods, antibiotics and hormones in animals used for food, and hidden food allergens (e.g., nuts, milk, or eggs) in prepared foods. People often fail to recognize that a prepared food contains an ingredient to which they are allergic (e.g., caseinates as milk protein), and sometimes an allergen may be an unintentional food additive (e.g., peanut material found in a milk chocolate candy might be residue left on machinery from earlier processing of peanut butter cups). Other, less frequently discussed food hazards include physical contamination with glass fragments and other sharp objects, heavy metals, and naturally occurring toxins in seafood and some agricultural products. (See **Figure 17.1**.)

Food Safety

Foodborne illness (food poisoning) is caused by consuming contaminated foods or beverages. The two most common types of foodborne illness are *intoxication* and *infection*. Intoxication occurs when toxins in food cause illness. Food toxins may be naturally occurring, produced by microorganisms, or introduced during processing. Infection occurs when a person becomes ill from consuming food that contains infectious microorganisms.

Although some people develop gastrointestinal symptoms after ingesting a pathogen, others never know that they are suffering from foodborne illness. Most cases of foodborne illness go unreported or are attributed to "24-hour flu." People most at risk for serious complications of foodborne illness are young children and those with compromised immune systems. For these individuals, an incident of foodborne illness can be life threatening.

Harmful Substances in Foods

Pathogens

In North America, most food safety experts agree that the chief cause of foodborne illness is pathogenic (disease-causing) microorganisms, including bacteria, viruses, and parasites. (See **Table 17.1** for a list of common foodborne microbes and the serious illnesses they cause.) Researchers at the Centers for Disease Control and Prevention (CDC) estimate that foodborne microbes cause 76 million illnesses, 325,000 hospitalizations, and 5,000 deaths in the United States each year.[1] These figures take into account the estimated number of unrecognized and unreported food-caused illnesses. The U.S. Department of Agriculture (USDA) estimates that the seven most common foodborne pathogens are responsible for $6.5 billion to $34.9 billion in medical costs and productivity losses each year.[2] Illnesses can range from relatively mild stomach upset to severe symptoms that can be fatal.

Development of foodborne illness results from the interaction of three factors: the pathogen, the host, and the environment in which they exist and interact.[3] Foodborne illnesses can result directly from infection with a pathogen or from toxins produced by a pathogenic microorganism. For example, the bacterium *Staphylococcus aureus* creates havoc with the gastrointestinal tract by producing a toxin. When food containing *S. aureus* stands unrefrigerated, the bacteria begin multiplying. After several hours

Quick Bites

Is It Stomach Flu or Food Poisoning?

Both can have similar symptoms—miserable vomiting, abdominal cramping, and diarrhea. Although we often do not know the exact cause, stomach flu tends to occur in the winter months and is preceded by other symptoms, such as sore throat. Food poisoning tends to occur in summer months, and symptoms usually appear suddenly without warning. Symptoms may not begin until 12 to 72 hours after eating tainted food. If many people who ate the same food get sick around the same time, it's probably food poisoning.

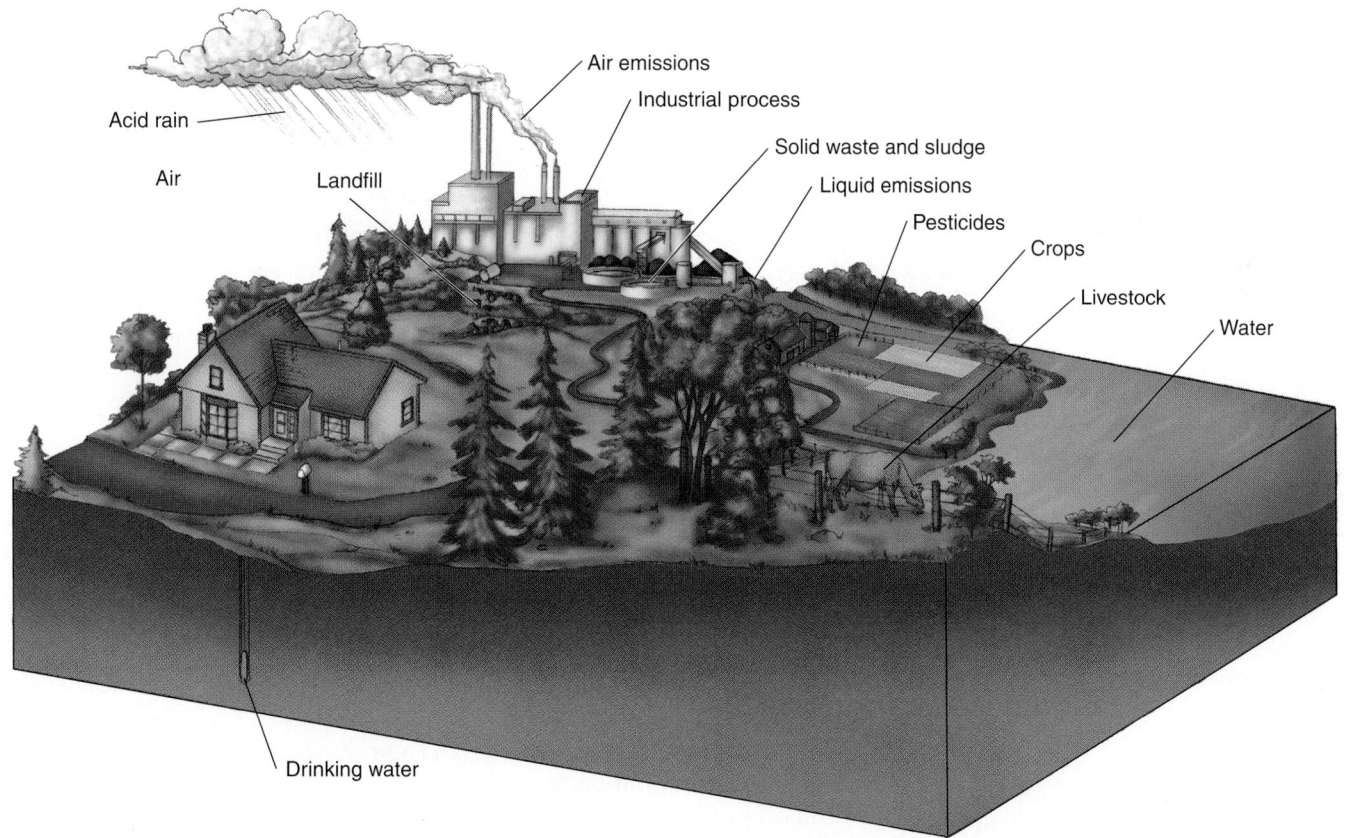

Acid rain
Air
Landfill
Air emissions
Industrial process
Solid waste and sludge
Liquid emissions
Pesticides
Crops
Livestock
Water
Drinking water

Figure 17.1 **Heavy metals and other contaminants can be found in foods.** Industrial plants and automobiles release heavy metals and other contaminants into the air. Rainfall carries these contaminants to the soil. Plants for food crops and animal feed absorb contaminants from the soil. Runoff can pick up contaminants from pesticides, fertilizers, and animal manure. This pollutes surface water (lakes and streams), groundwater, and coastal water. Polluted water contaminates seafood and other fish that people eat.

Table 17.1 Common Foodborne Pathogens and Illnesses

Organism	Sources	Diseases and Symptoms
Bacteria		
Campylobacter jejuni	Raw poultry and meat and unpasteurized milk	Campylobacteriosis **Onset:** usually 2 to 5 days after eating **Symptoms:** diarrhea, stomach cramps, fever, bloody stools; lasts 7 to 10 days
Clostridium botulinum—illness is caused by a toxin produced by this organism	Improperly canned foods, such as corn, green beans, soups, beets, asparagus, mushrooms, tuna, and liver pate; also, luncheon meats, ham, sausage, garlic in oil, lobster, and smoked and salted fish	Botulism **Onset:** usually 12 to 72 hours after eating **Symptoms:** nerve dysfunction, such as double vision, inability to swallow, speech difficulty, and progressive paralysis of respiratory system; can lead to death
Escherichia coli O157:H7	Raw or undercooked meat, raw vegetables, unpasteurized milk, minimally processed ciders and juices, contaminated water	*E. coli* infection **Onset:** 1 to 8 days after eating **Symptoms:** watery and bloody diarrhea, severe stomach cramps, dehydration, colitis, neurological symptoms, stroke, and hemolytic uremic syndrome (HUS); a particularly serious disease in young children that can cause kidney failure and death
Listeria monocytogenes	Soft cheeses, unpasteurized milk, imported seafood products, frozen cooked crab meat, cooked shrimp, surimi (imitation shellfish) **Note:** resists salt, heat, nitrites, and acidity better than most microorganisms	Listeriosis **Onset:** from 7 to 30 days after eating, but symptoms have been reported 9 to 48 hours after eating **Symptoms:** fever, headache, nausea, and vomiting; primarily affects pregnant women and their fetuses, newborns, older adults, people with cancer and compromised immune systems; can cause death in fetuses and babies
Salmonella	Meats, poultry; eggs; milk, ice cream, and other dairy products; seafood; fresh produce, including raw sprouts; coconut; pasta; chocolate; foods containing raw eggs	Salmonellosis **Onset:** usually 1 to 3 days after eating **Symptoms:** nausea, abdominal cramps, diarrhea, fever, and headache
Shigella	Undercooked liquid or moist food that has been handled by an infected person	Shigellosis (bacillary dysentery) **Onset:** 24 to 48 hours after eating **Symptoms:** stomach cramps; diarrhea; fever; sometimes vomiting; blood, pus, and mucus in stools

Quick Bites

Saucy *Salmonella*

Hollandaise and béarnaise sauces may pose health risks because of the infamous *Salmonella* bacteria. Cooks traditionally make these sauces with raw eggs, and even apparently pristine Grade A eggs may harbor the bacteria. Raw cookie dough and certain homemade salad dressings such as Caesar have the same problem.

the expanding bacterial population can produce enough of a nasty toxin to cause nausea, vomiting, and abdominal cramps. Staphylococcal food poisoning is extremely common, causing more than 1 million illnesses each year. Fortunately, the illness usually resolves after a day or so of vomiting and feeling miserable, with no further harmful effects. Another toxin-producing bacterium, *Clostridium botulinum*, causes the rare but deadly illness **botulism**. Improperly canned foods, as well as garlic in oil preparations, are sources of botulism. Honey can be contaminated with *C. botulinum*, but the acid in

Table 17.1 Common Foodborne Pathogens and Illnesses—*continued*

Organism	Sources	Diseases and Symptoms
Bacteria		
Staphylococcus aureus—illness is caused by a toxin produced by this organism	Meat and poultry; egg products; tuna, potato, and macaroni salads; cream-filled pastries and other foods left unrefrigerated for long periods **Note:** *S. aureus* is frequently found in cuts on skin and in nasal passages	Staphylococcal food poisoning **Onset:** 1 to 6 hours after eating **Symptoms:** diarrhea, vomiting, nausea, stomach pain, and cramps; lasts 1 to 2 days
Vibrio vulnificus	Raw seafood, especially raw oysters	*Vibrio* infection **Onset:** 1 to 7 days **Symptoms:** chills, fever, nausea and vomiting, and possibly death, especially in people with underlying health problems
Viruses		
Hepatitis A	Raw shellfish from polluted water, food handled by an infected person	Hepatitis A **Onset:** average about 1 month after exposure **Symptoms:** at first, malaise, loss of appetite, nausea, vomiting, and fever; after 3 to 10 days, jaundice and darkened urine; severe cases can result in liver damage and death
Noroviruses (Norwalk-like viruses)	Raw shellfish from polluted water; salads, sandwiches, and other ready-to-eat foods handled by an infected person	Gastroenteritis **Onset:** 1 to 3 days **Symptoms:** nausea, vomiting, diarrhea, stomach pain, headache, and low-grade fever
Parasites		
Anisakis	Raw fish	Anisakiasis **Onset:** 12 to 24 hours **Symptoms:** abdominal pain, can be severe
Cryptosporidium	Food that comes in contact with sewage-contaminated water; foods handled by a person who did not wash hands after using the toilet	Cryptosporidiosis **Onset:** 1 to 12 days **Symptoms:** profuse watery stools, stomach pain, loss of appetite, vomiting, and low-grade fever
Giardia lamblia	Consumption of contaminated water, contamination of food by an infected person	Giardiasis **Onset:** 1 to 3 days **Symptoms:** diarrhea, abdominal cramps, nausea
Toxoplasma gondii	Raw or undercooked meat and, under certain conditions, unwashed fruits and vegetables; also, cats shed cysts in their feces during acute infection—organism may be transmitted to humans, if feces are handled	Toxoplasmosis **Onset:** 10 to 13 days **Symptoms:** fever, headache, rash, sore muscles, diarrhea; can kill a fetus or cause severe defects, such as mental retardation

adult stomachs kills the bacteria. Infants produce insufficient amounts of stomach acid to kill *C. botulinum,* so even small amounts of contaminated honey can be fatal.

Salmonella bacteria cause an estimated 1.3 million cases of foodborne illness each year.[4] *Salmonella* bacteria are prevalent on poultry and in eggs as well as in a wide variety of other foods. Choosing eggs cooked "over easy" is potentially disastrous because inadequate cooking can leave you vulnerable to the misery of salmonellosis. (See the FYI feature "Safe Food

botulism An often fatal type of food poisoning caused by a toxin released from *Clostridium botulinum,* a bacterium that can grow in improperly canned low-acid foods.

Salmonella Rod-shaped bacteria responsible for many foodborne illnesses.

Escherichia coli (E. coli) Bacteria that are the most common cause of urinary tract infections. Because they release toxins, some types of *E. coli* can rapidly cause shock and death.

Practices" later in this chapter for more information on how to protect yourself from foodborne illness.)

Scientists long have known that pathogens such as *Salmonella* and *Clostridium botulinum* cause foodborne illness, but other microbes, such as **Escherichia coli (E. coli)** did not emerge as foodborne pathogens until the past decade. Also, some foods that weren't previously recognized as harboring pathogenic microorganisms are now recognized as potential sources. Unpasteurized fruit and vegetable juices, for example, can contain harmful bacteria. Contaminated water also has gained greater recognition as a source of foodborne pathogens.[5] Today we know that many foods, including eggs, dairy products, meat and poultry, seafood, fresh produce, juices, and cereal grains, can harbor disease-causing bacteria.

Because bacteria and other infectious organisms are pervasive in the environment, the contamination of food can occur anywhere from the farm to your plate. Many organisms capable of causing foodborne illness in humans are naturally present in food-producing animals and their environment. For example, *Salmonella enteritidis* bacteria enter eggs directly from the egg-laying hen,[6] and *E. coli* are normally present in the intestines of cattle. Microorganisms natural to the marine environment,

𝓕𝔂𝓲 Seafood Safety

Seafood can be a delicious and heart-healthy part of our diets. However, as with all food, contamination can have serious consequences. Seafood is one of the most rapidly perishable foods, so proper refrigeration and rapid processing and transport to the consumer are essential. Although certain types of microbial contaminants and toxins are unique to seafood, properly handled and cooked seafood is as safe to eat as most other foods.

Eating raw seafood, on the other hand, is risky business. Despite the popularity of such dishes as sashimi, sushi, and raw oysters, uncooked fish, no matter how carefully prepared, poses a risk for infection. People with liver disease, diabetes, cancer, or other diseases that impair immune function should be especially careful to stay away from raw seafood. Pregnant women also should avoid uncooked seafood; some physicians recommend that pregnant women avoid seafood altogether. The rest of us should think twice before enjoying those raw oysters and sashimi and, at the very least, should make sure they are fresh and from a reliable source before letting those slippery delicacies pass our lips.

Seafood-related illness falls into several categories. Sources of infection include bacteria, viruses, and parasites. Toxins occur naturally in some fish, and human pollution may contaminate seafood. The following are several examples of seafood-caused illness:

- Raw or undercooked shellfish such as oysters, clams, and mussels may be contaminated with bacteria such as *Salmonella, Vibrio* species, and *Staphylococcus aureus*. Hepatitis A (caused by a virus) and gastroenteritis are other illnesses that can be contracted by eating uncooked shellfish from polluted waters.
- Fish such as mahi-mahi, tuna, and bluefish that have begun to spoil can cause scombroid poisoning. A toxin in these decomposing fish causes flushing, itching, and headache. Cooking does not destroy the toxin, so the best prevention is proper refrigeration and rapid use of fresh fish.
- Some tropical fish, such as red snapper and barracuda, may contain ciguatera toxin, which can cause gastrointestinal and neurological problems in humans.

Larger warm-water fish are most often implicated in this illness. The toxin is actually produced by tiny plants that are eaten by small fish. When larger fish consume many small fish, the toxin can accumulate. The flesh of these large fish may contain enough of the toxin to make humans very ill. Heating or freezing does not destroy this toxin.

- *Anisakis* is a parasite found in raw fish. After a person eats an infected fish, the larvae of this roundworm can invade the human stomach, causing severe abdominal pain. Cooking or freezing the fish for at least 72 hours can kill this parasite.
- Red tide is a well-known phenomenon in which huge numbers of tiny toxic organisms called dinoflagellates infest seawater. Shellfish in the area become poisonous as a result. Respiratory paralysis and death are possible effects of eating shellfish from red tide areas.
- Human pollution is a serious problem, especially near population centers where industrial wastes and human sewage flow into the water. Heavy metals such as mercury can accumulate in

but toxic to humans, can contaminate seafood. (See the FYI feature "Seafood Safety.")

Exposure to animal manure or sewage runoff can contaminate crops. Sewage runoff into rivers and streams also can contaminate fish that live there. In the food-processing stage, contamination can occur from dirty equipment, rodent droppings, improper food storage, and infectious employees who fail to wash their hands adequately or take proper precautions when handling food. Poor food safety practices in retail facilities and at home also can contaminate food.

Patterns of foodborne illness have changed dramatically over the last several decades as our food production has become more centralized. When food animals and produce were grown, prepared, and eaten on the family farm, the consequences of errors in food handling were generally limited to a single family. Now, much of the food we eat is mass-produced at central locations and distributed widely to restaurant chains and supermarkets. Although most food poisoning cases arise from poor food handling in homes and restaurants, contamination at a processing plant can make hundreds or even thousands of people ill. This can have nationwide implications and therefore receives intense national media attention.

Quick Bites

How Many *Salmonella* Does It Take?

In 1994, 224,000 people in 41 states came down with *Salmonella* food poisoning from eating contaminated ice cream. The amazing part? The ice cream contained only about six *Salmonella* bacteria per serving.

larger fish (e.g., sharks and swordfish) that have been exposed to mercury in their environment for long periods. Since commercially caught fish generally contain minimal amounts of mercury, even large fish are safe to eat. However, the FDA has advised pregnant women not to eat shark, swordfish, King mackerel, or tile fish. These large fish have the highest levels of methylmercury, which poses a risk to the developing nervous system in the fetus.[1]

• Dioxin and polychlorinated biphenols (PCBs) also can accumulate in fish living in polluted water. Commercial seafood companies tend to avoid contaminated areas, but local fishers who frequently catch and eat fish from these waters may be at some risk.[2]

1 US Department of Health and Human Services and US Environmental Protection Agency. What you need to know about mercury in fish and shellfish. March 2004. http://www.cfsan.fda.gov/~dms/admehg3.html. Accessed 1/8/07.

2 US Food and Drug Administration. *FDA and Seafood Safety.* Washington, DC: FDA, 1991.

Table 1 **Understanding Seafood Safety**

Condition	Explanation
Scombroid poisoning	Scombroid poisoning is a type of foodborne intoxication caused by the consumption of scombroid and scombroidlike marine fish species that have begun to spoil with the growth of particular types of bacteria. Fish most commonly involved are members of the *Scombroidae* family (tuna and mackerel) and a few nonscombroid relatives (bluefish, mahi-mahi, and amberjack). The suspected toxin is an elevated level of histamine generated by bacterial degradation of substances in the muscle protein.
Anisakis	*Anisakis simplex* (herring worm) and *Pseudoterranova (Phocanema, Terranova) decipiens* (cod or seal worm) are anisakid nematodes (roundworms) that have been implicated in human infections caused by the consumption of raw or undercooked seafood. *Anisakiasis* is the term generally used to refer to the acute disease in humans.
Red tide	When temperature, salinity, and nutrients reach certain levels, algae grow very fast or "bloom" and accumulate into dense, visible patches near the surface of the water. *Red tide* is a common name for such a phenomenon where certain species of phytoplankton contain reddish pigments and "bloom" such that the water appears to be colored red. The term is a misnomer because the reddish color is not associated with tides. A small number of species produce potent neurotoxins that can cause illness and even death.
Polychlorinated biphenols (PCBs)	This group of toxic, persistent chemicals is used as insulation for electrical transformers and capacitors and as lubricants in gas pipeline systems. PCBs are a serious health problem because of their persistence in the environment, accumulation in the body, and potential for a long-term negative effect on health. In the United States, their manufacture was stopped in 1976.

Prions and Mad Cow Disease

Bovine spongiform encephalopathy (BSE), also known as **mad cow disease**, is a chronic degenerative disease that affects the central nervous system of cattle. Once thought to infect only cows, scientists have found that BSE can cause a rare, but fatal, brain-wasting disease in humans.

Researchers believe that **prions**—proteins found in the cells of humans and other mammals—are responsible. When mammals eat tissues contaminated with abnormal prions, they can develop BSE. Cooking and irradiation do not kill or deactivate abnormal prions.

The skull, brain, eyes, vertebral column, and spinal cord of cows at least 30 months of age are most likely to harbor abnormal prions. The tonsils and a portion of the small intestine of all cattle also may contain the agent. To protect the safety of meat, milk, and dairy products, Canadian and U.S. agencies prohibit these cow parts in the human food supply. Government agencies also regulate and provide guidance to manufacturers who produce cow-derived foods, such as gelatin and some dietary supplements.

Key Concepts: *Foodborne pathogens are a major cause of illness in the United States and Canada. Pathogenic (disease-causing) agents include bacteria, viruses, parasites, and prions. Contamination of food can occur at many points along the chain from farm to table.*

Chemical Contamination

Food safety experts view chemical contamination of food as a less significant public health hazard than contamination with pathogenic microorganisms. Yet surveys and retail trends suggest that consumers think otherwise. To avoid foods exposed to chemicals, more and more people are turning to **organic foods**. (See the section "Organic Alternatives" later in this chapter.) Chemical contaminants include pesticides, drugs, pollutants, and natural toxins.

Pesticides

Pesticides play an important role in food production—controlling plant diseases, weeds, insects, and other pests. Pesticides protect crops and ensure a substantial yield, thus assuring consumers of a wide variety of foods at affordable prices. Without these chemicals, many argue that crop production would fall and prices for food would rise.

Every year, the U.S. Food and Drug Administration (FDA) collects thousands of domestic and imported food samples and analyzes them for pesticide residues.[7] Since 1987, the FDA has found no illegal residues in more than 99 percent of domestic and more than 95 percent of imported samples. When a violation occurred, it usually involved the use of a pesticide on crops for which it was not approved, rather than an excessive level. In 2002, the FDA found no residues in over 65 percent of the samples.[8]

The FDA also samples and analyzes domestic and imported animal feeds for pesticide residues. This monitoring focuses on feeds for livestock and poultry—animals that become or produce foods for human consumption. In 2002, the FDA analyzed 445 domestic and 89 imported feed samples. Only 13 of these samples exceeded an established EPA tolerance or an FDA-requested maximum level.[9]

Despite these reassuring results, concerns about pesticides in food persist. Processing methods can either reduce or concentrate pesticide residues in foods. (See **Figure 17.2**.) Infants and young children are particularly susceptible to the hazards of pesticides. Their small size and rapid

bovine spongiform encephalopathy (BSE) A chronic degenerative disease, widely referred to as "mad cow disease," that affects the central nervous system of cattle.

mad cow disease See *bovine spongiform encephalopathy (BSE).*

prions Short for proteinaceous infectious particle. Self-reproducing protein particles that can cause disease.

organic foods Foods that originate from farms or handling operations that meet the standards set by the USDA National Organic Program.

pesticides Chemicals used to control insects, diseases, weeds, fungi, and other pests on plants, vegetables, fruits, and animals.

integrated pest management (IPM) Economically sound pest control techniques that minimize pesticide use, enhance environmental stewardship, and promote sustainable systems.

growth make them especially vulnerable to pesticide residues, which can accumulate in their bodies over their lifetimes. Enacted in 1996, the Food Quality Protection Act includes landmark protections for the young. For the first time, manufacturers must show that pesticide levels are safe for infants and children. In addition, when determining a safe level for a pesticide in a food, the Environmental Protection Agency (EPA) now must account for the cumulative effect of exposures to similar pesticides and toxic chemicals.[10]

Consumers Union (the nonprofit publisher of *Consumer Reports*) has issued a report stating that legally permitted pesticide levels in some foods are much higher than the levels that scientific data show are safe for children.[11] Consumers Union analyzed data collected by the USDA's Pesticide Data Program and concluded that a relatively small number of highly toxic insecticides accounted for most of the toxicity in foods. Consumers Union suggests that focusing on reducing or eliminating these high-risk pesticides may be the best way to reduce toxicity from our foods.

To decrease pesticide intake, Consumers Union recommends washing and peeling fruits and vegetables (if possible) and eating a variety of produce.[12] Because the benefits of these foods far outweigh the risks from the pesticides they might contain, Consumers Union emphasizes that it *does not* recommend eating fewer fruits and vegetables.

Excessive use of synthetic pesticides, herbicides, and fertilizers contributes substantially to the pollution of soil and water. Overuse can be particularly hazardous to farm workers, whose exposure to these chemicals typically is much higher than that of consumers. Overuse also threatens wildlife. Today, many farmers use **integrated pest management (IPM)** to reduce pesticide use. (See **Figure 17.3**.) IPM methods include crop rotation, use

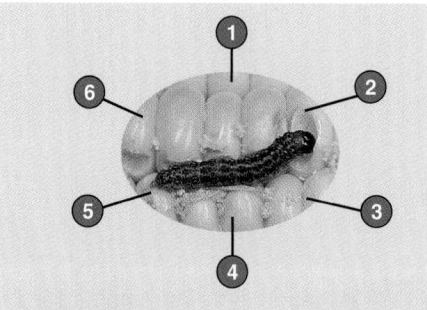

1. **Legal control**
   State and federal guidelines are designed to limit the spread of pests.

2. **Biological control**
   Beneficial organisms, such as predators, parasites, and viruses, are released into the environment to suppress pest organisms.

3. **Cultural control**
   Rotation, sanitation, and other good farming techniques are employed to help reduce pest populations.

4. **Physical control**
   Barriers, traps, and the location and timing of planting are all used to control pest infestations.

5. **Genetic control**
   Resistant plant strains are developed to reduce the impact of pests.

6. **Chemical control**
   Conventional pesticides, biopesticides, pheromones, and other chemicals are used to prevent or suppress pest outbreaks. The chemical controls are specific to a pest species and are ideally short-lived in the environment. In addition, the chemicals are used at their lowest effective rate and may be alternated to help prevent the development of pest resistance.

Figure 17.3 **Integrated pest management.** Integrated pest management is a sustainable approach that combines prevention, avoidance, monitoring, and suppression strategies in a way that minimizes economic, health, and environmental risks. It minimizes pesticide use and promotes economically sound practices.

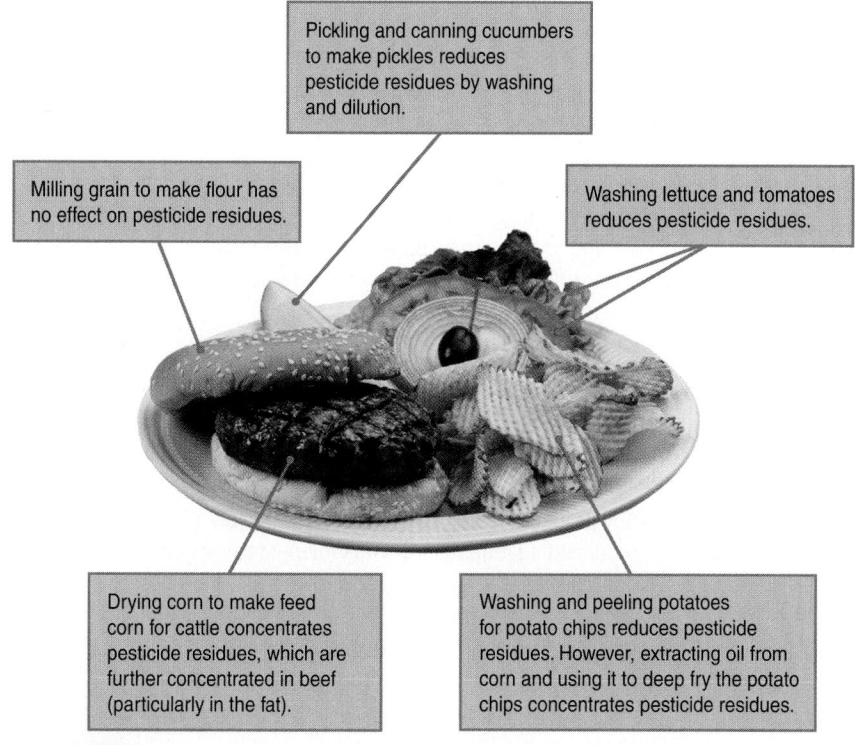

Pickling and canning cucumbers to make pickles reduces pesticide residues by washing and dilution.

Milling grain to make flour has no effect on pesticide residues.

Washing lettuce and tomatoes reduces pesticide residues.

Drying corn to make feed corn for cattle concentrates pesticide residues, which are further concentrated in beef (particularly in the fat).

Washing and peeling potatoes for potato chips reduces pesticide residues. However, extracting oil from corn and using it to deep fry the potato chips concentrates pesticide residues.

Figure 17.2 **Pesticide pathways to dinner.** Food processing and preparation methods can either reduce or concentrate pesticide residues in foods.

of natural rather than synthetic pesticides, and planting nonfood crops nearby that lure pests away from food crops. Releasing sterile fruit flies into orchards also allows reductions in pesticide use. Because fruit flies produce no offspring when they mate with sterile partners, the overall fruit fly population drops.

Organic Alternatives

Organic foods are grown or produced without synthetic pesticides and without synthetic fertilizer. More than 60 million households, or 30 percent of the U.S. population, use organic products.[13] Sales of organic foods exceed $10 billion annually and are growing.[14] Growth of the industry may reflect, in part, a distrust of technology and a desire to return to a simpler, more "natural" way of food production.

The Organic Foods Production Act and the National Organic Program (NOP) are intended to assure consumers that the organic foods they purchase are produced, processed, and certified to consistent national standards. The labeling requirements of this program apply to raw meats, fresh produce, and processed foods that contain organic ingredients. Foods that are sold, labeled, or represented as organic must be produced and processed in accordance with the NOP standards.[15] **Table 17.2** outlines the requirements for labeling organic food.

Under the NOP, farm and processing operations that grow and process organic foods must be certified by the USDA. The certification process includes an on-site inspection to verify that the applicant's operation com-

---

Table 17.2 **Labeling Requirements for Organic Food**

Labeling requirements are based on the percentage of a product's ingredients that are organic.

Foods labeled "100 percent organic" and "organic"

- Products labeled "100 percent organic" must contain only organically produced ingredients (excluding water and salt).
- Products labeled "organic" must consist of at least 95 percent organically produced ingredients (excluding water and salt). Any other ingredients must consist of nonagricultural substances approved on the National List maintained by the USDA National Organic Program or non–organically produced agricultural products that are not commercially available in organic form.
- Products that meet the requirements may display these terms and the percentage of organic content on their principal display panel.
- The USDA seal and the seal or mark of certifying agents may appear on product packages and in advertisements.
- Foods labeled "100 percent organic" and "organic" cannot be produced using excluded methods, sewage sludge, or ionizing radiation.

Processed products labeled "made with organic (specified ingredients)"

- Products that contain at least 70 percent organic ingredients can use the phrase "made with organic ingredients" and list up to three of the organic ingredients or food groups on the principal

display panel. For example, soup made with at least 70 percent organic ingredients and only organic vegetables may be labeled either "soup made with organic peas, potatoes, and carrots" or "soup made with organic vegetables."

- Foods labeled "made with organic ingredients" cannot be produced using excluded methods, sewage sludge, or ionizing radiation.
- The percentage of organic content and the certifying agent's seal or mark may be used on the package. However, the USDA seal cannot be used anywhere on the package.

Processed products that contain less than 70 percent organic ingredients

- The packaging of these products can make no organic claim, except on the information panel, where they may identify the specific ingredients that are organically produced.

Other labeling provisions

- Any product labeled as organic must identify each organically produced ingredient in the ingredient statement on the information panel.
- The name and address of the certifying agent of the final product must be displayed on the information panel.
- There are no restrictions on the use of other truthful labeling claims, such as "no drugs or growth hormones used," "free range," or "sustainably harvested."

Source: *USDA, National Organic Program. http://www.ams.usda.gov/nop/FactSheets/LabelingE.html. Accessed 8/7/06.*

plies with strict national organic standards. Certifying agents may collect and test soil, water, waste, plant and animal tissues, and processed products. A certified operation may label its products or ingredients as organic and may use the "USDA Certified Organic" seal.

Even though there is no scientific evidence that genetic engineering and irradiation of foods present unacceptable risks, public opposition led the NOP to prohibit use of these technologies with organic foods. Although irradiation and genetic engineering have been approved for use in agriculture and may offer certain benefits for the environment and human health, consumers strongly oppose their use in organically grown foods. Because of consumer opposition, foods produced with these techniques are prohibited from carrying the organic label.[16]

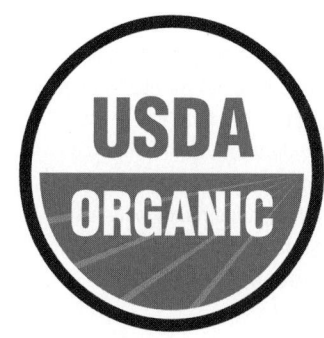

Organic food advocates claim that using natural fertilizer, such as manure, produces a soil that is richer in a range of nutrients than a soil treated with chemical fertilizers, which typically contain only a few basic nutrients. They reason that organically fertilized soils produce foods that contain more nutrients. A review of 41 studies comparing organic and conventionally produced crops supports this idea, finding more iron, magnesium, phosphorus, and vitamin C in organic crops.[17] However, many of the studies reviewed are more than 20 years old. Study limitations prevent conclusions about whether organic foods are nutritionally superior, inferior, or the same as conventionally grown foods.[18] Other research suggests that organic farming techniques may enhance beneficial antioxidant levels in fruits and vegetables.[19] Better research is needed to clarify differences between organic and nonorganic foods.

Organic farming has its drawbacks. The use of manure raises food safety concerns. The organic producer must manage animal and plant waste materials so they do not contribute to contamination of crops, soil, or water. Manure runoff can pollute nearby lakes and streams. Other critics charge that organic farming is "elitist," that synthetic fertilizers and pesticides are necessary to meet the food needs of an expanding world population. They also point out that complete freedom from pesticides cannot be guaranteed, no matter how carefully a food is produced, since pesticide residues may still exist in soil, water, and air.[20]

Organic foods are not pesticide-free foods. Organic farmers can use natural and approved synthetic pesticides to control weeds and insects.[21] Microbial contaminants that cause foodborne illness can be found in organic as well as conventional foods. Consumers must handle all food appropriately, whether organically or conventionally grown.

Animal Drugs

Current agricultural practice depends heavily on the use of drugs in food animals and food-producing animals raised specifically to provide meat, milk, and eggs. Producers use drugs to maintain animal health and well-being as well as to increase production. Keeping animals in good health reduces the chance that disease will spread from animals to humans, and healthy animals can use nutrients for growth and production rather than for fighting infection. But there is a possibility that drugs used in animals could enter human food and possibly increase the risk of ill health in humans. Many researchers fear that overuse of animal antibiotics will contribute to the emergence of antibiotic-resistant microorganisms that could threaten human health. Another potential problem, though with less widespread effects, is that humans with drug allergies could have reactions to drug residues in food-producing animals. Some people worry that the

pollutants Gaseous, chemical, or organic wastes that contaminate air, soil, or water.

dioxins Chemical compounds created in the manufacturing, combustion, and chlorine bleaching of pulp and paper and in other industrial processes.

natural toxins Poisons that are produced by or naturally occur in plants or microorganisms.

ciguatera A toxin found in more than 300 species of Caribbean and South Pacific fish. It is a nonbacterial source of food poisoning.

widespread use of hormones may impair animal health or the quality of the food obtained from treated animals.

Five major classes of drugs are used in animals raised for food:[22]

1. Topical antiseptics, bactericides, and fungicides used to treat skin or hoof infections, cuts, and abrasions

2. Ionophores, which alter stomach microorganisms to more efficiently digest feeds and to help protect against some parasites

3. Hormone and hormonelike production enhancers (anabolic hormones for meat production, and bovine somatotropin for increased milk production in dairy cows)

4. Antiparasitics

5. Antibiotics used to prevent infections, treat disease, and promote growth

The FDA is responsible for ensuring that drugs approved for use in animals are safe not only for the animals but also for humans who eat food produced from the animals. In addition, the FDA enforces regulations to ensure that drugs are used properly in cows, chickens, and seafood. However, FDA surveillance is not perfect; government investigations have revealed that a few U.S. veterinarians and farmers illegally use animal drugs that are known to be dangerous to humans.

Pollutants

Pollutants from animal manure and other wastes, factories, human sewage, and other runoff can contaminate food-production areas. For example, some scientists theorize that contamination of foods by **dioxins** may cause human cancer. Dioxins are chemical compounds created in the manufacturing, combustion, and chlorine bleaching of pulp and paper and in other industrial processes.[23] Dioxins can accumulate in the food chain and are potent animal carcinogens. Fish from dioxin-polluted waters can contain significant amounts of dioxin.[24] The commercial fishing industry avoids areas of known dioxin pollution. Dioxins in tiny amounts are found in food packages, paper plates, and coffee filters made of bleached paper. Because the quantity of this toxic chemical is minimal, however, the FDA has concluded that use of these products poses no significant risk to human health.

Natural Toxins

Other chemical contamination of food can occur from **natural toxins**.[25] Examples include the following:

- Aflatoxins, found in contaminated food or animal feed. Aflatoxins are produced by certain strains of *Aspergillus* fungi under certain conditions of temperature and humidity. The most pronounced contamination has been found in tree nuts, peanuts, and other oilseeds, such as corn and cottonseed. Aflatoxins have been implicated as a factor in the development of liver cancer, particularly in parts of the world where food and water are frequently contaminated with this fungus.

- **Ciguatera** and other marine toxins. These toxins can accumulate in seafood (mainly in large tropical fish) and, when ingested, can cause serious problems, including paralysis, amnesia, and nerve toxicity. Commercial fishers avoid waters known to harbor ciguatera toxin. Ciguatera poisoning sometimes occurs when these fish are caught as part of recreational fishing. Cooking does not destroy these toxins.

- **Methylmercury**. Mercury occurs naturally in the environment and is produced by human activities. It is soluble in water, where bacteria can cause chemical changes that transform mercury to methylmercury, a more toxic form that can be harmful, especially to unborn babies and young children whose nervous systems are still developing. Fish absorb methylmercury from water passing over their gills and by eating other contaminated aquatic species. Because larger predatory fish can consume many contaminated smaller fish, they accumulate higher levels of methylmercury. (See **Figure 17.4**.)

Fish and shellfish are an important part of a healthy diet. They contain high-quality protein, other essential nutrients and *omega*-3 fatty acids, and fish are low in saturated fat. A well-balanced diet that includes a variety of fish and shellfish can contribute to a healthy heart and to healthy, well-developed children. One week's consumption of fish does not change the level of mercury in the body much. If you eat a lot of fish one week, you can cut back for the next week or two. Just make sure to average the recommended amount per week.

Nearly all fish and shellfish contain traces of methylmercury, and some types of fish and shellfish contain higher levels of mercury. The risks depend on the amount of fish and shellfish eaten and the levels of mercury

methylmercury A toxic compound that results from the chemical transformation of mercury by bacteria. Mercury is water-soluble in trace amounts and contaminates many bodies of water.

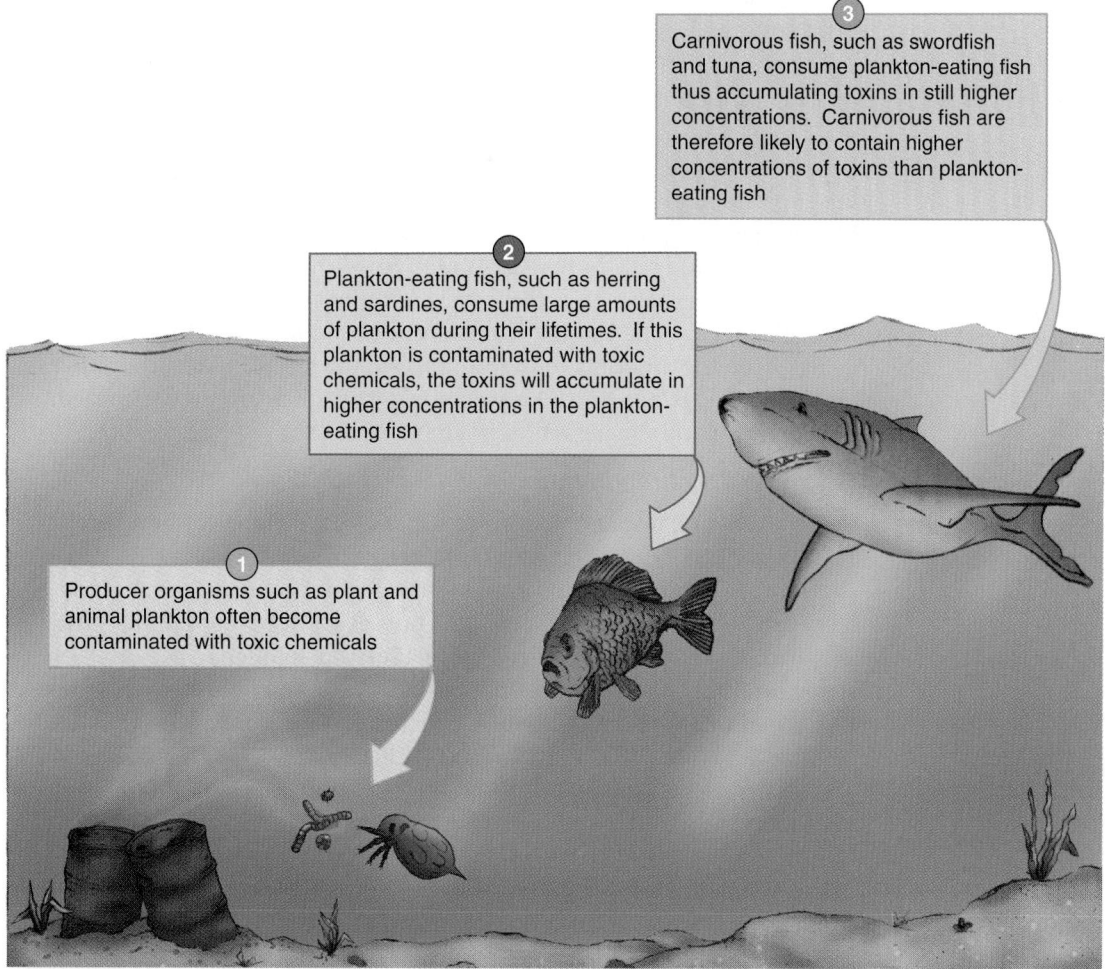

3 Carnivorous fish, such as swordfish and tuna, consume plankton-eating fish thus accumulating toxins in still higher concentrations. Carnivorous fish are therefore likely to contain higher concentrations of toxins than plankton-eating fish

2 Plankton-eating fish, such as herring and sardines, consume large amounts of plankton during their lifetimes. If this plankton is contaminated with toxic chemicals, the toxins will accumulate in higher concentrations in the plankton-eating fish

1 Producer organisms such as plant and animal plankton often become contaminated with toxic chemicals

Figure 17.4 **Toxins in the food chain.** As toxins travel up the food chain, they become concentrated in larger fish.

poisonous mushrooms Mushrooms that contain toxins that can cause stomach upset, dizziness, hallucinations, and other neurological symptoms.

solanine A potentially toxic alkaloid that is present with chlorophyll in the green areas on potato skins.

acrylamide A chemical produced in starchy foods by high-temperature cooking methods and found to be carcinogenic in animal tests.

Food Allergy & Anaphylaxis Network A nonprofit organization devoted to increasing public awareness of food allergy and anaphylaxis (a life-threatening allergic reaction), educating the public about food allergies, and advancing research on food allergies.

in the seafood. Because shark, swordfish, king mackerel, and tilefish contain high levels of mercury, the FDA and EPA recommend that women who may become pregnant, pregnant women, nursing mothers, and young children avoid eating these fish.[26] (See Chapter 15, "Life Cycle: Maternal and Infant Nutrition.")

- **Poisonous mushrooms**. These plants produce toxic substances that can cause stomach upset, dizziness, hallucinations, and other neurological symptoms.[27] The more lethal mushroom species can cause liver and kidney failure, coma, and death.
- **Solanine**, a toxic substance in raw potato skins.[28] Solanine develops in the greenish layer of improperly stored potatoes. It can be removed by thoroughly peeling the potato.

A variety of compounds in herbs and spices also can be toxic. However, foodborne illness caused by these and other natural toxins is relatively rare compared with illness from pathogenic microorganisms.

Acrylamide

On April 24, 2002, the Swedish National Food Administration announced that elevated levels of **acrylamide,** a known carcinogen in animal tests, had been found in starchy foods, such as potatoes and bread, cooked at high temperatures.[29] The FDA immediately began a testing program and found acrylamide in U.S. foods.

Because traditional high-temperature cooking methods, such as frying, roasting, or baking, can lead to formation of acrylamide in foods, researchers believe acrylamide has been present in cooked foods for thousands of years. In collaboration with other public health agencies, the FDA is studying the potential human health risk, seeking to better understand how acrylamide is formed in foods, and looking for ways to reduce acrylamide levels.[30]

In 2005, a study of more than 40,000 Swedish women found no significant association between breast cancer and dietary intake of acrylamide.[31] Although acrylamide is a toxic substance, the implications for public health from the amounts found in food are unclear. A better scientific understanding is needed to help determine whether, and to what extent, formal risk management action might be necessary.

Other Food Contaminants

Because labeling does not identify a substance inadvertently added to a food, people who are allergic to it are at risk of severe illness. The most common food allergens, according to the **Food Allergy & Anaphylaxis Network**, are milk, eggs, peanuts, tree nuts (e.g., cashews, walnuts), fish, shellfish, soy, and wheat.[32] (See **Figure 17.5**.) In an allergic person, these foods can cause a variety of reactions, including gastrointestinal problems, skin irritation, breathing difficulty, shock, and even death. (See Chapter 16, "Life Cycle: From Childhood Through Adulthood.")

Whether intentionally added through tampering or unintentionally during food production, contaminants such as glass, metal, and other objects can have serious health consequences. Lead can leach into tap water from old lead pipes or copper pipes soldered with lead. Lead also leaches from some imported ceramic plates, cups, and bowls that use a lead-based glaze. Lead toxicity is particularly dangerous for children. (See Chapter 16, "Life Cycle: From Childhood Through Adulthood.") Misuse of cleaning agents in food-contact areas such as refrigerator trucks, food-production lines, and storage units can introduce undesirable chemicals into food. Although generally not a health hazard, insects, dirt, and other undesirable items also can contaminate a food.

Key Concepts: *Chemical contaminants in foods include pesticides, natural toxins, and contamination related to pollution. Although organic foods are grown without synthetic pesticides or fertilizers, they still can contain chemical contaminants. Other potential food hazards are allergens and nonfood contaminants.*

Keeping Food Safe

Having safe foods to eat requires the efforts of a great many people along the way from the farm to your plate. Imagine yourself enjoying a piece of broiled chicken. Consider that harmful contamination of that chicken could have occurred at the farm, in the processing plant, or during transportation to the supermarket. Once at the supermarket, the chicken might have been underrefrigerated or kept too long before being sold. After buying the chicken, you might have left it in a warm car or kept it in a refrigerator that was not cold enough. Your kitchen hygiene might not have been the best; and finally, you could have undercooked the chicken. Considering the many opportunities for contamination, it is truly amazing that most of the time our food does not make us sick.

Keeping foods free from contamination is a job that falls to many parties. It is the responsibility not only of government officials at the national, state, and local levels, but also of everyone who comes in contact with food—the producer, the manufacturer, the retailer, and ultimately the consumer.

Government Agencies

The basis of modern food law is the Federal Food, Drug, and Cosmetic (FD&C) Act of 1938, which gives the Food and Drug Administration authority over food and food ingredients and defines requirements for truthful labeling of ingredients. Today at the federal level, six agencies (**Figure 17.6**) share responsibility for food safety.

1. *The Food and Drug Administration (FDA)* enforces laws governing the safety of domestic and imported food, except meat and poultry.

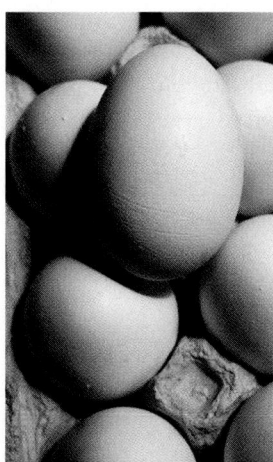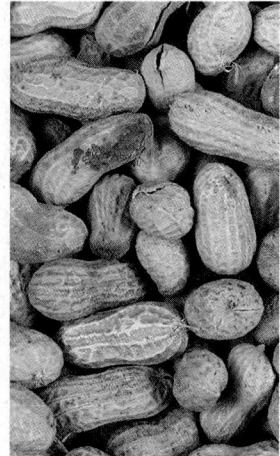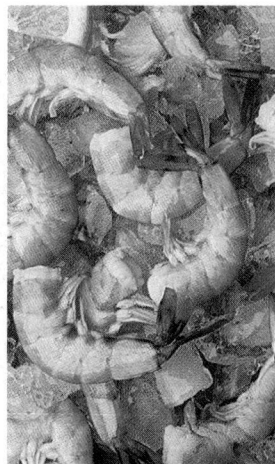

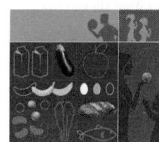

Dietary Guidelines for Americans, 2005
key recommendations

- To avoid microbial foodborne illness:
  - Clean hands, food contact surfaces, and fruits and vegetables. Meat and poultry should *not* be washed or rinsed.
  - Separate raw, cooked, and ready-to-eat foods while shopping, preparing, or storing foods.
  - Cook foods to a safe temperature to kill microorganisms.
  - Chill (refrigerate) perishable food promptly and defrost foods properly.
  - Avoid raw (unpasteurized) milk or any products made from unpasteurized milk, raw or partially cooked eggs or foods containing raw eggs, raw or undercooked meat and poultry, unpasteurized juices, and raw sprouts.

Key Recommendations for Specific Population Groups

- *Infants and young children, pregnant women, older adults, and those who are immunocompromised.* Do not eat or drink raw (unpasteurized) milk or any products made from unpasteurized milk, raw or partially cooked eggs or foods containing raw eggs, raw or undercooked meat and poultry, raw or undercooked fish or shellfish, unpasteurized juices, and raw sprouts.
- *Pregnant women, older adults, and those who are immunocompromised:* Only eat certain deli meats and frankfurters that have been reheated to steaming hot.

Figure 17.5 **Foods that commonly cause allergic reactions.** In sensitive people, an allergic reaction to food can be life threatening.

2. *The Centers for Disease Control and Prevention (CDC)* monitors outbreaks of foodborne diseases, investigates their causes, and determines proper prevention.

3. *The USDA Food Safety and Inspection Service (FSIS)* enforces laws governing the safety of domestic and imported meat and poultry products.

4. *The USDA Cooperative State Research, Education, and Extension Service (CSREES)* develops research and education programs on food safety for farmers and consumers.

5. *The USDA Agricultural Research Service (ARS)* conducts research to extend knowledge of various agricultural practices, including those involving animal and crop safety.

6. *The Environmental Protection Agency (EPA)* regulates public drinking water and approves pesticides and other chemicals used in the environment.

Figure 17.6 **Government agencies that help protect our food supply.** While the FDA has primary responsibility for the safety of much of our food supply, many government agencies provide oversight.

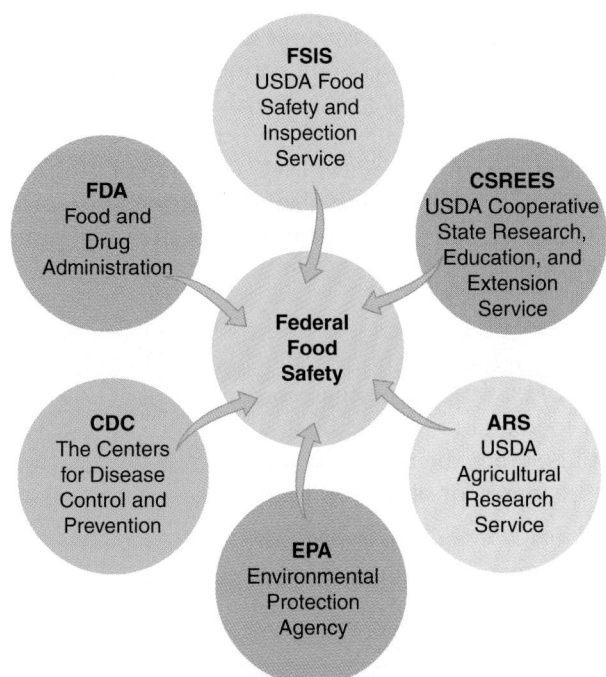

FSIS USDA Food Safety and Inspection Service

CSREES USDA Cooperative State Research, Education, and Extension Service

FDA Food and Drug Administration

Federal Food Safety

ARS USDA Agricultural Research Service

CDC The Centers for Disease Control and Prevention

EPA Environmental Protection Agency

OTHER AGENCIES WITH FOOD SAFETY RESPONSIBILITIES

Federal Trade Commission (FTC)
- Regulates the advertising and marketing of food products.
- Has the authority to take legal action against unwarranted advertising claims.

Department of Justice
- Seizes products when federal food safety laws are violated.
- Prosecutes suspected violators of food safety laws.

Bureau of Alcohol, Tobacco and Firearms (BATF)
- Enforces laws that involve the production, distribution, and labeling of most alcoholic beverages.
- Sometimes shares responsibilities with FDA when alcoholic beverages are adulterated or contain food or color additives, pesticides, or contaminants.

National Marine Fisheries Service (NMFS)
- Responsible for seafood quality and identification, fisheries management and development, habitat conservation, and aquaculture production.

State and Local Governments
- Inspect restaurants, retail food outlets, dairies, grain mills, and other food establishments within their areas of jurisdiction.
- Embargo illegal food products in many situations.

State and local health and agricultural departments oversee food safety in their jurisdictions, often in conjunction with federal agencies.

The public's heightened concern about food safety is evident in the creation of new consumer advocacy groups such as **S.T.O.P. (Safe Tables Our Priority)**, a national organization that works with government agencies and industry to prevent foodborne illnesses and deaths. In addition, the federal **Food Safety Initiative** calls on the federal government to take the lead in expanding research, training, and education about safety at all levels of food production.[33] The Food Safety Initiative has expanded the use of the food industry safety system called **Hazard Analysis Critical Control Point**, or HACCP (pronounced "hassip"). The Food Safety Initiative has also created a campaign to educate consumers, health professionals (such as doctors), and retail establishments about food safety. Other goals of the Food Safety Initiative include improved detection of foodborne pathogens and prevention of microbial growth during food production and distribution.[34]

Hazard Analysis Critical Control Point

Hazard Analysis Critical Control Point is a food industry program that focuses on preventing contamination by identifying areas in food production and retail where contamination could occur. HACCP also is an important line of defense against intentional contamination by bioterrorists. (See the FYI feature "At War with Bioterrorism.") HACCP is intended to replace the traditional system of spot checks at manufacturing sites and random sampling of final products. That system uncovered problems only after they had occurred, whereas HACCP works by preventing contamination.

Companies and retailers analyze their food-production processes and determine **critical control points (CCPs)**—points at which hazards could occur. They then determine measures that they can institute at these points to prevent, control, or eliminate the hazards. (See **Table 17.3.**)

Safe Tables Our Priority (S.T.O.P.) A national organization devoted to preventing illness and death from foodborne illness by working with government agencies and industry to encourage practices and policies that promote safe food.

Food Safety Initiative A 1996 presidential directive to three cabinet members to identify specific steps to improve the safety of the U.S. food supply.

Hazard Analysis Critical Control Point (HACCP) A modern food safety system that focuses on preventing contamination by identifying potential areas in food production and retail in which contamination could occur and taking steps to ensure contaminants are not introduced at these points.

critical control points (CCPs) Operational steps or procedures in a process, production method, or recipe, at which control can be applied to prevent, reduce, or eliminate a food safety hazard.

 **Table 17.3** HACCP: Hazard Analysis and Critical Control Point Systems

Step 1: Analyze hazards.	Identify the potential hazards associated with a food. The hazard could be biological (e.g., a microbe), chemical (e.g., mercury), or physical (e.g., ground glass or metal).
Step 2: Identify critical control points (CCPs).	Identify points in a food's production path—from its raw state through processing and shipping to consumption—where a potential hazard can be controlled or eliminated. Examples of CCPs are cooking, chilling, handling, cleaning, and storage.
Step 3: Establish preventive measures with critical limits for each control point.	An example is setting the minimum cooking temperature and time to ensure safety for a particular food (the temperature and time are critical limits).
Step 4: Establish procedures to monitor the control points.	Such procedures might include determining how and by whom cooking time and temperature should be monitored.
Step 5: Establish corrective actions to be taken when a critical limit has not been met.	For example, reprocessing or disposing of food if the minimum cooking temperature is not met.
Step 6: Establish procedures to verify that the system is working properly.	For example, testing time-recording and temperature-recording devises to verify that a cooking unit is working properly.
Step 7: Establish effective record keeping to document the HACCP system.	For example, recording hazards and their control methods, the monitoring of safety requirements, and action taken to correct potential problems.

The HACCP method focuses on preventing hazards, relies heavily on scientific principles, permits efficient government oversight, and places greater responsibility on food operations to ensure food safety.

Source: HACCP: A state-of-the-art approach to food safety. *FDA Backgrounder.* October, 2001. http://www.cfsan.fda.gov/~lrd/bghaccp.html. Accessed 1/12/07.

Critical control points can occur anywhere in a food's production—from its raw state through processing and shipping to purchase by the consumer. Preventive measures can include proper cooking, chilling, and sanitizing, as well as preventing cross-contamination and improving employee hygiene.

The USDA requires HACCP for meat and poultry, the food products that it regulates.[35] The FDA, which regulates all other foods, requires HACCP in the seafood and low-acid canned-food industries and recently added this requirement for the juice industry.[36] Also, the FDA has incorporated HACCP principles in its *Food Code,* a reference for restaurants, grocery stores, institutional food services, vending operations, and other retailers on how to store, prepare, and serve food to prevent foodborne illness.[37] The FDA updates and publishes the *Food Code* periodically as a model for states to adopt and use to regulate retail food establishments in their jurisdictions.

Food Code A reference published periodically by the Food and Drug Administration for restaurants, grocery stores, institutional food services, vending operations, and other retailers on how to store, prepare, and serve food to prevent foodborne illness.

Key Concepts: *Food safety is the responsibility of many agencies at the federal and state levels. The use of the Hazard Analysis Critical Control Point system allows government and industry to identify possible sites of food contamination and correct problems before they occur.*

Fyi At War with Bioterrorism

FOR YOUR INFORMATION

Late one afternoon, restaurant owner Dave Lutgens first felt nauseated, then experienced mild stomach cramps. By evening he was dizzy and disoriented. Suffering from diarrhea, he had to crawl to reach the toilet. Weak and dehydrated, he was wracked with chills, fever, and vomiting. Two days later his wife became ill with the same symptoms. By the end of the week, 13 employees were sick, as well as dozens of customers. The culprit was *Salmonella typhimurium,* a rod-shaped bacteria responsible for many foodborne illnesses. But this was not a simple case of food poisoning. Occurring in 1984, this was a bioterrorist assault on the small Oregon town of Dalles. The Rajaneesh religious cult deliberately perpetrated this terrifying food experience by contaminating a number of self-service salad bars and coffee creamers with home-grown *Salmonella.* Ten restaurants were affected and more than 700 people fell ill from the biological attack.

Biocriminals also have assaulted Canada. In 1970, four students in Montreal, Quebec, were admitted to the hospital after eating eggs inoculated with a parasitic nematode, *Ascaris suum.* They had signs of a parasitic infection and suffered from asthma and other lung problems. In 2000, 27 people suffered food poisoning after drinking coffee from a single vending machine at Lavalle University in Quebec City. The coffee had been laced with arsenic. In 2003, arsenic-laced coffee also poisoned more than a dozen people after a church service in New Sweden, Maine. One person died.

Food and water poisonings can be described by three categories:[1]

1. *Bioterrorism and biowarfare:* Terrorist acts by state-sponsored or hate groups. Few events have occurred to date.

2. *Biocrime:* Intent to harm for personal gain or revenge. A few dozen events have occurred during recent decades.

3. *Biomisfortune:* Naturally occurring foodborne disease. Virtually all foodborne disease falls into this category, which is a daily concern for public health agencies everywhere.

Bioterrorist attacks can range from making false statements or accusations to actively inflicting injury on people, animals, or crops. Threats can be as devastating as actual destruction. Just claiming that a product has been intentionally contaminated can be sufficient to trigger an expensive recall and harmful adverse publicity. Product tampering, whether a hoax or real, can provide notoriety to the perpetrator, who is attempting to terrorize people and businesses.

Our food supply is an obvious route for the delivery of certain chemical and biological agents. Food production and distribution is a complex system not protected easily from the deliberate introduction of toxic agents. The attacks on the World Trade Center and

The Consumer's Role in Food Safety

Food safety advice to consumers used to consist of a simple message: "Keep hot foods hot and cold foods cold." (See **Figure 17.7**.) Now food safety experts urge consumers to follow the following four rules (see **Figure 17.8**):

1. *Clean*. Wash hands and surfaces often. Clean fruits and vegetables. Meat and poultry should *not* be washed or rinsed.

2. *Separate*. Don't cross-contaminate. When shopping, preparing, or storing food, separate raw, cooked, and ready-to-eat foods.

3. *Cook*. Cook to proper temperatures. Avoid unpasteurized milk and juices, raw sprouts, raw or partially cooked eggs, and raw or undercooked meat and poultry.

4. *Chill*. Refrigerate promptly. Defrost foods properly and quickly refrigerate perishable foods.[38]

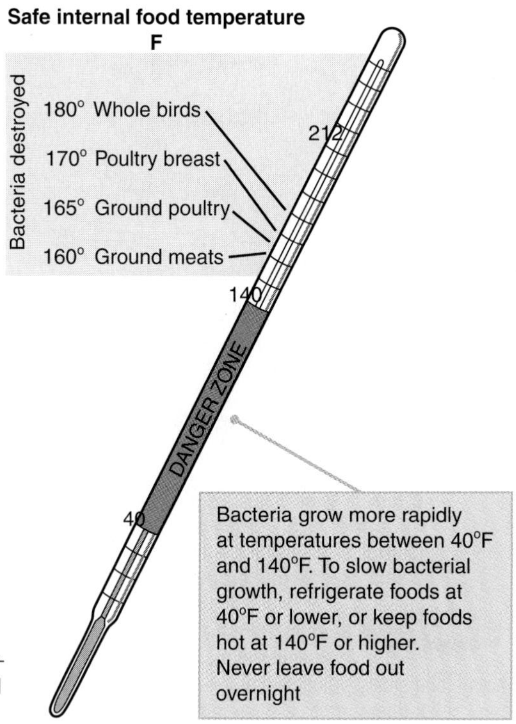

Safe internal food temperature
F

Bacteria destroyed

180° Whole birds
170° Poultry breast
165° Ground poultry
160° Ground meats
212
140

DANGER ZONE

40

Bacteria grow more rapidly at temperatures between 40°F and 140°F. To slow bacterial growth, refrigerate foods at 40°F or lower, or keep foods hot at 140°F or higher. Never leave food out overnight

Figure 17.7 **Temperature guide.** To prevent bacterial growth, keep hot food hot and cold food cold.

Pentagon and the anthrax assault have increased the concern and vigilance of the U.S. and Canadian governments, which are acutely aware that public food and water supplies are among the most vulnerable avenues for terrorist attacks.

At ports of entry, food inspection facilities, and research labs and buildings, government personnel are at a heightened state of alert. To prevent the entry of animal or plant pests and diseases, they are carrying out intensified product and cargo inspections of travelers and baggage. Food safety inspectors have been given a mandate to be alert to any irregularities at food-processing facilities. Within processing facilities, specific plans for security should be developed. Such plans can be based on HACCP principles.[2]

The FDA has adopted five broad strategies to counter bioterrorism:[3]

1. *Awareness:* Increasing awareness through collecting, analyzing, and spreading information and knowledge.

2. *Prevention:* Identifying specific threats or attacks that involve biological, chemical, radiological, or nuclear agents.

3. *Preparedness:* Developing and making available medical countermeasures such as drugs, devices, and vaccines.

4. *Response:* Ensuring rapid and coordinated response to any terrorist attacks.

5. *Recovery:* Ensuring rapid and coordinated treatment for any illness that may result from a terrorist attack.

What can we as consumers do to protect ourselves from food contamination? We must be the final judges of the safety of the food we buy. At minimum we should do the following:

- Make sure the food package or can is intact before opening it. If it has been damaged or dented or opened prior to purchase, call it to the attention of the appropriate person.
- Be alert to abnormal color, taste, and appearance of a food item. If you have any doubt, don't eat it.

- If the food appears to have been tampered with, report it immediately.
- Follow safe handling food practices. (See the FYI feature "Safe Food Practices.")

1 Sobel J. Epidemiologic preparedness and response to terrorist events involving the nation's food supply. Paper presented at: Centers for Disease Control Health Preparedness Conference; February 2005.

2 Bledsoe GE, Rasco BA. Addressing the risk of bioterrorism in food production. *Food Technol.* 2002;56(2):43–47.

3 Meadows M. The FDA and the fight against terrorism. *FDA Consumer.* 2004;38(1). http://www.fda.gov/fdac/features/2004/104_terror.html. Accessed 8/6/06.

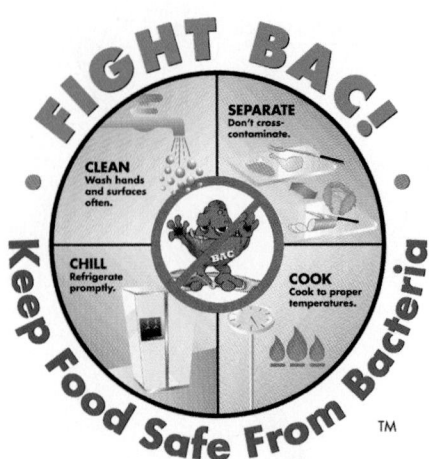

Clean: Wash hands and surfaces often
Separate: Dont cross-contaminate
Cook: Cook to proper temperatures
Chill: Refrigerate properly

Figure 17.8 **Keeping harmful bacteria at bay.**
While our food supply generally is safe, home food safety practices are the weakest link in the food chain from farm to kitchen table. Be sure to follow the four basic practices: clean, separate, cook, and chill. Reprinted with permission from Partnership for Food Safety Education, www.fightbac.org.

Quick Bites

How Good Are Your Food Safety Habits?

Do Americans practice food safety in their own kitchens? Apparently not. A study conducted by the FDA and the Centers for Disease Control and Prevention showed that one-half of people surveyed ate undercooked eggs in the past year. Twenty percent of people ate undercooked hamburger, and 25 percent of men and 14 percent of women failed to wash their hands with soap after handling raw meat.

Once a consumer takes possession of a food, food safety becomes his or her responsibility. (See **Table 17.4**.) Unfortunately, studies show that many consumers fail to follow safe food practices in the home. Current public health efforts focus on teaching consumers—from young children to older Americans—safe food practices in the home. (See the FYI feature "Safe Food Practices.")

Some food-handling practices are so important that the federal government requires specific instructions or warnings on labels of certain foods. Following outbreaks of illness from *E. coli* O157:H7 in contaminated hamburger in 1993, the USDA mandated instructions on labels of raw meat and poultry to encourage consumers to follow recommendations for the safe handling and cooking of these products.[39]

Because of a 1998 FDA rule, labels of unpasteurized or otherwise untreated packaged juice products carry a statement about the product's possible danger to children, older adults, and people with weakened immune systems.[40] The warning states that the product has not been pasteurized and therefore may contain harmful bacteria that can cause serious illness in these high-risk groups. This requirement was made after a number of people became seriously ill from drinking unpasteurized apple juice that was contaminated with *E. coli*.

In 2000 the FDA finalized rules requiring safe handling statements on egg cartons.[41] The required statement reads

SAFE HANDLING INSTRUCTIONS: To prevent illness from bacteria: keep eggs refrigerated, cook eggs until yolks are firm, and cook foods containing eggs thoroughly.

Food manufacturers may voluntarily place other safe handling instructions on the label, such as those for proper cooking and storage of the item. Consumers should always follow these instructions.

Who's at Increased Risk for Foodborne Illness?

Infants and young children, pregnant women, older adults, and those who are immunocompromised or have certain chronic conditions need to be especially careful about following safe food practices. In particular, they should not eat or drink raw (unpasteurized) milk or any products made from raw milk. They also should not eat raw or partially cooked eggs or foods containing raw eggs, raw or undercooked meat and poultry, raw or undercooked fish or shellfish, unpasteurized juices, and raw sprouts.

People who are at risk include individuals with these conditions:

- Immune disorders, such as HIV infection
- Cancer
- Diabetes
- Long-term steroid use, such as for asthma or arthritis
- Liver disease
- Hemochromatosis, an iron storage disorder that affects the liver
- Stomach problems, including previous stomach surgery and low stomach acid (for example, from chronic antacid use)

Because these conditions are more common in older adults, seniors have an increased risk of foodborne illness. Young children do not have fully developed immune systems, so they are particularly vulnerable to serious illness from foodborne pathogens. Also, pregnant women and their fetuses are at special risk from the bacterium *Listeria monocytogenes* and the parasite

Table 17.4 Moldy Food: When to Use and When to Discard

Food	Handling	Reason
Luncheon meats, bacon, or hot dogs	Discard.	Foods with high moisture content can be contaminated below the surface. Moldy foods may also have bacteria growing along with the mold.
Hard salami and dry-cured country hams	Use. Scrub mold off surface.	It is normal for these shelf-stable products to have surface mold.
Cooked leftover meat and poultry	Discard.	Foods with high moisture content can be contaminated below the surface. Moldy foods may also have bacteria growing along with the mold.
Cooked casseroles	Discard.	Foods with high moisture content can be contaminated below the surface. Moldy foods may also have bacteria growing along with the mold.
Cooked grain and pasta	Discard.	Foods with high moisture content can be contaminated below the surface. Moldy foods may also have bacteria growing along with the mold.
Hard cheese (not cheese where mold is part of the processing)	Use. Cut off at least 1 inch around and below the mold spot (keep the knife out of the mold itself so it will not cross-contaminate other parts of the cheese). After trimming off the mold, re-cover the cheese in fresh wrap.	Mold generally cannot penetrate deep into the product.
Cheese made with mold (such as Roquefort, blue, Gorgonzola, Stilton, Brie, Camembert)	Discard soft cheeses such as Brie and Camembert if they contain molds that are not a part of the manufacturing process. If surface mold is on hard cheeses such as Gorgonzola and Stilton, cut off mold at least 1 inch around and below the mold spot and handle like hard cheese (see above).	Molds that are not a part of the manufacturing process can be dangerous.
Soft cheese (such as cottage, cream cheese, Neufchatel, chevre, Bel Paese, etc.) Crumbled, shredded, and sliced cheeses (all types)	Discard.	Foods with high moisture content can be contaminated below the surface. Shredded, sliced, or crumbled cheese can be contaminated by the cutting instrument. Moldy soft cheese can also have bacteria growing along with the mold.
Yogurt and sour cream	Discard.	Foods with high moisture content can be contaminated below the surface. Moldy foods may also have bacteria growing along with the mold.
Jams and jellies	Discard.	The mold could be producing a mycotoxin. Microbiologists recommend against scooping out the mold and using the remaining condiment.
Fruits and vegetables, firm (such as cabbage, bell peppers, carrots, etc.)	Use. Cut off at least 1 inch around and below the mold spot (keep the knife out of the mold itself so it will not cross-contaminate other parts of the produce).	Small mold spots can be cut off fruits and vegetables with low moisture content. It's difficult for mold to penetrate dense foods.
Fruits and vegetables, soft (such as cucumbers, peaches, tomatoes, etc.)	Discard.	Fruits and vegetables with high moisture content can be contaminated below the surface.
Bread and baked goods	Discard.	Porous foods can be contaminated below the surface.
Peanut butter, legumes, and nuts	Discard.	Foods processed without preservatives are at high risk for mold.

Source: USDA Food Safety and Inspection Service. Molds on foods: are they dangerous? September 2005.
http://www.fsis.usda.gov/Fact_Sheets/Molds_On_Food/index.asp. Accessed 8/7/06.

pasteurization A process for destroying pathogenic bacteria by heating liquid foods to a prescribed temperature for a specified time.

preservatives Chemicals or other agents that slow the decomposition of a food.

Toxoplasma gondii. Both of these microorganisms can harm—even kill—fetuses and young babies.

A Final Word on Food Safety

A totally risk-free system of food production is an unreasonable and unattainable goal. The United States and Canada enjoy a reputation for having food supplies that are among the safest in the world. We expect our food to be clean, fresh, and uncontaminated with debris, chemicals, or organisms that cause sickness or discomfort. To make sure it stays that way, food safety experts are continually trying to ensure that every participant in the food production chain—from the farmer who produces the food to the manufacturer who processes it to the retailer who sells it and to the consumer who buys it—undertakes measures to help reduce and perhaps even eliminate foodborne disease. That's one reason food safety advice today is turning up in so many places—to ensure that everyone gets the word on food safety.

Key Concepts: Consumers play a huge role in food safety. They can avoid foodborne illness by following a few simple food-handling and preparation rules: Keep hands and food-preparation areas clean, avoid cross-contamination of foods, cook foods adequately, and refrigerate foods promptly. People who have weak or less-developed immune systems are at higher risk for foodborne illnesses.

Fyi Safe Food Practices

FOR YOUR INFORMATION

Because bacteria grow rapidly between 40°F and 140°F (4°C–60°C), most food should be kept out of this temperature range, known as the Danger Zone. Cold temperatures keep bacteria from multiplying; the fewer bacteria, the less the risk of illness. Proper cooking (or other heat treatment, such as pasteurization) kills the bacteria. These principles serve as the basis for many of the following recommended food-handling practices.

Buying Food

- Buy from reputable dealers and grocers who keep their selling areas and facilities clean and sanitary and maintain food at the appropriate temperature—for example, holding dairy foods, eggs, meats, seafood, and certain produce such as cut melons and raw sprouts at refrigerator temperatures.
- Don't buy canned goods with dents or bulges. Avoid torn, crushed, or open food packages. Also, avoid buying packages that are above the frost line in the store's freezer. If the package cover is transparent, avoid those with

frost or ice crystals, signs that the product has been stored for a long time or thawed and refrozen.

Storing Food

- Refrigerate perishable items as quickly as possible after purchase. The refrigerator temperature should be 40°F or colder. Check it periodically with a thermometer to make sure the correct temperature is being maintained.
- Keep eggs in their original carton and store them in the refrigerator itself, not the door, where the temperature is warmer.
- If raw meat, poultry products, or fresh seafood will be used within two days, store them in the coldest part of the refrigerator, usually under the freezer compartment or in a special "meat keeper." Store the packages loosely to allow air to circulate freely around each package, and be sure to wrap them tightly so that raw juices can't leak out and contaminate other foods.
- If raw meat, poultry, and seafood will not be used within two days, store

them in the freezer, which should have a temperature of 0°F. Check this temperature periodically too, and adjust as needed.
- Read label directions for storing other foods; for example, mayonnaise and ketchup need to be refrigerated after they have been opened.
- Store potatoes and onions in a cool, dark place, but not under the sink because leakage from pipes can contaminate and damage them. Keep them away from household cleaning products and other chemicals as well.

Preparing Food

- Wash hands thoroughly with warm, soapy water for at least 20 seconds before beginning food preparation and every time you handle raw foods, including fresh produce.
- Defrost meat, poultry, and seafood products in the refrigerator, microwave oven, or in a water-tight plastic bag submerged in cold water (the water must be changed every 30 minutes). Never defrost at room temperature—an

Food Technology

Technology is having a larger and larger impact on the food we eat. Our use of preservatives, other preservation techniques, and genetic engineering has implications for our food supply in the years to come and has triggered debates about the risks and benefits of these technologies.

Food Preservation

In our modern society, few people grow their own vegetables, fruits, and grains or keep livestock as a source of meat and milk. Rather, we shop for our food, typically at a large, full-service supermarket. Because we don't consume our food at the point of harvest or slaughter, we use food preservation methods to help maintain the quality of the foods we purchase. Among food preservation methods are the addition of chemical preservatives, canning or freezing, **pasteurization**, and more recent methods such as irradiation.

Preservatives

Preservatives are added to foods to prevent spoilage and increase shelf life. The most common antimicrobial agents are salt and sugar. Other preservatives, such as potassium sorbate and sodium propionate, extend the shelf life of baked goods and many other products. Antioxidants are a type of

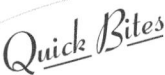

Quick Bites

Wood Versus Plastic: The Cutting Controversy

Which type of cutting board is safer to use while cutting meat: wood or plastic? Both have drawbacks. A wood cutting board tends to absorb bacteria, sucking them down into the wood fibers. This may be safer than a plastic board, which keeps bacteria on the surface, in an easy position to rub off onto food and other objects. But with use, wooden cutting boards tend to keep more on the surface than new wooden boards, acting more like plastic boards. What's the solution? Keep cutting boards clean by heating wooden boards in the microwave or putting plastic boards in the dishwasher.

---

ideal temperature for bacteria to grow and multiply.

- Marinate foods in the refrigerator. Discard the marinade after use because it contains raw juices, which may harbor bacteria; make a separate batch for basting food while cooking.
- Always use a clean cutting board. Wash cutting boards with hot water, soap, and a scrub brush. Then sanitize them in an automatic dishwasher or by rinsing with a solution of 5 milliliters (1 teaspoon) chlorine bleach to about 1 liter (1 quart) of water. If possible, use one cutting board for fresh produce and a separate one for raw meat, poultry, and seafood. Once cutting boards become excessively worn or develop hard-to-clean grooves, you should replace them.
- Before opening canned foods, wash the top of the can to prevent dirt from coming in contact with the food.
- Wash fresh fruits and vegetables thoroughly with water only.
- Avoid eating dough or batter containing raw eggs because of the risk of

Salmonella enteritidis, a bacterium that can live in eggs. Cook eggs until both the yolk and the white are firm. Scrambled eggs should not be runny. Casseroles and other dishes containing eggs should be cooked to 160°F as measured with a food thermometer.

Cooking Food

- Cook foods to the appropriate minimum internal temperature:
  Beef, lamb, and pork   160°F (71°C)
  Poultry   165°F (74°C)
- Always use a thermometer to ensure that the product has reached the correct minimum internal temperature throughout. Color is not always a good guide.
- Cook seafood according to the following guidelines:
  Fin fish
    Cook until opaque and flakes easily with a fork.
  Shrimp, lobster, crab
    Should turn red, and flesh should become pearly opaque.

Scallops
  Should turn milky white or opaque and firm.
Clams, mussels, oysters
  Cook until shells open.
- When microwaving foods, rotate the dish and stir its contents several times to ensure even cooking. Follow recommended standing times, then check meat, poultry, and seafood products with a thermometer to make sure they have reached the correct internal temperature.

Serving Food

- Keep hot foods at 140°F (60°C) or higher and cold foods at 40°F (4°C) or lower.
- Do not keep leftovers at room temperature for more than two hours. Refrigerate as quickly as possible.
- Date leftovers so that they can be used within a safe time—generally, three to five days in the refrigerator.

irradiation A food preservation technique in which foods are exposed to measured doses of radiation to reduce or eliminate pathogens and kill insects, reduce spoilage, and, in certain fruits and vegetables, inhibit sprouting and delay ripening.

genetically modified (GM) foods Foods produced using plant or animal ingredients that have been modified using gene technology.

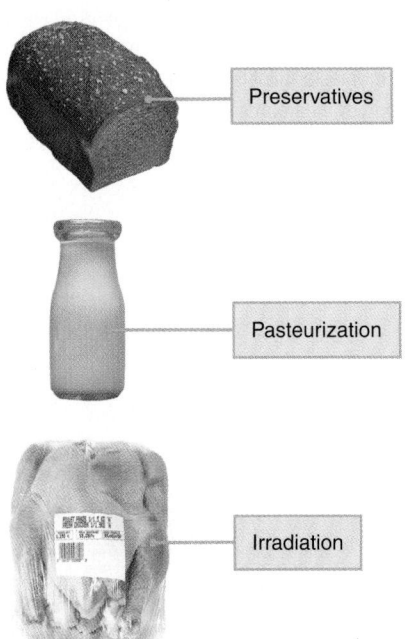

Preservatives

Pasteurization

Irradiation

Preparing food for safe consumption.

Quick Bites

Where Do *E. coli* Hang Out?

Ground beef is the most common source of *E. coli* bacteria, but *E. coli* also have been found on apples and lettuce.

preservative that prevents the changes in color and flavor caused by exposure to air. Common antioxidants include vitamin C and vitamin E, sulfites, and BHA and BHT.

Preparation for Preservation

Some preservation techniques, such as salting and fermenting, date to ancient times and are still practiced along with their modern counterparts—freezing, canning, pasteurization, and the like. Salting, drying, or fermenting foods creates an environment in which bacteria cannot multiply and therefore cannot cause food spoilage. Canned foods are heated quickly to a temperature that kills microbes and then are sealed airtight to prevent both contamination and oxidative damage. Freezing temperatures not only keep bacteria from multiplying but also prevent normal enzymatic changes in food that would cause spoilage. Pasteurization of milk or other beverages uses a very high temperature for a very short time to kill bacteria, but minimizes changes that would result from longer heating. The food industry and the North American public readily accept these food preservation methods. One of the most modern preservation techniques—irradiation—is also the most controversial, in part because of our fear of anything that has to do with radiation.

Irradiation

Before it received official approval, food **irradiation** underwent more than 40 years of scientific research and testing—more than any other food technology.[42] During irradiation, foods are exposed to a measured dose of radiation to reduce or eliminate pathogenic bacteria, including *E. coli* O157:H7, *Salmonella*, and *Campylobacter*, the chief causes of foodborne illness today.[43] Irradiation also can destroy insects and parasites, reduce spoilage, and inhibit sprouting and delay ripening of certain fruits and vegetables. Irradiated strawberries, for example, stay unspoiled for up to three weeks versus three to five days for untreated berries. Irradiation can reduce pathogens in raw poultry or meat by 99.9 percent.[44] Some people fear irradiation will make the food radioactive. This concern is unfounded. The energy used to irradiate foods passes through the food and leaves no residue—in the same way that microwaves pass through food. Despite its benefits, use of irradiation remains rare in the North America.

Because food manufacturers fear consumer rejection, they have been reluctant to use irradiation on their products.[45] Some consumers and advocacy groups protest its use because they are concerned that irradiation may compromise a food's nutritional value and change its texture, taste, or appearance. According to the American Dietetic Association (ADA), the nutritive loss associated with irradiation is actually less than for most conventional methods of food preservation.[46] The ADA also states that at appropriate doses, irradiation of food does not significantly change its flavor, texture, or appearance. Many organizations, including the ADA, the American Medical Association, and the World Health Organization, endorse irradiation as a means of providing the public with a safer food supply.

The FDA has approved irradiation for the following:

- Spices and dry vegetable seasoning to decontaminate and control insects and microorganisms

- Dry or dehydrated enzyme preparations to control insects and microorganisms

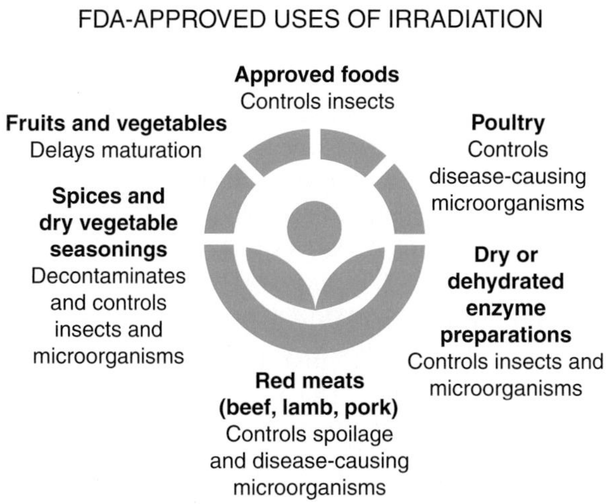

FDA-APPROVED USES OF IRRADIATION

Approved foods
Controls insects

Fruits and vegetables
Delays maturation

**Spices and
dry vegetable
seasonings**
Decontaminates
and controls
insects and
microorganisms

Poultry
Controls
disease-causing
microorganisms

**Dry or
dehydrated
enzyme
preparations**
Controls insects and
microorganisms

**Red meats
(beef, lamb, pork)**
Controls spoilage
and disease-causing
microorganisms

Figure 17.9 **Irradiation.** Irradiation can retard spoilage and reduce risk of foodborne illness.

- Fruits and vegetables to inhibit maturation
- Poultry and red meat to control spoilage and pathogenic microorganisms
- All the foods listed above, to control insects, mites, and other arthropod pests

The FDA requires labels of irradiated foods to state that the product was "treated with irradiation" or "treated by irradiation" and to display the international symbol for irradiation, the radura. (See **Figure 17.9.**)

Some experts believe the time is right for food irradiation to become more widespread. News stories about deaths related to foodborne illness have made the public more aware of the need for protection against contamination of food. As more consumers become aware of the benefits of irradiation, the demand for irradiated foods is expected to increase. Studies have shown that education about irradiation significantly improves customers' attitudes.[47]

Key Concepts: Various processing methods help protect us from contamination of food by pathogens. Drying, salting, canning, freezing, and pasteurizing are methods that consumers accept. Irradiation is a process in which foods are exposed to a measured dose of radiation to reduce or eliminate pathogenic bacteria. Although government and professional organizations deem irradiation a safe procedure, consumers are still wary.

Genetically Modified Foods

Genetically modified (GM) foods have arrived, and most of us are already dining on them. When you prepare a dinner of broccoli and tofu, some of the soybeans used to make the tofu probably came from plants genetically modified to resist herbicide sprays or insect pests or both. And although your broccoli is currently "natural," you can be sure that in a lab somewhere genetically modified broccoli seeds are sprouting, perhaps with enhanced nutrient or other phytochemical levels. If you are eating tenderloin tonight, the steak probably came from a steer fed on genetically modified corn that had its DNA altered by the addition of foreign genes to allow the plant to resist insect pests and herbicides.

Quick Bites

Bacteria at the Supermarket

Bacteria abound on the surface of supermarket meat. A piece of pork, on average, may harbor a few hundred bacteria per cubic centimeter, and a piece of chicken may have 10,000 in the same area.

Should you be indignant that these new foods are showing up on your table without any indication on the label, or should you be grateful that these high-tech methods are keeping crop yields high and food costs low? An informed answer to this question requires some understanding of how genetic engineering works, how new crops and foods are regulated, and how gene modification of crops and animals differs from the classical methods of agricultural breeding that have been practiced for thousands of years.

A Short Course in Plant Genetics

How do GM food plants differ from those developed through traditional cross-pollination and hybridization? The answer, surprisingly, is that most crop modifications achieved by DNA manipulation and associated techniques of **biotechnology** could also be achieved with classical techniques, but the time scale and expense are very different.[48]

The classical techniques for breeding a plant with new characteristics have been practiced for hundreds of years. They involve crossing two plants with different characteristics, then growing the resulting hybrid seeds and looking for plants with the desired combination of characteristics. Hybrid plants get half of their genes from one parent and half from the other. Though the hybrid may combine favorable qualities from both parents, a lot of undesirable genetic baggage must be sorted out after formation of such a hybrid. It usually takes dozens of additional crosses, and many years, to separate the desirable genes from the undesirable, and the process has a large element of chance. Due to human intervention, today virtually every domesticated crop plant species differs greatly from its original, wild form.[49]

Genetic engineering, on the other hand, allows scientists to transform a plant one gene at a time, using well-established methods for manipulating DNA sequences and integrating them into the plant **genome** (its set of genes). (See **Figure 17.10**.) Because many plant genes have already been identified, and complete DNA sequences of plant genomes will be available soon, we can anticipate that the genetic engineering of plants will become increasingly powerful and precise. Designing a new GM plant should come to resemble a manufacturing process rather than the tedious guessing game of classical genetics. In some cases, a gene can be selected and introduced into plant cells, and new GM seeds can be prepared within a year or two. When we consider that it took centuries of selection and breeding to transform the weedy wild maize plant of pre-Columbian Mexico into our modern varieties of corn, the scale and speed of the gene revolution in agriculture is both astounding and a little frightening.

Genetically Modified Foods: An Unstoppable Experiment?

How extensive is the shift to gene-modified crops, and how many different crops are involved? The United States accounts for nearly two-thirds of all biotechnology crops planted globally. GM food crops grown by U.S. farmers include corn, cotton, soybeans, canola, squash, and papaya. About 85 percent of the U.S. soybean crop and over 75 percent of the cotton crop are genetically modified.[50] Other major producers of GM crops are Argentina, which plants primarily biotech soybeans; Canada, whose principal biotech crop is canola; Brazil, which recently approved the planting of GM soybeans; China, where the acreage of GM cotton continues to increase; and South Africa, where cotton is also the principle biotech crop. The increased

biotechnology The set of laboratory techniques and processes used to modify the genome of plants or animals and thus create desirable new characteristics. Genetic engineering in the broad sense.

genetic engineering Manipulation of the genome of an organism by artificial means for the purpose of modifying existing traits or adding new genetic traits.

genome The total genetic information of an organism, stored in the DNA of its chromosomes.

Quick Bites

Biotechnology in the 1930s

One of the first examples of genetic theory successfully applied to food production was hybrid corn. When first introduced, it seemed miraculous and convinced skeptical farmers of the potential benefits of this emerging agricultural science. To this day, tougher and healthier new hybrids continue to outyield their predecessors.

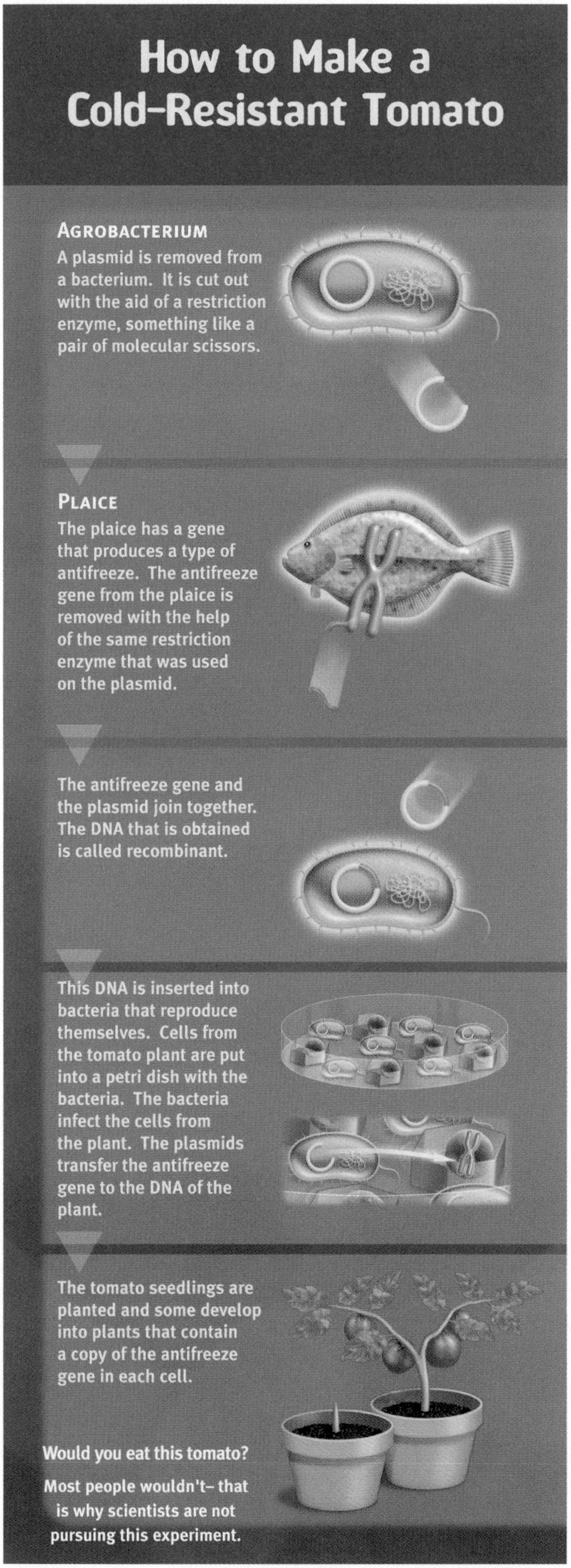

How to Make a Cold-Resistant Tomato

AGROBACTERIUM
A plasmid is removed from a bacterium. It is cut out with the aid of a restriction enzyme, something like a pair of molecular scissors.

PLAICE
The plaice has a gene that produces a type of antifreeze. The antifreeze gene from the plaice is removed with the help of the same restriction enzyme that was used on the plasmid.

The antifreeze gene and the plasmid join together. The DNA that is obtained is called recombinant.

This DNA is inserted into bacteria that reproduce themselves. Cells from the tomato plant are put into a petri dish with the bacteria. The bacteria infect the cells from the plant. The plasmids transfer the antifreeze gene to the DNA of the plant.

The tomato seedlings are planted and some develop into plants that contain a copy of the antifreeze gene in each cell.

Would you eat this tomato?

Most people wouldn't– that is why scientists are not pursuing this experiment.

Figure 17.10 **Genetically Modifying a Tomato.** Scientists may use recombinant DNA technology to create a genetically modified plant whose genetic code has been altered to give it new features, such as a tomato resistant to cold temperatures.
Source: Canadian Museum of Nature. Using genomics: The science behind GMOs. http://www.nature.ca/genome/03/d/30/03d_33_e.cfm. Accessed 12/11/06. Reprinted with permission from the Canadian Museum of Nature, Ottawa, Canada.

yields and lower costs associated with GM crops make them attractive to farmers. There is now strong, perhaps unstoppable, momentum to continue and expand GM crop plantings.

European countries, however, have been slow to accept gene-modified crops. They are concerned about possible ecological damage from such crops and fear potential unintended consequences of genetic "tampering" with the food supply. Although some U.S. consumer groups voice similar concerns, agribusiness and the U.S. federal government have been quite supportive of the trend toward GM foods.

The GM crops mentioned earlier are just the tip of the genetic modification iceberg; hundreds more are under development in university laboratories and in the labs of giant agribusinesses such as Monsanto, Novartis, and DuPont. The goals of these modifications are higher yields, increased amounts of critical nutrients, and a healthier mix of plant oils. Many of these goals would be achievable with classical selection techniques; however, with genetic engineering, they move from laboratory to table in decades rather than centuries.

Genetic engineering also has affected the food-processing industry. The cheese-making industry uses genetically modified bacteria to produce the widely used enzyme chymosin. Chymosin has virtually replaced the natural milk-clotting enzyme rennet, which is extracted from the stomachs of calves.

In the future we will probably see GM plants that have been modified to yield better textile fibers, including colored cotton, or specialized proteins for use in human pharmaceuticals—or even plants that produce the starting materials for manufacture of plastics. In economic terms, these nonfood GM crops may become even more important than GM foods.

If only plant genes were involved in GM food production, there would be much less controversy. However, *any* gene, including genes from bacteria and animals, can be introduced into a plant genome. Some people find this frightening, and an imaginative term, *Frankenfoods,* has been coined to express the "unnatural" nature of some GM products. But how unnatural is the exchange of DNA between species? It may be reassuring to realize that organisms have been swapping DNA for eons, with no help from humans. Foreign DNA can be carried from one species to another by a variety of viruses, for example. Nature has already performed millions of "gene modifications" on its own, and exchange of DNA is an established part of the evolutionary process. Now that we can do our own experiments with DNA manipulation, we hope the benefits will be increased.

Benefits of Genetic Engineering

Whatever the risks, no one can argue with the success of these GM techniques. For instance, a bacterial gene was used to create Monsanto's insect-resistant varieties of corn, potatoes, and soybeans. This gene, the **Bt gene**, was taken from the soil bacterium *Bacillus thuringiensis.* When inserted into a plant genome, the Bt gene directs the production of a protein in the plant that makes the plant toxic to insects. Such crops have been extremely successful and produce high yields without use of insecticides.

Bt-modified crops, which are now grown in the United States over an area larger than Rhode Island, are a boon to both the economy and the environment. Because chemical insecticides are not necessary, many benign insects are spared, and insect **biodiversity** is preserved. Similarly, other

Bt gene *Bacillus thuringiensis* (Bt) is a bacterium that produces a protein called the Bt toxin. One of the bacterium's genes, the Bt gene, carries the information for the Bt toxin. Inserting a copy of the Bt gene into plants enables them to produce Bt toxin protein and resist some insect pests. The Bt protein is not toxic to humans.

biodiversity The countless species of plants, animals, and insects that exist on the earth. An undisturbed tropical forest is an example of the biodiversity of a healthy ecosystem.

plants can be genetically modified to resist the effects of common herbicides. Chemical sprays that are lethal to most plant life have no effect on these GM plants. The crop plant grows larger in the absence of weeds, and the farmer gets a better yield with less effort and expense.

The economic benefits of GM foods are clearly substantial. Increased yields of important food plants can help feed increasing populations without the need for putting more land under the plow or increasing the use of toxic insecticides. In the coming century, this may be the difference between starvation and adequate nutrition in many developing countries.

It is easy to imagine how manipulation of plant amino acids and plant oils could yield superior foods, which not only would be able to satisfy calorie requirements, but also would address protein and vitamin needs. A strain of rice, genetically modified to be rich in beta-carotene, could benefit the more than 1 million children in developing countries who die or are weakened by vitamin A deficiency.[51] In developed countries, where heart disease and cancer loom as greater risks than malnutrition, the ability to adjust the saturation level of plant lipids or to boost beneficial phytochemicals would be of great value to public health. But do these undoubted benefits outweigh the risks?

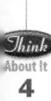

Risks

What are the specific risks of GM foods? Many consumers are concerned about whether these new foods are safe to eat. The answer to this concern is a fairly unequivocal yes. When a new protein or other substance is introduced into a food, the FDA requires substantial testing to demonstrate its safety. With GM foods, the principal risk appears to be the possibility of introducing a new allergen into a GM food.[52] To be cautious, the FDA has focused on allergy issues. Under the law and the FDA's biotech food policy, companies must tell consumers on the food label when a product includes a gene from a food that commonly causes an allergic reaction. The only exception is when the company can show that the protein produced by the added gene does not make the genetically modified food allergenic.[53]

Of greater concern, and more difficult to predict, are environmental effects, though no ecological disasters have occurred thus far. What if the Bt-containing plants lead to the development of insects resistant to Bt-modified plants and to other insecticides? Would the appearance of Bt-resistant insects spell the doom of a large portion of our crops of soybeans or maize? In a study of Bt cotton plants, scientists estimated that 1 in 350 pests carried resistance to the Bt gene,[54] but further research shows that genetic engineering can also be used to overcome or at least delay development of Bt resistance.[55] Scientists suggest that planting a certain percentage of normal plants alongside the Bt-modified plants should delay the appearance of such resistant mutants. If populations of such mutants became significant, farmers could fall back on conventional pest-control techniques. Meanwhile, we could have better crop yields with a reduction in pesticide use.

A related concern is the development of herbicide-resistant weeds, or "superweeds." When herbicide-resistant crops are planted in proximity to related wild plants, pollen may drift from food plant to weed, and the resistant genes might be passed to the weedy cousins of the GM plants. In the presence of herbicide, this might lead to the rapid selection of herbicide-resistant weeds. Although transfer of the herbicide-resistant gene

 **GM Concerns and Current Research**

1. GM crops will hurt innocent creatures.

Will crops engineered to contain insecticides harm nondestructive species important to biodiversity? While laboratory studies show that genetic modifications to plants can harm nontarget insects, such as monarch butterflies, field studies suggest the risk is small.

2. GM crops will lead to the emergence of superweeds.

Will genetic modifications that give crops the ability to kill insect pests or withstand certain herbicides migrate to weeds? Almost every crop has weedy relatives somewhere in the world. Despite anecdotal reports, studies have not found superweeds. Yet to avoid pollen spreading from modified genes to weeds, scientists warn that GM crops should not be grown near weedy relatives.

3. GM crops will have sudden failures.

Will target insect pests become tolerant to insecticides in GM plants and will weeds become immune to herbicides sprayed on herbicide-resistant GM crops? Could these threats become unstoppable? While there are no documented GM crop failures, scientists believe they are likely. Are current prevention measures adequate? Critics and proponents disagree.

to a related weed can occur, so far the effects have been minor, and the "superweeds" have rapidly lost the resistance gene once the herbicide was removed.

A final concern is that the herbicide-resistant food plants may become so successful that they are planted over a vast acreage in developing countries and sprayed with excessive amounts of herbicides. In the worst scenario, this could lead to a loss of many species of unmodified plants as well as the insect and animal communities that depend on them. Many scientists feel that the loss of biodiversity is one of the greatest threats to the planet today. Because of the complexity and interdependence of the biosphere, this is perhaps the greatest unknown and the greatest danger of unmonitored use of GM crops. **Table 17.5** summarizes current concerns and scientific research areas.

Regulation

The FDA regulates foods and food safety, and it oversees genetically modified foods as well as conventional foods. For foods derived from new varieties of plants, the FDA takes the position that whether modified by traditional breeding or genetic engineering, testing for safe human consumption is the legal responsibility of the producer or manufacturer of the foods. Crops such as Bt-modified soybeans do not require special testing, labeling, or FDA approval. Although the plant expresses the Bt protein, the beans do not contain it. Except for some foreign DNA sequences, the beans are identical to unmodified soybeans. However, when a new substance is added to a food, FDA review and approval are necessary. Thus, if a new substance is produced or introduced into a food by genetic means, it must be tested as though it were a food additive. (See the "Spotlight on Complementary and Alternative Nutrition.")

Some consumer groups are pushing for mandatory labeling of GM foods. They believe consumers have the right to know whether a food is bioengineered. Other groups desire labeling so they can adhere to cultural or religious beliefs that may ban certain animal foods. Because the FDA believes that the way a food is developed or produced is irrelevant information, current FDA policy does not require labeling of GM foods. In its 1992 policy statement "Foods Derived from New Plant Varieties," the FDA describes four situations in which changes in labels would be important to "reveal all material facts about the food":[56]

- If a bioengineered food is significantly different from its traditional counterpart, such that the common or usual name no longer adequately describes the food, the name must be changed to describe the difference.

- If an issue exists for the food or a constituent of the food regarding how the food is used or consequences of its use, a statement must be made on the labeling to describe the issue.

- If a bioengineered food has a significantly different nutritional property, its labeling must reflect the difference.

- If a new food includes an allergen that consumers would not expect to be present based on the name of the food, the presence of that allergen must be disclosed in the labeling.

In its 2001 draft guidance for industry regarding voluntary labeling, the FDA asked for comments on how the terms "biotech free," "GM free," or "no genetically engineered materials" could be used without being false or misleading, and how these claims could be substantiated.[57] Considering that most, if not all, food crops have been genetically modified in some way, it would be very difficult to have a completely "GM-free" food. Also, saying that a food or ingredient is not bioengineered may be misleading if there are no marketed bioengineered foods of that type. Before finalizing any further policy on labeling of foods that contain genetically engineered ingredients, additional work clearly needs to be done.

Similar to U.S regulations, Health Canada requires special labeling for genetically modified foods where there is a potential for allergic reactions, and a different name must be used for a GM food that is different in composition or nutritional value. Voluntary positive ("does contain") and voluntary negative ("does not contain") labeling is permitted provided the statements are factual and not misleading or deceptive.[58]

The generally conservative approach of the FDA is based on decades of experience with food plants, which contain thousands of different substances. The plants we eat every day produce a variety of compounds that, if eaten in sufficient quantity, are toxic to humans. Potatoes, for instance, produce variable amounts of solanine, a fairly toxic alkaloid. These naturally occurring toxins may be inadvertently increased by classical breeding, so monitoring levels of toxins in plants is neither new nor unusual. If there are unexpected consequences of gene modification, the FDA is in an excellent position to evaluate them and alter food-testing procedures where necessary. Many groups, from government agencies such as the FDA to professional organizations such as the ADA to consumer advocacy groups, are monitoring developments in biotechnology. Web sites for these organizations can be a source of policy statements and breaking news in this area. Regardless of our views on genetic manipulation of food plants, research and development will continue. It remains to be seen how consumers will accept new GM foods in the coming years.

Key Concepts: *Genetic engineering allows scientists to transform a plant one gene at a time, using well-established methods for manipulating DNA sequences. The goals of genetic modification of foods are higher yields, lower costs, increased amounts of critical nutrients, and a healthier mix of plant oils. Because of the complexity and interdependence of the biosphere, loss of genetic biodiversity is perhaps the greatest unknown and the greatest danger of unmonitored GM crops.*

American Dietetic Association

Agricultural and Food Biotechnology

It is the position of the American Dietetic Association that agricultural and food biotechnology techniques can enhance the quality, safety, nutritional value, and variety of food available for human consumption and increase the efficiency of food production, food processing, food distribution, and environmental and waste management. The ADA encourages the government, food manufacturers, food commodity groups, and qualified food and nutrition professionals to work together to inform consumers about this new technology and encourage availability of these products in the marketplace.

J Am Diet Assoc. 2006;106:285–293. Reprinted with permission.

LEARNING *Portfolio* c h a p t e r 1 7

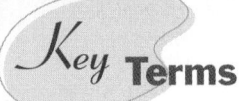

Key Terms

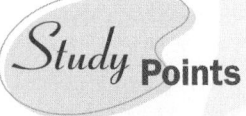

Study Points

➤ Foodborne illness is extremely common; it affects millions of Americans each year. Estimates of the frequency of foodborne illness are difficult because the vast majority of foodborne illnesses go unreported.

➤ The incidence of foodborne illness may be on the rise in the United States and Canada. Many factors are responsible, including the increased centralization of food preparation, food imports, an increasing population of especially susceptible individuals (such as the elderly and those with weakened immune systems), and failure of consumers and retail establishments to follow appropriate food safety measures.

➤ Microorganisms cause most foodborne diseases in the United States and Canada. Most of these illnesses are preventable.

➤ *Staphylococcus aureus* is one of the most common causes of foodborne illness. Onset of illness is rapid, typically occurring between 30 minutes and a few hours after consuming the contaminated food.

➤ Common symptoms of foodborne illness are diarrhea, nausea, abdominal cramps, and sometimes fever. The severity of the illness depends on the type of organism and the amount of contaminant eaten.

➤ Ensuring a safe food supply is a farm-to-table continuum involving producers, manufacturers, retailers, and consumers.

➤ Pesticides, animal drugs, natural toxins, and pollutants are the major forms of chemical food contamination.

➤ The government monitors imported and domestic foods for pesticide residues by testing food samples for both amounts and types of pesticides. Efforts are underway to reduce the allowable amounts of certain pesticides to avoid harm to infants and children.

➤ The FDA evaluates drugs used in food-producing animals for safety in both animals and humans. Overuse of animal antibiotics could contribute to the emergence of antibiotic-resistant microorganisms that could threaten human health.

➤ The government and the food industry use the Hazard Analysis Critical Control Point system to prevent food contamination.

➤ Consumers must take responsibility for food safety in their homes. Cleaning hands and surfaces, avoiding cross-contamination, cooking adequately, and refrigerating foods promptly are important steps that prevent foodborne illness.

➤ Food preservation techniques inhibit growth of microorganisms. Canning, drying, freezing, fermentation, and pasteurization are common.

➤ Although the FDA has approved food irradiation for numerous uses, it is rarely used, mostly because of consumer fears. Food irradiation does not make foods radioactive. It can kill insects and most microorganisms. Appropriate doses of radiation extend the shelf life of many foods.

➤ Genetically modified (GM) foods are most likely already on your table. Soybeans, corn, and potatoes are some of the GM foods being commercially produced. Concerns about GM foods include worries about decreasing biodiversity and the development of herbicide-resistant weeds.

Study Questions

1. **What are the two main ways that pathogenic bacteria can cause foodborne illness?**

2. **Why shouldn't your 97-year-old great-grandmother drink homemade eggnog made from raw eggs?**

3. **How can you limit your intake of pesticides, according to the Consumers Union?**

4. **List four naturally occurring toxins.**

5. **List the most common food allergens. What are some symptoms of a food allergy?**

6. **What does "HACCP" stand for and what is its purpose?**

7. **The home kitchen can be a breeding ground for pathogenic bacteria; what are some ways to keep food safe at home?**

8. **List the most common food preservation techniques.**

9. **What are three major concerns about genetically engineered crops?**

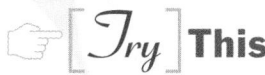

Bacterial Detective

What sources of bacteria do you encounter in your everyday activities? Here's an experiment to find out.

First, you'll need …
Cotton swabs
Six or more Petri dishes with agar
If you are unable to obtain a set of agar-filled Petri dishes from your school or local health department, you can make your own culture medium. Here's how:

- Add 2 teaspoons of unflavored gelatin (1 packet) and 2 teaspoons of sugar to $^2/_3$ cup of water.
- Bring the solution to a boil and stir for 1 minute until everything is dissolved. Pour $^1/_4$ inch of the solution into each Petri dish or other suitable container.

Then, using separate Petri dishes,

1. Pluck a hair and lay it in one Petri dish, labeled "Hair."
2. Sneeze or cough into another Petri dish, labeled "Cough."
3. Run a cotton swab around a nostril and carefully zigzag it across the agar in another Petri dish, labeled "Nose."
4. Run a cotton swab across a dampened kitchen sink sponge and carefully zigzag it across the agar in another Petri dish, labeled "Sponge."
5. Run a cotton swab around a clean kitchen countertop and carefully zigzag it across the agar in another Petri dish, labeled "Countertop."
6. Use the same procedure to collect additional samples from any other area in which bacteria may be present.
7. Store the Petri dishes in a warm environment, at a constant temperature around 80°F. Check your specimens periodically. Within a week, you should see something growing!

Organic Foods

Organic foods are increasing in popularity. Are organic foods widely available in your neighborhood? What types of organic produce can you find? Go to either a natural food store or the local grocery store and look at the array of organic produce. Compare the prices of organic produce and nonorganic produce. Do you think the cost differences outweigh possible benefits? Compare the look of the organic and nonorganic produce. Do you see any differences? What other organic products can you find?

References

1 Mead PS, Slutsker L, Dietz V, et al. Food-related illness and death in the United States. *Emerg Infect Dis.* 1999;5:607–625; and Centers for Disease Control and Prevention. Preliminary FoodNet data on the incidence of foodborne illnesses—selected sites, United States, 2000. *MMWR.* 2001;50:241–246.

2 US Environmental Protection Agency and US Departments of Health and Human Services and Agriculture. *Food Safety from Farm to Table: A National Food-Safety Initiative.* Washington, DC: Food and Drug Administration, 1997.

3 Institute of Food Technologists. *IFT Expert Report on Emerging Microbiological Food Safety Issues: Implications for Control in the 21st Century.* Chicago, IL: Institute of Food Technologists, 2002. http://www.ift.org/cms/?pid=1000379. Accessed 8/7/06.

4 Ibid.

5 Position of the American Dietetic Association: food and water safety. *J Am Diet Assoc.* 2003;103:1203–1218.

6 Advance notice of proposed rulemaking. *Salmonella enteritidis* in eggs. *Federal Register.* 1998;63:27502–27511.

7 US Food and Drug Administration. *Pesticide Program Residue Monitoring 2003.* June 2005. http://www.cfsan.fda.gov /~acrobat/pes03rep.pdf. Accessed 8/7/06.

8 Ibid.

9 Ibid.

10 Food Quality Protection Act: Title III of Public Law 104-170; 1996.

11 Consumers Union. *Do You Know What You're Eating? Pesticide Residues in Food.* Yonkers, NY: Consumers Union of United States, 1999.

12 Ibid.

13 Natural Marketing Institute. *Organic Consumer Trends Report 2005.* Harleysville, PA: Natural Marketing Institute, 2005.

14 Ibid.

15 US Department of Agriculture. Labeling and marketing information. National Organic Program fact sheet; March 2000.

16 US Department of Agriculture. The National Organic Program. Agricultural Marketing Service fact sheet; June 2000.

17 Worthington V. Nutritional quality of organic versus conventional fruits, vegetables, and grains. *J Altern Complement Med.* 2001;7(2):161–173.

18 Williams CM. Nutritional quality of organic foods: shades of grey or shades of green? *Proc Nutr Soc.* 2002;61:19–24.

19 Benbrook CM. Elevating antioxidant levels in food through organic farming and food processing. The Organic Center for Education and Promotion, January 2005. http://www .organic-center.org/reportfiles/Antioxidant_SSR.pdf. Accessed 8/7/06.

20 Greener greens? *Consumer Reports.* January 1998:12–18.

21 US Department of Agriculture. The National Organic Program. Op. cit.; and US Department of Agriculture. Questions and answers about the National Organic Program proposed rule. USDA press release; December 1997.

22 Institute of Medicine, Committee on Drug Use in Food Animals. *The Use of Drugs in Food Animals: Benefits and Risks.* Washington, DC: National Academy Press, 1999.

23 US Food and Drug Administration. FDA stops distribution of some eggs and catfish because of dioxin-contaminated animal feed. http://www.cfsan.fda.gov/~lrd/hhsdiox.html. Accessed 8/7/06.

24 Schecter A, Cramer P, Boggess K, et al. Intake of dioxins and related compounds from food in the U.S. population. *J Toxicol Environ Health A.* 2001;63:1–18.

25 US Food and Drug Administration. *Foodborne Pathogenic Microorganisms and Natural Toxins Handbook.* Washington, DC: Food and Drug Administration, 1992.

26 US Department of Health and Human Services and US Environmental Protection Agency. What you need to know about mercury in fish and shellfish. March 2004. http://www .cfsan.fda.gov/~dms/admehg3.html. Accessed 8/7/06.

27 Segal M. Stalking the wild mushroom. *FDA Consumer.* October 1994;20–24.

28 US Food and Drug Administration. 1992. Op. cit.

29 Swedish National Food Administration. Acrylamide is formed during the preparation of food and occurs in many foodstuffs. http://www.konsumentverket.se/html-sidor/livsmedelsverket /engakrylpressmeddelande.htm. Accessed 8/7/06; and World Health Organization. WHO to hold urgent expert consultation on acrylamide in food after findings of Swedish National Food Administration. http://www.who.int/mediacentre/releases /release32/en/print.html. Accessed 8/7/06.

30 US Food and Drug Administration. Acrylamide questions and answers. February 25, 2003. http://www.cfsan.fda.gov /~dms/acryfaq.html. Accessed 8/7/06.

31 Mucci LA, Sandin S, Magnussen C. Acrylamide intake and breast cancer risk in Swedish women: research letter. *JAMA.* 2005;293(11):1326–1327.

32 The Food Allergy & Anaphylaxis Network. Common food allergens. www.foodallergy.org/allergens.html. Accessed 8/7/06.

33 US Environmental Protection Agency and US Departments of Health and Human Services and Agriculture. Op. cit.

34 Ibid.

35 Pathogen reduction: Hazard Analysis and Critical Control Point (HACCP) systems; final rule. *Federal Register.* 1996; 61:38805–38989.

36 Hazard Analysis and Critical Control Point (HAACP); Procedures for the safe and sanitary processing and importing of juice; final rule. *Federal Register.* 2001;66:6137–6202.

37 US Department of Health and Human Services, Food and Drug Administration. *Food Code.* Washington, DC: Food and Drug Administration, 2005.

38 Partnership for Food Safety Education. Fight bac! Four simple steps to food safety. www.fightbac.org Accessed 8/7/06; and US Department of Agriculture and US Department of Health and Human Services. *Dietary Guidelines for Americans.* 6th ed. Washington, DC: US Government Printing Office, 2005.

39 US Department of Agriculture. USDA issues final rule on safe handling labels for meat and poultry products. USDA press release 0860.93; October 8, 1993.

40 Food labeling: warning and notice statement: labeling of juice products; final rule. *Federal Register*. 1998;63:37029–37056.

41 Food labeling, safe handling statements, labeling of shell eggs; refrigeration of shell eggs held for retail distribution, final rule. *Federal Register*. 2000;65:76091–76114.

42 Wood OB, Bruhn CM. Position of the American Dietetic Association: food irradiation, *J Am Diet Assoc*. 2000;100:246–253.

43 US Environmental Protection Agency and US Departments of Health and Human Services and Agriculture. Op. cit.

44 Wood OB, Bruhn CM. Op. cit.

45 Henkle J. Irradiation: a safe measure for safer food. *FDA Consumer*. May/June 1998.

46 Wood OB, Bruhn CM. Op. cit.

47 Pohlman A, Wood OB, Mason AC. Influence of audiovisuals and food samples on consumer acceptance of food irradiation. *Food Technol*. 1994;48(12):46–49.

48 Henkle J. Genetic engineering: fast forwarding to future foods. *FDA Consumer*. February 1998 update.

49 Formanek R Jr. Proposed rules issued for bioengineered foods. *FDA Consumer*. March/April 2001;35:9–11.

50 Pew Initiative on Food and Biotechnology. *Genetically Modified Crops in the United States*. Washington, DC: Pew Charitable Trust, 2004. http://pewagbiotech.org/resources/factsheets /display.php3?FactsheetID=2. Accessed 8/7/06.

51 Nash MJ. Grains of hope. *Time*. July 31, 2000;39–46; and Greger JL. Response: genetically engineered "golden" rice unlikely to overcome vitamin A deficiency. *J Am Diet Assoc*. 2001;101:289–290.

52 Shewry PR, Tatham AS, Halford NG. Genetic modification and plant food allergies. *J Chromatogr B Biomed Sci Appl*. 2001; 756:327–335; and Taylor SL, Hefle SL. Will genetically modified foods be allergenic? *J Allergy Clin Immunol*. 2001; 107:765–771.

53 Thompson L. Are bioengineered foods safe? *FDA Consumer*. January/February 2000.

54 Gould F, Anderson A, Jones A, et al. Initial frequency of alleles for resistance to *Bacillus thuringiensis* toxins in field populations of *Heliothis virescens*. *Proc Natl Acad Sci*. 1997; 94:3519–3523.

55 Kota M, Daniell H, Varma S, et al. Overexpression of the *Bacillus thuringiensis* (Bt) Cry2Aa2 protein in chloroplasts confers resistance to plants against susceptible and Bt-resistant insects. *Proc Natl Acad Sci*. 1999;96:1840–1845.

56 Statement of policy: foods derived from new plant varieties. *Federal Register*. 1992;57:22984.

57 Draft guidance for industry: voluntary labeling indicating whether foods have or have not been developed using bioengineering: availability. *Federal Register*. 2001;66:4839–4842.

58 Health Canada. Novel foods (GMF). http://www.hc-sc.gc.ca /english/protection/novel_foods.html. Accessed 8/7/06.

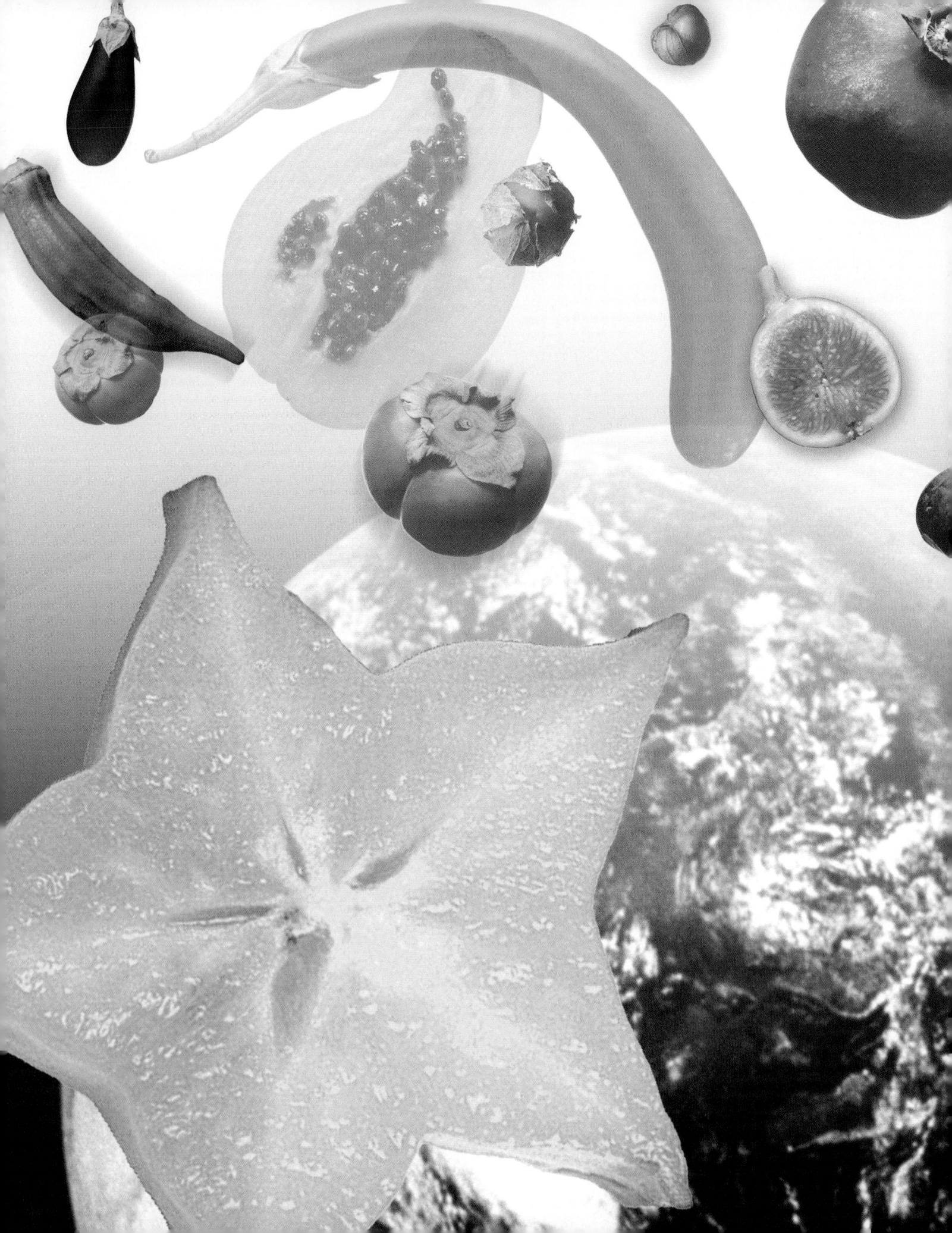

Chapter 18

World View of Nutrition

Think About It

1   Have you ever experienced hunger without being able to satisfy it within a day?

2   Have you seen evidence of hunger or malnutrition in your community?

3   What can you do to help eliminate hunger in North America?

4   How do you feel about the United States sending food to impoverished nations?

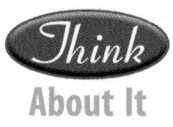

Fyi for your Information

This chapter's FYI boxes include practical information on the following topics:

• Hungry and Homeless

• AIDS and Malnutrition

• Tough Choices

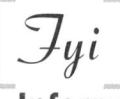

The Web site for this book offers many useful tools and is a great source for additional nutrition information for both students and instructors. For information on the world view of nutrition, visit the site at nutrition.jbpub.com. You'll find exercises that explore the following topics:

• The ADA and World Hunger

• U.S. Food Insecurity

• UNICEF

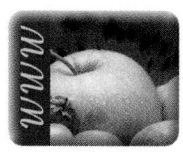

*E*ach day on your way to class, you pass a soup kitchen. You look at the long line of men and women waiting to get their meals and wonder what brought them to this point. You wonder how many similar soup lines exist in your community and how many people need food assistance but can't get it. If **hunger** exists in our rich country, what about people living in poor countries?

More than 800 million people in developing countries do not have enough to eat.[1] The challenge of reaching the World Food Summit goal of reducing this number to 400 million by 2015 remains daunting. Hunger and **malnutrition** are the underlying cause of more than half of all child deaths, killing nearly 6 million children each year.[2] Relatively few die of starvation; most are killed by diseases that often are treatable, including diarrhea, pneumonia, malaria, and measles.

In this chapter, we look at hunger and malnutrition. By *hunger* we don't mean that mildly empty feeling one gets before mealtime. We mean the inability, day after day, to satisfy basic nutrition needs, the gnawing emptiness that creates a constant focus on eating and how to obtain food. In contrast to the hunger dieters feel from cutting calories, this deprivation is involuntary and unwanted.

Technically speaking, *malnutrition* can be any kind of unhealthy nutritional status, including the result of imbalance and excess—obesity or toxicity from oversupplementation, for example. And although we touch on obesity as an emerging issue, even in developing countries, by and large in this chapter *malnutrition* means undernutrition resulting from hunger.

Along the spectrum of malnutrition and hunger is the less extreme condition of **food insecurity**, the ongoing worry about having enough to eat. At the opposite end of the spectrum is **food security**, access to nutritionally adequate and safe food. Most people in the industrialized world are food-secure. Overabundance and obesity are the primary problems in these populations, but malnutrition is a serious problem among certain groups, such as the homeless and urban poor.

Malnutrition in the United States

The Face of American Malnutrition

In the food-rich United States, food insecurity remains a problem.[3] (See **Figure 18.1.**) It is characterized by anxiety about having enough to eat and about running out of food and having no money to purchase more. Some people actually go hungry in the United States: During 2004, 38.2 million people, including 13.9 million children, lived in a household in which at least one person experienced hunger.[4]

Households that are struggling to meet basic food needs tend to follow a typical pattern as their plight worsens. First, adults worry about having enough food. Then, they stretch resources and juggle other necessities, with more of the budget going for fixed expenses than for food. The quality and variety of the diet declines. Next, the adults eat less and less often. And finally, as food becomes more limited, the children also eat less.

hunger The uneasy or painful sensation caused by a lack of food; the recurrent and involuntary lack of access to food that may produce malnutrition over time.

malnutrition Failure to achieve nutrient requirements, which can impair physical and/or mental health. It may result from consuming too little food or a shortage or imbalance of key nutrients.

food insecurity (1) Limited or uncertain availability of nutritionally adequate and safe foods or (2) limited or uncertain ability to acquire acceptable foods in socially acceptable ways.

food security Access to enough food for an active, healthy life, including (1) the ready availability of nutritionally adequate and safe foods and (2) an assured ability to acquire acceptable foods in socially acceptable ways.

Think About It

1

PREVALENCE OF FOOD INSECURITY

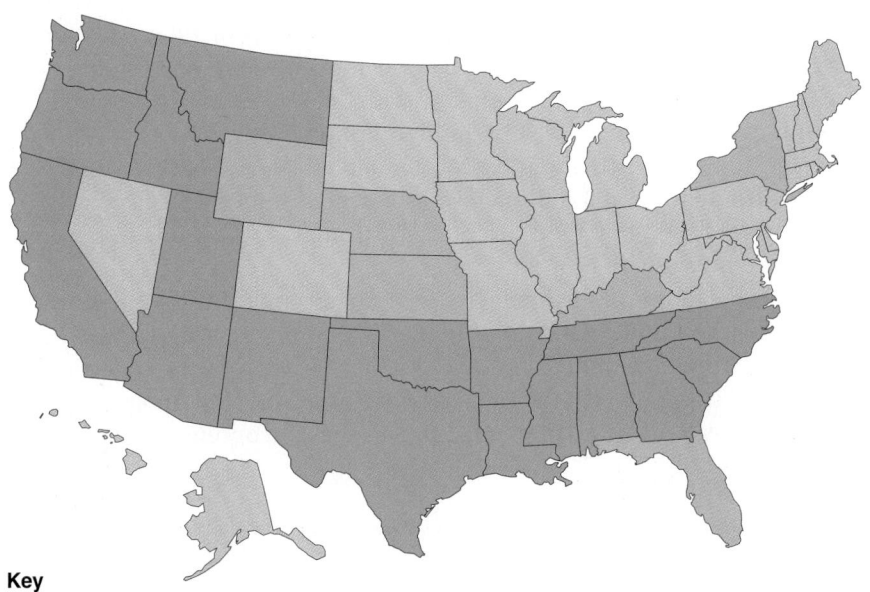

Key

▢ Below national average
▢ Near national average
▢ Above national average

Figure 18.1 **Prevalence of food insecurity.** Food insecurity is as common among the working poor as the unemployed. Food insecurity is more common in southern and western states.
Source: Nord M, Andrews M, Carlsen S. *Household Food Security in the United States, 2004.* Washington, DC: US Department of Agriculture, October 2005. Economic Research Report No. 11. http://www.ers.usda.gov/Publications/err11/. Accessed 8/5/06.

Surprisingly, there is more obesity among low-income, food-insecure groups than among those with higher incomes. But the quality of those low-income diets is typically poor, and worsening food insecurity is accompanied by progressively more disordered eating patterns. Patterns such as binge eating can become habitual and contribute to obesity.[5]

Those who live in a state of food insecurity consume significantly fewer healthful foods and micronutrients. Although such suboptimal diets usually do not lead to overt deficiency diseases, more subtle effects are serious and costly, showing up years later as chronic illness or more immediately as reduced immune function. More illness, more medicines, more doctor visits and hospital stays, more missed days and poorer performance at school and work, poor pregnancy outcome, delayed growth and development—suboptimal nutrition contributes to them all.

Prevalence and Distribution

How much hunger and food insecurity exist in the United States? Until recently, it was difficult to measure. Estimates were based on the percentage of the population living in poverty (see **Table 18.1**), with the assumption that they were at risk of undernutrition. Such estimates are somewhat flawed because being *at risk* does not necessarily mean that people *are* poorly nourished. Many people with limited financial resources manage to eat well. On the other hand, under certain circumstances, such as loss of a job, people who live well above the poverty line may be food-insecure.

Quick Bites

Food Recovery and Gleaning

*E*ach year more than 96 billion pounds of food produced in this country go to waste. Programs throughout the country are rescuing much of this wholesome food and distributing it to people in need. "Gleaning" is harvesting excess food from farms, orchards, and packing houses. Perishable items are also salvaged from wholesale and retail markets; fresh foods that are wholesome but will spoil before they can be sold are given to local food pantries and meal providers. Canned goods and other staples are collected from groceries, distributors, food processors, and individual homes. Even surplus food from restaurants, caterers, and other food services is collected by some charities for local food programs.

The U.S. Department of Agriculture (USDA) tracks hunger with an annual **Food Security Supplement Survey**, which asks about food availability and hunger in the household. (See **Table 18.2**.) In 2004, 38.2 million people (13.2 percent of the U.S. population) lived in households experiencing food insecurity, compared with 36.3 million in 2003 and 31 million in 1999. In 2004, 13.5 million households (11.9 percent of all households) worried about having enough to eat, and of these food-insecure households, 4.5 million also experienced hunger.[6]

The survey found that food insecurity is strongly associated with poverty and is interlinked with economic and social factors. Food insecurity and hunger were highest in the inner city, in Hispanic and African American households, and in households with young children, as well as those headed by women and those headed by a person with limited education. (See **Figure 18.2**.) Clearly, then, to end food insecurity and hunger, nutrition programs must be accompanied by social and economic efforts.

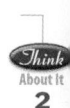

Think About It
2

The Working Poor

Employment does not guarantee that families always have enough to eat. The third National Health and Nutrition Examination Survey (NHANES III) found that food insecurity is as common among the working poor as the unemployed. Since the 1996 **Personal Responsibility and Work Opportunity Reconciliation Act**, commonly called welfare reform, thousands have left the welfare rolls for jobs. Often the pay is too little to lift households above poverty level, and work-related expenses such as transportation or child care further deplete family budgets.[7] Low-paid workers may be unaware that they still qualify for food-assistance programs. On the other hand, their work hours may preclude program participation.

Food Security Supplement Survey A federally funded survey that measures the prevalence and severity of food insecurity and hunger.

Personal Responsibility and Work Opportunity Reconciliation Act A 1996 federal welfare reform plan that dramatically changed the nation's welfare system into one that requires work in exchange for time-limited assistance. Also called the Welfare Reform Act.

Table 18.1 Poverty Guidelines: Income Levels Defined as Poverty for a Given Household Size

Persons in Family or Household	Income ($)		
	48 Contiguous States and D.C.	Alaska	Hawaii
1	9,800	12,250	11,270
2	13,200	16,500	15,180
3	16,600	20,750	19,090
4	20,000	25,000	23,000
5	23,400	29,250	26,910
6	26,800	33,500	30,820
7	30,200	37,750	34,730
8	33,600	42,000	38,640
For each additional person, add	3,400	4,250	3,910

Note: Despite the limits to the use of household income as a proxy for estimating food insecurity, poverty remains an intuitively reasonable indicator. Keep in mind that in addition to food, income must cover housing, clothing, transportation, medical care, and other essentials.

Source: *Federal Register.* 2006;71(15):3848–3849. http://aspe.hhs.gov/poverty/06poverty .shtml.

Table 18.2 Sample Questions from the Food Security Questionnaire

Light Food Insecurity

"We worried whether our food would run out before we got money to buy more."
   Was that often, sometimes, or never true for you in the last 12 months?

"The food that we bought just didn't last and we didn't have money to get more."
   Was that often, sometimes, or never true for you in the last 12 months?

Moderate Food Insecurity

In the last 12 months did you or other adults in the household ever cut the size of your meals or skip meals because there wasn't enough money for food?

In the last 12 months, were you ever hungry but didn't eat because you couldn't afford enough food?

Severe Food Insecurity

In the last 12 months did you or other adults in the household ever not eat for a whole day because there wasn't enough money for food?

(For households with children) In the last 12 months did any of the children ever not eat for a whole day because there wasn't enough money for food?

Source: Nord M, Andrews M, Carlsen S. *Household Food Security in the United States, 2004.* Washington, DC: US Department of Agriculture, October 2005. Economic Research Report No. 11. http://www.ers.usda.gov/Publications/err11/. Accessed 8/5/06.

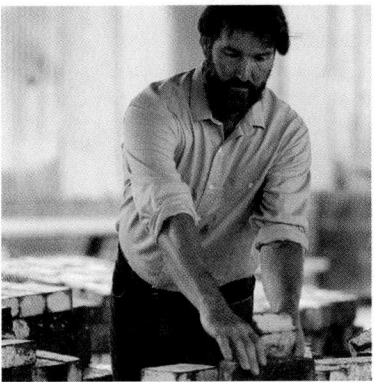
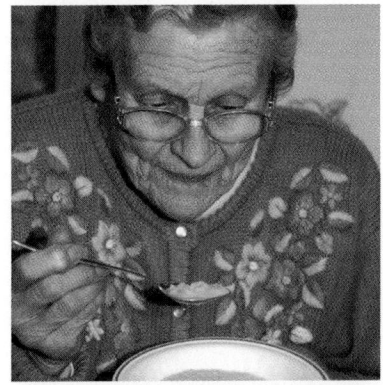
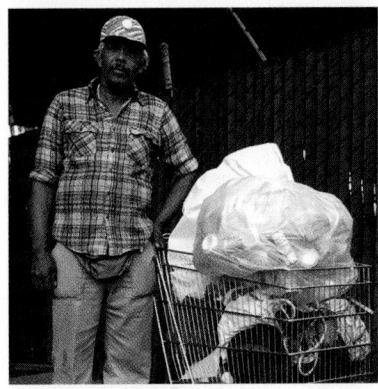
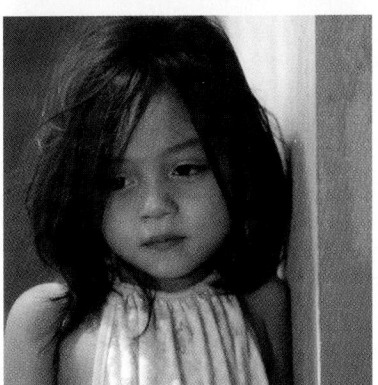

The Isolated

People in remote rural areas may live far from food resources and lack access to transportation. Other people become isolated despite living in populated cities. Even though they live in a crowded neighborhood or apartment building, they are alone and are physically or mentally unable to obtain adequate food.

Elders

The infirmities of age, along with feelings of vulnerability, keep some elderly people homebound and lonely, conditions hardly conducive to a healthy appetite. Physical ailments may make cooking and eating difficult, while actually increasing nutrient needs. Elders often have small incomes, with little prospect for improvement. Like others with limited resources, they cut food purchases to pay for other necessities. Although food assistance may be available, pride or shame may keep an older person from participating in such programs.[8]

The Homeless or Inadequately Housed

The homeless rely on soup kitchens and other public programs for much of their food. Some resort to handouts and even forage through garbage. Many are mentally ill or substance abusers. The addict often has little interest in eating and may sell available food to buy more drugs. Many other people live in welfare hotels, single-room-occupancy facilities, or rooming houses without storage or cooking facilities. Budget-stretching strategies such as buying food in bulk and carefully using leftovers are out of the question for these people; as the monthly budget dwindles, they often rely on fast food meals and then soup kitchens.

Figure 18.2 **Americans at risk.** Americans most at risk for hunger include working poor, elders, homeless people, and children.

Food Research and Action Center (FRAC)
Founded in 1970 as a public interest law firm, this nonprofit child advocacy group works to improve public policies to eradicate hunger and undernutrition in the United States.

Children

Perhaps no group is more vulnerable to hunger than the young. Growth and development are delayed in poorly nourished children. They get sick more often. It is harder for them to concentrate in school. Children are captives of their family circumstances; poverty and lack of nutritious food in the household are beyond a child's control. In 2004, one or more children were hungry at times during the year in 274,000 households.[9] The prevalence of food insecurity is substantially higher among families with single parents. Children living with a single mother are more likely to be affected by hunger, as are children living in low-income households.

Attacking Hunger in America

Government efforts to fight hunger began during the Great Depression of the 1930s. From that modest beginning, federal efforts have grown to include at least 14 programs that address hunger. (See **Table 18.3**.) The School Lunch Program was created in 1946, after many young men had failed the physical requirements for military service in World War II because of poor nutrition. The Food Stamp Program, begun on a small scale years earlier, was greatly expanded in the early 1970s following an exposé of hunger in Appalachia and the Mississippi Delta and the television documentary "Hunger in America." The federal government initiated the Special Supplemental Nutrition Program for Women, Infants, and Children (WIC) in the 1970s as a response to concerns about maternal and child health. Other government programs have since been added to meet the special needs of the young, the elderly, the disadvantaged, and the disabled.

Table 18.3 **U.S. Programs That Address Food Insecurity and Hunger**

Food Stamp Program

Nutrition Assistance Program for Puerto Rico

National School Lunch Program

School Breakfast Program

Child and Adult Care Food Program

Summer Food Service Program

Special Milk Program

Special Supplemental Nutrition Program for Women, Infants, and Children (WIC)

Commodity Supplemental Food Program

Food Distribution Program on Indian Reservations

Older Americans Act Nutrition Program

Disaster Feeding Program

The Emergency Food Assistance Program (TEFAP)

Food Distribution Program for Charitable Institutions and Summer Camps

Source: Position of American Dietetic Association: domestic food and nutrition security. *J Am Diet Assoc.* 2002;102:1840–1847.

The **Food Research and Action Center (FRAC)** is a national nonprofit advocacy group that fights hunger and undernutrition at the national, state, and local levels. Nonprofit community agencies, charities, religious organizations, and similar groups create a large network of food pantries, soup kitchens, and services for home-delivered meals. Most of the federal government's programs for direct distribution of food or meals operate at the local level through these networks. Both laypeople and professionals, such as dietitians, work in these programs, either as volunteers or as staff, to fight hunger and malnutrition.

Food assistance programs have greatly reduced the prevalence of hunger, but not of food insecurity, which requires social and economic change. The following are among the federal government's most far-reaching programs against hunger.

Fyi Hungry and Homeless

FOR YOUR INFORMATION

A shabbily dressed man slowly pushes a shopping cart along the sidewalk. It is laden with bottles and cans that he can redeem for cash. In front of a supermarket, a woman and child clutch a sign scrawled with the words "Hungry. Please help." On a street corner, a man confronts every passing car with a sign that says "Will work for food." When confronted by a homeless person, do you feel uncomfortable? Do you turn away? Or do you try to help?

Who are the homeless? Single men and families with children are the largest homeless groups. Roughly equal in size, they make up about 81 percent of the homeless population. Single women (14 percent) and unaccompanied minors (5 percent) account for the remainder. About 23 percent of the homeless are mentally ill, 30 percent are substance abusers, 17 percent are unemployed, and 10 percent are veterans.[1]

Hunger in the homeless is caused by a number of interrelated factors, including high housing costs, poverty or lack of income, substance abuse, mental health problems, and food stamp cuts. Family members—children and their parents—most frequently request emergency food assistance. Thirty-eight percent of the adults requesting food assistance are employed.[2]

Complex challenges face the homeless, who may sleep in the streets or in emergency shelters. The homeless get food from many sources—shelters, drop-in centers, fast food restaurants, and garbage bins. Soup kitchens are a primary source of meals, yet navigating this system to obtain adequate food can be a formidable and time-consuming task. Also, while homeless people often are eligible for food stamps, they are extremely limited in their ability to store and prepare food, and few restaurants are authorized to accept food stamps.

A major public health concern for homeless people is not only whether they are getting enough to eat but also the nutritional quality of their diet. This concern is complicated by the special needs of infants, children, and women, especially pregnant women. Diets of the homeless often are nutritionally inadequate. Studies of homeless women and children indicate that they consume less than half of the RDA for iron, zinc, magnesium, and folate daily.[3] Homeless adult males have diets low in calcium, zinc, vitamin B_6, and calories. Homeless adults consume less than 50 percent of the RDA for calcium. Poor diets put the homeless at an increased risk for illness and chronic conditions. Pregnant women, children, and people with compromised health status are particularly vulnerable.

Homeless families and individuals rely on emergency food assistance facilities not only during emergencies but also for extended periods. Unfortunately, these facilities are strained beyond their capacities—over 52 percent cannot provide an adequate quantity of food.[4] Some shelters have resorted to rationing to extend their food resources to a greater number of people. Because of a lack of resources, over half may be forced to turn people away. Addressing hunger is a top priority. Once access to food is secure, obtaining a nutritionally adequate diet and dealing with health issues become reasonable goals.

1 The United States Conference of Mayors. Hunger homelessness survey summary. January 2005. http://www .usmayors.org/uscm/us_mayor_newspaper/documents /01_10_05/hunger_survey.asp. Accessed 8/6/06.

2 Ibid.

3 Silliman K, Yamanoha M, Morrissey A. Evidence of nutritional risk in a population of homeless adults in rural Northern California. *J Am Diet Assoc.* 1998;98:908–910.

4 The United States Conference of Mayors. Op. cit.

Electronic Benefits Transfer (EBT) Electronic delivery of government benefits by a single plastic card that allows access to food benefits at point-of-sale locations.

Child and Adult Care Food Program A federally funded program that reimburses approved family child-care providers for USDA-approved foods served to preschool children; also provides funds for meals and snacks served at after-school programs for school-aged children and to adult day care centers serving chronically impaired adults or people over age 60.

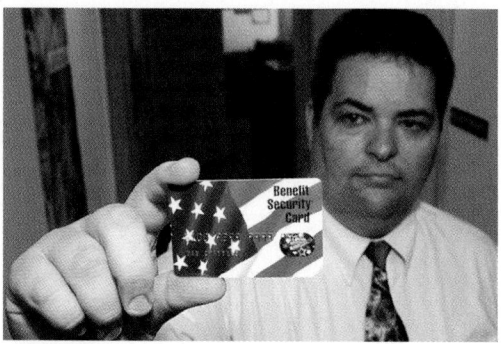

Figure 18.3 **Electronic Benefits Transfer card.**
Electronic Benefits Transfer (EBT) is an electronic system that allows recipients to authorize transfer of their government benefits from a federal account to a retailer account to pay for products received.

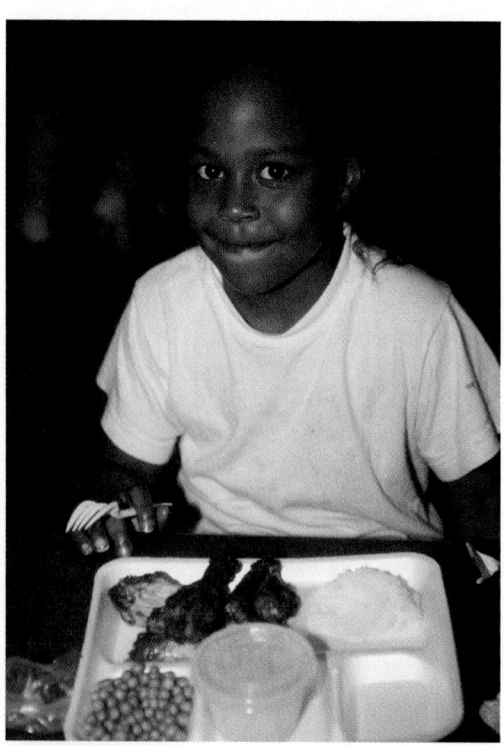

Figure 18.4 **National School Lunch Program.**

The Food Stamp Program

The Food Stamp Program is our main food security program. Recipients can use food stamp benefits to purchase food, but not nonfood items such as paper goods, pet food, and alcohol. The benefit amount varies according to household size and income level.

Actually, the term *food stamp* is becoming a misnomer. Almost half of the people who receive benefits use **Electronic Benefits Transfer (EBT)** cards. (See **Figure 18.3**.) The card resembles and functions like a debit card. Each month the household's benefit amount is credited to the card, which is then used at participating groceries.

Special Supplemental Nutrition Program for Women, Infants, and Children

The WIC program provides food to pregnant and breastfeeding women, infants, and preschoolers. More than 8 million women and children receive WIC benefits each month.[10] To be eligible, the participant must be at nutritional risk, and household income must be less than 185 percent of the poverty level. For 2006–2007, the gross annual income for a family of four could not exceed $37,000.[11]

Nutrition assessment and nutrition education are important components of the WIC program. Participants receive coupons, or "checks," for specific categories of healthful foods, and they "cash" them at participating groceries. Unlike food stamps, the amount of the WIC benefit varies with nutritional need, not income.

National School Lunch Program

The National School Lunch Program ensures that children in primary and secondary schools receive at least one healthy meal every school day (supplemented in many areas by the School Breakfast Program). For a family of four for the year 2006–2007, the child's meals were free if the household income was less than $26,000; the meals were reduced in price if household income was less than $37,000.[12] The lunch must provide one-third or more of dietary requirements for key nutrients. The program operates in nearly 100,000 public and nonprofit private schools and residential child-care institutions. It provides nutritionally balanced, low-cost or free lunches to more than 28 million children each school day.[13] (See **Figure 18.4**.)

Child and Adult Care Food Program

The **Child and Adult Care Food Program** provides funds for children's meals and snacks at nonprofit licensed child-care centers, day care homes, after-school programs, and similar settings. Nutritious meals for elderly or disabled people are also funded at nonprofit facilities such as adult day care centers and recreation centers.

Key Concepts: *Overt malnutrition in the United States is uncommon. Food insecurity and hunger are interlinked with poverty. Groups at risk include the working poor, the isolated, the homeless, children, and elders. A large network of individual volunteers, nonprofit agencies, and charities, together with major government programs such as Food Stamps, WIC, and School Lunch, have done much to reduce hunger. However, food insecurity, which continues among an unacceptably large number of people, must be overcome by social and economic improvements.*

Malnutrition in the Developing World

"Proper nutrition and health are fundamental human rights," according to the **World Health Organization (WHO)**. "Nutrition is a cornerstone that affects and defines the health of all people, rich and poor. It paves the way for us to grow, develop, work, play, resist infection and aspire to realization of our fullest potential as individuals and societies. Conversely, malnutrition makes us all more vulnerable to disease and premature death."[14]

Hunger is a global problem. (See **Figure 18.5**.) "It is debilitating. It blights the lives of all who are affected and undermines national economies and development processes where it is found on a large scale," says the **Food and Agriculture Organization (FAO)** of the United Nations.[15] Although food shortages severe enough to cause endemic starvation or famine have lessened significantly, natural disasters, epidemics, economic or political upheaval, or war can quickly precipitate famine.

The FAO reports three irrefutable facts and three inescapable conclusions:

1. Efforts to reduce chronic hunger in the developing world have fallen far short of the pace required to cut the number of hungry people by half no later than the year 2015. We must do better.

2. Despite slow and faltering progress on a global scale, numerous countries in all regions of the developing world have proven that

World Health Organization (WHO) A global organization that directs and coordinates international health work. Its goal is the attainment by all peoples of the highest possible level of health, defined as a state of complete physical, mental, and social well-being and not merely the absence of disease or infirmity.

Food and Agriculture Organization (FAO) The largest autonomous UN agency; the FAO works to alleviate poverty and hunger by promoting agricultural development, improved nutrition, and the pursuit of food security.

Figure 18.5 **Global hunger.** Although the proportion of the world's population that is chronically undernourished has been decreasing over the last few decades, undernutrition is still widespread, particularly in certain regions. Furthermore, projections to the year 2010 suggest that there will be little change in the absolute number of chronically undernourished people.
Source: Food and Agriculture Organization of the United Nations, Luxembourg Income Study; First World Hunger, USDA; Second Harvest. http://www.fao.org/es/ess/faostat/foodsecurity/FSMap/map14_en.htm.

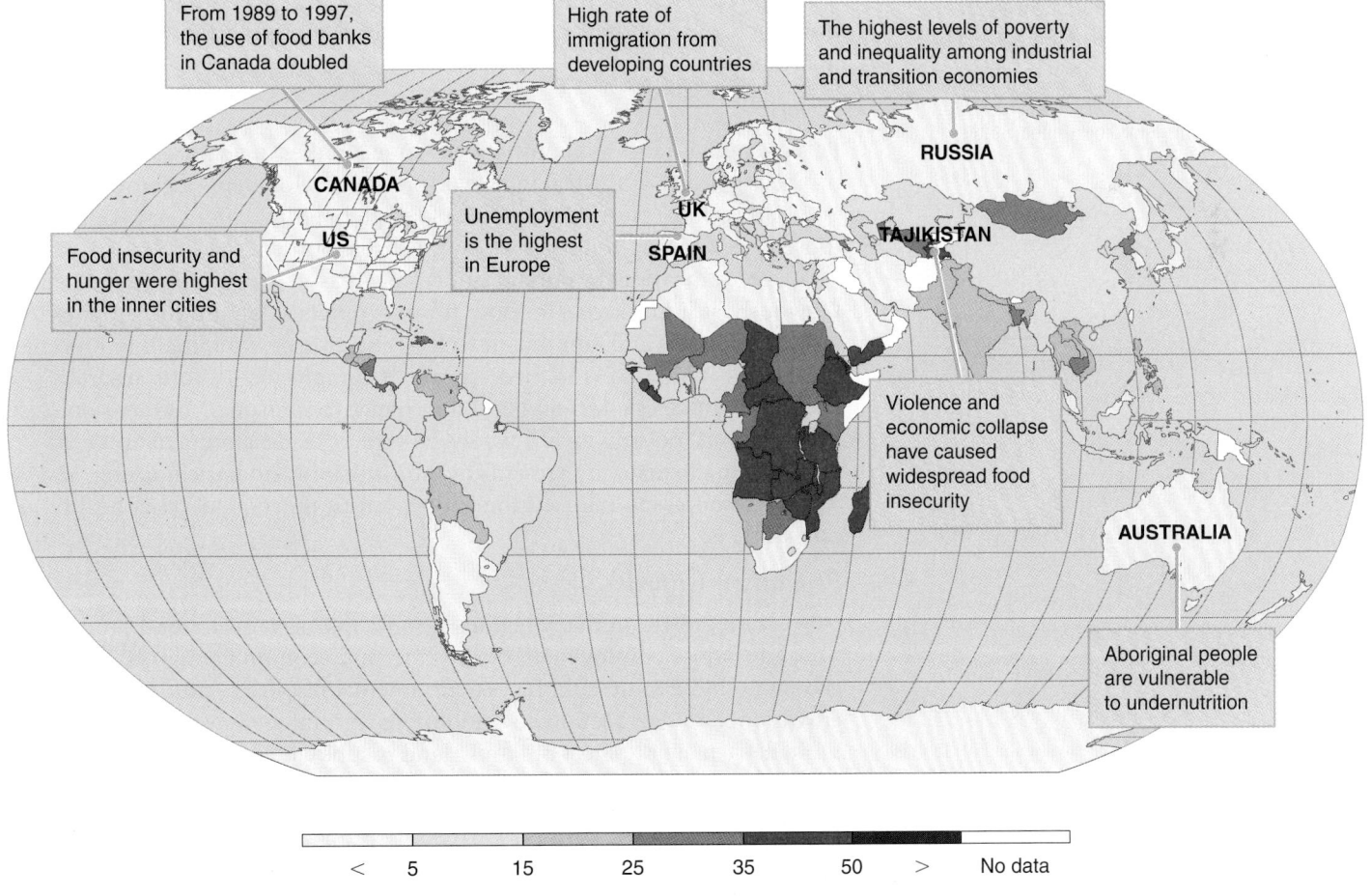

From 1989 to 1997, the use of food banks in Canada doubled

High rate of immigration from developing countries

The highest levels of poverty and inequality among industrial and transition economies

Unemployment is the highest in Europe

Food insecurity and hunger were highest in the inner cities

Violence and economic collapse have caused widespread food insecurity

Aboriginal people are vulnerable to undernutrition

CANADA · US · UK · SPAIN · RUSSIA · TAJIKISTAN · AUSTRALIA

| < | 5 | 15 | 25 | 35 | 50 | > | No data |

% Undernourished population

Quick Bites

Where Were You Born?

Your survival was greatly influenced by the location of your birth. Angola has the highest infant mortality rate (195 deaths per 1,000 live births), according to estimates for 2000. Other countries with high infant mortality rates include Sierra Leone (148 per 1,000), Afghanistan (149 per 1,000), and Liberia (134 per 1,000). At the other end of the spectrum is Finland (4 per 1,000). Canada (5 per 1,000) has a lower infant mortality rate than the United States (7 per 1,000).

success is possible. More than 30 countries, with a total population of over 2.2 billion people, have reduced the prevalence of undernourishment by 25 percent and have made significant progress toward reducing the number of hungry people by half by the year 2015. We can do better.

3. The costs of not taking immediate and strenuous action to reduce hunger at comparable rates worldwide are staggering. Every year that hunger continues at present levels costs more than 5 million children their lives and costs developing countries billions of dollars in lost productivity and earnings. The costs of interventions that could sharply reduce hunger are trivial in comparison. We cannot afford to fail.[16]

Why Hunger?

Why, in a world of plenty, does hunger still exist? The causes are simple, but the solutions are tremendously complex; they require economic, political, and social change, as well as improvements in nutrition, food production, and environmental safeguards. As you study the critical nutrient deficiencies in the developing world, you will see that poverty, infection, poor sanitation, and social upheaval interact with nutrient shortages to bring about the deficiencies.

Social and Economic Factors

Poverty, overpopulation, and migration to overcrowded cities are closely interrelated causes of hunger. (See **Figure 18.6.**) Each situation worsens the effects of the others as they steadily drive a population toward malnutrition.

Poverty

Poverty, hunger, and malnutrition stalk one another in a vicious circle, compromising health and wreaking havoc on the development of entire countries and regions. Nearly 30 percent of the global population—especially those in developing countries—bear this triple burden.[17]

Poverty is the most important underlying reason for chronic hunger. Obviously, it limits access to food. It limits purchase of farming supplies to grow food, boats and equipment to fish, and storage equipment to prevent spoilage. It limits access to medical care. It compromises efforts at sanitation. It discourages education and the chance for personal advancement.

For nations, poverty means paralyzed economic development and too few jobs; inadequate investments in infrastructure and basic housing; and too few resources to train doctors, nutritionists, nurses, and other health care workers.

Population Growth

Population growth in many regions is outstripping gains in food production, education, employment, health care, and economic progress. The burgeoning numbers stress limited environmental resources, contributing to environmental degradation and pollution. In rural areas where farmland is limited, each small parcel of family land is subdivided with each generation, until there is too little land to support each family.

You might think that poverty would pressure parents to limit family size, but ironically, poverty and sickness do just the reverse. Where child mortality rates are high, having many babies is a guarantee some children will survive. In countries that have no economic safeguards for disability,

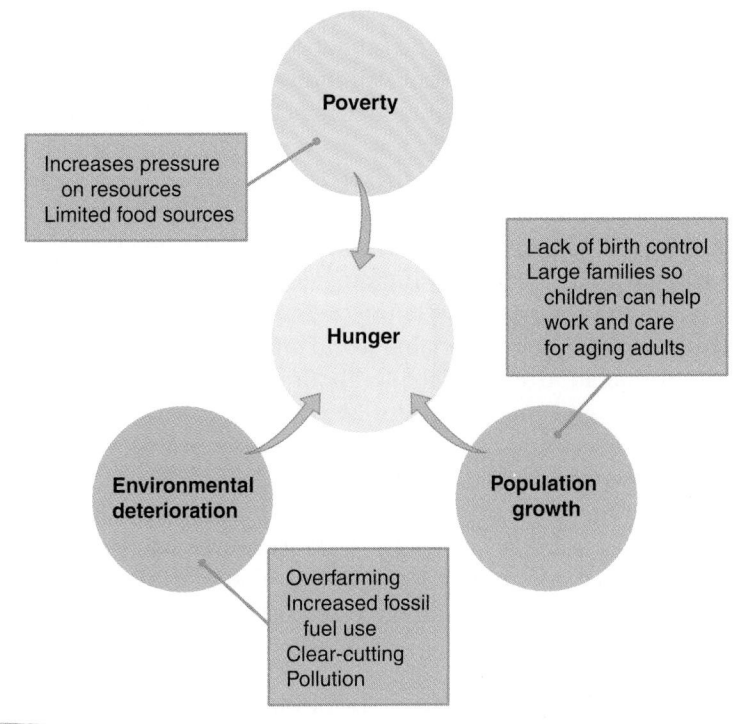

Figure 18.6 **Major problems causing hunger.** Poverty, population growth, and environmental degradation interact to make hunger worse.

unemployment, or old age, parents consider their children a source of security and support in times of need. Many other factors contribute to large families, from ignorance of birth control methods to the attitude that big families reflect the father's masculinity. Some political groups also encourage high birth rates and fast population growth as a way to achieve political or military dominance.

To slow population growth, socioeconomic and cultural changes that make smaller family size acceptable, even desirable, must accompany access to birth control.

Urbanization

Urbanization is a worldwide trend. As rural lands become too crowded or exhausted farmland no longer supports good crops, rural people migrate to the city in hopes of jobs and a better life. Unfortunately, in fast-growing cities, social disorder, sanitary conditions, and living standards may be much worse. Hunting, fishing, foraging, and gardening—sources of accessible food in the rural setting—are seldom an option in the city. Breastfeeding becomes impractical for many mothers who could nurse their babies while doing farm work, but cannot do so with jobs in the city.

Infection and Disease

Infection interacts with malnutrition, each making its victim more vulnerable to the other and each making the other worse, in a downward spiral. Nutrient deficiencies lower resistance to infections.[18] In turn, the fever of infection speeds depletion of calories and nutrients. Other symptoms (e.g., loss of appetite, weakness, nausea, and mouth lesions) limit ability to eat. Infectious diarrhea is especially dangerous, quickly wasting what few nutrients are consumed; infants and young children can die quickly from loss of

Quick Bites

Food Supply Versus Food Safety

Sometimes obtaining food is more important than safety. Food from street vendors is important in the diets of many urban populations, particularly the socially disadvantaged. Health authorities responsible for food safety should balance their risk management with issues of food availability and hunger. Rigorous application of codes and regulations suited to larger and permanent food-service establishments may cause the disappearance of the street vendors, with consequent aggravation of hunger and malnutrition. WHO encourages the development of regulations that empower vendors to take greater responsibility for the preparation of safe food.

Quick Bites

Rehydration Therapy for Diarrhea

Simple and inexpensive packets of carbohydrate and salts diluted with sterile water replace lost fluids and electrolytes. These packets are saving thousands of people each year.

American Dietetic Association

Nutrition Intervention in the Care of Persons with Human Immunodeficiency Virus Infection

It is the position of the American Dietetic Association and Dietitians of Canada that efforts to optimize nutritional status, including medical nutrition therapy, assurance of food and nutrition security, and nutrition education, are essential components of the total health care available to people with human immunodeficiency virus infection throughout the continuum of care.

J Am Diet Assoc. 2004;104:1425–1441.
Reprinted with permission.

electrolytes. Programs that prevent or control infection (e.g., immunizations, improvements in hygiene and sanitation, safe water supplies, and access to medicine and medical care) all indirectly improve nutrition status.

Infection with the human immunodeficiency virus (HIV) provides a dramatic demonstration of the interaction between malnutrition and infection. Transmission of the virus from mother to fetus is greater when the mother is deficient in vitamin A.[19] The infection progresses fastest in people who are poorly nourished.[20] And severe loss of weight and muscle are hallmarks of the advanced disease, acquired immune deficiency syndrome (AIDS). An estimated 38.6 million people were infected with HIV in 2005—more than 90 percent of them in the developing world and more than 24.5 million of them in sub-Saharan Africa.[21] Globally, about one-third of adults living with HIV are young people aged 15 to 24 years.

In the United States and Canada, HIV medications available since 1997 have changed the face of AIDS. People with HIV are not progressing to AIDS as quickly and, if current trends continue, can expect to live at least another 20 years without advancing to AIDS. However, many of these medications, as well as the virus itself, are causing other nutrition-related problems, such as high triglycerides, an increased risk for diabetes, and abnormal body fat distribution.

Political Disruptions and Natural Disasters

Social upheavals and natural disasters such as floods and drought can leave famine in their wake. The resulting displacement of populations and inequitable food distribution usually lead to hunger and malnutrition.

War

Whereas poverty is the underlying cause of chronic mild to moderate malnutrition, war and its aftermath cause severe malnutrition and famine. War diverts limited financial resources from development efforts to expenditures for fighting and destruction. Men and women no longer farm, fish, or bring

Fyi **AIDS and Malnutrition**

FOR YOUR INFORMATION

Like other infections, HIV interacts with malnutrition in a vicious, devastating cycle. Left untreated, HIV infection progresses to acquired immune deficiency syndrome (AIDS). The virus attacks by destroying its victim's immune system. When a person is unable to fight infections and malignancies, disease quickly depletes marginal nutrient stores, speeding the way to severe malnutrition and death. But malnutrition and HIV interact on several other levels:

- Low vitamin A levels in pregnant women increase the rate of HIV transmission to their unborn babies.[1]

- HIV is transmitted to infants in breast milk; but in impoverished regions, substitutions for breast milk typically increase infantile diarrhea, malnutrition, and death.[2]
- AIDS leaves mothers too weak to feed and care for their children. Eventually AIDS turns children into orphans.
- AIDS disables parents so they cannot work to support and feed their families.
- Reduced intake of micronutrients in an HIV-infected person is associated with faster progression of HIV disease and AIDS.[3]

- Weight loss and muscle wasting in an infected person are associated with faster progression of HIV disease and AIDS.[4]
- Infections that accompany AIDS cause fever and diarrhea, making malnutrition worse. Nausea and loss of appetite also contribute to malnutrition.
- Severe protein-energy malnutrition (PEM) is characteristic of untreated AIDS and frequently the ultimate cause of death.

home a paycheck—they are in the army. Households become fatherless and sometimes motherless, often permanently. Crops and croplands are destroyed, along with irrigation systems, food-processing facilities, and transportation infrastructure, which may have taken decades to develop.

Refugees

Masses of refugees—many very young or old, infirm, and already weakened by chronic hunger—find themselves without the basic elements of sustenance. The resulting famine has become an all too common sight on the evening news. International relief agencies have learned to respond to these emergencies quickly and with great determination, but logistic difficulties (e.g., mobilizing manpower, obtaining foods, transporting supplies, setting up feeding stations) may slow relief until it is too late for the sickest or weakest. Some refugee groups are inaccessible, hidden, or intentionally kept hungry as part of a political plan; emergency food may never reach many of them.

Sanctions

International sanctions and embargoes create food shortages, both directly and indirectly, by limiting access to agricultural supplies, fuel, and food-processing supplies. Some people argue that shortages created by embargoes hurt powerless people rather than government officials; others say that such actions are preferable to war.

Floods, Droughts, Mudslides, and Hurricanes

Many countries are not equipped to deal with food shortages and hunger from natural disasters. International relief agencies and other governments step in to help when possible. Some U.S. agencies involved are the USDA, the U.S. State Department through its Agency for International Development, and the Centers for Disease Control and Prevention (CDC) through the Center for Communicable Diseases. These agencies offer both short-term emergency efforts and long-term programs for repair and rebuilding.

Quick Bites

Accidental Solution

Sometimes a solution to undernutrition is not planned. On October 9, 1998, the *Wall Street Journal* carried the headline "In Guatemala, Organic Farms Sprout on Civil War Turf." During the country's 35-year civil war, local farmers abandoned their land. As the farmlands reverted to jungle and pesticide levels diminished, wild spices thrived. With the trend toward "organic" spices, coffee, and natural dyes, the premium prices commanded by these new crops could be significant for the farmers' incomes.

Quick Bites

Emergency Management

Imagine a civil war in a developing country that displaces tens of thousands of people. What are the most important measures for preventing sickness and death among these refugees? Protection from violence heads the list, closely followed by adequate food rations, clean water and sanitation, diarrheal disease control, measles immunization, and maternal and child health care.

As of 2004, 39.4 million people were living with HIV. Sub-Saharan Africa had 25.4 million people infected with HIV. Southeast Asia had 8.2 million people infected with HIV, Latin America had 1.7 million, and eastern Europe and Central Asia had 1.4 million.[5] Without treatment or a cure, these people are doomed to die, usually within 10 years of the initial infection. The fate of severe PEM in millions of people appears unavoidable. If we do not arrest the continued transmission of HIV, the number of PEM victims will climb even higher.

1 Semba RD, Miotti PG, Chiphangwi JD. Maternal vitamin A deficiency and mother-to-child transmission of HIV-1. *Lancet.* 1994;343:1593–1597.

2 Desclaux A, Taverne B, Alfieri C, et al. Socio-cultural obstacles in the prevention of HIV transmission through breast-milk in West Africa. Program and abstracts of the 13th International AIDS Conference; July 9–14, 2000; Durban, South Africa. Abstract MoOrD205.

3 Tang AM, Graham NMH, Kirby AJ, et al. Dietary micronutrient intake and risk of progression to acquired immunodeficiency syndrome (AIDS) in human immunodeficiency virus type-1 (HIV-1)–infected homosexual men. *Am J Epidemiol.* 1993;138:937–951.

4 Coodley GO, Loveless MO, Merrill TM. The HIV wasting syndrome: a review. *J Acq Immune Defic Syndr.* 1994;7:681–694.

5 UNAIDS. *Global Facts and Figures.* Geneva, Switzerland: UNAIDS, 2005.

Inequitable Food Distribution

Advances in agriculture have increased food production worldwide. Enough calories are now produced to supply the energy needs of every person on earth.[22] But distribution of these calories is uneven—among the continents, among nations, within nations, and even within families.

In some societies, the father of the family may be wrongly perceived as having the greatest nutrition needs and will be given priority for the most nutritious, high-protein foods. In those societies, older boys will have second priority; pregnant and breastfeeding women, women in general, and small children will have the lowest priority. Nations may follow a similar pattern, ensuring that their soldiers or men of fighting age receive the scarce foodstuffs.

Regional Trends

In sub-Saharan Africa, where the population is growing at an unprecedented rate of 3 percent per year, food production cannot keep pace; in fact, food availability per capita is declining.[23] Economic factors, violent regional conflicts, and the tremendous cost of the AIDS epidemic contribute to widespread, worsening hunger.

Among the former Communist countries of eastern Europe and Eurasia, abrupt economic transition and political upheaval have led to severe food shortages, often made worse by violent conflicts. In Latin America, despite great progress, hunger remains in pockets of rural poverty and in inner-city slums.

There has been progress, however. Improved national economies have led to reduction in hunger in the Middle East. In the Asia-Pacific region, per capita food supplies have increased, partly because of austere birth control measures in China as well as improved food production. However, even in nations that have achieved food sufficiency, regions of impoverishment or isolation have food shortages.

Agriculture and Environment: A Tricky Balance

Advances in agriculture increase food supplies and reduce food costs. Because the economies of most developing countries are based on agriculture, improvements boost rural incomes and buying power, increase demand for agricultural labor, stimulate commerce among small vendors and food processors, and ultimately help a nation's economy.

Dramatic gains in agricultural productivity took place in the 1960s and 1970s with the development of new seed varieties, especially rice and corn. The seeds greatly increased crop yields. Expectations were so strong that these seeds would finally solve the world's food shortage that their development and use was dubbed the "Green Revolution." Despite its successes, the Green Revolution had limitations. The seeds required irrigation and heavy use of pesticides and fertilizers, which poor farmers could not afford. The farming techniques were sometimes hard on the environment. Gains from the Green Revolution have now about reached their limit and, if current trends continue, threaten to be lost to the population explosion.

Proponents of agricultural biotechnology see it as another step along the continuum of plant-breeding techniques and a promising tool to increase crop production. Some uses of biotechnology are well accepted—for example, diagnostic kits that identify plants and insects by DNA and tissue culture for plant reproduction, a technique already in widespread commercial use. More controversial is the modification of plant genetic material. The technology has the potential to improve plants' resistance to disease, tolerance to adverse conditions, yield, and nutritional quality. Chapter 17, "Food Safety and Technology," describes the techniques and controversies surrounding this application of biotechnology.

At the other end of the technology spectrum is a renewed appreciation and conservation of traditional seed varieties, those selected over the generations by local farmers because they do well in local conditions. In developing countries, farmers typically save some of these seeds at each harvest to use the next planting season. The seeds grow well in the regions where they've evolved, whereas imported seeds, no matter how carefully bred, often fail.

In addition to seed selection, strategies to optimize agriculture include irrigation, soil preparation, improved planting and harvest methods, erosion prevention, fertilization, pest control, and flood control. The methods should be affordable, suitable for the level of local development, and protective of the environment. For example, where there is an abundant supply of willing farm laborers and gasoline is expensive, using heavy-duty farm machinery makes little sense. Other examples include mulching to conserve water and control weeds, and using manure (after composting to kill pathogens) to reduce the need for fertilizer.

Environmental Degradation

Environmental degradation is a growing concern in both the developing and the industrialized world. In developing countries, there is pressure for more land to support rapidly expanding populations. In industrialized countries, there is pressure from the affluent for more land, more houses, larger properties, more recreation areas, and so on. Residents of the industrialized world consume vast amounts of resources (e.g., water, fuel, wood, paper, textiles, and food) without a thought and often without making the small effort to conserve or recycle. Residents of the developing world consume much less per person, but the impact of their numbers is greater.

Environmental degradation has nutritional consequences because it threatens food production. Urbanization and the expansion of cities reduce the acreage available for farming. The pressure to supply food to growing populations leads to clear-cutting marginal land, eventually eroding hilly

Quick Bites

Who Produces the World's Soybeans?

*B*efore 1900, the soybean was rarely grown in the United States. Today, it is the largest American crop. The United States produces 75 percent of the world's soybeans.

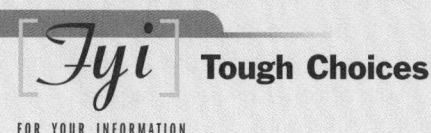

Tough Choices

FOR YOUR INFORMATION

Imagine you live in a poor village of a developing country. How would you make these choices?

- You've learned you must boil your drinking water to prevent diarrhea. But that means cutting young trees for firewood. You recently planted those trees to stop erosion. What do you do?
- You've recently given birth to your fourth child. Your husband was injured in an accident and is unable to work. But you can work at a nearby factory and use

your pay to buy food and clothes for the older children. How would you feed the new baby?

- Your small herd of goats provides milk for your young children. You like the goats because they can survive in the rough, hilly countryside. But the goats are overgrazing the grasses on the hillside. What can you do?
- Insects have destroyed your crop. In the past, you burned fields after harvest to control insects, but you've learned that

"slash and burn" is bad for the land. You've thought about using a chemical pesticide, but it is too expensive. You could clear the jungle for another growing field. Do you have other choices? What should you do?

- You can grow either vegetables to feed your family or a "cash crop" to sell for export. The cash crop would help pay for medicine and other necessities. Which should you grow?

terrain or quickly exhausting fragile rain forest soils. Overdependence on irrigation can drain water, eventually creating deserts. The destruction of vast areas of natural ground cover can lead to global climate changes. Overuse of pesticides and fertilizers pollutes waterways, destroying fish and seafood.

Key Concepts: *Despite gains in eradicating malnutrition, 30 percent of the global population—especially people in the developing world—continue to suffer from chronic hunger. Although world food supplies are adequate, factors that allow hunger to continue include poverty, poor sanitation, urbanization, and inefficient food distribution. Infection (especially AIDS), rapid population growth, wars, and environmental degradation threaten to reverse hard-won gains.*

Malnutrition: Its Nature, Its Victims, and Its Eradication

Previous chapters discussed the diseases of nutritional deficiency. Most of these diseases exist throughout the developing world, but seldom in isolation. Typically, the malnourished person has two or more coexisting deficiencies, each increasing the severity of the other. Keep the potential for this deadly synergy in mind as we discuss some of the major categories of malnutrition.

Protein-Energy Malnutrition

As you learned in Chapter 6, "Proteins and Amino Acids," lack of protein and energy can have devastating consequences, especially on the young. In kwashiorkor, the body and face swell with excess fluid, the hair turns wispy and red, and a terrible rash develops; without treatment, the person dies. Marasmus paints an even more dramatic picture of sunken eyes, shriveled limbs, and a clearly visible outline of the skeleton; it is as deadly as kwashiorkor.

Protein-energy malnutrition (PEM) is by far the most lethal form of malnutrition, and children are its most visible victims.[24] Their fast growth creates high nutrient demands, leaving them especially vulnerable to inappropriate food distribution in the family, inappropriate infant and child feeding practices, and interactions of infection with malnutrition. PEM typically develops after a child is weaned from the breast. Men in the household may have priority for nutritious food. In big families, the young child must also compete for food with many siblings.

In the developing world, breastfeeding is almost always essential to an infant's survival. Inappropriate bottle-feeding puts a baby at grave risk. Relative to income, formula is usually very expensive and is often diluted to make it stretch. Contaminated water and lack of other hygienic requirements for bottle preparation cause diarrhea. The combination of diarrhea and nutritional deficiency from watered-down formula is often fatal.

A tremendous educational effort, including promotion of breastfeeding, has reduced the global prevalence and severity of infant and childhood PEM. Severe PEM typified by kwashiorkor or marasmus has become more sporadic, occurring mainly as a result of war or natural disaster. However, mild to moderate PEM continues to pose a grave problem in the developing world, putting children at risk of delayed growth, impaired psychological development, and the deadly interactions of disease and malnutrition. In fact, almost half of all deaths of children younger than 5 are still associated with PEM. Most of these deaths are from mild to moderate PEM interacting with other illness, rather than from severe malnutrition.[25]

Quick Bites

Is Breastfeeding Always Best?

An HIV-positive mother can transmit the virus to her baby through breast milk. HIV-positive women whose infants were spared HIV transmission during pregnancy face the dilemma of how to feed those babies. In developing countries, the WHO is working to prevent HIV transmission through breastfeeding while continuing to protect, promote, and support breastfeeding as the best way to feed babies of women who are HIV-negative and women who do not know their status. Unfortunately, alternatives such as formula feeding are expensive, carry the risk of food poisoning from contaminated water, and often carry a social stigma.

Moreover, with an epidemic of HIV infection raging in many developing countries, the return of widespread severe PEM threatens.

Iodine Deficiency Disorders

Iodine deficiency is the developing world's most common cause of preventable brain damage and impaired psychomotor development.[26] Its impairment of intellectual ability and work performance is potentially so widespread that **iodine deficiency disorders (IDD)** can actually slow a nation's social and economic development.

Iodine deficiency is most devastating during pregnancy, causing spontaneous abortions, stillbirths, and birth defects, including cretinism, a disease of mental retardation that is often severe. Deafness and spastic paralysis are likely to accompany the retardation. In regions of Africa, dwarfism also occurs where diets rich in goitrogen-containing vegetables (e.g., cassava or cabbage) make the deficiency worse. Moreover, iodine deficiency is damaging at all ages, limiting mental development in infants and children and producing apathy and marginal mental function in adults. (See **Figure 18.7**.)

Iodine deficiency disorders are endemic throughout much of the developing world where the soil is low in iodine. These areas typically are mountainous or far from the oceans. They often are isolated and impoverished. Although imported food is a potential source of iodine, it often is not consumed.

Disturbing though these figures may be, great strides have been made in IDD prevention, mainly through iodizing salt: The proportion of households in the developing world consuming adequately iodized salt has risen from less than 20 percent in 1990 to over 70 percent today. China has been one of the most phenomenal success stories of the 1990s, with iodization rates rising from 39 percent to 95 percent in a span of 10 years. Others include Jordan, which has increased coverage from 5 percent to nearly 90 percent, and Bangladesh, where iodization has increased from 20 to 70 percent. Latin American countries such as Peru have a long history of commitment to salt iodization, and notable African successes include Nigeria and Kenya.[27]

Vitamin A Deficiency

Vitamin A deficiency is the leading cause of preventable childhood blindness and is the leading cause of needless visual impairment in women and children. It also predisposes its victims to infection, and it worsens existing infections. Vitamin A deficiency is most damaging to infants, children, and pregnant or lactating women. At least 100 million children younger than 5 suffer from vitamin A deficiency, high levels of which can cause blindness and greatly increase the risk that a child may die from diseases such as measles, diarrhea, and acute respiratory infections.[28]

In communities where vitamin A deficiency exists, pregnant and breastfeeding women often experience night blindness, an early symptom of deficiency. Maternal death, poor pregnancy outcome, and failure to lactate are all increased with vitamin A deficiency. Vitamin A levels in the breast milk of these women are likely to be low as well, putting their infants at later risk of deficiency.

Many countries are taking a multipronged approach to vitamin A deficiency that includes promotion of breastfeeding, fortification of foods, supplementation, and nutrition education. Foods such as eggs, dairy foods, and liver are promoted as important for women and children; educational programs also encourage growing and eating fruits and vegetables high in

iodine deficiency disorders (IDD) A wide range of disorders due to iodine deficiency that affect growth and development.

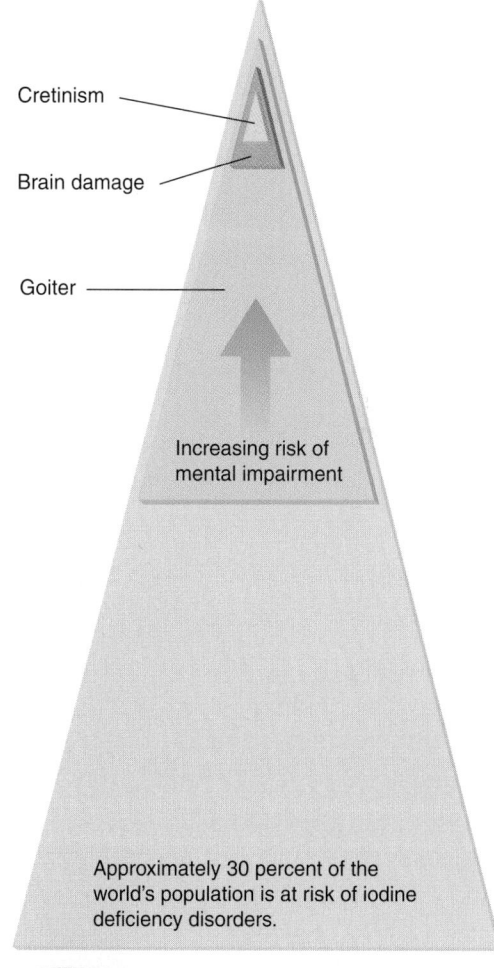

Cretinism

Brain damage

Goiter

Increasing risk of mental impairment

Approximately 30 percent of the world's population is at risk of iodine deficiency disorders.

Figure 18.7 **The toll of iodine deficiency.** Iodine deficiency remains the single greatest cause of preventable brain damage and mental retardation worldwide.
Source: World Health Organization.

beta-carotene. However, dietary change can be difficult and slow. The best sources of vitamin A are often the most expensive or inaccessible. For absorption and conversion to vitamin A, beta-carotene requires dietary fat—another expensive item in many areas—and other factors that are not completely understood. Meanwhile, periodic single, large-dose vitamin A supplements, often given in tandem with maternal-child immunizations, are proving an effective short-term measure.

Vitamin A supplements, costing only two cents per capsule, can improve a child's chance of survival by up to 25 percent. Providing vitamin A to pregnant women can also reduce maternal deaths. Today the majority of children in more than 40 countries are receiving at least one vitamin A supplement yearly. UNICEF estimates that as many as 300,000 child deaths are prevented each year because of vitamin A supplementation.[29]

Biotechnology may have a significant impact on vitamin A deficiency. Through genetic engineering, scientists have developed a strain of rice that is rich in beta-carotene. When these rice plants are crossed with locally grown strains of rice, they become suited to a particular region's climate and growing conditions. If local farmers and consumers accept such crops, bioengineered rice may play a critical role in feeding the world's burgeoning population and alleviating widespread vitamin A deficiency.[30]

Iron-Deficiency Anemia

Iron deficiency is the most pervasive nutritional problem in the world. Between 4 and 5 billion people suffer from iron deficiency, and an estimated 2 billion are anemic. Women and young children are most vulnerable: 50 percent of pregnant women and 40 to 50 percent of children younger than 5 in developing countries are iron deficient.[31] Fast growth in young children and reproductive blood loss in women make them especially vulnerable to low-iron diets. However, iron deficiency occurs in all age groups. Like deficiencies discussed previously, anemia impairs psychomotor development, work capacity, learning capacity, and resistance to disease. Anemia during pregnancy increases illness and death rates for mother and baby. For all groups of people, anemia can cause profound fatigue, and severe anemia causes death.

Iron-deficient diets are typically high in starch and cereal grains. During digestion, cereals may bind with the very limited iron the diet provides, preventing its absorption. Other blood-building nutrients, such as vitamins B_6 and B_{12} and folate, are in short supply as well.

The anemias of the developing world demonstrate the interaction of multiple nutrient deficiencies, which in turn interact with infection, sanitation, and poverty. Supplying iron alone is seldom enough to correct the problem. Anemia-producing parasites are common in areas of iron deficiency, aggravating the effects of poor diet. Blood cells are destroyed by malarial infections. Intestinal malabsorption and intestinal bleeding are caused by hookworm, prevalent where human waste contaminates the fields where people walk barefoot, and by other parasites, acquired when human waste contaminates the water that people drink or in which people bathe.

People debilitated by anemia may be too weak to build outhouses, too poor to buy shoes or fuel to boil water, or too apathetic to clear standing water where malaria-carrying mosquitoes breed. Moreover, they often do not understand the connection between sanitation, infection, and malnutrition. Added to this mix are excessive blood loss from repeated pregnancies, inherited blood disorders such as sickle cell disease, and chronic bacterial or viral infections such as HIV.

Quick Bites

The Importance of Rice

Rice is the principal food crop for one-half of the world's population.

Efforts to increase intake of iron-rich foods have limited effectiveness because these foods are costly and dietary improvements are likely to come too slowly. When iron-rich foods—liver, red meats, eggs, fish, whole-grain bread, legumes—are not widely available or affordable, fortifying staples such as flour is an alternative for reaching a large portion of the population. Finally, in malaria-endemic countries, antimalarial interventions, such as bed nets, are critical for preventing anemia because malaria is often the major underlying factor.

Deficiencies of Other Micronutrients

Deficiencies of zinc and calcium often coexist with other deficiencies, contributing to illness and death during periods of growth and threatening immune function and skeletal health in people who survive to old age.

Selenium deficiency, although limited to only a few countries, has serious consequences. It occurs in distinct regional patterns in China and Russia where the soil is selenium-poor. In China, where the deficiency is most severe, it predisposes individuals to the fatal Keshan disease, in which heart muscle is destroyed. Keshan disease affects mainly women and children. The condition can be prevented by selenium supplementation or by fortification, as in programs undertaken in New Zealand, where the soil is also low in selenium.

The classic deficiency diseases beriberi, pellagra, and scurvy still occur among the world's poorest and most underprivileged people. Most often, however, these diseases strike the victims of war and political strife—the refugees. Diets based on milled cereals and starchy roots, all poor thiamin sources, predispose refugee populations to beriberi. People who rely on corn-based diets low in niacin and tryptophan are susceptible to pellagra. The disruption of refugee life can easily tip the balance from marginal deficiency to overt deficiency disease.

Overweight and Obesity

In some developing countries, obesity exists right alongside undernutrition. Obesity is more likely in areas of economic advancement and urban areas, less so in rural populations. Its prevalence is rising rapidly in Latin America and the Caribbean, but obesity still is relatively uncommon in Asia and Africa.

The factors leading to obesity in poor communities are different from those in affluent societies. Cultural attitudes toward overweight may be more accepting, even admiring. Calorie-dense foods that have few other nutrients are often cheap, satisfying, convenient, and heavily promoted; some are foreign brands that have become affordable status symbols. With urbanization and modernization, trends that typically reduce physical activity, comes a reduction in caloric expenditure that can be dramatic. Malnutrition itself may actually play a role; there is evidence that malnutrition during fetal development and early childhood predisposes people to obesity in adulthood.[32]

Key Concepts: *The most critical nutritional deficiencies in today's developing world are deficiencies of protein, calories, iodine, vitamin A, and iron. Breastfeeding promotion, nutrition education, and improvements in food supplies have produced some gains in reducing the severity and prevalence of protein-energy malnutrition. Fortification and supplementation programs are effectively attacking iodine and vitamin A deficiencies but have had less success in overcoming iron deficiency. All of the underlying causes of malnutrition must be addressed to reduce and eliminate these and other deficiencies.*

Quick Bites

Undernutrition Cannot Be Blamed for Everything

In all populations in the developing world, low weight- and height-for-age affect 10 to 15 percent of preschool and school-aged children. Most experts attribute this shortfall to insufficiency of food. A study of African schoolchildren, however, found no significant difference between well-fed and underfed pupils on measures such as their class position, aptitude for games, and interest in education. Among children of school age, one must be careful not to overrate the effects of undernutrition or the health disadvantages from mild to moderate malnutrition.

LEARNING *Portfolio*   c h a p t e r   1 8

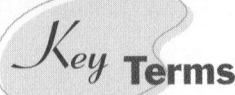

Key Terms

Study Points

- Hunger and malnutrition continue to be problems in both industrialized and developing countries.

- Although most people in the United States are food-secure, malnutrition is a serious problem among the working poor, the rural poor, the homeless, elders, and children.

- The Food Stamp Program; the Special Supplemental Nutrition Program for Women, Infants, and Children (WIC); the National School Lunch and Breakfast Programs; and the Child and Adult Care Food Program are among the many federal programs that address hunger in the United States.

- Although the rates of malnutrition and hunger in the developing world declined in the last three decades of the twentieth century, progress is still too slow and uneven. It is estimated that more than 800 million people in the developing world do not have enough to eat.

- Social and economic factors, infection, disease, political disruptions, natural disasters, and inequitable food distribution all contribute to hunger in the developing world.

- Advances in agricultural practices have increased food supplies and reduced food costs in the developing world; however, the increase in production has led to environmental degradation as a result of urbanization, clear-cutting, overirrigation, and soil erosion.

- Protein-energy malnutrition (PEM) refers to conditions, such as kwashiorkor and marasmus, that result from not having enough to eat.

- Infants and children are most likely to suffer from PEM. However, nutrition education efforts, including promotion of breastfeeding, have reduced the severity and prevalence of PEM.

- Iodine deficiency is the largest cause of preventable brain damage and impaired psychomotor development in the developing world. It can cause damage to people of all ages.

- Great strides have been made in preventing iodine deficiency disorders (IDD) through salt iodization programs. More than two-thirds of households in IDD-affected countries now use iodized salt.

- Vitamin A deficiency is the leading cause of preventable childhood blindness. It also makes its victims more vulnerable to infection, diarrheal diseases, and PEM.

- Pregnant and breastfeeding women with vitamin A deficiency are at increased risk of death, poor pregnancy outcomes, and lactation failure.

- Many countries are taking a multipronged approach to vitamin A deficiency that includes promotion of breastfeeding, fortification of foods, supplementation, and nutrition education.

- The best sources of vitamin A often are expensive and inaccessible to people in developing countries. Scientists have developed new bioengineered strains of rice that are rich in beta-carotene and that may play a critical role in alleviating widespread vitamin A deficiency.

- The anemias of the developing world demonstrate the interaction of multiple nutrient deficiencies, which in turn interact with infection, poor sanitation, and poverty.

➤ **Food fortification and iron supplementation for women and children are the mainstays of anemia prevention and treatment, along with efforts to overcome poverty and improve sanitation.**

➤ **The classic deficiency diseases beriberi, pellagra, and scurvy still occur among the world's poorest and most underprivileged people.**

➤ **In some developing countries, obesity exists right alongside undernutrition.**

Study Questions

1. **What's the difference between food insecurity and hunger?**
2. **What is food security?**
3. **List four common nutritional deficiencies worldwide.**
4. **List four causes of malnutrition worldwide.**
5. **List some of the organizations and programs fighting hunger and food insecurity in the United States.**
6. **What populations are at increased risk of nutritional deficiencies, and why?**

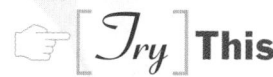
Try This

Try Giving Up Your Stove and Refrigerator

A homeless person has no kitchen facilities to store or prepare food. For one day, eat a balanced diet without resorting to cooking or using your refrigerator. Some of the foods you could eat include the following:

breads, bagels, tortillas, rolls

cereals

crackers

milk—canned, evaporated, or aseptically packaged

cheese—hard cheeses keep well

pudding cups (single-serve, nonrefrigerated type)

tuna/chicken—canned

sardines, salmon—canned

nuts, peanut butter

beans—canned

fruits and vegetables—fresh, canned, dried fruits

How satisfying did you find this eating pattern? What did you miss most? What would it be like to eat this way for an extended time?

Community Food Programs

The purpose of this exercise is to see how you can contribute to decreasing or eliminating food insecurity in your community. Look in the phone book (under "Food Programs" and "Human Services") to see what programs are available. Consider volunteering at your local food bank or another community program to help feed people who do not have the means to feed themselves.

References

1 Food and Agriculture Organization of the United Nations. *Undernourishment Around the World 2005.* http://www.fao.org/docrep/008/a0200e/a0200e00.htm. Accessed 8/5/06.

2 Ibid.; and Position of the American Dietetic Association: addressing world hunger, malnutrition, and food insecurity. *J Am Diet Assoc.* 2003;103:1046–1057.

3 Kendall A, Kennedy E. Position of the American Dietetic Association: food insecurity and hunger in the United States. *J Am Diet Assoc.* 2006;106:446–458.

4 US Department of Agriculture. *Food Security in the United States.* http://www.ers.usda.gov/Briefing/FoodSecurity/. Accessed 8/5/06.

5 Scheier LM. What is the hunger-obesity paradox? *J Am Diet Assoc.* 2005;105:883–884, 886.

6 Nord M, Andrews M, Carlsen S. *Household Food Security in the United States, 2004.* Washington, DC: US Department of Agriculture, October 2005. Economic Research Report No. 11. http://www.ers.usda.gov/Publications/err11/. Accessed 8/5/06.

7 Schlesinger JM. Working full time is no longer enough. *Wall Street Journal.* June 29, 2000:A2, A12.

8 Wellman NS, Weddle DO, Kranz S, Brain CT. Elder insecurities: poverty, hunger, and malnutrition. *J Am Diet Assoc.* 1997;97(suppl):S120–S122.

9 Nord M, Andrews M, Carlsen S. Op. cit.

10 USDA Food and Nutrition Service Online. WIC fact sheet. http://www.fns.usda.gov/wic/WIC-Fact-Sheet.pdf. Accessed 8/5/06.

11 USDA Food and Nutrition Service Online. WIC income eligibility guidelines. http://www.fns.usda.gov/wic/howtoapply/eligibilityrequirements.htm. Accessed 8/5/06.

12 USDA Food and Nutrition Service Online. School programs: income eligibility guidelines. http://www.fns.usda.gov/cnd/governance/notices/iegs/iegs.htm. Accessed 8/5/06.

13 USDA Food and Nutrition Service Online. National School Lunch Program. September 2006. http://www.fns.usda.gov/cnd/lunch/AboutLunch/NSLPFactSheet.pdf. Accessed 8/5/06.

14 Brundtland GH. Nutrition, health, and human rights. World Health Organization, 2003. http://www.who.int/director-general/speeches/1999/english/19990412_nutrition.html. Accessed 1/3/07.

15 Food and Agriculture Organization of the United Nations. Op. cit.

16 Ibid.

17 Brundtland GH. Op. cit.

18 Mata LJ, Urrutia JJ, Albertazzi C. Influence of recurrent infections on nutrition and growth of children in Guatemala. *Am J Clin Nutr.* 1972;25:1267–1275.

19 Semba RD, Miotti PG, Chipangwi JD, et al. Maternal vitamin A deficiency and mother-to-child transmission of HIV-1. *Lancet.* 1994;343:1593–1597.

20 Tang AM, Graham NMH, Kirby AJ, et al. Dietary micronutrient intake and risk of progression to acquired immunodeficiency syndrome (AIDS) in human immunodeficiency virus type 1 (HIV-1)–infected homosexual men. *Am J Epidemiol.* 1993; 138:937–951.

21 Joint United Nations Programme on HIV/AIDS. *2006 Report on the Global HIV/AIDS Epidemic.* Geneva, Switzerland: UNAIDS, 2006. http://www.who.int/hiv/mediacentre/news60/en/index.html. Accessed 8/5/06.

22 Position of the American Dietetic Association: addressing world hunger. Op. cit.

23 Ibid.

24 World Health Organization. Protein energy malnutrition. http://www.wpro.who.int/health_topics/protein_energy/general_info.htm. Accessed 8/5/06.

25 World Health Organization. Alleviating protein-energy malnutrition. www.who.int/nut/pem.htm. Accessed 3/27/05.

26 UNICEF. Micronutrients—iodine, iron, vitamin A. http://www.unicef.org/nutrition/index_iodine.html. Accessed 8/6/06.

27 Ibid.

28 Ibid.

29 Ibid.

30 Nash M. Grains of hope. *Time.* 156:5(July 31, 2000):38–46; and Greger JL. Response: genetically engineered "golden" rice unlikely to overcome vitamin A deficiency. *J Am Diet Assoc.* 2001;101:289–290.

31 UNICEF. Op. cit.

32 Pena M, Bacallao J. *Obesity and Poverty: A New Public Health Challenge.* PAHO scientific publication 576. Geneva, Switzerland: World Health Organization, 2000.

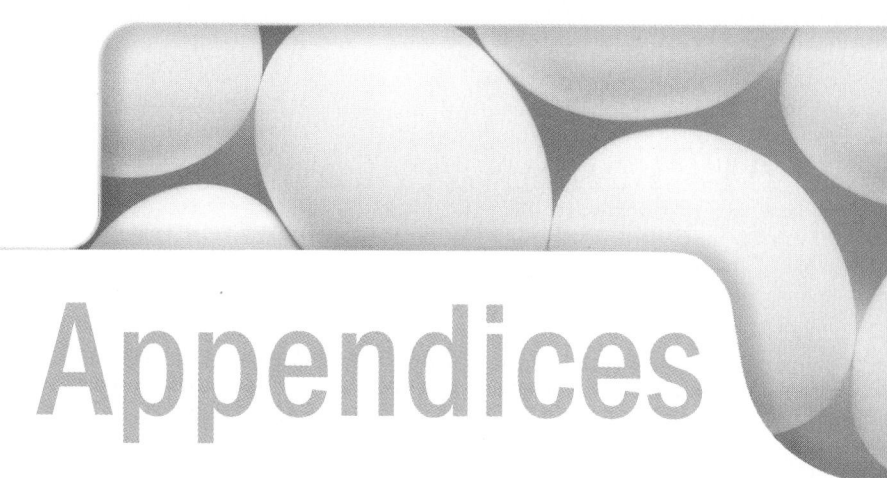

Appendices

APPENDIX A Food Composition Tables

Baking Ingredients, p. A-1; Bars, p. A-1; Beverages, p. A-2; Condiments & Accompaniments, p. A-6; Dairy Products & Non-Dairy
Substitutes, p. A-10; Desserts, p. A-16; Eggs & Egg Substitutes, p. A-26; Fats & Fat Substitutes, p. A-26; Fruits, p. A-28;
Grain Products, p. A-32; Infant Foods, p. A-44; Meats & Meat Substitutes, p. A-44; Nuts & Seeds, p. A-54; Prepared Packaged
Foods, p. A-56; Prepared Homemade Dishes, p. A-60; Restaurant Food, p. A-66; Vegetables & Legumes, p. A-74

ESHA CODE	FOOD DESCRIPTION	AMT	UNIT	WT (g)	CAL (kcal)	WTR (g)	PROT (g)	CARB (g)	FIBR (g)	FAT (g)	SATF (g)	MONO (g)	POLY (g)
Baking	**Ingredients**												
23010	Baking Chocolate-Square	1	ea	28.35	142	<1	4	8	5	15	9.2	4.6	0.4
28003	Baking Soda	1	tsp	4.6	0	<1	0	0	0	0	0	0	0
23012	Chocolate Chips-Semisweet	1	cup	168	805	1	7	106	10	50	29.8	16.7	1.6
28200	Cocoa Powder	1	Tbs	5.38	12	<1	1	3	2	1	0.4	0.2	<0.1
30000	Cornstarch	1	Tbs	8	30	1	<1	7	<1	<1	<0.1	<0.1	<0.1
53002	Soy Sauce	1	Tbs	16	8	11	1	1	<1	<1	<0.1	<0.1	<0.1
53267	Soy Sauce-Lite	1	Tbs	18	15		1	2	0	<1	0		
27205	Vinegar-Malt Ale	1	Tbs	16	0	16	0	0	0	0	0	0	0
53099	Worcestershire Sauce	1	Tbs	17	11	13	0	3	0	0	0	0	0
28000	Yeast-Dry-Active-Baker's	1	tsp	4	12	<1	2	2	1	<1	<0.1	0.1	<0.1
Sugars & Syrups													
63655	Agave Nectar	1	Tbs	21	60	0		16	0	0	0	0	0
31183	Blackstrap Molasses	1	Tbs	20.5	53	5	1	13	1	<1	<0.1	<0.1	<0.1
25010	Corn Syrup-Dark	1	cup	328	938	72	0	254	0	0	0	0	0
25000	Corn Syrup-Light	1	cup	328	928	75	0	252	0	1	0	0	0
25001	Honey-Strained/Extracted	1	Tbs	21.2	64	4	<1	17	<1	0	0	0	0
25002	Maple Syrup	1	Tbs	20	52	6	0	13	0	<1	<0.1	<0.1	<0.1
23042	Pancake Syrup	1	Tbs	20	47	8	0	12	<1	0	0	0	0
23090	Pancake Syrup+Butter	1	Tbs	19.69	58	5	0	15	0	<1	0.2	0.1	<0.1
23172	Pancake Syrup-Reduced Cal	1	Tbs	15	25	8	0	7	0	0	0	0	0
25005	Sugar-Brown	1	tsp	4.6	17	<1	0	4	0	0	0	0	0
63348	Sugar-Turbinado	1	tsp	4	15	0	0	4	0	0	0	0	0
25006	Sugar-White-Granulated	1	tsp	4.167	16	<1	0	4	0	0	0	0	0
25009	Sugar-White-Powdered	1	tsp	2.5	10	<1	0	2	0	<1	<0.1	<0.1	<0.1
Bars													
53227	Cereal Bar-Nutrigrain-MixBerry	1	ea	37	137	5	2	27	1	3	0.6	1.9	0.4
23100	Granola Bar-Almond-Hard	1	ea	23.6	117	1	2	15	1	6	3	1.8	0.9
23105	Granola Bar-Choc Chip-Soft	1	ea	42.52	178	3	2	30	2	7	2.6	3	0.7
23108	Granola Bar-PeanutButter-Soft	1	ea	28.35	121	2	3	18	1	4	1	1.9	1.2
23059	Granola Bar-Plain-Hard	1	ea	24.5	115	1	2	16	1	5	0.6	1.1	3
23097	Granola Bar-Raisin-Soft	1	ea	42.52	190	3	3	28	2	8	4.1	1.2	1.4
23104	Granola Bar-Soft	1	ea	28.35	126	2	2	19	1	5	2.1	1.1	1.5
23065	Kudos Bar-Nutty Fudge	1	ea	28.35	120	2	1	20	1	4	2		
62640	SlimFast NutriBar-DutchChoc	1	ea	34	140		5	20	2	5	3		
62205	Tiger Sport Bar	1	ea	35	140		6	18	1	5	1		
62643	UltrSlmFstBar-ChwyCarmlCrnch	1	svg	28	120		1	22	2	4	2.5		
62641	UltrSlmFstBar-PntCarmlCrnch	1	svg	28	120		1	21	1	4	2.5		

< = Trace amount present   Blank = Not available

ESHA, EatRight Analysis CD-ROM; **AMT,** amount; **WT,** weight; **CAL,** calories; **WTR,** water; **PROT,** protein; **CARB,** carbohydrate; **FIBR,** fiber; **FAT,** fat; **SATF,** saturated fat; **MONO,** monounsaturated fat; **POLY,** polyunsaturated fat; **CHOL,** cholesterol; **V,** vitamin; **THI,** thiamin; **RIB,** riboflavin; **NIA,** niacin; **FOL,** folate; **CALC,** calcium; **PHOS,** phosphorus; **SOD,** sodium; **POT,** potassium; **MAG,** magnesium

CHOL (g)	V-A (RE)	THI (mg)	RIB (mg)	NIA (mg)	V-B6 (mg)	FOL (µg)	V-B12 (µg)	V-C (mg)	V-E (mg)	CALC (mg)	PHOS (mg)	SOD (mg)	POT (mg)	MAG (mg)	IRON (mg)	ZINC (mg)
0	0	<0.1	<0.1	0.4	<0.1	8	0	0	0.1	29	113	7	235	93	4.9	2.7
0	0	0	0	0	0	0	0	0	0	0	0	1259	0	0	0	0
0	0	0.1	0.2	0.7	0.1	22	0	0	0.4	54	222	18	613	193	5.3	2.7
0	0	<0.1	<0.1	0.1	<0.1	2	0	0	<0.1	7	39	1	82	27	0.7	0.4
0	0	0	0	0	0	0	0	0	0	<1	1	1	<1	<1	<0.1	<0.1
0	0	<0.1	<0.1	0.4	<0.1	2	0	0	0	3	20	902	35	7	0.3	0.1
0	0							0		3		505			0.1	
0	0							0		0		0	5		0	
0	2	<0.1	<0.1	0.1	0	1	0	2	<0.1	18	10	167	136	2	0.9	<0.1
0	0	0.1	0.2	1.6	0.1	94	<0.1	<1	0	3	52	2	80	4	0.7	0.3
0	0							0		0		0			0	
<1	<1	<0.1	<0.1	0.5				<1		213		70	431		3.2	
0	0	<0.1	<0.1	0.1	<0.1	0	0	0	0	59	36	508	144	26	1.2	0.1
0	0	0.2	0	0	0	0	0	0	0	43	0	203	3	3	0	1.4
0	0	0	<0.1	<0.1	<0.1	<1	0	<1	0	1	1	1	11	<1	0.1	<0.1
0	0	<0.1	<0.1	<0.1	<0.1	0	0	0	0	13	<1	2	41	3	0.2	0.8
0	0	<0.1	<0.1	<0.1	<0.1	0	0	0	0	1	2	16	3	<1	<0.1	<0.1
1	3	<0.1	<0.1	<0.1	0	0	0	0	<0.1	<1	2	19	1	<1	<0.1	<0.1
0	0	<0.1	<0.1	<0.1	0	0	0	0	0	<1	6	30	<1	0	<0.1	<0.1
0	0	<0.1	<0.1	<0.1	<0.1	<1	0	0	0	4	1	2	16	1	0.1	<0.1
0	0							0		0		0			0	
0	0	0	<0.1	0	0	0	0	0	0	<1	0	0	<1	0	<0.1	0
0	0	0	<0.1	0	0	0	0	0	0	<1	0	<1	<1	0	<0.1	0
0	150	0.4	0.4	5	0.5	40	0	0	0	14	36	110	70	10	1.8	1.5
0	1	0.1	<0.1	0.1	<0.1	3	0	0	0.4	8	54	60	64	19	0.6	0.4
0	0	0.1	<0.1	0.3	<0.1	7	0	0	0.1	17	75	76	101	27	0.9	0.6
<1	1	0.1	<0.1	0.9	<0.1	9	0.1	0	0.3	26	71	116	82	24	0.6	0.5
0	4	0.1	<0.1	0.4	<0.1	6	0	<1	0.3	15	68	72	82	24	0.7	0.5
<1	0	0.1	0.1	0.5	<0.1	9	0.1	0	0.5	43	94	120	154	31	1	0.6
<1	0	0.1	<0.1	0.1	<0.1	7	0.1	0	0.3	30	65	79	92	21	0.7	0.4
0	20							1		200		75		8	0.4	
5	250	0.4	0.4	5	0.4	40	1.5	15	3.4	100	100	80	160	16	4.5	3.8
0	150	1.3	0.6	3	0.6		1.5	6		300	100	75		100	2.7	
5	150	0.2	0.3	3	0.3	60	0.9	9	2	250	100	75			2.7	
3	150	0.2	0.3	3	0.3	60	0.9	9	2	250	100	80			2.7	

ESHA, EatRight Analysis CD-ROM; **AMT,** amount; **WT,** weight; **CAL,** calories; **WTR,** water; **PROT,** protein; **CARB,** carbohydrate; **FIBR,** fiber; **FAT,** fat; **SATF,** saturated fat; **MONO,** monosaturated fat; **POLY,** polyunsaturated fat

ESHA CODE	FOOD DESCRIPTION	AMT	UNIT	WT (g)	CAL (kcal)	WTR (g)	PROT (g)	CARB (g)	FIBR (g)	FAT (g)	SATF (g)	MONO (g)	POLY (g)
Beverages													
Alcoholic Beverages and Mixes													
22500	Beer	12	floz	356.4	153	328	2	13	0	0	0	0	0
22512	Beer-Light	12	floz	354	103	336	1	6	0	0	0	0	0
20276	Beer-Non-Alcoholic	12	floz	340.5	56		<1	12		0	0	0	0
22519	Coffee Liqueur, 53 proof	1	floz	34.8	117	11	<1	16	0	<1	<0.1	<0.1	<0.1
22521	De Menthe Liqueur 72 proof	1	floz	33.6	125	10	0	14	0	<1	<0.1	<0.1	0.1
22543	Gin-Rum-Vodka-Whiskey, 100prf	1	floz	27.8	82	16	0	0	0	0	0	0	0
22514	Gin-Rum-Vodka-Whiskey, 80prf	1	floz	27.8	64	19	0	0	0	0	0	0	0
22516	Gin-Rum-Vodka-Whiskey, 86prf	1	floz	27.8	70	18	0	<1	0	0	0	0	0
22542	Gin-Rum-Vodka-Whiskey, 94prf	1	floz	27.8	76	17	0	0	0	0	0	0	0
22601	Sangria Wine Drink	6	floz	177	118	153	<1	16	<1	<1	<0.1	<0.1	<0.1
22518	Wine-Dessert, Dry	1	floz	29.5	45	21	<1	3	0	0	0	0	0
22507	Wine-Dessert, Sweet	1	floz	29.5	47	21	<1	4	0	0	0	0	0
20077	Wine-Light-Non Alcoholic	6	floz	174	10	171	1	2	0	0	0	0	0
20076	Wine-Non Alcoholic	6	floz	174	10	171	1	2	0	0	0	0	0
22501	Wine-Red	6	floz	177	150	153	<1	5	0	0	0	0	0
22862	Wine-Riesling	6	floz	177	143	153	<1	7		0			
22638	Wine-Sherry-Spray Dried	1	g	1	4	<1	0	1	0	0	0	0	0
22504	Wine-White, Medium	6	floz	177	147	154	<1	5	0	0	0	0	0
Carbonated Drinks													
20006	Club Soda	1	cup	236.8	0	237	0	0	0	0	0	0	0
90615	Cola	1	cup	248	92	224	<1	24	0	<1	0	0	0
20054	Cola-Caffeine Free	1	cup	240	107	212	0	27	0	0	0	0	0
20056	Cola-Diet-Caffeine Free	1	cup	240	0		0	0	0	0	0	0	0
90617	Cola-Diet-w/asp	1	cup	236.8	5	236	<1	1	0	<1	0	0	0
20028	Cream Soda	1	cup	247.2	126	214	0	33	0	0	0	0	0
20189	Creme Soda, Diet	1	cup	240	0	240	0	0	0	0	0	0	0
20007	Diet Soda, Assorted Flavors	1	cup	236.8	0	236	0	<1	0	0	0	0	0
20027	Dr. Pepper Type Soda	1	cup	245.6	101	220	0	26	0	<1	0.2	0	0
20008	Ginger Ale	1	cup	244	83	223	0	21	0	0	0	0	0
20031	Grape Soda	1	cup	248	107	220	0	28	0	0	0	0	0
20032	Lemon-Lime Soda	1	cup	245.6	98	220	<1	25	0	<1	0	0	0
20029	Orange Soda	1	cup	248	119	217	0	31	0	0	0	0	0
20009	Root Beer	1	cup	246.4	101	220	0	26	0	0	0	0	0
Coffees & Coffee Substitutes													
20592	Cappuccino, LowFat Milk-Tall	1.5	cup	244	110		8	11	0	4	2.5		
20639	Cappuccino, Whole Milk-Tall	1.5	cup	244	140		7	11	0	7	4.5		
20659	Coffee Latte, Iced, LowFat Milk-Tall	1.5	cup	392	90		7	10	0	3	2		
20662	Coffee Latte, Iced, Whole Milk-Tall	1.5	cup	392	120		6	10	0	6	4		
20668	Coffee Latte, LowFat Milk-Tall	1.5	cup	366	170		12	17	0	6	4		
20671	Coffee Latte, Whole Milk-Tall	1.5	cup	366	210		11	17	0	11	7		
20677	Coffee Mocha, LowFat Milk-Tall	1.5	cup	392	300		12	33	1	15	9		
20680	Coffee Mocha, Whole Milk-Tall	1.5	cup	392	340		12	33	1	20	12		
20093	Coffee+Chicory-Prep from Instant	1	cup	179	5	177	<1	1	0	0	<0.1	0	<0.1
20012	Coffee-Brewed	1	cup	237	2	236	<1	0	0	<1	<0.1	<0.1	<0.1

< = Trace amount present   Blank = Not available

CHOL, cholesterol; **V,** vitamin; **THI,** thiamin; **RIB,** riboflavin; **NIA,** niacin; **FOL,** folate;
CALC, calcium; **PHOS,** phosphate; **SOD,** sodium; **POT,** potassium; **MAG,** magnesium

CHOL (g)	V-A (RE)	THI (mg)	RIB (mg)	NIA (mg)	V-B6 (mg)	FOL (μg)	V-B12 (μg)	V-C (mg)	V-E (mg)	CALC (mg)	PHOS (mg)	SOD (mg)	POT (mg)	MAG (mg)	IRON (mg)	ZINC (mg)
0	0	<0.1	0.1	1.8	0.2	21	0.1	0	0	14	50	14	96	21	0.1	<0.1
0	0	<0.1	0.1	1.4	0.1	21	0.1	0	0	14	42	14	74	18	0.1	<0.1
0												3				
0	0	<0.1	<0.1	0.1	0	0	0	0	0	<1	2	3	10	1	<0.1	<0.1
0	0	0	0	<0.1	0	0	0	0	0	0	0	2	0	0	<0.1	<0.1
0	0	<0.1	<0.1	<0.1	<0.1	0	0	0	0	0	1	<1	1	0	<0.1	<0.1
0	0	<0.1	<0.1	<0.1	<0.1	0	0	0	0	0	1	<1	1	0	<0.1	<0.1
0	0	<0.1	<0.1	<0.1	<0.1	0	0	0	0	0	1	<1	1	0	<0.1	<0.1
0	0	<0.1	<0.1	<0.1	<0.1	0	0	0	0	0	1	<1	1	0	<0.1	<0.1
0	3	<0.1	<0.1	0.1	<0.1	5	<0.1	8	<0.1	8	8	12	63	6	0.2	0.1
0	0	<0.1	<0.1	0.1	0	0	0	0	0	2	3	3	27	3	0.1	<0.1
0	0	<0.1	<0.1	0.1	0	0	0	0	0	2	3	3	27	3	0.1	<0.1
0	0	0	<0.1	0.2	<0.1	2	0	0	0	16	26	12	153	17	0.7	0.1
0	0	0	<0.1	0.2	<0.1	2	0	0	0	16	26	12	153	17	0.7	0.1
0	0	<0.1	0.1	0.4	0.1	2	0	0	0	14	41	7	225	21	0.8	0.2
0	0							0	0	<1		<1			<0.1	
0	0	<0.1	<0.1	0.2	0.1	2	0	0	0	16	32	9	126	18	0.5	0.2
0	0	0	0	0	0	0	0	0	0	12	0	50	5	2	<0.1	0.2
0	0	0	0	0	0	0	0	0	0	5	25	10	5	0	0.3	<0.1
0							0				33	30	0				
0							0				33	37	36				
0	0	<0.1	0.1	0	0	0	0	0	0	7	21	19	19	2	0.3	<0.1
0	0	0	0	0	0	0	0	0	0	12	0	30	2	2	0.1	0.2
0							0				0	37	0				
0	0	0	0	0	0	0	0	0	0	9	26	38	9	2	<0.1	0.1
0	0	0	0	0	0	0	0	0	0	7	27	25	2	0	0.1	0.1
0	0	0	0	0	0	0	0	0	0	7	0	17	2	2	0.4	0.1
0	0	0	0	0	0	0	0	0	0	7	0	37	2	2	0.2	0.2
0	0	0	0	<0.1	0	0	0	0	0	5	0	22	2	2	0.3	0.1
0	0	0	0	0	0	0	0	0	0	12	2	30	5	2	0.1	0.2
0	0	0	0	0	0	0	0	0	0	12	0	32	2	2	0.1	0.2
15	80							2		250		110			0	
30	60							2		250		105			0	
15	60							1		250		100			0	
25	40							1		250		95			0	
25	100							4		400		170			0	
45	80							4		400		170			0	
55	150							2		400		160			2.7	
70	150							2		400		150			2.7	
0	0	0	<0.1	0.4	0	0	0	0	0	5	5	9	61	5	0.1	<0.1
0	0	<0.1	0.2	0.5	<0.1	5	0	0	<0.1	5	7	5	116	7	<0.1	<0.1

ESHA, EatRight Analysis CD-ROM; **AMT,** amount; **WT,** weight; **CAL,** calories; **WTR,** water; **PROT,** protein; **CARB,** carbohydrate; **FIBR,** fiber; **FAT,** fat; **SATF,** saturated fat; **MONO,** monosaturated fat; **POLY,** polyunsaturated fat

ESHA CODE	FOOD DESCRIPTION	AMT	UNIT	WT (g)	CAL (kcal)	WTR (g)	PROT (g)	CARB (g)	FIBR (g)	FAT (g)	SATF (g)	MONO (g)	POLY (g)
Beverages (continued)													
Coffees & Coffee Substitutes (continued)													
20686	Coffee-Decaf	1	cup	236.8	0	235	<1	0	0	0	<0.1	0	<0.1
20091	Coffee-Decaf-Prep from Instant	1	cup	179	4	177	<1	1	0	0	<0.1	0	<0.1
20023	Coffee-Prep from Instant	1	cup	238.4	5	236	<1	1	0	0	<0.1	0	<0.1
20439	Espresso	1	cup	237	5	232	<1	0	0	<1	0.2	0	0.2
20972	Espresso-Decaf	1	cup	237	0	232	<1	0	0	<1	0.2	0	0.2
22517	French Van Coffee, dry mix	1	svg	14	65	<1	<1	10	<1	3	0.6		
20048	Postum Coffee Substitute	1	cup	240	14	236	<1	3	1	<1	<0.1	<0.1	<0.1
Fruit Flavored Drinks													
20052	Five Alive Citrus Drink	1	cup	248	124	217	<1	30	<1	<1	0	0	0
20131	Fruit Punch-Prep w/Water	1	cup	262	97	237	0	25	0	<1	<0.1	<0.1	<0.1
20967	Fruit Drink-LowCal-Pwd	1	tsp	2	5	<1	<1	2	<1	<1	<0.1	<0.1	<0.1
20024	Fruit Punch Drink, Canned	1	cup	248	117	218	0	30	<1	0	0	<0.1	<0.1
20035	Fruit Punch Drink, Prep from Frzn	1	cup	247.2	114	218	<1	29	<1	0	<0.1	<0.1	<0.1
20101	Grape Drink-Canned	1	cup	250.4	153	211	0	39	0	0	0	0	0
3064	Grape Juice-FrznConc+Water	1	cup	250	128	217	<1	32	<1	<1	0.1	<0.1	0.1
20158	Hi-C Fruit Punch-Box	1	ea	250.1	130		0	34	0	0	0	0	0
20000	Lemonade, Prep from Frozen	1	cup	248	131	213	<1	34	<1	<1	<0.1	<0.1	<0.1
20045	Lemonade, Prep from Mix	1	cup	266	112	237	0	29	0	0	<0.1	<0.1	<0.1
20047	Lemonade-LoCal, Prep from Mix	1	cup	236.8	5	235	<1	1	0	0	0	0	<0.1
20002	Limeade, Prep from Frozen	1	cup	247.2	104	220	<1	26	0	<1	0	0	0
20004	Orange Drink, Prep from Mix	1	cup	248	122	216	0	31	<1	0	0	0	0
20025	Pineapple Orange Drink, Canned	1	cup	250.4	125	218	3	30	<1	0	0	0	0
20117	Pink Lemonade, Prep from Frzn	1	cup	247.2	99	221	<1	26	0	0	<0.1	<0.1	<0.1
20070	Sunny Delight Orange Ade	1	cup	248	122	217	0	31	0	<1	<0.1	<0.1	<0.1
Juices													
3008	Apple Juice-Canned/Bottled	1	cup	248	117	218	<1	29	<1	<1	<0.1	<0.1	0.1
3010	Apple Juice-FrznConc+Water	1	cup	239	112	210	<1	28	<1	<1	<0.1	<0.1	0.1
3015	Apricot Nectar-Canned	1	cup	251	141	213	1	36	2	<1	<0.1	0.1	<0.1
5226	Carrot Juice-Canned	1	cup	236	94	210	2	22	2	<1	0.1	<0.1	0.2
20042	Clam and Tomato Juice	1	cup	241.6	116	211	1	26	1	<1	0	0	0
3042	Cranberry Juice Cocktail	1	cup	252.8	137	218	0	34	0	<1	<0.1	<0.1	0.1
3276	CranberryJce Cocktail-LowCal	1	cup	236.8	45	225	<1	11	0	<1	0	0	0
3062	Grape Juice-Canned/Bottled	1	cup	253	154	213	1	38	<1	<1	0.1	<0.1	0.1
3052	Grapefruit Juice-Canned	1	cup	247	94	223	1	22	<1	<1	<0.1	<0.1	0.1
3053	Grapefruit Juice-FrznConc+Water	1	cup	247	101	221	1	24	<1	<1	<0.1	<0.1	0.1
3304	Guava Nectar	1	cup	250	149	211	<1	38	2	<1	0.1	<0.1	0.1
3069	Lemon Juice-Bottled	1	Tbs	15.25	3	14	<1	1	<1	<1	<0.1	<0.1	<0.1
3073	Lime juice-bottled	1	Tbs	15.4	3	14	<1	1	<1	<1	<0.1	<0.1	<0.1
4949	Mango Nectar	1	cup	250	120		0	29	0	0	0	0	0
3046	Orange Juice+Calcium	1	cup	247.2	110	219	2	26	0	0	0	0	0
3092	Orange Juice-Chilled	1	cup	249	110	220	2	25	<1	1	0.1	0.1	0.2
3090	Orange Juice-Fresh	1	cup	248	112	219	2	26	<1	<1	0.1	0.1	0.1
3091	Orange Juice-FrznConc+Water	1	cup	249	112	219	2	27	<1	<1	<0.1	<0.1	<0.1
3226	OrangeStrawberryBanana Juice	1	cup	247.2	110		1	27	0	0	0	0	0

< = Trace amount present   Blank = Not available

CHOL, cholesterol; **V,** vitamin; **THI,** thiamin; **RIB,** riboflavin; **NIA,** niacin; **FOL,** folate; **CALC,** calcium; **PHOS,** phosphate; **SOD,** sodium; **POT,** potassium; **MAG,** magnesium

CHOL (g)	V-A (RE)	THI (mg)	RIB (mg)	NIA (mg)	V-B6 (mg)	FOL (µg)	V-B12 (µg)	V-C (mg)	V-E (mg)	CALC (mg)	PHOS (mg)	SOD (mg)	POT (mg)	MAG (mg)	IRON (mg)	ZINC (mg)
0	0	0	0	0.5	0	0	0	0	0	5	2	5	128	12	0.1	<0.1
0	0	0	<0.1	0.5	0	0	0	0	0	5	7	4	82	9	0.1	0
0	0	0	<0.1	0.6	0	0	0	0	0	10	7	5	72	7	0.1	<0.1
0	0	<0.1	0.4	12.3	<0.1	2	0	<1	<0.1	5	17	33	273	190	0.3	0.1
0	0	<0.1	0.4	12.3	<0.1	2	0	<1	0	5	17	33	273	190	0.3	0.1
0	0									0	2	28	56	76		<0.1
0	0	<0.1	<0.1	0.7	<0.1	2	0	0	<0.1	7	24	10	98	12	0.2	<0.1
0	5	<0.1	<0.1	0.2	<0.1	7	0	36	<0.1	12	10	5	122	10	0.1	<0.1
0	0	0	<0.1	<0.1	0	0	0	9	0	47	0	8	3	3	<0.1	<0.1
0	120	<0.1	0.1	1.6	0.2	<1	0	48	<0.1	16	10	<1	50	5	<0.1	<0.1
0	10	<0.1	0.1	0.1	<0.1	2	0	73	<0.1	20	7	94	77	7	0.2	<0.1
0	3	<0.1	<0.1	0.1	<0.1	2	0	108	0	10	2	10	32	5	0.2	<0.1
0	0	<0.1	<0.1	<0.1	<0.1	0	0	79	0	130	0	40	30	3	0.2	0.3
0	2	<0.1	0.1	0.3	0.1	2	0	60	0	10	10	5	52	10	0.2	0.1
	0						0	100				30				
0	<1	<0.1	0.1	0.1	<0.1	2	0	13	<0.1	10	7	7	50	5	0.5	0.1
0	0	0	<0.1	0	0	0	0	34	0	29	3	19	3	3	0.1	0.1
0	0	0	0	0	0	0	0	6	0	52	24	5	0	2	0.1	<0.1
0	<1	<0.1	<0.1	<0.1	<0.1	2	0	6	0	7	2	5	22	2	<0.1	<0.1
0	191	0	0.2	2.5	0.3	0	0	73	0	126	47	10	60	2	<0.1	<0.1
0	5	0.1	<0.1	0.5	0.1	23	0	56	0.1	13	10	8	115	15	0.7	0.2
0	<1	<0.1	0.1	<0.1	<0.1	5	0	10	0	7	5	7	37	5	0.4	0.1
0	5	0	0	<0.1	0	5	0	142	<0.1	12	2	7	45	5	0.1	<0.1
0	<1	0.1	<0.1	0.2	0.1	0	0	2	<0.1	17	17	7	295	7	0.9	0.1
0	0	<0.1	<0.1	0.1	0.1	0	0	1	<0.1	14	17	17	301	12	0.6	0.1
0	331	<0.1	<0.1	0.7	0.1	3	0	2	0.8	18	23	8	286	13	1	0.2
0	4512	0.2	0.1	0.9	0.5	9	0	20	2.7	57	99	68	689	33	1.1	0.4
0	34	0.1	<0.1	0.6	0.1	19	0.1	12	0.3	19	27	875	215	12	0.4	0.2
0	2	0	0	0.1	0	0	0	107	0.6	8	3	5	35	3	0.3	0.1
0	<1	0	<0.1	<0.1	<0.1	0	0	76	0.1	21	2	7	59	5	0.1	<0.1
0	2	0.1	0.1	0.7	0.2	8	0	<1	0	23	28	8	334	25	0.6	0.1
0	2	0.1	<0.1	0.6	<0.1	25	0	72	0.1	17	27	2	378	25	0.5	0.2
0	2	0.1	0.1	0.5	0.1	10	0	83	0.1	20	35	2	336	27	0.3	0.1
0	21	<0.1	<0.1	0.4	<0.1	3	0	47	0.4	11	10	7	93	5	0.1	0.1
0	<1	<0.1	<0.1	<0.1	<0.1	2	0	4	<0.1	2	1	3	16	1	<0.1	<0.1
0	<1	<0.1	<0.1	<0.1	<0.1	1	0	1	<0.1	2	2	2	12	1	<0.1	<0.1
0	100									12	40		10	105		0.7
0	0	0.2		0.8	0.1	60		108	0	350		0	450		0	
0	20	0.3	0.1	0.7	0.1	45	0	82	0.5	25	27	2	473	27	0.4	0.1
0	50	0.2	0.1	1	0.1	74	0	124	0.1	27	42	2	496	27	0.5	0.1
0	25	0.2	<0.1	0.5	0.1	110	0	97	0.5	22	40	2	473	25	0.2	0.1
0	0	0		0	0	0		6	0	20		5	380		0	

ESHA, EatRight Analysis CD-ROM; **AMT,** amount; **WT,** weight; **CAL,** calories; **WTR,** water; **PROT,** protein; **CARB,** carbohydrate; **FIBR,** fiber; **FAT,** fat; **SATF,** saturated fat; **MONO,** monosaturated fat; **POLY,** polyunsaturated fat

ESHA CODE	FOOD DESCRIPTION	AMT	UNIT	WT (g)	CAL (kcal)	WTR (g)	PROT (g)	CARB (g)	FIBR (g)	FAT (g)	SATF (g)	MONO (g)	POLY (g)
Beverages (continued)													
Juices (continued)													
3095	Papaya Nectar-Canned	1	cup	250	142	213	<1	36	2	<1	0.1	0.1	0.1
3120	Pineapple Juice-Canned-Unswt	1	cup	250	132	216	1	32	1	<1	<0.1	<0.1	0.1
3128	Prune Juice-Bottled	1	cup	256	182	208	2	45	3	<1	<0.1	0.1	<0.1
3102	TangerineOrange Juice	1	cup	247.2	110	220	2	25	0	0	0	0	0
5397	Tomato Juice-Canned-LowSod	1	cup	243	41	228	2	10	1	<1	<0.1	<0.1	0.1
5188	Tomato Juice-Canned-Regular	1	cup	243	41	228	2	10	1	<1	<0.1	<0.1	0.1
20080	V-8 Juice-LowSodium	1	cup	242	46	226	2	11	2	<1	<0.1	<0.1	0.1
Other Beverages													
20421	All Sport Drink, Fruit Punch	1	cup	240	53		0	15	0	0	0	0	0
21	Cocoa, Prep w/Whole Milk	1	cup	250	192	206	9	27	2	6	3.6	1.7	0.1
46	Cocoa-SugarFree, Prep from Mix	1	cup	256	74	236	3	14	1	1	0	0.2	<0.1
62599	Diet Drink-Straw Supreme-PwdScp	1	ea	33	120		5	25	4	<1	0	0	0
20648	Gatorade	1	cup	240.9	63	225	0	15	0	<1	0	0	0
48	Hot Cocoa-Prep w/water	1	cup	274.67	151	237	2	32	1	2	0.9	0.5	<0.1
27	Instant Breakfast+ Skim Milk	1	cup	282	216	225	16	36		1	0.7		
101	Instant Breakfast+1% Milk	1	cup	281	233	223	15	36	<1	3	1.8		
26	Instant Breakfast+2% Milk	1	cup	281	280	217	15	36	<1	9	5.3		
25	Instant Breakfast+Whole Milk	1	cup	281	253	220	15	36	<1	5	3.1		
41	Nestle's Quik-Strawberry+Milk	1	cup	266	234	215	8	33	0	8	5.1	2.4	0.3
38	Ovaltine Drink-Choc Flavor	1	cup	265	223	216	9	29	1	9	5	2.2	0.5
20925	Soy Eggnog, Silk, LowFat	0.5	cup	127	90		3	15	0	2	0		
Teas													
20118	Camomile Tea, Brewed	1	cup	236.8	2	236	0	<1	0	0	<0.1	<0.1	<0.1
20924	Chai Tea, Soy Milk-Silk	1	cup	248	140		6	19	0	4	0		
20036	Herbal Tea, Brewed	1	cup	236.8	2	236	0	<1	0	0	<0.1	<0.1	<0.1
20014	Tea-Brewed	1	cup	236.8	2	236	0	1	0	0	<0.1	<0.1	<0.1
20079	Tea-Decaf-LoCal-Prep from Frzn	1	cup	245	6	243	<1	2	0	<1	<0.1	<0.1	<0.1
20040	Tea-Lemon-LoCal-Prep from Inst	1	cup	236.8	5	235	<1	1	0	0	0	0	<0.1
20020	Tea-Prep from Instant	1	cup	236.8	2	236	<1	<1	0	0	0	0	0
20022	Tea-Sweet-Prep from Instant	1	cup	259	91	236	<1	22	<1	<1	<0.1	<0.1	<0.1
62652	UltraSlimFast Choc Pwdr Scoop	1	svg	33	120		5	23	5	2	0.5	0	0
Waters													
20050	Bottled Water-Perrier	1	cup	236.5	0	236	0	0	0	0	0	0	0
20051	Bottled Water-PolandSprings	1	cup	237	0	237	0	0	0	0	0	0	0
20010	Tonic / Quinine Water	1	cup	244	83	222	0	21	0	0	0	0	0
4793	Tonic Water-Diet	1	cup	244	0	244	0	0	0	0	0	0	0
20041	Water	1	cup	236.5	0	236	0	0	0	0	0	0	0
Condiments & Accompaniments													
Condiments													
27000	Catsup/Ketchup	1	Tbs	15	15	10	<1	4	<1	<1	<0.1	<0.1	<0.1
27001	Catsup/Ketchup-Packet	1	ea	6	6	4	<1	2	<1	<1	<0.1	<0.1	<0.1
27004	Horseradish-Prepared	1	tsp	5	2	4	<1	1	<1	<1	<0.1	<0.1	<0.1
8046	Mayonnaise	1	Tbs	13.8	99	2	<1	1	0	11	1.6	2.7	5.9

< = Trace amount present   Blank = Not available

CHOL, cholesterol; **V,** vitamin; **THI,** thiamin; **RIB,** riboflavin; **NIA,** niacin; **FOL,** folate;
CALC, calcium; **PHOS,** phosphate; **SOD,** sodium; **POT,** potassium; **MAG,** magnesium

CHOL (g)	V-A (RE)	THI (mg)	RIB (mg)	NIA (mg)	V-B6 (mg)	FOL (µg)	V-B12 (µg)	V-C (mg)	V-E (mg)	CALC (mg)	PHOS (mg)	SOD (mg)	POT (mg)	MAG (mg)	IRON (mg)	ZINC (mg)
0	90	<0.1	<0.1	0.4	<0.1	5	0	8	0.6	25	0	12	78	8	0.9	0.4
0	1	0.1	0.1	0.5	0.2	45	0	25	<0.1	32	20	5	325	30	0.8	0.3
0	1	<0.1	0.2	2	0.6	0	0	10	0.3	31	64	10	707	36	3	0.5
0	0	0.2		0.8	0.1	60		27	0	20		0	450		0	
0	112	0.1	0.1	1.6	0.3	49	0	44	0.8	24	44	24	556	27	1	0.4
0	112	0.1	0.1	1.6	0.3	49	0	44	0.8	24	44	654	556	27	1	0.4
0	378	0.1	0.1	1.8	0.3	51	0	67	0.8	27	41	653	467	27	1	0.5
0	0						0	0		0	7	37	37		0	
20	128	0.1	0.5	0.3	0.1	12	1	1	0.1	262	262	110	492	58	1.2	1.6
0	36	0.1	0.3	0.2	0.1	3	0.3	<1	0.1	120	179	228	540	44	1	0.7
5	150	0.4	0.2	10	0.6	100	2.1	27	13.6	150	100	130	170	100	6.3	4.5
0		<0.1		0.5	0.1			1	0	2	22	94	34	2	0.5	0.6
3	1	<0.1	0.2	0.2	<0.1	0	0.5	1	0.2	60	118	195	269	33	0.5	0.6
9	469	0.4	0.4	5.5	0.5	118	1.6	31	5.3	407	406	268	755	112	4.8	4.1
14	469	0.4	0.5	5.5	0.5	118	1.5	31	5.4	406	392	267	731	119	4.9	4.1
38	630	0.4	0.5	5.5	0.5	118	1.5	31	5.5	396	386	262	721	117	4.9	4.1
24	469	0.4	0.5	5.5	0.5	118	1.5	31	5.5	403	390	264	726	119	4.9	4.1
32	69	0.1	0.4	0.2	0.1	13	0.9	2	0.3	293	229	128	370	32	0.2	0.9
26	904	0.8	1.3	11.1	1	19	1.1	32	0.2	339	289	231	578	45	3.8	1.2
0	0							0		20		75			0.7	
0	5	<0.1	<0.1	0	0	2	0	0	0	5	0	2	21	2	0.2	0.1
0	60		0.3				0.9	0		300		50			1.1	0.9
0	0	<0.1	<0.1	0	0	2	0	0	0	5	0	2	21	2	0.2	0.1
0	0	0	<0.1	0	0	12	0	0	0	0	2	7	88	7	<0.1	<0.1
0	0	0	<0.1	0	0	13	0	0	0	<1	2	7	90	7	<0.1	<0.1
0	0	0	<0.1	<0.1	<0.1	0	0	0	0	7	2	9	31	2	0.1	<0.1
0	0	0	<0.1	0.1	<0.1	0	0	0	0	7	2	5	43	2	<0.1	<0.1
0	0	<0.1	0	<0.1	<0.1	0	0	0	0	5	0	5	39	3	0.1	<0.1
5	150	0.4	0.2	10	0.6	100	2.1	27	13.6	150	100	100	200	100	6.3	4.5
0	0	0	0	0	0	0	0	0	0	33	0	2	0	0	0	0
0	0	0	0	0	0	0	0	0	0	2	0	2	0	2	<0.1	0
0	0	0	0	0	0	0	0	0	0	2	0	29	0	0	<0.1	0.2
0								0				35				
0	0	0	0	0	0	0	0	0	0	7	0	7	2	2	0	0
0	14	<0.1	<0.1	0.2	<0.1	2	0	2	0.2	3	5	167	57	3	0.1	<0.1
0	6	<0.1	<0.1	0.1	<0.1	1	0	1	0.1	1	2	67	23	1	<0.1	<0.1
0	<1	<0.1	<0.1	<0.1	<0.1	3	0	1	<0.1	3	2	16	12	1	<0.1	<0.1
5	11	0	0	<0.1	0.1	1	<0.1	0	0.7	2	4	78	5	<1	0.1	<0.1

ESHA, EatRight Analysis CD-ROM; **AMT,** amount; **WT,** weight; **CAL,** calories; **WTR,** water; **PROT,** protein; **CARB,** carbohydrate; **FIBR,** fiber; **FAT,** fat; **SATF,** saturated fat; **MONO,** monosaturated fat; **POLY,** polyunsaturated fat

ESHA CODE	FOOD DESCRIPTION	AMT	UNIT	WT (g)	CAL (kcal)	WTR (g)	PROT (g)	CARB (g)	FIBR (g)	FAT (g)	SATF (g)	MONO (g)	POLY (g)
Condiments & Accompaniments (continued)													
Condiments (continued)													
8069	Mayonnaise-FatFree	1	Tbs	16	11	13	<1	2	<1	<1	0.1		
8032	Mayonnaise-Imitation	1	Tbs	15	35	9	<1	2	0	3	0.5	0.7	1.6
44462	Mayonnaise-LowSod-LowCal	1	Tbs	14	32	9	<1	2	0	3	0.5	0.6	1.5
8021	Miracle Whip	1	Tbs	14.7	57	6	<1	4	0	5	0.7	1.3	2.6
8122	Miracle Whip-Light	1	Tbs	14	37	8	<1	3	0	3	0.4	0.6	1.5
435	Mustard-Yellow-Prepared	1	tsp	5	3	4	<1	<1	<1	<1	<0.1	0.1	<0.1
Gravies													
53023	Beef Gravy-Canned	.5	cup	116.5	62	102	4	6	<1	3	1.3	1.1	0.1
53006	Beef Gravy-Homemade	0.5	cup	135	107	115	3	7	1	8	1.9	3.4	2
53022	Chicken Gravy-Canned	.5	cup	119	94	102	2	6	<1	7	1.7	3	1.8
53005	Chicken Gravy-Homemade	0.5	cup	130	97	110	6	6		5	1.4	2.2	1.3
53026	Mushroom Gravy-Canned	.5	cup	119	60	106	1	7	<1	3	0.5	1.4	1.2
53033	Turkey Gravy-Canned	.5	cup	119.2	61	106	3	6	<1	3	0.7	1.1	0.6
Jams													
23000	Apple Butter	1	Tbs	18	31	10	<1	8	<1	0	0	0	0
23278	Fruit Spread-LowCal-Strawberry	1	Tbs	17	25	11	0	6	0	0	0	0	0
23054	Jam/Preserves	1	Tbs	20	56	6	<1	14	<1	<1	<0.1	<0.1	0
23003	Jelly	1	Tbs	19	51	6	<1	13	<1	<1	<0.1	<0.1	<0.1
23165	Jelly-Reduced Sugar	1	Tbs	18.8	34	10	<1	9	<1	<1	<0.1	<0.1	<0.1
23005	Marmalade-Orange	1	Tbs	20	49	7	<1	13	<1	0	0	0	0
Salad Dressings													
8024	1000 Island Dressing	1	Tbs	15.6	58	7	<1	2	<1	5	0.8	1.2	2.8
8023	1000 Island Dressing-LowCal	1	Tbs	15.3	31	9	<1	3	<1	2	0.1	1	0.4
8013	Blue Cheese Dressing	2	Tbs	30.6	154	10	1	2	0	16	3	3.8	8.5
44705	Caesar Dressing	2	Tbs	29.4	155	10	<1	1	<1	17	2.6	4	9.7
8498	Catalina Dressing-FatFree	2	Tbs	33	35		0	8	1	0	0	0	0
8015	French Dressing	1	Tbs	15.6	71	6	<1	2	0	7	0.9	1.3	3.3
44467	French Dressing-FatFree	1	Tbs	16	21	10	<1	5	<1	<1	<0.1	<0.1	<0.1
8014	French Dressing-LowCal	1	Tbs	16.3	38	9	<1	5	<1	2	0.2	1	0.8
8504	HoneyDijon Dressing-FatFree	2	Tbs	34	50		1	10	1	0	0	0	0
8530	Honey Mustard Dressing	2	Tbs	30	160		0	8	<1	15	2		
8020	Italian Dressing	1	Tbs	14.7	43	8	<1	2	0	4	0.7	0.9	1.9
8491	Italian Dressing-FatFree	2	Tbs	33	20	27	<1	4	<1	<1	0.2		
8016	Italian Dressing-LowCal	1	Tbs	15	11	13	<1	1	0	1	0.1	0.3	0.3
8035	Oil & Vinegar Dressing	1	Tbs	15.6	70	7	0	<1	0	8	1.4	2.3	3.8
8555	Ranch Dressing	2	Tbs	29	148	11	<1	1	<1	16	2.4		
8493	Ranch Dressing-FatFree	2	Tbs	35	48	22	<1	11	<1	<1	0.1		
8022	Russian Dressing	1	Tbs	15.3	54	6	<1	5	<1	4	0.6	0.9	2.3
8123	Yogurt Dressing	1	Tbs	15.4	11	13	<1	1	<1	1	0.3	0.2	0.1
Sauces													
53388	Alfredo Sauce-DiGiorno	0.25	cup	62	180		3	3	0	18	7		
53000	Barbecue Sauce	.25	cup	62.5	94	38	0	23	<1	<1	0	<0.1	0.1
9570	Creamy Garlic Alfredo Sauce	0.25	cup	61	100	45	2	3	0	10	4		
53016	Curry Sauce	0.5	cup	115	74	102	3	3	<1	6	1		

< = Trace amount present   Blank = Not available

CHOL, cholesterol; **V,** vitamin; **THI,** thiamin; **RIB,** riboflavin; **NIA,** niacin; **FOL,** folate;
CALC, calcium; **PHOS,** phosphate; **SOD,** sodium; **POT,** potassium; **MAG,** magnesium

CHOL (g)	V-A (RE)	THI (mg)	RIB (mg)	NIA (mg)	V-B6 (mg)	FOL (µg)	V-B12 (µg)	V-C (mg)	V-E (mg)	CALC (mg)	PHOS (mg)	SOD (mg)	POT (mg)	MAG (mg)	IRON (mg)	ZINC (mg)
2	3							0	0.5	1	4	120	8		<0.1	
4	0	0	0	0	0	0	0	0	0.3	0	0	75	2	0	0	<0.1
3	0	0	<0.1	0	0	0	<0.1	0	0.9	0	0	15	1	0	0	<0.1
4	4	<0.1	<0.1	<0.1	<0.1	1	<0.1	0	0.3	2	4	105	1	<1	<0.1	<0.1
4	4	<0.1	<0.1	0	<0.1	1	<0.1	0	0.4	2	4	97	3	<1	<0.1	<0.1
0	<1	<0.1	<0.1	<0.1	<0.1	<1	0	<1	<0.1	3	5	57	7	2	0.1	<0.1
3	1	<0.1	<0.1	0.8	<0.1	2	0.1	0	<0.1	7	35	652	94	2	0.8	1.2
3	150	<0.1	0.1	0.6	<0.1	3	0.1	0	0.2	27	39	779	147	3	0.6	1.1
2	1	<0.1	0.1	0.5	<0.1	2	0.1	0	0.2	24	35	687	130	2	0.6	1
55	326	<0.1	0.2	1.6	0.1	49	2.3	1	0.3	16	62	683	151	5	1.5	1.5
0	0	<0.1	0.1	0.8	<0.1	14	0	0	0.1	8	18	678	126	2	0.8	0.8
2	0	<0.1	0.1	1.5	<0.1	2	0.1	0	0.1	5	35	688	130	2	0.8	1
0	<1	<0.1	<0.1	<0.1	<0.1	<1	0	<1	<0.1	3	1	3	16	1	0.1	<0.1
0	0							0		0		0			0	
0	0	<0.1	<0.1	<0.1	<0.1	2	0	2	<0.1	4	4	6	15	1	0.1	<0.1
0	<1	<0.1	<0.1	<0.1	<0.1	<1	0	<1	0	1	1	6	10	1	<0.1	<0.1
0	<1	<0.1	<0.1	<0.1	<0.1	<1	0	0	0	1	1	<1	13	1	<0.1	<0.1
0	1	<0.1	<0.1	<0.1	<0.1	2	0	1	<0.1	8	1	11	7	<1	<0.1	<0.1
4	4	0.2	<0.1	0.1	0	0	0	0	0.6	3	4	135	17	1	0.2	<0.1
<1	5	<0.1	<0.1	0.1	0	0	0	0	0.2	2	2	127	31	1	0.1	<0.1
5	21	<0.1	<0.1	<0.1	<0.1	9	0.1	1	1.8	25	23	335	11	0	0.1	0.1
1	1	<0.1	<0.1	<0.1	0	1	<0.1	0	1.5	7	6	317	9	1	0.1	<0.1
0	0							0		0		320			0	
0	7	<0.1	<0.1	<0.1	0	0	<0.1	0	0.8	4	3	130	10	1	0.1	<0.1
0	1	<0.1	<0.1	<0.1	0	2	0	0	<0.1	1	0	128	13	<1	0.1	<0.1
0	9	<0.1	<0.1	0.1	<0.1	<1	0	0	<0.1	2	3	131	17	1	0.1	<0.1
0	0							0		0		340			0	
5	0							0		0		160			0	
0	1	<0.1	<0.1	0	<0.1	0	0	0	0.7	1	1	243	7	<1	0.1	<0.1
1	11							<1		14	68	430	38		0.1	
1	<1	0	<0.1	0	<0.1	0	0	0	<0.1	1	2	205	13	1	0.1	<0.1
0	0	0	0	0	0	0	0	0	0.7	0	0	<1	1	0	0	0
8	2							<1		8	26	287	14		0.1	
<1	1							<1		9	28	354	31		<0.1	
0	13	<0.1	<0.1	0.1	<0.1	1	0	1	0.5	3	3	144	26	2	0.1	<0.1
2	4	<0.1	<0.1	<0.1	<0.1	1	<0.1	<1	<0.1	15	12	6	22	2	<0.1	0.1
25	0							0		0		600			0	
0	15	<0.1	<0.1	0.3	<0.1	1	0	<1	0.4	8	11	699	130	8	0.1	0.1
30	40							0		40		360			0	
0	44	<0.1	<0.1	1.6	<0.1	5	0.1	<1	0.8	9	38	392	103	3	0.5	0.1

ESHA, EatRight Analysis CD-ROM; **AMT**, amount; **WT**, weight; **CAL**, calories; **WTR**, water; **PROT**, protein; **CARB**, carbohydrate; **FIBR**, fiber; **FAT**, fat; **SATF**, saturated fat; **MONO**, monosaturated fat; **POLY**, polyunsaturated fat

ESHA CODE	FOOD DESCRIPTION	AMT	UNIT	WT (g)	CAL (kcal)	WTR (g)	PROT (g)	CARB (g)	FIBR (g)	FAT (g)	SATF (g)	MONO (g)	POLY (g)
Condiments & Accompaniments (continued)													
Sauces (continued)													
9054	Enchilada Sauce	0.25	cup	61	20	56	0	3	0	1	0		
53233	Enchilada Sauce-Mild Green Chili	0.25	cup	61	30	55	1	3	0	2	0		
27135	French Onion Dip	2	Tbs	31	60		1	3	0	4	3		
53406	Horseradish Sauce	1	tsp	5	20		0	1	0	2	0		
53524	Marinara Sauce	0.5	cup	125	92	103	2	14	1	3	0.5	1	1.3
7563	Miso Sauce	1	cup	248	389	141	13	73	6	7	1	1.5	3.8
53106	Pesto Sauce	2	Tbs	29	155	6	6	2	1	14	3.8	8.7	1
53466	Salsa Ready-to-Serve	.25	cup	64.8	17	58	1	4	1	<1	<0.1	<0.1	0.1
53718	Spaghetti Sauce w/Meat-Cnd	0.5	cup	125	60	105	3	14	3	1	0		
53010	Spaghetti Sauce w/Meat-Recipe	1	cup	248	287	189	16	21		17	4.5	6.2	4.3
51018	Spaghetti Sauce w/Mushroom-Cnd	0.5	cup	125	60	106	2	14	2	1	0		
53085	Tabasco Sauce/PepperSauce	1	Tbs	15.6	2	15	<1	<1	<1	<1	<0.1	<0.1	<0.1
53415	Tartar Sauce-NonFat-Kraft	2	Tbs	32	25		0	5	0	0	0	0	0
53004	Teriyaki Sauce	1	Tbs	18	15	12	1	3	<1	0	0	0	0
53468	White Sauce	1	cup	250	368	187	10	23	1	27	7.1	11.1	7.2
Spices & Seasonings													
26001	Basil-Dried	1	tsp	1.4	4	<1	<1	1	1	<1	<0.1	<0.1	<0.1
26040	Celery Seed	1	tsp	2	8	<1	<1	1	<1	1	<0.1	0.3	0.1
26002	Chili Powder	1	tsp	2.6	8	<1	<1	1	1	<1	0.1	0.1	0.2
26003	Cinnamon	1	tsp	2.3	6	<1	<1	2	1	<1	<0.1	<0.1	<0.1
26038	Coriander/Cilantro-Fresh	0.25	cup	4	1	4	<1	<1	<1	<1	<0.1	<0.1	<0.1
26004	Curry Powder	1	tsp	2	6	<1	<1	1	1	<1	<0.1	0.1	0.1
26021	Dill Weed-Dried	1	tsp	1	3	<1	<1	1	<1	<1	<0.1		
26007	Garlic Powder	1	tsp	2.8	9	<1	<1	2	<1	<1	<0.1	<0.1	<0.1
26023	Ginger-Ground	1	tsp	1.8	6	<1	<1	1	<1	<1	<0.1	<0.1	<0.1
26008	Onion Powder	1	tsp	2.1	7	<1	<1	2	<1	<1	<0.1	<0.1	<0.1
26009	Oregano-Ground	1	tsp	1.5	5	<1	<1	1	1	<1	<0.1	<0.1	0.1
26010	Paprika	1	tsp	2.1	6	<1	<1	1	1	<1	<0.1	<0.1	0.2
26016	Pepper-Black	1	tsp	2.1	5	<1	<1	1	1	<1	<0.1	<0.1	<0.1
26037	Pepper-White	1	tsp	2.4	7	<1	<1	2	1	<1	<0.1	<0.1	<0.1
26031	Sage-Ground	1	tsp	0.7	2	<1	<1	<1	<1	<1	<0.1	<0.1	<0.1
26014	Salt	.25	tsp	1.5	0	<1	0	0	0	0	0	0	0
26091	Salt Substitute (Morton)	0.25	tsp	1.1	1	<1	<1	<1	0	<1			
26048	Salt-Light (Morton)	0.25	tsp	1.4	<1	<1	0	<1		<1			
Spreads & Pastes													
90737	Chicken Salad, cnd	1	svg	118	171	87	6	12		11	2.3	3.5	4.2
13034	Ham Salad Spread	1	Tbs	15	32	9	1	2	0	2	0.8	1.1	0.4
7081	Hummous/Hummus	2	Tbs	30.75	54	20	1	6	1	3	0.3	1.5	0.6
56007	Tuna Salad	.5	cup	102.5	192	65	16	10	0	9	1.6	3	4.2
Dairy Products & Non-Dairy Substitutes													
Cheese - Natural													
1003	Blue Cheese	.25	cup	33.75	119	14	7	1	0	10	6.3	2.6	0.3
1037	Brick Cheese-Shredded	.25	cup	28.25	105	12	7	1	0	8	5.3	2.4	0.2

< = Trace amount present   Blank = Not available

CHOL, cholesterol; V, vitamin; THI, thiamin; RIB, riboflavin; NIA, niacin; FOL, folate; CALC, calcium; PHOS, phosphate; SOD, sodium; POT, potassium; MAG, magnesium

CHOL (g)	V-A (RE)	THI (mg)	RIB (mg)	NIA (mg)	V-B6 (mg)	FOL (µg)	V-B12 (µg)	V-C (mg)	V-E (mg)	CALC (mg)	PHOS (mg)	SOD (mg)	POT (mg)	MAG (mg)	IRON (mg)	ZINC (mg)
0	75							1		0		380			0	
0	0							6		0		330			0	
0	0							0		0		210			0	
5	0							0		0		35			0	
0	68	<0.1	0.1	4.9	0.2	14	0	4	2.5	34	45	601	470	26	1.1	0.7
0	10	0.1	0.3	1	0.2	37	0	0	<0.1	77	173	4062	208	53	3.2	3.7
10	42	<0.1	0.1	0.2	<0.1	7	0.2	2	1.4	220	113	238	91	16	1.1	0.5
0	19	<0.1	<0.1	<0.1	0.1	3	0	1	0.8	17	20	389	192	10	0.3	0.2
0	150							9		40		720			1.4	
46	487	0.2	0.3	6	0.5	30	1.4	37	5.3	59	173	868	1099	62	3.5	3.4
0	75							9		40		630			1.4	
<1	65							<1	0.1	4	3	93	20	1	0.4	<0.1
0	0							0		0		200			0	
0	0	<0.1	<0.1	0.2	<0.1	4	0	0	0	4	28	690	40	11	0.3	<0.1
18	230	0.2	0.5	1	0.1	20	0.7	2	0.7	295	245	885	390	35	0.8	1
0	13	<0.1	<0.1	0.1	<0.1	4	0	1	0.1	30	7	<1	48	6	0.6	0.1
0	<1	<0.1	<0.1	0.1	<0.1	<1	0	<1	<0.1	35	11	3	28	9	0.9	0.1
0	77	<0.1	<0.1	0.2	0.1	3	0	2	0.8	7	8	26	50	4	0.4	0.1
0	1	<0.1	<0.1	<0.1	<0.1	1	0	1	<0.1	28	1	1	12	1	0.9	<0.1
0	27	<0.1	<0.1	<0.1	<0.1	2	0	1	0.1	3	2	2	21	1	0.1	<0.1
0	2	<0.1	<0.1	0.1	<0.1	3	0	<1	0.4	10	7	1	31	5	0.6	0.1
0	6	<0.1	<0.1	<0.1	<0.1		0	<1		18	5	2	33	5	0.5	<0.1
0	0	<0.1	<0.1	<0.1	0.1	<1	0	1	<0.1	2	12	1	31	2	0.1	0.1
0	<1	<0.1	<0.1	0.1	<0.1	1	0	<1	0.3	2	3	1	24	3	0.2	0.1
0	0	<0.1	<0.1	<0.1	<0.1	3	0	<1	<0.1	8	7	1	20	3	0.1	<0.1
0	10	<0.1	<0.1	0.1	<0.1	4	0	1	0.3	24	3	<1	25	4	0.7	0.1
0	111	<0.1	<0.1	0.3	0.1	2	0	1	0.6	4	7	1	49	4	0.5	0.1
0	1	<0.1	<0.1	<0.1	<0.1	<1	0	<1	<0.1	9	4	1	26	4	0.6	<0.1
0	0	<0.1	<0.1	<0.1	<0.1	<1	0	1	0.1	6	4	<1	2	2	0.3	<0.1
0	4	<0.1	<0.1	<0.1	<0.1	2	0	<1	0.1	12	1	<1	7	3	0.2	<0.1
0	0	0	0	0	0	0	0	0	0	<1	0	581	<1	<1	<0.1	<0.1
0							0					<1	476			
							0			1		276	354	1		
31	0											552				
6	0	0.1	<0.1	0.3	<0.1	<1	0.1	0	0.3	1	18	137	22	2	0.1	0.2
0	<1	<0.1	<0.1	0.1	0.1	18	0	2	0.2	15	34	74	53	9	0.5	0.3
13	27	<0.1	0.1	6.9	0.1	8	1.2	2	1	17	182	412	182	19	1	0.6
25	69	<0.1	0.1	0.3	0.1	12	0.4	0	0.1	178	131	471	86	8	0.1	0.9
27	84	<0.1	0.1	<0.1	<0.1	6	0.4	0	0.1	190	127	158	38	7	0.1	0.7

ESHA, EatRight Analysis CD-ROM; **AMT,** amount; **WT,** weight; **CAL,** calories; **WTR,** water; **PROT,** protein; **CARB,** carbohydrate; **FIBR,** fiber; **FAT,** fat; **SATF,** saturated fat; **MONO,** monosaturated fat; **POLY,** polyunsaturated fat

ESHA CODE	FOOD DESCRIPTION	AMT	UNIT	WT (g)	CAL (kcal)	WTR (g)	PROT (g)	CARB (g)	FIBR (g)	FAT (g)	SATF (g)	MONO (g)	POLY (g)
Dairy Products & Non-Dairy Substitutes (continued)													
Cheese - Natural (continued)													
1004	Brie Cheese-Sliced	.25	cup	36	120	17	7	<1	0	10	6.3	2.9	0.3
1006	Camembert Cheese	2	Tbs	30.75	92	16	6	<1	0	7	4.7	2.2	0.2
1423	Cheddar Cheese-LowFat	1	oz	28.35	70	13	8	1	0	4	3		
1448	Cheddar Cheese-LowFat-Shred	0.25	cup	28.25	49	18	7	1	0	2	1.2	0.6	0.1
1451	Cheddar Cheese-LowSod-Shred	0.25	cup	28.25	112	11	7	1	0	9	5.9	2.6	0.3
1008	Cheddar Cheese-Shredded	0.25	cup	28.25	114	10	7	<1	0	9	6	2.7	0.3
1010	Colby Cheese-Shredded	0.25	cup	28.25	111	11	7	1	0	9	5.7	2.6	0.3
1047	Cottage Cheese-1% Lowfat	0.5	cup	113	81	93	14	3	0	1	0.7	0.3	<0.1
1014	Cottage Cheese-2% lowfat	0.5	cup	113	102	90	16	4	0	2	1.4	0.6	0.1
1013	CottageCheese-Crm-Lg Curd	0.5	cup	105	108	83	13	3	0	5	3	1.3	0.1
1012	CottageCheese-Crm-Sm Curd	0.5	cup	112.5	116	89	14	3	0	5	3.2	1.4	0.2
1015	Cream Cheese	1	Tbs	14.5	51	8	1	<1	0	5	3.2	1.4	0.2
1115	Cream Cheese-FatFree	1	Tbs	16.5	15	13	2	1	0	0	0	0	0
1098	Cream Cheese-LowFat	1	Tbs	15	35	10	2	1	0	3	1.7	0.7	0.1
1083	Cream Cheese-Soft	1	Tbs	15	50	8	1	<1	0	5	3.5		
1050	Edam Cheese	1	oz	28.35	101	12	7	<1	0	8	5	2.3	0.2
1016	Feta Cheese-Shredded	0.25	cup	37.5	99	21	5	2	0	8	5.6	1.7	0.2
1052	Fontina Cheese-Shredded	0.25	cup	27	105	10	7	<1	0	8	5.2	2.3	0.4
1078	Goat cheese-hard	1	oz	28.35	128	8	9	1	0	10	7	2.3	0.2
1080	Goat cheese-soft type	1	oz	28.35	76	17	5	<1	0	6	4.1	1.4	0.1
1054	Gouda Cheese	1	oz	28.35	101	12	7	1	0	8	5	2.2	0.2
1074	Gruyere Cheese-Shredded	0.25	cup	27	112	9	8	<1	0	9	5.1	2.7	0.5
1017	Monterey Jack Cheese-Shredded	0.25	cup	28.25	105	12	7	<1	0	9	5.4	2.5	0.3
48289	Mozzarella Cheese-LowSod-1"Cube	1	ea	18	50	9	5	1	0	3	2	0.9	0.1
1056	Mozzarella Cheese-Whole-Shred	0.25	cup	28	84	14	6	1	0	6	3.7	1.8	0.2
1058	Mozzarella-PartSkim-Shredded	0.25	cup	28.25	72	15	7	1	0	4	2.9	1.3	0.1
13348	Mozzarella-String-Sticks	1	ea	28	50	16	8	1	0	2	1		
1021	Muenster Cheese-Shredded	0.25	cup	28.25	104	12	7	<1	0	8	5.4	2.5	0.2
1060	Neufchatel Cheese	1	oz	28.35	74	18	3	1	0	7	4.2	1.9	0.2
1075	Parmesan Cheese-Grated	1	Tbs	5	22	1	2	<1	0	1	0.9	0.4	0.1
1112	Parmesan Cheese-Shredded	1	Tbs	5	21	1	2	<1	0	1	0.9	0.4	<0.1
1062	Port du Salut Cheese-Shredded	0.25	cup	28.25	99	13	7	<1	0	8	4.7	2.6	0.2
1023	Provolone Cheese-Diced	0.25	cup	33	116	14	8	1	0	9	5.6	2.4	0.3
1024	Ricotta Cheese-Part Skim	0.5	cup	124	171	92	14	6	0	10	6.1	2.9	0.3
1064	Ricotta Cheese-Whole Milk	0.5	cup	124	216	89	14	4	0	16	10.3	4.5	0.5
1428	Swiss Cheese-LowFat	1	oz	28.35	90	12	8	1	0	6	4		
1027	Swiss Cheese-Shredded	0.25	cup	27	103	10	7	1	0	8	4.8	2	0.3
Cheese - Processed													
1001	American Cheese Food	1	oz	28.35	94	12	6	2	0	7	4.4	2	0.2
47928	American Cheese Spread-Slice	1	ea	34	99	16	6	3	0	7	4.5	2.1	0.2
1287	American Cheese-Nonfat	1	pce	21.2625	31	12	5	2	<1	<1	0.1		
1000	American Processed Cheese	1	pce	21.26	80	8	5	<1	0	7	4.2	1.9	0.2
1002	Cheez Whiz/Cheese Spread	2	Tbs	30.5	88	15	5	3	0	6	4.1	1.9	0.2
1069	Pimento Proc Cheese-Shred	0.25	cup	28.25	106	11	6	<1	<1	9	5.6	2.5	0.3

< = Trace amount present   Blank = Not available

CHOL, cholesterol; **V**, vitamin; **THI,** thiamin; **RIB,** riboflavin; **NIA,** niacin; **FOL,** folate;
CALC, calcium; **PHOS,** phosphate; **SOD,** sodium; **POT,** potassium; **MAG,** magnesium

CHOL (g)	V-A (RE)	THI (mg)	RIB (mg)	NIA (mg)	V-B6 (mg)	FOL (μg)	V-B12 (μg)	V-C (mg)	V-E (mg)	CALC (mg)	PHOS (mg)	SOD (mg)	POT (mg)	MAG (mg)	IRON (mg)	ZINC (mg)
36	63	<0.1	0.2	0.1	0.1	23	0.6	0	0.1	66	68	226	55	7	0.2	0.9
22	74	<0.1	0.2	0.2	0.1	19	0.4	0	0.1	119	107	259	58	6	0.1	0.7
15	60							0		200		170		0		
6	17	<0.1	0.1	<0.1	<0.1	3	0.1	0	<0.1	117	137	173	19	5	0.1	0.5
28	77	<0.1	0.1	<0.1	<0.1	5	0.2	0	0.1	199	137	6	32	8	0.2	0.9
30	77	<0.1	0.1	<0.1	<0.1	5	0.2	0	0.1	204	145	175	28	8	0.2	0.9
27	77	<0.1	0.1	<0.1	<0.1	5	0.2	0	0.1	194	129	171	36	7	0.2	0.9
5	12	<0.1	0.2	0.1	0.1	14	0.7	0	<0.1	69	151	459	97	6	0.2	0.4
9	24	<0.1	0.2	0.2	0.1	15	0.8	0	<0.1	78	171	459	108	7	0.2	0.5
16	47	<0.1	0.2	0.1	0.1	13	0.7	0	<0.1	63	139	425	88	5	0.1	0.4
17	51	<0.1	0.2	0.1	0.1	14	0.7	0	<0.1	68	148	456	94	6	0.2	0.4
16	54	<0.1	<0.1	<0.1	<0.1	2	0.1	0	<0.1	12	15	43	17	1	0.2	0.1
2	50		<0.1				0.1	0		75	100	100	38	0	0	0.2
8	28	<0.1	<0.1	<0.1	<0.1	3	0.1	0	<0.1	17	22	44	25	1	0.3	0.1
15	30		<0.1				0	0		10	20	50	20	0	0	0
25	69	<0.1	0.1	<0.1	<0.1	5	0.4	0	0.1	207	152	274	53	9	0.1	1.1
33	47	0.1	0.3	0.4	0.2	12	0.6	0	0.1	185	126	418	23	7	0.2	1.1
31	71	<0.1	0.1	<0.1	<0.1	2	0.5	0	0.1	148	93	216	17	4	0.1	0.9
30	140	<0.1	0.3	0.7	<0.1	1	<0.1	0	0.1	254	207	98	14	15	0.5	0.5
13	83	<0.1	0.1	0.1	0.1	3	0.1	0	0.1	40	73	104	7	5	0.5	0.3
32	47	<0.1	0.1	<0.1	<0.1	6	0.4	0	0.1	198	155	232	34	8	0.1	1.1
30	74	<0.1	0.1	<0.1	<0.1	3	0.4	0	0.1	273	163	91	22	10	<0.1	1.1
25	58	<0.1	0.1	<0.1	<0.1	5	0.2	0	0.1	211	125	151	23	8	0.2	0.8
10	25	<0.1	0.1	<0.1	<0.1	2	0.2	0	<0.1	132	94	3	17	5	<0.1	0.6
22	52	<0.1	0.1	<0.1	<0.1	2	0.6	0	0.1	141	99	176	21	6	0.1	0.8
18	37	<0.1	0.1	<0.1	<0.1	3	0.2	0	<0.1	221	131	175	24	6	0.1	0.8
5	40							0		200		220			0	
27	84	<0.1	0.1	<0.1	<0.1	3	0.4	0	0.1	203	132	177	38	8	0.1	0.8
22	87	<0.1	0.1	<0.1	<0.1	3	0.1	0	0.3	21	39	113	32	2	0.1	0.1
4	6	<0.1	<0.1	<0.1	<0.1	<1	0.1	0	<0.1	55	36	76	6	2	<0.1	0.2
4	7	<0.1	<0.1	<0.1	<0.1	<1	0.1	0	<0.1	63	37	85	5	3	<0.1	0.2
35	90	<0.1	0.1	<0.1	<0.1	5	0.4	0	0.1	184	102	151	38	7	0.1	0.7
23	80	<0.1	0.1	0.1	<0.1	3	0.5	0	0.1	249	164	289	46	9	0.2	1.1
38	135	<0.1	0.2	0.1	<0.1	16	0.4	0	0.1	337	227	155	155	19	0.5	1.7
63	153	<0.1	0.2	0.1	0.1	15	0.4	0	0.1	257	196	104	130	14	0.5	1.4
20	60							0		250		35			0	
25	61	<0.1	0.1	<0.1	<0.1	2	0.9	0	0.1	214	153	52	21	10	0.1	1.2
18	48	<0.1	0.1	<0.1	<0.1	1	0.4	0	0.2	141	113	274	103	9	0.2	0.9
19	61	<0.1	0.1	<0.1	<0.1	2	0.1	0	0.1	191	242	457	82	10	0.1	0.9
3	92		0.1					<1		151	196	276	50		<0.1	0.5
20	55	<0.1	0.1	<0.1	<0.1	2	0.1	0	0.1	117	109	317	36	6	<0.1	0.6
17	54	<0.1	0.1	<0.1	<0.1	2	0.1	0	0.1	171	217	410	74	9	0.1	0.8
27	74	<0.1	0.1	<0.1	<0.1	2	0.2	1	0.1	173	210	403	46	6	0.1	0.8

ESHA, EatRight Analysis CD-ROM; **AMT,** amount; **WT,** weight; **CAL,** calories; **WTR,** water; **PROT,** protein; **CARB,** carbohydrate; **FIBR,** fiber; **FAT,** fat; **SATF,** saturated fat; **MONO,** monosaturated fat; **POLY,** polyunsaturated fat

ESHA CODE	FOOD DESCRIPTION	AMT	UNIT	WT (g)	CAL (kcal)	WTR (g)	PROT (g)	CARB (g)	FIBR (g)	FAT (g)	SATF (g)	MONO (g)	POLY (g)
Dairy Products & Non-Dairy Substitutes (continued)													
Cheese - Processed (continued)													
1071	Swiss Cheese Food	1	oz	28.35	92	12	6	1	0	7	4.4	1.9	0.2
1272	Velveeta Cheese Spread	1	oz	28.35	86	13	5	3	0	6	4.1		
Creams													
501	Cream-Coffee/Table	2	Tbs	30	58	22	1	1	0	6	3.6	1.7	0.2
500	Cream-Half & Half	2	Tbs	30	39	24	1	1	0	3	2.1	1	0.1
502	Cream-Heavy Whipping-Liq	2	Tbs	29.75	103	17	1	1	0	11	6.9	3.2	0.4
503	Cream-Hvy Whipping-Whipped	2	Tbs	14.94	52	9	<1	<1	0	6	3.4	1.6	0.2
511	Cream-Light Whipping-Liq	2	Tbs	29.88	87	19	1	1	0	9	5.8	2.7	0.3
540	Cremora NonDairy Creamer	1	tsp	2	10	0	0	1	0	1	1	0	0
517	Mocha Mix Creamer	1	Tbs	14.2	19	11	<1	1	0	2			
504	Sour Cream-Cultured	2	Tbs	28.75	62	20	1	1	0	6	3.8	1.7	0.2
505	Sour Cream-Imitation	2	Tbs	28.75	60	20	1	2	0	6	5.1	0.2	<0.1
515	Sour Cream-LowCal	2	Tbs	30	40	24	1	1	0	4	2.2	1	0.1
54316	Soy Creamer-French Vanilla	1	Tbs	16	20		0	3	0	1	0		
54317	Soy Creamer-Hazlenut	1	Tbs	16	16		0	1	0	1	0		
54315	Soy Creamer-Plain	1	Tbs	15.38	15		0	1	0	1	0		
Milks & Non-Dairy Milk Substitutes													
7	Buttermilk-Cultured-Skim	1	cup	245	98	221	8	12	0	2	1.3	0.6	0.1
21109	Chocolate Milk+Calc-LowFat	1	cup	250	195	205	7	30	2	5	2.9	1.1	0.2
19	Chocolate Milk-1% Fat	1	cup	250	158	211	8	26	1	2	1.5	0.8	0.1
18	Chocolate Milk-2% Fat	1	cup	250	190	205	7	30	2	5	2.9	1.1	0.2
20	Chocolate Milk-Whole	1	cup	250	208	206	8	26	2	8	5.3	2.5	0.3
72	Eggnog-Prep w/milk	1	cup	272	258	215	8	39	0	8	4.6	2.1	0.5
17	Eggnog-Whole Milk	1	cup	254	343	189	10	34	0	19	11.3	5.7	0.9
10	Evaporated Milk-Skim	2	Tbs	32	25	25	2	4	0	<1	<0.1	<0.1	<0.1
23	Goat Milk	1	cup	244	168	212	9	11	0	10	6.5	2.7	0.4
54	Lactose Reduced Milk-1% Fat	1	cup	246	103	222	8	12	0	3	1.6	0.8	0.1
81	Milk Substitute, fluid, w/hydrog veg oil	1	cup	244	149	215	4	15	0	8	1.9	4.9	1.2
164	Milk, evaporated, low fat	2	Tbs	31.7	25	26	2	3	0	<1	0.5	0	0
21097	Milk, skim, lactose free w/ Vit A&D	1	cup	245	80	223	8	12	0	0	0	0	0
4	Milk-1% Fat	1	cup	244	102	219	8	12	0	2	1.5	0.7	0.1
2	Milk-2% Fat	1	cup	244	122	218	8	11	0	5	3.1	1.4	0.2
6	Milk-NonFat	1	cup	245	83	223	8	12	0	<1	0.1	0.1	<0.1
1	Milk-Whole, 3.25%	1	cup	244	146	216	8	11	0	8	4.6	2	0.5
57	Nonfat Dry Milk Powder+Water	1	cup	245	82	223	8	12	0	<1	0.1	<0.1	<0.1
20145	So Good Lite Soy Drink	1	cup	260	114	229	9	17	2	2	0.3	0.5	1
20144	So Good Soy Drink	1	cup	255	158	222	8	13	2	8	0.8	2	4.6
20033	Soy Milk	1	cup	245	127	216	11	12	3	5	0.6	0.9	1.9
7801	Soy Milk Bev-Carob (Eden)	1	cup	244	170		7	27	0	4	0.5	1	2
7775	Soy Milk Bev-Vanilla (VitaSoy)	1	cup	228.3	190		7	27		6	1	1	3
20920	Soy Milk-Chocolate	1	cup	250	140		5	23	0	4	0		
20916	Soy Milk-Plain-organic	1	cup	245	100	225	7	8	0	4	0		
20918	Soy Milk-Van-organic	1	cup	246	100	226	6	10	0	4	0		
11	Sweetened Condensed Milk	2	Tbs	38.25	123	10	3	21	0	3	2.1	0.9	0.1

< = Trace amount present   Blank = Not available

CHOL, cholesterol; **V**, vitamin; **THI**, thiamin; **RIB**, riboflavin; **NIA**, niacin; **FOL**, folate;
CALC, calcium; **PHOS**, phosphate; **SOD**, sodium; **POT**, potassium; **MAG**, magnesium

CHOL (g)	V-A (RE)	THI (mg)	RIB (mg)	NIA (mg)	V-B6 (mg)	FOL (µg)	V-B12 (µg)	V-C (mg)	V-E (mg)	CALC (mg)	PHOS (mg)	SOD (mg)	POT (mg)	MAG (mg)	IRON (mg)	ZINC (mg)
23	68	<0.1	0.1	<0.1	<0.1	2	0.7	0	0.2	205	149	440	81	8	0.2	1
23	63		0.1					<1		132	245	425	95		0.1	0.5
20	55	<0.1	<0.1	<0.1	<0.1	1	0.1	<1	0.2	29	24	12	37	3	<0.1	0.1
11	30	<0.1	<0.1	<0.1	<0.1	1	0.1	<1	0.1	32	28	12	39	3	<0.1	0.2
41	124	<0.1	<0.1	<0.1	<0.1	1	0.1	<1	0.3	19	18	11	22	2	<0.1	0.1
20	62	<0.1	<0.1	<0.1	<0.1	1	<0.1	<1	0.2	10	9	6	11	1	<0.1	<0.1
33	85	<0.1	<0.1	<0.1	<0.1	1	0.1	<1	0.3	21	18	10	29	2	<0.1	0.1
0	0					0		0		0		10	15		0	
0											8		20	0		
13	52	<0.1	<0.1	<0.1	<0.1	3	0.1	<1	0.2	33	24	15	41	3	<0.1	0.1
0	0	0	0	0	0	0	0	0	0.2	1	13	29	46	2	0.1	0.3
12	31	<0.1	<0.1	<0.1	<0.1	3	0.1	<1	0.1	31	28	12	39	3	<0.1	0.2
0	0							0		0		5			0	
0	0							0		0		5			0	
0	0							0		0		5			0	
10	17	0.1	0.4	0.1	0.1	12	0.5	2	0.1	284	218	257	370	27	0.1	1
20	162	0.1	1.4	0.4	0.1	5	0.8	0	0.1	485	190	165	308	35	0.6	1
8	145	0.1	0.4	0.3	0.1	12	0.9	2	<0.1	288	258	152	425	32	0.6	1
20	162	0.1	0.5	0.4	0.1	5	0.8	0	0.1	272	255	165	422	35	0.6	1
30	65	0.1	0.4	0.3	0.1	12	0.8	2	0.1	280	252	150	418	32	0.6	1
30	71	0.1	0.5	0.3	0.1	14	1.1	0	0.2	250	209	150	329	27	0.3	1
150	114	0.1	0.5	0.3	0.1	3	1.1	4	0.5	330	277	137	419	48	0.5	1.2
1	38	<0.1	0.1	0.1	<0.1	3	0.1	<1	0	93	62	37	106	9	0.1	0.3
27	142	0.1	0.3	0.7	0.1	2	0.2	3	0.2	327	271	122	498	34	0.1	0.7
10	145	0.1	0.4	0.2	0.1	13	0.9	2	0.1	303	237	124	384	34	0.1	1
0	0	<0.1	0.2	0	0	0	0	0	0.7	81	181	190	278	15	1	2.9
5	20		0.1						0	80	60	35	100		0	
5	150								0	500		125	460		0	
12	142	<0.1	0.5	0.2	0.1	12	1.1	0	<0.1	290	232	107	366	27	0.1	1
20	134	0.1	0.5	0.2	0.1	12	1.1	<1	0.1	285	229	100	366	27	0.1	1
5	149	0.1	0.4	0.2	0.1	12	1.3	0	<0.1	306	247	103	382	27	0.1	1
24	68	0.1	0.4	0.3	0.1	12	1.1	0	0.1	276	222	98	349	24	0.1	1
4	162	0.1	0.4	0.2	0.1	11	0.9	1	<0.1	285	224	132	388	29	0.1	1.1
0	203	0.2	0.5		0.2	26	0.8	5		257		94	322		2.1	0.5
0	199	0.2	0.5		0.2	26	0.8	5		252		92	316		2	0.5
0	152	0.1	0.1	0.7	0.2	39	3	0	3.3	93	135	135	304	61	2.7	1.1
0	0	0.3	0.1	2	0.2	80		0		75	125	95	350	58	1.3	0.8
0		0.2	0.2							80		130	210		0.7	
0	100		0.5			24	3	0		300		75	350		1.4	0.6
0	100		0.5			24	3	0		300		75	280		1.1	0.6
0	100		0.5			24	3	0		300		95	280		1.1	0.6
13	29	<0.1	0.2	0.1	<0.1	4	0.2	1	0.1	109	97	49	142	10	0.1	0.4

ESHA, EatRight Analysis CD-ROM; **AMT,** amount; **WT,** weight; **CAL,** calories; **WTR,** water; **PROT,** protein; **CARB,** carbohydrate;
FIBR, fiber; **FAT,** fat; **SATF,** saturated fat; **MONO,** monosaturated fat; **POLY,** polyunsaturated fat

ESHA CODE	FOOD DESCRIPTION	AMT	UNIT	WT (g)	CAL (kcal)	WTR (g)	PROT (g)	CARB (g)	FIBR (g)	FAT (g)	SATF (g)	MONO (g)	POLY (g)
Dairy Products & Non-Dairy Substitutes (continued)													
Yogurts													
7546	Tofu Yogurt	1	cup	262	246	203	9	42	1	5	0.7	1	2.7
2001	Yogurt-LowFat-Fruit	1	cup	245	250	182	11	47	0	3	1.7	0.7	0.1
2000	Yogurt-LowFat-Plain	1	cup	245	154	208	13	17	0	4	2.5	1	0.1
2012	Yogurt-NonFat-Plain	1	cup	245	137	209	14	19	0	<1	0.3	0.1	<0.1
11982	Yogurt-Nonfat-Vanilla	1	cup	226	220		12	40	0	0	0	0	0
72086	Yogurt-Nonfat-Vanilla+LoCalSwtnr	1	cup	225	106	197	9	17	0	<1	0.3	0.1	<0.1
2428	Yogurt-Strawberry-Light	1	cup	227	250	165	9	48	0	2	1.5		
2013	Yogurt-Whole Milk-Plain	1	cup	245	149	215	9	11	0	8	5.1	2.2	0.2
Desserts													
Brownies & Dessert Bars													
47000	Brownie+Nuts+Icing-Commerc	1	ea	61	247	8	3	39	1	10	2.6	5.5	1.4
47019	Brownie-FudgeNut-Recipe	1	ea	24	112	3	1	12	1	7	1.8	2.6	2.3
47078	Lemon Bar Cookie	1	ea	16	69	2	1	10	<1	3	0.6	1.4	0.8
44219	Rice Krispies Treats-Square	1	ea	22	91	1	1	18	<1	2	0.3	0.6	1.1
Cakes													
46004	Angelfood Cake-1/12	1	pce	28.35	73	9	2	16	<1	<1	<0.1	<0.1	0.1
46098	Applesauce Cake-No Icing	1	pce	87	313	20	3	52	2	12	2.4	5	3.5
46103	Banana Cake-No Icing	1	pce	87	262	29	3	46	1	8	1.6	3.6	2.1
49004	Cheesecake (pce=1/12)	1	pce	80	257	36	4	20	<1	18	7.9	6.9	1.3
49001	Cheesecake-Mix-Prepared	1	pce	99	271	44	5	35	2	13	6.6	4.5	0.8
46275	Choc Fudge Cake-Frzn	1	pce	69	250		3	31	1	11	3		
71626	Choc Ganache Cheesecake-1/13	1	pce	153	580	51	9	52		39	20		
46013	Chocolate Cake+Choc Icing	1	pce	64	235	15	3	35	2	10	3.1	5.6	1.2
46118	Chocolate Cake+Van Icing	1	pce	103	367	29	3	53	1	17	4.3		
46093	CoffeeCake-Cinn+Crumb Top	1	pce	63	263	14	4	29	1	15	3.7	8.2	2
46097	CoffeeCake-Fruit	1	pce	50	156	16	3	26	1	5	1.2	2.8	0.7
46106	Date Pudding Cake	1	pce	42	131	14	2	19	1	6	3	1.9	0.3
46000	Gingerbread Cake-Homemade	1	pce	74	263	21	3	36	1	12	3.1	5.3	3.1
71650	Lemon Layer Cake-Frzn	1	pce	88	290		2	43	0	12	3.5		
46070	Pineapple UpsideDown Cake-1/9	1	pce	115	367	37	4	58	1	14	3.4	6	3.8
46107	Plum Pudding Cake	1	pce	42	131	14	2	19	1	6	3	1.9	0.3
46016	Pound Cake w/Butter	1	pce	28.35	110	7	2	14	<1	6	3.3	1.7	0.3
46011	Snack Cake/Choc+Filling	1	ea	50	200	9	2	30	2	8	2.4	4.3	0.9
46116	Spice Cake w/Icing	1	pce	109	368	29	5	62	1	12	3.2	5.9	1.9
46078	Sponge Cake-Recipe	1	pce	63	187	19	5	36	<1	3	0.8	1	0.4
46008	Twinkie Snack Cake	1	ea	42.5	155	9	1	27	<1	5	1.1	1.7	1.4
46007	White Cake+Choc Frosting	1	pce	100	428	6	2	75	1	14	7.2		
46012	Yellow Cake w/Choc Icing	1	pce	64	243	14	2	35	1	11	3	6.1	1.4
Candies													
23136	100 Grand Candy Bar-Fun Size	1	ea	42.52	188	3	1	31	<1	7	5.1	1.4	0.3
23125	5th Avenue Candy Bar	1	ea	56.7	273	1	5	36	2	14	3.8	6	1.9
23049	Almond Joy Candy Bar	1	ea	48.19	231	4	2	29	2	13	8.5	2.5	0.6
23110	Baby Ruth Candy Bar	1	ea	59.53	273	4	3	39	1	13	7.2	3.3	1.6

< = Trace amount present   Blank = Not available

CHOL, cholesterol; V, vitamin; THI, thiamin; RIB, riboflavin; NIA, niacin; FOL, folate;
CALC, calcium; PHOS, phosphate; SOD, sodium; POT, potassium; MAG, magnesium

CHOL (g)	V-A (RE)	THI (mg)	RIB (mg)	NIA (mg)	V-B6 (mg)	FOL (µg)	V-B12 (µg)	V-C (mg)	V-E (mg)	CALC (mg)	PHOS (mg)	SOD (mg)	POT (mg)	MAG (mg)	IRON (mg)	ZINC (mg)
0	10	0.2	0.1	0.6	0.1	16	0	7	0.8	309	100	92	123	105	2.8	0.8
10	24	0.1	0.4	0.2	0.1	22	1.2	2	<0.1	372	292	142	478	37	0.2	1.8
15	34	0.1	0.5	0.3	0.1	27	1.4	2	0.1	448	353	172	573	42	0.2	2.2
5	5	0.1	0.6	0.3	0.1	29	1.5	2	0	488	385	189	625	47	0.2	2.4
5	100							4		450		180			0	
4	0	0.1	0.4	0.2	0.1	18	1	2	0	322	245	133	398	29	0.3	1.5
15	200	0.1	0.3					0		250	200	130	390		0	
32	66	0.1	0.3	0.2	0.1	17	0.9	1	0.1	296	233	113	380	29	0.1	1.4
10	12	0.2	0.1	1	<0.1	29	<0.1	0	0.1	18	62	190	91	19	1.4	0.4
18	46	<0.1	<0.1	0.2	<0.1	7	<0.1	<1	0.7	14	32	82	42	13	0.4	0.2
12	32	<0.1	<0.1	0.2	<0.1	2	<0.1	1	0.4	7	12	42	11	1	0.2	0.1
0	71	0.3	0.3	3.6	0.2	24	0	0	0	1	9	77	9	3	0.3	0.1
0	0	<0.1	0.1	0.3	<0.1	10	<0.1	0	<0.1	40	92	212	26	3	0.1	<0.1
22	10	0.1	0.1	1.1	0.1	6	<0.1	1	1.6	17	45	141	145	11	1.4	0.2
32	83	0.1	0.2	1.2	0.2	11	0.1	3	1.2	26	50	181	168	15	1.1	0.3
44	118	<0.1	0.2	0.2	<0.1	14	0.1	<1	1.3	41	74	166	72	9	0.5	0.4
29	99	0.1	0.3	0.5	0.1	30	0.3	<1	1.1	170	232	376	209	19	0.5	0.5
30	0							0			0	160			1.1	
135	30							0			60	330			0.4	
27	17	<0.1	0.1	0.4	<0.1	11	0.1	<1	<0.1	28	78	214	128	22	1.4	0.4
23	52	0.1	0.1	1	<0.1	33	0.1	<1	0.9	23	47	232	61	11	1	0.3
20	21	0.1	0.1	1.1	<0.1	38	0.1	<1	2.1	34	68	221	77	14	1.2	0.5
4	7	<0.1	0.1	1.3	<0.1	24	<0.1	<1	0.4	22	59	192	45	8	1.2	0.3
15	10	0.1	0.1	0.5	0.1	3	0.1	<1	0.2	46	36	66	199	23	1	0.2
24	10	0.1	0.1	1.3	0.1	24	<0.1	<1	1.8	53	40	242	325	52	2.1	0.3
35												250				
25	75	0.2	0.2	1.4	<0.1	30	0.1	1	1.5	138	94	367	129	15	1.7	0.4
15	10	0.1	0.1	0.5	0.1	3	0.1	<1	0.2	46	36	66	199	23	1	0.2
63	44	<0.1	0.1	0.4	<0.1	12	0.1	0	0.2	10	39	113	34	3	0.4	0.1
0	<1	<0.1	<0.1	0.5	0.1	13	<0.1	1	0.5	58	44	194	88	18	1.8	0.5
50	39	0.1	0.2	1.1	<0.1	9	0.1	<1	2.2	76	209	281	136	13	1.5	0.4
107	49	0.1	0.2	0.8	<0.1	25	0.2	0	0.3	26	63	144	89	6	1	0.4
7	2	0.1	0.1	0.5	<0.1	17	<0.1	<1	0.5	19	79	155	37	3	0.5	0.1
21	56	0.1	0.1	1.1	<0.1	30	<0.1	<1	0.5	43	148	356	80	19	0.9	0.3
35	21	0.1	0.1	0.8	<0.1	14	0.1	0	1.5	24	103	216	114	19	1.3	0.4
6	15	<0.1	0.1	0.1	<0.1	2	0.1	<1	0.4	32	36	86	69	11	0.1	0.4
3	8	0.1	0.1	2.2	0.1	20	0.1	<1	1.5	41	80	128	197	35	0.7	0.6
2	4	<0.1	0.1	0.2	<0.1		0.1	<1	<0.1	31	54	68	122	32	0.6	0.4
0	0	<0.1	0.1	0.7	<0.1	7	<0.1	0	0.6	28	56	137	148	26	0.4	0.4

ESHA, EatRight Analysis CD-ROM; **AMT,** amount; **WT,** weight; **CAL,** calories; **WTR,** water; **PROT,** protein; **CARB,** carbohydrate; **FIBR,** fiber; **FAT,** fat; **SATF,** saturated fat; **MONO,** monosaturated fat; **POLY,** polyunsaturated fat

ESHA CODE	FOOD DESCRIPTION	AMT	UNIT	WT (g)	CAL (kcal)	WTR (g)	PROT (g)	CARB (g)	FIBR (g)	FAT (g)	SATF (g)	MONO (g)	POLY (g)
Desserts (continued)													
Candies (continued)													
4148	Bit-O-Honey Candy	1	ea	48.1	180	4	1	38	<1	4	2.6	0.5	0.2
23226	Breathsaver Mints-Spearmint	1	pce	2	10	0	0	2	0	0	0	0	0
23066	Butterfinger Candy Bar	1	ea	61.23	281	1	3	45	1	12	5.8	3.1	1.9
23115	Butterscotch Candy	5	pce	30	117	2	<1	27	0	1	0.6	0.3	<0.1
92671	Cadbury Almond Candy Bar	10	pce	40	220	1	4	21	1	13	7		
23116	Caramello Candy Bar	1	ea	45.36	210	3	3	29	1	10	5.8	2.4	0.3
23015	Caramel-Plain/Chocolate	1	pce	10.1	39	1	<1	8	0	1	0.3	0.2	0.4
23082	Chewing Gum	1	pce	3	7	<1	0	2	<1	<1	<0.1	<0.1	<0.1
92196	Chewing Gum-NoSugar	1	pce	2	5	<1	0	2	<1	<1	<0.1	<0.1	<0.1
92197	Choc Candy-Dietetic	1	oz	28.35	163	1	4	12	1	11	6.2	3.1	1.2
90658	ChocCvrd Fondant Candy-Lrg	1	ea	43	157	3	1	34	1	4	2.3	1.3	0.1
23063	Chocolate Candy Kisses	6	pce	28.35	145	<1	2	17	1	9	5.2	2.8	0.3
23021	Chocolate Coated Peanuts	1	cup	149	773	3	20	74	7	50	21.8	19.3	6.5
23022	Chocolate Covered Raisins	1	cup	190	741	21	8	130	8	28	16.7	9	1
23123	Demet's Turtles Candy	1	oz	28.35	137	2	2	16	1	8	3.1	3.1	1.3
23074	Dietetic Hard Candy	1	pce	3	11	<1	0	3	0	0	0	0	0
90808	Divinity Candy-f/Recipe	1	pce	41.51	113	12	<1	29	0	<1	<0.1		
23036	English Toffee Candy Bar	1	ea	39.69	212	1	1	24	1	13	7.5	3.7	0.5
23024	Fondant Candy	1	pce	16	60	1	0	15	0	<1	0	0	0
23025	Fudge-Chocolate	1	pce	17	70	2	<1	13	<1	2	1	0.5	<0.1
23026	Fudge-Chocolate-Nuts	1	pce	19	88	1	1	13	<1	4	1.1	0.7	1.4
23129	Golden AlmondChoc Bar	1	ea	79.38	458		10	37	3	31	13.2		
23130	Golden AlmondChoc Candies	1	ea	78	445		9	37	3	29	11.9		
23132	Goobers Choc Peanut-Pce	10	pce	10	51	<1	1	5	1	3	1.2		
92647	Good & Plenty Candy-SnackSz	1	ea	17	60		0	14	0	0	0	0	0
23029	Gumdrops Candy-Small	10	pce	36	143	<1	0	36	<1	0	0	0	0
23030	Gummy Bears Candy	10	pce	22	87	<1	0	22	<1	0	0	0	0
23031	Hard Candy, all flavors	1	pce	6	24	<1	0	6	0	<1	0	0	0
23033	Jelly Beans Candy	10	pce	11	41	1	0	10	<1	<1	0	0	0
23060	Kit Kat candy bar	1	ea	42.52	220	1	3	27	<1	11	7.6	2.5	0.4
23061	Krackle candy bar	1	ea	42.52	218	<1	3	27	1	11	6.8	2.7	0.2
23048	M&M's Peanut Choc Candy	10	pce	20	103	<1	2	12	1	5	2	1.6	0.7
23047	M&M's Peanut Choc Candy-pkg	1	cup	170	876	4	16	103	6	44	17.3	13.7	5.9
23046	M&M's Plain Choc Candy	10	pce	7	34	<1	<1	5	<1	1	0.9	0.2	<0.1
23037	Mars Candy Bar-Fun Size	1	ea	50	234	2	4	31	1	12	3.6	5.3	2
23007	Marshmallows	1	ea	7.2	23	1	<1	6	<1	<1	<0.1	<0.1	<0.1
23018	Milk Choc Bar+Almonds	1	ea	41.10	216	1	4	22	3	14	7	5.5	0.9
23058	Milk Choc Bar+RiceCereal	1	ea	39.69	197	1	3	25	1	11	6.3	3.4	0.3
23192	Milk Choc Candy Bar	1	ea	41.1	220		2	26	1	13	8		
23016	Milk Chocolate Candy Bar	1	ea	43.94	235	1	3	26	1	13	6.3	5.8	0.4
23038	Milky Way Candy Bar	1	ea	59.53	269	4	2	42	1	10	7.2	1.3	0.2
23035	Mounds Candy Bar	1	ea	53.86	262	5	2	32	2	14	11.1	0.2	0.1
23062	Mr. Goodbar Candy Bar	1	ea	49.61	267	<1	5	27	2	16	7	4.1	2.2
23135	Oh Henry! Candy Bar	1	ea	56.7	262	1	4	37	1	13	5.4	3.1	1.5
23081	Peanut Brittle-Homemade	1.5	oz	42.53	207	<1	3	30	1	8	1.8	3.4	1.9

< = Trace amount present   Blank = Not available

CHOL, cholesterol; V, vitamin; THI, thiamin; RIB, riboflavin; NIA, niacin; FOL, folate;
CALC, calcium; PHOS, phosphate; SOD, sodium; POT, potassium; MAG, magnesium

CHOL (g)	V-A (RE)	THI (mg)	RIB (mg)	NIA (mg)	V-B6 (mg)	FOL (µg)	V-B12 (µg)	V-C (mg)	V-E (mg)	CALC (mg)	PHOS (mg)	SOD (mg)	POT (mg)	MAG (mg)	IRON (mg)	ZINC (mg)
0	0	<0.1	<0.1	<0.1	<0.1	1	<0.1	<1	0.1	17	13	142	21	3	0.1	0.2
0												0	0			
0	0	0.1	<0.1	1.6	<0.1	17	<0.1	0	1.1	22	59	141	135	29	0.5	0.6
3	9	<0.1	<0.1	<0.1	0	0	0	0	<0.1	1	<1	117	1	0	<0.1	<0.1
10	0							0		100		80			0.4	
12	28	<0.1	0.2	0.5	<0.1		0.3	1	0.1	97	68	55	155	19	0.5	0.4
1	1	<0.1	<0.1	<0.1	<0.1	<1	<0.1	<1	<0.1	14	12	25	22	2	<0.1	<0.1
0	0	0	0	0	0	0	0	0	0	0	0	<1	<1	0	0	0
0	0	0	0	0	0	0	0	0	0	<1	0	<1	0	0	0	0
6	16	0.1	0.1	0.6	<0.1	7	0.2	<1	0.8	86	94	31	172	28	0.4	0.8
0	0	<0.1	<0.1	0.2	<0.1	1	0	0	0.1	7	41	11	72	27	0.7	0.2
6	16	<0.1	0.1	0.1	<0.1	2	0.1	<1	0.4	54	61	23	109	17	0.4	0.4
13	51	0.2	0.3	6.3	0.3	12	0.7	0	5.2	155	316	61	748	143	2	3.6
6	46	0.2	0.3	0.8	0.2	13	0.3	<1	1.9	163	272	68	977	86	3.2	1.5
6	9	<0.1	0.1	0.1	<0.1	3	0.1	<1		45	56	27	87	15	0.4	0.4
0	0	0	0	0	0	0	0	0	0	0	0	0	0	0	0	0
0	0	<0.1	<0.1	<0.1	<0.1	<1	<0.1	0	0	1	1	49	6	1	<0.1	<0.1
21	57	<0.1	<0.1	0.1	<0.1	1	0.1	<1	<0.1	52	24	126	61	4	0.2	0.1
0	0	<0.1	<0.1	<0.1	<0.1	0	0	0	0	<1	0	3	1	0	<0.1	0
2	8	<0.1	<0.1	<0.1	<0.1	1	<0.1	0	<0.1	8	12	8	22	6	0.3	0.2
2	7	<0.1	<0.1	0.1	<0.1	3	<0.1	<1	<0.1	10	21	8	34	10	0.4	0.3
10		<0.1	0.4	0.8	<0.1		0.3	0	0.5	152	214	51	374	88	1.5	1.3
10	0	<0.1	0.4	0.8	<0.1		0.4	0	1.8	158	234	41	393	92	2	1.4
1	1	<0.1	<0.1	0.5	<0.1	1	<0.1	<1	0.3	9	30	4	50	12	0.1	0.2
0	0							0		0		40			0.1	
0	0	<0.1	<0.1	<0.1	<0.1	0	0	0	0	1	<1	16	2	<1	0.1	0
0	0	<0.1	<0.1	<0.1	<0.1	0	0	0	0	1	<1	10	1	<1	0.1	0
0	0	<0.1	<0.1	<0.1	<0.1	0	0	0	0	<1	<1	2	<1	<1	<0.1	<0.1
0	0	<0.1	<0.1	<0.1	<0.1	0	0	0	0	<1	<1	6	4	<1	<0.1	<0.1
5	10	<0.1	0.1	0.2	<0.1	6	0.2	0	0.1	53	57	23	98	16	0.4	<0.1
5	9	<0.1	0.1	0.1	<0.1	3	0.2	<1	<0.1	67	52	83	138	6	0.5	0.2
2	4	<0.1	<0.1	0.7	<0.1	11	0.1	0	0.6	20	38	10	69	14	0.2	0.4
14	37	0.1	0.2	5.7	0.2	94	0.5	0	4.8	173	323	85	590	117	2	3
1	4	<0.1	<0.1	<0.1	<0.1	1	<0.1	<1	0.1	7	10	4	19	3	0.1	0.1
8	8	<0.1	0.2	0.5	<0.1	4	0.2	<1	3.9	84	117	85	162	36	0.6	0.6
0	0	<0.1	<0.1	<0.1	<0.1	<1	0	0	0	<1	1	6	<1	<1	<0.1	<0.1
8	18	<0.1	0.2	0.3	<0.1	6	0.1	<1	1.8	92	109	30	182	37	0.7	0.6
8	25	<0.1	0.1	0.2	<0.1	6	0.2	<1	0.8	68	77	58	136	19	0.3	0.4
10	0							0		60		25			0	
10	22	<0.1	0.1	0.2	<0.1	5	0.3	0	0.9	83	91	35	163	28	1	0.9
5	20	<0.1	0.1	0.1	<0.1	2	0.1	<1	0.5	68	40	99	74	12	0.3	0.4
1	0	0	0	0	0	0	0	<1	0.1	11	0	78	173	0	1.1	0
5	17	0.1	0.1	1.7	<0.1	19	0.2	<1	1.6	55	81	20	195	23	0.7	0.5
4	0	0.1	0.1	1.4	<0.1	25	0.1	0	1.3	39	79	109	147	29	0.3	0.7
5	17	0.1	<0.1	1.1	<0.1	20	<0.1	0	1.1	11	45	189	71	18	0.5	0.4

ESHA, EatRight Analysis CD-ROM; **AMT,** amount; **WT,** weight; **CAL,** calories; **WTR,** water; **PROT,** protein; **CARB,** carbohydrate; **FIBR,** fiber; **FAT,** fat; **SATF,** saturated fat; **MONO,** monosaturated fat; **POLY,** polyunsaturated fat

ESHA CODE	FOOD DESCRIPTION	AMT	UNIT	WT (g)	CAL (kcal)	WTR (g)	PROT (g)	CARB (g)	FIBR (g)	FAT (g)	SATF (g)	MONO (g)	POLY (g)
Desserts (continued)													
Candies (continued)													
90803	Praline Candy-f/Recipe	1	pce	39.94	174	7	1	22	1	10	2.7		
23043	Reese's Peanut Butter Cup	1	ea	45.36	234	1	5	25	2	14	4.9	5.9	2.5
23140	Reese's Pieces Candy	10	pce	8	40	<1	1	5	<1	2	1.3	0.4	0.2
23141	Rolo Caramel Candy	1	pce	3	14	<1	<1	2	<1	1	0.4	0.1	<0.1
23142	Sesame Crunch Candy	20	pce	35	181	1	4	18	3	12	1.6	4.4	5.1
23431	Skittles Candy	1.5	oz	42.53	172	2	<1	39	0	2	1.8	0	0
23040	Snickers Candy Bar	1	ea	56.7	269	3	4	34	1	14	5.1	4.5	1.7
23057	Special Dark Candy Bar	1	ea	41.10	218	<1	2	24	3	13		2.1	0.2
23144	Starburst Fruit Candy	1	pce	5	20	<1	<1	4	0	<1	0.4	0	0
91520	Sugar Coated Almonds	1	ea	3.5	17	<1	<1	2	<1	1	0.1	0.4	0.1
23146	Symphony Candy Bar	1	ea	42.52	226	<1	4	25	1	13	7.8	3.4	0.3
90806	Taffy Candy-f/Rec	1	pce	33.95	99	12	1	17	<1	3	1		
23075	Three Muskateers Candy Bar	1	ea	60.38	258	4	2	47	1	8	5.2	1.4	0.2
23076	Three Musketeer-Fun Size	1	ea	16.5	71	1	<1	13	<1	2	1.4	0.4	0.1
23117	Tootsie Roll Candy-BiteSz	7	ea	49	190	3	1	43	<1	2	0.5	0.9	0.1
23154	Twizzlers-Small Pkg	1	ea	70.87	248		2	57	0	2	0		
23151	Whatchamacallit Candy Bar	1	ea	48.2	238	1	4	30	1	11	8.2	1.8	0.4
23507	Yogurt Covered Raisins	35	pce	40	160	5	1	28	1	5	1		
23152	York Peppermint Patty-Lrg	1	ea	42	161	4	1	34	1	3	1.8	0.2	<0.1
Cookies													
91664	Almond Cookie	2	ea	29	170		2	19	0	10	3		
47005	Butter Cookie-Thin	5	ea	25	117	1	2	17	<1	5	2.8	1.4	0.2
47075	Butterscotch Brownie	1	ea	34	152	4	2	20	<1	8	1.4	3.3	2.5
47032	Choc Chip Cookie-Commerc	1	ea	10	45	<1	1	7	<1	2	0.4	0.6	0.5
47002	Choc Chip Cookie-Recipe-Marg	1	ea	16	78	1	1	9	<1	5	1.3	1.7	1.3
43728	Choc Mint Cake Cookie	1	ea	16	50		1	12	0	<1	0		
47041	Chocolate Wafer Cookie	2	ea	12	52	1	1	9	<1	2	0.5	0.6	0.5
47042	Coconut Macaroons-Recipe	1	ea	24	97	3	1	17	<1	3	2.7	0.1	<0.1
47012	Fig Bar Cookie	1	ea	16	56	3	1	11	1	1	0.2	0.5	0.4
47043	Fortune Cookie	1	ea	8	30	1	<1	7	<1	<1	0.1	0.1	<0.1
47376	Fruit Cookie-NoFat (Archway)	1	ea	28	90		2	21	0	0	0	0	0
47324	Fudge Brownie Cookie-SugFree	1	ea	24	90		1	17	0	4	1	1	0
47045	Gingersnap Cookie	1	ea	7	29	<1	<1	5	<1	1	0.2	0.4	0.1
47009	Lady Finger Cookie	4	ea	44	161	9	5	26	<1	4	1.5	1.9	0.7
47046	Marshmallow Cookie-ChocDip	1	ea	13	55	1	1	9	<1	2	0.6	1.2	0.3
47109	Molasses Cookie	1	ea	15	64	1	1	11	<1	2	0.5	1.1	0.3
47171	NillaWafer Cookie (Nabisco)	8	ea	32	140	2	1	24	1	5	1	1.5	0
47054	Oatmeal Cookie-Homemade	1	ea	15	67	1	1	10	<1	3	0.5	1.2	0.8
47496	Oatmeal Raisin Cookie (Archway)	1	ea	26	106	3	1	18	1	3	0.7	1.3	0.3
53689	Peanut Butter Sandwich Cookie	1	ea	43	210	1	3	28	1	10	2.5		
47010	PeanutButter Cookie-Homemade	1	ea	20	95	1	2	12	<1	5	0.9	2.2	1.4
47062	Pecan Shortbread Cookie	1	ea	14	76	<1	1	8	<1	5	1.1	2.6	0.6
47038	Sandw Cookie-Choc-ChocDip	1	ea	17	82	<1	1	11	1	4	1.3	2.5	0.5
47006	Sandwich Cookie-all types	4	ea	40	186	1	2	29	1	8	1.5	4.3	0.9
47180	Sandwich Cookie-Oreo	3	ea	33	155	1	1	23	1	7	1.5		

< = Trace amount present   Blank = Not available

CHOL, cholesterol; **V,** vitamin; **THI,** thiamin; **RIB,** riboflavin; **NIA,** niacin; **FOL,** folate; **CALC,** calcium; **PHOS,** phosphate; **SOD,** sodium; **POT,** potassium; **MAG,** magnesium

CHOL (g)	V-A (RE)	THI (mg)	RIB (mg)	NIA (mg)	V-B6 (mg)	FOL (µg)	V-B12 (µg)	V-C (mg)	V-E (mg)	CALC (mg)	PHOS (mg)	SOD (mg)	POT (mg)	MAG (mg)	IRON (mg)	ZINC (mg)
10	30	0.1	<0.1	0.1	<0.1	2	<0.1	<1	0.4	20	33	40	67	13	0.3	0.4
3	8	0.1	<0.1	2	<0.1	23	0.3	<1	0.1	35	73	142	156	28	0.5	0.6
0	0	<0.1	<0.1	0.5	<0.1	4	<0.1	0	0.1	6	17	16	29	7	<0.1	0.1
<1	1	<0.1	<0.1	<0.1	0	0	<0.1	<1	<0.1	4	2	6	6	0	<0.1	0
0	<1	0.2	0.1	1.3	0.2	18	0	<1	0.1	229	148	58	113	88	1.5	1.3
0	0	0	<0.1	<0.1	<0.1	0	0	28	0.1	0	<1	6	5	<1	0	<0.1
7	27	<0.1	0.1	2	0.1	15	0.1	<1	0.9	53	108	139	183	41	0.4	1.4
2	0	<0.1	0	0	0	0	0	0	0.1	12	21	2	206	13	0.9	<0.1
0	<1	<0.1	<0.1	<0.1	0	<1	0	3	<0.1	0	<1	<1	<1	<1	<0.1	0
0	<1	<0.1	<0.1	<0.1	<0.1	1	0	0	0.4	4	6	<1	9	5	0.1	0.1
10	20	<0.1	0.2	0.1	<0.1		0.2	1	0.1	107	88	43	186	23	0.4	0.5
4		<0.1	<0.1	0.1	<0.1	1	<0.1	0	0.6	9	16	152	19	9	<0.1	0.1
3	12	<0.1	<0.1	0.1	<0.1	2	0.1	<1	0.6	33	42	117	80	18	0.4	0.3
1	3	<0.1	<0.1	<0.1	<0.1	1	<0.1	<1	0.2	9	11	32	22	5	0.1	0.1
1	<1	<0.1	<0.1	0.1	<0.1	4	0	0	0.3	18	28	22	57	11	0.4	0.2
0	0							0		0		203			0.4	
6	19	0.1	0.1	1.2	<0.1	9	0.2	<1	0.6	57	67	144	146	13	0.5	0.2
0	1							1		30		10			0	
<1	<1	<0.1	<0.1	0.4	<0.1		<0.1	0	<0.1	5	0	12	47	26	0.4	0.3
0	0							0		0		75			0	
29	42	0.1	0.1	0.8	<0.1	19	0.1	0	0.1	7	26	88	28	3	0.6	0.1
21	67	0.1	0.1	0.5	<0.1	5	<0.1	<1	1	24	31	90	72	10	0.8	0.2
0	<1	<0.1	<0.1	0.3	<0.1	7	0	0	0.2	2	8	38	12	3	0.3	0.1
5	25	<0.1	<0.1	0.2	<0.1	5	<0.1	<1	0.5	6	16	58	36	9	0.4	0.1
0	0							0		0		40			0.4	
<1	<1	<0.1	<0.1	0.3	<0.1	7	<0.1	0	0.1	4	16	70	25	6	0.5	0.1
0	0	<0.1	<0.1	<0.1	<0.1	1	<0.1	0	<0.1	2	10	59	37	5	0.2	0.2
0	1	<0.1	<0.1	0.3	<0.1	6	<0.1	<1	0.1	10	10	56	33	4	0.5	0.1
<1	<1	<0.1	<0.1	0.1	<0.1	5	<0.1	0	<0.1	1	3	22	3	1	0.1	<0.1
0	0							0	<0.1	0		95			0.4	
0	0							0		0		130			1.1	
0	<1	<0.1	<0.1	0.2	<0.1	6	0	0	0.1	5	6	46	24	3	0.4	<0.1
97	3	0.1	0.2	0.9	0.1	26	0.3	2	0.3	21	76	65	50	5	1.6	0.5
0	<1	<0.1	<0.1	0.1	<0.1	3	<0.1	<1	<0.1	6	13	22	24	5	0.3	0.1
0	0	0.1	<0.1	0.5	<0.1	13	0	0	<0.1	11	14	69	52	8	1	0.1
5										20		100	30		1.1	
5	26	<0.1	<0.1	0.2	<0.1	5	<0.1	<1	0.4	16	25	90	27	6	0.4	0.1
2	1	0.1	<0.1	0.4		12		0		10		88	74		0.6	
0	0							0		0		200			1.1	
6	30	<0.1	<0.1	0.7	<0.1	11	<0.1	<1	0.8	8	23	104	46	8	0.4	0.2
5	<1	<0.1	<0.1	0.3	<0.1	9	<0.1	0	0.5	4	12	39	10	3	0.3	0.1
0	<1	<0.1	<0.1	0.2	<0.1	3	<0.1	0	<0.1	6	15	55	41	7	0.5	0.1
0	<1	0.1	0.1	1.1	0	21	<0.1	0	0.7	8	37	193	75	19	1.6	0.4
0	0							0		0		175			1.4	

ESHA, EatRight Analysis CD-ROM; **AMT**, amount; **WT**, weight; **CAL**, calories; **WTR**, water; **PROT**, protein; **CARB**, carbohydrate; **FIBR**, fiber; **FAT**, fat; **SATF**, saturated fat; **MONO**, monosaturated fat; **POLY**, polyunsaturated fat

ESHA CODE	FOOD DESCRIPTION	AMT	UNIT	WT (g)	CAL (kcal)	WTR (g)	PROT (g)	CARB (g)	FIBR (g)	FAT (g)	SATF (g)	MONO (g)	POLY (g)
Desserts (continued)													
Cookies (continued)													
47059	Sandwich Cookie-Peanut Butter	1	ea	14	67	<1	1	9	<1	3	0.7	1.6	0.5
47071	Sandwich Cookie-Vanilla	1	ea	10	48	<1	<1	7	<1	2	0.3	0.8	0.8
47007	Shortbread Cookie	4	ea	32	161	1	2	21	1	8	2	4.3	1
47153	Snackwell DevFd Cookie-Svg	1	ea	16	49	3	1	12	<1	<1	0.1	<0.1	<0.1
47160	Snackwell VanSanCookie-Svg	2	ea	26	110		1	20	0	3	0.5		
47011	Snickerdoodle Cookie	1	ea	20	80	4	1	12	<1	3	2.1		
47064	Sugar Cookie	1	ea	15	72	1	1	10	<1	3	0.8	1.8	0.4
47065	Sugar Cookie, no sodium	1	ea	7	30	<1	<1	5	<1	1	0.1	0.4	0.3
47068	Sugar Cookie-Made w/Marg	1	ea	14	66	1	1	8	<1	3	0.7	1.4	1
47069	Sugar Wafers-CremeFilled	1	ea	9	46	<1	<1	6	<1	2	0.3	0.9	0.8
Doughnuts & Pastries													
45516	Baklava-2x2x2.5 in piece	1	pce	78	336	19	5	29	2	23	9.3	8.1	4.2
45505	Cake Doughnut	1	ea	47	196	11	3	21	1	11	3.3	6	1.2
45524	Cake Doughnut-Choc Icing	1	ea	43	194	7	2	22	1	11	5.8	3.7	0.8
45523	Cheese Croissant	1	ea	57	236	12	5	27	1	12	6.1	3.7	1.4
42164	Cheese Sweet Roll	1	ea	66	238	19	5	29	1	12	4	6	1.3
45557	Chinese Pastry	2	oz	56.7	136	26	1	26	1	3	0.5	0.9	1.7
45508	Chocolate Eclair+Custard	1	ea	100	262	52	6	24	1	16	4.1	6.5	3.9
42166	Cinnamon Roll-Bkd-Frosted	1	ea	30	109	7	2	17	1	4	1	2.2	0.5
45509	Cream Puff + Custard	1	ea	130	335	70	9	30	1	20	4.8	8.5	5.4
45563	Crm Filled Yeast Doughnut	1	ea	85	307	32	5	26	1	21	4.6	10.3	2.6
45527	French Cruller Doughnut	1	ea	41	169	7	1	24	<1	8	1.9	4.3	0.9
45562	Funnel Cake-6 inch diam	1	pce	90	278	38	7	29	1	14	2.7	4.4	6.3
45555	Guava Turnover	1	ea	78	234	34	2	28	3	13	2.5	5.5	3.9
45507	Jelly Filled Doughnut	1	ea	85	289	30	5	33	1	16	4.1	8.7	2
45560	Oriental Doughnu/Okinawan	1	ea	18	76	3	1	10	<1	4	0.9	2	0.5
42094	Pan Dulce w/Topping	1	ea	79	291	17	5	48	1	9	1.8	4	2.5
45504	Poptart-Fruit Filled	1	ea	52	203	8	2	36	1	5	1.4	3.3	0.6
45604	Poptart-Fruit Filled-Frosted	1	ea	52	205	6	2	37	1	6	1	3.2	1.3
42071	Scone	1	ea	42	150	12	4	19	1	6	2	2.6	1.3
42072	Scone-Whole Wheat	1	ea	42	144	11	5	18	3	7	2.1	2.6	1.4
46077	Shortcake Biscuit-Recipe	2	oz	56.7	196	16	3	27	1	8	2.1	3.4	2.1
45506	Yeast Doughnut-Plain	1	ea	60	239	14	4	30	1	11	3.3	6	1.7
Frozen Desserts													
2070	Banana Split w/WhipCream	1	ea	425	1089	217	15	124	1	65	37.5	18.7	5.3
72207	Caramel Crunch Ice Cream Bar	1	ea	93	270		3	26	0	17	13		
72208	Choc Choc Ice Cream Bar	1	ea	91	280		3	23	1	19	14		
71819	Choc Frozen Yogurt-Nonfat	1	cup	186	199	137	8	37	2	1	0.9	0.4	0.1
46110	Choc Ice Cream Cake Roll	1	pce	34	101	13	1	14	<1	5	2.1	1.8	0.8
72330	Cookies & Cream Ice Cream Bar	1	ea	60	190		2	21	1	12	6		
72191	Creamsicle Ice Cream Bar	1	ea	65	100	43	1	18	0	2	1.5		
72255	Creamsicle Ice Cream Bar-Rasp	1	ea	65	100	43	1	18	0	2	1.5		
72448	Frozen Dessert Pop-NoAddSug	1	ea	44	25	36	1	6	<1	<1	0.2		
23174	Frozen Fruit Juice Bar	1	ea	77	67	60	1	16	1	<1	0	0	<0.1

< = Trace amount present   Blank = Not available

CHOL, cholesterol; **V,** vitamin; **THI,** thiamin; **RIB,** riboflavin; **NIA,** niacin; **FOL,** folate;
CALC, calcium; **PHOS,** phosphate; **SOD,** sodium; **POT,** potassium; **MAG,** magnesium

CHOL (g)	V-A (RE)	THI (mg)	RIB (mg)	NIA (mg)	V-B6 (mg)	FOL (µg)	V-B12 (µg)	V-C (mg)	V-E (mg)	CALC (mg)	PHOS (mg)	SOD (mg)	POT (mg)	MAG (mg)	IRON (mg)	ZINC (mg)
0	<1	<0.1	<0.1	0.5	<0.1	9	<0.1	<1	0.3	7	26	52	27	7	0.4	0.1
0	0	<0.1	<0.1	0.3	<0.1	5	0	0	0.2	3	8	35	9	1	0.2	<0.1
6	6	0.1	0.1	1.1	<0.1	22	<0.1	0	0.1	11	35	146	32	5	0.9	0.2
0	<1	<0.1	<0.1	0.2	<0.1	3	<0.1	<1		5	11	28	18	4	0.4	0.1
0	0							0		0		130			0.4	
9	25	0.1	<0.1	0.4	<0.1	14	<0.1	<1	0.1	8	10	75	23	2	0.5	0.1
8	4	<0.1	<0.1	0.4	<0.1	8	<0.1	<1	<0.1	3	12	54	9	2	0.3	0.1
0	0	<0.1	<0.1	0.3	<0.1	5	0	0	0.1	2	5	<1	7	1	0.3	<0.1
4	35	<0.1	<0.1	0.3	<0.1	9	<0.1	<1	0.4	10	13	69	11	2	0.3	0.1
0	0	<0.1	<0.1	0.2	<0.1	5	0	0	0.2	2	5	13	5	1	0.2	<0.1
36	124	0.2	0.2	1.4	<0.1	11	<0.1	1	2	33	93	293	144	35	1.7	0.5
4	1	0.1	0.1	0.9	<0.1	38	<0.1	1	0.9	12	123	262	53	8	1.4	0.3
8	2	0.1	0.1	0.7	<0.1	28	<0.1	1	0.9	10	90	178	86	13	1.7	0.4
32	120	0.3	0.2	1.2	<0.1	42	0.2	<1	0.8	30	74	316	75	14	1.2	0.5
50	34	0.1	0.1	0.5	<0.1	28	0.2	<1	1.3	78	65	236	90	13	0.5	0.4
0	<1	<0.1	<0.1	0.5	0.1	2	0	0	0.5	12	31	5	51	15	0.4	0.3
127	209	0.1	0.3	0.8	0.1	43	0.3	<1	2	63	107	337	117	15	1.2	0.6
0	<1	0.1	0.1	1.1	<0.1	16	<0.1	<1	0.5	10	104	250	19	4	0.8	0.1
174	194	0.2	0.4	1.1	0.1	48	0.5	<1	1.9	86	142	443	150	16	1.5	0.8
20	9	0.3	0.1	1.9	0.1	60	0.1	0	0.2	21	65	263	68	17	1.6	0.7
5	1	0.1	0.1	0.9	<0.1	17	<0.1	0	0.1	11	50	141	32	5	1	0.1
63	58	0.2	0.3	1.9	0.1	14	0.2	<1	2.4	128	137	117	155	18	1.9	0.6
<1	32	0.1	0.1	1.5	0.1	6	<0.1	48	2	13	33	13	120	9	1.1	0.2
22	15	0.3	0.1	1.8	0.1	58	0.2	0	0.4	21	72	249	67	17	1.5	0.6
13	7	<0.1	0.1	0.4	<0.1	2	<0.1	<1	0.5	24	22	38	15	2	0.4	0.1
26	67	0.2	0.2	2	<0.1	19	0.1	<1	1.2	13	56	75	57	9	1.8	0.4
0	160	0.2	0.3	2.7	0.2	27	0	0	0.4	6	37	174	39	6	2	0.2
0	100	0.2	0.2	2	0.2	52	0	0	0	11	46	211	44	8	1.8	0.6
49	69	0.1	0.2	1.2	<0.1	8	0.1	<1	0.7	80	74	171	49	7	1.3	0.3
50	71	0.1	0.1	1.3	0.1	11	0.1	<1	0.9	86	126	175	114	33	1.1	0.8
2	11	0.2	0.2	1.5	<0.1	30	<0.1	<1	1.1	116	81	287	60	9	1.4	0.3
18	3	0.2	0.1	1.6	<0.1	65	0.1	1	0.9	28	83	232	60	11	2.2	0.8
204	531	0.1	0.9	0.5	0.2	19	1.4	2	0.5	466	485	360	783	92	1.6	2.7
25	40							0		100		80			0	
20	40							0		80		55			1.1	
7	6	0.1	0.3	0.4	0.1	22	0.9	1	0.1	296	240	151	631	74	0.1	0.9
15	22	<0.1	0.1	0.3	<0.1	2	0.1	<1	0.3	42	40	45	57	9	0.5	0.2
10	20							0		60		120			0.4	
5	0							0		40		30			0	
5	0							0		40		30			0	
1	2							<1		60		18			0.1	
0	2	<0.1	<0.1	0.1	<0.1	5	0	7	0	4	5	3	41	3	0.1	<0.1

ESHA, EatRight Analysis CD-ROM; **AMT,** amount; **WT,** weight; **CAL,** calories; **WTR,** water; **PROT,** protein; **CARB,** carbohydrate;
FIBR, fiber; **FAT,** fat; **SATF,** saturated fat; **MONO,** monosaturated fat; **POLY,** polyunsaturated fat

ESHA CODE	FOOD DESCRIPTION	AMT	UNIT	WT (g)	CAL (kcal)	WTR (g)	PROT (g)	CARB (g)	FIBR (g)	FAT (g)	SATF (g)	MONO (g)	POLY (g)
Desserts (continued)													
Frozen Desserts (continued)													
2043	Frozen Yogurt Bar-Choc Coat	1	ea	41	109	21	1	12	<1	7	5.3	0.8	0.2
2035	Frozen Yogurt-Choc-Soft	0.5	cup	72	115	46	3	18	2	4	2.6	1.3	0.2
2064	Frozen Yogurt-Vanilla	0.5	cup	72	117	47	3	17	0	4	2.5	1.1	0.2
72188	Fudgsicle Ice Cream Bar	1	ea	61	90	40	3	16	1	2	1		
2216	Ice Cream-ChChipCookDo-Rich	0.5	cup	105	273		4	32	0	15	10.1		
49013	Ice Cream Cone-Cake/Wafer	1	ea	4	17	<1	<1	3	<1	<1	<0.1	0.1	0.1
49014	Ice Cream Cone-Sugar/Rolled	1	ea	10	40	<1	1	8	<1	<1	0.1	0.1	0.1
2105	Ice Cream-Cookies&Crm-LowFat	0.5	cup	71	120		3	21	1	2	1	1	0
2050	Ice Cream-Hard-Choc	0.5	cup	66	143	37	3	19	1	7	4.5	2.1	0.3
71809	Ice Cream-Orange Float Sherbet	0.5	cup	65	120		2	21	0	4	2.5		
2008	Ice Cream-Soft-French Vanilla	0.5	cup	86	191	51	4	19	1	11	6.4	3	0.4
2063	Ice Cream-Strawberry	0.5	cup	66	127	40	2	18	1	6	3.4		
2004	Ice Cream-Vanilla	0.5	cup	66	133	40	2	16	<1	7	4.5	2	0.3
2006	Ice Cream-Vanilla-Rich	0.5	cup	74	184	42	3	16	0	12	7.6	3.3	0.5
2057	Ice Milk-Chocolate	0.5	cup	65.5	95	43	3	17	<1	2	1.3	0.6	0.1
2009	Ice Milk-Hard-Vanilla	0.5	cup	66	109	42	3	17	<1	3	1.9	0.8	0.1
23051	Ice Slushy	1	cup	193	247	129	1	63	0	0	0	0	0
49198	Lemon Sorbet	0.5	cup	70	90		0	22	0	0	0	0	0
2011	Orange Sherbet	0.5	cup	74	107	49	1	22	2	1	0.9	0.4	0.1
23050	Popsicle/Ice Pops-Double	1	ea	128	101	103	0	25	0	<1	<0.1	0.1	<0.1
72709	StrawBanana FrznYogurt-LowFat	0.5	cup	106	160		3	30	<1	2	1		
70675	Strawberry Frozen Yogurt-Nonfat	0.5	cup	95	140		5	31	0	0	0	0	0
49197	Strawberry Sorbet	0.5	cup	70	80		0	19	0	0	0	0	0
2592	Vanilla Rasp Frzn Yogurt-LowFat	0.5	cup	108	170		4	32	0	2	1.5		
Pies													
70536	Apple Pie-1/10	1	pce	130	300	73	2	39	2	15	3		
48022	Apple Pie-Homemade	1	ea	1240	3286	587	30	460	17	155	37.8	66.9	41.4
49015	Apple Strudel	1	pce	71	195	31	2	29	2	8	1.5	2.3	3.8
70557	Boston Cream Pie-1/10	1	pce	78	220		2	32	0	9	2.5		
70538	Cherry Pie-1/10	1	pce	130	330	63	3	48	1	15	3		
70554	Chocolate Cream Pie-1/10	1	pce	130	370	61	3	44	1	21	13		
49018	Fruit Filled Blintz	1	ea	70	124	44	4	17	<1	4	1.3	1.8	0.9
70562	Lemon Meringue Pie-1/9	1	pce	120	250		2	46	0	6	1.5		
49063	Peach Cobbler-Ckd f/Frzn	0.25	ea	120.5	360		3	47	0	18	6		
70559	Pecan Pie-1/8	1	pce	128	550	19	7	75	2	26	6		
70561	Pumpkin Pie-1/10th	1	pce	125	310		5	47	2	12	3		
Puddings													
57915	Bread Pudding-f/Recipe	1	svg	270.9	475	169	15	66	2	17	8		
2613	Egg Custard-Mix+Whl Milk	0.5	cup	133	161	98	5	23	0	5	2.8	1.6	0.3
2625	Flan CarmCustardMix+WhMlk	0.5	cup	133	150	99	4	25	0	4	2.4	1.1	0.1
23052	Gelatin/Jello-Prepared	0.5	cup	135	84	114	2	19	0	0	0	0	0
23093	Gelatin/Jello-SugFree-Prepared	0.5	cup	117	23	111	1	5	0	0	0	0	0
2628	Pudding-Instant+2%Milk	0.5	cup	147	154	110	4	29	0	2	1.4	0.7	0.2
58203	Pudding-Inst-LowCal	1	svg	8	28	1	<1	7	<1	<1	<0.1	<0.1	<0.1

< = Trace amount present   Blank = Not available

CHOL, cholesterol; **V**, vitamin; **THI**, thiamin; **RIB**, riboflavin; **NIA**, niacin; **FOL**, folate;
CALC, calcium; **PHOS**, phosphate; **SOD**, sodium; **POT**, potassium; **MAG**, magnesium

CHOL (g)	V-A (RE)	THI (mg)	RIB (mg)	NIA (mg)	V-B6 (mg)	FOL (μg)	V-B12 (μg)	V-C (mg)	V-E (mg)	CALC (mg)	PHOS (mg)	SOD (mg)	POT (mg)	MAG (mg)	IRON (mg)	ZINC (mg)
1	18	<0.1	0.1	0.1	<0.1	2	0.1	<1	<0.1	46	43	28	74	6	0.1	0.2
4	32	<0.1	0.2	0.2	0.1	8	0.2	<1	0.1	106	100	71	188	19	0.9	0.4
1	43	<0.1	0.2	0.2	0.1	4	0.2	1	0.1	103	93	63	152	10	0.2	0.3
5	0							0		80		65			0.4	
66	101							0		151		91			0.7	
0	0	<0.1	<0.1	0.2	<0.1	7	0	0	<0.1	1	4	6	4	1	0.1	<0.1
0	0	0.1	<0.1	0.5	<0.1	14	0	0	<0.1	4	10	32	14	3	0.4	0.1
5	40	<0.1	0.2					0		100	141	90	254			
22	79	<0.1	0.1	0.1	<0.1	11	0.2	<1	0.2	72	71	50	164	19	0.6	0.4
15	20							1			60		40		0	
78	142	<0.1	0.2	0.1	<0.1	8	0.4	1	0.5	113	100	52	152	10	0.2	0.4
19	63	<0.1	0.2	0.1	<0.1	8	0.2	5	<0.1	79	66	40	124	9	0.1	0.2
29	79	<0.1	0.2	0.1	<0.1	3	0.3	<1	0.2	84	69	53	131	9	0.1	0.5
68	137	<0.1	0.1	0.1	<0.1	6	0.3	0	0.4	87	78	45	116	8	0.3	0.3
6	18	<0.1	0.1	0.1	<0.1	4	0.3	<1	0.1	94	78	41	155	13	0.2	0.4
18	85	<0.1	0.2	0.1	<0.1	4	0.3	1	0.1	106	68	49	137	9	0.1	0.5
0	0	<0.1	0	<0.1	<0.1	0	0	2	0	4	2	42	6	2	0.3	<0.1
0												33	3			
0	8	<0.1	0.1	0.1	<0.1	5	0.1	4	<0.1	40	30	34	71	6	0.1	0.4
0	0	0	0	0	0	0	0	1	0	0	0	9	19	1	0.7	0.2
30	0							6		80		25			0	
3	0							6		150		40			0	
0												1	34			
25	0							1		100		35			0	
0	0	<0.1	<0.1	0.4	0.1			0		0		390	96		0.4	
0	161	1.8	1.3	15.3	0.4	298	0	21	23.6	87	347	2616	980	87	13.9	2.4
4	4	<0.1	<0.1	0.2	<0.1	20	0.2	1	1	11	23	191	106	6	0.3	0.1
30	0	<0.1	0.1	0.2	<0.1			0		20		170	77		0.4	
0	80	<0.1	<0.1	0.2	0.1			0		80		360	112		0.4	
20	20	<0.1	0.1	1.4	<0.1			0		35		359	176		0.9	
53	73	0.1	0.1	0.4	<0.1	8	0.2	1	0.5	35	59	93	78	7	0.8	0.3
0	0							0		0		290	23		0	
0	0							4		0		240			1.1	
85	40							0		0		510	90		0.7	
45	700	0.1	0.2	0.5				0		80		390	193		1.4	
243	171	0.3	0.6	2.2	0.2	78	1	2	1	241	267	666	406	39	2.7	1.4
70	51	0.1	0.3	0.2	0.1	12	0.6	1	0.1	190	181	117	294	25	0.5	0.7
16	40	<0.1	0.2	0.1	<0.1	5	0.3	1	0.1	148	112	149	213	16	0.1	0.5
0	0	0	<0.1	<0.1	0	1	0	0	0	4	30	101	1	1	<0.1	<0.1
0	0	0	0	0	0	0	0	0	0	4	80	56	1	1	<0.1	0
9	68	<0.1	0.2	0.1	0.1	6	0.4	1	0.1	150	318	435	193	18	0.1	0.5
0	0	<0.1	<0.1	<0.1	<0.1	<1	<0.1	0	<0.1	11	189	340	2	<1	<0.1	<0.1

ESHA, EatRight Analysis CD-ROM; **AMT,** amount; **WT,** weight; **CAL,** calories; **WTR,** water; **PROT,** protein; **CARB,** carbohydrate;
FIBR, fiber; **FAT,** fat; **SATF,** saturated fat; **MONO,** monosaturated fat; **POLY,** polyunsaturated fat

ESHA CODE	FOOD DESCRIPTION	AMT	UNIT	WT (g)	CAL (kcal)	WTR (g)	PROT (g)	CARB (g)	FIBR (g)	FAT (g)	SATF (g)	MONO (g)	POLY (g)
Desserts (continued)													
Puddings (continued)													
2636	Pudding-RegMix+2% Milk	0.5	cup	142	155	105	5	28	<1	3	1.7	0.8	0.1
2604	Pudding-RegMix+Whole Milk	0.5	cup	142	169	104	5	28	1	4	2.6	1.2	0.3
48044	Pumpkin Pie Mix-Canned	0.5	cup	135	140	97	1	36	11	0.1	<0.1	<0.1	<0.1
2653	TapiocaPudding + 2% Milk	0.5	cup	141	148	106	4	28	0	2	1.4	0.6	0.1
Toppings													
23069	Butterscotch Topping	2	Tbs	41	103	13	1	27	<1	<1	<0.1	<0.1	0
23070	Caramel Topping	2	Tbs	41	103	13	1	27	<1	<1	<0.1	<0.1	0
23013	Chocolate syrup-Thin	2	Tbs	37.5	105	12	1	24	1	<1	0.2	0.1	<0.1
509	Dessert Topping/DreamWhip	2	Tbs	10	19	7	<1	2	0	1	1.1	0.1	<0.1
569	Dream Whip Topping-Dry Mix	1	svg	2	10	0	0	2		0	0	0	0
508	FrznDessertTopping/Cool Whip	2	Tbs	9.375	30	5	<1	2	0	2	2	0.2	<0.1
23014	HotFudge ChocolateTopping	2	Tbs	38	133	8	2	24	1	3	1.5	1.5	0.1
23064	Marshmallow Creme	2	Tbs	12	40	2	0	10	0	0	0	0	0
23071	Marshmallow Creme Topping	1	oz	28.35	91	6	<1	22	<1	<1	<0.1	<0.1	<0.1
23162	Nuts in Syrup Topping	2	Tbs	41	184	6	2	24	1	9	0.8	2	5.6
510	Whipped Cream-Pressurized	2	Tbs	7.5	19	5	<1	1	0	2	1	0.5	0.1
Eggs & Egg Substitutes													
19581	Egg Beaters-Egg Substitute	0.25	cup	61	30	53	6	1	0	0	0	0	0
19522	Egg White-Cooked	1	ea	33.4	17	29	4	<1	0	0	0	0	0
19507	Egg White-Raw-Fresh	0.25	cup	60.75	32	53	7	<1	0	<1	0	0	0
19506	Egg White-Raw-Fresh-Large	1	ea	33.4	17	29	4	<1	0	<1	0	0	0
19523	Egg Yolk-Cooked	1	ea	16.6	59	8	3	<1	0	5	1.6	1.9	0.7
19508	Egg Yolk-Raw-Fresh-Large	1	ea	16.6	53	9	3	1	0	4	1.6	1.9	0.7
19511	Egg-Hard Boiled-Chopped	0.33	cup	45.33	70	34	6	1	0	5	1.5	1.8	0.6
19510	Egg-Hard Cooked/Boiled	1	ea	50	78	37	6	1	0	5	1.6	2	0.7
19509	Egg-Large-Fried in Marg	1	ea	46	90	32	6	<1	0	7	2	2.9	1.2
19517	Egg-Poached-Large	1	ea	50	71	38	6	<1	0	5	1.5	1.9	0.7
19500	Egg-Whole-Raw-Fresh-Large	0.25	cup	60.75	87	46	8	<1	0	6	1.9	2.3	0.8
Fats & Fat Substitutes													
Butters & Margarines													
250	Benecol Spread	1	Tbs	14	70	6	0	0	0	8	1	4.5	2
8825	Benecol Spread-Light	1	Tbs	14	50	9	0	0	0	5	0.5	2.5	2
8001	Butter-Pat	1	ea	5	36	1	<1	<1	0	4	2.6	1.1	0.2
8000	Butter-Regular-Salted	1	Tbs	14	100	2	<1	<1	0	11	7.2	2.9	0.4
8025	Butter-Unsalted	1	Tbs	14	100	3	<1	<1	0	11	7.2	2.9	0.4
8142	Butter-Whipped	1	Tbs	9.44	68	1	<1	<1	0	8	4.8	2.2	0.3
44466	Butter Substitute-LowFat-Pwd	1	Tbs	5	19	<1	<1	4	0	<1	<0.1	<0.1	<0.1
8698	I Can't Believe It's Not Butter	1	Tbs	14	90	4	0	0	0	10	2		
90226	Margarine-Hard	1	Tbs	14.1	101	2	<1	<1	0	11	1.8	5.3	3.7
8165	Margarine-Liquid	1	Tbs	14.2	102	2	<1	0	0	11	1.9	4	5.1
8790	Margarine-Soft	1	Tbs	14	100	3	0	0	0	11	2		
90233	Margarine-Unsalt-Hard	1	Tbs	14.1	101	3	<1	<1	0	11	2.1	5.2	3.5
8176	Shedd's Spread	1	Tbs	14.5	62	7	0	0	0	7	1.6		

< = Trace amount present   Blank = Not available

CHOL, cholesterol; **V,** vitamin; **THI,** thiamin; **RIB,** riboflavin; **NIA,** niacin; **FOL,** folate;
CALC, calcium; **PHOS,** phosphate; **SOD,** sodium; **POT,** potassium; **MAG,** magnesium

CHOL (g)	V-A (RE)	THI (mg)	RIB (mg)	NIA (mg)	V-B6 (mg)	FOL (µg)	V-B12 (µg)	V-C (mg)	V-E (mg)	CALC (mg)	PHOS (mg)	SOD (mg)	POT (mg)	MAG (mg)	IRON (mg)	ZINC (mg)
10	68	<0.1	0.2	0.1	0.1	6	0.4	1	0.1	159	136	148	237	30	0.5	0.7
13	34	0.1	0.3	0.2	<0.1	6	0.4	0	0.1	136	124	139	213	28	0.5	0.7
0	1120	<0.1	0.2	0.5	0.2	47	0	5	1.1	50	61	281	186	22	1.4	0.4
8	68	<0.1	0.2	0.1	<0.1	6	0.4	1	0.1	148	116	171	188	17	0.1	0.5
<1	11	<0.1	<0.1	<0.1	<0.1	1	<0.1	<1	0	22	19	143	34	3	0.1	0.1
<1	11	<0.1	<0.1	<0.1	<0.1	1	<0.1	<1	0	22	19	143	34	3	0.1	0.1
0	0	<0.1	<0.1	0.1	<0.1	2	0	<1	<0.1	5	48	27	84	24	0.8	0.3
1	3	<0.1	<0.1	<0.1	<0.1	<1	<0.1	<1	<0.1	9	9	7	15	1	<0.1	<0.1
0	0							0		0		0			0	
0	1	0	0	0	0	0	0	0	0.1	1	1	2	2	<1	<0.1	<0.1
1	2	<0.1	0.1	0.1	<0.1	2	0.1	<1	0.9	38	64	131	171	24	0.6	0.3
0	0							0		0		10			0	
0	<1	<0.1	<0.1	<0.1	<0.1	<1	0	0	0	1	2	23	1	1	0.1	<0.1
0	<1	0.1	<0.1	0.2	0.1	11	0	<1	0.1	14	48	17	62	22	0.4	0.4
6	14	<0.1	<0.1	<0.1	<0.1	<1	<0.1	0	<0.1	8	7	10	11	1	<0.1	<0.1
0	60		0.9		0.1	32	0.6	0	0.8	20		125	85		1.1	0.6
0	0	<0.1	0.1	<0.1	<0.1	1	0.1	0	0	2	4	55	48	4	<0.1	<0.1
0	0	<0.1	0.3	0.1	<0.1	2	0.1	0	0	4	9	101	99	7	<0.1	<0.1
0	0	<0.1	0.1	<0.1	<0.1	1	<0.1	0	0	2	5	55	54	4	<0.1	<0.1
213	97	<0.1	0.1	<0.1	0.1	18	0.4	0	0.5	23	81	7	16	1	0.6	0.5
205	65	<0.1	0.1	<0.1	0.1	24	0.3	0	0.4	21	65	8	18	1	0.5	0.4
192	77	<0.1	0.2	<0.1	0.1	20	0.5	0	0.5	23	78	56	57	5	0.5	0.5
212	85	<0.1	0.3	<0.1	0.1	22	0.6	0	0.5	25	86	62	63	5	0.6	0.5
210	93	<0.1	0.2	<0.1	0.1	23	0.6	0	0.6	27	96	94	68	6	0.9	0.6
211	70	<0.1	0.2	<0.1	0.1	24	0.6	0	0.5	26	95	147	66	6	0.9	0.6
257	86	<0.1	0.3	<0.1	0.1	29	0.8	0	0.6	32	116	85	81	7	1.1	0.7
0	100							0	2.7	0		110		0		
0	100							0	2.7	0		110		0		
11	35	<0.1	<0.1	<0.1	<0.1	<1	<0.1	0	0.1	1	1	29	1	<1	<0.1	<0.1
30	98	<0.1	<0.1	<0.1	<0.1	<1	<0.1	0	0.3	3	3	81	3	<1	<0.1	<0.1
30	98	<0.1	<0.1	<0.1	<0.1	<1	<0.1	0	0.3	3	3	2	3	<1	<0.1	<0.1
21	66	<0.1	<0.1	<0.1	<0.1	<1	<0.1	0	0.2	2	2	78	2	<1	<0.1	<0.1
<1	0	0	0	0	0	0	0	0	0	1	<1	60	<1	0	0.1	0
0	100							0		0		90		0		
0	123	<0.1	<0.1	<0.1	<0.1	<1	<0.1	<1	0.4	4	3	133	6	<1	0	
0	124	<0.1	<0.1	<0.1	<0.1	<1	<0.1	<1	0.7	9	7	111	13	1	0	0
0	100							0		0		95		0		
0	123	<0.1	<0.1	<0.1	<0.1	<1	<0.1	<1	1.8	2	2	<1	4	<1	0	0
0	104							0				114		0		

ESHA, EatRight Analysis CD-ROM; **AMT,** amount; **WT,** weight; **CAL,** calories; **WTR,** water; **PROT,** protein; **CARB,** carbohydrate; **FIBR,** fiber; **FAT,** fat; **SATF,** saturated fat; **MONO,** monosaturated fat; **POLY,** polyunsaturated fat

ESHA CODE	FOOD DESCRIPTION	AMT	UNIT	WT (g)	CAL (kcal)	WTR (g)	PROT (g)	CARB (g)	FIBR (g)	FAT (g)	SATF (g)	MONO (g)	POLY (g)
Fats & Fat Substitutes (continued)													
Fats & Oils													
8004	Beef Fat/Tallow-Drippings	1	Tbs	12	108	0	0	0	0	12	6	5	0.5
8031	Butter Oil/Ghee	1	Tbs	12.8	112	<1	<1	0	0	13	7.9	3.7	0.5
8084	Canola Oil	1	Tbs	14	124	0	0	0	0	14	1	8.2	4.1
8005	Chicken Fat	1	Tbs	12.8	115	<1	0	0	0	13	3.8	5.7	2.7
8037	Coconut Oil	1	Tbs	13.6	117	0	0	0	0	14	11.8	0.8	0.2
8067	Cod Liver Oil (Fish Oil)	1	Tbs	13.6	123	0	0	0	0	14	3.1	6.4	3.1
8009	Corn Oil	1	Tbs	13.6	120	0	0	0	0	14	1.8	3.8	7.4
8081	Cottonseed Oil	1	Tbs	13.6	120	0	0	0	0	14	3.5	2.4	7.1
8012	Crisco/Wesson Oil	1	Tbs	13.6	120	0	0	0	0	14	2	3.2	7.9
8008	Olive Oil	1	Tbs	13.5	119	0	0	0	0	14	1.9	9.8	1.4
8083	Palm Kernel Oil	1	Tbs	13.6	117	0	0	0	0	14	11.1	1.6	0.2
8082	Palm Oil	1	Tbs	13.6	120	0	0	0	0	14	6.7	5	1.3
8002	Pam CkingSpray-BtrFlav-1/3sec	1	ea	0.266	2	0	0	0	0	<1			
8026	Peanut Oil	1	Tbs	13.5	119	0	0	0	0	14	2.3	6.2	4.3
8010	Safflower Oil	1	Tbs	13.6	120	0	0	0	0	14	0.8	2	10.1
8027	Sesame Oil	1	Tbs	13.6	120	0	0	0	0	14	1.9	5.4	5.7
8007	Shortening (Crisco)	1	Tbs	12.8	113	0	0	0	0	13	3.2	5.7	3.3
8028	Soybean + Cottonseed Oil	1	Tbs	13.6	120	0	0	0	0	14	2.4	4	6.5
8085	Walnut Oil	1	Tbs	13.6	120	0	0	0	0	14	1.2	3.1	8.6
8011	Wesson Sunlite/Sunflower Oil	1	Tbs	13.6	120	0	0	0	0	14	1.4	2.7	8.9
8038	Wheat Germ Oil-Tablespoon	1	Tbs	13.6	120	0	0	0	0	14	2.6	2.1	8.4
Fruits													
Canned Fruits													
3147	Applesauce-Canned-Sweet	1	cup	255	194	203	<1	51	3	<1	0.1	<0.1	0.1
3006	Applesauce-Canned-Unsweet	1	cup	244	105	216	<1	28	3	<1	<0.1	<0.1	<0.1
3152	Apricot Halves+Juice-Canned	0.5	cup	122	59	106	1	15	2	<1	<0.1	<0.1	<0.1
3040	Cranberry Sauce-Strained	1	cup	277	418	168	1	108	3	<1	<0.1	0.1	0.2
3045	Fruit Cocktail+HeavySyrup	1	cup	248	181	199	1	47	2	<1	<0.1	<0.1	0.1
3163	Fruit Cocktail+LiteSyrup	1	cup	242	138	204	1	36	2	<1	<0.1	<0.1	0.1
3164	Fruit Cocktail-Juice Pack	1	cup	237	109	207	1	28	2	<1	<0.1	<0.1	<0.1
3313	Fruit Cocktail-Water Pack	1	cup	237	76	215	1	20	2	<1	<0.1	<0.1	<0.1
3089	Oranges-Mandarin-Canned	1	cup	249	92	223	2	24	2	<1	<0.1	<0.1	<0.1
3174	Peach Halves+LtSyrup-Canned	0.5	cup	125.5	68	106	1	18	2	<1	<0.1	<0.1	<0.1
3098	Peaches-Canned+Heavy Syrup	1	cup	262	194	208	1	52	3	<1	<0.1	0.1	0.1
3107	Pears-Canned+Heavy Syrup	1	cup	266	197	214	1	51	4	<1	<0.1	0.1	0.1
3179	Pears-Canned+Juice	1	cup	248	124	214	1	32	4	<1	<0.1	<0.1	<0.1
3177	Pears-Canned+Light Syrup	1	cup	251	143	212	<1	38	4	<1	<0.1	<0.1	<0.1
3115	Pineapple-Canned+HeavySyrup	1	cup	254	198	201	1	51	2	<1	<0.1	<0.1	0.1
3183	Pineapple-Canned+Juice	1	cup	249	149	208	1	39	2	<1	<0.1	<0.1	0.1
3181	Pineapple-Canned+Light Syrup	1	cup	252	131	216	1	34	2	<1	<0.1	<0.1	0.1
Dried Fruits													
3005	Apple Rings-Dried	10	ea	64	156	20	1	42	6	<1	<0.1	<0.1	0.1
3013	Apricot Halves-Dried-Each	1	ea	3.5	8	1	<1	2	<1	<1	<0.1	<0.1	<0.1

< = Trace amount present   Blank = Not available

CHOL, cholesterol; **V,** vitamin; **THI,** thiamin; **RIB,** riboflavin; **NIA,** niacin; **FOL,** folate;
CALC, calcium; **PHOS,** phosphate; **SOD,** sodium; **POT,** potassium; **MAG,** magnesium

CHOL (g)	V-A (RE)	THI (mg)	RIB (mg)	NIA (mg)	V-B6 (mg)	FOL (µg)	V-B12 (µg)	V-C (mg)	V-E (mg)	CALC (mg)	PHOS (mg)	SOD (mg)	POT (mg)	MAG (mg)	IRON (mg)	ZINC (mg)
13	0	0	0	0	0	0	0	0	0.3	0	0	0	0	0	0	0
33	110	<0.1	<0.1	<0.1	<0.1	0	<0.1	0	0.4	1	<1	<1	1	0	0	<0.1
0	0	0	0	0	0	0	0	0	2.4	0	0	0	0	0	0	0
11	0	0	0	0	0	0	0	0	0.3	0	0	0	0	0	0	0
0	0	0	0	0	0	0	0	0	<0.1	0	0	0	0	0	<0.1	0
78	4080	0	0	0	0	0	0	0	0.4	0	0	0	0	0	0	0
0	0	0	0	0	0	0	0	0	1.9	0	0	0	0	0	0	0
0	0	0	0	0	0	0	0	0	4.8	0	0	0	0	0	0	0
0	0	0	0	0	0	0	0	0	1.3	0	0	0	0	0	<0.1	0
0	0	0	0	0	0	0	0	0	1.9	<1	0	<1	<1	0	0.1	0
0	0	0	0	0	0	0	0	0	0.5	0	0	0	0	0	0	0
0	0	0	0	0	0	0	0	0	2.2	0	0	0	0	0	<0.1	0
0	0							0		0		0			0	
0	0	0	0	0	0	0	0	0	2.1	0	0	0	0	0	<0.1	<0.1
0	0	0	0	0	0	0	0	0	4.6	0	0	0	0	0	0	0
0	0	0	0	0	0	0	0	0	0.2	0	0	0	0	0	0	0
0	0	0	0	0	0	0	0	0	0.1	0	0	0	0	0	0	0
0	0	0	0	0	0	0	0	0	1.6	0	0	0	0	0	0	0
0	0	0	0	0	0	0	0	0	0.1	0	0	0	0	0	0	0
0	0	0	0	0	0	0	0	0	5.6	0	0	0	0	0	0	0
0	0	0	0	0	0	0	0	0	20.3	0	0	0	0	0	0	0
0	5	<0.1	0.1	0.5	0.1	3	0	4	0.5	10	18	8	156	8	0.9	0.1
0	5	<0.1	0.1	0.5	0.1	2	0	3	0.5	7	17	5	183	7	0.3	0.1
0	207	<0.1	<0.1	0.4	0.1	2	0	6	0.7	15	24	5	201	12	0.4	0.1
0	11	<0.1	0.1	0.3	<0.1	3	0	6	2.3	11	17	80	72	8	0.6	0.1
0	50	<0.1	<0.1	0.9	0.1	7	0	5	1	15	27	15	218	12	0.7	0.2
0	48	<0.1	<0.1	0.9	0.1	7	0	5	1.2	15	27	15	215	12	0.7	0.2
0	71	<0.1	<0.1	1	0.1	7	0	6	0.9	19	33	9	225	17	0.5	0.2
0	62	<0.1	<0.1	0.9	0.1	7	0	5	0.9	12	26	9	223	17	0.6	0.2
0	214	0.2	0.1	1.1	0.1	12	0	85	0.2	27	25	12	331	27	0.7	1.3
0	45	<0.1	<0.1	0.7	<0.1	4	0	3	0.6	4	14	6	122	6	0.5	0.1
0	89	<0.1	0.1	1.6	<0.1	8	0	7	1.3	8	29	16	241	13	0.7	0.2
0	0	<0.1	0.1	0.6	<0.1	3	0	3	0.2	13	19	13	173	11	0.6	0.2
0	1	<0.1	<0.1	0.5	<0.1	2	0	4	0.2	22	30	10	238	17	0.7	0.2
0	0	<0.1	<0.1	0.4	<0.1	3	0	2	0.2	13	18	13	166	10	0.7	0.2
0	5	0.2	0.1	0.7	0.2	13	0	19	<0.1	36	18	3	264	41	1	0.3
0	10	0.2	<0.1	0.7	0.2	12	0	24	<0.1	35	15	2	304	35	0.7	0.2
0	10	0.2	0.1	0.7	0.2	13	0	19	<0.1	35	18	3	265	40	1	0.3
0	0	0	0.1	0.6	0.1	0	0	2	0.3	9	24	56	288	10	0.9	0.1
0	13	<0.1	<0.1	0.1	<0.1	<1	0	<1	0.2	2	2	<1	41	1	0.1	<0.1

ESHA, EatRight Analysis CD-ROM; **AMT**, amount; **WT**, weight; **CAL**, calories; **WTR**, water; **PROT**, protein; **CARB**, carbohydrate; **FIBR**, fiber; **FAT**, fat; **SATF**, saturated fat; **MONO**, monosaturated fat; **POLY**, polyunsaturated fat

ESHA CODE	FOOD DESCRIPTION	AMT	UNIT	WT (g)	CAL (kcal)	WTR (g)	PROT (g)	CARB (g)	FIBR (g)	FAT (g)	SATF (g)	MONO (g)	POLY (g)
Fruits (continued)													
Dried Fruits (continued)													
3307	Banana Chips	1	oz	28.35	147	1	1	17	2	10	8.2	0.6	0.2
3043	Dates-Chopped	1	cup	178	502	37	4	134	14	1	0.1	0.1	<0.1
3044	Dates-Whole-Each	10	ea	83	234	17	2	62	7	<1	<0.1	<0.1	<0.1
3162	Dried Figs	1	ea	19	47	6	1	12	2	<1	<0.1	<0.1	0.1
3126	Prunes-Dried	10	ea	84	202	26	2	54	6	<1	0.1	<0.1	0.1
3129	Raisins-Seedless-Packed	1	cup	165	493	25	5	131	6	1	0.1	0.1	0.1
3130	Raisins-Seedless-Unpacked	1	cup	145	434	22	4	115	5	1	0.1	0.1	0.1
61372	Strawberry Fruit Leather	1	ea	14	45	3	0	11	1	0	0	0	0
Fresh Fruits													
3000	Apple+Peel-Medium	1	ea	138	72	118	<1	19	3	<1	<0.1	<0.1	0.1
3003	Apple-Peeled-Medium	1	ea	128	61	111	<1	16	2	<1	<0.1	<0.1	<0.1
3388	Apple Slices-Peeled-Cooked	0.5	cup	85.5	45	73	<1	12	2	<1	<0.1	<0.1	0.1
3157	Apricots-Fresh-Pitted	1	ea	35	17	30	<1	4	1	<1	<0.1	0.1	<0.1
3016	Avocado-Fresh	1	ea	201	322	147	4	17	13	29	4.3	19.7	3.7
3020	Banana-Fresh	1	ea	118	105	88	1	27	3	<1	0.1	<0.1	0.1
3024	Blackberries-Fresh	1	cup	144	62	127	2	14	8	1	<0.1	0.1	0.4
3029	Blueberries-Fresh	1	cup	145	83	122	1	21	3	<1	<0.1	0.1	0.2
3663	Breadfruit-Fresh	0.25	ea	96	99	68	1	26	5	<1	<0.1	<0.1	0.1
3076	Cantaloupe Melon	1	ea	552	188	498	5	45	5	1	0.3	<0.1	0.4
3075	Cantaloupe Melon-Cubes	1	cup	160	54	144	1	13	1	<1	0.1	<0.1	0.1
3240	Carambola/Starfruit-Fresh	1	ea	127	39	116	1	9	4	<1	<0.1	<0.1	0.2
3079	Casaba/Crenshaw Melon	1	ea	1640	459	1506	18	108	15	2	0.4	<0.1	0.6
3078	Casaba/Crenshaw Melon-Cubes	1	cup	170	48	156	2	11	2	<1	<0.1	<0.1	0.1
3036	Cherries-Fresh	0.5	cup	72.5	46	60	1	12	2	<1	<0.1	<0.1	<0.1
71089	Concord Grapes	10	ea	24	16	20	<1	4	<1	<1	<0.1	<0.1	<0.1
3039	Cranberries-Fresh	1	cup	95	44	83	<1	12	4	<1	<0.1	<0.1	0.1
3271	Feijoa Fruit-Raw	1	ea	50	24	43	1	5	2	<1			
3160	Figs-Medium-Fresh	1	ea	50	37	40	<1	10	1	<1	<0.1	<0.1	0.1
3048	Grapefruit-Fresh-Pieces	1	cup	230	74	209	1	19	3	<1	<0.1	<0.1	0.1
3047	Grapefruit-Fresh-White	0.5	ea	118	39	107	1	10	1	<1	<0.1	<0.1	<0.1
3207	Guava-Fresh	1	ea	90	61	73	2	13	5	1	0.2	0.1	0.4
3081	Honeydew Melon (1/10th)	1	pce	160	58	144	1	15	1	<1	0.1	<0.1	0.1
3080	Honeydew Melon-Cubes	1	cup	170	61	153	1	15	1	<1	0.1	<0.1	0.1
3065	Kiwifruit	1	ea	76	46	63	1	11	2	<1	<0.1	<0.1	0.2
3066	Lemon-Fresh-Peeled	1	ea	58	17	52	1	5	2	<1	<0.1	<0.1	0.1
3071	Lime-Fresh-Peeled	1	ea	67	20	59	<1	7	2	<1	<0.1	<0.1	<0.1
3257	Lychees	1	ea	9.6	6	8	<1	2	<1	<1	<0.1	<0.1	<0.1
3221	Mango-Fresh-Whole	1	ea	207	135	169	1	35	4	1	0.1	0.2	0.1
3215	Nectarine-Fresh	1	ea	136	60	119	1	14	2	<1	<0.1	0.1	0.2
3082	Orange-Fresh-Medium	1	ea	131	62	114	1	15	3	<1	<0.1	<0.1	<0.1
3083	Orange-Fresh-Sections-Cup	1	cup	180	85	156	2	21	4	<1	<0.1	<0.1	<0.1
3171	Papaya-Fresh	1	ea	304	119	270	2	30	5	<1	0.1	0.1	0.1
3096	Peach-Fresh-Medium	1	ea	98	38	87	1	9	1	<1	<0.1	0.1	0.1
3103	Pears-Bartlett-Fresh-Med	1	ea	166	96	139	1	26	5	<1	<0.1	<0.1	<0.1

< = Trace amount present   Blank = Not available

CHOL, cholesterol; **V,** vitamin; **THI,** thiamin; **RIB,** riboflavin; **NIA,** niacin; **FOL,** folate;
CALC, calcium; **PHOS,** phosphate; **SOD,** sodium; **POT,** potassium; **MAG,** magnesium

CHOL (g)	V-A (RE)	THI (mg)	RIB (mg)	NIA (mg)	V-B6 (mg)	FOL (μg)	V-B12 (μg)	V-C (mg)	V-E (mg)	CALC (mg)	PHOS (mg)	SOD (mg)	POT (mg)	MAG (mg)	IRON (mg)	ZINC (mg)
0	2	<0.1	<0.1	0.2	0.1	4	0	2	0.1	5	16	2	152	22	0.4	0.2
0	<1	0.1	0.1	2.3	0.3	34	0	1	0.1	69	110	4	1168	77	1.8	0.5
0	<1	<0.1	0.1	1.1	0.1	16	0	<1	<0.1	32	51	2	544	36	0.8	0.2
0	<1	<0.1	<0.1	0.1	<0.1	2	0	<1	0.1	31	13	2	129	13	0.4	0.1
0	66	<0.1	0.2	1.6	0.2	3	0	1	0.4	36	58	2	615	34	0.8	0.4
0	0	0.2	0.2	1.3	0.3	8	0	4	0.2	82	167	18	1236	53	3.1	0.4
0	0	0.2	0.2	1.1	0.3	7	0	3	0.2	72	146	16	1086	46	2.7	0.3
0	0									0		0	110		0	
0	8	<0.1	<0.1	0.1	0.1	4	0	6	0.2	8	15	1	148	7	0.2	0.1
0	5	<0.1	<0.1	0.1	<0.1	0	0	5	0.1	6	14	0	115	5	0.1	0.1
0	3	<0.1	<0.1	0.1	<0.1	1	0	<1	<0.1	4	7	1	75	3	0.2	<0.1
0	67	<0.1	<0.1	0.2	<0.1	3	0	4	0.3	5	8	<1	91	4	0.1	0.1
0	28	0.1	0.3	3.5	0.5	163	0	20	4.2	24	105	14	975	58	1.1	1.3
0	7	<0.1	0.1	0.8	0.4	24	0	10	0.1	6	26	1	422	32	0.3	0.2
0	32	<0.1	<0.1	0.9	<0.1	36	0	30	1.7	42	32	1	233	29	0.9	0.8
0	9	0.1	0.1	0.6	0.1	9	0	14	0.8	9	17	1	112	9	0.4	0.2
0	0	0.1	<0.1	0.9	0.1	13	0	28	0.1	16	29	2	470	24	0.5	0.1
0	1866	0.2	0.1	4.1	0.4	116	0	203	0.3	50	83	88	1474	66	1.2	1
0	541	0.1	<0.1	1.2	0.1	34	0	59	0.1	14	24	26	427	19	0.3	0.3
0	8	<0.1	<0.1	0.5	<0.1	15	0	44	0.2	4	15	3	169	13	0.1	0.2
0	0	0.2	0.5	3.8	2.7	131	0	358	0.8	180	82	148	2985	180	5.6	1.1
0	0	<0.1	0.1	0.4	0.3	14	0	37	0.1	19	8	15	309	19	0.6	0.1
0	4	<0.1	<0.1	0.1	<0.1	3	0	5	0.1	9	15	0	161	8	0.3	0.1
0	2	<0.1	<0.1	0.1	<0.1	1	0	1	<0.1	3	2	<1	46	1	0.1	<0.1
0	6	<0.1	<0.1	0.1	0.1	1	0	13	1.1	8	12	2	81	6	0.2	0.1
0	0	<0.1	<0.1	0.1	<0.1	19	0	10		8	10	2	78	4	<0.1	<0.1
0	7	<0.1	<0.1	0.2	0.1	3	0	1	0.1	18	7	<1	116	8	0.2	0.1
0	212	0.1	<0.1	0.6	0.1	23	0	79	0.3	28	18	0	320	18	0.2	0.2
0	5	<0.1	<0.1	0.3	0.1	12	0	39	0.2	14	9	0	175	11	0.1	0.1
0	56	0.1	<0.1	1	0.1	44	0	205	0.7	16	36	2	375	20	0.2	0.2
0	10	0.1	<0.1	0.7	0.1	30	0	29	<0.1	10	18	29	365	16	0.3	0.1
0	10	0.1	<0.1	0.7	0.1	32	0	31	<0.1	10	19	31	388	17	0.3	0.2
0	6	<0.1	<0.1	0.3	<0.1	19	0	70	1.1	26	26	2	237	13	0.2	0.1
0	1	<0.1	<0.1	0.1	<0.1	6	0	31	0.1	15	9	1	80	5	0.3	<0.1
0	3	<0.1	<0.1	0.1	<0.1	5	0	19	0.1	22	12	1	68	4	0.4	0.1
0	0	<0.1	<0.1	0.1	<0.1	1	0	7	<0.1	<1	3	<1	16	1	<0.1	<0.1
0	157	0.1	0.1	1.2	0.3	29	0	57	2.3	21	23	4	323	19	0.3	0.1
0	46	<0.1	<0.1	1.5	<0.1	7	0	7	1	8	35	0	273	12	0.4	0.2
0	29	0.1	0.1	0.4	0.1	39	0	70	0.2	52	18	0	237	13	0.1	0.1
0	40	0.2	0.1	0.5	0.1	54	0	96	0.3	72	25	0	326	18	0.2	0.1
0	334	0.1	0.1	1	0.1	116	0	188	2.2	73	15	9	781	30	0.3	0.2
0	31	<0.1	<0.1	0.8	<0.1	4	0	6	0.7	6	20	0	186	9	0.2	0.2
0	3	<0.1	<0.1	0.3	<0.1	12	0	7	0.2	15	18	2	198	12	0.3	0.2

ESHA, EatRight Analysis CD-ROM; **AMT**, amount; **WT**, weight; **CAL**, calories; **WTR**, water; **PROT**, protein; **CARB**, carbohydrate; **FIBR**, fiber; **FAT**, fat; **SATF**, saturated fat; **MONO**, monosaturated fat; **POLY**, polyunsaturated fat

ESHA CODE	FOOD DESCRIPTION	AMT	UNIT	WT (g)	CAL (kcal)	WTR (g)	PROT (g)	CARB (g)	FIBR (g)	FAT (g)	SATF (g)	MONO (g)	POLY (g)
Fruits (continued)													
Fresh Fruits (continued)													
3113	Pineapple-Fresh-Slices	1	pce	84	40	73	<1	11	1	<1	<0.1	<0.1	<0.1
5632	Plantain-Fried-Ripe	1	cup	169	425	81	2	61	4	22	3	6.8	11.5
3121	Plum-Medium-Fresh	1	ea	66	30	58	<1	8	1	<1	<0.1	0.1	<0.1
3648	Raspberries-Fresh	10	ea	19	10	16	<1	2	1	<1	<0.1	<0.1	0.1
3056	Red Grapes	10	ea	50	34	40	<1	9	<1	<1	<0.1	<0.1	<0.1
3209	Rhubarb-raw-diced	1	cup	122	26	114	1	6	2	<1	0.1	<0.1	0.1
3664	Starfruit-Raw-Cube-Cup	1	cup	137	42	125	1	9	4	<1	<0.1	<0.1	0.3
3136	Strawberries-Medium Size	1	ea	12	4	11	<1	1	<1	<1	<0.1	<0.1	<0.1
3135	Strawberries-Sliced-Cup	1	cup	166	53	151	1	13	3	<1	<0.1	0.1	0.3
71991	Tangelo-Fresh-Medium	1	ea	109	50	92	1	15	3	<1	0		
3138	Tangerine-Fresh	1	ea	84	45	72	1	11	2	<1	<0.1	0.1	0.1
3055	Thompson Seedless Grapes	10	ea	50	34	40	<1	9	<1	<1	<0.1	<0.1	<0.1
3142	Watermelon-Fresh Pieces	1	cup	152	46	139	1	11	1	<1	<0.1	0.1	0.1
Frozen Fruits													
3028	Blackberries-Frozen	1	cup	151	97	124	2	24	8	1	<0.1	0.1	0.4
3031	Blueberries-Frozen	1	cup	155	79	134	1	19	4	1	0.1	0.1	0.4
3232	Blueberries-Swtnd-Frzn	0.5	cup	115	93	89	<1	25	3	<1	<0.1	<0.1	0.1
71120	Raspberries-Swtnd-Frzn	0.5	cup	125	129	91	1	33	6	<1	<0.1	<0.1	0.1
3133	Rhubarb-Fzn-Cooked+Sugar	1	cup	240	278	163	1	75	5	<1	<0.1	<0.1	0.1
3236	Strawberries-Frzn/Sweet/Thaw	1	cup	255	245	187	1	66	5	<1	<0.1	<0.1	0.2
3158	Sweet Cherries-frozen	1	cup	259	231	196	3	58	5	<1	0.1	0.1	0.1
Grain Products													
Breads													
42100	Bagel-Cinnamon Raisin	1	ea	71	194	23	7	39	2	1	0.2	0.1	0.5
42041	Bagel-Egg-3.5 inch diam	1	ea	71	197	23	8	38	2	1	0.3	0.3	0.5
42103	Bagel-Oat Bran	1	ea	71	181	23	8	38	3	1	0.1	0.2	0.3
42000	Bagel-Plain-3.5in diam	1	ea	71	182	26	7	36	2	1	0.3	0.4	0.5
72307	Bagel-Whole Wheat	1	ea	95	260	28	11	52	9	2	0.5		
42206	Biscuit-Cheese-2" diam	1	ea	30	113	8	3	13	<1	6	1.7	2.3	1.4
42110	Biscuit-LowFat Dough-Baked	1	ea	21	63	6	2	12	<1	1	0.3	0.6	0.2
42002	Biscuit-Prep f/Dry	1	oz	28.35	95	8	2	14	1	3	0.8	1.2	1.2
42001	Biscuit-Prep f/Recipe	1	ea	60	212	17	4	27	1	10	2.6	4.2	2.5
42205	Biscuit-Whole Wheat-3inch	1	ea	63	199	18	6	30	5	7	1.7	3	2.2
42039	Banana Bread-Recipe w/Marg	1	pce	60	196	18	3	33	1	6	1.3	2.7	1.9
42052	Boston Brown Bread-Canned	1	pce	45	88	21	2	19	2	1	0.1	0.1	0.3
42004	Bread Crumbs-Dry-Grated	1	cup	108	427	7	14	78	5	6	1.3	1.1	2.2
42144	Bread Crumbs-Seasoned-Dry	1	cup	120	460	8	17	82	6	7	1.7	1.4	2.8
42090	Challah/Egg Bread	1	pce	40	113	14	4	19	1	2	0.6	0.9	0.4
42648	Cornbread	1	pce	52	140		3	26	1	2	1	1	0
42115	Cornbread-Dry Mix-Prep	1	ea	60	188	19	4	29	1	6	1.6	3.1	0.7
42116	Cornbread-Recipe w/2%Milk	1	ea	65	173	25	4	28	2	5	1	1.2	2.1
42042	Cracked Wheat Bread-Slice	1	pce	25	65	9	2	12	1	1	0.2	0.5	0.2
42015	Croissant-4.5x4x2	1	ea	57	231	13	5	26	1	12	6.6	3.1	0.6

< = Trace amount present   Blank = Not available

CHOL, cholesterol; **V,** vitamin; **THI,** thiamin; **RIB,** riboflavin; **NIA,** niacin; **FOL,** folate; **CALC,** calcium; **PHOS,** phosphate; **SOD,** sodium; **POT,** potassium; **MAG,** magnesium

CHOL (g)	V-A (RE)	THI (mg)	RIB (mg)	NIA (mg)	V-B6 (mg)	FOL (µg)	V-B12 (µg)	V-C (mg)	V-E (mg)	CALC (mg)	PHOS (mg)	SOD (mg)	POT (mg)	MAG (mg)	IRON (mg)	ZINC (mg)
0	5	0.1	<0.1	0.4	0.1	13	0	30	<0.1	11	7	1	97	10	0.2	0.1
0	162	0.1	0.1	1.2	0.5	21	0	25	4.7	5	65	8	858	71	1.1	0.3
0	22	<0.1	<0.1	0.3	<0.1	3	0	6	0.2	4	11	0	104	5	0.1	0.1
0	1	<0.1	<0.1	0.1	<0.1	4	0	5	0.2	5	6	<1	29	4	0.1	0.1
0	3	<0.1	<0.1	0.1	<0.1	1	0	5	0.1	5	10	1	96	4	0.2	<0.1
0	12	<0.1	<0.1	0.4	<0.1	9	0	10	0.5	105	17	5	351	15	0.3	0.1
0	8	<0.1	<0.1	0.5	<0.1	16	0	47	0.2	4	16	3	182	14	0.1	0.2
0	<1	<0.1	<0.1	<0.1	<0.1	3	0	7	<0.1	2	3	<1	18	2	<0.1	<0.1
0	3	<0.1	<0.1	0.6	0.1	40	0	98	0.5	27	40	2	254	22	0.7	0.2
0	0						0	30		40		0			0	
0	57	<0.1	<0.1	0.3	0.1	13	0	22	0.2	31	17	2	139	10	0.1	0.1
0	3	<0.1	<0.1	0.1	<0.1	1	0	5	0.1	5	10	1	96	4	0.2	<0.1
0	85	0.1	<0.1	0.3	0.1	5	0	12	0.1	11	17	2	170	15	0.4	0.2
0	18	<0.1	0.1	1.8	0.1	51	0	5	1.8	44	45	2	211	33	1.2	0.4
0	6	<0.1	0.1	0.8	0.1	11	0	4	0.7	12	17	2	84	8	0.3	0.1
0	5	<0.1	0.1	0.3	0.1	8	0	1	0.6	7	8	1	69	2	0.4	0.1
0	8	<0.1	0.1	0.3	<0.1	32	0	21	0.9	19	21	1	142	16	0.8	0.2
0	19	<0.1	0.1	0.5	<0.1	12	0	8	0.6	348	19	2	230	29	0.5	0.2
0	5	<0.1	0.1	1	0.1	38	0	106	0.6	28	33	8	250	18	1.5	0.2
0	47	0.1	0.1	0.5	0.1	10	0	3	0.2	31	41	3	515	26	0.9	0.1
0	15	0.3	0.2	2.2	<0.1	79	0	<1	0.2	13	71	229	105	20	2.7	0.8
17	23	0.4	0.2	2.4	0.1	62	0.1	<1	0.1	9	60	359	48	18	2.8	0.5
0	1	0.2	0.2	2.1	<0.1	70	0	<1	0.2	9	78	360	82	22	2.2	0.6
0	0	0.4	0.2	2.8	<0.1	103	0	1	0.1	63	62	318	53	16	4.3	1.3
0	0	0.2	0.1	4		32		0		100		450			2.7	
4	16	0.1	0.1	0.8	<0.1	3	0.1	<1	0.6	91	68	150	46	6	0.8	0.3
0	0	0.1	<0.1	0.7	<0.1	17	0	0	<0.1	4	98	305	39	4	0.6	0.1
1	8	0.1	0.1	0.9	<0.1	15	0.1	<1	0.1	52	133	271	53	7	0.6	0.2
2	14	0.2	0.2	1.8	<0.1	37	<0.1	<1	0.8	141	98	348	73	11	1.7	0.3
2	14	0.1	0.1	2.2	0.1	13	0.1	<1	1.3	155	199	210	200	57	1.7	1.2
26	69	0.1	0.1	0.9	0.1	20	0.1	1	1.1	13	35	181	80	8	0.8	0.2
<1	11	<0.1	0.1	0.5	<0.1	5	<0.1	0	0.1	32	50	284	143	28	0.9	0.2
0	0	1	0.4	7.2	0.1	116	0.4	0	0.1	198	178	791	212	46	5.2	1.6
1	23	1.2	0.5	7.4	0.2	143	<0.1	3	0.3	218	212	2111	277	55	5.9	1.7
20	25	0.2	0.2	1.9	<0.1	42	<0.1	0	0.1	37	42	197	46	8	1.2	0.3
5	0							0		26	130	400	60		0.6	
37	28	0.1	0.2	1.2	0.1	33	0.1	<1	0.7	44	226	467	77	12	1.1	0.4
26	36	0.2	0.2	1.5	0.1	50	0.1	<1	0.6	162	110	428	96	16	1.6	0.4
0	0	0.1	0.1	0.9	0.1	15	<0.1	0	0.1	11	38	134	44	13	0.7	0.3
38	120	0.2	0.1	1.2	<0.1	50	0.1	<1	0.5	21	60	424	67	9	1.2	0.4

ESHA, EatRight Analysis CD-ROM; **AMT**, amount; **WT**, weight; **CAL**, calories; **WTR**, water; **PROT**, protein; **CARB**, carbohydrate; **FIBR**, fiber; **FAT**, fat; **SATF**, saturated fat; **MONO**, monosaturated fat; **POLY**, polyunsaturated fat

ESHA CODE	FOOD DESCRIPTION	AMT	UNIT	WT (g)	CAL (kcal)	WTR (g)	PROT (g)	CARB (g)	FIBR (g)	FAT (g)	SATF (g)	MONO (g)	POLY (g)
Grain Products (continued)													
Breads (continued)													
42016	Croutons	1	cup	30	122	2	4	22	2	2	0.5	0.9	0.4
42148	Croutons-Seasoned	1	cup	40	186	1	4	25	2	7	2.1	3.8	0.9
42325	Crumpet-Whole Wheat	1	oz	28.35	48	15	2	10	1	<1			
42173	Cuban/Spanish/Portug Bread	1	pce	20	55	7	2	10	1	1	0.1	0.2	0.1
42157	Dinner Roll/Bun	1	ea	28	87	8	3	15	1	2	0.4	0.5	0.7
42160	Dinner Roll/Bun-Wheat	1	ea	28.35	77	10	2	13	1	2	0.4	0.9	0.3
42070	Dinner Roll-Oat Bran	1	ea	33	78	15	3	13	1	2	0.2	0.5	0.5
42091	Egg Bread/Challah-Toasted	1	pce	37	117	10	4	19	1	2	0.6	1.1	0.4
42043	French/Vienna Bread	1	pce	32	92	9	4	18	1	1	0.2	0.1	0.3
42368	Garlic Bread-Frozen PPF	1	pce	47	160	14	5	20	1	8	1.9		
42184	Garlic Roll	1	ea	35	105	11	3	18	1	3	0.6	1.3	0.4
42020	Hamburger Bun	1	ea	43	120	15	4	21	1	2	0.5	0.5	0.8
42022	Hard Roll-White	1	ea	57	167	18	6	30	1	2	0.3	0.6	1
42381	Hoagie Roll	1	ea	69	200		7	33	2	5	1.5		
42021	Hotdog/Frankfurter Bun	1	ea	43	120	15	4	21	1	2	0.5	0.5	0.8
49012	Hush Puppies-Recipe	1	ea	22	74	6	2	10	1	3	0.5	0.7	1.6
72411	Indian Fry Bread	2	oz	56.7	187	18	4	27		7	2.6	2.5	0.6
42046	Italian Bread	1	pce	30	81	11	3	15	1	1	0.3	0.2	0.4
42185	Mexican Bolillo Roll	1	ea	117	307	43	10	61	2	2	0.5	0.2	0.6
42047	Mixed Grain Bread-Slice	1	pce	26	65	10	3	12	2	1	0.2	0.4	0.2
62746	Multigrain Bread-Low Fat	1	pce	31	60		3	14	5	1	0		
42190	Pannetone-Italian Sweetbread	1	pce	27	87	8	2	15	1	2	1.2	0.7	0.2
71227	Pita Bread-4"	1	ea	28	77	9	3	16	1	<1	<0.1	<0.1	0.1
42007	Pita Pocket Bread-White	1	ea	60	165	19	5	33	1	1	0.1	0.1	0.3
42080	Pita Pocket Bread-Whole Wheat	1	ea	64	170	20	6	35	5	2	0.3	0.2	0.7
42006	Pumpernickel Bread-Slice	1	pce	26	65	10	2	12	2	1	0.1	0.2	0.3
42051	Raisin Bread	1	pce	26	71	9	2	14	1	1	0.3	0.6	0.2
42005	Rye Bread	1	pce	32	83	12	3	15	2	1	0.2	0.4	0.3
42045	Sourdough Bread-Med Slice	1	pce	32	92	9	4	18	1	1	0.2	0.1	0.3
12485	Sprouted Multigrain Bread	2	oz	56.7	130	23	6	26	4	0	0	0	0
42037	Stuffing Mix-Bread-Prep	0.5	cup	100	177	65	3	22	3	9	1.7	3.8	2.6
42147	Stuffing Mix-Cornbread-Prep	0.5	cup	100	179	65	3	22	3	9	1.8	3.9	2.7
42168	Taco Shell-Bkd	1	ea	13.3	62	1	1	8	1	3	0.6	1.6	0.5
42023	Tortilla-Corn-Enr-Reg-6in	1	ea	26	57	12	1	12	2	1	0.1	0.2	0.4
42025	Tortilla-Flour-8 inch	1	ea	72	225	22	6	37	2	6	1.4	2.8	1.1
71938	Tortilla-Whole Wheat	1	ea	47	140		4	22	2	3	0		
42012	Wheat Berry Bread	1	pce	25	66	9	3	12	1	1	0.2	0.2	0.4
42136	Wheat Bran Bread	1	pce	36	89	14	3	17	1	1	0.3	0.6	0.2
42012	Wheat Bread	1	pce	25	66	9	3	12	1	1	0.2	0.2	0.4
42095	Wheat Bread-LowCal	1	pce	23	46	10	2	10	3	1	0.1	0.1	0.2
42216	White Bread	1	pce	30	80	11	2	15	1	1	0.2	0.2	0.4
42084	White Bread-LowCal	1	pce	23	48	10	2	10	2	1	0.1	0.2	0.1
42014	Whole Wheat Bread	1	pce	28	69	11	4	12	2	1	0.2	0.4	0.2
42057	Whole Wheat Roll	1	ea	28.35	75	9	2	14	2	1	0.2	0.3	0.6

< = Trace amount present   Blank = Not available

CHOL, cholesterol; **V**, vitamin; **THI**, thiamin; **RIB**, riboflavin; **NIA**, niacin; **FOL**, folate; **CALC**, calcium; **PHOS**, phosphate; **SOD**, sodium; **POT**, potassium; **MAG**, magnesium

CHOL (g)	V-A (RE)	THI (mg)	RIB (mg)	NIA (mg)	V-B6 (mg)	FOL (µg)	V-B12 (µg)	V-C (mg)	V-E (mg)	CALC (mg)	PHOS (mg)	SOD (mg)	POT (mg)	MAG (mg)	IRON (mg)	ZINC (mg)
0	0	0.2	0.1	1.6	<0.1	40	0	0	0.1	23	34	209	37	9	1.2	0.3
3	3	0.2	0.2	1.9	<0.1	42	0.1	0	0.2	38	56	495	72	17	1.1	0.4
	0	<0.1	0	0.4				0		21		245	32	8	0.5	0.1
0	0	0.1	0.1	0.9	<0.1	6	0	0	<0.1	9	21	122	23	5	0.5	0.2
1	<1	0.1	0.1	1.5	<0.1	28	<0.1	<1	0.1	50	34	150	39	7	1	0.3
0	0	0.1	0.1	1.2	<0.1	17	0	0	0.1	50	29	96	33	10	1	0.3
0	0	0.1	0.1	1.6	<0.1	31	0	0	0.2	28	38	136	40	11	1.4	0.3
21	26	0.1	0.2	1.8	<0.1	36	<0.1	0	0.1	38	43	200	47	8	1.2	0.3
0	0	0.1	0.1	1.5	<0.1	47	0	<1	0.1	14	36	208	41	9	1.2	0.3
6	38							3		38		291			1	
<1	0	0.2	0.1	1.4	<0.1	10	<0.1	<1	0.3	42	41	181	47	8	1.1	0.3
0	0	0.2	0.1	1.8	<0.1	48	0.1	0	<0.1	59	27	206	40	9	1.4	0.3
0	0	0.3	0.2	2.4	<0.1	54	0	0	0.2	54	57	310	62	15	1.9	0.5
0	0	0.2	0.1	2		40		0		80		320			1.4	
0	0	0.2	0.1	1.8	<0.1	48	0.1	0	<0.1	59	27	206	40	9	1.4	0.3
10	10	0.1	0.1	0.6	<0.1	20	<0.1	<1	0.3	61	42	147	32	5	0.7	0.1
4		0.2	0.1	2.6	<0.1	69	0		0	32	70	187	44	10	2.3	0.2
0	0	0.1	0.1	1.3	<0.1	57	0	0	0.1	23	31	175	33	8	0.9	0.3
1	4	0.7	0.5	6.6	<0.1	41	<0.1	<1	0.1	14	90	7	98	22	3.8	0.8
0	0	0.1	0.1	1.1	0.1	31	<0.1	<1	0.1	24	46	127	53	14	0.9	0.3
0	0	0.2	0.2	2	0.2	40	0.9	0		60		90		40	1.1	2.2
19	23	0.1	0.1	1	<0.1	19	0.1	<1	0.1	16	40	28	54	5	0.8	0.2
0	0	0.2	0.1	1.3	<0.1	30	0	0	0.1	24	27	150	34	7	0.7	0.2
0	0	0.4	0.2	2.8	<0.1	64	0	0	0.2	52	58	322	72	16	1.6	0.5
0	0	0.2	0.1	1.8	0.2	22	0	0	0.4	10	115	340	109	44	2	1
0	0	0.1	0.1	0.8	<0.1	24	0	0	0.1	18	46	174	54	14	0.7	0.4
0	0	0.1	0.1	0.9	<0.1	28	0	<1	0.1	17	28	101	59	7	0.8	0.2
0	<1	0.1	0.1	1.2	<0.1	35	0	<1	0.1	23	40	211	53	13	0.9	0.4
0	0	0.1	0.1	1.5	<0.1	47	0	<1	0.1	14	36	208	41	9	1.2	0.3
0	0							0		20		3			1.8	
0	125	0.1	0.1	1.5	<0.1	39	<0.1	0	1.4	32	42	543	74	12	1.1	0.3
0	83	0.1	0.1	1.2	<0.1	97	<0.1	1	0.9	26	34	455	62	13	0.9	0.2
0	<1	<0.1	<0.1	0.2	<0.1	9	0	0	0.1	13	30	52	30	11	0.2	0.2
0	<1	<0.1	<0.1	0.4	0.1	1	0	0	0.1	21	82	12	48	19	0.3	0.3
0	0	0.4	0.2	2.6	<0.1	75	0	0	0.1	93	89	458	112	16	2.4	0.4
0	0							0		0		170			1.1	
0	0	0.1	0.1	1.3	<0.1	21	0	<1	<0.1	36	39	130	46	12	0.9	0.3
0	0	0.1	0.1	1.6	0.1	38	0	0	0.1	27	67	175	82	29	1.1	0.5
0	0	0.1	0.1	1.3	<0.1	21	0	<1	<0.1	36	39	130	46	12	0.9	0.3
0	0	0.1	0.1	0.9	<0.1	21	0	<1	0.1	18	23	118	28	9	0.7	0.3
0	0	0.1	0.1	1.3	<0.1	33	0	0	0.1	45	30	204	30	7	1.1	0.2
0	<1	0.1	0.1	0.8	<0.1	22	0.1	<1	<0.1	22	28	104	17	5	0.7	0.3
0	<1	0.1	0.1	1.3	0.1	14	0	0	0.1	30	57	132	69	23	0.7	0.5
0	0	0.1	<0.1	1	0.1	9	0	0	0.3	30	64	136	77	24	0.7	0.6

ESHA, EatRight Analysis CD-ROM; **AMT**, amount; **WT**, weight; **CAL**, calories; **WTR**, water; **PROT**, protein; **CARB**, carbohydrate; **FIBR**, fiber; **FAT**, fat; **SATF**, saturated fat; **MONO**, monosaturated fat; **POLY**, polyunsaturated fat

ESHA CODE	FOOD DESCRIPTION	AMT	UNIT	WT (g)	CAL (kcal)	WTR (g)	PROT (g)	CARB (g)	FIBR (g)	FAT (g)	SATF (g)	MONO (g)	POLY (g)
Grain Products (continued)													
Cereals - Cooked & Dry Mixes													
40178	Corn Grits-Unenrich-Ckd	1	cup	242	143	207	3	31	1	<1	0.1	0.1	0.2
40094	Corn Grits-White, cooked	1	cup	242	143	207	3	31	1	<1	0.1	0.1	0.2
40093	Corn Grits-White-Enr, cooked	1	cup	242	143	207	3	31	1	<1	0.1	0.1	0.2
40078	Cream of Rice Cereal, cooked	1	cup	244	127	214	2	28	<1	<1	0.1	0.1	0.1
40006	Farina Cereal-Enrich-Cooked	1	cup	233	112	205	3	24	1	<1	<0.1	<0.1	0.1
40239	Maypo Cereal-Ckd w/Salt	1	cup	240	170	198	6	32	5	2	0.4	0.6	0.5
40015	Maypo Cereal-Cooked	0.75	cup	180	128	149	4	24	4	2	0.3	0.5	0.7
38014	Multigrain Cereal-Dry	0.5	cup	40	133	4	5	29	5	1	0.2	0.2	0.5
40431	Oat Bran Cereal-Hot-Dry	0.5	cup	40	146	4	7	25	6	3	0.6	1	1.2
40000	Oatmeal-Cooked-No Salt	1	cup	234	147	200	6	25	4	2	0.4	0.7	0.9
40072	Oatmeal-Instant-Pkt-Prepared	1	cup	234	129	202	5	22	4	2	0.3	0.7	0.8
40075	Oatmeal-Inst-Flavored-Pkt-Prep	1	ea	155	157	116	4	31	3	2	0.3	0.7	0.6
40088	Ralston Cereal-Cooked	1	cup	253	134	218	6	28	6	1	0.1	0.1	0.4
38008	Rolled Oats-Dry	1	cup	81	311	7	13	54	8	5	0.9	1.6	1.9
40002	Rolled wheat-cooked	1	cup	242	160	202	5	33	4	1	0.1	0.1	0.5
40016	Roman Meal Cereal-Cooked	0.75	cup	181	110	150	5	25	6	1	0.1		
40191	Wheatena Cereal-Ckd w/Salt	1	cup	243	143	208	5	29	5	1	0.2	0.2	0.6
40080	Wheatena Cereal-Cooked	1	cup	243	136	208	5	29	7	1	0.2	0.2	0.6
Cereals - Ready to Eat													
40063	100% Natural Cereal	0.5	cup	48	218	1	5	32	4	9	4	2.1	0.9
40065	100% Natural Cereal-RaisinDate	0.5	cup	105	474	4	11	69	7	19	13	3.5	1.6
60959	7 Whole Grain Puffs Cereal	1	cup	25	98	1	3	20	2	1	0.2	0.2	0.3
40246	AlphaBits Cereal-Frosted	1	cup	32	130	<1	3	27	1	1	0.3		
40123	Amaranth Flakes Cereal	1	cup	38	134	1	6	27	4	3	0.5	0.8	1
40035	Apple Zaps Cereal-Cup	0.75	cup	30	118	1	1	27	1	1	0.3	0.2	0.2
61388	Autumn Wheat Cereal	1	cup	54	181	2	5	45	8	1	0.2	0.2	0.6
40029	Bran Buds Cereal	0.33	cup	30	75	1	2	24	13	1	0.1	0.2	0.4
40259	Bran Flakes Cereal	0.75	cup	30	96	1	3	24	5	1	0.1		
40032	Cap'n Crunch Cereal	0.75	cup	27	108	1	1	23	1	2	0.4	0.3	0.2
40026	Cap'n Crunch, AllBerry	1	cup	32	129	1	2	27	1	2	0.4	0.4	0.3
40034	Cap'n Crunch, Peanut Butter	0.75	cup	27	112	1	2	21	1	3	0.5	1.1	0.6
40033	Cap'n Crunchberries	0.75	cup	26	104	1	1	22	1	1	0.4	0.3	0.2
40335	Chex Wheat Cereal	1	cup	30	108	1	3	24	3	1	0.1	0.1	0.2
61645	Cinnamon Harvest Cereal	1	cup	54	202	3	4	44	6	1	0.2	0.2	0.6
60927	Cinnamon Oat Crunch Cereal	1	cup	60	228	2	6	48	5	3	0.5	0.9	0.8
40037	Cocoa Pebbles Cereal	1	cup	33	130	1	1	29	1	1	0.3	0.2	0.2
40036	Corn Bran Cereal	0.75	cup	27	90	<1	1	23	5	1	0.2	0.2	0.3
61393	Cranberry Sunshine Cereal	1	cup	29	116	1	2	26	3	1	0.1	0.2	0.5
40040	Crispy Wheat`n Raisins Cereal	1	cup	55	183	4	4	45	5	1	0.2	0.1	0.4
40217	Frosted Flakes Cereal	0.75	cup	31	114	1	1	28	1	<1	0.1	<0.1	0.1
40043	Frosted Mini Wheats Cereal	1	cup	51	175	3	5	41	5	1	0.2	0.1	0.5
60932	Frosted Oats Cereal	0.75	cup	28	111	1	2	23	1	2	0.4	0.5	0.3
40038	Fruitangy Ohs Cereal	1	cup	31	122	1	2	27	1	1	0.3	0.5	0.3
40245	Golden Crisp Cereal	0.75	cup	27	107	1	1	25	0	<1	0.1		

< = Trace amount present   Blank = Not available

CHOL, cholesterol; **V,** vitamin; **THI,** thiamin; **RIB,** riboflavin; **NIA,** niacin; **FOL,** folate;
CALC, calcium; **PHOS,** phosphate; **SOD,** sodium; **POT,** potassium; **MAG,** magnesium

CHOL (g)	V-A (RE)	THI (mg)	RIB (mg)	NIA (mg)	V-B6 (mg)	FOL (µg)	V-B12 (µg)	V-C (mg)	V-E (mg)	CALC (mg)	PHOS (mg)	SOD (mg)	POT (mg)	MAG (mg)	IRON (mg)	ZINC (mg)
0	10	<0.1	<0.1	0.4	0.1	2	0	0	<0.1	7	27	540	51	12	0.4	0.2
0	<1	<0.1	<0.1	0.4	0.1	2	0	0	<0.1	7	27	5	51	12	0.4	0.2
0	0	0.2	0.1	1.7	0.1	80	0	0	<0.1	7	27	5	51	12	1.5	0.2
0	0	0	0	1	0.1	7	0	0	<0.1	7	41	2	49	7	0.5	0.4
0	0	0.1	0.1	1.1	<0.1	79	0	0	<0.1	9	28	5	30	5	1.2	0.2
0	701	0.7	0.8	9.4	0.9	12	2.8	28	0.2	130	247	259	211	53	8.4	1.5
0	526	0.5	0.5	7	0.7	7	2.2	22	0.1	94	185	7	158	38	6.3	1.1
0	1	0.1	0.1	1.4	0.1	10	0	0	0.2	14	138	1	165	46	1.2	1.3
0	8	0.4	0.1	0.3	<0.1	15	0	0	0.2	32	278	2	232	96	3.2	1.7
0	0	0.3	<0.1	0.3	<0.1	9	0	0	0.2	19	178	2	131	56	1.6	1.1
0	377	0.3	0.4	4.8	0.5	101	0	0	0.2	131	126	105	124	54	10.2	1.1
0	319	0.3	0.3	4	0.4	85	0	0	0.2	108	129	253	107	39	3.8	0.9
0	0	0.2	0.2	2	0.1	18	0.1	0	0.3	13	147	5	154	58	1.6	1.4
0	0	0.6	0.1	0.6	0.1	26	0	0	0.6	42	384	3	284	120	3.4	2.5
0	<1	0.2	0.1	2.1	0.2	34	0	0	0.6	22	167	0	172	56	1.5	1.2
0	0	0.2	0.1	2.3	0.1	18	0	0	0.3	22	161	2	226	81	1.6	1.3
0	1	<0.1	0.1	1.3	<0.1	22	0	0	1.3	15	146	578	187	51	1.4	1.7
0	0	<0.1	<0.1	1.3	<0.1	17	0	0	0.9	10	146	5	187	49	1.4	1.7
1	1	0.2	0.1	1	0.1	17	0.1	<1	1	57	165	23	238	53	1.2	1.1
0	12	0.3	0.6	2	0.2	43	0.1	0	0.7	152	332	45	513	119	3	2
0	<1	<0.1	<0.1	0.8	0.1	8	0	0	0.2	10	60	2	83	38	0.7	0.8
0	150	0.4	0.4	5	0.5	100	1.5	0		10	67	212	62	25	2.7	1.5
0	0	<0.1	<0.1	1	<0.1	4	0	1	0.5	6	126	13	134	10	0.7	0.1
0	165	0.4	0.5	5.5	0.5	420	0	7	0.2	3	45	135	52	15	4.9	4.1
0	0									31	122	2	183	44	1.6	0.8
0	153	0.4	0.4	5.1	2	404	6	6	0.5	19	150	203	300	62	4.5	1.5
0	150	0.4	0.4	5	0.5	100	1.5	0		17	152	220	185	64	8.1	1.5
0	4	0.4	0.5	5.7	0.6	420	0	0	0.2	4	45	202	54	15	5.2	4.3
<1	8	0.6	0.7	7.8	0.8	155	<0.1	<1	0.3	11	55	183	67	17	7	5.8
0	4	0.6	0.5	5.8	1.3	420	0	0	0.3	4	40	187	51	15	5.3	4.5
0	4	0.4	0.5	5.5	0.5	405	<0.1	<1	0.2	5	44	182	54	15	4.9	4.1
0	90	0.2	0.3	3	0.3	240	0.9	4	0.2	60	90	252	114	24	8.6	2.2
0													169		1.5	
0	1	0.2	0.2	1.4	0.1	22	0	<1	1.2	44	215	251	322	64	2.2	1.5
0	158	0.4	0.5	5.5	0.5	420	0	7	0.3	2	50	135	62	17	4.9	4.1
0	4	0.1	0.5	5.5	0.5	400	0	0	0.2	19	36	232	56	14	8.3	4.1
0												21	83		0.4	
0	150	0.7	0.9	10	1	200	3	0	0.3	0	140	251	227	42	7.5	7.5
0	160	0.4	0.5	5	0.5	101	1.5	6	<0.1	2	11	148	23	2	4.5	0.1
0	0	0.4	0.4	5	0.5	100	1.5	0	0.3	16	150	5	173	60	14.8	1.6
0	178	0.3	0.5	5.9	0.6	448	0	7	0.1	7	68	242	52	17	5.3	4.4
0	311	0.4	0.4	5.2	0.5	104	0	12	0.3	3	55	152	59	18	4.7	3.9
0	150	0.4	0.4	5	0.5	100	1.5	0		4	37	40	34	16	1.8	1.5

ESHA, EatRight Analysis CD-ROM; **AMT,** amount; **WT,** weight; **CAL,** calories; **WTR,** water; **PROT,** protein; **CARB,** carbohydrate; **FIBR,** fiber; **FAT,** fat; **SATF,** saturated fat; **MONO,** monosaturated fat; **POLY,** polyunsaturated fat

ESHA CODE	FOOD DESCRIPTION	AMT	UNIT	WT (g)	CAL (kcal)	WTR (g)	PROT (g)	CARB (g)	FIBR (g)	FAT (g)	SATF (g)	MONO (g)	POLY (g)
Grain Products (continued)													
Cereals - Ready to Eat (continued)													
38361	Granola Cereal-Low Fat	0.5	cup	55	209	2	5	44	3	3	0.6	1.4	0.5
40045	Granola-LowFat w/Raisins	0.66	cup	55	213	2	5	44	3	3	0.8	1.3	0.6
40009	Granola-Oats-Honey-Raisin	0.5	cup	51	225	2	5	34	3	9	3.6	3.8	1.1
40265	GrapeNut Flakes Cereal	0.75	cup	29	106	1	3	24	3	1	0.2		
60928	Groovy Grahams Cereal	0.75	cup	28	104	1	2	24	1	<1	0.1	0.1	0.2
40004	Harvest Oat Flakes Cereal	0.75	cup	29	109	1	3	23	2	1	0.2	0.4	0.4
40005	Harvest Oat Flakes-AppleAlmnd	0.75	cup	30	115	1	3	24	2	2	0.2	0.8	0.5
60967	Honey Crisp Cereal	0.75	cup	30	112	1	2	27	1	<1	<0.1	0.1	0.1
40051	Honey Nut Cheerios Cereal	1	cup	30	118	1	3	23	2	2	0	0.5	0.5
60966	Honey Nut Oats Cereal	0.75	cup	28	108	1	2	24	1	1	0.2	0.4	0.3
60965	Honey Roundups Cereal	0.75	cup	28	107	1	2	25	1	1	0.1	0.2	0.2
40108	Just Right Cereal	1	cup	55	204	2	4	46	3	1	0.1	0.3	1
40055	Kashi Breakfast Pilaf Cereal	0.5	cup	140	170		6	30	6	3	0		
60961	Kashi Good Friends Cereal	0.75	cup	30	95	1	3	25	7	1	0.1	0.3	0.5
60960	Kashi Honey Puffed Cereal	1	cup	30	120	1	3	25	2	1	0.1	0.2	0.3
60963	Kashi Medley Cereal	0.5	cup	30	106	1	3	24	3	1	0.1	0.3	0.4
60962	Kashi Pillows Cereal	0.75	cup	55	204	2	3	46	2	1			
40054	King Vitamin Cereal	1.5	cup	31	120	1	2	26	1	1	0.2	0.2	0.3
40010	Kix Cereal	1.33	cup	30	120	1	2	25	1	1	0.1	0.3	0.4
40011	Life Cereal	0.75	cup	32	120	1	3	25	2	1	0.3	0.5	0.5
40451	Maple Buckwheat Flakes Cereal	1	cup	43	170		4	35	1	1	0	0.5	0.5
40046	Marshmallow Safari Cereal	0.75	cup	30	119	1	2	25	1	2	0.4	0.8	0.4
40418	Mueslix Cereal	0.66	cup	55	196	5	5	40	4	3	0.4	1.6	1
61168	Oat Bran Flakes Cereal	1	cup	47	166	2	5	37	6	1	0.1	0.2	0.2
61310	Oat Bran Granola Cereal	0.5	cup	50	210	4	6	31	5	8	1		
40018	Puffed Rice Cereal	1	cup	14	54	1	1	12	<1	<1	<0.1	<0.1	<0.1
40023	Puffed Wheat Cereal	1.25	cup	15	55	1	2	11	1	<1	0.1	<0.1	0.2
40066	Quisp Cereal	1	cup	27	109	1	1	23	1	2	0.4	0.3	0.2
61554	Raisin Bran Cereal	1	cup	59	190	5	4	46	8	1	0		
40488	Raisin Bran Cereal	1	cup	56	210	3	4	45	6	2	0		
40393	Raisin Nut Bran Cereal	1	cup	55	200	4	4	42	5	3	0.5	1.5	0.5
40019	Rice Crisps Cereal	1.25	cup	30	113	1	2	26	<1	<1	<0.1	0.1	0.1
40017	Rice Krispies Cereal	1	cup	28	102	1	2	24	<1	<1	0.1	0.1	0.1
40020	Shredded Wheat Cereal-Biscuits	1	ea	21	72	1	2	17	2	<1	0.1	0.1	0.2
40062	Shredded Wheat-Lg Biscuit	2	ea	47.2	159	3	5	37	6	1	0.2	0.2	0.6
40022	Shredded Wheat-Sm Biscuit	0.75	cup	32	114	2	4	26	3	1	0.1	0.1	0.3
40068	Sugar Smacks Cereal	0.75	cup	27	104	1	2	24	1	<1	0.1	0.2	0.2
40047	Sweet Puffs Cereal	1	cup	34	133	1	2	30	1	1	0.1	0.1	0.3
12430	Synergy 8 Grain Cereal	0.75	cup	30	100		3	24	5	1	0		
40070	Tasteeos Cereal	1	cup	24	96	1	3	18	3	1	0.2	0.4	0.4
60926	Toasted Oat Bran Cereal+BrwnSug	0.75	cup	32	119	1	4	24	3	2	0.3	0.5	0.6
60935	Toasted Oats Cereal	1	cup	30	114	1	3	23	2	2	0.3	0.5	0.4
40021	Total Wheat Cereal	0.75	cup	30	100	1	2	23	3	1	0.1	0.1	0.2
40128	Uncle Sam's Fiber Cereal	1	cup	55	237	2	9	36	11	6	0.7	1.1	4.6

< = Trace amount present   Blank = Not available

CHOL, cholesterol; **V**, vitamin; **THI**, thiamin; **RIB**, riboflavin; **NIA**, niacin; **FOL**, folate;
CALC, calcium; **PHOS**, phosphate; **SOD**, sodium; **POT**, potassium; **MAG**, magnesium

CHOL (g)	V-A (RE)	THI (mg)	RIB (mg)	NIA (mg)	V-B6 (mg)	FOL (µg)	V-B12 (µg)	V-C (mg)	V-E (mg)	CALC (mg)	PHOS (mg)	SOD (mg)	POT (mg)	MAG (mg)	IRON (mg)	ZINC (mg)
0	262	0.4	0.5	5.9	2.3	449	6.7	3	0.6	23	131	135	138	45	2	4.2
1	2	0.2	0.1	1	0.1	13	0	<1	0.3	33	130	145	189	44	1.4	1
1	1	0.1	0.1	0.8	0.1	14	0.1	<1	0.5	59	152	19	250	49	1.2	1
0	150	0.4	0.4	5	0.5	100	1.5	0	0.1	11	88	140	99	30	8.1	1.2
0	4	<0.1	0.2	0.4	<0.1	4	0	0	0.4	39	45	243	211	16	1.4	0.3
0	2	0.1	0.1	0.7	0.1	11	0	0	0.5	16	102	204	99	32	0.9	0.8
0	2	0.1	0.1	0.7	0.1	10	0	<1	0.6	18	94	174	122	32	0.9	0.7
0	150	0.4	0.4	5	0.5	100	0	15	<0.1	<1	14	261	27	5	4.5	0.1
0	161	0.4	0.5	5.4	0.5	214	1.6	6	0.3	107	107	204	123	34	4.8	4
0	110	0.3	0.5	5.5	0.5	420	0	7	0.1	8	71	225	53	18	5	4.1
0	8	0.1	<0.1	0.3	<0.1	5	0	0	0.6	6	55	164	66	18	0.5	0.4
0	376	0.4	0.4	5	0.5	102	1.5	0	1.5	14	106	338	121	34	16.2	0.9
0	0							0		20		15			1.4	
0	4	0.1	<0.1	1.2	0.1	13	0	0	0.3	10	71	73	148	34	0.9	0.8
0	<1	0.1	<0.1	0.8	<0.1	8	0	0	0.3	9	79	6	79	34	0.7	0.8
0	<1	0.1	0.1	1.2	<0.1	8	0		0.2	8	24	69	98	5	0.6	0.1
0		<0.1	0.1	1.2	0.1	8				20	100	50	280	100	0.7	
0	299	0.4	0.4	5.2	0.5	413	1.5	12	1.4	4	79	260	86	26	9	3.9
0	141	0.4	0.4	5	0.5	200	1.5	6	0.1	150	40	220	40	8	8.4	3.8
0	1	0.4	0.5	5.5	0.6	416	0	0	0.2	112	133	164	91	31	9	4.1
0	0	0.2	<0.1	1.6				6		20		190	100		0.7	
0	300	0.4	0.4	5	0.5	100	0	12	0.1	26	58	192	42	17	4.5	3.8
0	90	0.4	0.4	5.5	2	406	6.1	<1	4	32	100	170	240	49	4.5	3.7
0	<1	0.2	0.2	3.2	0.1	22	0	<1	0.2	18	238	17	151	79	2.3	1.2
0	20							1		20		0			1.4	
0	0	0.1	<0.1	0.5	0	22	0	0	<0.1	1	17	1	16	4	0.4	0.2
0	0	0.1	0.1	0.8	<0.1	23	0	0	0	4	50	1	55	20	0.7	0.5
0	11	0.4	0.5	5.5	0.6	420	0	3	0.2	3	45	200	51	15	5	4.1
0	150							0		20		300			10.8	
0	150							6		40		320	300		18	
0	<1	0.4	0.4	5	0.5	100	1.5	0	0.9	20	150	250	200	40	4.5	3.8
0	150	0.4	0.4	5	0.5	100	0	15	0	<1	<1	293	26	0	1.8	0
0	197	0.6	0.8	8.1	0.5	170	1.5	18	<0.1	1	27	214	31	6	9.2	0.4
0	0	<0.1	<0.1	1.1	0.1	10		0		9	75	1	74	36	0.7	0.5
0	0	0.1	0.1	2.5	0.5	20	0	5	0	24	175	3	177	63	1.4	1.4
0	0	0.1	0.1	1.7	0.1	16	0	0	0.2	12	113	3	116	42	1.4	1.1
0	153	0.4	0.4	5	0.5	101	1.5	6	0.1	6	46	50	41	16	0.4	0.4
0	<1	<0.1	<0.1	1.5	<0.1	6	0.1	0	0.4	3	48	80	50	19	0.6	0.4
0	0							0		20		0			2.7	
0	123	0.4	0.5	5.8	0.5	160	1.3	4	0.1	86	126	205	74	30	7.2	3.4
	4	0.1	0.1	0.6	<0.1	13	0	0	0.7	21	147	202	157	46	1.3	1
0	165	0.2	0.5	5.5	0.5	420	0	7	0	12	116	286	86	29	8.9	4.1
0	150	1.5	1.7	20	2	400	6	60	13.5	1000	80	190	90	24	18	15
0	0	1.2	1.5	9	0.5	29	0	34	0.4	52	206	113	245	113	2.2	2.1

ESHA, EatRight Analysis CD-ROM; **AMT**, amount; **WT**, weight; **CAL**, calories; **WTR**, water; **PROT**, protein; **CARB**, carbohydrate; **FIBR**, fiber; **FAT**, fat; **SATF**, saturated fat; **MONO**, monosaturated fat; **POLY**, polyunsaturated fat

ESHA CODE	FOOD DESCRIPTION	AMT	UNIT	WT (g)	CAL (kcal)	WTR (g)	PROT (g)	CARB (g)	FIBR (g)	FAT (g)	SATF (g)	MONO (g)	POLY (g)
Grain Products (continued)													
Crackers													
139	Butter Crackers (Club)	2	ea	8	40	<1	1	5	<1	2	0.3	0.9	0.8
43771	Cheese Crackers	22	ea	30	150	0	3	18	1	8	2		
43500	Cheese Crackers-Cheez-its	10	ea	10	50	<1	1	6	<1	3	0.9	1.2	0.2
43501	CheeseCrackers-PnutButter Filled	6	ea	42	208	1	5	24	1	11	1.9	5.5	2.1
43527	Graham Cracker-Chocolate	1	ea	14	68	<1	1	9	<1	3	1.9	1.1	0.1
43502	Graham Cracker-Plain	2	ea	14	59	1	1	11	<1	1	0.2	0.6	0.5
43534	Matzoh Crackers-Plain	1	ea	28.35	112	1	3	24	1	<1	0.1	<0.1	0.2
43509	Melba Toast-Plain	1	pce	5	20	<1	1	4	<1	<1	<0.1	<0.1	0.1
43507	Oyster Crackers	1	cup	45	193	2	4	32	1	5	0.7	3.2	0.6
43505	Oyster crackers-crushed	1	cup	70	300	4	6	50	2	8	1.2	4.9	0.9
43543	Round Crackers (Ritz)	10	ea	30	151	1	2	18	<1	8	1.1	3.2	2.9
43541	Rye Crackers-Cheese Filled	6	ea	42	202	2	4	26	2	9	2.5	5.1	1.2
43532	Rye Crispbread	1	ea	10	37	1	1	8	2	<1	<0.1	<0.1	0.1
43506	Saltine Crackers	4	ea	12	51	1	1	9	<1	1	0.2	0.8	0.1
43586	Saltine Crackers-UnsaltedTops	2	ea	6	28	<1	<1	4	0	1	0		
72335	Stoned Wheat Crackers-LowFat	5	ea	14	60	<1	2	10	1	1	0		
43508	Triscuits WhlWheatCracker	2	ea	8	35	<1	1	5	1	1	0.3	0.5	0.5
44677	Wheat Crackers	1	svg	15	62	<1	1	12	1	2			
43547	Wheat Crackers	5	ea	10	47	<1	1	6	<1	2	0.5	1.1	0.3
43548	Wheat Crackers-Cheese Filled	6	ea	42	209	1	4	24	1	10	1.7	4.3	3.8
43747	Wheat Thins Crackers-LowSod	16	ea	31	150	<1	3	21	1	6	1		
43549	WheatCrackers-PnutBtr Filled	1	ea	7	35	<1	1	4	<1	2	0.3	0.8	0.6
43818	Whole Wheat Saltine Crackers	5	ea	15	60		1	11	<1	2	0.5	0.5	0
43695	Zesty Cheese Crackers	1	svg	30	129	1	2	23	1	3	0.7	0.8	0.4
Muffins													
44520	Blueberry Muffin-made w/2% Milk	1	ea	57	162	23	4	23	1	6	1.2	1.5	3.1
44524	Corn Muffin-made w/2%Milk	1	ea	57	180	19	4	25	2	7	1.3	1.7	3.5
42059	English Muffin	1	ea	57	129	25	5	25	2	1	0.4	0.2	0.3
42082	English Muffin-100% Wheat	1	ea	66	134	30	6	27	4	1	0.2	0.3	0.6
42214	English Muffin-Cheese	1	ea	63	153	26	5	28	2	2	0.8	0.5	0.6
42060	English Muffin-Sourdough	1	ea	57	129	25	5	25	2	1	0.4	0.2	0.3
44515	Muffin-Plain-Made w/2% Milk	1	ea	57	169	21	4	24	2	6	1.2	1.6	3.3
44656	Muffin-Whole Wheat-LowFat	1	ea	56.7	150		3	32	1	1	0	0.5	0.5
44514	Oat Bran Muffin	1	ea	57	154	20	4	28	3	4	0.6	1	2.4
44522	Toasted Muffin-Corn	1	ea	33	114	8	2	19	1	4	0.6	0.9	2.1
44518	Toaster Muffin-Blueberry	1	ea	33	103	10	2	18	1	3	0.5	0.7	1.8
44536	Zucchini Muffin w/Nuts	1	ea	58	219	16	3	27	1	11	1.5	3.4	5.3
Pancakes, French Toast, & Waffles													
45194	Crepe	1	ea	12.8	30	6	1	5	0	<1	0		
42156	French Toast-Rec w/2%Milk	1	pce	65	149	36	5	16	1	7	1.8	2.9	1.7
45023	Pancake-Blueberry-Recipe	1	ea	38	84	20	2	11	<1	3	0.8	0.9	1.6
45025	Pancake-Buttermilk-Recipe	1	ea	38	86	20	3	11	<1	4	0.7	0.9	1.7
45044	Pancake-Chinese	1	ea	28	58	14	1	13	<1	<1	<0.1	<0.1	<0.1
45067	Pancake-Frozen-Heated-6in	1	ea	73	164	35	4	29	2	4	0.6	1.4	0.8

< = Trace amount present   Blank = Not available

CHOL, cholesterol; **V,** vitamin; **THI,** thiamin; **RIB,** riboflavin; **NIA,** niacin; **FOL,** folate; **CALC,** calcium; **PHOS,** phosphate; **SOD,** sodium; **POT,** potassium; **MAG,** magnesium

CHOL (g)	V-A (RE)	THI (mg)	RIB (mg)	NIA (mg)	V-B6 (mg)	FOL (μg)	V-B12 (μg)	V-C (mg)	V-E (mg)	CALC (mg)	PHOS (mg)	SOD (mg)	POT (mg)	MAG (mg)	IRON (mg)	ZINC (mg)
0	0	<0.1	<0.1	0.3	<0.1	7	0	0	0.2	10	18	68	11	2	0.3	0.1
3	0							0		20		360			1.1	
1	3	0.1	<0.1	0.5	0.1	15	<0.1	0	<0.1	15	22	100	14	4	0.5	0.1
0	<1	0.2	0.1	2.4	0.1	39	0.1	0	1	21	113	298	92	24	1.1	0.4
0	1	<0.1	<0.1	0.3	<0.1	3	0	0	<0.1	8	19	41	29	8	0.5	0.1
0	<1	<0.1	<0.1	0.6	<0.1	6	0	0	<0.1	3	15	85	19	4	0.5	0.1
0	0	0.1	0.1	1.1	<0.1	5	0	0	<0.1	4	25	1	32	7	0.9	0.2
0	0	<0.1	<0.1	0.2	<0.1	6	0	0	<0.1	5	10	41	10	3	0.2	0.1
0	0	<0.1	0.2	2.4	<0.1	63	0	0	0.4	31	45	482	69	10	2.5	0.4
0	0	0.1	0.3	3.7	0.1	97	0	0	0.7	48	71	750	108	15	3.9	0.6
0	0	0.1	0.1	1.2	<0.1	27	0	0	0.6	36	68	254	40	8	1.1	0.2
4	17	0.3	0.2	1.5	<0.1	34	0.1	<1	0.8	93	142	438	144	16	1	0.3
0	0	<0.1	<0.1	0.1	<0.1	5	0	0	0.1	3	27	26	32	8	0.2	0.2
0	0	<0.1	0.1	0.6	<0.1	17	0	0	0.1	8	12	129	18	3	0.7	0.1
0	0							0		0		46			0.3	
0	0							0		20		140			0.4	
0	0	<0.1	<0.1	0.4	<0.1	2	0	0	0.1	4	24	53	24	8	0.2	0.2
	0	<0.1	0.1					0	0	22	50	150	28	7	0.6	0.3
0	0	0.1	<0.1	0.5	<0.1	12	0	0	0.1	5	22	80	18	6	0.4	0.2
3	8	0.2	0.2	1.3	0.1	27	0.1	1	0.3	86	160	383	129	23	1.1	0.4
0	0							0		0		80			1.1	
0	0	<0.1	<0.1	0.4	<0.1	5	0	0	<0.1	12	24	56	21	3	0.2	0.1
0	0							0		0		230			0.4	
1	10	0.1	0.1	1.1	<0.1	17	<0.1	<1		13	60	315	47	10	1	0.4
21	22	0.2	0.2	1.3	<0.1	27	0.1	1	1	108	83	251	70	9	1.3	0.3
24	27	0.2	0.2	1.4	0.1	43	0.1	<1	1	148	101	333	83	13	1.5	0.3
0	0	0.3	0.1	2.3	<0.1	54	<0.1	1	0.2	93	52	242	62	14	2.3	0.6
0	<1	0.2	0.1	2.3	0.1	32	0	0	0.3	175	186	312	139	47	1.6	1.1
3	9	0.3	0.2	2.3	<0.1	23	<0.1	<1	0.1	127	96	297	82	13	1.5	0.5
0	0	0.3	0.1	2.3	<0.1	54	<0.1	1	0.2	93	52	242	62	14	2.3	0.6
22	23	0.2	0.2	1.3	<0.1	29	0.1	<1	1	114	87	266	69	10	1.4	0.3
0	0							0		70	150	380	70		0.6	
0	0	0.1	0.1	0.2	0.1	51	<0.1	0	0.4	36	214	224	289	89	2.4	1
4	7	0.1	0.1	0.8	<0.1	19	<0.1	0	0.5	6	50	142	30	5	0.5	0.1
2	31	0.1	0.1	0.7	<0.1	21	<0.1	0	0.3	4	19	158	27	4	0.2	0.1
38	22	0.1	0.1	1	<0.1	9	0.1	1	2	39	48	113	66	8	1.2	0.3
5	0							0		0		50			0	
75	84	0.1	0.2	1.1	<0.1	28	0.2	<1	0.7	65	76	311	87	11	1.1	0.4
21	20	0.1	0.1	0.6	<0.1	14	0.1	1		78	57	157	52	6	0.7	0.2
22	12	0.1	0.1	0.6	<0.1	14	0.1	<1	0.5	60	53	198	55	6	0.6	0.2
0	0	<0.1	<0.1	0.3	<0.1	1	0	0	<0.1	5	18	1	18	4	0.1	0.2
13	47	0.3	0.4	2.1	0.1	52	0.1	<1	0.2	52	214	369	91	10	1.6	0.3

ESHA, EatRight Analysis CD-ROM; **AMT,** amount; **WT,** weight; **CAL,** calories; **WTR,** water; **PROT,** protein; **CARB,** carbohydrate; **FIBR,** fiber; **FAT,** fat; **SATF,** saturated fat; **MONO,** monosaturated fat; **POLY,** polyunsaturated fat

ESHA CODE	FOOD DESCRIPTION	AMT	UNIT	WT (g)	CAL (kcal)	WTR (g)	PROT (g)	CARB (g)	FIBR (g)	FAT (g)	SATF (g)	MONO (g)	POLY (g)
Grain Products (continued)													
Pancakes, French Toast, & Waffles (continued)													
45002	Pancake-Mix-Prepared	1	ea	38	74	20	2	14	<1	1	0.2	0.3	0.3
45001	Pancake-Plain-Recipe	1	ea	38	86	20	2	11	1	4	0.8	0.9	1.7
45008	Pancake-Whole Wheat	1	ea	44	92	23	4	13	1	3	0.8	0.8	1.1
45036	Rye Pancakes-4 inch	1	ea	21	63	7	1	10	1	2	0.5	0.9	0.6
45035	Sourdough Pancakes-4 inch	1	ea	21	46	11	1	7	<1	1	0.3	0.4	0.6
45094	Waffle-Blueberry-Frzn	2	ea	70	190	28	4	30	1	6	1.5		
45093	Waffle-Buttermilk-Eggo	2	ea	70	180	31	5	26	1	6	1.5		
45005	Waffle-Frozen-Toasted	1	ea	33	103	10	2	16	1	3	0.5	1.6	0.7
45003	Waffles-From Recipe	1	ea	75	218	32	6	25	1	11	2.1	2.6	5.1
45083	Waffles-Whole Grain-Frzn	2	ea	71	154	30	6	29	3	3	0.9	1.1	0.6
Pastas													
38048	Chow Mein Noodles-dry	1	cup	45	237	<1	4	26	2	14	2	3.5	7.8
38076	Couscous-Cooked	1	cup	157	176	114	6	36	2	<1	<0.1	<0.1	0.1
38260	Egg Noodles-Cooked	1	cup	160	221	108	7	40	2	3	0.7	0.9	0.9
38047	Egg Noodles-Enr-Cooked	1	cup	160	221	108	7	40	2	3	0.7	0.9	0.9
38102	Macaroni-Enriched-Cooked	1	cup	140	221	87	8	43	3	1	0.2	0.2	0.4
38092	Pasta/Noodles-Fresh-Cooked	3	oz	85.05	111	58	4	21	1	1	0.1	0.1	0.4
38067	Ramen Noodles-Cooked	1	cup	227	154	195	3	20	1	7	1.7	1.2	3.3
38551	Rice Noodles-Cooked	0.5	cup	88	96	65	1	22	1	<1	<0.1	<0.1	<0.1
38105	Shells Pasta-Small-Cooked	1	cup	115	182	71	7	35	2	1	0.2	0.2	0.4
38118	Spaghetti Noodles-Enr-Cooked	1	cup	140	221	87	8	43	3	1	0.2	0.2	0.4
38121	SpagNoodles-Enr-Ckd+Salt	1	cup	140	220	87	8	43	3	1	0.2	0.2	0.4
38066	SpagNoodles-Spinach-Cooked	1	cup	140	182	95	6	37	5	1	0.1	0.1	0.4
38060	SpagNoodles-WhlWheat-Cooked	1	cup	140	174	94	7	37	6	1	0.1	0.1	0.3
Snack Foods													
44039	BBQ Flavor Pork Skin	1	oz	28.35	153	1	16	<1		9	3.3	4.3	1
44029	Bugles Corn Chips-Plain	1	oz	28.35	145	1	2	18	<1	8	6.4	0.5	0.2
44032	Chex Party Mix	1	cup	42.5	181	1	5	28	2	7	2.4		
44033	Combos Pretzels w/Cheese	10	pce	30	139	1	3	20		5			
44031	Cornnuts-Toasted Corn Nuggets	1	oz	28.35	126	<1	2	20	2	4	0.7	2.7	0.9
44037	Cracker Jacks Snack	1	cup	42.5	170	1	3	34	2	3	0.4	1.2	1.4
44012	Popcorn-Air Popped-Plain	1	cup	8	31	<1	1	6	1	<1	<0.1	0.1	0.2
44014	Popcorn-Caramel Corn	1	oz	28.35	122	1	1	22	1	4	1	0.8	1.3
44038	Popcorn-Cheese	1	cup	11	58	<1	1	6	1	4	0.7	1.1	1.7
44013	Popcorn-Cooked in Oil+Salt	1	cup	11	64	<1	1	5	1	5	0.8	1.1	2.6
44006	Potato Chips	1	oz	28.35	155	1	2	14	1	11	3.1	2.8	3.5
44043	Potato Chips-Light	1	oz	28.35	134	<1	2	19	2	6	1.2	1.4	3.1
44015	Pretzels-Dutch Twist	10	pce	60	228	2	6	48	2	2	0.2	0.8	0.5
42454	Pretzel-Soft	1	ea	138	391		12	83	3	1	0		
42456	Pretzel-Soft-Whole Wheat	1	ea	140	408		13	84	8	2	0		
44017	Rice Cake-CarmelCorn-Mini	1	ea	3.2	13	<1	<1	3	<1	<1	0.1	<0.1	<0.1
44028	Rice Cake-Plain	1	ea	9	34	<1	1	7	<1	<1	0.1	0.1	0.1
44016	Rice Cake-Plain-Regular Size	1	ea	9	35	<1	1	7	<1	<1	0.1	0.1	0.1
61056	Sweet Potato Chips-Spiced	1	oz	28.35	140		1	16	3	7	1		

< = Trace amount present   Blank = Not available

CHOL, cholesterol; **V,** vitamin; **THI,** thiamin; **RIB,** riboflavin; **NIA,** niacin; **FOL,** folate;
CALC, calcium; **PHOS,** phosphate; **SOD,** sodium; **POT,** potassium; **MAG,** magnesium

CHOL (g)	V-A (RE)	THI (mg)	RIB (mg)	NIA (mg)	V-B6 (mg)	FOL (µg)	V-B12 (µg)	V-C (mg)	V-E (mg)	CALC (mg)	PHOS (mg)	SOD (mg)	POT (mg)	MAG (mg)	IRON (mg)	ZINC (mg)
5	4	0.1	0.1	0.7	<0.1	14	0.1	<1	0.3	48	127	239	66	8	0.6	0.1
22	21	0.1	0.1	0.6	<0.1	14	0.1	<1	0.4	83	60	167	50	6	0.7	0.2
27	29	0.1	0.2	1	<0.1	13	0.1	<1	<0.1	110	164	252	123	20	1.4	0.5
8	4	<0.1	<0.1	0.3	<0.1	2	<0.1	<1	0.3	22	25	58	97	15	0.5	0.2
8	4	0.1	0.1	0.6	<0.1	7	<0.1	<1	0.3	3	16	53	17	3	0.5	0.1
15	200	0.3	0.3	4	0.4	40	1.2	0		100	200	370	55		3.6	
15	200	0.3	0.3	4	0.4	40	1.2	0		100	200	420	60		3.6	
5	131	0.2	0.2	2.9	0.3	25	1	0	0.3	101	142	241	48	8	2.3	0.2
52	50	0.2	0.3	1.6	<0.1	34	0.2	<1	1.7	191	142	383	119	14	1.7	0.5
5	0							0		221	406	676	176	34	5.8	0.6
0	<1	0.3	0.2	2.7	<0.1	40	0	0	1.6	9	72	198	54	23	2.1	0.6
0	0	0.1	<0.1	1.5	0.1	24	0	0	0.2	13	35	8	91	13	0.6	0.4
46	10	<0.1	<0.1	0.6	0.1	11	0.1	0	0.3	19	122	8	61	34	1	1
46	10	0.5	0.2	3.3	0.1	134	0.1	0	0.3	19	122	8	61	34	2.4	1
0	0	0.4	0.2	2.4	0.1	102	0	0	0.1	10	81	1	62	25	1.8	0.7
28	5	0.2	0.1	0.8	<0.1	54	0.1	0	0.1	5	54	5	20	15	1	0.5
<1	2	<0.1	<0.1	0.3	<0.1	3	<0.1	<1	2.3	13	24	802	49	10	0.4	0.2
0	0	<0.1	<0.1	0.1	<0.1	3	0	0		4	18	17	4	3	0.1	0.2
0	0	0.3	0.2	1.9	0.1	84	0	0	0.1	8	67	1	51	21	1.5	0.6
0	0	0.4	0.2	2.4	0.1	102	0	0	0.1	10	81	1	62	25	1.8	0.7
0	0	0.4	0.2	2.4	0.1	102	0	0	0.1	10	81	183	62	25	1.8	0.7
0	22	0.1	0.1	2.1	0.1	17	0	0	<0.1	42	151	20	81	87	1.5	1.5
0	<1	0.2	0.1	1	0.1	7	0	0	0.4	21	125	4	62	42	1.5	1.1
33	26	<0.1	0.1	1	<0.1	9	<0.1	<1		12	62	756	51	0	0.3	0.2
0	9	0.1	0.1	0.4	<0.1	1	0	0	0.5	1	12	290	23	3	0.7	0.1
0	6	0.7	0.2	7.2	0.7	21	5.3	20	0.1	15	79	432	114	27	10.5	0.9
2	2	0.1	0.2	1	<0.1	2	<0.1	0	0.1	59	43	335	39	7	0.3	0.2
0	0	<0.1	<0.1	0.5	0.1	0	0	0	0.6	3	78	156	79	32	0.5	0.5
0	3	<0.1	0.1	0.8	0.1	7	0	0	0.4	28	54	125	151	34	1.7	0.5
0	2	<0.1	<0.1	0.2	<0.1	2	0	0	<0.1	1	29	1	26	12	0.3	0.2
1	1	<0.1	<0.1	0.6	<0.1	1	<0.1	0	0.3	12	24	58	31	10	0.5	0.2
1	5	<0.1	<0.1	0.2	<0.1	1	0.1	<1	<0.1	12	40	98	29	10	0.2	0.2
0	2	<0.1	<0.1	0.1	<0.1	3	0	<1	0.3	<1	22	116	20	9	0.2	0.3
0	0	<0.1	0.1	1.2	0.2	21	0	5	1.9	7	44	149	466	20	0.5	0.7
0	0	0.1	0.1	2	0.2	8	0	7	1.6	6	55	139	494	25	0.4	<0.1
0	0	0.3	0.2	3.1	<0.1	112	0	0	0.2	11	68	814	82	17	3.1	0.9
0	0							0			34	1035			2.7	
0	0							0			35	1283			2.3	
<1	1	<0.1	<0.1	0.1	<0.1	1	0	<1	<0.1	1	6	14	6	3	<0.1	<0.1
0	0	0	<0.1	0.7	<0.1	2	0	0	<0.1	1	32	1	25	11	0.1	0.2
0	0	<0.1	<0.1	0.6	0.1	2	0	0	<0.1	1	33	14	25	14	0.1	2
0	400							5		60		105			1.1	

ESHA, EatRight Analysis CD-ROM; **AMT,** amount; **WT,** weight; **CAL,** calories; **WTR,** water; **PROT,** protein; **CARB,** carbohydrate; **FIBR,** fiber; **FAT,** fat; **SATF,** saturated fat; **MONO,** monosaturated fat; **POLY,** polyunsaturated fat

ESHA CODE	FOOD DESCRIPTION	AMT	UNIT	WT (g)	CAL (kcal)	WTR (g)	PROT (g)	CARB (g)	FIBR (g)	FAT (g)	SATF (g)	MONO (g)	POLY (g)
Grain Products (continued)													
Snack Foods (continued)													
44266	Tortilla Chips-Low Fat	13	pce	28	109	1	2	24	2	1	0	0.3	0.7
44054	Tortilla Chips-Nacho-LowFat	1	oz	28.35	126	<1	2	20	1	4	0.8	2.5	0.6
44267	Tortilla Chips-No Salt	13	pce	28	109		3	24	2	1	0		
44058	Trail Mix-Regular	1	cup	150	693	14	21	67	8	44	8.3	18.8	14.5
44085	Trail Mix-Regular-Unsalted	1	cup	150	693	14	21	67	8	44	8.3	18.8	14.5
44060	Trail Mix-Tropical	1	cup	140	570	13	9	92	9	24	11.9	3.5	7.2
Grains & Flours													
38030	AllPurpose WhiteFlour-Enrich	1	cup	125	455	15	13	95	3	1	0.2	0.1	0.5
38003	Barley-Pearled-Cooked	1	cup	157	193	108	4	44	6	1	0.1	0.1	0.3
38001	Barley-Whole-Cooked	1	cup	200	270	130	7	59	14	2	0.4	0.3	1.2
38010	Brown Rice-LongGrain-Cooked	1	cup	195	216	143	5	45	4	2	0.4	0.6	0.6
38082	Brown Rice-MedGrain-Cooked	0.5	cup	97.5	109	71	2	23	2	1	0.2	0.3	0.3
38028	Bulgar Wheat-Cooked	1	cup	182	151	142	6	34	8	<1	0.1	0.1	0.2
38039	Cake Flour-Baked Value	1	cup	109	395	14	9	85	2	1	0.1	0.1	0.4
38041	Cornmeal-Enrich-BakedValu	1	cup	138	505	16	12	107	10	2	0.3	0.6	1
38083	Glutinous Sticky Rice-Ckd	1	cup	174	169	133	4	37	2	<1	0.1	0.1	0.1
38044	Light RyeFlour-BakedValue	1	cup	102	374	9	9	82	15	1	0.1	0.2	0.6
38052	Millet-Cooked	1	cup	174	207	124	6	41	2	2	0.3	0.3	0.9
38078	Oat Bran-Cooked	1	cup	219	88	184	7	25	6	2	0.4	0.6	0.7
38064	Oat Bran-Dry	1	cup	94	231	6	16	62	14	7	1.2	2.2	2.6
38043	Rolled Oats-Baked Value	1	cup	80	307	7	13	54	8	5	0.9	1.6	1.8
38438	Unbleach Enrich White Flour	0.25	cup	34	120	2	5	26	1	<1	0		
38024	Wheat Bran-Crude	0.5	cup	29	63	3	5	19	12	1	0.2	0.2	0.6
38055	Wheat Germ-HoneyCrunch	1.66	Tbs	14	52	<1	4	8	1	1	0.2	0.1	0.7
38026	Wheat Germ-Toasted	1	cup	113	432	6	33	56	17	12	2.1	1.7	7.5
38037	White Flour-Enr-Baked	1	cup	125	455	15	13	95	3	1	0.2	0.1	0.5
38013	White Rice-LongGrain-Cooked	1	cup	158	205	108	4	45	1	<1	0.1	0.1	0.1
38019	White Rice-LongGrain-Inst-Ckd	1	cup	165	193	119	4	41	1	1	<0.1	0.1	<0.1
38097	White Rice-MedGrain-Cooked	1	cup	186	242	128	4	53	1	<1	0.1	0.1	0.1
38032	Whole Wheat Flour	1	cup	120	407	12	16	87	15	2	0.4	0.3	0.9
38040	Whole Wheat Flour-Baked	1	cup	120	407	12	16	87	15	2	0.4	0.3	0.9
38021	Wild Rice-Cooked	1	cup	164	166	121	7	35	3	1	0.1	0.1	0.3
Infant Foods													
60491	BabyFd Beef Stew-Toddler	1	Tbs	16	8	14	1	1	<1	<1	0.1	0.1	<0.1
60500	BabyFd Carrots	1	Tbs	14	4	13	<1	1	<1	<1	<0.1	<0.1	<0.1
60616	BabyFd Cereal-Rice+MixFruit	1	Tbs	15	12	12	<1	3	<1	<1	<0.1	<0.1	<0.1
60632	BabyFd Sweet Potatoes	1	Tbs	14	8	12	<1	2	<1	<1	<0.1	<0.1	<0.1
60638	BabyFd Turkey Meat Sticks	1	ea	10	18	7	1	<1	<1	1	0.4	0.5	0.4
62893	BabyFd Veg Beef Dinner-Jr	1	Tbs	16	10	14	<1	1	<1	<1	0.1	0.1	<0.1
Meats & Meat Substitutes													
Beef & Veal													
10015	Beef Heart-Simmered	3	oz	85.05	140	56	24	<1	0	4	1.2	0.9	0.8
10051	Beef Jerky-Large Piece	1	ea	19.8	81	5	7	2	<1	5	2.1	2.2	0.2

< = Trace amount present   Blank = Not available

CHOL, cholesterol; **V,** vitamin; **THI,** thiamin; **RIB,** riboflavin; **NIA,** niacin; **FOL,** folate;
CALC, calcium; **PHOS,** phosphate; **SOD,** sodium; **POT,** potassium; **MAG,** magnesium

CHOL (g)	V-A (RE)	THI (mg)	RIB (mg)	NIA (mg)	V-B6 (mg)	FOL (µg)	V-B12 (µg)	V-C (mg)	V-E (mg)	CALC (mg)	PHOS (mg)	SOD (mg)	POT (mg)	MAG (mg)	IRON (mg)	ZINC (mg)
0	0	<0.1	<0.1	0.4				0		37	79	198	84		0.4	0
1	12	0.1	0.1	0.1	0.1	7	0	<1	0.2	45	90	284	77	27	0.5	
0												0				
0	3	0.7	0.3	7.1	0.4	106	0	2	5.3	117	518	344	1028	237	4.6	4.8
0	3	0.7	0.3	7.1	0.4	106	0	2	5.3	117	518	15	1028	237	4.6	4.8
0	6	0.6	0.2	2.1	0.5	59	0	11	3.1	80	260	14	993	134	3.7	1.6
0	0	1	0.6	7.4	0.1	229	0	0	0.1	19	135	2	134	28	5.8	0.9
0	1	0.1	0.1	3.2	0.2	25	0	0	<0.1	17	85	5	146	35	2.1	1.3
0	0	0.2	0.1	2.8	0.2	16	0	0	1.2	26	230	1	230	44	2.1	1.6
0	0	0.2	<0.1	3	0.3	8	0	0	0.1	20	162	10	84	84	0.8	1.2
0	0	0.1	<0.1	1.3	0.1	4	0	0	0.2	10	75	1	77	43	0.5	0.6
0	<1	0.1	0.1	1.8	0.2	33	0	0	<0.1	18	73	9	124	58	1.7	1
0	0	0.7	0.4	7	<0.1	84	0	0	0.1	15	93	2	114	17	8	0.7
0	57	0.7	0.5	6.6	0.3	52	0	0	0.5	7	116	4	224	55	5.7	1
0	0	<0.1	<0.1	0.5	<0.1	2	0	0	0.1	3	14	9	17	9	0.2	0.7
0	0	0.3	0.1	0.8	0.2	11	0	0	0.6	21	198	2	238	71	1.8	1.8
0	1	0.2	0.1	2.3	0.2	33	0	0	<0.1	5	174	3	108	77	1.1	1.6
0	0	0.4	0.1	0.3	0.1	13	0	0	0.2	22	261	2	201	88	1.9	1.2
0	0	1.1	0.2	0.9	0.2	49	0	0	0.9	55	690	4	532	221	5.1	2.9
0	8	0.4	0.1	0.6	0.1	13	0	0	0.6	42	379	3	280	118	3.4	2.5
0	0	0.1	0.1	1.2				0		0		0	35		1.1	
0	<1	0.2	0.2	3.9	0.4	23	0	0	0.4	21	294	1	343	177	3.1	2.1
0	0	0.2	0.1	0.7	0.1	85	0	0	2.8	7	142	2	135	38	1.1	1.9
0	11	1.9	0.9	6.3	1.1	398	0	7	18.1	51	1295	5	1070	362	10.3	18.8
0	0	0.7	0.5	7	<0.1	96	0	0	0.1	19	135	2	134	28	5.8	0.9
0	0	0.3	<0.1	2.3	0.1	92	0	0	0.1	16	68	2	55	19	1.9	0.8
0	0	0.1	<0.1	2.9	0.1	116	0	0	<0.1	13	61	7	15	8	2.9	0.8
0	0	0.3	<0.1	3.4	0.1	108	0	0	0.1	6	69	0	54	24	2.8	0.8
0	1	0.5	0.3	7.6	0.4	53	0	0	1	41	415	6	486	166	4.7	3.5
0	0	0.4	0.2	7.3	0.3	26	0	0	1.5	41	415	6	486	166	4.7	3.5
0	<1	0.1	0.1	2.1	0.2	43	0	0	0.4	5	134	5	166	52	1	2.2
2	26	<0.1	<0.1	0.2	<0.1	1	0.1	<1	0.1	1	7	55	23	2	0.1	0.1
0	165	<0.1	<0.1	0.1	<0.1	2	0	1	0.1	3	3	7	28	2	0.1	<0.1
0	<1	<0.1	<0.1	0.3	<0.1	<1	<0.1	1	<0.1	2	3	2	8	1	0.4	<0.1
0	93	<0.1	<0.1	0.1	<0.1	1	0	1	0.1	2	3	3	34	2	0.1	<0.1
6	1	<0.1	<0.1	0.2	<0.1	1	0.1	<1	<0.1	7	10	48	9	2	0.1	0.2
1	41	<0.1	<0.1	0.1	<0.1	1	<0.1	<1	0.1	2	6	12	20	2	0.1	0.1
180	0	0.1	1	5.7	0.2	4	9.2	0	0.2	4	216	50	186	18	5.4	2.4
10	0	<0.1	<0.1	0.3	<0.1	27	0.2	0	0.1	4	81	438	118	10	1.1	1.6

ESHA, EatRight Analysis CD-ROM; **AMT,** amount; **WT,** weight; **CAL,** calories; **WTR,** water; **PROT,** protein; **CARB,** carbohydrate; **FIBR,** fiber; **FAT,** fat; **SATF,** saturated fat; **MONO,** monosaturated fat; **POLY,** polyunsaturated fat

ESHA CODE	FOOD DESCRIPTION	AMT	UNIT	WT (g)	CAL (kcal)	WTR (g)	PROT (g)	CARB (g)	FIBR (g)	FAT (g)	SATF (g)	MONO (g)	POLY (g)
Meats & Meat Substitutes (continued)													
Beef & Veal (continued)													
10010	Beef Liver-fried	3	oz	85.05	149	53	23	4	0	4	1.3	0.6	0.5
11237	Beef Roast-Brsd	3	oz	85.05	190	49	29	0	0	8	2.7	3.2	0.3
10089	Beef Tripe-Cooked	1	cup	140	132	114	16	3	0	6	1.9	2.2	0.3
11280	Beef-Filet Mignon-Brld	3	oz	85.05	164	54	24	0	0	7	2.5	2.7	0.2
10020	Beef-Flank Steak-Brld	3	oz	85.05	165	54	24	0	0	7	2.9	2.8	0.3
10268	Beef-Lean-Ckd	3	oz	85.05	179	50	25	0	0	8	3	3.3	0.3
10706	Beef-Rib Eye Steak-Lean-Brld	3	oz	85.05	174	52	25	0	0	8	2.9	3.1	0.3
58327	Beef-Sirloin Steak-Lean-Brld	3	oz	85.05	159	54	25	0	0	6	2.2	2.3	0.2
11286	Beef-Strip Steak-Brld	3	oz	85.05	155	55	25	0	0	5	2.1	2.2	0.2
11162	Beef-Top Round Steak-Fried	3	oz	85.05	236	44	28	0	0	13	4.5	5	1.5
11170	Beef-TopRoundSteak-Lean-Fried	3	oz	85.05	193	47	30	0	0	7	2.1	2.4	1.4
10008	Corned Beef-Canned	3	oz	85.05	213	49	23	0	0	13	5.3	5.1	0.5
58117	Grnd Beef Patty-15%Fat-Brld	1	ea	77	192	45	20	0	0	12	4.5	5.1	0.4
58122	Grnd Beef Patty-20% fat-Brld	1	ea	77	209	43	20	0	0	14	5.2	6.1	0.4
58107	Grnd Beef Patty-5%Fat-Brld	1	ea	82	140	54	22	0	0	5	2.4	2.2	0.3
10028	Porterhouse Steak-Broiled-Ln	1	ea	170	366	102	44	0	0	20	6.7	9.6	0.6
10624	ShortRibs-Braised	3	oz	85.05	401	30	18	0	0	36	15.1	16.1	1.3
10035	Sizzlean Formed Bacon-Cooked	3	ea	34	153	9	11	<1	0	12	4.9	5.7	0.5
10007	TBoneSteak-Broiled-Lean	3	oz	85.05	174	52	23	0	0	9	3.1	4.2	0.3
11530	Veal- Ground-Broiled	3	oz	85.05	146	57	21	0	0	6	2.6	2.4	0.5
11517	Veal Loin Cutlet-Brsd-Lean+Fat	1	ea	80	227	42	24	0	0	14	5.4	5.4	0.9
11519	Veal Rib-Roasted-Lean+Fat	3	oz	85.05	194	51	20	0	0	12	4.6	4.6	0.8
11527	Veal Sirloin-Roasted	3	oz	85.05	172	53	21	0	0	9	3.8	3.5	0.6
Fish, Seafood, & Shellfish													
19086	Abalone-Cooked	1	cup	150	315	74	51	18	0	2	0.4	0.3	0.3
17124	Anchovies+Oil-Canned	5	ea	20	42	10	6	0	0	2	0.4	0.8	0.5
17106	Butterfish Fillet-Baked/Broiled	1	ea	25	47	17	6	0	0	3			
17179	Catfish-Brld	3	oz	85.05	129	61	16	0	0	7	1.5	3.5	1.2
17034	Caviar-Granular-Black/Red	1	Tbs	16	40	8	4	1	0	3	0.6	0.7	1.2
19002	Clams-Canned-Drained	1	cup	160	237	102	41	8	0	3	0.3	0.3	0.9
19036	Crab Leg-Alaska King-Boiled	1	ea	134	130	104	26	0	0	2	0.2	0.2	0.7
19038	Crayfish/Crawdads-Steam/Boiled	3	oz	85.05	70	68	14	0	0	1	0.2	0.2	0.3
19022	Crayfish/Crawfish-raw	8	ea	27	21	22	4	0	0	<1	<0.1	<0.1	0.1
19004	Dungeness Crab-Stmd	3	oz	85.05	94	62	19	1	0	1	0.1	0.2	0.3
17071	Grouper Fillet-Bkd/Brld	1	ea	202	238	148	50	0	0	3	0.6	0.5	0.8
17090	Haddock Fillet-Bkd/Brld	1	ea	150	168	111	36	0	0	1	0.3	0.2	0.5
17047	Herring Fillet-Baked/Broiled	1	ea	143	290	92	33	0	0	17	3.7	6.8	3.9
17012	Herring-Pickled	1	pce	20	52	11	3	2	0	4	0.5	2.4	0.3
19006	Lobster-Northern-Stmd	3	oz	85.05	83	65	17	1	0	1	0.1	0.1	0.1
19044	Mussels-Steamed/Boiled	3	oz	85.05	146	52	20	6	0	4	0.7	0.9	1
19048	Octopus-Cooked-Moist	3	oz	85.05	139	51	25	4	0	2	0.4	0.3	0.4
19025	Octopus-Raw	4	oz	113.4	93	91	17	2	0	1	0.3	0.2	0.3
17121	Orange Roughy-Baked/Broiled	3	oz	85.05	89	57	19	0	0	1	<0.1	0.4	0.2
19027	Oysters-Eastern-Boiled/Steamed	6	ea	42	58	30	6	3	0	2	0.6	0.3	0.8

< = Trace amount present   Blank = Not available

CHOL, cholesterol; **V,** vitamin; **THI,** thiamin; **RIB,** riboflavin; **NIA,** niacin; **FOL,** folate;
CALC, calcium; **PHOS,** phosphate; **SOD,** sodium; **POT,** potassium; **MAG,** magnesium

CHOL (g)	V-A (RE)	THI (mg)	RIB (mg)	NIA (mg)	V-B6 (mg)	FOL (µg)	V-B12 (µg)	V-C (mg)	V-E (mg)	CALC (mg)	PHOS (mg)	SOD (mg)	POT (mg)	MAG (mg)	IRON (mg)	ZINC (mg)
324	6600	0.2	2.9	14.9	0.9	221	70.7	1	0.4	5	412	65	299	19	5.2	4.4
84	0	0.1	0.2	5	0.4	9	1.6	0	0.4	7	177	37	230	19	2.3	4.8
220	0	0	<0.1	0.6	0	4	1	0	0.2	113	92	95	59	21	0.9	2.4
67	0	0.1	0.1	6.9	0.5	9	1.4	0	0.3	15	191	50	308	20	1.5	4.5
47	0	0.1	0.1	7	0.5	8	1.5	0	0.3	13	179	48	287	20	1.6	4.3
73	0	0.1	0.2	3.4	0.3	7	2.2	0	0.1	7	196	56	302	22	2.5	5.8
77	0	0.1	0.1	7.2	0.5	9	1.5	0	0.3	14	193	51	309	21	1.7	4.7
54	0	0.1	0.1	6.6	0.5	8	1.4	0	0.3	14	196	52	314	21	1.7	4.7
54	0	0.1	0.1	7.1	0.5	9	1.4	0	0.3	16	195	51	315	21	1.6	4.6
82	0	0.1	0.2	4.3	0.5	10	2.7	0	0.2	5	228	58	400	27	2.5	3.6
82	0	0.1	0.2	4.7	0.5	11	2.9	0	0.1	4	248	60	436	30	2.7	3.9
73	0	<0.1	0.1	2.1	0.1	8	1.4	0	0.1	10	94	856	116	12	1.8	3
69	0	<0.1	0.1	4.1	0.3	7	2	0	0.3	14	152	55	245	16	2	4.9
70	0	<0.1	0.1	3.9	0.3	8	2.1	0	0.4	18	149	58	234	15	1.9	4.8
62	0	<0.1	0.1	4.9	0.3	6	2	0	0.3	6	169	53	285	18	2.3	5.3
117	0	0.2	0.4	7.9	0.7	14	3.9	0	0.2	10	359	117	512	42	5.5	8.6
80	0	<0.1	0.1	2.1	0.2	4	2.2	0	0.2	10	138	43	191	13	2	4.2
40	0	<0.1	0.1	2.2	0.1	3	1.2	0	0.1	3	80	766	140	9	1.1	2.2
50	0	0.1	0.2	3.9	0.3	7	1.9	0	0.1	5	183	65	278	22	3.1	4.3
88	0	0.1	0.2	6.8	0.3	9	1.1	0	0.1	14	185	71	287	20	0.8	3.3
94	0	<0.1	0.2	7.2	0.2	11	1	0	0.3	22	176	64	224	19	0.9	2.9
94	0	<0.1	0.2	5.9	0.2	11	1.2	0	0.3	9	168	78	251	19	0.8	3.5
87	0	0.1	0.3	7.5	0.3	13	1.2	0	0.4	11	190	71	299	22	0.8	2.8
255	5	0.5	0.2	3.4	0.4	11	1.3	4	12	88	399	768	525	122	8.6	2.5
17	2	<0.1	0.1	4	<0.1	3	0.2	0	0.7	46	50	734	109	14	0.9	0.5
21	8	<0.1	<0.1	1.4	0.1	4	0.5	0	0.2	7	77	28	120	8	0.2	0.2
54	13	0.4	0.1	2.1	0.1	6	2.4	1	1.1	8	208	68	273	22	0.7	0.9
94	90	<0.1	0.1	<0.1	0.1	8	3.2	0	1.1	44	57	240	29	48	1.9	0.2
107	290	0.2	0.7	5.4	0.2	46	158.2	35	1	147	541	179	1005	29	44.7	4.4
71	12	0.1	0.1	1.8	0.2	68	15.4	10	1.2	79	375	1436	351	84	1	10.2
113	13	<0.1	0.1	1.9	0.1	37	1.8	1	1.3	51	230	80	252	28	0.7	1.5
31	4	<0.1	<0.1	0.6	<0.1	10	0.5	<1	0.8	7	69	16	82	7	0.2	0.4
65	26	<0.1	0.2	3.1	0.1	36	8.8	3	1	50	149	321	347	49	0.4	4.7
95	101	0.2	<0.1	0.8	0.7	20	1.4	0	1.3	42	289	107	960	75	2.3	1
111	28	0.1	0.1	6.9	0.5	20	2.1	0	0.7	63	362	130	598	75	2	0.7
110	51	0.2	0.4	5.9	0.5	17	18.8	1	2	106	433	164	599	59	2	1.8
3	52	<0.1	<0.1	0.7	<0.1	<1	0.9	0	0.3	15	18	174	14	2	0.2	0.1
61	22	<0.1	0.1	0.9	0.1	9	2.6	0	0.9	52	157	323	299	30	0.3	2.5
48	77	0.3	0.4	2.6	0.1	65	20.4	12	1.2	28	242	314	228	31	5.7	2.3
82	77	<0.1	0.1	3.2	0.6	20	30.6	7	1	90	237	391	536	51	8.1	2.9
54	51	<0.1	<0.1	2.4	0.4	18	22.7	6	1.4	60	211	261	397	34	6	1.9
68	20	<0.1	0.1	1.5	0.1	4	0.4	0	1.6	9	87	59	154	15	1	0.3
44	23	0.1	0.1	1	<0.1	6	14.7	3	0.7	38	85	177	118	40	5	76.3

ESHA, EatRight Analysis CD-ROM; **AMT,** amount; **WT,** weight; **CAL,** calories; **WTR,** water; **PROT,** protein; **CARB,** carbohydrate; **FIBR,** fiber; **FAT,** fat; **SATF,** saturated fat; **MONO,** monosaturated fat; **POLY,** polyunsaturated fat

ESHA CODE	FOOD DESCRIPTION	AMT	UNIT	WT (g)	CAL (kcal)	WTR (g)	PROT (g)	CARB (g)	FIBR (g)	FAT (g)	SATF (g)	MONO (g)	POLY (g)
Meats & Meat Substitutes (continued)													
Fish, Seafood, & Shellfish (continued)													
19026	Oysters-Eastern-Raw	1	cup	248	169	211	17	10	0	6	1.9	0.8	2.4
17107	Pacific Cod Fish-Fillet-Bkd/Brld	3	oz	85.05	89	65	20	0	0	1	0.1	0.1	0.3
19012	Prawns/Lrg Shrimp-Steamed	4	ea	22	22	17	5	0	0	<1	0.1	<0.1	0.1
17123	Salmon Fillet-Baked/Broiled	0.5	ea	154	280	92	39	0	0	13	1.9	4.2	5
17060	Sardines+Oil-Cnd-Drained	1	ea	12	25	7	3	0	0	1	0.2	0.5	0.6
19011	Scallops-Stmd	3	oz	85.05	95	62	20	0	0	1	0.1	0.1	0.4
17086	Sea Bass Fillet-Baked/Broiled	1	ea	101	125	73	24	0	0	3	0.7	0.5	1
19000	Small Clams-Steamed/Boild	20	ea	190	281	121	49	10	0	4	0.4	0.3	1
17022	Snapper Fillet-Baked/Broiled	1	ea	170	218	120	45	0	0	3	0.6	0.5	1
17068	Sole/Flounder-Fillet-Broiled	1	ea	127	149	93	31	0	0	2	0.5	0.4	0.8
19068	Squid/Calamari-Baked	1	cup	140	194	99	26	5	0	7	1.4	2.2	2.1
17104	Striped Bass-Baked/Broiled	1	ea	124	154	91	28	0	0	4	0.8	1	1.2
17072	Striped Mullet Fillet- Baked	1	ea	93	140	66	23	0	0	5	1.3	1.3	0.9
17080	Surimi	3	oz	85.05	84	65	13	6	0	1	0.2	0.1	0.4
17066	Swordfish Broiled/Baked	1	ea	106	164	73	27	0	0	5	1.5	2.1	1.3
17024	Tuna Fish+Oil-Canned	0.5	cup	73	145	44	21	0	0	6	1.1	2.2	2.1
17026	Tuna Fish+Wtr-Canned	0.5	cup	77	89	57	20	0	0	1	0.2	0.1	0.3
17101	Tuna-Bluefin-Baked/Broiled	3	oz	85.05	156	50	25	0	0	5	1.4	1.7	1.6
19040	Whelk-Steamed/Boiled	3	oz	85.05	234	27	41	13	0	1	0.1	<0.1	<0.1
Game Meats													
14008	Beefalo Meat-Roasted	3	oz	85.05	160	52	26	0	0	5	2.3	2.3	0.2
14009	Bison/Buffalo Meat-Roasted	3	oz	85.05	122	57	24	0	0	2	0.8	0.8	0.2
14013	Deer/Venison-Roasted	3	oz	85.05	134	55	26	0	0	3	1.1	0.7	0.5
40570	Deer-Round Steak-Lean-Brld	3	oz	85.05	129	56	27	0	0	2	0.9	0.4	0.1
14014	Elk Meat-Roasted	3	oz	85.05	124	56	26	0	0	2	0.6	0.4	0.3
14029	Frog Legs-Steamed	2	ea	100	106	74	24	0	0	<1	0.1	0.1	0.1
14004	Rabbit-Roasted	3	oz	85.05	168	52	25	0	0	7	2	1.8	1.3
14030	Turtle Meat-Cooked	1	cup	140	220	96	33	<1	0	9	1.8	4.1	2.6
Goat & Lamb													
13623	Goat-Rstd	3	oz	85.05	122	58	23	0	0	3	0.8	1.2	0.2
13524	Ground Lamb-Broiled	3	oz	85.05	241	47	21	0	0	17	6.9	7.1	1.2
13522	Lamb Kabob Meat-Broiled-Lean	3	oz	85.05	158	54	24	0	0	6	2.2	2.5	0.6
13501	Leg of Lamb-Roasted-Lean	3	oz	85.05	162	54	24	0	0	7	2.3	2.9	0.4
13513	Lamb Loin Chop Broiled-Lean	1	ea	46	99	28	14	0	0	4	1.6	2	0.3
13523	Lamb Stew Meat-Braised-Lean	3	oz	85.05	190	48	29	0	0	7	2.7	3	0.7
Lunchmeats													
13000	Beef lunchmeat-thin slice	5	pce	21	31	14	4	<1	0	1	0.6	0.7	0.1
13010	Beef+Pork Hotdog	1	ea	45	137	25	5	1	0	12	4.8	6.2	1.2
13006	Bologna-Beef & Pork	1	pce	28.35	87	15	4	2	0	7	2.6	3	0.3
13007	Bologna-Turkey	2	pce	56.7	119	37	6	3	<1	9	2.5	3.9	2.2
13079	Bratwurst Sausage Link-Cooked	1	ea	85	283	44	12	2	0	25	8.6	12.5	2.2
13066	Braunschweiger Sausage	1	pce	18	59	9	3	1	0	5	1.7	2.3	0.6
13052	Breakfast Sausage-Turkey	1	pce	28.4	65	17	6	0	0	5	1.6	1.8	1.2
13099	Chinese Pork Sausage	3	oz	85.05	302	33	18	6	0	25			

< = Trace amount present   Blank = Not available

CHOL, cholesterol; V, vitamin; THI, thiamin; RIB, riboflavin; NIA, niacin; FOL, folate;
CALC, calcium; PHOS, phosphate; SOD, sodium; POT, potassium; MAG, magnesium

CHOL (g)	V-A (RE)	THI (mg)	RIB (mg)	NIA (mg)	V-B6 (mg)	FOL (µg)	V-B12 (µg)	V-C (mg)	V-E (mg)	CALC (mg)	PHOS (mg)	SOD (mg)	POT (mg)	MAG (mg)	IRON (mg)	ZINC (mg)
131	74	0.2	0.2	3.4	0.2	25	48.3	9	2.1	112	335	523	387	117	16.5	225.2
40	9	<0.1	<0.1	2.1	0.4	7	0.9	3	0.3	8	190	77	440	26	0.3	0.4
43	15	<0.1	<0.1	0.6	<0.1	1	0.3	<1	0.3	9	30	49	40	7	0.7	0.3
109	20	0.4	0.7	15.5	1.5	45	4.7	0	1.9	23	394	86	967	57	1.6	1.3
17	4	<0.1	<0.1	0.6	<0.1	1	1.1	0	0.2	46	59	61	48	5	0.4	0.2
45	26	0.1	0.1	1.1	0.1	10	1.1	0	1.3	98	287	225	405	47	2.6	2.6
54	65	0.1	0.2	1.9	0.5	6	0.3	0	0.6	13	250	88	331	54	0.4	0.5
127	325	0.3	0.8	6.4	0.2	55	187.9	42	3.7	175	642	213	1193	34	53.1	5.2
80	60	0.1	<0.1	0.6	0.8	10	5.9	3	1.1	68	342	97	887	63	0.4	0.7
86	17	0.1	0.1	2.8	0.3	11	3.2	0	0.8	23	367	133	437	74	0.4	0.8
395	57	<0.1	0.6	3.5	0.1	8	2.1	8	2.7	56	376	124	420	56	1.2	2.6
128	38	0.1	<0.1	3.2	0.4	12	5.5	0	0.8	24	315	109	407	63	1.3	0.6
59	39	0.1	0.1	5.9	0.5	9	0.2	1	1.1	29	227	66	426	31	1.3	0.8
26	17	<0.1	<0.1	0.2	<0.1	2	1.4	0	0.5	8	240	122	95	37	0.2	0.3
53	43	<0.1	0.1	12.5	0.4	2	2.1	1	0.7	6	357	122	391	36	1.1	1.6
13	17	<0.1	0.1	9.1	0.1	4	1.6	0	0.6	9	227	258	151	23	1	0.7
23	13	<0.1	0.1	10.2	0.3	3	2.3	0	0.3	8	126	260	182	21	1.2	0.6
42	644	0.2	0.3	9	0.4	2	9.3	0	1.1	9	277	43	275	54	1.1	0.7
111	42	<0.1	0.2	1.7	0.6	9	15.4	6	0.2	96	240	350	590	146	8.6	2.8
49	0	<0.1	0.1	4.2	0.3	15	2.2	8	0.2	20	213	70	390	<1	2.6	5.4
70	0	0.1	0.2	3.2	0.3	7	2.4	0	0.3	7	178	48	307	22	2.9	3.1
95	0	0.2	0.5	5.7	0.3	4	2.7	0	0.2	6	192	46	285	20	3.8	2.3
72	0	0.2	0.4	7.1	0.6	9	1.9	0	0.5	3	231	38	321	26	3.6	3.1
62	0					8	5.5	0	<0.1	4	153	52	279	20	3.1	2.7
72	20	0.2	0.3	1.6	0.2	16	0.5	0	1.4	26	160	84	372	29	2	1.4
70	0	0.1	0.2	7.2	0.4	9	7.1	0	0.7	16	224	40	326	18	1.9	1.9
82	126	0.2	0.3	1.7	0.2	21	1.5	<1	2.1	197	299	209	383	33	2.3	1.6
64	0	0.1	0.5	3.4	0	4	1	0	0.3	14	171	73	344	0	3.2	4.5
82	0	0.1	0.2	5.7	0.1	16	2.2	0	0.1	19	171	69	288	20	1.5	4
77	0	0.1	0.3	5.6	0.1	20	2.6	0	0.2	11	191	65	285	26	2	4.9
76	0	0.1	0.2	5.4	0.1	20	2.2	0	0.2	7	175	58	287	22	1.8	4.2
44	0	0.1	0.1	3.2	0.1	11	1.2	0	0.1	9	104	39	173	13	0.9	1.9
92	0	0.1	0.2	5.1	0.1	18	2.3	0	0.2	13	174	60	221	24	2.4	5.6
15	0	<0.1	<0.1	0.9	0.1	2	0.5	0	<0.1	2	35	297	90	4	0.4	0.8
22	8	0.1	0.1	1.2	0.1	2	0.6	0	0.1	5	39	504	75	4	0.5	0.8
17	7	0.1	0.1	0.7	0.1	2	0.5	<1	0	24	46	209	89	5	0.3	0.7
43	5	<0.1	0.1	1.5	0.1	5	0.1	8	0.3	70	65	710	77	9	1.7	0.7
63	1	0.5	0.2	3.9	0.3	3	0.7	0	<0.1	24	191	719	220	18	0.5	2.1
32	760	<0.1	0.3	1.5	0.1	8	3.6	0	0.1	2	30	209	36	2	2	0.5
23	0	<0.1	0.1	1.4	0.1	1	0.5	0	0.1	5	52	191	76	6	0.5	1
	0	0.4	0.2	4				0		20	184	748				2.6

ESHA, EatRight Analysis CD-ROM; **AMT**, amount; **WT**, weight; **CAL**, calories; **WTR**, water; **PROT**, protein; **CARB**, carbohydrate; **FIBR**, fiber; **FAT**, fat; **SATF**, saturated fat; **MONO**, monosaturated fat; **POLY**, polyunsaturated fat

ESHA CODE	FOOD DESCRIPTION	AMT	UNIT	WT (g)	CAL (kcal)	WTR (g)	PROT (g)	CARB (g)	FIBR (g)	FAT (g)	SATF (g)	MONO (g)	POLY (g)
Meats & Meat Substitutes (continued)													
Lunchmeats (continued)													
13070	Chorizo Sausage-Link	1	ea	60	273	19	14	1	0	23	8.6	11	2.1
13250	Hot Dog-Beef-Fat Free	1	ea	50	39	39	7	3	0	<1	0.1	0.1	<0.1
13008	Hotdog-Beef-2oz	1	ea	57	188	30	6	2	0	17	6.7	8.2	0.7
13012	Hotdog-Turkey	1	ea	45	102	28	6	1	0	8	2.7	2.5	2.2
13015	Italian Pork Sausage Link-Ckd	1	ea	67	230	32	13	3	<1	18	6.4	8	2.2
13043	Kielbasa Sausage	1	pce	26	81	14	3	1	0	7	2.6	3.4	0.8
13019	Liverwurst-Pork	1	pce	18	59	9	3	<1	0	5	1.9	2.4	0.5
13020	Pastrami-Turkey	2	pce	56.7	70	41	9	2	<1	2	0.7	0.8	0.6
13021	Pepperoni Sausage	1	pce	5.5	26	2	1	<1	<1	2	0.9	1	0.1
13051	Pickle & Pimento Loaf	2	pce	56.7	128	34	6	5	<1	9	3	4	1.6
13022	Polish Sausage-Pork	1	ea	227	740	121	32	4	0	65	23.4	30.7	7
13023	Salami-Beef-Cooked	1	pce	23	60	14	3	<1	0	5	2.3	2.4	0.2
13026	Salami-Dry-Beef & Pork	2	pce	20	77	7	5	1	0	6	2.1	3	0.6
11913	Spam	2	oz	56.7	176	30	8	2	0	15	5.6	7.8	1.7
13328	Turkey Lunchmeat-Roasted	1	ea	28	28	21	5	1	0	1	0.1	0.2	0.1
13112	TurkeyBreast-Smkd-FatFree	1	pce	28	23	22	4	1	0	<1	0.1	0.1	<0.1
Meat Substitutes													
7726	BlackBean Burger	1	ea	78	150	44	12	15	3	5	0.6	1.2	2.4
7752	Breakfast Strip-Frozen	2	ea	16	60		2	2	<1	4	0.5	1	3
7724	Deli Franks	1	ea	45	60	29	9	5	2	1	0.1	0.1	0.3
7518	Firm Tofu-Raw	0.5	cup	126	88	107	10	2	1	5	1.1	1.5	2.3
7673	HarvestBurger-Italian-Frozen	1	ea	90	140		17	8	5	4	1.5	0.5	0.5
7674	HarvestBurger-Original-Frozen	1	ea	90	138	58	18	7	6	4	1	2.1	0.3
7718	Soy Burger-BlackBean&Salsa	1	ea	142	200		19	20	3	4	1.5		
7564	Tempeh	.5	cup	83	160	50	15	8		9	1.8	2.5	3.2
8835	Tofu Franks/Wiener-Each	1	ea	38	45		9	2	0	<1	0		
7520	Tofu-Fried	1	pce	13	35	7	2	1	1	3	0.4	0.6	1.5
7500	Tofu-Regular	1	cup	248	151	216	16	4	<1	9	1.3	2	5.2
7670	Vegan Burger	1	ea	85	120	55	16	9	6	2	0.3	0.6	0.9
7665	Vege Chicken Patties-Frozen	1	ea	71	150		9	16	2	6	1	1.5	2.5
7727	Vege ChickenNugget Frozen	5	pce	85	250		13	14	2	15	2	4.5	8
7722	Vege Patties	1	ea	67	111	41	12	10	3	3	0.4	0.7	1.6
8169	Veget Baloney-Pce LLF	1	pce	14.33	20	10	3	1	0	1	0.3		
8127	Veget Frank/Wiener-Jumbo	1	ea	76	80	55	16	4	1	0	0	0	0
8166	Veget Sausage-Lean-Breakfast	1	ea	35	60	24	4	4	0	3	1		
92033	Vegetarian Beef-Herb Crusted	1	ea	71	170		10	12	2	9	1		
7511	Vegetarian BreakfastLinks	1	ea	25	64	13	5	2	1	5	0.7	1.1	2.3
7512	Vegetarian BreakfastPatty	1	ea	38	98	19	7	4	1	7	1.1	1.7	3.5
7732	Vegetarian Burger	0.25	cup	55	70		10	3	1	2	0	0	1
7548	Vegetarian Chicken-BreadFried	1	pce	57	133	32	12	5	2	7	0.6	1.8	2.6
7636	Vegetarian Chicken-Frozen	2	pce	57	90		9	2	1	4	1	1	2.5
7610	Vegetarian Choplets-Canned	2	pce	92	90		18	4	2	1	0	0	0.5
7642	Vegetarian Fillets-Frozen	2	pce	85	180		16	8	4	9	1	3.5	4.5
7549	Vegetarian Fish Sticks	2	ea	57	165	26	13	5	3	10	1.6	2.5	5.3
7746	Vegetarian Grillers	1	ea	64	140		15	5	2	6	1	2	3

< = Trace amount present   Blank = Not available

CHOL, cholesterol; **V,** vitamin; **THI,** thiamin; **RIB,** riboflavin; **NIA,** niacin; **FOL,** folate;
CALC, calcium; **PHOS,** phosphate; **SOD,** sodium; **POT,** potassium; **MAG,** magnesium

CHOL (g)	V-A (RE)	THI (mg)	RIB (mg)	NIA (mg)	V-B6 (mg)	FOL (µg)	V-B12 (µg)	V-C (mg)	V-E (mg)	CALC (mg)	PHOS (mg)	SOD (mg)	POT (mg)	MAG (mg)	IRON (mg)	ZINC (mg)
53	0	0.4	0.2	3.1	0.3	1	1.2	0	0.1	5	90	741	239	11	1	2
15	0							0		10	64	464	234	10	1	1.2
30	0	<0.1	0.1	1.4	0.1	3	1	0	0.1	8	91	650	89	8	0.9	1.4
48	0	<0.1	0.1	1.9	0.1	4	0.1	0	0.3	48	60	642	81	6	0.8	1.4
38	7	0.4	0.2	2.8	0.2	3	0.9	<1	0.2	14	114	809	204	12	1	1.6
17	0	0.1	0.1	0.7	<0.1	1	0.4	0	0.1	11	38	280	70	4	0.4	0.5
28	1495	<0.1	0.2	0.8	<0.1	5	2.4	0	0.1	5	41	155	31	2	1.2	0.4
39	2	<0.1	0.1	2	0.2	3	0.1	9	0.1	6	113	556	196	8	2.4	1.2
6	<1	<0.1	<0.1	0.3	<0.1	<1	0.1	<1	0	1	10	98	17	1	0.1	0.2
33	59	0.3	0.1	1.9	0.2	9	0.4	4	0.2	62	81	739	179	12	0.8	1.1
159	0	1.1	0.3	7.8	0.4	5	2.2	2	0.5	27	309	1989	538	32	3.3	4.4
16	0	<0.1	<0.1	0.7	<0.1	<1	0.7	0	<0.1	1	47	262	43	3	0.5	0.4
20	0	0.1	0.1	1	0.1	<1	0.4	0	0.1	2	28	402	76	3	0.3	0.6
40	0					2		1		8		776	130	8	0.5	1
11	0					2		0		2	70	270	62	6	0.3	0.3
10	0							0		3	69	300	61	8	0.2	0.2
2	28	7.4	0.3	0	0.2		0.1	0	0.4	44	162	458	314	44	3.4	0.8
0	0	0.8	<0.1	0.4	0.1		0.2	0		0		220	15		0.4	
0	0	0.1	0.1	0	<0.1		<0.1	0	1.3	10	42	481	54	4	0.7	0.4
0	0	0.1	0.1	0.1	0.1	24	0	<1	<0.1	253	152	15	186	47	2	1
0	0	0.3	0.1	4	0.3		1.5	0		80		370			2.7	6.8
0	0	0.3	0.2	6.3	0.4	22	0	0	1.6	102	225	411	432	70	3.9	8.1
0											660					
0	0	0.1	0.3	2.2	0.2	20	0.1	0	<0.1	92	221	7	342	67	2.2	0.9
0	0	0.2					0.6	0		20		240	90	8	2.2	0.6
0	<1	<0.1	<0.1	<0.1	<0.1	4	0	0	<0.1	48	37	2	19	8	0.6	0.3
0	2	0.1	0.1	1.3	0.1	109	0	<1	<0.1	275	228	20	298	67	2.8	1.6
0	0	0.3	0.6	4.1	0.2	246	0	0	<0.1	26	181	547	297	16	2.4	0.4
0	0	1.8	0.2	2	0.2		1.2	0		0		540	210		1.8	
0	0	0.4	0.2	6	0.8		3	0		20		490	210		1.4	
1	42	7.5	0.2	0	0	59	0	0	0.5	40	110	349	142	29	1.5	0.7
0	0							1		7		80			0.2	
0	0							1		40		590			0.7	
0	0							2		20		130			0.9	
0	0							0		40		510			1.4	
0	0	0.6	0.1	2.8	0.2	6	0	0	0.5	16	56	222	58	9	0.9	0.4
0	0	0.9	0.2	4.3	0.3	10	0	0	0.8	24	86	337	88	14	1.4	0.6
0	0	0.1	0.1	1.6	0.2		2.4	0		0		250	25		1.4	
0	0	0.7	0.2	7.3	0.5	32	2.9	0	1.1	24	140	228	171	7	2.2	0.4
0	0	0.4	0.1	4	0.3		1.8	0		250		250	250		1.8	
0	0							0		0		500	40		0.4	
0	0	0.4	0.1	0.8	0.4		2.7	0		20		650	130		1.8	
0	0	0.6	0.5	6.8	0.9	58	2.4	0	2.3	54	256	279	342	13	1.1	0.8
0	0	1.8	0.2	2	0.4		2.7	0		40		260	130		1.1	

ESHA, EatRight Analysis CD-ROM; **AMT,** amount; **WT,** weight; **CAL,** calories; **WTR,** water; **PROT,** protein; **CARB,** carbohydrate;
FIBR, fiber; **FAT,** fat; **SATF,** saturated fat; **MONO,** monosaturated fat; **POLY,** polyunsaturated fat

ESHA CODE	FOOD DESCRIPTION	AMT	UNIT	WT (g)	CAL (kcal)	WTR (g)	PROT (g)	CARB (g)	FIBR (g)	FAT (g)	SATF (g)	MONO (g)	POLY (g)
Meats & Meat Substitutes (continued)													
Meat Substitutes (continued)													
91501	Vegetarian Ground Beef	0.5	cup	57	60	36	13	6	3	<1	0	0	0
8173	Vegetarian Ham-Country-Piece	1	pce	14.33	17	10	3	1	0	0	0	0	0
92148	Vegetarian Hot Dog	1	ea	70	163	41	14	5	3	10	1.4	2.7	5.5
8159	Vegetarian Italian Sausage-Lean	1	ea	40	60	27	5	5	0	2	1		
7734	Vegetarian Leanies-Frozen	1	ea	40	100		8	2	1	7	1	1.5	4.5
7551	Vegetarian Luncheon Meat	1	pce	67	127	44	12	3	0	7	0.9	1.4	2.9
7561	Vegetarian Meat Patties	1	ea	71	140	41	15	6	3	6	1	1.6	3.3
7552	Vegetarian Meatballs	7	ea	70	138	41	15	6	3	6	1	1.5	3.3
91059	Vegetarian Pizza Burger	1	ea	67	130		11	7	3	6	1.5	1.5	3
7618	Vegetarian Salami-Frozen	3	pce	57	120		12	3	2	7	1	1	5
7555	Vegetarian Sandwich Spread	1	Tbs	15	22	10	1	1	<1	1	0.2	0.3	0.7
7554	Vegetarian Soyburger	1	ea	71	138	41	15	5	3	6	0.8	1.2	2.5
7624	Vegetarian Tuno-Frozen	0.5	cup	55	90		7	3	2	6	1	2	3
Pork & Ham													
12000	Bacon-Regular-Cooked	3	pce	19	103	2	7	<1	0	8	2.6	3.5	0.9
12002	Canadian Bacon-Grilled	2	pce	46.5	86	29	11	1	0	4	1.3	1.9	0.4
12175	Cured Ham-Rstd	3	oz	85.05	145	54	21	0	0	6	2	2.7	0.7
12225	Ham-Canned-Unheated-XLean	1	cup	140	202	100	25	0	0	10	3.4	5	1.1
12006	Ham-Whole-Rstd-Lean Only	1	cup	140	220	92	35	0	0	8	2.6	3.5	0.9
12236	Pork Country Rib-Lean-Rstd	3	oz	85.05	210	49	23	0	0	13	4.5	5.5	0.9
12035	Pork Loin Chop-Broiled-Lean	1	ea	79	166	48	23	0	0	8	2.9	3.5	0.6
12031	Pork Loin-Roasted Slice	1	pce	89	221	51	24	0	0	13	4.8	5.8	1.1
12098	Spareribs-Braised-Lean	3	oz	85.05	199	51	22	0	0	12	4.2	5	0.9
Poultry													
15016	Chicken+Broth-Can	1	ea	142	234	97	31	0	0	11	3.1	4.5	2.5
15050	Chicken Back-Meat-Fried	1	ea	116	334	56	35	7	0	18	4.8	6.6	4.2
15001	Chicken Breast+Skin-Roastd	1	ea	98	193	61	29	0	0	8	2.1	3	1.6
15057	Chicken Breast-NoSkin-Fried	1	ea	86	161	52	29	<1	0	4	1.1	1.5	0.9
15004	Chicken Breast-NoSkin-Roasted	1	ea	86	142	56	27	0	0	3	0.9	1.1	0.7
15042	Chicken Drumstick-Fried	1	ea	42	82	26	12	0	0	3	0.9	1.2	0.8
15035	Chicken Drumstick-NoSkin-Roast	1	ea	44	76	29	12	0	0	2	0.7	0.8	0.6
15008	Chicken Drumstick-Roasted	1	ea	52	112	33	14	0	0	6	1.6	2.2	1.3
15025	Chicken Gizzards-Simmered	1	cup	145	212	98	44	0	0	4	1	0.8	0.5
15028	Chicken Meat-All-Fried	1	cup	140	307	81	43	2	<1	13	3.4	4.7	3
15000	Chicken Meat-All-Roasted	1	cup	140	266	89	41	0	0	10	2.9	3.7	2.4
15006	Chicken Meat-All-Stewed	1	cup	140	248	94	38	0	0	9	2.6	3.3	2.2
15010	Chicken Thigh+Skin-Roasted	1	ea	62	153	37	16	0	0	10	2.7	3.8	2.1
15011	Chicken Thigh-NoSkin-Fried	1	ea	52	113	31	15	1	0	5	1.4	2	1.3
15012	Chicken Thigh-NoSkin-Roast	1	ea	52	109	33	13	0	0	6	1.6	2.2	1.3
15002	Chicken Wing+Skin-Roasted	1	ea	34	99	19	9	0	0	7	1.9	2.6	1.4
15027	Chicken-Dark Meat-Roasted	1	cup	140	287	88	38	0	0	14	3.7	5	3.2
15032	Chicken-Light Meat-Roasted	1	cup	140	242	91	43	0	0	6	1.8	2.2	1.4
15240	Cornish Game Hen+Skin-Rstd	3	oz	85.05	221	50	19	0	0	15	4.3	6.8	3.1
16295	Duck+Skin-Rstd	3	oz	85.05	287	44	16	0	0	24	8.2	11	3.1
14000	Duck-Meat Only-Roasted	3	oz	85.05	171	55	20	0	0	10	3.5	3.1	1.2

< = Trace amount present   Blank = Not available

CHOL, cholesterol; **V,** vitamin; **THI,** thiamin; **RIB,** riboflavin; **NIA,** niacin; **FOL,** folate; **CALC,** calcium; **PHOS,** phosphate; **SOD,** sodium; **POT,** potassium; **MAG,** magnesium

CHOL (g)	V-A (RE)	THI (mg)	RIB (mg)	NIA (mg)	V-B6 (mg)	FOL (µg)	V-B12 (µg)	V-C (mg)	V-E (mg)	CALC (mg)	PHOS (mg)	SOD (mg)	POT (mg)	MAG (mg)	IRON (mg)	ZINC (mg)
0	0						0			60		270			1.8	
0	0							<1		0		100			1.8	
0	0	0.3	0.6	2.2	0.1	55	1.6	0	1.3	23	241	330	69	13	1	0.8
0	0							2		20		160			1.1	
0	0	0.2	0.1	0.8	0.2		0.9	0		20		430	40		0.7	
0	0	2.7	0.2	7.4	0.6	67	2.7	0	2	27	296	476	134	15	1.2	1.1
0	0	0.6	0.4	7.1	0.9	55	1.7	0	1.2	21	244	390	128	13	1.5	1.3
0	0	0.7	0.1	1.8	0.1	55	1	0	1.2	18	241	385	126	13	1.5	1.3
10	40							6		60		280	200		1.8	
0	0	0.8	0.2	4	0.2		0.6	0		0		800	95		1.1	
0	2	0.1	0.1	2	0.2	15	0.5	0	0.3	7	33	94	51	19	0.2	0.2
0	0	0.6	0.4	7.1	0.9	55	1.7	0	1.2	21	244	390	128	13	1.5	1.3
0	0	0.2	<0.1	4	0.3		2.1	0		20		300	45		1.8	
21	2	0.1	0.1	2.1	0.1	<1	0.2	0	0.1	2	101	439	107	6	0.3	0.7
27	0	0.4	0.1	3.2	0.2	2	0.4	0	0.2	5	138	719	181	10	0.4	0.8
41	0	0.6	0.2	4.1	0.3	3	0.9	0	0.2	9	207	1047	248	14	0.9	2.5
53	0	1.2	0.3	6.4	0.6	8	1.1	0	0.3	8	290	1786	468	22	1.3	2.6
77	0	1	0.4	7	0.7	6	1	0	0.4	10	318	1858	442	31	1.3	3.6
79	2	0.5	0.3	4	0.4	4	0.7	<1	0.4	25	188	25	297	20	1.1	3.2
62	2	0.7	0.3	4.1	0.4	5	0.6	1	0.2	13	200	51	346	23	0.7	2
73	3	0.9	0.3	5	0.5	5	0.6	1	0.2	17	215	53	363	23	0.9	2.1
73	2	0.5	0.2	3.5	0.3	3	0.6	1	0.4	21	143	54	293	15	1.2	3.4
88	48	<0.1	0.2	9	0.5	6	0.4	3	0.4	20	158	714	196	17	2.2	2
108	34	0.1	0.3	8.9	0.4	10	0.4	0	0.7	30	204	115	291	29	1.9	3.2
82	27	0.1	0.1	12.5	0.5	4	0.3	0	0.3	14	210	70	240	26	1	1
78	6	0.1	0.1	12.7	0.6	3	0.3	0	0.4	14	212	68	237	27	1	0.9
73	5	0.1	0.1	11.8	0.5	3	0.3	0	0.2	13	196	64	220	25	0.9	0.9
39	8	<0.1	0.1	2.6	0.2	4	0.1	0	0.2	5	78	40	105	10	0.6	1.4
41	8	<0.1	0.1	2.7	0.2	4	0.1	0	0.2	5	81	42	108	11	0.6	1.4
47	16	<0.1	0.1	3.1	0.2	4	0.2	0	0.1	6	91	47	119	12	0.7	1.5
536	0	<0.1	0.3	4.5	0.1	7	1.5	0	0.3	25	274	81	260	4	4.6	6.4
132	25	0.1	0.3	13.5	0.7	10	0.5	0	0.6	24	287	127	360	38	1.9	3.1
125	22	0.1	0.2	12.8	0.7	8	0.5	0	0.4	21	273	120	340	35	1.7	2.9
116	21	0.1	0.2	8.6	0.4	8	0.3	0	0.4	20	210	98	252	29	1.6	2.8
58	31	<0.1	0.1	3.9	0.2	4	0.2	0	0.2	7	108	52	138	14	0.8	1.5
53	11	<0.1	0.1	3.7	0.2	5	0.2	0	0.3	7	103	49	135	14	0.8	1.5
49	10	<0.1	0.1	3.4	0.2	4	0.2	0	0.1	6	95	46	124	12	0.7	1.3
29	16	<0.1	<0.1	2.3	0.1	1	0.1	0	0.1	5	51	28	63	6	0.4	0.6
130	31	0.1	0.3	9.2	0.5	11	0.4	0	0.4	21	251	130	336	32	1.9	3.9
119	13	0.1	0.2	17.4	0.8	6	0.5	0	0.4	21	302	108	346	38	1.5	1.7
111	27	0.1	0.2	5	0.3	2	0.2	<1	0.3	11	124	54	208	15	0.8	1.3
71	54	0.1	0.2	4.1	0.2	5	0.3	0	0.6	9	133	50	174	14	2.3	1.6
76	20	0.2	0.4	4.3	0.2	9	0.3	0	0.6	10	173	55	214	17	2.3	2.2

ESHA, EatRight Analysis CD-ROM; **AMT**, amount; **WT**, weight; **CAL**, calories; **WTR**, water; **PROT**, protein; **CARB**, carbohydrate; **FIBR**, fiber; **FAT**, fat; **SATF**, saturated fat; **MONO**, monosaturated fat; **POLY**, polyunsaturated fat

ESHA CODE	FOOD DESCRIPTION	AMT	UNIT	WT (g)	CAL (kcal)	WTR (g)	PROT (g)	CARB (g)	FIBR (g)	FAT (g)	SATF (g)	MONO (g)	POLY (g)
Meats & Meat Substitutes (continued)													
Poultry (continued)													
81166	Emu-Top Loin-Brld	3	oz	85.05	129	57	25	0	0	3	0.7	1.1	0.4
16048	Goose Liver Pate-Cnd	1	Tbs	13	60	5	1	1	0	6	1.9	3.3	0.1
14002	Goose Meat-NoSkin-Roasted	3	oz	85.05	202	49	25	0	0	11	3.9	3.7	1.3
14003	Goose+Skin-Domestic-Roast	3	oz	85.05	259	44	21	0	0	19	5.8	8.7	2.1
81180	Ostrich-Tenderloin-Raw	4	oz	113.4	139	84	25	0	0	4	1.3	1.4	0.9
16040	Tom Turkey-NoSkin-Roasted	1	cup	140	235	91	41	0	0	7	2.2	1.4	1.9
16003	Turkey- Ground Patty-Cooked	1	ea	82	193	49	22	0	0	11	2.8	4	2.6
16000	Turkey Meat-All-Roasted	1	cup	140	238	91	41	0	0	7	2.3	1.4	2
51101	Turkey-Dark Meat-Rstd	3	oz	85.05	159	54	24	0	0	6	2.1	1.4	1.8
51152	Turkey-Light+Water-Canned	2	oz	56.7	80		16	0	0	1	0.5		
16001	Turkey-White Meat-Roasted	1	cup	140	196	96	42	0	0	2	0.5	0.3	0.4
Nuts & Seeds													
4534	Almond Butter-Plain	1	Tbs	16	101	<1	2	3	1	9	0.9	6.1	2
4572	Almond Butter-Salted	1	Tbs	16	101	<1	2	3	1	9	0.9	6.1	2
4503	Almonds-Slivered/Pkd Measure	1	cup	108	624	6	23	21	13	55	4.2	34.7	13.2
4525	Black Walnuts-Chopped	1	cup	125	772	6	30	12	9	74	4.2	18.8	43.8
4519	Cashews-Dry Roasted+Salt	1	cup	137	786	2	21	45	4	63	12.5	37.4	10.7
4621	Cashews-Dry Roast-No Salt	1	cup	137	786	2	21	45	4	63	12.5	37.4	10.7
4596	Cashews-Oil Roasted	1	cup	130	755	3	22	39	4	62	11	33.7	11.1
4622	Cashews-Oil Roast-No Salt	1	cup	130	754	5	22	39	4	62	11	33.7	11.1
4538	Chestnuts-Roasted	1	cup	143	350	58	5	76	7	3	0.6	1.1	1.2
4649	Coconut Cream-Canned	1	cup	296	568	211	8	25	7	52	46.5	2.2	0.6
4528	Coconut Milk-Raw	1	cup	240	552	162	5	13	5	57	50.7	2.4	0.6
4511	Coconut-Dried-Sweet-Shred	1	cup	93	466	12	3	44	4	33	29.3	1.4	0.4
4510	Coconut-Dried-Unsweet	2	Tbsp	9.25	61	<1	1	2	2	6	5.3	0.3	0.1
4508	Coconut-Raw Piece-2.5x2in	1	pce	45	159	21	1	7	4	15	13.4	0.6	0.2
4556	English Walnuts-Chopped	1	cup	120	785	5	18	16	8	78	7.4	10.7	56.6
4557	English Walnuts-Halves	1	cup	100	654	4	15	14	7	65	6.1	8.9	47.2
4514	Filberts/Hazelnuts-Chopped	1	cup	115	722	6	17	19	11	70	5.1	52.5	9.1
4513	Filberts/Hazelnuts-Whole	1	cup	135	848	7	20	23	13	82	6	61.6	10.7
4533	Mixed Nuts+Pnuts-Oil Roast	1	cup	142	876	3	24	30	14	80	12.4	45	18.9
4594	MixedNuts-NoPnts-Oil Roast	1	cup	144	886	5	22	32	8	81	13.1	47.7	16.5
4576	Peanut Butter-Chunky-NoSalt	2	Tbs	32	188	<1	8	7	3	16	2.6	7.9	4.7
4626	Peanut Butter-Smooth-Salted	2	Tbs	32	188	<1	8	7	3	16	2.6	7.9	4.7
4542	Peanuts-Oil Roasted-Unsalted	1	cup	133	773	3	35	25	9	66	9.1	32.5	20.7
4578	Pecans-Dried Halves	1	cup	108	746	4	10	15	10	78	6.7	44.1	23.3
4577	Pecans-Dried-Chopped	1	cup	119	822	4	11	16	11	86	7.4	48.6	25.7
4554	Pine Nuts/Pinon-Dried	10	ea	1	6	<1	<1	<1	<1	1	0.1	0.2	0.3
4521	Pistachios	47	ea	28.35	158	1	6	8	3	13	1.5	6.6	3.8
4564	PumpkinSeeds-Roasted+Salt	1	cup	64	285	3	12	34		12	2.3	3.9	5.7
4523	Sesame Seeds-Whole-Dried	1	cup	144	825	7	26	34	17	72	10	27	31.4
4545	Sunflower Seeds-Dry	1	cup	144	821	8	33	27	15	71	7.5	13.6	47.1
4552	SunflowerSeeds-Oil Roasted	1	cup	135	799	2	27	31	14	69	9.5	10.9	46.3
4532	Tahini (Sesame Butter)	1	Tbs	14	85	<1	3	3	1	8	1.1	3	3.5

< = Trace amoudnt present   Blank = Not available

CHOL, cholesterol; **V,** vitamin; **THI,** thiamin; **RIB,** riboflavin; **NIA,** niacin; **FOL,** folate;
CALC, calcium; **PHOS,** phosphate; **SOD,** sodium; **POT,** potassium; **MAG,** magnesium

CHOL (g)	V-A (RE)	THI (mg)	RIB (mg)	NIA (mg)	V-B6 (mg)	FOL (µg)	V-B12 (µg)	V-C (mg)	V-E (mg)	CALC (mg)	PHOS (mg)	SOD (mg)	POT (mg)	MAG (mg)	IRON (mg)	ZINC (mg)
75	0	0.3	0.5	7.8	0.7	8	7.4	0	0.2	8	233	49	318	26	4.3	2.9
20	130	<0.1	<0.1	0.3	<0.1	8	1.2	<1	0.2	9	26	91	18	2	0.7	0.1
82	10	0.1	0.3	3.5	0.4	10	0.4	0	1.3	12	263	65	330	21	2.4	2.7
77	18	0.1	0.3	3.5	0.3	2	0.3	0	1.5	11	230	60	280	19	2.4	2.2
91	0	0.2	0.3	5.4	0.6	9	5.7	0	0.2	7	249	98	363	25	5.5	4.4
108	0	0.1	0.3	7.4	0.7	11	0.5	0	0.6	35	300	104	421	36	2.5	4.4
84	0	<0.1	0.1	4	0.3	6	0.3	0	0.3	20	161	88	221	20	1.6	2.3
106	0	0.1	0.3	7.6	0.6	10	0.5	0	0.5	35	298	98	417	36	2.5	4.3
72	0	0.1	0.2	3.1	0.3	8	0.3	0	0.5	27	174	67	247	20	2	3.8
55	0							0		0		150			0	
120	0	0.1	0.2	9.7	0.8	8	0.5	0	0.1	21	302	78	388	39	2.2	2.9
0	0	<0.1	0.1	0.5	<0.1	10	0	<1	3.2	43	84	2	121	48	0.6	0.5
0	<1	<0.1	0.1	0.5	<0.1	10	0	<1	4.2	43	84	72	121	48	0.6	0.5
0	1	0.3	0.9	4.2	0.1	31	0	0	27.9	268	512	1	786	297	4.6	3.6
0	5	0.1	0.2	0.6	0.7	39	0	2	2.2	76	641	2	654	251	3.9	4.2
0	0	0.3	0.3	1.9	0.4	95	0	0	1.3	62	671	877	774	356	8.2	7.7
0	0	0.3	0.3	1.9	0.4	95	0	0	1.3	62	671	22	774	356	8.2	7.7
0	0	0.5	0.3	2.3	0.4	32	0	<1	1.2	56	690	400	822	355	7.9	7
0	0	0.5	0.3	2.3	0.4	32	0	<1	1.2	56	690	17	822	355	7.9	7
0	3	0.3	0.3	1.9	0.7	100	0	37	0.7	41	153	3	847	47	1.3	0.8
0	0	0.1	0.1	0.1	0.1	41	0	5	0.4	3	65	148	299	50	1.5	1.8
0	0	0.1	0	1.8	0.1	38	0	7	0.4	38	240	36	631	89	3.9	1.6
0	0	<0.1	<0.1	0.4	0.3	7	0	1	0.4	14	100	244	313	46	1.8	1.7
0	0	<0.1	<0.1	0.1	<0.1	1	0	<1	<0.1	2	19	3	50	8	0.3	0.2
0	0	<0.1	<0.1	0.2	<0.1	12	0	1	0.1	6	51	9	160	14	1.1	0.5
0	2	0.4	0.2	1.4	0.6	118	0	2	0.8	118	415	2	529	190	3.5	3.7
0	2	0.3	0.2	1.1	0.5	98	0	1	0.7	98	346	2	441	158	2.9	3.1
0	2	0.7	0.1	2.1	0.6	130	0	7	17.3	131	334	0	782	187	5.4	2.8
0	3	0.9	0.2	2.4	0.8	153	0	9	20.3	154	392	0	918	220	6.3	3.3
0	3	0.7	0.3	7.2	0.3	118	0	1	8.5	153	659	16	825	334	4.6	7.2
0	3	0.7	0.7	2.8	0.3	81	0	1	8.6	153	647	16	783	361	3.7	6.7
0	0	<0.1	<0.1	4.4	0.1	29	0	0	2	14	102	5	238	51	0.6	0.9
0	0	<0.1	<0.1	4.4	0.1	29	0	0	2	14	102	156	238	51	0.6	0.9
0	0	0.3	0.1	19	0.3	168	0	0	9.2	117	688	8	907	246	2.4	8.8
0	6	0.7	0.1	1.3	0.2	24	0	1	1.5	76	299	0	443	131	2.7	4.9
0	7	0.8	0.2	1.4	0.2	26	0	1	1.7	83	330	0	488	144	3	5.4
0	<1	<0.1	<0.1	<0.1	<0.1	1	0	<1	<0.1	<1	<1	1	6	2	<0.1	<0.1
0	16	0.2	<0.1	0.4	0.5	14	0	1	0.7	30	139	<1	291	34	1.2	0.6
0	4	<0.1	<0.1	0.2	<0.1	6	0	<1	0.3	35	59	368	588	168	2.1	6.6
0	1	1.1	0.4	6.5	1.1	140	0	0	0.4	1404	906	16	674	505	21	11.2
0	9	3.3	0.4	6.5	1.1	327	0	2	49.7	167	1015	4	992	510	9.7	7.3
0	1	0.4	0.4	5.6	1.1	316	0	1	49	117	1538	554	652	171	5.8	7
0	1	0.2	<0.1	0.8	<0.1	14	0	0	0.3	20	111	<1	64	49	0.9	1.5

ESHA, EatRight Analysis CD-ROM; **AMT**, amount; **WT**, weight; **CAL**, calories; **WTR**, water; **PROT**, protein; **CARB**, carbohydrate; **FIBR**, fiber; **FAT**, fat; **SATF**, saturated fat; **MONO**, monosaturated fat; **POLY**, polyunsaturated fat

ESHA CODE	FOOD DESCRIPTION	AMT	UNIT	WT (g)	CAL (kcal)	WTR (g)	PROT (g)	CARB (g)	FIBR (g)	FAT (g)	SATF (g)	MONO (g)	POLY (g)
Prepared Packaged Foods													
Canned Dishes													
7040	Baked Beans w/Pork-Canned	1	cup	253	268	181	13	51	14	4	1.5	1.7	0.5
50000	Bean+Bacon Soup w/Water	1	cup	253	172	213	8	23	9	6	1.5	2.2	1.8
20057	Beef Broth+TomatoJce-Cnd	1	tsp	30.5	11	27	<1	3	<1	<1	<0.1	<0.1	<0.1
50183	Beef Broth-Canned-LowSodium	1	cup	240	38	230	5	1	0	1	0.4	0.7	0.3
50198	Beef MushroomSoup+Wat-Can	1	cup	244	73	226	6	6	<1	3	1.5	1.2	0.1
50003	Beef Noodle Soup + Water	1	cup	244	83	224	5	9	1	3	1.1	1.2	0.5
50066	Beef Soup-Chunky-Prepared	1	cup	240	170	200	12	20	1	5	2.5	2.1	0.2
57659	Beef Stew-Canned	1	svg	232	220	189	11	16	3	12	5.2	5.5	0.5
50060	Black Bean Soup + Water	1	cup	247	116	216	6	20	4	2	0.4	0.5	0.5
50204	Bouillabaise Soup/Chowder	1	cup	227	241	177	34	5	1	9	2	3.9	1.5
50071	Cheese Soup + Milk	1	cup	251	231	207	9	16	1	15	9.1	4.1	0.5
50004	Chicken Broth-Can + Water	1	cup	244	39	234	5	1	0	1	0.4	0.6	0.3
50005	Chicken Noodle Soup+Water	1	cup	241	75	222	4	9	1	2	0.7	1.1	0.6
50020	Chicken Rice Soup+Water	1	cup	241	60	226	4	7	1	2	0.5	0.9	0.4
50091	Chicken Veget Soup+Water	1	cup	241	75	223	4	9	1	3	0.8	1.3	0.6
50074	ChickenDumplingSoup+Water	1	cup	241	96	221	6	6	<1	6	1.3	2.5	1.3
56001	Chili + Beans-Canned	1	cup	256	287	193	15	30	11	14	6	6	0.9
50007	Chili Beef Soup + Water	1	cup	250	170	212	7	21	9	7	3.4	2.8	0.3
50145	Chunky Vegetable Soup	1	cup	240	122	210	4	19	1	4	0.6	1.6	1.4
50008	Clam Chowder-NewEng+Milk	1	cup	248	164	211	9	17	1	7	3	2.3	1.1
50093	ClamChowder-Manhattan-Prep	1	cup	240	134	206	7	19	3	3	2.1	1	0.1
50098	Consomme+Gelatin+Water	1	cup	241	29	232	5	2	0	0	0	0	0
50011	Cream Mushroom Soup+Milk	1	cup	248	203	210	6	15	<1	14	5.1	3	4.6
50049	Cream Mushroom Soup+Water	1	cup	244	129	220	2	9	<1	9	2.4	1.7	4.2
50402	Cream of Broccoli Soup-Cnd	1	cup	244	88	224	2	13	2	3	0.7	0.9	0.6
50006	Cream of ChickenSoup+Milk	1	cup	248	191	210	7	15	<1	11	4.6	4.5	1.6
50018	Cream of ChickenSoup+Water	1	cup	244	117	221	3	9	<1	7	2.1	3.3	1.5
50026	Cream Potato Soup + Milk	1	cup	248	149	215	6	17	<1	6	3.8	1.7	0.6
50103	Gazpacho Soup-Prepared	1	cup	244	46	229	7	4	<1	<1	<0.1	<0.1	0.1
50105	Lentil & Ham Soup-Prepared	1	cup	248	139	213	9	20		3	1.1	1.3	0.3
28181	Lobster Bisque Soup-Semi Cond	0.67	cup	152.5	160		4	12	1	11	5		
50009	Minestrone Soup + Water	1	cup	241	82	220	4	11	1	3	0.6	0.7	1.1
50024	Oyster Stew + Milk	1	cup	245	135	218	6	10	0	8	5	2.1	0.3
7023	Pork & Beans, Sweet Sauce	1	cup	253	283	179	13	53	11	4	1.2	1.3	1
7004	Pork & Beans, Tomato Sauce	1	cup	253	238	186	13	47	10	2	0.7	1.2	0.3
50025	Split Pea+Ham Soup+Water	1	cup	253	190	207	10	28	2	4	1.8	1.8	0.6
50135	Tomato Bisque Soup-Prep f/Cnd	1	cup	247	124	215	2	24	<1	3	0.5	0.7	1.1
50012	Tomato Soup + Milk	1	cup	248	161	210	6	22	3	6	2.9	1.6	1.1
50028	Tomato Soup + Water	1	cup	244	85	220	2	17	<1	2	0.4	0.4	1
50186	Vege Soup-LowSod+Water	1	cup	241	53	225	2	12	<1	1	0.5	0.1	0.1
91659	Vegetarian Chili-Pkg	1	ea	300	230		21	37	14	1	0		
7559	Vegetarian Stew	1	cup	247	304	173	42	17	3	7	1.2	1.8	3.8
50013	Vegetarian Vege Soup+Water	1	cup	241	72	223	2	12	<1	2	0.3	0.8	0.7
50027	Vichyssoise Soup	1	cup	248	149	215	6	17	<1	6	3.8	1.7	0.6

< = Trace amount present   Blank = Not available

CHOL, cholesterol; **V,** vitamin; **THI,** thiamin; **RIB,** riboflavin; **NIA,** niacin; **FOL,** folate;
CALC, calcium; **PHOS,** phosphate; **SOD,** sodium; **POT,** potassium; **MAG,** magnesium

CHOL (g)	V-A (RE)	THI (mg)	RIB (mg)	NIA (mg)	V-B6 (mg)	FOL (µg)	V-B12 (µg)	V-C (mg)	V-E (mg)	CALC (mg)	PHOS (mg)	SOD (mg)	POT (mg)	MAG (mg)	IRON (mg)	ZINC (mg)
18	0	0.1	0.1	1.1	0.2	91	0	5	1	134	273	1047	782	86	4.3	3.7
3	91	0.1	<0.1	0.6	<0.1	33	0.1	2	0.8	81	132	951	402	46	2	1
0	4	<0.1	<0.1	0.1	<0.1	1	<0.1	<1	0.1	3	4	40	29	1	0.2	<0.1
0	0	0	0.1	3.3	<0.1	5	0.2	0	<0.1	10	72	72	206	2	0.5	0.2
7	0	<0.1	0.1	1	<0.1	10	0.2	5		5	34	942	154	10	0.9	1.5
5	12	0.1	0.1	1.1	<0.1	20	0.2	<1	0.7	15	46	952	100	5	1.1	1.5
14	259	0.1	0.2	2.7	0.1	14	0.6	7	0.7	31	120	866	336	5	2.3	2.6
37	408	0.2	0.1	2.9	0.3	26	0.9	10	0.3	28	128	947	404	32	1.6	1.9
0	49	0.1	0.1	0.5	0.1	25	<0.1	1	0.2	44	106	1198	274	42	2.1	1.4
90	89	0.2	0.2	5	0.4	28	10.4	12	2	83	340	416	733	74	3.9	1.9
48	361	0.1	0.3	0.5	0.1	10	0.4	1	0.3	289	251	1019	341	20	0.8	0.7
0	0	<0.1	0.1	3.3	<0.1	5	0.2	0	<0.1	10	73	776	210	2	0.5	0.2
7	70	0.1	0.1	1.4	<0.1	22	0.1	<1	0.1	17	36	1106	55	5	0.8	0.4
7	43	<0.1	<0.1	1.1	<0.1	0	0.1	<1	0.1	17	22	815	101	0	0.7	0.3
10	193	<0.1	0.1	1.2	<0.1	5	0.1	1	0.4	17	41	945	154	7	0.9	0.4
34	70	<0.1	0.1	1.8	<0.1	2	0.2	0	0.6	14	60	860	116	5	0.6	0.4
44	87	0.1	0.3	0.9	0.3	59	0	4	1.5	120	394	1336	934	115	8.8	5.1
12	150	0.1	0.1	1.1	0.2	18	0.3	4	1.5	42	148	1035	525	30	2.1	1.4
0	581	0.1	0.1	1.2	0.2	17	0	6	1.3	55	72	1010	396	7	1.6	3.1
22	57	0.1	0.2	1	0.1	10	10.2	3	0.4	186	156	992	300	22	1.5	0.8
14	329	0.1	0.1	1.8	0.3	10	7.9	12	1.6	67	84	1001	384	19	2.6	1.7
0	0	<0.1	<0.1	0.7	<0.1	2	0	1	<0.1	10	31	636	154	0	0.5	0.4
20	35	0.1	0.3	0.9	0.1	10	0.5	2	1.2	179	156	918	270	20	0.6	0.6
2	17	<0.1	0.1	0.7	<0.1	5	<0.1	1	1	46	49	881	100	5	0.5	0.6
5	59	<0.1	0.1	0.3	0.1	29	0	6	0.4	41	39	578	161	15	1.2	0.3
27	186	0.1	0.3	0.9	0.1	7	0.5	1	0.2	181	151	1047	273	17	0.7	0.7
10	166	<0.1	0.1	0.8	<0.1	2	0.1	<1	0.2	34	37	986	88	2	0.6	0.6
22	67	0.1	0.2	0.6	0.1	10	0.5	1	0.1	166	161	1061	322	17	0.5	0.7
0	29	<0.1	<0.1	0.9	0.1	20	0	7	0.4	24	37	739	224	7	1	0.2
7	35	0.2	0.1	1.4	0.2	50	0.3	4	0.2	42	184	1319	357	22	2.7	0.7
40	40							0		40		1090			0.7	
2	236	0.1	<0.1	0.9	0.1	36	0	1	0.1	34	55	911	313	7	0.9	0.7
32	59	0.1	0.2	0.3	0.1	10	2.6	4	0.5	167	162	1041	235	20	1.1	10.3
18	2	0.1	0.1	0.9	0.1	20	0	7	0.1	149	258	845	653	83	4.2	3.5
18	20	0.1	0.1	1.2	0.2	38	0	8	0.3	142	293	1106	746	86	8.2	13.9
8	46	0.1	0.1	1.5	0.1	3	0.3	2	0.2	23	213	1007	400	48	2.3	1.3
5	79	0.1	0.1	1.1	0.1	15	0	6	0.7	40	59	1047	417	10	0.8	0.6
17	79	0.1	0.2	1.5	0.2	17	0.4	68	1.2	159	149	744	449	22	1.8	0.3
0	49	0.1	0.1	1.4	0.1	15	0	66	2.3	12	34	695	264	7	1.8	0.2
0	19	<0.1	<0.1	0.7	<0.1	24	0	6	0.2	51	48	125	400	19	0.6	0.2
0	160							30		150		850	1010		7.2	
0	232	1.7	1.5	29.6	2.7	254	5.4	0	1.2	77	543	988	296	314	3.2	2.7
0	231	0.1	<0.1	0.9	0.1	10	0	1	0.4	22	34	822	210	7	1.1	0.5
22	67	0.1	0.2	0.6	0.1	10	0.5	1	0.1	166	161	1061	322	17	0.5	0.7

ESHA, EatRight Analysis CD-ROM; **AMT,** amount; **WT,** weight; **CAL,** calories; **WTR,** water; **PROT,** protein; **CARB,** carbohydrate; **FIBR,** fiber; **FAT,** fat; **SATF,** saturated fat; **MONO,** monosaturated fat; **POLY,** polyunsaturated fat

ESHA CODE	FOOD DESCRIPTION	AMT	UNIT	WT (g)	CAL (kcal)	WTR (g)	PROT (g)	CARB (g)	FIBR (g)	FAT (g)	SATF (g)	MONO (g)	POLY (g)
Prepared Packaged Foods (continued)													
Canned Dishes (continued)													
50181	Wonton Soup	1	cup	241	182	203	14	14	1	7	2.3	3	1
50999	Zesty Gumbo Soup-Cnd	1	cup	244	100	216	6	15	3	2	1		
Dry/Prepared Dishes													
50033	Beef Broth-Cube + Water	1	cup	241	7	236	1	1	0	<1	0.1	0.1	0
90738	Cheeseburger Macaroni-DryMix	1	svg	42.53	168	3	5	27		4	1.2		
50035	Chicken Broth-Cube + Water	1	cup	243	12	237	1	2	0	<1	0.1	0.1	0.1
50193	Chicken Broth-Dry Cube	1	ea	4.8	10	<1	1	1	0	<1	0.1	0.1	0.1
50037	Chicken Noodle Soup-Dry+Water	1	cup	252.3	58	238	2	9	<1	1	0.3	0.5	0.4
50038	ChickenVegSoup-dry+water	1	cup	250.7	50	237	3	8		1	0.2	0.3	0.2
38613	Herb & Butter Rice-Dry Mix	1	oz	28.35	99	3	2	21	1	1	0.2	0.2	0.1
50040	Onion Soup-Dry Mix+Water	1	cup	246	27	237	1	5	1	1	0.1	0.3	0.1
38618	Oriental Stir Fry Rice-Dry Mix	1	oz	28.35	97	3	2	22	1	<1	0.1	0.1	0.1
57323	Pasta&Sc-CreamBrocc (Lipton)	0.66	cup	69	270		8	47	1	5	3.5		
5276	Potatoes-Au Gratin from Mix	1	svg	137	127	108	3	18	1	6	3.5	1.6	0.2
5464	Potatoes-Mashed-Flakes-Prep	0.5	cup	105	102	85	2	11	1	5	3.3	1.4	0.2
5271	Potatoes-Scalloped from Mix	1	svg	137	127	108	3	17	2	6	3.6	1.7	0.3
38619	Red Beans & Rice-Dry Mix	1	oz	28.35	95	2	3	20	2	1	0.1	0.1	0.1
38163	Rice & Pasta-Cooked	1	cup	202	246	145	5	43	5	6	1.1	2.3	1.9
57331	Rice Pilaf-Dry Mix	0.5	cup	61	220	5	6	46	1	1	0		
66097	Romanoff Pasta-Dry Mix	1	oz	28.35	109	3	4	18	1	3	0.9	1.3	0.2
57333	Spanish Rice-Dry Mix	0.5	cup	67	240		6	51	2	1	0		
57534	Stroganoff-Prep f/Dry	1	cup	124	390		22	30	2	20			
Frozen/Refrigerated Dishes													
11118	BeefPotRoast Din-HealthyChoice	1	ea	312	300		20	41	8	6	2		
70688	Beef Chow Mein-Frzn	1	cup	247	105		9	15	3	2	0.8		
16234	Beef Pot Pie-Banquet	1	ea	198.5	400		9	38	1	23	11		
70893	Beef Pot Pie-Frzn	1	ea	198	449	113	13	44	2	24	8.5	9.7	2.7
70734	Beef Pot Pie-Swansons	1	ea	198	415	120	11	41	2	23	9		
11050	Beef Stroganoff-Frzn	1	svg	276.4	370		21	32	3	17	7		
56737	Cheese Cannelloni-LeanCuisine	1	svg	258.7	220		21	27	3	3	2	1	0.5
56901	Cheese Ravioli-LeanCuisine	1	svg	241	260		12	38	4	7	3.5	1.5	0.5
56996	Cheese Sausage-BagelBites	4	pce	88	200		10	24	3	7	2.5		
4120	Chicken & Dumplings-Frozen	1	svg	283.5	340		21	35	3	13	5		
15974	Chicken & Noodles, escalloped, fzn	1	svg	283	419	206	17	31		25	6	7	12.3
15964	Chicken Chow Mein+Rice-LnCuis	1	svg	255	240		14	37	3	3	1	1.5	0.5
70692	Chicken Chow Mein-Frzn	1	svg	250	91		5	11	2	4	0.9		
16198	Chicken Enchilada Entrée	1	svg	283	424	188	15	61	4	13	7.4	2.7	0.9
82030	Chicken Enchilada Suiza	1	svg	284	280		14	43	5	6	3		
16200	Chicken Parmigiana-Frzn	1	svg	340.2	460		24	54	5	16	4		
15967	Chicken Parmesan-LeanCuisine	1	svg	308	300		21	46	5	6	2	2	1.5
16260	ChickenBroc Alfredo-HealthyChce	1	svg	326	300		25	34	2	7	3		
82034	ChickenEnchiladaDin-HlthyChce	1	svg	320	352	239	12	58	5	8	3.3	2.3	2.1
16252	ChickenFettucAlfred-HealthyChce	1	svg	241	280		25	30	4	7	2.5		
92888	ChickTomaSpinach Pizza-DiGiorno	1	pce	133	260		16	33	2	8	3.5		

< = Trace amount present   Blank = Not available

CHOL, cholesterol; **V**, vitamin; **THI**, thiamin; **RIB**, riboflavin; **NIA**, niacin; **FOL**, folate;
CALC, calcium; **PHOS**, phosphate; **SOD**, sodium; **POT**, potassium; **MAG**, magnesium

CHOL (g)	V-A (RE)	THI (mg)	RIB (mg)	NIA (mg)	V-B6 (mg)	FOL (µg)	V-B12 (µg)	V-C (mg)	V-E (mg)	CALC (mg)	PHOS (mg)	SOD (mg)	POT (mg)	MAG (mg)	IRON (mg)	ZINC (mg)
53	99	0.4	0.3	4.6	0.2	19	0.4	3	0.4	31	153	543	316	21	1.8	1.1
10	40							4		40		480			0.7	
0	<1	<0.1	<0.1	0.2	0	2	0	0	<0.1	2	12	1157	19	2	0.1	0
4												863				
0	2	<0.1	<0.1	0.3	0	2	<0.1	0	<0.1	12	12	792	24	2	0.1	<0.1
1	<1	<0.1	<0.1	0.2	<0.1	2	<0.1	<1	<0.1	9	9	1152	18	3	0.1	<0.1
10	5	0.2	0.1	1.1	<0.1	18	0.1	0	0.1	5	30	578	33	8	0.5	0.2
3	2	0.1	<0.1	0.7	0.1	3	0.1	1		15	33	807	68	23	0.6	0.2
<1	9	0.1	<0.1	1	0.1	38	<0.1	1	0.3	10	38	432	44	9	0.8	0.3
0	0	<0.1	0.1	0.5	0	2	0	<1	0	12	30	849	64	5	0.1	<0.1
<1	15	0.1	<0.1	0.8	0.1	34	<0.1	1	0.2	12	36	471	50	10	0.8	0.3
10	0	0.5	0.2	4		120		0		40		740	0		1.8	
21	75	<0.1	0.1	1.3	0.1	10	0	4	1.6	114	130	601	300	21	0.4	0.3
15	46	0.1	0.1	0.8	0.1	6	0.1	11	0.1	34	43	171	173	12	0.2	0.2
15	51	<0.1	0.1	1.4	0.1	14	0	5	0.2	49	77	467	278	19	0.5	0.3
<1	21	0.1	<0.1	0.7	0.1	57	<0.1	6	<0.1	25	66	449	143	21	1	0.4
2	0	0.2	0.2	3.6	0.2	89	0.1	<1	0.3	16	75	1147	85	24	1.9	0.6
0	0	0.4	0.1	4		100		0		20		880	0		1.8	
2	4	0.2	0.1	1.2	<0.1	39	0.1	<1	<0.1	18	68	367	97	13	0.6	0.4
0	40	0.4	0.1	4		100		5		20		880	0		2.7	
90				5												
40	250							18		20		600			1.8	
12	12							11		30		756			0.6	
30	150							0		20		1000			1.1	
38	102										737					
25	150							0		20		740			1.8	
65	20	0	0.1	1.1	0.1			0		40		950	570		1.4	
15	60	0.1	0.3	1.6	0.1		0	6		350		550	440	36	0.7	1.6
35	100	0.1	0.3	1.2	0.2	48	0.3	5		150	168	590	450	42	1.4	1.5
15	80							12		100		500	140		0.7	
65	500							1		200		1320	510		1.8	
76	0							0		116		1211	329		1.1	
35	20	0.1	0.2	5				0		40		590	300	30	0.7	1.1
9	5							4		43		865			0.7	
51	96							4		300		855	243		2.2	
40	60							2		150		440			1.1	
45	150							12		150		1060	670		2.7	
35	100	0.2	0.3	7				9		100		689	919	59	1.8	1.3
50	20							12		100		530			1.8	
35	80							18		58	237	573	384		1	
35	0							2		100		600			1.1	
25	100							1		200		550			1.4	

ESHA, EatRight Analysis CD-ROM; **AMT**, amount; **WT**, weight; **CAL**, calories; **WTR**, water; **PROT**, protein; **CARB**, carbohydrate; **FIBR**, fiber; **FAT**, fat; **SATF**, saturated fat; **MONO**, monosaturated fat; **POLY**, polyunsaturated fat

ESHA CODE	FOOD DESCRIPTION	AMT	UNIT	WT (g)	CAL (kcal)	WTR (g)	PROT (g)	CARB (g)	FIBR (g)	FAT (g)	SATF (g)	MONO (g)	POLY (g)
Prepared Packaged Foods (continued)													
Frozen/Refrigerated Dishes (continued)													
70961	Chimichanga, fzn beef&bean,FiestaCafé	1	ea	227	422	132	24	56	6	12	2.2	3.9	3.5
83000	Egg Roll-Chicken-ChunKing	6	pce	205.5	210		6	25	2	9	2.5		
83009	Egg Roll-Pork	1	ea	170.1	220		5	24	2	11	2.5		
56704	Egg Roll-Pork&Shrimp-ChunKing	6	pce	205.5	210		6	27	2	9	2.5		
83001	Egg Roll-Shrimp-ChunKing	6	pce	205.5	190		5	28	2	6	1.5		
70379	Fish & Chips-Batter Fried	1	svg	284	490	181	19	59	5	20	4		
56733	FrBread Cheese Pizza-LnCuisine	1	ea	145	264		14	41	3	5	3	1.3	0.4
56736	FrBread Deluxe Pizza-LnCuisine	1	ea	174	291		16	43	3	6	2.5	2	1
56735	FrBread PepperoniPizza-LnCuisn	1	ea	149	300		15	43	3	8	3.5	3	1
70697	Fried Rice	1	svg	139	236		5	53	2	1	0.2		
70954	Herb Bkd Fish Dinner-Frzn	1	ea	309	340		16	54	5	7	1.5		
56740	Lasagna w/Meat Sauce-LnCuisne	1	svg	298	300		19	38	4	8	4.5	2	1
18825	Lemon Pepper Fish-HealthyChc	1	ea	303	320		14	50	5	7	2		
7758	Lentil Rice Loaf	1	pce	90	160		8	16	4	7	1	1.5	4.5
66047	Macaroni & Cheese-HealthyChce	1	svg	255	240		12	36	3	5	2.5		
81080	Manicotti-3 Cheese HealthyChce	1	svg	312	300		15	40	5	9	3		
14072	Meatloaf-Beef+Pork	3	oz	85.05	169	55	15	5	<1	9	3.3	4.1	0.6
11093	Meatloaf-LeanCuisine	1	svg	265.8	260		20	28	4	7	2.8	1.8	0.4
70767	MexicanStyleDinner-HungryMan	1	ea	567	690	420	26	87	13	27	9		
7669	Nine Bean Loaf	1	ea	91	150		8	15	4	7	1.5	2	3.5
1874	Noodle Bowl-Honey Ginger Chicken	1	ea	340.2	430		25	69	3	5	1.5		
971	Noodle Bowl-Thai Chicken	1	ea	340.2	400		21	60	6	8	5		
70696	Oriental Beef Pepper-Frzn	1	cup	246	104		10	12	4	2	0.6		
57866	Oriental Chicken-Frzn	1	svg	396.9	370		21	66	4	2	0.5	0.5	0.5
70693	Pork Chow Mein-Frzn	1	svg	250	89		6	11	3	3	1.2		
70916	Pot Pie-Chicken	1	ea	198	380	127	11	36	3	21	8.3	9.2	3.7
56868	Ravioli-Cheese+Tomato Sauce	1	svg	301.2	230		10	38	2	4	2.5		
52165	Rice Bowl-Chicken-Sweet+Sour	1	ea	340.2	360		17	65	2	3	0.5		
11063	Salisbury Steak Dinner-Swansons	1	ea	312	340	242	16	35	6	15	6		
70700	Shrimp Chow Mein-Frzn	1	svg	141.75	35		2	6	2	1	0		
56732	Spaghetti w/Meatballs-LnCuisine	1	svg	269	250	210	18	33	4	5	2	1.9	0.8
56076	Spinach Souffle	1	cup	136	233	96	11	8	1	18	8.3	4.1	0.8
4110	Stuffed Bell Pepper-Frzn	1	svg	226.8	200		9	21	2	9	3		
56738	Stuffed Cabbage-LeanCuisine	1	svg	269	196	224	11	24	4	6	1.7	3	0.9
5154	Succotash-Frozen-Boiled	0.5	cup	85	79	63	4	17	3	1	0.1	0.1	0.4
977	Teriyaki Beef Dish+Rice-Frzn	1	svg	340.2	320		16	52	4	5	1.5	1.5	1
57140	Three Cheese Tortellini-DiGiorno	1	svg	81	250	25	11	37	2	7	3.5		
18820	Tuna Noodle Casserole	1	svg	283.5	360		18	36	2	16	5		
16928	Turkey Pot Pie-Banquet	1	ea	198	370	127	10	38	3	20	8		
70698	Vegetable Chop Suey-Frzn	1	cup	85	11		1	2	1	<1	0		
Prepared Homemade Dishes													
Breakfast Dishes													
19516	Egg-Scrambled+Milk+Marg	1	ea	61	102	45	7	1	0	7	2.2	2.9	1.3
19543	Omelette-1Egg+Mushroom	1	ea	69	88	54	6	2	<1	6	1.8	2.4	1

< = Trace amount present   Blank = Not available

CHOL, cholesterol; **V,** vitamin; **THI,** thiamin; **RIB,** riboflavin; **NIA,** niacin; **FOL,** folate;
CALC, calcium; **PHOS,** phosphate; **SOD,** sodium; **POT,** potassium; **MAG,** magnesium

CHOL (g)	V-A (RE)	THI (mg)	RIB (mg)	NIA (mg)	V-B6 (mg)	FOL (µg)	V-B12 (µg)	V-C (mg)	V-E (mg)	CALC (mg)	PHOS (mg)	SOD (mg)	POT (mg)	MAG (mg)	IRON (mg)	ZINC (mg)
36	0							6				804			6.8	
15	20	0.2	0.1	1.4				0		20	174	650	233		1.1	
10	60							0		20		390			1.1	
15	20	0.4	0.2	1.4				0		20	136	540	252		1.1	
10	100	0.2	0.1	0.8				0		20	97	730	155		1.1	
45	20							2		60		1030			1.4	
13	34							3		298		443	375		1.2	
25	40							6		150		551	441		1.8	
25	40							1		100		590	410		1.8	
0	0							0		2		1024			4.6	
35	600							0		40		480			0.7	
30	100	0.2	0.3	3.1	0.3			6		250		590	610	45	1.4	3
30	100							30		20		480			1.1	
0	100							0		20		350	150		1.1	
20	0							0		200		600			1.1	
35	150							0		250		550			1.8	
69	16	0.1	0.2	3.2	0.1	9	1.1	1	0.1	35	138	101	250	18	1.4	2.5
55	20							0		80		690	920		2.7	
35	300							36		300		2170			3.6	
5	100							1		40		320	200		0.7	
85												1700				
80												980				
12	87							7		24		969			0.5	
35	450							27		60		850	870		1.4	
10	8							4		3		1242			8.1	
30	273							0		30		842			1	
60	20							1		200		790	360		0.4	
30												620				
30	1000							6		80		920			2.7	
18	10							13		2		547			2.4	
24	51	0.2	0.2	4.3				3		100		568	511		2.2	
160	494	0.1	0.4	0.7	0.1	99	0.5	10	1.3	224	192	770	318	41	1.6	1.2
20	40							18		20		1130	400		1.4	
13	22	0.2	0.1	2.6				1		89		710	732		1.5	
0	17	0.1	0.1	1.1	0.1	28	0	5	0.2	13	60	38	225	20	0.8	0.4
20	500							9		40		890	860		1.1	
35	0							0		0		300			0	
30	20	0	0.1	1.4				0		150		1060	360		0.7	
45	150							0		40		850			1.1	
0	0							3		15		439			0.1	
215	89	<0.1	0.3	<0.1	0.1	18	0.5	<1	0.5	43	104	171	84	7	0.7	0.6
177	102	<0.1	0.2	0.3	0.1	17	0.4	<1	0.7	43	100	147	97	9	0.7	0.6

ESHA, EatRight Analysis CD-ROM; **AMT**, amount; **WT**, weight; **CAL**, calories; **WTR**, water; **PROT**, protein; **CARB**, carbohydrate; **FIBR**, fiber; **FAT**, fat; **SATF**, saturated fat; **MONO**, monosaturated fat; **POLY**, polyunsaturated fat

ESHA CODE	FOOD DESCRIPTION	AMT	UNIT	WT (g)	CAL (kcal)	WTR (g)	PROT (g)	CARB (g)	FIBR (g)	FAT (g)	SATF (g)	MONO (g)	POLY (g)
Prepared Homemade Dishes (continued)													
Breakfast Dishes (continued)													
19548	Omelette-Ham & Cheddar	1	ea	397	743		36	24	2	55	10		
19534	Omelette-Plain (1 Lrg Egg)	1	ea	61	96	46	6	<1	0	7	2.1	3	1.3
56612	Omelette-Veggie Cheese	1	ea	454	714		28	29	4	53	10		
Main & Side Dishes													
15907	Almond Chicken	1	cup	242	280	186	22	16	3	15	1.9	6.1	5.6
57428	Beef Cannelloni	2	ea	170.1	391		20	28	1	22	7.8		
10081	Beef Cube Steak-FlourFried	1	ea	165	460	79	44	18	1	22	6.2	8.2	5.8
57411	Beef Ravioli	9	pce	146.3	300		14	40	1	8	3.8		
57416	Beef Ravioli	1	cup	214	450		22	48	3	19	9		
57400	Beef Ravioli-Breaded	1	cup	120	270		11	43	2	6	2		
57407	Beef Tortellini	1	cup	128	250		11	38	2	6	3.5		
15930	Cashew Chicken	1	cup	162	431	88	29	11	2	31	5.2	13.9	9.7
56075	Cheese Souffle-Recipe	1	cup	112	192	80	11	6	<1	14	5.1		
15003	Chicken Breast+Skin-FlourFried	1	ea	98	218	55	31	2	<1	9	2.4	3.4	1.9
15978	Chicken Enchilada Suiza	1	svg	255	311	185	14	45	3	8	3.6	2.3	1.3
81223	Chicken Patty-Ckd f/Frzn	1	ea	90	210	52	13	10	0	13	3		
57420	Chicken Ravioli	1	cup	214	450		21	52	2	17	10		
8954	Chicken Ravioli, jalapeno filled	6	pce	137.4	316		15	49	2	7	2.7		
15915	Chicken Teriyaki-Breast	1	ea	128	178	86	27	7	<1	4	0.9	1.1	0.9
15916	Chicken Teriyaki-Drumstick	1	ea	68	94	45	14	4	<1	2	0.5	0.6	0.5
15009	Chicken Thigh+Skin-FlourFried	1	ea	62	162	34	17	2	<1	9	2.5	3.6	2.1
15029	Chicken Wing-Flour Fried	1	ea	32	103	16	8	1	<1	7	1.9	2.8	1.6
56112	Chiles Rellenos	1	ea	143	365	84	17	8	1	30	12.5	9	6.7
57618	Chow Mein, pork, w/ndles	1	cup	220	448	136	22	31	4	27	4.8	7.7	12.8
19080	Clams-Breaded-Fried-Sml	3	oz	85.05	172	52	12	9	<1	9	2.3	3.9	2.4
18805	Codfish Ball	1	ea	63	125	39	9	8	1	7	1.4	2.8	1.9
18806	Codfish Cake	1	ea	120	237	75	16	15	1	13	2.7	5.3	3.7
19420	Crab Cakes-Blue Crab	1	ea	60	93	43	12	<1	0	5	0.9	1.7	1.4
19539	Deviled Egg-1/2+Filling	1	ea	31	63	22	4	<1	0	5	1.2	1.7	1.5
56132	Egg Foo Yung Patty	1	ea	86	113	67	6	3	1	8	2	3.4	2.1
70259	Fish Fillet-Battered-Frzn	1	ea	75	180	42	8	12	0	11			
17003	Fish Patty/FrozenSq-Heated	1	ea	57	142	30	6	12	1	8	1.6	2.4	3.2
17002	Fish Sticks-Frozen-Heated	1	ea	28	70	15	3	6	<1	4	0.8	1.2	1.6
56119	Flauta-Beef	1	ea	113	354	57	14	13	2	28	4.8	11.8	9.4
56120	Flauta-Chicken	1	ea	113	330	62	13	12	2	26	4.2	10.7	9.3
17040	Fried Fish Cakes-Frzn-Heated	1	ea	85	231	45	8	15		15	6	3.4	3.4
17103	Gefiltefish-Sweet-Commercial	1	pce	42	35	34	4	3	0	1	0.2	0.3	0.1
56242	Gumbo w/Rice	1	cup	244	193	203	14	17	2	8	1.6	2.6	2.7
56150	Hash-Roast Beef	1	cup	190	312	131	21	21	2	16	4.9	5.7	3.3
5621	Hawaiian Vegetables-Pickled	0.5	cup	75	19	68	1	4	2	<1	0.1	<0.1	0.1
56239	Jambalaya-Shrimp	1	cup	243	310	176	27	28	1	9	1.8	3.8	2.8
56296	Knish-Meat	1	ea	50	175	19	7	13	1	11	2.6	4.9	2.3
56294	Knish-Potato	1	ea	61	215	22	5	21	1	12	2.6	5.8	3.3
13900	Lamb Curry	1	cup	236	256	189	28	3	1	14	3.9	4.9	3.4

< = Trace amount present   Blank = Not available

CHOL, cholesterol; **V,** vitamin; **THI,** thiamin; **RIB,** riboflavin; **NIA,** niacin; **FOL,** folate;
CALC, calcium; **PHOS,** phosphate; **SOD,** sodium; **POT,** potassium; **MAG,** magnesium

CHOL (g)	V-A (RE)	THI (mg)	RIB (mg)	NIA (mg)	V-B6 (mg)	FOL (µg)	V-B12 (µg)	V-C (mg)	V-E (mg)	CALC (mg)	PHOS (mg)	SOD (mg)	POT (mg)	MAG (mg)	IRON (mg)	ZINC (mg)
657	580							7		290		1518			3.1	
217	96	<0.1	0.2	<0.1	0.1	24	0.7	0	0.6	29	99	98	70	6	0.9	0.6
644	610							35		290		955			3.2	
40	37	0.1	0.2	9.5	0.4	26	0.3	7	3.8	69	252	526	549	60	2	1.6
137											149	672			2.1	
125	5	0.3	0.5	7	0.7	17	4.7	<1	1.7	80	380	316	653	54	6.4	8.4
77											119	400			2.1	
135	20							0		100		930			3.6	
25	0							1		60		660			2.7	
40	20							1		60		490			1.8	
64	58	0.2	0.1	13.2	0.6	43	0.3	8	3.9	49	263	907	428	63	2	1.5
195	118	0.1	0.4	0.3	0.1	27	0.8	<1	1.3	191	191	274	146	16	0.8	1
87	15	0.1	0.1	13.5	0.6	6	0.3	0	0.6	16	228	74	254	29	1.2	1.1
33	0							4		189		727			0.8	
45	0							0		0		400			0.7	
115	60							0		200		420			2.7	
48											83	841			3	
82	16	0.1	0.2	8.8	0.5	12	0.3	3	0.4	27	199	1683	309	35	1.7	2
44	8	<0.1	0.1	4.7	0.2	6	0.2	2	0.2	14	105	894	164	19	0.9	1
60	18	0.1	0.2	4.3	0.2	7	0.2	0	0.5	9	116	55	147	16	0.9	1.6
26	12	<0.1	<0.1	2.1	0.1	2	0.1	0	0.2	5	48	25	57	6	0.4	0.6
168	250	0.1	0.4	0.9	0.3	29	0.5	113	4.7	1	307	522	386	36	1.7	2.1
48	19	0.8	0.4	6.2	0.4	42	0.4	20	2.7	45	249	848	489	53	3.3	2.6
52	77	0.1	0.2	1.8	0.1	31	34.2	9	2.1	54	160	310	277	12	11.8	1.2
35	13	0.1	0.1	1.3	0.2	7	0.3	2	0.9	18	108	175	275	20	0.4	0.3
67	25	0.1	0.1	2.5	0.3	13	0.6	5	1.6	34	206	334	523	38	0.8	0.7
90	37	0.1	<0.1	1.7	0.1	32	3.6	2	0.9	63	128	198	194	20	0.6	2.5
122	50	<0.1	0.1	<0.1	<0.1	13	0.3	0	0.6	15	50	50	37	3	0.4	0.3
185	86	<0.1	0.3	0.4	0.1	30	0.4	5	1.2	31	93	317	117	12	1	0.7
20											200		190			
18	18	0.1	0.1	0.9	<0.1	18	0.7	0	0.7	15	104	240	123	16	0.6	0.3
9	9	<0.1	<0.1	0.4	<0.1	9	0.4	0	0.3	7	51	118	60	8	0.3	0.1
37	21	0.1	0.1	1.9	0.2	10	1.2	19	4.7	51	179	68	313	28	1.9	3.4
35	26	0.1	0.1	3.1	0.2	8	0.1	18	4.4	50	140	71	269	27	1	1.1
22		<0.1	0.1	1.4	<0.1	11	0.9	0	0.5	9	143		298	15	0.3	0.3
13	11	<0.1	<0.1	0.4	<0.1	1	0.4	<1	0.1	10	31	220	38	4	1	0.3
40	63	0.2	0.2	4.5	0.2	46	2.4	14	1.4	71	152	542	446	40	2.6	15.2
57	<1	0.2	0.2	3.7	0.5	16	1.8	7	1.2	19	204	470	587	36	2.5	5
0	25	<0.1	<0.1	0.4	0.1	25	0	0	<0.1	30	17	795	148	7	0.4	0.2
181	133	0.3	0.1	4.8	0.2	12	1.2	17	2.3	104	300	370	439	64	4.4	1.7
52	89	0.1	0.2	1.5	<0.1	8	0.3	<1	1.2	12	61	107	88	8	1.2	1
59	130	0.2	0.2	1.5	0.1	10	0.1	1	1.7	16	60	140	96	10	1.3	0.4
89	2	0.1	0.3	8.1	0.2	28	2.9	1	1.2	36	284	323	496	40	3	6.6

ESHA, EatRight Analysis CD-ROM; **AMT,** amount; **WT,** weight; **CAL,** calories; **WTR,** water; **PROT,** protein; **CARB,** carbohydrate; **FIBR,** fiber; **FAT,** fat; **SATF,** saturated fat; **MONO,** monosaturated fat; **POLY,** polyunsaturated fat

ESHA CODE	FOOD DESCRIPTION	AMT	UNIT	WT (g)	CAL (kcal)	WTR (g)	PROT (g)	CARB (g)	FIBR (g)	FAT (g)	SATF (g)	MONO (g)	POLY (g)
Prepared Homemade Dishes (continued)													
Main & Side Dishes (continued)													
56108	Lasagna w/Meat-Recipe	1	pce	245	392	164	23	40		16	8	5.2	0.8
7086	Lentil Loaf-3/4 in slice	1	pce	47	83	29	4	10	3	4	0.4	0.9	2.1
18800	Lobster Newburg	1	cup	244	611	150	30	11	<1	50	29.6	14.7	2.3
81411	Meatloaf-Angus+Sauce	1	svg	156	310		22	16	1	19	8		
56250	Moo Goo Gai Pan	1	cup	216	272	168	15	12	3	19	3.8	6.7	7
56080	Moussaka-Lamb/Eggplant	1	cup	250	238	204	17	13	4	13	4.6		
5514	Mushroom-Batter Fried	5	ea	70	156	44	2	11	1	12	1.5	3.6	6
5644	Okra-Batter Fried	1	cup	92	175	62	2	14	2	13	1.7	3.1	7.1
27042	Olives-Green-Stuffed	10	ea	40	41	32	1	1	<1	4	0.6	3.2	0.4
5190	Onion Rings-Frozen-Heated	10	ea	71	289	20	4	27	1	19	6.1	7.7	3.6
19403	Oysters Rockefeller	1	cup	224	301	165	16	21	3	17	7.7	5.7	2.4
19009	Oysters-BreadFried-East	6	ea	88	173	57	8	10	<1	11	2.8	4.1	2.9
56234	Pork Chop Suey+Noodles	1	cup	220	448	136	22	31	4	27	4.8	7.7	12.8
12082	Pork Chop-Breaded-Baked	1	ea	80	184	44	21	5	<1	8	2.9	3.7	0.9
56292	Pork Dumpling-Fried	1	ea	100	341	41	13	25	1	21	4.8	9.1	5.7
56288	Pork Egg Foo Yung-Patty	1	ea	86	124	65	8	4	1	8	2.1	3	2.3
5569	Potatoes-Mashed w/Milk+Butter	0.5	cup	105	119	79	2	18	2	4	2.2	0.9	0.2
56098	Quiche Lorraine-1/8 Pie	1	pce	176	526	93	15	25	1	41	18.9	14.3	5.2
56303	Ravioli-Meat w/Tomato Sauce	2	ea	70	110	48	6	10	1	5	1.7	2.1	0.5
40067	Salisbury Stk-Flame Brld	1	ea	72.3	162		16	2		10	3.9		
18807	Salmon Croquette	1	ea	63	137	38	9	7	1	8	1.9	3.4	2.4
5270	Scalloped potatoes-recipe	0.5	cup	122.5	108	99	4	13	2	5	1.7	1.7	0.9
57517	Shrimp Creole w/Rice	1	cup	243	310	176	27	28	1	9	1.8	3.8	2.8
57408	Spinach & Cheese Tortellini-PreCkd	1	cup	128	280		13	40	2	8	5		
2995	Spring Roll-Thai Veg-f/Recipe	1	pce	63.22	158	31	4	20	1	7	0.9		
56236	Stuffed Grape Leaves-Lamb	1	ea	21	56	12	2	2	1	4	1.1	2.5	0.5
5251	Succotash-Boiled	0.5	cup	96	110	66	5	23	4	1	0.1	0.1	0.4
56244	Sukiyaki	1	cup	162	172	126	19	7	1	8	2.9	3.1	0.7
91818	Sushi-California Roll	1	ea	198	292		8	49	3	3	1		
91912	Sushi-Crab Salad Roll	1	ea	198	306		8	49	3	5	1		
91814	Sushi-Cucumber Roll	6	pce	85	120	55	3	25	2	1	0		
91816	Sushi-Tuna Roll	6	pce	105	150	66	8	30	1	0	0	0	0
92384	Sushi-Vegetarian Roll	4.5	pce	110	140		4	27	1	2	0		
15921	SweetSour Chicken Breast	1	ea	131	118	103	8	15	1	3	0.5	0.9	1.4
56061	Taco-Chicken	1	ea	77.3	175	44	15	9	1	9	2.8		
91464	Tamale-Beef-w/Sauce	2	ea	190	310		6	26	4	23	10		
56062	Tostada-Bean+Chicken	1	ea	156.2	242	109	19	16	3	11	4.5		
11902	Veal Scallopini	1	pce	96	238	57	18	1	<1	17	4.8	7.4	3.2
11583	Veal Steak-Breaded-Fried	3	oz	85.05	194	44	23	8	<1	8	2.6	2.9	1.3
Salads													
4826	Chicken Salad+Dressing	1	svg	445	272		29	27	6	5	1		
52035	Cucumber Salad	0.5	cup	100	50		1	13	0	0	0	0	0
52066	Egg Salad	0.5	cup	100	230		9	8	0	18	4		
56005	Potato Salad+Mayo + Eggs	1	cup	250	358	190	7	28	3	20	3.6	6.2	9.3

< = Trace amount present   Blank = Not available

CHOL, cholesterol; **V,** vitamin; **THI,** thiamin; **RIB,** riboflavin; **NIA,** niacin; **FOL,** folate;
CALC, calcium; **PHOS,** phosphate; **SOD,** sodium; **POT,** potassium; **MAG,** magnesium

CHOL (g)	V-A (RE)	THI (mg)	RIB (mg)	NIA (mg)	V-B6 (mg)	FOL (µg)	V-B12 (µg)	V-C (mg)	V-E (mg)	CALC (mg)	PHOS (mg)	SOD (mg)	POT (mg)	MAG (mg)	IRON (mg)	ZINC (mg)
58	158	0.2	0.3	4.2	0.2	20	1	14	1.2	270	299	391	460	50	3.1	3.3
0	<1	0.1	<0.1	0.7	0.1	61	<0.1	1	2.2	18	88	44	156	27	1.5	0.6
369	523	0.1	0.4	1.6	0.2	32	4	1	2	241	398	647	607	55	1.2	4.1
75												650				
35	142	0.2	0.3	4.4	0.3	42	0.3	34	3.7	131	199	304	488	34	1.7	1.6
97	109	0.2	0.3	4.1	0.2	46	1.5	6	1	75	185	460	565	40	1.7	2.6
2	6	0.1	0.3	2.3	<0.1	8	<0.1	1	2.3	15	119	112	154	7	1.2	0.4
2	39	0.2	0.1	1.4	0.1	38	<0.1	10	3	61	122	122	190	36	1.3	0.5
0	25	<0.1	<0.1	<0.1	<0.1	1	0	5	1.1	21	7	826	28	8	0.6	0.1
0	16	0.2	0.1	2.6	0.1	47	0	1	0.5	22	58	266	92	13	1.2	0.3
87	805	0.4	0.4	4	0.3	122	21	27	2.2	195	254	708	583	115	10.3	97.9
71	80	0.1	0.2	1.5	0.1	27	13.8	3	2	55	140	367	215	51	6.1	76.7
48	19	0.8	0.4	6.2	0.4	42	0.4	20	2.7	45	249	848	489	53	3.3	2.6
57	1	0.7	0.3	3.9	0.4	5	0.5	1	0.4	17	197	333	331	22	0.8	1.8
27	11	0.5	0.3	3.6	0.2	9	0.3	<1	2.3	33	131	86	198	18	1.8	1.1
167	86	0.1	0.2	0.8	0.1	22	0.4	3	1.1	27	105	131	157	12	0.8	0.9
12	38	0.1	<0.1	1.1	0.2	8	0.1	6	0.1	25	48	333	300	19	0.3	0.3
221	279	0.3	0.5	2	0.1	19	0.6	1	2	231	261	221	239	24	1.9	1.5
48	49	0.1	0.1	1.7	0.1	8	0.5	2	0.7	20	62	50	148	11	1.2	1
	18							1		29		503			2	
30	14	<0.1	0.1	2.9	0.2	10	1.2	2	1.3	95	145	266	203	17	0.5	0.5
7	44	0.1	0.1	1.3	0.2	13	0	13	0.4	70	77	410	463	23	0.7	0.5
181	133	0.3	0.1	4.8	0.2	12	1.2	17	2.3	104	300	370	439	64	4.4	1.7
30	120							0			150	320			1.8	
3	140	0.2	0.1	1.9	<0.1	32	<0.1	1	1.3	58	42	263	75	12	1.8	0.4
5	145	<0.1	<0.1	0.6	<0.1	6	0.1	2	0.5	22	19	14	41	8	0.4	0.3
0	29	0.2	0.1	1.3	0.1	32	0	8	0.3	16	112	16	394	51	1.5	0.6
148	256	0.1	0.4	3.1	0.4	61	1.5	5	0.7	62	204	675	463	47	3.2	3.6
3	90							5		20		952			1.1	
6	90							5		20		968			1.1	
0	50							0		0		90			0.4	
5	10							1		0		120			0.7	
0	200							2		0		105			0.7	
23	22	0.1	0.1	3.1	0.2	6	0.1	12	0.7	15	75	506	185	21	0.8	0.7
45	38	0.1	0.1	4.1	0.3	13	0.2	1	0.6	82	156	132	157	28	1	1.3
20	200							2		40		870			1.1	
55	63	0.1	0.1	4.3	0.3	25	0.3	5	0.7	146	220	387	263	41	1.6	1.9
65	101	<0.1	0.2	5.1	0.2	12	0.9	1	1.7	54	172	278	253	19	1	2.8
95	9	0.1	0.3	8.8	0.3	23	1.1	0	0.5	33	213	386	316	26	1.4	2.3
47	416							16		36		1475			4	
0												580				
240	0							0			40	570			1.4	
170	88	0.2	0.1	2.2	0.4	18	0	25	4.7	48	130	1322	635	38	1.6	0.8

ESHA, EatRight Analysis CD-ROM; **AMT,** amount; **WT,** weight; **CAL,** calories; **WTR,** water; **PROT,** protein; **CARB,** carbohydrate;
FIBR, fiber; **FAT,** fat; **SATF,** saturated fat; **MONO,** monosaturated fat; **POLY,** polyunsaturated fat

ESHA CODE	FOOD DESCRIPTION	AMT	UNIT	WT (g)	CAL (kcal)	WTR (g)	PROT (g)	CARB (g)	FIBR (g)	FAT (g)	SATF (g)	MONO (g)	POLY (g)
Prepared Homemade Dishes (continued)													
Salads (continued)													
52065	Seafood Salad	0.5	cup	100	230		6	14	8	17	2.5		
52064	Shrimp Salad	0.5	cup	100	170		7	5	3	14	2		
5537	Spinach Salad-No Dressing	1	cup	74	108	51	5	11	2	5	1.4	2.2	0.7
56917	Tabouli Salad	1	cup	160	589	15	17	122	13	4	0.8	0.6	2.1
6255	Three Bean Salad	0.5	cup	121	90		3	20	4	0	0	0	0
56006	Waldorf salad	1	cup	137	411	79	4	12	3	41	4.3		
Sandwiches													
57544	BBQ Beef Hot Pocket-Frzn	1	ea	128	340	56	10	47	2	12	5		
56009	BLT Sandwich	1	ea	123.8	318	64	10	29	2	18	4.1		
56281	Bologna Sandwich	1	ea	83	256	34	7	26	1	13	4.1	6.3	2.1
69154	Chicken Club Sandwich-Chargrld	1	ea	202	360		30	31	2	13	5		
13093	Chicken Hotdog on Bun	1	ea	85	235	38	9	24	1	11	3	5	2.2
56020	Corned Beef+Swiss on Rye	1	ea	156	427	73	28	22	6	26	9.5		
56013	Grilled Cheese Sandwich	1	ea	119	399	44	17	30	1	23	11.9		
56033	Ham & Swiss on Rye Sandwich	1	ea	149.5	385	72	22	30	4	19	6.5		
56066	Ham Salad Sandwich on Wheat	1	ea	130.6	357	63	11	33	2	20	4.7		
56031	Ham Sandwich on Wheat	1	ea	156.3	356	84	25	26	2	17	3.6		
56267	Pastrami Sandwich	1	ea	134	331	71	14	27	2	18	6.2	8.7	1
56038	Patty Melt Sandwich on Rye	1	ea	181.9	561	83	37	22	6	37	12.7		
56040	PeanutButter&Jelly on White	1	ea	101	348	28	11	47	3	14	2.7		
81477	Roast Beef Gyro Sandwich	1	ea	240	541		23	48	2	29	7.6		
56046	Roast Beef Sandwich on Wheat	1	ea	155.8	397	73	30	30	2	17	3.2		
56670	Steak Sandwich	1	ea	204	459	104	30	52		14	3.8	5.3	3.3
56048	Tuna Salad Sandwich	1	ea	121.8	326	56	13	35	1	14	1.9		
56053	Turkey Sandwich-Whole Wheat	1	ea	168.8	360	92	27	29	4	16	2.3		
56103	TurkeyHam Sandwich on Rye	1	ea	149.5	279	90	21	20	6	13	2.5		
56059	TurkeyHam+Cheese on Wheat	1	ea	156.3	396	78	23	28		22	8.2		
Soups, Stews, & Chilis													
50190	Egg Drop Soup	1	cup	244	73	229	8	1	0	4	1.1	1.5	0.6
50211	Fish Chowder	1	cup	244	194	201	24	12	1	5	2.4	1.9	0.6
50182	Hot & Sour Soup	1	cup	244	162	211	15	5	1	8	2.7	3.4	1.2
50207	Pork Rice Vegetable Soup	1	cup	244	124	219	12	8	1	4	1.5	2.1	0.4
50209	Sweet & Sour Soup	1	cup	244	72	222	3	14	2	1	0.3	0.3	0.1
Restaurant Food													
Arby's													
6432	Arby's Curly Fries	1	svg	99.22	310	40	4	39	3	15	3.5		
81476	Arby's Melt Sandwich	1	ea	147	303		15	36	1	12	4.5		
53256	Arby's Sauce	1	svg	14	15		0	4	0	0	0	0	0
69056	Beef'nCheddar Sandwich	1	ea	198	460		23	43	2	23	9		
48162	Cherry Turnover-Iced	1	ea	128	410	44	4	63	1	16	4.5		
69048	Italian Sub Sandwich	1	ea	312	699		26	55	2	37	7.9		
69055	Phily Beef'nSwiss Sandwich	1	ea	311	678		35	47	4	36	10.9		
56336	Roast Beef Sandwch-Reg	1	ea	157	330		21	35	2	14	7		

< = Trace amount present   Blank = Not available

CHOL, cholesterol; **V**, vitamin; **THI**, thiamin; **RIB**, riboflavin; **NIA**, niacin; **FOL**, folate; **CALC**, calcium; **PHOS**, phosphate; **SOD**, sodium; **POT**, potassium; **MAG**, magnesium

CHOL (g)	V-A (RE)	THI (mg)	RIB (mg)	NIA (mg)	V-B6 (mg)	FOL (µg)	V-B12 (µg)	V-C (mg)	V-E (mg)	CALC (mg)	PHOS (mg)	SOD (mg)	POT (mg)	MAG (mg)	IRON (mg)	ZINC (mg)
20	0							0		20		770			0.4	
85	0							0		4		620			0.7	
77	176	0.1	0.3	1.7	0.1	60	0.2	7	0.9	46	83	227	242	27	1.5	0.6
	253							6		105		54			4.9	
0	80							0		60		490			1.4	
21	36	0.1	0.1	0.5	0.4	34	0.1	5	8.6	44	89	235	258	37	1	0.7
15	0							0		150		740			4.5	
20	49	0.4	0.3	3.7	0.2	66	0.3	6	2.3	68	123	631	239	22	2.2	1
16	37	0.3	0.2	2.7	0.1	19	0.4	<1	0.8	60	74	598	112	15	2	0.9
80	40							4		150		1370			2.7	
45	17	0.2	0.1	2.7	0.2	17	0.1	0	0.1	83	82	819	76	13	2	0.8
83	58	0.2	0.3	2.8	0.2	32	1.7	<1	2.6	267	269	1470	232	28	3	3.6
53	167	0.3	0.4	2.4	0.1	60	0.4	<1	1	407	470	1155	162	26	2	2
56	51	0.6	0.4	5	0.3	55	1	<1	2.5	240	345	1392	369	42	2.7	3
30	6	0.5	0.2	3.6	0.2	44	0.5	0	3.7	65	164	947	212	32	2.3	1.3
56	7	0.9	0.4	6.9	0.4	44	0.6	<1	2.7	68	307	1254	439	43	3.1	2.9
51	3	0.3	0.3	4.8	0.1	21	1	2	0.3	68	135	1335	243	23	2.6	2.7
113	95	0.2	0.5	6.1	0.4	37	2.4	<1	3.5	221	324	714	391	39	4.2	7
1	<1	0.3	0.2	5.4	0.1	79	<0.1	2	2.6	76	143	429	240	52	2.3	1.1
59	100							11		100		1504			5.4	
45	8	0.3	0.3	6.9	0.4	51	2.3	0	3.6	67	232	1640	492	41	4.2	4.1
73	39	0.4	0.4	7.3	0.4	90	1.6	6		92	298	798	524	49	5.2	4.5
13	15	0.3	0.2	5.9	0.1	63	0.7	1	2.8	76	152	588	168	25	2.4	0.7
47	8	0.3	0.2	10.1	0.5	35	1.9	0	3.9	53	356	1734	417	71	2.5	2.2
55	7	0.2	0.3	4.3	0.3	29	0.3	<1	2.9	51	211	1175	342	26	4	2.9
64	74	0.3	0.4	4.4	0.3	30	0.4	0	3.2	246	411	1389	354	44	3.7	3.2
103	41	<0.1	0.2	3	0.1	15	0.5	0	0.3	21	108	729	220	5	0.8	0.5
56	63	0.2	0.3	2.9	0.4	16	1.3	7	0.4	148	298	180	711	49	0.7	1.1
34	2	0.3	0.3	5	0.2	13	0.4	1	0.1	29	188	1011	384	29	1.9	1.5
41	295	0.3	0.1	2.5	0.2	6	0.3	1	0.2	16	96	55	206	15	1.1	2
5	31	0.1	0.1	0.9	0.1	16	<0.1	17	0.5	27	43	1292	227	15	0.6	0.3
0	0	0.1	0.1	2			0	12		0		770	724		1.4	0.6
30	20							0		60		921			2.9	
0								1		0		180	28		0	
50		0.4	0.6	10				1		100		1170	328		3.6	3
0		<0.1	0.1	0.6				7		10		250	102		1.6	
57	135							14		315		2237			3.6	
91	51							9		314		1968			4.7	
45	0							0		60	122	890	427	16	3.6	3.8

ESHA, EatRight Analysis CD-ROM; **AMT,** amount; **WT,** weight; **CAL,** calories; **WTR,** water; **PROT,** protein; **CARB,** carbohydrate; **FIBR,** fiber; **FAT,** fat; **SATF,** saturated fat; **MONO,** monosaturated fat; **POLY,** polyunsaturated fat

ESHA CODE	FOOD DESCRIPTION	AMT	UNIT	WT (g)	CAL (kcal)	WTR (g)	PROT (g)	CARB (g)	FIBR (g)	FAT (g)	SATF (g)	MONO (g)	POLY (g)
Restaurant Food (continued)													
Arby's (continued)													
56337	Roast Beef Sandwich-Jr	1	ea	129	290		16	34	2	12	5		
69049	Roast Beef Sub Sandwich	1	ea	334	807		38	53	3	47	12.6		
69044	Turkey Sub Sandwich	1	ea	306	681		38	52	2	32	6.1		
Burger King													
57002	BK Broiler Chicken Sandwich	1	ea	258	550		30	52	3	25	5		
56360	Chicken Sandwich-Burger King	1	ea	224	660		25	53	3	39	8		
57001	Double Cheeseburger	1	ea	197	570		35	32	2	34	17		
56362	Ocean Catch Fish Filet	1	ea	263	710		24	67	4	38	14		
56363	Onion Rings-Serving	1	svg	91	320		4	40	3	16	4		
56999	Whopper Jr Sandwich	1	ea	167	410	91	18	32	2	23	7		
57000	Whopper Jr Sandwich+Cheese	1	ea	180	460		21	33	2	27	10		
56354	Whopper Sandwich	1	ea	278	648	157	30	52	5	36	11.8	13	9.4
56355	Whopper Sandwich+Cheese	1	ea	303	758	166	34	51	3	46	17.5	15.3	11.5
Carl's Junior													
91408	Chicken Sandwich-Charbroiled Club	1	ea	239	460		32	33	2	22	7		
91410	Chicken Sandwich-Crispy Ranch	1	ea	266	730		29	77	4	34	7.1		
91413	Fish Sandwich-Carl's Catch	1	ea	201	510	103	18	50	1	27	7		
Dairy Queen													
2131	Banana Split	1	ea	369	510		8	96	3	12	8		
72141	Banana Split Blizzard	1	ea	382	580		12	97	1	17	11		
2133	Buster Bar	1	ea	149	450		10	41	2	28	12		
69069	Chili Cheese Hot Dog	1	ea	262	710		27	42	3	47	18		
2222	Cone-Chocolate-Reg	1	ea	198	340		8	53	0	11	7		
2135	Dilly Bar	1	ea	85	210	47	3	21	0	13	7		
2136	Dipped Cone-Regular	1	ea	220	490		8	59	1	24	13		
69027	Double Bacon Cheeseburger	1	ea	269	670		40	29	2	43	19		
13236	Hot Dog-Super-1/4lb	1	ea	198	580		20	39	2	37	13		
56374	Hotdog	1	ea	99	240	55	9	19	1	14	5		
2134	Ice Cream Sandwich	1	ea	85	200	43	4	31	1	6	3		
2348	Ice Cream-Soft Serve-Choc	0.5	cup	94	150		4	22	0	5	3.5		
2368	Oreo Blizzard	1	ea	326	640		12	97	1	23	11		
2151	Peanut Buster Parfait	1	ea	305	730		16	99	2	31	17		
2224	Shake-Chocolate-Reg	1	ea	539	770		17	130	0	20	13		
56371	Single Cheeseburger	1	ea	152	340	83	20	29	2	17	8		
56368	Single Hamburger	1	ea	138	290	78	17	29	2	12	5		
2154	Sundae-Chocolate-Regular	1	ea	234	400		8	71	0	10	6		
Dunkin' Donuts													
42636	Apple Fritter	1	ea	95	300		5	41	2	13	3		
45749	Apple Turnover	1	ea	109	350		5	49	2	15	4		
45736	Cake Doughnut	1	ea	60	260		3	29	2	14	3		
45746	Lemon Tart	1	ea	98	280		5	43	1	11	3		
44616	Muffin-Chocolate Chip	1	ea	95	400		5	63	2	16	6		

< = Trace amount present   Blank = Not available

CHOL, cholesterol; **V,** vitamin; **THI,** thiamin; **RIB,** riboflavin; **NIA,** niacin; **FOL,** folate; **CALC,** calcium; **PHOS,** phosphate; **SOD,** sodium; **POT,** potassium; **MAG,** magnesium

CHOL (g)	V-A (RE)	THI (mg)	RIB (mg)	NIA (mg)	V-B6 (mg)	FOL (µg)	V-B12 (µg)	V-C (mg)	V-E (mg)	CALC (mg)	PHOS (mg)	SOD (mg)	POT (mg)	MAG (mg)	IRON (mg)	ZINC (mg)
40		0.3	0.4	9.6	0.1	10				60	87	700	291	12	2.7	2.2
98	101							7		313		2470			2.3	
81	97							8		302		2186	595		3.7	
105	60							6		60		1110			3.6	
70	20							0		80		1330			2.7	
110	100							0		250		1020			4.5	
50	20							0		80		1200			3.6	
0	0						0	0		100		460			0	
50	40							5		80		520			3.6	
60	80							5		150		740			3.6	
83		0.6	0.5	8	0.3	131		1	0.4	108	250	870	470	50	12.1	7.9
109		0.6	0.6	7.8	0.2	155		1	0.2	248	342	1373	512	55	6.1	4.8
90	80							6		200		1110			2.7	
59	71							6		177		1436			4.2	
80	60							2		150		1030			1.8	
30	200							15		250		180			1.8	
50	250							9		400		260			1.8	
15	80							0		150		280			1.1	
105	150							2		250		2270			4.5	
30	150							1		250		160			1.8	
10	60							0		100		75			0.4	
30	150							2		250		190			1.8	
135	150							9		250		1210			4.5	
75	0							0		250		1710			4.5	
25	20							4		60		730			1.8	
10	40							0		80		140			1.1	
15	100							0		100		75			0.7	
45	250							1		400		500			2.7	
35	150							1		300		400			1.8	
70	400							2		600		420			2.7	
55	100							4		150		850			3.6	
45	40							4		60		630			2.7	
30	150							0		250		210			1.4	
0	0							0		0		320			1.4	
0	0							2		0		340			0.7	
0	0							0		20		300			0.7	
0	0							2		0		340			0.7	
35	0							0		40		190			1.8	

ESHA, EatRight Analysis CD-ROM; **AMT**, amount; **WT**, weight; **CAL**, calories; **WTR**, water; **PROT**, protein; **CARB**, carbohydrate;
FIBR, fiber; **FAT**, fat; **SATF**, saturated fat; **MONO**, monosaturated fat; **POLY**, polyunsaturated fat

ESHA CODE	FOOD DESCRIPTION	AMT	UNIT	WT (g)	CAL (kcal)	WTR (g)	PROT (g)	CARB (g)	FIBR (g)	FAT (g)	SATF (g)	MONO (g)	POLY (g)
Restaurant Food (continued)													
Hardees													
56411	Biscuit 'n Gravy	1	ea	221	530	123	10	56		30	9		
2247	Cool Twist Cone-Van/Choc	1	ea	118	180		4	34		2	1		
69061	Frisco Hamburger	1	ea	219	717		33	37	2	49	13.9		
56420	Hot Ham 'n Cheese Sandwich	1	ea	201	421		23	43	3	17	9.6		
56418	RoastBeef Sandwich-Regular	1	ea	123	310		17	26	2	16	6		
Jack in the Box													
69032	Bacon Cheeseburger	1	ea	274	783		32	48	2	52	17.7		
56430	Breakfast Jack Sandwich	1	ea	126	292		17	29	1	12	4.5		
56441	Chicken Fajita Pita	1	ea	230	317		24	33	3	11	4.7		
69035	Chicken Sandwich-Jack in the Box	1	ea	164	452		17	43	2	24	5.1		
69033	Grilled Sourdough Burger	1	ea	233	675		26	34	3	49	17.1		
56436	Jumbo Jack Burger	1	ea	271	623		22	53	3	36	12.5		
56437	Jumbo Jack Burger+Cheese	1	ea	296	714		26	56	3	43	16.6		
69040	Sourdough Breakfast Sandwich	1	ea	162	436		21	32	2	25	8.3		
11919	Southwest Pita Sandwich	1	ea	179	260		20	35	4	4	1		
Kentucky Fried Chicken													
15169	Chicken Breast-ExtraCrispy	1	ea	168	477	80	35	20	0	29	8.3		
15163	Chicken Breast-Original	1	ea	153	361	84	38	10	0	18	5.7		
81293	Chicken Drumstick	1	ea	59	140	32	14	4	0	8	2		
81291	Chicken Drumstick-Extra Crispy	1	ea	60	160	32	12	5	0	10	2.5		
15177	Hot Wings-Pieces	6	pce	135	453		24	23	1	29	6		
15184	Hot&Spicy Chicken Drumstick	1	ea	64	160	35	14	4	0	10	2.7		
15187	Hot&Spicy Chicken Wing	1	ea	55	180	23	11	9	0	11	3		
McDonalds													
69010	Big Mac Sandwich	1	ea	216	555	111	26	43	3	32	8.2	7.5	0.7
42332	Biscuit+BiscuitSpread	1	ea	69	240	23	4	30	1	11	2.5		
56675	Breakfast Burrito	1	ea	113	296	56	13	24	1	17	6.1	6.5	2.4
69009	Cheeseburger	1	ea	121	318	54	16	34	1	14	5.4	4.4	0.4
15174	Chicken McNuggets	4	pce	72	190	36	11	12	0	11	2.4	4.5	3.6
42335	Danish-Apple	1	ea	105	340		5	47	2	15	3		
69005	Egg McMuffin	1	ea	136	292	75	17	28	1	12	4.4	3.7	2.5
69013	Filet-O-Fish Sandwich	1	ea	156	443	69	16	45	1	23	4	4.7	7.8
2166	FrozenYogurt Cone-Vanilla	1	ea	90	146	57	4	24	<1	4	2.2	1.1	0.3
4732	Grill Chick Dlxe Sand w/oMayo	1	ea	215	340		26	45	2	7	1.5		
69008	Hamburger	1	ea	107	270	49	13	33	1	10	3.1	3.4	0.2
6155	Hashbrown Potatoes	1	svg	53	136	28	1	13	2	9	1.6	3.9	2.2
45069	Hotcakes+Marg+Syrup	1	svg	228	600		9	104	0	17	3		
47147	McDonaldland Cookies	1	ea	57	255	2	4	41	1	9	1.8	4.6	1.2
69011	Quarter Pounder	1	ea	172	420	87	24	38	3	20	6.9	7.2	0.5
69012	Quarter Pounder+Cheese	1	ea	200	516	98	29	40	3	28	11.3	9.2	0.9
69006	Sausage McMuffin	1	ea	112	373	44	14	27	2	24	8.1	8.7	3.6
19579	Scrambled Eggs	1	svg	102	197	68	15	2		15	4.1	5.3	2.2
2167	Shake-LowFat-Choc	1	ea	294.6	480	186	11	82	1	13	6.8	3.3	0.6
2168	Shake-LowFat-Strawberrry	1	ea	294	465	189	10	79	0	13	6.6	3.2	0.6
2169	Shake-LowFat-Vanilla	1	ea	293.4	458	190	10	78	0	13	6.6	3.2	0.6

< = Trace amount present   Blank = Not available

CHOL, cholesterol; **V,** vitamin; **THI,** thiamin; **RIB,** riboflavin; **NIA,** niacin; **FOL,** folate;
CALC, calcium; **PHOS,** phosphate; **SOD,** sodium; **POT,** potassium; **MAG,** magnesium

CHOL (g)	V-A (RE)	THI (mg)	RIB (mg)	NIA (mg)	V-B6 (mg)	FOL (µg)	V-B12 (µg)	V-C (mg)	V-E (mg)	CALC (mg)	PHOS (mg)	SOD (mg)	POT (mg)	MAG (mg)	IRON (mg)	ZINC (mg)
15												1550				
10												120				
100												1079				
78												1831				
43												804				
89												1500	391			
222												766	212			
69												928	475			
40												826	271			
71												1170	409			
47												976	395			
72												1356	424			
239												1018	239			
40												880	450			
140	0							0		0		1276			1.5	
138	0							0		0		1093			1.7	
75	0							0		0		440			0.7	
70	0							0		0		420			0.7	
146	60							4		81		1128			1.8	
69	0							0		0		405			0.8	
60	0							0		0		420			0.7	
78	81	0.4	0.5	7.3	0.4	99	1.9	1	0.1	251	264	994	391	43	4.3	4.1
0	2			2		4		0	0.7	40	321	640	95	8	1.8	0.3
173	101	0.2	0.3	1.9	0.4	70	0.6	1	0.2	203	247	763	155	19	1.8	1.3
42	59	0.3	0.3	4.9	0.1	71	1	1	0.1	202	169	757	242	24	2.8	2.3
28	14	0.1	0.1	5.3	0.3	20	0.2	1		10	239	503	181	16	0.6	0.4
20	100	0.3	0.2	2				15		60	0	340	113		1.4	
224	107	0.4	0.5	4.2	0.2	107	0.9	2	0.8	269	264	842	214	26	2.9	1.6
44	28	0.4	0.3	3.8	0.1	78	1.1	0	1.8	181	184	700	273	31	2.3	0.8
14	58	<0.1	0.2	0.4	<0.1	8	0.5		<0.1	116	100	60	174	12	0.3	0.4
50	40							6			200		890		2.7	
29	12	0.3	0.3	4.9	0.1	68	0.9	1	0.1	129	114	542	217	21	2.8	2
0	0	0.1	<0.1	1.2	0.1	20		2	1	10	57	289	207	11	0.4	0.2
20	80					<1		<1	1.2	100	516	770	292	28	4.5	0.5
	0	0.2	0.2	2.1	0.1	58			1.1	10	63	275	56	10	1.9	0.3
67	19	0.3	0.6	7.7	0.3	96	2.2	2	0.1	144	213	734	390	38	4.1	4.6
94	112	0.3	0.7	7.7	0.2	102	2.5	2	0.4	288	322	1158	438	44	4.2	5.3
44	58	0.4	0.3	4.7	0.2	77	0.5	0	0.3	251	183	776	211	24	2.3	1.4
436	186	0.1	0.6	0.1	0.2	71	1.1		1.5	67	266	196	142	12	2.1	1.5
41	268	0.1	0.6	0.4	0.1	3	1.6		0	359	309	209	666	47	1.6	1.5
41	268	0.1	0.6	0.4	0.1	9	1.6	1	0	359	294	144	541	35	0.3	1.3
41	179	0.1	0.6	0.3	0.1	0	1.6		0	355	293	156	516	35	0.2	1.3

ESHA, EatRight Analysis CD-ROM; **AMT**, amount; **WT**, weight; **CAL**, calories; **WTR**, water; **PROT**, protein; **CARB**, carbohydrate; **FIBR**, fiber; **FAT**, fat; **SATF**, saturated fat; **MONO**, monosaturated fat; **POLY**, polyunsaturated fat

ESHA CODE	FOOD DESCRIPTION	AMT	UNIT	WT (g)	CAL (kcal)	WTR (g)	PROT (g)	CARB (g)	FIBR (g)	FAT (g)	SATF (g)	MONO (g)	POLY (g)
Restaurant Food (continued)													
Pizza Hut													
56481	Cheese Pizza-Pan Style	1	pce	110	308	48	13	33	2	14	5.7	3.5	3
56490	Pepperoni Pizza-HandTossed	1	pce	116	325	48	15	37	2	13	6	4.7	2.4
56482	Pepperoni Pizza-Pan Style	1	pce	106	316	43	13	32	2	15	5.6	4.7	3.7
56493	Pepperoni Pizza-Pers Pan	1	ea	257	716		29	76	4	34	12.6		
56486	Pepperoni Pizza-Thin/Crispy	1	pce	81	221	37	11	22	1	11	4.7		
56483	Supreme Pizza-Pan Style	1	pce	133	335		14	31	2	17	6.3		
56487	Supreme Pizza-Thin/Crispy	1	pce	117	265		12	24	2	12	5.5		
Subway													
69117	Club Sandwich (6-inch)	1	ea	255	320		24	46	4	6	2		
52120	Cold Cut Salad	1	svg	316	230		14	11	3	15	6		
69129	Meatball Sandwich (6-inch)	1	ea	287	530		24	53	6	26	10		
52116	Seafood/Crab Salad	1	svg	314	200		9	17	4	11	3.5		
52118	Tuna Salad	1	svg	314	240		13	10	3	16	4		
69107	Tuna Sandwich (6-inch)	1	ea	168	330		13	36	3	16	4.5		
52113	Veggie Delite Salad	1	ea	233	50		2	9	3	1	0		
69109	Veggie Sandwich (6-inch)	1	ea	166	230		9	44	4	3	1		
Taco Bell													
56691	7 Layer Burrito	1	ea	283	530		18	67	10	22	8		
56522	Burrito-Beef Supreme	1	ea	248	469	150	20	52	8	20	7.6	8.1	2
56688	Chicken Burrito	1	ea	171	306	104	17	35	4	11	4	4.4	1.4
56689	Chicken Soft Taco	1	ea	121	244	68	17	24	2	9	3.2	3.4	1.3
45585	Cinnamon Twists	1	svg	28	128		1	22	0	4	0.8		
56531	Mexican Pizza	1	ea	220	560		21	47	7	32	11.2		
56534	Nachos Bellgrande	1	svg	312	790		20	81	12	44	13.2		
56684	Nachos Supreme	1	svg	198	487	106	15	46	8	27	7.9	13.9	2.8
56536	Pintos+Cheese+Red Sauce	1	svg	120	169	83	9	19	6	7	3.3		
56526	Soft Taco Supreme	1	ea	142	276		12	23	3	15	7.4		
56693	Steak Soft Taco	1	ea	128	288	73	15	22	2	15	4.3	5	4.5
56524	Taco	1	ea	78	184	44	8	14	3	11	3.6	4.2	1.6
56692	Taco Supreme	1	ea	113	220		9	14	3	14	7		
56525	Taco-Beef-Soft	1	ea	99	217	55	12	20	3	10	4.2	4.3	1
21037	Tea-Lemon-Btl/Cnd	1	cup	245	86	223	0	22	0	0	0	0	
Taco Time													
12418	Cheddar Tator Tots	1	svg	198.45	519		12	40		35			
7273	Chicken Taco Salad	1	ea	255.15	370		19	27	3	21	7		
56540	Crispy Bean Burrito	1	ea	164.2	471		17	58	10	20	5.5		
56541	Crispy Meat Burrito	1	ea	162.8	604		37	43	8	33	10.9		
56553	Mexi-Fries	1	svg	114.2	268		3	27		17			
50979	Quesadilla-Cheddar Melt	1	ea	92.14	205		11	17	1	11	6		
56544	Soft Combo Burrito	1	ea	272	623		39	67	18	23	10.1		
Wendy's													
56571	Bacon Cheeseburger	1	ea	165	380		20	34	2	19	7		
56574	Big Classic Burger+Cheese	1	ea	282	570		34	46	3	29	12		
2177	Frosty Dairy Dessert-Med	1	ea	298	393	206	10	70	10	8	4.9	2.1	0.3
69059	Grilled Chicken Sandwich	1	ea	188	300		24	36	2	7	1.5		

< = Trace amount present   Blank = Not available

CHOL, cholesterol; **V,** vitamin; **THI,** thiamin; **RIB,** riboflavin; **NIA,** niacin; **FOL,** folate;
CALC, calcium; **PHOS,** phosphate; **SOD,** sodium; **POT,** potassium; **MAG,** magnesium

CHOL (g)	V-A (RE)	THI (mg)	RIB (mg)	NIA (mg)	V-B6 (mg)	FOL (µg)	V-B12 (µg)	V-C (mg)	V-E (mg)	CALC (mg)	PHOS (mg)	SOD (mg)	POT (mg)	MAG (mg)	IRON (mg)	ZINC (mg)
23	80	0.3	0.3	4.3	0.1		0.7	0	1.2	229	265	686	185	23	2	1.8
30	67	0.4	0.3	4.7	0.2		0.8	0	0.9	180	253	929	240	27	2.5	1.9
26	51	0.3	0.3	4.1	0.1		0.7	0	0.8	155	217	734	211	23	2.3	1.6
63	169							5		337		1432			6.1	
26	63							3		158		579			1.5	
26	63							6		157		681			2.8	
28	66							10		166		706			2	
35	60							21		60		1300			5.4	
55	200							30		150		1370			1.8	
55	150							27		150		1360			5.4	
25	200							30		100		970			1.1	
40	200							30		100		880			1.1	
25	80							12		150		830			3.6	
0	150							30		40		310			1.1	
0	60							21		60		510			3.6	
25	100							5		300		1360			3.6	
40	20	0.4	0.4	4.3	0.3	112	1.2		1.1	231	337	1424	608	62	5.6	2.6
36	14	0.3	0.3	6.7	0.2	82	0.6		0.7	161	279	964	451	48	2.7	1.1
45	3	0.3	0.2	7.7	0.2	58	0.4		0.4	127	271	733	287	27	2.1	1
0	0							0		0		120			0.3	
46	153							6		356		1049			3.7	
35	101							6		203		1317			2.7	
38	16	0.2	0.3	1.9	0.3	57	0.8		1.4	145	390	851	479	91	4.2	2.7
14	94							3		141		656			1	
42	106							5		159		668			1.9	
40	3	0.4	0.2	3.8	0.1	47	1.2		0.6	150	198	705	234	27	2.8	2.8
24	6	0.1	0.1	1.5	0.1	15	0.7		0.5	62	139	349	168	26	1.5	1.7
40	100							5		80		360			1.4	
28	8	0.2	0.2	2.6	0.1	51	0.8		0.4	115	161	626	179	20	2.4	1.6
0										2	64	51	47	0	0	<0.1
												1372				
48												861				
13												500				
63												1094				
												805				
30												255				
64												1356				
55	80							9		150		890	320		3.6	
100	150							15		200		1460	580		5.4	
48		0.2	2.1	1	0		1.8	0		381	334	292	551	60	3.1	1.3
55	40							9		80		740	430		2.7	

ESHA, EatRight Analysis CD-ROM; **AMT,** amount; **WT,** weight; **CAL,** calories; **WTR,** water; **PROT,** protein; **CARB,** carbohydrate; **FIBR,** fiber; **FAT,** fat; **SATF,** saturated fat; **MONO,** monosaturated fat; **POLY,** polyunsaturated fat

ESHA CODE	FOOD DESCRIPTION	AMT	UNIT	WT (g)	CAL (kcal)	WTR (g)	PROT (g)	CARB (g)	FIBR (g)	FAT (g)	SATF (g)	MONO (g)	POLY (g)
Restaurant Food (continued)													
Wendy's (continued)													
69058	Junior Cheeseburger Deluxe	1	ea	179	350		17	37	2	15	6		
69057	Junior Hamburger	1	ea	117	284	56	15	33	2	10	4.1	4.1	1.3
56566	Single Burger-Deluxe	1	ea	218	464	127	28	37	3	23	8	8.9	3.4
71596	Spring Mix Salad-No Dressing	1	ea	315	180		11	12	5	11	6		
81443	Ultimate Grill Chicken Sandwich	1	ea	225	403	134	33	42	2	11	2.3	3.3	4.1
Generic Fast Foods													
66025	Burrito-Bean	1	ea	108.5	224	57	7	36	4	7	3.4	2.4	0.6
56629	Burrito-Bean+Cheese	1	ea	93	189	50	8	27		6	3.4	1.2	0.9
66024	Burrito-Beef	1	ea	110	262	55	13	29	1	10	5.2	3.7	0.4
66021	Cheese enchilada	1	ea	163	319	103	10	29		19	10.6	6.3	0.8
56628	Chef Style Salad	1.5	cup	326	267	269	26	5		16	8.2	5.2	1.4
91370	Chicken Buffalo Wings-Hot	1	ea	24.9	45		5	1	<1	2	0.6		
56656	Chicken Fillet Sandwich+Cheese	1	ea	228	632	105	29	42		39	12.4	13.7	9.9
56634	Chimichanga-Beef	1	ea	174	425	88	20	43	2	20	8.5	8.1	1.1
56668	Corndog (hotdog+coating)	1	ea	175	460	82	17	56		19	5.2	9.1	3.5
56606	Croissant + Egg & Cheese	1	ea	127	368	58	13	24		25	14.1	7.5	1.4
66020	Enchirito-Bean+Beef+Cheez	1	ea	193	344	121	18	34		16	7.9	6.5	0.3
42064	English Muffin+Butter	1	ea	63	189	21	5	30	2	6	2.4	1.5	1.3
56461	Fish-Batter Fried	1	pce	92.14	230	50	11	16	0	13	4		
17187	Fish Fillet-Batter Fried	3	oz	85.05	197	46	12	14	<1	10	2.4	2.2	5.3
69030	Fish Sandwich Batter Dip	1	ea	174.3	434		17	46	3	21	4.9		
66011	FishSandwich+Cheese+TartarSc	1	ea	183	523	83	21	48	<1	29	8.1	8.9	9.4
5460	French Fries-Veg Oil-Serving	1	svg	169	539	67	6	63	6	29	6.7	16.7	5.1
56638	Frijoles + Cheese	1	cup	167	225	115	11	29		8	4.1	2.6	0.7
5463	Hashbrown Potatoes-Svg	0.5	cup	72	235	30	2	23	2	16			
2032	Hot Fudge Sundae	1	ea	158	284	94	6	48	0	9	5	2.3	0.8
56667	Hotdog + Chili	1	ea	114	296	54	14	31		13	4.9	6.6	1.2
66004	Hotdog/Frankfurter & Bun	1	ea	98	242	53	10	18		15	5.1	6.9	1.7
2020	Milkshake-Chocolate	1	cup	166.4	211	119	6	34	3	6	3.8	1.8	0.2
2117	Mikshake-Chocolate Malt	1	ea	284	579		12	77	0	27	17		
56639	Nachos-Chips + Cheese	7	pce	113	346	46	9	36		19	7.8	8	2.2
6176	Onion Rings-Serving	8.5	pce	83	276	31	4	31		16	7	6.7	0.7
56672	Roast Beef Submarine Sandwich	1	ea	216	410	127	29	44		13	7.1	1.8	2.6
19114	Scallops-Bread-Fried	3	oz	85.05	228	41	9	23		11	2.9	7.4	0.4
2022	Strawberry Milkshake	1	cup	283	320	210	10	53	1	8	4.9		
2033	Strawberry sundae	1	ea	153	268	93	6	45	0	8	3.7	2.7	1
56671	Submarine Sandwich w/Coldcuts	1	ea	228	456	132	22	51	2	19	6.8	8.2	2.3
56643	Taco Salad	1.5	cup	198	279	143	13	24		15	6.8	5.2	1.7
56645	Tostada-Beef+Cheese	1	ea	163	315	101	19	23		16	10.4	3.3	1
56623	Vegetable Salad-No Dressing	1.5	cup	207	33	198	3	7		<1	<0.1	<0.1	0.1
Vegetables & Legumes													
Canned													
5191	Artichoke Hearts-Marinated-Cnd	0.5	cup	65	58	52	2	7	2	3	0		
5842	Asparagus-Canned+Liq-LowSod	0.5	cup	122	18	115	2	3	1	<1	0.1	<0.1	0.1

< = Trace amount present   Blank = Not available

CHOL, cholesterol; **V,** vitamin; **THI,** thiamin; **RIB,** riboflavin; **NIA,** niacin; **FOL,** folate;
CALC, calcium; **PHOS,** phosphate; **SOD,** sodium; **POT,** potassium; **MAG,** magnesium

CHOL (g)	V-A (RE)	THI (mg)	RIB (mg)	NIA (mg)	V-B6 (mg)	FOL (µg)	V-B12 (µg)	V-C (mg)	V-E (mg)	CALC (mg)	PHOS (mg)	SOD (mg)	POT (mg)	MAG (mg)	IRON (mg)	ZINC (mg)
45	100							9		150		890	320		3.6	
32		0.5	0.3	4.5	0.1		1.5	1		53	125	631	205	25	3.9	2.5
76		0.6	0.4	7	0.2		3.2	1		74	225	861	425	39	6	5.4
30	1700							30		300		230	620		1.8	
90		0.9	0.6	9.4	0.3		0.7	2		56	378	961	497	54	3.5	1.3
2	17	0.3	0.3	2	0.2	43	0.5	1	0.9	56	49	493	327	43	2.3	0.8
14	77	0.1	0.4	1.8	0.1	37	0.4	1		107	90	583	248	40	1.1	0.8
32	13	0.1	0.5	3.2	0.2	65	1	1	0.6	42	87	746	370	41	3	2.4
44	150	0.1	0.4	1.9	0.4	65	0.7	1	1.5	324	134	784	240	51	1.3	2.5
140	183	0.4	0.4	6	0.4	101	0.8	16		235	401	743	401	49	2	3.1
26	27							1		5		354			0.3	
78	169	0.4	0.5	9.1	0.4	109	0.5	3		258	406	1238	333	43	3.6	2.9
9	14	0.5	0.6	5.8	0.3	84	1.5	5		63	124	910	586	63	4.5	5
79	61	0.3	0.7	4.2	0.1	103	0.4	0	0.7	102	166	973	262	18	6.2	1.3
216	282	0.2	0.4	1.5	0.1	47	0.8	<1		244	348	551	174	22	2.2	1.8
50	131	0.2	0.7	3	0.2	95	1.6	5	1.5	218	224	1251	560	71	2.4	2.8
13	33	0.3	0.3	2.6	<0.1	57	<0.1	1	0.1	103	85	386	69	13	1.6	0.4
30	0							5		20		701			1.8	
29	9	0.1	0.1	1.8	0.1	14	0.9	0		15	145	452	272	20	1.8	0.4
39	59							9		59		1105			3.6	
68	130	0.5	0.4	4.2	0.1	92	1.1	3	1.8	185	311	939	353	37	3.5	1.2
0	0	0.3	0.1	4.2	0.6	51	0	5	1.3	22	233	328	930	57	2.3	1.2
37	55	0.1	0.3	1.5	0.2	112	0.7	2		189	175	882	605	85	2.2	1.7
0	0	0.1	0.1	1.2	0.2	14	0	2	0.7	12	79	373	256	14	0.5	0.2
21	62	0.1	0.3	1.1	0.1	9	0.6	2	0.7	207	228	182	395	33	0.6	0.9
51	7	0.2	0.4	3.7	<0.1	73	0.3	3		19	192	480	166	10	3.3	0.8
44	0	0.2	0.3	3.6	<0.1	48	0.5	<1	0.3	24	97	670	143	13	2.3	2
22	45	0.1	0.4	0.3	0.1	8	0.6	1	0.2	188	170	161	333	28	0.5	0.7
108	280							6		380		278			1.1	
18	154	0.2	0.4	1.5	0.2	10	0.8	1		272	276	816	172	55	1.3	1.8
14	2	0.1	0.1	0.9	0.1	55	0.1	1	0.3	73	86	430	129	16	0.8	0.3
73	50	0.4	0.4	6	0.3	71	1.8	6		41	192	845	330	67	2.8	4.4
64	25	0.1	0.5	0	<0.1	31	0.3	0		11	173	543	174	19	1.2	0.6
31	74	0.1	0.6	0.5	0.1	8	0.9	2	0.4	320	283	235	515	37	0.3	1
21	60	0.1	0.3	0.9	0.1	18	0.6	2	0.8	161	155	92	271	24	0.3	0.7
36	82	1	0.8	5.5	0.1	87	1.1	12		189	287	1651	394	68	2.5	2.6
44	93	0.1	0.4	2.5	0.2	83	0.6	4		192	143	762	416	51	2.3	2.7
41	83	0.1	0.6	3.1	0.2	75	1.2	3		217	179	896	572	64	2.9	3.7
0	236	0.1	0.1	1.1	0.2	77	0	48		27	81	54	356	23	1.3	0.4
0	0							14		0		244			0	
0	95	0.1	0.1	1	0.1	104	0	20	0.4	18	46	32	210	11	0.7	0.6

ESHA, EatRight Analysis CD-ROM; **AMT**, amount; **WT**, weight; **CAL**, calories; **WTR**, water; **PROT**, protein; **CARB**, carbohydrate; **FIBR**, fiber; **FAT**, fat; **SATF**, saturated fat; **MONO**, monosaturated fat; **POLY**, polyunsaturated fat

ESHA CODE	FOOD DESCRIPTION	AMT	UNIT	WT (g)	CAL (kcal)	WTR (g)	PROT (g)	CARB (g)	FIBR (g)	FAT (g)	SATF (g)	MONO (g)	POLY (g)
Vegetables & Legumes (continued)													
Canned (continued)													
5007	Asparagus-Spears-Canned	1	pce	18	3	17	<1	<1	<1	<1	<0.1	<0.1	0.1
7038	BakedBeans-Vegetarian-Cnd	0.5	cup	127	119	91	6	27	5	<1	0.1	0.1	0.2
5401	Bamboo Shoots-Canned Slices	1	cup	131	25	124	2	4	2	1	0.1	<0.1	0.2
5231	Beans-Green-Cannd+Liq-LowSod	1	cup	240	36	227	2	8	4	<1	0.1	<0.1	0.1
7087	Beans-Kidney-Canned+Liquid	0.5	cup	128	108	100	7	19	6	1	0.2	0.6	0.4
7051	Beans-Pinto-Canned+Liquid	0.5	cup	120	103	93	6	18	6	1	0.2	0.2	0.3
7135	Beans-Red Kidney-Canned-Drain	1	cup	256	302	176	19	55	23	1			
5310	Beets-Pickled-Slices	1	cup	227	148	186	2	37	6	<1	<0.1	<0.1	0.1
5515	Corn w/Red Pepper-Mexican	1	cup	227	170	176	5	41	5	1	0.2	0.4	0.6
5201	Corn-Canned + Liquid	0.5	cup	128	82	104	2	20	2	1	0.1	0.2	0.3
5066	Corn-Canned-Drained	0.5	cup	82	66	63	2	15	2	1	0.1	0.2	0.4
5562	Corn-White-Canned+Liquid	0.5	cup	128	82	104	2	20	1	1	0.1	0.2	0.3
5563	Corn-White-Canned-Drained	0.5	cup	82	66	63	2	15	2	1	0.1	0.2	0.4
5068	Creamed Corn-Canned	0.5	cup	128	92	101	2	23	2	1	0.1	0.2	0.3
27012	Dill Pickle	1	ea	65	8	61	<1	2	1	<1	<0.1	<0.1	<0.1
27013	Dill Pickle-Slices	10	ea	70	8	66	<1	2	1	<1	<0.1	<0.1	<0.1
7055	Fava/Broadbeans-Canned+Liq	0.5	cup	128	91	103	7	16	5	<1	<0.1	0.1	0.1
7088	GarbanzoBeans/Chickpeas+Liq	0.5	cup	120	143	84	6	27	5	1	0.1	0.3	0.6
6751	Green Beans-Canned	0.5	cup	67.5	14	63	1	3	2	<1	<0.1	<0.1	<0.1
38077	Hominy-White-Canned	1	cup	165	119	136	2	24	4	1	0.2	0.4	0.7
5470	Hominy-Yellow-Canned	1	cup	160	115	132	2	23	4	1	0.2	0.4	0.6
5293	Jalapeno Peppers-Chop-Can	0.5	cup	68	18	60	1	3	2	1	0.1	<0.1	0.3
5305	Mixed Vegetable-Canned-Drain	1	cup	163	80	142	4	15	5	<1	0.1	<0.1	0.2
5197	Mung Bean Sprouts-Canned	1	cup	125	15	120	2	3	1	<1	<0.1	<0.1	<0.1
5094	Mushroom Pieces-Canned	0.5	cup	78	20	71	1	4	2	<1	<0.1	<0.1	0.1
27009	Olives-Large-Ripe-Pitted	10	ea	44	51	35	<1	3	1	5	0.6	3.5	0.4
5281	Peas+Carrots-Canned+Liquid	1	cup	255	97	225	6	22	5	1	0.1	0.1	0.3
7016	Peas-Cowpea/Blackeye-Canned	1	cup	240	185	191	11	33	8	1	0.3	0.1	0.6
5214	Peas-Green-Canned+Liquid	0.5	cup	124	66	107	4	12	4	<1	0.1	<0.1	0.2
5267	Peas-Green-LowSod-Cnd+Liq	0.5	cup	85	45	73	3	8	3	<1	<0.1	<0.1	0.1
27016	Pickle-Sweet-Medium	1	ea	35	28	27	<1	7	<1	<1	<0.1	<0.1	0.1
5227	Pimento-Canned	1	Tbs	12	3	11	<1	1	<1	<1	<0.1	<0.1	<0.1
5228	Pimiento Slices-Canned	20	pce	20	5	19	<1	1	<1	<1	<0.1	<0.1	<0.1
5352	Potato Pieces-Canned	0.5	cup	90	54	76	1	12	2	<1	<0.1	<0.1	0.1
7024	RefriedBeans/Frijoles-Canned	1	cup	252.8	238	192	14	39	13	3	1.2	1.4	0.4
5145	Sauerkraut-Canned+Liquid	0.5	cup	118	22	109	1	5	3	<1	<0.1	<0.1	0.1
5531	Sauerkraut-Canned-LowSod	0.5	cup	71	16	66	1	3	2	<1	<0.1	<0.1	<0.1
5601	Succotash-Whole Corn-Canned	0.5	cup	127.5	80	104	3	18	3	1	0.1	0.1	0.3
5476	Tomato Puree-Canned	1	cup	250	95	220	4	22	5	1	0.1	0.1	0.2
5179	Tomatoes-Canned	0.5	cup	120	20	113	1	5	1	<1	<0.1	<0.1	0.1
5474	Tomatoes-Stewed-Cnd-LowSod	0.5	cup	127.5	33	117	1	8	1	<1	<0.1	<0.1	0.1
9522	Vegetables-Unsalt-Canned	0.5	cup	96	36	87	1	7	3	<1	<0.1	<0.1	0.1
5387	WaterChestnuts-Canned-Slices	0.5	cup	70	35	60	1	9	2	<1	<0.1	<0.1	<0.1
5553	Yams-Orange+Syrup-Canned	1	cup	228	203	176	2	48	6	<1	0.1	<0.1	0.2

< = Trace amount present   Blank = Not available

CHOL, cholesterol; **V,** vitamin; **THI,** thiamin; **RIB,** riboflavin; **NIA,** niacin; **FOL,** folate;
CALC, calcium; **PHOS,** phosphate; **SOD,** sodium; **POT,** potassium; **MAG,** magnesium

CHOL (g)	V-A (RE)	THI (mg)	RIB (mg)	NIA (mg)	V-B6 (mg)	FOL (µg)	V-B12 (µg)	V-C (mg)	V-E (mg)	CALC (mg)	PHOS (mg)	SOD (mg)	POT (mg)	MAG (mg)	IRON (mg)	ZINC (mg)
0	15	<0.1	<0.1	0.2	<0.1	17	0	3	0.1	3	8	52	31	2	0.3	0.1
0	13	0.1	<0.1	0.5	0.1	15	0	0	0.2	43	94	436	284	34	1.5	2.9
0	3	<0.1	<0.1	0.2	0.2	4	0	1	0.8	10	33	9	105	5	0.4	0.9
0	77	0.1	0.1	0.5	0.1	43	0	8	0.3	58	46	34	221	31	2.2	0.5
0	0	0.1	0.1	0.5	0.1	46	0	2	<0.1	44	115	379	303	35	1.5	0.6
0	0	0.1	0.1	0.4	0.1	72	0	1	0.7	52	110	353	292	32	1.8	0.8
0	1	0.4	0.3	1.6	0.1	179	0				333			99		2
0	5	<0.1	0.1	0.6	0.1	61	0	5	0.3	25	39	599	336	34	0.9	0.6
0	54	<0.1	0.2	2.2	0.2	77	0	20	2.5	11	141	788	347	57	1.8	0.8
0	8	<0.1	0.1	1.2	<0.1	49	0	7	<0.1	5	65	273	210	20	0.5	0.5
0	3	<0.1	<0.1	0.3	0.1	35	0	1	0.1	4	39	244	111	12	0.6	0.3
0	<1	<0.1	0.1	1.2	<0.1	49	0	7	<0.1	5	65	15	210	20	0.5	0.5
0	<1	<0.1	0.1	1	<0.1	40	0	7	0.1	4	53	265	160	16	0.7	0.3
0	10	<0.1	0.1	1.2	0.1	58	0	6	0.1	4	65	365	172	22	0.5	0.7
0	12	<0.1	<0.1	0.1	<0.1	1	0	1	0.1	27	8	569	60	5	0.2	0.1
0	13	<0.1	<0.1	0.1	<0.1	1	0	1	0.1	29	8	612	64	5	0.3	0.1
0	3	<0.1	0.1	1.2	0.1	42	0	2	0.1	33	101	580	310	41	1.3	0.8
0	2	<0.1	<0.1	0.2	0.6	80	0	5	0.2	38	108	359	206	35	1.6	1.3
0	24	<0.1	<0.1	0.1	<0.1	22	0	3	<0.1	19	14	177	75	9	0.6	0.2
0	<1	<0.1	<0.1	0.1	<0.1	2	0	0	0.1	16	58	346	15	26	1	1.7
0	19	<0.1	<0.1	0.1	<0.1	2	0	0	0.2	16	56	336	14	26	1	1.7
0	116	<0.1	<0.1	0.3	0.1	10	0	7	0.5	16	12	1136	131	10	1.3	0.2
0	1897	0.1	0.1	0.9	0.1	39	0	8	0.6	44	68	243	474	26	1.7	0.7
0	1	<0.1	0.1	0.3	<0.1	12	0	<1	<0.1	18	40	175	34	11	0.5	0.3
0	0	0.1	<0.1	1.2	<0.1	9	0	0	<0.1	9	51	332	101	12	0.6	0.6
0	18	<0.1	0	<0.1	<0.1	0	0	<1	0.7	39	1	384	4	2	1.5	0.1
0	1474	0.2	0.1	1.5	0.2	46	0	17	0.5	59	117	663	255	36	1.9	1.5
0	5	0.2	0.2	0.8	0.1	122	0	6	0.2	48	168	718	413	67	2.3	1.7
0	179	0.1	0.1	1	0.1	36	0	12	<0.1	22	66	310	124	21	1.3	0.9
0	122	0.1	0.1	0.7	0.1	25	0	8	<0.1	15	45	8	85	14	0.9	0.6
0	27	<0.1	<0.1	<0.1	<0.1	<1	0	<1	0.1	21	6	160	35	2	0.1	<0.1
0	32	<0.1	<0.1	0.1	<0.1	1	0	10	0.1	1	2	2	19	1	0.2	<0.1
0	53	<0.1	<0.1	0.1	<0.1	1	0	17	0.1	1	3	3	32	1	0.3	<0.1
0	0	0.1	<0.1	0.8	0.2	5	0	5	<0.1	4	25	197	206	13	1.1	0.3
20	0	0.1	<0.1	0.8	0.4	28	0	15	0	88	217	756	675	83	4.2	3
0	2	<0.1	<0.1	0.2	0.2	28	0	17	0.2	35	24	780	201	15	1.7	0.2
0	1	<0.1	<0.1	0.1	0.1	17	0	10	0.1	21	14	219	121	9	1	0.1
0	18	<0.1	0.1	0.8	0.1	41	0	6	1.2	14	70	282	208	24	0.7	0.6
0	130	0.1	0.2	3.7	0.3	28	0	27	4.9	45	100	998	1098	58	4.4	0.9
0	14	0.1	0.1	0.9	0.1	10	0	11	0.8	37	23	172	226	13	1.2	0.2
0	23	0.1	<0.1	0.9	<0.1	6	0	10	1.1	43	26	282	264	15	1.7	0.2
0	1117	<0.1	<0.1	0.5	0.1	17	0	4	0.3	20	36	25	132	14	0.6	0.5
0	0	<0.1	<0.1	0.3	0.1	4	0	1	0.3	3	13	6	83	4	0.6	0.3
0	1719	0.1	0.1	1	0.1	16	0	24	2.1	34	62	100	422	30	1.8	0.4

ESHA, EatRight Analysis CD-ROM; **AMT,** amount; **WT,** weight; **CAL,** calories; **WTR,** water; **PROT,** protein; **CARB,** carbohydrate; **FIBR,** fiber; **FAT,** fat; **SATF,** saturated fat; **MONO,** monosaturated fat; **POLY,** polyunsaturated fat

ESHA CODE	FOOD DESCRIPTION	AMT	UNIT	WT (g)	CAL (kcal)	WTR (g)	PROT (g)	CARB (g)	FIBR (g)	FAT (g)	SATF (g)	MONO (g)	POLY (g)
Vegetables & Legumes (continued)													
Cooked													
5314	Acorn Squash-Baked	0.5	cup	102.5	57	85	1	15	5	<1	<0.1	<0.1	0.1
5000	Artichoke-Globe-Cooked	1	ea	120	60	101	4	13	6	<1	<0.1	<0.1	0.1
5004	Asparagus-Spears-Cooked	4	pce	60	13	56	1	2	1	<1	<0.1	0	0.1
7037	Baked Beans-Homemade	1	cup	253	382	165	14	54	14	13	4.9	5.4	1.9
5249	Bamboo Shoots-Cooked Slices	1	cup	120	14	115	2	2	1	<1	0.1	<0.1	0.1
5250	Bamboo Shoots-Whole-Boiled	1	ea	144	17	138	2	3	1	<1	0.1	<0.1	0.1
7084	Bean Cake	1	ea	32	130	7	2	16	1	7	1	2.9	2.6
5319	Beans-Baby Limas-Boiled	0.5	cup	85	105	57	6	20	5	<1	0.1	<0.1	0.1
7058	Beans-Baby Limas-Dry-Boiled	0.5	cup	91	115	61	7	21	7	<1	0.1	<0.1	0.2
7012	Beans-Black-Dry-Ckd	1	cup	172	227	113	15	41	15	1	0.2	0.1	0.4
7021	Beans-Great Northern-Boiled	1	cup	177	209	122	15	37	12	1	0.2	<0.1	0.3
5011	Beans-Green-Fresh-Boiled	0.5	cup	62.5	22	56	1	5	2	<1	<0.1	<0.1	0.1
5013	Beans-Green-Frozen-Boiled	1	cup	135	38	123	2	9	4	<1	0.1	<0.1	0.1
7022	Beans-Navy-Dry-Cooked	1	cup	182	255	116	15	47	19	1	0.2	0.3	0.9
7013	Beans-Pinto-Dry-Cooked	1	cup	171	245	108	15	45	15	1	0.2	0.2	0.4
7047	Beans-Red Kidney-Boiled	1	cup	177	225	118	15	40	13	1	0.1	0.1	0.5
5022	Beets-Fresh-Diced-Cooked	0.5	cup	85	37	74	1	8	2	<1	<0.1	<0.1	0.1
5679	Broccoflower-Cooked	1	cup	156	50	140	5	10	5	<1	0.1	<0.1	0.2
5653	Broccoli Pieces-Steamed	1	cup	156	44	141	5	8	5	1	0.1	<0.1	0.3
5029	Broccoli Spear-Cooked	1	ea	180	63	161	4	13	6	1	0.1	0.1	0.3
5028	Broccoli-Pieces-Boiled	0.5	cup	78	27	70	2	6	3	<1	0.1	<0.1	0.1
5030	Broccoli-Pieces-Frozen-Cooked	1	cup	184	52	167	6	10	6	<1	<0.1	<0.1	0.1
5033	Brussels Sprouts-Cooked	1	cup	156	56	139	4	11	4	1	0.2	0.1	0.4
5035	Brussels Sprouts-Frozen-Cooked	1	cup	155	65	134	6	13	6	1	0.1	<0.1	0.3
5237	Cabbage-Bok Choy-Boiled	1	cup	170	20	162	3	3	2	<1	<0.1	<0.1	0.1
5671	Cabbage-Chinese-Steamed	0.5	cup	85	11	81	1	2	1	<1	<0.1	<0.1	0.1
5038	Cabbage-Cooked	1	cup	150	34	139	2	8	3	<1	0	<0.1	<0.1
5235	Cabbage-Pe-Tsai-Boiled	1	cup	119	17	113	2	3	2	<1	<0.1	<0.1	0.1
5047	Carrots-Cooked	0.5	cup	78	27	70	1	6	2	<1	<0.1	<0.1	0.1
5358	Carrots-Frozen-Cooked	0.5	cup	73	27	66	<1	6	2	<1	0.1	<0.1	0.2
5625	Cassava/Yuca Blanca-Cooked	1	cup	137	221	81	2	53	2	<1	0.1	0.1	0.1
5052	Cauliflower Flowerets-Boiled	3	ea	54	12	50	1	2	1	<1	<0.1	<0.1	0.1
5053	Cauliflower-Frozen-Cooked	1	cup	180	34	169	3	7	5	<1	0.1	<0.1	0.2
5061	Collard Greens-Boiled	1	cup	190	49	175	4	9	5	1	0.1	<0.1	0.3
5062	Collard Greens-Frozen-Boiled	1	cup	170	61	150	5	12	5	1	0.1	<0.1	0.4
5364	CornOnCob-Small-Frozen-Ckd	1	ea	63	59	46	2	14	2	<1	0.1	0.1	0.2
5560	CornOnCob-White-Boiled	1	ea	77	83	54	3	19	2	1	0.2	0.3	0.5
5380	CornOnCob-Yellow-Med-Boiled	1	ea	77	83	54	3	19	2	1	0.2	0.3	0.5
5393	Corn-White-Frozen-Cooked	0.5	cup	82	66	63	2	16	2	<1	0.1	0.1	0.2
5379	Corn-Yellow-Boiled	0.5	cup	82	89	57	3	21	2	1	0.2	0.3	0.5
5065	Corn-Yellow-Frozen-Boiled	0.5	cup	82	66	63	2	16	2	1	0.1	0.2	0.3
5673	Eggplant Pieces-Steamed	1	cup	96	25	88	1	6	2	<1	<0.1	<0.1	0.1
5674	Eggplant Pieces-Stir Fried	1	cup	96	25	88	1	6	2	<1	<0.1	<0.1	0.1
7027	Fava/Broadbeans-Dry-Cooked	1	cup	170	187	122	13	33	9	1	0.1	0.1	0.3
5139	French Fries-Frozen-Heated	10	pce	50	166	18	2	20	2	9	3	5.7	0.7

< = Trace amount present   Blank = Not available

CHOL, cholesterol; **V,** vitamin; **THI,** thiamin; **RIB,** riboflavin; **NIA,** niacin; **FOL,** folate;
CALC, calcium; **PHOS,** phosphate; **SOD,** sodium; **POT,** potassium; **MAG,** magnesium

CHOL (g)	V-A (RE)	THI (mg)	RIB (mg)	NIA (mg)	V-B6 (mg)	FOL (μg)	V-B12 (μg)	V-C (mg)	V-E (mg)	CALC (mg)	PHOS (mg)	SOD (mg)	POT (mg)	MAG (mg)	IRON (mg)	ZINC (mg)
0	43	0.2	<0.1	0.9	0.2	19	0	11	0.1	45	46	4	448	44	1	0.2
0	22	0.1	0.1	1.2	0.1	61	0	12	0.2	54	103	114	425	72	1.5	0.6
0	60	0.1	0.1	0.7	<0.1	89	0	5	0.9	14	32	8	134	8	0.5	0.4
13	0	0.3	0.1	1	0.2	121	0	3	1.3	154	276	1068	906	109	5	1.8
0	0	<0.1	0.1	0.4	0.1	2	0	0	0.8	14	24	5	640	4	0.3	0.6
0	0	<0.1	0.1	0.4	0.1	3	0	0	1	17	29	6	768	4	0.3	0.7
0	0	0.1	<0.1	0.5	<0.1	9	0	0	1.2	3	21	1	58	6	0.7	0.2
0	32	0.1	0.1	0.9	0.2	22	0	9	0.1	27	110	14	484	63	2.1	0.7
0	0	0.1	0.1	0.6	0.1	136	0	0	0.2	26	116	3	365	48	2.2	0.9
0	1	0.4	0.1	0.9	0.1	256	0	0	0.1	46	241	2	611	120	3.6	1.9
0	<1	0.3	0.1	1.2	0.2	181	0	2	0.5	120	292	4	692	88	3.8	1.6
0	44	<0.1	0.1	0.4	<0.1	21	0	6	0.3	28	18	1	91	11	0.4	0.2
0	76	<0.1	0.1	0.5	0.1	31	0	6	0.1	57	39	1	215	26	0.9	0.3
0	0	0.4	0.1	1.2	0.3	255	0	2	<0.1	126	262	0	708	96	4.3	1.9
0	0	0.3	0.1	0.5	0.4	294	0	1	1.6	79	251	2	746	86	3.6	1.7
0	0	0.3	0.1	1	0.2	230	0	2	1.5	50	251	4	713	80	5.2	1.9
0	3	<0.1	<0.1	0.3	0.1	68	0	3	<0.1	14	32	65	259	20	0.7	0.3
0	11	0.1	0.1	1.2	0.3	76	0	98	0.5	50	100	36	502	31	1.1	0.8
0	228	0.1	0.2	0.9	0.2	94	0	123	0.7	75	103	42	505	39	1.4	0.6
0	277	0.1	0.2	1	0.4	194	0	117	2.6	72	121	74	527	38	1.2	0.8
0	120	<0.1	0.1	0.4	0.2	84	0	51	1.1	31	52	32	229	16	0.5	0.4
0	206	0.1	0.1	0.8	0.2	103	0	74	2.4	61	90	20	261	24	1.1	0.5
0	122	0.2	0.1	0.9	0.3	94	0	97	0.7	56	87	33	495	31	1.9	0.5
0	143	0.2	0.2	0.8	0.4	157	0	71	0.8	40	87	23	450	28	0.7	0.4
0	721	0.1	0.1	0.7	0.3	70	0	44	0.2	158	49	58	631	19	1.8	0.3
0	242	<0.1	0.1	0.4	0.1	47	0	33	0.1	89	31	55	214	16	0.7	0.2
0	12	0.1	0.1	0.4	0.2	45	0	56	0.2	72	50	12	294	22	0.3	0.3
0	114	0.1	0.1	0.6	0.2	63	0	19	0.1	38	46	11	268	12	0.4	0.3
0	1342	0.1	<0.1	0.5	0.1	11	0	3	0.8	23	23	45	183	8	0.3	0.2
0	1213	<0.1	<0.1	0.3	0.1	8	0	2	0.7	26	23	43	140	8	0.4	0.3
0	2	0.1	0.1	1.1	0.1	24	0	19	0.3	21	34	18	338	28	0.4	0.4
0	1	<0.1	<0.1	0.2	0.1	24	0	24	<0.1	9	17	8	77	5	0.2	0.1
0	9	0.1	0.1	0.6	0.2	74	0	56	0.1	31	43	32	250	16	0.7	0.2
0	1543	0.1	0.2	1.1	0.2	177	0	35	1.7	266	57	30	220	38	2.2	0.4
0	1955	0.1	0.2	1.1	0.2	129	0	45	2.1	357	46	85	427	51	1.9	0.5
0	15	0.1	<0.1	1	0.1	20	0	3	0.1	2	47	3	158	18	0.4	0.4
0	<1	0.2	0.1	1.2	<0.1	35	0	5	0.1	2	79	13	192	25	0.5	0.4
0	20	0.2	0.1	1.2	<0.1	35	0	5	0.1	2	79	13	192	25	0.5	0.4
0	<1	0.1	0.1	1.1	0.1	25	0	3	0.1	3	47	4	121	16	0.3	0.3
0	21	0.2	0.1	1.3	<0.1	38	0	5	0.1	2	84	14	204	26	0.5	0.4
0	16	<0.1	0.1	1.1	0.1	29	0	3	0.1	2	65	1	191	23	0.4	0.5
0	8	<0.1	<0.1	0.5	0.1	16	0	1	<0.1	7	21	3	208	13	0.3	0.1
0	7	<0.1	<0.1	0.5	0.1	15	0	1	<0.1	7	21	3	208	13	0.3	0.1
0	3	0.2	0.2	1.2	0.1	177	0	1	<0.1	61	212	8	456	73	2.5	1.7
0	0	<0.1	<0.1	1.3	0.1	11	0	3	0.2	6	48	306	270	12	0.8	0.2

ESHA, EatRight Analysis CD-ROM; **AMT**, amount; **WT**, weight; **CAL**, calories; **WTR**, water; **PROT**, protein; **CARB**, carbohydrate; **FIBR**, fiber; **FAT**, fat; **SATF**, saturated fat; **MONO**, monosaturated fat; **POLY**, polyunsaturated fat

ESHA CODE	FOOD DESCRIPTION	AMT	UNIT	WT (g)	CAL (kcal)	WTR (g)	PROT (g)	CARB (g)	FIBR (g)	FAT (g)	SATF (g)	MONO (g)	POLY (g)
Vegetables & Legumes (continued)													
Cooked (continued)													
5791	French Fries-Cottage Cut-Frzn	10	pce	65	99	43	2	16	2	4	1.8	1.5	0.3
5536	Fried Green Tomatoes	1	ea	144	284	97	5	19	1	22	4.6	9.4	6.4
7001	GarbanzoBeans/Chickpeas-Ckd	1	cup	164	269	99	15	45	12	4	0.4	1	1.9
5140	HashBrownPotatoes-Frzn-Ckd	1	cup	78	170	44	2	22	2	9	3.5	4	1
5141	HashBrowns-Frozen-FriedPatty	1	ea	29	63	16	1	8	1	3	1.3	1.5	0.4
5640	Hominy-Cooked	1	cup	165	119	136	2	24	4	1	0.2	0.4	0.7
5075	Kale-Cooked	1	cup	130	36	119	2	7	3	1	0.1	<0.1	0.3
7006	Lentils-Cooked	1	cup	198	230	138	18	40	16	1	0.1	0.1	0.3
7503	Miso (soybean)	1	cup	275	547	118	32	73	15	17	3.1	3.4	8.8
5187	Mixed Vegetables-Frzn-Cooked	1	cup	182	118	151	5	24	8	<1	0.1	<0.1	0.1
5021	Mung Bean Sprouts-Boiled	1	cup	124	26	116	3	5	1	<1	<0.1	<0.1	<0.1
5092	Mushroom Pieces-Boiled	0.5	cup	78	22	71	2	4	2	<1	<0.1	<0.1	0.1
5096	Mustard Greens-Boiled	1	cup	140	21	132	3	3	3	<1	<0.1	0.2	0.1
7508	Natto-Soybean-Fermented	1	cup	175	371	96	31	25	9	19	2.8	4.3	10.9
5098	Okra Pods-Boiled	8	ea	85	19	79	2	4	2	<1	<0.1	<0.1	<0.1
5100	Okra Pods-Frozen-Boiled	0.5	cup	92	26	84	2	5	3	<1	0.1	<0.1	0.1
5099	Okra Slices-Boiled	0.5	cup	80	18	74	1	4	2	<1	<0.1	<0.1	<0.1
5108	Onions-Boiled	0.5	cup	105	46	92	1	11	1	<1	<0.1	<0.1	0.1
5212	Parsnips-Boiled	1	cup	156	111	125	2	27	6	<1	0.1	0.2	0.1
5123	Peas+Carrots-Frozen-Boiled	0.5	cup	80	38	69	2	8	2	<1	0.1	<0.1	0.2
7018	Peas-Cowpea/Blackeye-Dry-Boil	1	cup	172	200	120	13	36	11	1	0.2	0.1	0.4
5117	Peas-Green-Boiled	0.5	cup	80	67	62	4	13	4	<1	<0.1	<0.1	0.1
5118	Peas-Greens-Frozen-Boiled	0.5	cup	80	62	64	4	11	4	<1	<0.1	<0.1	0.1
5126	Pepper-Sweet Green-Cooked	0.5	cup	68	19	62	1	5	1	<1	<0.1	<0.1	0.1
5265	Potato Puffs-Heated f/Frzn	1	cup	128	243	76	3	36	3	11	2.3	7.7	0.6
5339	Potato Skin-Oven Baked	1	ea	58	115	27	2	27	5	<1	<0.1	<0.1	<0.1
5130	Potato-Baked-Flesh-Medium	0.5	cup	61	57	46	1	13	1	<1	<0.1	<0.1	<0.1
5947	Potato-Baked-Salted w/Skin	1	ea	202	188	151	5	43	4	<1	0.1	<0.1	0.1
5269	Potatoes-O'brien-Frozen-Cooked	0.5	cup	97	198	60	2	21	2	13	3.2	5.6	3.4
5136	Potato-Peeled-Boiled-Pieces	0.5	cup	78	67	60	1	16	1	<1	<0.1	<0.1	<0.1
5238	Red Cabbage-Boiled	0.5	cup	75	22	68	1	5	2	<1	<0.1	<0.1	0.1
5969	Rutabaga-Mashed-w/Salt	0.5	cup	120	47	107	2	10	2	<1	<0.1	<0.1	0.1
5385	Shiitake Mushroom-Boiled Piece	1	cup	145	81	121	2	21	3	<1	0.1	0.1	<0.1
5122	Snow Pea Pods-Boiled	1	cup	160	67	142	5	11	4	<1	0.1	<0.1	0.2
5296	Snow Pea Pods-Frozen-Boiled	0.5	cup	80	42	69	3	7	2	<1	0.1	<0.1	0.1
7015	Soybeans-Dry-Cooked	1.25	cup	215	372	134	36	21	13	19	2.8	4.3	10.9
5147	Spinach-Boiled	0.5	cup	90	21	82	3	3	2	<1	<0.1	<0.1	0.1
7020	Split Peas-Cooked	1	cup	196	231	136	16	41	16	1	0.1	0.2	0.3
5317	Squash-Butternut-Baked	0.5	cup	102.5	41	90	1	11	3	<1	<0.1	<0.1	<0.1
5453	Squash-Hubbard-Baked	0.5	cup	120	60	102	3	13	3	1	0.2	0.1	0.3
5455	Squash-Spaghetti-Boiled	0.5	cup	77.5	21	72	1	5	1	<1	<0.1	<0.1	0.1
5152	Squash-Summer-Boiled	0.5	cup	90	18	84	1	4	1	<1	0.1	<0.1	0.1
5303	Squash-Winter-Baked	0.5	cup	102.5	38	91	1	9	3	<1	0.1	<0.1	0.2
5155	Sweet Potato-Baked+Skin	1	ea	114	103	86	2	24	4	<1	<0.1	<0.1	0.1
5166	Sweet Potatoes-Candied	1	pce	105	151	70	1	29	3	3	1.4	0.7	0.2

< = Trace amount present   Blank = Not available

CHOL, cholesterol; **V,** vitamin; **THI,** thiamin; **RIB,** riboflavin; **NIA,** niacin; **FOL,** folate;
CALC, calcium; **PHOS,** phosphate; **SOD,** sodium; **POT,** potassium; **MAG,** magnesium

CHOL (g)	V-A (RE)	THI (mg)	RIB (mg)	NIA (mg)	V-B6 (mg)	FOL (μg)	V-B12 (μg)	V-C (mg)	V-E (mg)	CALC (mg)	PHOS (mg)	SOD (mg)	POT (mg)	MAG (mg)	IRON (mg)	ZINC (mg)
0	0	0.1	<0.1	1.2	0.1	10	0	5	0.1	5	30	21	220	10	0.7	0.2
41	82	0.2	0.2	1.4	0.1	13	0.1	21	3	101	102	134	254	17	1.5	0.4
0	3	0.2	0.1	0.9	0.2	282	0	2	0.6	80	276	11	477	79	4.7	2.5
0	0	0.1	<0.1	1.9	0.1	5	0	5	0.1	12	56	27	340	13	1.2	0.2
0	0	<0.1	<0.1	0.7	<0.1	2	0	2	0.1	4	21	10	126	5	0.4	0.1
0	0	<0.1	<0.1	0.1	<0.1	2	0	0	0.1	16	58	346	15	26	1	1.7
0	1771	0.1	0.1	0.6	0.2	17	0	53	1.1	94	36	30	296	23	1.2	0.3
0	2	0.3	0.1	2.1	0.4	358	0	3	0.2	38	356	4	731	71	6.6	2.5
0	22	0.3	0.6	2.5	0.5	52	0.2	0	<0.1	157	437	10252	578	132	6.8	7
0	779	0.1	0.2	1.5	0.1	35	0	6	0.8	46	93	64	308	40	1.5	0.9
0	2	0.1	0.1	1	0.1	36	0	14	0.1	15	35	12	125	17	0.8	0.6
0	0	0.1	0.2	3.5	0.1	14	0	3	<0.1	5	68	2	278	9	1.4	0.7
0	885	0.1	0.1	0.6	0.1	102	0	35	1.7	104	57	22	283	21	1	0.2
0	0	0.3	0.3	0	0.2	14	0	23	<0.1	380	304	12	1276	201	15.1	5.3
0	24	0.1	<0.1	0.7	0.2	39	0	14	0.2	65	27	5	115	31	0.2	0.4
0	31	0.1	0.1	0.7	<0.1	134	0	11	0.3	88	42	3	215	47	0.6	0.6
0	22	0.1	<0.1	0.7	0.1	37	0	13	0.2	62	26	5	108	29	0.2	0.3
0	<1	<0.1	<0.1	0.2	0.1	16	0	5	<0.1	23	37	3	174	12	0.3	0.2
0	0	0.1	0.1	1.1	0.1	90	0	20	1.6	58	108	16	573	45	0.9	0.4
0	749	0.2	0.1	0.9	0.1	21	0	6	0.4	18	39	54	126	13	0.8	0.4
0	3	0.3	0.1	0.9	0.2	358	0	1	0.5	41	268	7	478	91	4.3	2.2
0	64	0.2	0.1	1.6	0.2	50	0	11	0.1	22	94	2	217	31	1.2	1
0	168	0.2	0.1	1.2	0.1	47	0	8	<0.1	19	62	58	88	18	1.2	0.5
0	20	<0.1	<0.1	0.3	0.2	11	0	51	0.4	6	12	1	113	7	0.3	0.1
0	1	0.2	<0.1	1.9	0.2	18	0	8	0.3	18	132	614	399	22	0.8	0.4
0	1	0.1	0.1	1.8	0.4	13	0	8	<0.1	20	59	12	332	25	4.1	0.3
0	0	0.1	<0.1	0.9	0.2	5	0	8	<0.1	3	30	3	239	15	0.2	0.2
0	4	0.1	0.1	2.8	0.6	57	0	19	0.1	30	141	493	1081	57	2.2	0.7
0	17	0.1	0.1	1.4	0.4	12	0	10	0.2	19	90	42	459	33	0.9	0.5
0	<1	0.1	<0.1	1	0.2	7	0	6	<0.1	6	31	4	256	16	0.2	0.2
0	3	0.1	<0.1	0.3	0.2	18	0	26	0.1	32	25	21	196	13	0.5	0.2
0	<1	0.1	<0.1	0.9	0.1	18	0	23	0.4	58	67	305	391	28	0.6	0.4
0	0	0.1	0.2	2.2	0.2	30	0	<1	<0.1	4	42	6	170	20	0.6	1.9
0	166	0.2	0.1	0.9	0.2	46	0	77	0.6	67	88	6	384	42	3.2	0.6
0	106	0.1	0.1	0.5	0.1	28	0	18	0.4	47	46	4	174	22	1.9	0.4
0	10	0.3	0.6	0.9	0.5	116	0	4	0.8	219	527	2	1107	185	11.1	2.5
0	943	0.1	0.2	0.4	0.2	131	0	9	1.9	122	50	63	419	78	3.2	0.7
0	7	0.4	0.1	1.7	0.1	127	0	1	0.1	27	194	4	710	71	2.5	2
0	1144	0.1	<0.1	1	0.1	19	0	15	1.3	42	28	4	291	30	0.6	0.1
0	725	0.1	0.1	0.7	0.2	19	0	11	0.1	20	28	10	430	26	0.6	0.2
0	9	<0.1	<0.1	0.6	0.1	6	0	3	0.1	16	11	14	91	9	0.3	0.2
0	20	<0.1	<0.1	0.5	0.1	18	0	5	0.1	24	35	1	173	22	0.3	0.4
0	535	<0.1	0.1	0.5	0.2	20	0	10	0.1	23	19	1	247	13	0.5	0.2
0	2191	0.1	0.1	1.7	0.3	7	0	22	0.8	43	62	41	542	31	0.8	0.4
8	0	<0.1	<0.1	0.4	<0.1	12	0	7	4	27	27	74	198	12	1.2	0.2

ESHA, EatRight Analysis CD-ROM; **AMT,** amount; **WT,** weight; **CAL,** calories; **WTR,** water; **PROT,** protein; **CARB,** carbohydrate; **FIBR,** fiber; **FAT,** fat; **SATF,** saturated fat; **MONO,** monosaturated fat; **POLY,** polyunsaturated fat

ESHA CODE	FOOD DESCRIPTION	AMT	UNIT	WT (g)	CAL (kcal)	WTR (g)	PROT (g)	CARB (g)	FIBR (g)	FAT (g)	SATF (g)	MONO (g)	POLY (g)
Vegetables & Legumes (continued)													
Cooked (continued)													
5059	Swiss Chard-Boiled	0.5	cup	87.5	18	81	2	4	2	<1	<0.1	<0.1	<0.1
5302	Taro Slices-Cooked	0.5	cup	66	94	42	<1	23	3	<1	<0.1	<0.1	<0.1
5183	Turnip Cubes-Boiled	0.5	cup	78	17	73	1	4	2	<1	<0.1	<0.1	<0.1
5185	Turnip Greens-Boiled	0.5	cup	72	14	67	1	3	3	<1	<0.1	<0.1	0.1
5186	Turnip Greens-Frozen-Boiled	0.5	cup	82	24	74	3	4	3	<1	0.1	<0.1	0.1
7490	Wasabi Radish-Cooked	0.5	cup	73.5	12	70	<1	3	1	<1	0.1	<0.1	0.1
7053	White Beans-Boiled	1	cup	179	249	113	17	45	11	1	0.2	0.1	0.3
5160	Yams-Orange-Peeled-Boiled	1	cup	328	249	263	4	58	8	<1	0.1	0	0.2
5667	Zucchini Slices-Steamed	0.5	cup	90	13	86	1	3	1	<1	<0.1	<0.1	0.1
5327	Zucchini Squash-Boiled	0.5	cup	90	14	85	1	4	1	<1	<0.1	<0.1	<0.1
Fresh													
5010	Alfalfa Sprouts	0.5	cup	16.5	4	15	1	<1	<1	<1	<0.1	<0.1	0.1
6033	Arugula-Chopped-Raw	0.5	cup	10	2	9	<1	<1	<1	<1	<0.1	<0.1	<0.1
5678	Broccoflower-Raw	1	cup	100	32	90	3	6	3	<1	<0.1	<0.1	0.1
5041	Cabbage-Bok Choy-Raw	1	cup	70	9	67	1	2	1	<1	<0.1	<0.1	0.1
5040	Cabbage-Pe Tsai-Raw-Pieces	1	cup	76	12	72	1	2	1	<1	<0.1	<0.1	0.1
5036	Cabbage-Raw-Shredded	1	cup	70	18	65	1	4	2	<1	<0.1	<0.1	<0.1
5042	Cabbage-Red-Raw	1	cup	70	22	63	1	5	1	<1	<0.1	<0.1	0.1
5046	Carrot-Raw-Grated	0.5	cup	55	23	49	1	5	2	<1	<0.1	<0.1	0.1
5045	Carrot-Raw-Whole	1	ea	72	30	64	1	7	2	<1	<0.1	<0.1	0.1
5439	Carrots-Baby-Raw-2.75inch	1	ea	10	4	9	<1	1	<1	<1	<0.1	<0.1	<0.1
5049	Cauliflower-Raw-Cup	0.5	cup	50	12	46	1	3	1	<1	<0.1	<0.1	<0.1
5054	Celery-Raw-Chopped	0.5	cup	60	10	57	<1	2	1	<1	<0.1	<0.1	<0.1
5055	Celery-Raw-Large Outer Stalk	1	ea	40	6	38	<1	1	1	<1	<0.1	<0.1	<0.1
5399	Chili Peppers-Hot Green-Raw	0.5	cup	75	30	66	2	7	1	<1	<0.1	<0.1	0.1
5288	Chili Peppers-Red-Raw Pieces	0.5	cup	75	30	66	1	7	1	<1	<0.1	<0.1	0.2
9667	Chinese Stir Fry Vegetables-Frzn	1	cup	85	25		2	6	2	0	0	0	0
6811	Cornsalad-Fresh	0.5	cup	28	6	26	1	1	<1	<1			
5071	Cucumber-Raw-Pieces w/Peel	0.5	cup	52	8	50	<1	2	<1	<1	<0.1	<0.1	<0.1
5070	Cucumber-Whole-8 inch	1	ea	301	45	287	2	11	2	<1	0.1	<0.1	0.1
5202	Escarole/Curly Endive	1	cup	50	8	47	1	2	2	<1	<0.1	<0.1	<0.1
26005	Garlic Cloves-Fresh	1	ea	3	4	2	<1	1	<1	<1	<0.1	<0.1	<0.1
9181	Jicama-Fresh	0.5	cup	65	25	59	<1	6	3	<1	<0.1	<0.1	<0.1
5206	Leeks-Raw	1	ea	89	54	74	1	13	2	<1	<0.1	<0.1	0.1
5080	Lettuce-Butterhead-Chopped	1	cup	55	7	53	1	1	1	<1	<0.1	<0.1	0.1
5083	Lettuce-Iceberg-Chopped	1	cup	55	8	53	<1	2	1	<1	<0.1	<0.1	<0.1
5084	Lettuce-Iceberg-Leaf	1	pce	15	2	14	<1	<1	<1	<1	<0.1	<0.1	<0.1
5086	Lettuce-Looseleaf-Chopped	1	cup	56	8	53	1	2	1	<1	<0.1	<0.1	<0.1
5087	Lettuce-Looseleaf-Leaf	1	pce	10	2	10	<1	<1	<1	<1	<0.1	<0.1	<0.1
5090	Mushroom Slices-Raw	0.5	cup	35	8	32	1	1	<1	<1	<0.1	0	<0.1
5091	Mushroom-Raw-Whole	1	ea	23	5	21	1	1	<1	<1	<0.1	0	<0.1
5106	Onion Slices-Raw	1	pce	38	15	34	<1	4	1	<1	<0.1	<0.1	<0.1
5104	Onion-Raw-Medium-Whole	1	ea	110	44	98	1	10	2	<1	<0.1	<0.1	<0.1
5101	Onions-Chopped-Raw	1	cup	160	64	143	2	15	3	<1	0.1	<0.1	<0.1
26012	Parsley-Fresh-Chopped	0.5	cup	30	11	26	1	2	1	<1	<0.1	0.1	<0.1

< = Trace amount present   Blank = Not available

CHOL, cholesterol; **V,** vitamin; **THI,** thiamin; **RIB,** riboflavin; **NIA,** niacin; **FOL,** folate; **CALC,** calcium; **PHOS,** phosphate; **SOD,** sodium; **POT,** potassium; **MAG,** magnesium

CHOL (g)	V-A (RE)	THI (mg)	RIB (mg)	NIA (mg)	V-B6 (mg)	FOL (μg)	V-B12 (μg)	V-C (mg)	V-E (mg)	CALC (mg)	PHOS (mg)	SOD (mg)	POT (mg)	MAG (mg)	IRON (mg)	ZINC (mg)
0	536	<0.1	0.1	0.3	0.1	8	0	16	1.7	51	29	157	480	75	2	0.3
0	5	0.1	<0.1	0.3	0.2	13	0	3	1.9	12	50	10	319	20	0.5	0.2
0	0	<0.1	<0.1	0.2	0.1	7	0	9	<0.1	26	20	12	138	7	0.1	0.1
0	549	<0.1	0.1	0.3	0.1	85	0	20	1.4	99	21	21	146	16	0.6	0.1
0	882	<0.1	0.1	0.4	0.1	32	0	18	2.2	125	28	12	184	21	1.6	0.3
0	0	0	<0.1	0.1	<0.1	12	0	11	0	12	18	10	209	7	0.1	0.1
0	0	0.2	0.1	0.3	0.2	145	0	0	1.7	161	202	11	1004	113	6.6	2.5
0	5163	0.2	0.2	1.8	0.5	20	0	42	3.1	89	105	89	754	59	2.4	0.7
0	29	0.1	<0.1	0.3	0.1	17	0	7	0.1	14	29	3	223	20	0.4	0.2
0	101	<0.1	<0.1	0.4	0.1	15	0	4	0.1	12	36	3	228	20	0.3	0.2
0	3	<0.1	<0.1	0.1	<0.1	6	0	1	<0.1	5	12	1	13	4	0.2	0.2
0	24	<0.1	<0.1	<0.1	<0.1	10	0	2	<0.1	16	5	3	37	5	0.1	<0.1
0	7	0.1	0.1	0.8	0.2	57	0	74	0.3	32	64	23	322	20	0.1	0.5
0	312	<0.1	<0.1	0.3	0.1	46	0	32	0.1	74	26	46	176	13	0.6	0.1
0	24	<0.1	<0.1	0.3	0.2	60	0	21	0.1	59	22	7	181	10	0.2	0.2
0	7	<0.1	<0.1	0.2	0.1	30	0	26	0.1	28	18	13	119	8	0.3	0.1
0	78	<0.1	<0.1	0.3	0.1	13	0	40	0.1	32	21	19	170	11	0.6	0.2
0	925	<0.1	<0.1	0.5	0.1	10	0	3	0.4	18	19	38	176	7	0.2	0.1
0	1211	<0.1	<0.1	0.7	0.1	14	0	4	0.5	24	25	50	230	9	0.2	0.2
0	138	<0.1	<0.1	0.1	<0.1	3	0	<1	<0.1	3	3	8	24	1	0.1	<0.1
0	1	<0.1	<0.1	0.3	0.1	28	0	23	<0.1	11	22	15	152	8	0.2	0.1
0	26	<0.1	<0.1	0.2	<0.1	22	0	2	0.2	24	14	48	156	7	0.1	0.1
0	18	<0.1	<0.1	0.1	<0.1	14	0	1	0.1	16	10	32	104	4	0.1	0.1
0	88	0.1	0.1	0.7	0.2	17	0	182	0.5	14	34	5	255	19	0.9	0.2
0	72	0.1	0.1	0.9	0.4	17	0	108	0.5	10	32	7	242	17	0.8	0.2
0	350							18		20		15	160		0.4	
0	199	<0.1	<0.1	0.1	0.1	4	0	11	<0.1	11	15	1	129	4	0.6	0.2
0	5	<0.1	<0.1	0.1	<0.1	4	0	1	<0.1	8	12	1	76	7	0.1	0.1
0	30	0.1	0.1	0.3	0.1	21	0	8	0.1	48	72	6	442	39	0.8	0.6
0	108	<0.1	<0.1	0.2	<0.1	71	0	3	0.2	26	14	11	157	8	0.4	0.4
0	0	<0.1	<0.1	<0.1	<0.1	<1	0	1	<0.1	5	5	1	12	1	0.1	<0.1
0	1	<0.1	<0.1	0.1	<0.1	8	0	13	0.3	8	12	3	98	8	0.4	0.1
0	148	0.1	<0.1	0.4	0.2	57	0	11	0.8	53	31	18	160	25	1.9	0.1
0	183	<0.1	<0.1	0.2	<0.1	40	0	2	0.1	19	18	3	131	7	0.7	0.1
0	28	<0.1	<0.1	0.1	<0.1	16	0	2	0.1	10	11	6	78	4	0.2	0.1
0	8	<0.1	<0.1	<0.1	<0.1	4	0	<1	<0.1	3	3	2	21	1	0.1	<0.1
0	414	<0.1	<0.1	0.2	0.1	21	0	10	0.2	20	16	16	109	7	0.5	0.1
0	74	<0.1	<0.1	<0.1	<0.1	4	0	2	<0.1	4	3	3	19	1	0.1	<0.1
0	0	<0.1	0.1	1.3	<0.1	6	<0.1	1	<0.1	1	30	2	111	3	0.2	0.2
0	0	<0.1	0.1	0.8	<0.1	4	<0.1	<1	<0.1	1	20	1	73	2	0.1	0.1
0	<1	<0.1	<0.1	<0.1	<0.1	7	0	3	<0.1	9	11	2	55	4	0.1	0.1
0	<1	0.1	<0.1	0.1	0.1	21	0	8	<0.1	25	32	4	161	11	0.2	0.2
0	<1	0.1	<0.1	0.2	0.2	30	0	12	<0.1	37	46	6	234	16	0.3	0.3
0	253	<0.1	<0.1	0.4	<0.1	46	0	40	0.2	41	17	17	166	15	1.9	0.3

ESHA, EatRight Analysis CD-ROM; **AMT,** amount; **WT,** weight; **CAL,** calories; **WTR,** water; **PROT,** protein; **CARB,** carbohydrate; **FIBR,** fiber; **FAT,** fat; **SATF,** saturated fat; **MONO,** monosaturated fat; **POLY,** polyunsaturated fat

ESHA CODE	FOOD DESCRIPTION	AMT	UNIT	WT (g)	CAL (kcal)	WTR (g)	PROT (g)	CARB (g)	FIBR (g)	FAT (g)	SATF (g)	MONO (g)	POLY (g)
Vegetables & Legumes (continued)													
Fresh (continued)													
5124	Peppers-Sweet Green-Fresh	0.5	cup	74.5	15	70	1	3	1	<1	<0.1	<0.1	<0.1
5125	Pepper-Sweet Green-Whole	1	ea	74	15	69	1	3	1	<1	<0.1	<0.1	<0.1
5128	Pepper-Sweet Red- Raw-Chpd	0.5	cup	74.5	19	69	1	4	2	<1	<0.1	<0.1	0.1
5441	Pepper-Sweet Yellow-Large	1	ea	186	50	171	2	12	2	<1	0.1		
5451	Radicchio-Raw-Shredded	1	cup	40	9	37	1	2	<1	<1	<0.1	<0.1	<0.1
5144	Radish-Red-Slices	0.5	cup	58	9	55	<1	2	1	<1	<0.1	<0.1	<0.1
5143	Radish-Red-Whole	10	ea	45	7	43	<1	2	1	<1	<0.1	<0.1	<0.1
5088	Romaine Lettuce-Chopped	1	cup	56	10	53	1	2	1	<1	<0.1	<0.1	0.1
5427	Shallots-Raw-Chopped	1	Tbs	10	7	8	<1	2	<1	<1	<0.1	<0.1	<0.1
5146	Spinach-Raw-Chopped	1	cup	30	7	27	1	1	1	<1	<0.1	<0.1	<0.1
5114	Spring/Green Onion-Pieces	0.5	cup	50	16	45	1	4	1	<1	<0.1	<0.1	<0.1
5178	Tomatoes-Cooked	0.5	cup	120	22	113	1	5	1	<1	<0.1	<0.1	0.1
5170	Tomatoes-Fresh-Chopped	0.5	cup	90	16	85	1	4	1	<1	<0.1	<0.1	0.1
90530	Tomatoes-Red Cherry-Fresh	1	ea	17	3	16	<1	1	<1	<1	<0.1	<0.1	<0.1
5169	Tomato-Fresh-Medium	0.5	ea	74.5	13	70	1	3	1	<1	<0.1	<0.1	0.1
5173	Tomato-Fresh-Slices	2	pce	40	7	38	<1	2	<1	<1	<0.1	<0.1	<0.1
5174	Tomato-Fresh-Wedge	1	pce	31	6	29	<1	1	<1	<1	<0.1	<0.1	<0.1
5172	Tomato-Italian/Plum-Fresh	1	ea	62	11	59	1	2	1	<1	<0.1	<0.1	0.1
5446	Tomatoes-Sun Dried	0.5	cup	27	70	4	4	15	3	1	0.1	0.1	0.3
5223	Watercress Sprigs-Fresh	10	ea	25	3	24	1	<1	<1	<1	<0.1	<0.1	<0.1
5222	Watercress-Fresh	1	cup	34	4	32	1	<1	<1	<1	<0.1	<0.1	<0.1
5326	Zucchini Squash-Raw	0.5	cup	62	10	59	1	2	1	<1	<0.1	<0.1	<0.1

< = Trace amount present   Blank = Not available

CHOL, cholesterol; **V,** vitamin; **THI,** thiamin; **RIB,** riboflavin; **NIA,** niacin; **FOL,** folate;
CALC, calcium; **PHOS,** phosphate; **SOD,** sodium; **POT,** potassium; **MAG,** magnesium

CHOL (g)	V-A (RE)	THI (mg)	RIB (mg)	NIA (mg)	V-B6 (mg)	FOL (µg)	V-B12 (µg)	V-C (mg)	V-E (mg)	CALC (mg)	PHOS (mg)	SOD (mg)	POT (mg)	MAG (mg)	IRON (mg)	ZINC (mg)
0	27	<0.1	<0.1	0.4	0.2	7	0	60	0.3	7	15	2	130	7	0.3	0.1
0	27	<0.1	<0.1	0.4	0.2	7	0	59	0.3	7	15	2	130	7	0.3	0.1
0	234	<0.1	0.1	0.7	0.2	34	0	95	1.2	5	19	3	157	9	0.3	0.2
0	37	0.1	<0.1	1.7	0.3	48	0	341	1.3	20	45	4	394	22	0.9	0.3
0	1	<0.1	<0.1	0.1	<0.1	24	0	3	0.9	8	16	9	121	5	0.2	0.2
0	<1	<0.1	<0.1	0.1	<0.1	14	0	9	0	14	12	23	135	6	0.2	0.2
0	<1	<0.1	<0.1	0.1	<0.1	11	0	7	0	11	9	18	105	4	0.2	0.1
0	325	<0.1	<0.1	0.2	<0.1	76	0	13	0.1	18	17	4	138	8	0.5	0.1
0	12	<0.1	<0.1	<0.1	<0.1	3	0	1	<0.1	4	6	1	33	2	0.1	<0.1
0	281	<0.1	0.1	0.2	0.1	58	0	8	0.6	30	15	24	167	24	0.8	0.2
0	50	<0.1	<0.1	0.3	<0.1	32	0	9	0.3	36	18	8	138	10	0.7	0.2
0	58	<0.1	<0.1	0.6	0.1	16	0	27	0.7	13	34	13	262	11	0.8	0.2
0	76	<0.1	<0.1	0.5	0.1	14	0	11	0.5	9	22	4	213	10	0.2	0.2
0	14	<0.1	<0.1	0.1	<0.1	3	0	2	0.1	2	4	1	40	2	<0.1	<0.1
0	63	<0.1	<0.1	0.4	0.1	11	0	9	0.4	7	18	4	177	8	0.2	0.1
0	34	<0.1	<0.1	0.2	<0.1	6	0	5	0.2	4	10	2	95	4	0.1	0.1
0	26	<0.1	<0.1	0.2	<0.1	5	0	4	0.2	3	7	2	73	3	0.1	0.1
0	52	<0.1	<0.1	0.4	<0.1	9	0	8	0.3	6	15	3	147	7	0.2	0.1
0	24	0.1	0.1	2.4	0.1	18	0	11	<0.1	30	96	566	925	52	2.5	0.5
0	118	<0.1	<0.1	0.1	<0.1	2	0	11	0.2	30	15	10	82	5	0.1	<0.1
0	160	<0.1	<0.1	0.1	<0.1	3	0	15	0.3	41	20	14	112	7	0.1	<0.1
0	12	<0.1	0.1	0.3	0.1	18	0	11	0.1	9	24	6	162	11	0.2	0.2

Starch List

Cereals, grains, pasta, breads, crackers, snacks, starchy vegetables, and cooked beans, peas, and lentils are starches. In general, one starch is:

- ½ cup of cooked cereal, grain, or starchy vegetable
- ⅓ cup of cooked rice or pasta
- 1 ounce of a bread product, such as 1 slice of bread
- ¾ to 1 ounce of most snack foods (some snack foods may also have added fat)

One starch exchange equals

**15 grams carbohydrate,
3 grams protein,
0–1 gram fat,
and 80 calories.**

Bread

Bagel	¼ (1 oz)
Bread, reduced-calorie	2 slices (1½ oz)
Bread, white, whole-wheat, pumpernickel, rye	1 slice (1 oz)
Bread sticks, crisp, 4 in. long x ½ in.	4 (⅔ oz)
English muffin	½
Hot dog or hamburger bun	½ (1 oz)
Naan, 8 × 2 in.	¼
Pancake, 4 in. across, ¼ in. thick	1
Pita, 6 in. across	½
Roll, plain, small	1 (1 oz)
Raisin bread, unfrosted	1 slice (1 oz)
Tortilla, corn, 6 in. across	1
Tortilla, flour, 6 in. across	1
Tortilla, flour, 10 in. across	⅓
Waffle, 4 in. square, reduced-fat	1

Cereals and Grains

Bran cereals	½ cup
Bulgur	½ cup
Cereals, cooked	½ cup
Cereals, unsweetened, ready-to-eat	¾ cup
Cornmeal (dry)	3 Tbsp
Couscous	⅓ cup
Flour (dry)	3 Tbsp
Granola, low-fat	¼ cup
Grape-Nuts®	¼ cup
Grits	½ cup
Kasha	½ cup
Millet	⅓ cup
Muesli	¼ cup
Oats	½ cup

Pasta	⅓ cup
Puffed cereal	1½ cups
Rice, white or brown	⅓ cup
Shredded Wheat®	½ cup
Sugar-frosted cereal	½ cup
Wheat germ	3 Tbsp

Starchy Vegetables

Baked beans	⅓ cup
Corn	½ cup
Corn on cob, large	½ cob (5 oz)
Mixed vegetables with corn, peas, or pasta	1 cup
Peas, green	½ cup
Plantain	½ cup
Potato, baked with skin	¼ large (3 oz)
Potato, boiled	½ cup or ½ medium (3 oz)
Potato, mashed	½ cup
Squash, winter (acorn, butternut, pumpkin)	1 cup
Yam, sweet potato, plain	½ cup

Crackers and Snacks

Animal crackers	8
Graham crackers, 2½ in. square	3
Matzoh	¾ oz
Melba toast	4 slices
Oyster crackers	24
Popcorn (popped, no fat added, or low-fat microwave)	3 cups
Pretzels	¾ oz
Rice cakes, 4 in. across	2
Saltine-type crackers	6
Snack chips, fat-free or baked (tortilla, potato)	15–20 (¾ oz)
Whole-wheat crackers, no fat added	2–5 (¾ oz)

Beans, Peas, and Lentils

(Count as 1 starch exchange, plus 1 very lean meat exchange.)

Beans and peas (garbanzo, pinto, kidney, white, split, black-eyed)	½ cup
Lima beans	⅔ cup
Lentils	½ cup
Miso ◥	3 Tbsp

Starchy Foods Prepared with Fat

(Count as 1 starch exchange, plus 1 fat exchange.)

Biscuit, 2½ in. across	1
Chow mein noodles	½ cup
Cornbread, 2 in. cube	1 (2 oz)
Crackers, round butter type	6
Croutons	1 cup
French-fried potatoes (oven-baked)	1 cup (2 oz)

◥ = 400 mg or more of sodium per serving.

Granola . . . . ¼ cup

Hummus . . . . ⅓ cup

Muffin, 5 oz . . . . ⅕ (1 oz)

Popcorn, microwave . . . . 3 cups

Sandwich crackers, cheese or peanut butter filling 3

Snack chips (potato, tortilla) . . . . 9–13 (¾ oz)

Stuffing, bread (prepared) . . . . ⅓ cup

Taco shell, 6 in. across 2

Waffle, 4 in. square or across 1

Whole-wheat crackers, fat added . . . . 4–6 (1 oz)

Fruit Juice, Unsweetened

Fresh, frozen, canned, and dried fruits and fruit juices are on this list. In general, one fruit exchange is:

- 1 small fresh fruit (4 oz)
- ½ cup of canned or fresh fruit or unsweetened fruit juice
- ¼ cup of dried fruit

One fruit exchange equals

15 grams carbohydrate and 60 calories.
The weight includes skin, core, seeds, and rind.

Fruit

Apple, unpeeled, small . . . . 1 (4 oz)

Applesauce, unsweetened . . . . ½ cup

Apples, dried . . . . 4 rings

Apricots, fresh . . . . 4 whole (5½ oz)

Apricots, dried . . . . 8 halves

Apricots, canned . . . . ½ cup

Banana, small . . . . 1 (4 oz)

Blackberries . . . . ¾ cup

Blueberries . . . . ¾ cup

Cantaloupe, small . . . . ⅓ melon (11 oz) or 1 cup cubes

Cherries, sweet, fresh . . . . 12 (3 oz)

Cherries, sweet, canned . . . . ½ cup

Dates 3

Figs, fresh . . . . 1½ large or 2 medium (3½ oz)

Figs, dried 1½

Fruit cocktail . . . . ½ cup

Grapefruit, large . . . . ½ (11 oz)

Grapefruit sections, canned . . . . ¾ cup

Grapes, small . . . . 17 (3 oz)

Honeydew melon . . . . 1 slice (10 oz) or 1 cup cubes

Kiwi . . . . 1 (3½ oz)

Mandarin oranges, canned . . . . ¾ cup

Mango, small . . . . ½ fruit (5½ oz) or ½ cup

Nectarine, small . . . . 1 (5 oz)

Orange, small . . . . 1 (6½ oz)

Papaya . . . . ½ fruit (8 oz) or 1 cup cubes

Peach, medium, fresh . . . . 1 (4 oz)

Peaches, canned . . . . ½ cup

Pear, large, fresh . . . . ½ (4 oz)

Pears, canned . . . . ½ cup

Pineapple, fresh . . . . ¾ cup

Pineapple, canned . . . . ½ cup

Plums, small . . . . 2 (5 oz)

Plums, canned . . . . ½ cup

Plums, dried (prunes) 3

Raisins . . . . 2 Tbsp

Raspberries . . . . 1 cup

Strawberries . . . . 1¼ cup whole berries

Tangerines, small . . . . 2 (8 oz)

Watermelon . . . . 1 slice (13½ oz) or 1¼ cup cubes

Fruit Juice

Apple juice/cider . . . . ½ cup

Cranberry juice cocktail . . . . ⅓ cup

Cranberry juice cocktail, reduced-calorie . . . . 1 cup

Fruit juice blends, 100% juice . . . . ⅓ cup

Grape juice . . . . ⅓ cup

Grapefruit juice . . . . ½ cup

Orange juice . . . . ½ cup

Pineapple juice . . . . ½ cup

Prune juice . . . . ⅓ cup

Milk List

Different types of milk and milk products are on this list. Cheeses are on the Meat and Meat Substitutes List, and cream and other dairy fats are on the Fat List. Based on the amount of fat they contain, milks are divided into fat-free/low-fat milk, reduced-fat milk, and whole milk. One choice of these includes the following.

	Carbohydrate (grams)	Protein (grams)	Fat (grams)	Calories
Fat-free/ low-fat (½% or 1%)	12	8	0–3	90
Reduced-fat (2%)	12	8	5	120
Whole	12	8	8	150

One milk exchange equals

12 grams carbohydrate and 8 grams protein.

Fat-Free and Low-Fat Milk

(0–3 grams fat per serving)

½% milk . . . . 1 cup

1% milk . . . . 1 cup

Buttermilk, fat-free or low-fat . . . . 1 cup

Evaporated fat-free milk . . . . ½ cup

Fat-free dry milk . . . . ⅓ cup dry

Fat-free milk . . . . 1 cup

Nonfat flavored yogurt sweetened with non-nutritive
sweetener and fructose . . . . ⅔ cup (6 oz)

Plain nonfat yogurt . . . . ⅔ cup (6 oz)

Soy milk, low-fat or fat-free . . . . 1 cup

Reduced-Fat Milk

(5 grams fat per serving)

2% milk	1 cup
Plain low-fat yogurt	¾ cup
Soy milk	1 cup
Sweet acidophilus milk	1 cup

Whole Milk

(8 grams fat per serving)

Evaporated whole milk	½ cup
Goat's milk	1 cup
Kefir	1 cup
Whole milk	1 cup
Yogurt, plain (made from whole milk)	¾ cup

Sweets, Desserts, and Other Carbohydrates List

Substitute food choices from this list for a starch, fruit, or milk choice on your meal plan. Some choices will also count as one or more fat choices.

One exchange equals

15 grams carbohydrate,
or 1 starch,
or 1 fruit,
or 1 milk.

Food	Serving Size	Exchanges per Serving
Angel food cake, unfrosted	1/12th cake (about 2 oz)	2 carbohydrates
Brownie, small, unfrosted	2 in. square (about 1 oz)	1 carbohydrate, 1 fat
Cake, unfrosted	2 in. square (about 1 oz)	1 carbohydrate, 1 fat
Cake, frosted	2 in. square (about 2 oz)	2 carbohydrates, 1 fat
Cookie or sandwich cookie with creme filling	2 small (about ⅔ oz)	1 carbohydrate, 1 fat
Cookie, sugar-free	3 small or 1 large (¾–1 oz)	1 carbohydrate, 1–2 fats
Cranberry sauce, jellied	¼ cup	1½ carbohydrates
Cupcake, frosted	1 small (about 2 oz)	2 carbohydrates, 1 fat
Doughnut, plain cake	1 medium (1½ oz)	1½ carbohydrates, 2 fats
Doughnut, glazed	3¾ in. across (2 oz)	2 carbohydrates, 2 fats
Energy, sport, or breakfast bar	1 bar (1⅓ oz)	1½ carbohydrates, 0–1 fat
Energy, sport, or breakfast bar	1 bar (2 oz)	2 carbohydrates, 1 fat
Fruit cobbler	½ cup (3½ oz)	3 carbohydrates, 1 fat
Fruit juice bars, frozen, 100% juice	1 bar (3 oz)	1 carbohydrate
Fruit snacks, chewy (pureed fruit concentrate)	1 roll (¾ oz)	1 carbohydrate
Fruit spreads, 100% fruit	1½ Tbsp	1 carbohydrate
Gelatin, regular	½ cup	1 carbohydrate
Gingersnaps	3	1 carbohydrate
Granola or snack bar, regular or low fat	1 bar (1 oz)	1½ carbohydrates
Honey	1 Tbsp	1 carbohydrate
Ice cream	½ cup	1 carbohydrate, 2 fats
Ice cream, light	½ cup	1 carbohydrate, 1 fat
Ice cream, low-fat	½ cup	1½ carbohydrates
Ice cream, fat-free, no sugar added	½ cup	1 carbohydrate
Jam or jelly, regular	1 Tbsp	1 carbohydrate
Milk, chocolate, whole	1 cup	2 carbohydrates, 1 fat
Pie, fruit, 2 crusts	⅙ pie of 8 in. commercially prepared pie	3 carbohydrates, 2 fats
Pie, pumpkin or custard	⅛ pie of 8 in. commercially prepared pie	2 carbohydrates, 2 fats
Pudding, regular (made with reduced-fat milk)	½ cup	2 carbohydrates
Pudding, sugar-free or sugar-free and fat-free (made with fat-free milk)	½ cup	1 carbohydrate
Reduced-calorie meal replacement (shake)	1 can (10–11 oz)	1½ carbohydrates, 0–1 fat
Rice milk, low-fat or fat-free, plain	1 cup	1 carbohydrate
Rice milk, low-fat, flavored	1 cup	1½ carbohydrates

Salad dressing, fat-free ✎	¼ cup	1 carbohydrate
Sherbet, sorbet	½ cup	2 carbohydrates
Spaghetti or pasta sauce, canned ✎	½ cup	1 carbohydrate, 1 fat
Sports drinks	8 oz (1 cup)	1 carbohydrate
Sugar	1 Tbsp	1 carbohydrate
Sweet roll or Danish	1 (2½ oz)	2½ carbohydrates, 2 fats
Syrup, light	2 Tbsp	1 carbohydrate
Syrup, regular	1 Tbsp	1 carbohydrate
Syrup, regular	¼ cup	4 carboydrates
Vanilla wafers	5	1 carbohydrate, 1 fat
Yogurt, frozen	½ cup	1 carbohydrate, 0–1 fat
Yogurt, frozen fat-free	⅓ cup	1 carbohydrate
Yogurt, low-fat with fruit	1 cup	3 carbohydrates, 0–1 fat

Nonstarchy Vegetable List

Vegetables that contain small amounts of carbohydrates and calories are on this list. In general, one vegetable exchange is:

- ½ cup of cooked vegetables or vegetable juice
- 1 cup of raw vegetables

If you eat 3 cups or more of raw vegetables or 1½ cups of cooked vegetables at one meal, count them as 1 carbohydrate choice.

One vegetable exchange equals

5 grams carbohydrate,
2 grams protein,
0 grams fat, and
25 calories.

Artichoke
Artichoke hearts
Asparagus
Beans (green, wax, Italian)
Bean sprouts
Beets
Broccoli
Brussels sprouts
Cabbage
Carrots
Cauliflower
Celery
Cucumber
Eggplant
Green onions or scallions
Greens (collard, kale, mustard, turnip)
Kohlrabi
Leeks
Mixed vegetables (without corn, peas, or pasta)

Mushrooms
Okra
Onions
Pea pods
Peppers (all varieties)
Radishes
Salad greens (endive, escarole, lettuce, romaine, spinach)
Sauerkraut ✎
Spinach
Summer squash
Tomato
Tomatoes, canned
Tomato sauce ✎
Tomato/vegetable juice ✎
Turnips
Water chestnuts
Watercress
Zucchini

Meat and Meat Substitutes List

Meat and meat substitutes that contain both protein and fat are on this list. In general, one meat exchange is:

- 1 oz meat, fish, poultry, or cheese
- ½ cup beans, peas, or lentils

Based on the amount of fat they contain, meats are divided into very lean, lean, medium-fat, and high-fat lists. One ounce (one exchange) of each of these includes the following.

	Carbohydrate (grams)	Protein (grams)	Fat (grams)	Calories
Very lean	0	7	0–1	35
Lean	0	7	3	55
Medium-fat	0	7	5	75
High-fat	0	7	8	100

✎ = 400 mg or more of sodium per exchange.

Very Lean Meat and Substitutes List

One exchange equals

0 grams carbohydrate,

7 grams protein,

0–1 gram fat,

and 35 calories.

One very lean meat exchange is equal to any one of the following items.

Poultry: Chicken or turkey (white meat, no skin), Cornish hen
(no skin) . . . . 1 oz
Fish: Fresh or frozen cod, flounder, haddock, halibut, lox
(smoked salmon)✎, trout; tuna, fresh or canned in water . . . 1 oz
Shellfish: Clams, crab, lobster, scallops, shrimp, imitation
shellfish . . . . 1 oz
Game: Duck or pheasant (no skin), venison, buffalo, ostrich . . . . 1 oz
Cheese with 1 gram or less fat per ounce:
Fat-free or low-fat cottage cheese . . . . ¼ cup
Fat-free cheese . . . . 1 oz
Other:
Processed sandwich meats with 1 gram or less fat per ounce, such
as deli thin, shaved meats, chipped beef✎, turkey ham . . . . 1 oz
Egg whites 2
Egg substitutes, plain . . . . ¼ cup
Hot dogs with 1 gram or less fat per ounce✎ . . . . 1 oz
Kidney (high in cholesterol) . . . . 1 oz
Sausage with 1 gram or less fat per ounce . . . . 1 oz
Count as one very lean meat and one starch exchange:
Beans, peas, lentils (cooked) . . . . ½ cup

Lean Meat and Substitutes List

One exchange equals

0 grams carbohydrate,

7 grams protein,

3 grams fat,

and 55 calories.

One lean meat exchange is equal to any one of the following items.

Beef: USDA Select or Choice grades of lean beef trimmed of fat, such
as round, sirloin, and flank steak; tenderloin; roast (rib, chuck,
rump); steak (T-bone, porterhouse, cubed); ground round . . . 1 oz
Pork: Lean pork, such as fresh ham; canned, cured, or boiled ham;
Canadian bacon✎; tenderloin, center loin chop . . . . 1 oz
Lamb: Roast, chop, leg . . . . 1 oz
Veal: Lean chop, roast . . . . 1 oz

Poultry: Chicken, turkey (dark meat, no skin), chicken (white meat with
skin), domestic duck or goose (well-drained of fat, no skin) . . 1 oz
Fish:
Herring (uncreamed or smoked) . . . . 1 oz
Oysters . . . . 6 medium
Salmon (fresh or canned), catfish . . . . 1 oz
Sardines (canned) . . . . 2 medium
Tuna (canned in oil, drained) . . . . 1 oz
Game: Goose (no skin), rabbit . . . . 1 oz
Cheese:
4.5%-fat cottage cheese . . . . ¼ cup
Grated Parmesan . . . . 2 Tbsp
Cheeses with 3 grams or less fat per ounce . . . . 1 oz
Other:
Hot dogs with 3 grams or less fat per ounce✎ . . . . 1½ oz
Processed sandwich meat with 3 grams or less fat per
ounce, such as turkey pastrami or kielbasa . . . . 1 oz
Liver, heart (high in cholesterol) . . . . 1 oz

Medium-Fat Meat and Substitutes List

One exchange equals

0 grams carbohydrate,

7 grams protein,

5 grams fat,

and 75 calories.

One medium-fat meat exchange is equal to any one of the
following items.

Beef: Most beef products fall into this category (ground beef,
meatloaf, corned beef, short ribs, Prime grades of meat trim-
med of fat, such as prime rib) . . . . 1 oz
Pork: Top loin, chop, Boston butt, cutlet . . . . 1 oz
Lamb: Rib roast, ground . . . . 1 oz
Veal: Cutlet (ground or cubed, unbreaded) . . . . 1 oz
Poultry: Chicken dark meat (with skin), ground turkey or ground
chicken, fried chicken (with skin) . . . . 1 oz
Fish: Any fried fish product . . . . 1 oz
Cheese: With 5 grams or less fat per ounce
Feta . . . . 1 oz
Mozzarella . . . . 1 oz
Ricotta . . . . ¼ cup (2 oz)
Other:
Egg (high in cholesterol, limit to 3 per week) 1
Sausage with 5 grams or less fat per ounce . . . . 1 oz
Tempeh . . . . ¼ cup
Tofu . . . . 4 oz or ½ cup

✎ = *400 mg or more of sodium per serving.*

High-Fat Meat and Substitutes List
One exchange equals

0 grams carbohydrate,
7 grams protein,
8 grams fat,
and 100 calories.

One high-fat meat exchange is equal to any one of the following items.

Pork: Spareribs, ground pork, pork sausage . . . . 1 oz
Cheese: All regular cheeses, such as American ✎ , cheddar,
   Monterey Jack, Swiss. . . . . 1 oz
Other:
   Processed sandwich meats with 8 grams or less fat per ounce,
   such as bologna, pimento loaf, salami . . . . 1 oz
   Sausage, such as bratwurst, Italian, knockwurst, Polish,
   smoked . . . . 1 oz
   Hot dog (turkey or chicken) ✎ 1 (10/lb)
   Bacon . . . . 3 slices (20 slices/lb)
Count as one high-fat meat plus one fat exchange:
Hot dog (beef, pork, or combination) ✎ 1 (10/lb)

Fat List

Fats are divided into three groups, based on the main type of fat they contain: monounsaturated, polyunsaturated, and saturated. Monounsaturated and polyunsaturated fats in the foods we eat are linked with good health benefits. Saturated fats and fats called *trans* fatty acids or *trans* unsaturated fatty acids are linked with heart disease. In general, one fat exchange is:

- 1 teaspoon of regular margarine or vegetable oil
- 1 tablespoon of regular salad dressing

Monounsaturated Fats List
One fat exchange equals

5 grams fat and
45 calories.

Avocado, medium . . . . 2 Tbsp (1 oz)
Oil (canola, olive, peanut) . . . . 1 tsp
Olives: ripe (black) . . . . 8 large
   green, stuffed ✎ . . . . 10 large
Nuts
   almonds, cashews . . . . 6 nuts
   mixed (50% peanuts) . . . . 6 nuts
   peanuts . . . . 10 nuts
   pecans . . . . 4 halves
Peanut butter, smooth or crunchy . . . . ½ Tbsp
Sesame seeds . . . . 1 Tbsp
Tahini or sesame paste . . . . 2 tsp

Polyunsaturated Fats List
One fat exchange equals

5 grams fat and
45 calories.

Margarine: stick, tub, or squeeze . . . . 1 tsp
   lower-fat spread (30% to 50% vegetable oil) . . . . 1 Tbsp
Mayonnaise: regular . . . . 1 tsp
   reduced-fat . . . . 1 Tbsp
Nuts, walnuts, English . . . . 4 halves
Oil (corn, safflower, soybean) . . . . 1 tsp
Salad dressing: regular ✎ . . . . 1 Tbsp
   reduced-fat . . . . 2 Tbsp
Miracle Whip Salad Dressing®: regular . . . . 2 tsp
   reduced-fat . . . . 1 Tbsp
Seeds: pumpkin, sunflower . . . . 1 Tbsp

Saturated Fats List
One fat exchange equals

5 grams of fat
and 45 calories.

Bacon, cooked . . . . 1 slice (20 slices/lb)
Bacon, grease . . . . 1 tsp
Butter: stick . . . . 1 tsp
   whipped . . . . 2 tsp
   reduced-fat . . . . 1 Tbsp
Chitterlings, boiled . . . . 2 Tbsp (½ oz)
Coconut, sweetened, shredded . . . . 2 Tbsp
Coconut milk . . . . 1 Tbsp
Cream, half and half . . . . 2 Tbsp
Cream cheese: regular . . . . 1 Tbsp (½ oz)
   reduced-fat . . . . 1½ Tbsp (¾ oz)
Fatback or salt pork ✎ , see below†
Shortening or lard . . . . 1 tsp
Sour cream: regular . . . . 2 Tbsp
   reduced-fat . . . . 3 Tbsp

†Use a piece 1 in. × 1 in. × ¼ in. if you plan to eat the fatback cooked with vegetables. Use a piece 2 in. × 1 in. × ½ in. when eating only the vegetables with the fatback removed.

Free Foods List

A *free food* is any food or drink that contains less than 20 calories or less than 5 grams of carbohydrate per serving. Foods with a serving size listed should be limited to three servings per day. Foods listed without a serving size can be eaten as often as you like.

Fat-Free or Reduced-Fat Foods

Cream cheese, fat-free . . . . 1 Tbsp (½ oz)
Creamers, nondairy, liquid . . . . 1 Tbsp
Creamers, nondairy, powdered . . . . 2 tsp

✎ = 400 mg or more of sodium per exchange.

Mayonnaise, fat-free . . . . 1 Tbsp
Mayonnaise, reduced-fat . . . . 1 tsp
Margarine spread, fat-free . . . . 4 Tbsp
Margarine spread, reduced-fat . . . . 1 tsp
Miracle Whip®, fat-free. . . . . 1 Tbsp
Miracle Whip®, reduced-fat. . . . . 1 tsp
Nonstick cooking spray
Salad dressing, fat-free or low-fat . . . . 1 Tbsp
Salad dressing, fat-free, Italian . . . . 2 Tbsp
Sour cream, fat-free, reduced-fat. . . . . 1 Tbsp
Whipped topping, regular. . . . . 1 Tbsp
Whipped topping, light or fat-free . . . . 2 Tbsp

Sugar-Free Foods

Candy, hard, sugar-free . . . . 1 candy
Gelatin dessert, sugar-free
Gelatin, unflavored
Gum, sugar-free
Jam or jelly, light . . . . 2 tsp
Sugar substitutes†
Syrup, sugar-free . . . . 2 Tbsp

†*Sugar substitutes, alternatives, or replacements that are approved by the Food and Drug Administration (FDA) are safe to use. Common brand names include:*

> *Equal® (aspartame)*
> *Splenda® (sucralose)*
> *Sprinkle Sweet® (saccharin)*
> *Sweet One® (acesulfame K)*
> *Sweet-10® (saccharin)*
> *Sugar Twin® (saccharin)*
> *Sweet 'n Low® (saccharin)*

Drinks

Bouillon, broth, consommé ☙
Bouillon or broth, low-sodium
Carbonated or mineral water

Club soda
Cocoa powder, unsweetened . . . . 1 Tbsp
Coffee
Diet soft drinks, sugar-free
Drink mixes, sugar-free
Tea
Tonic water, sugar-free

Condiments

Ketchup . . . . 1 Tbsp
Horseradish
Lemon juice
Lime juice
Mustard
Pickle relish . . . . 1 Tbsp
Pickles, dill ☙ . . . . 1½ medium
Pickles, sweet (bread and butter) . . . . 2 slices
Pickles, sweet (gherkin). . . . . ¾ oz
Salsa. . . . . ¼ cup
Soy sauce, regular or light ☙ . . . . 1 Tbsp
Taco sauce . . . . 1 Tbsp
Vinegar
Yogurt . . . . 2 Tbsp

Seasonings

Be careful with seasonings that contain sodium or are salts, such as garlic or celery salt, and lemon pepper.

Flavoring extracts
Garlic
Herbs, fresh or dried
Pimento
Spices
Tabasco® or hot pepper sauce
Wine, used in cooking
Worcestershire sauce

Combination Foods List

Many of the foods we eat are mixed together in various combinations. These combination foods do not fit into any one exchange list. This is a list of exchanges for some typical combination foods.

Entrees	Serving Size	Exchanges per Serving
Tuna noodle casserole, lasagna, spaghetti with meatballs, chili with beans, macaroni and cheese ☙	1 cup (8 oz)	2 carbohydrates, 2 medium-fat meats
Chow mein (without noodles or rice) ☙	2 cups (16 oz)	1 carbohydrate, 2 lean meats
Tuna or chicken salad	½ cup (3½ oz)	½ carbohydrate, 2 lean meats, 1 fat

Frozen Entrees and Meals		
Dinner-type meal ☙	generally 14–17 oz	3 carbohydrates, 3 medium-fat meats, 3 fats
Meatless burger, soy based	3 oz	½ carbohydrate, 2 lean meats

☙ = *400 mg or more of sodium per serving.*

Meatless burger, vegetable and starch based . . . . 3 oz. . . . . 1 carbohydrate, 1 lean meat
Pizza, cheese, thin crust ✎ . . . . ¼ of 12 in. (6 oz) . . . . 2 carbohydrates, 2 medium-fat meats, 1 fat
Pizza, meat topping, thin crust ✎ . . . . ¼ of 12 in. (6 oz) . . . . 2 carbohydrates, 2 medium-fat meats, 2 fats
Pot pie ✎ . . . . 1 (7 oz) . . . . 2½ carbohydrates, 1 medium-fat meat, 3 fats
Entree or meal with less than 340 calories ✎ . . . . about 8–11 oz . . . . 2–3 carbohydrates, 1–2 lean meats

Soups

Bean ✎ . . . . 1 cup . . . . 1 carbohydrate, 1 very lean meat
Cream (made with water) ✎ . . . . 1 cup (8 oz) . . . . 1 carbohydrate, 1 fat
Instant ✎ . . . . 6 oz prepared. . . . . 1 carbohydrate
Instant with beans/lentils ✎ . . . . 8 oz prepared. . . . . 2½ carbohydrates, 1 very lean meat
Split pea (made with water) ✎ . . . . ½ cup (4 oz) . . . . 1 carbohydrate
Tomato (made with water) ✎ . . . . 1 cup (8 oz). . . . . 1 carbohydrate
Vegetable beef, chicken noodle,
or other broth-type ✎ . . . . 1 cup (8 oz). . . . . 1 carbohydrate

Fast Foods List*

Food	Serving Size	Exchanges per Serving
Burritos with beef ✎	1 (5–7 oz)	3 carbohydrates, 1 medium-fat meat, 1 fat
Chicken nuggets ✎	6	1 carbohydrate, 2 medium-fat meats, 1 fat
Chicken breast and wing, breaded and fried ✎	1 each	1 carbohydrate, 4 medium-fat meats, 2 fats
Chicken sandwich, grilled ✎	1	2 carbohydrates, 3 very lean meats
Chicken wings, hot ✎	6 (5 oz)	1 carbohydrate, 3 medium-fat meats, 4 fats
Fish sandwich/tartar sauce ✎	1	3 carbohydrates, 1 medium-fat meat, 3 fats
French fries ✎	1 medium serving (5 oz)	4 carbohydrates, 4 fats
Hamburger, regular	1	2 carbohydrates, 2 medium-fat meats
Hamburger, large ✎	1	2 carbohydrates, 3 medium-fat meats, 1 fat
Hot dog with bun ✎	1	1 carbohydrate, 1 high-fat meat, 1 fat
Individual pan pizza ✎	1	5 carbohydrates, 3 medium-fat meats, 3 fats
Pizza, cheese, thin crust ✎	¼ of 12 in. (about 6 oz)	2½ carbohydrates, 2 medium-fat meats
Pizza, meat, thin crust ✎	¼ of 12 in. (about 6 oz)	2½ carbohydrates, 2 medium-fat meats, 1 fat
Soft-serve cone.	1 small (5 oz)	2½ carbohydrates, 1 fat
Submarine sandwich ✎	1 sub (6 in)	3 carbohydrates, 1 vegetable, 2 medium-fat meats, 1 fat
Submarine sandwich ✎ (less than 6 grams fat)	1 sub (6 in)	2½ carbohydrates, 2 lean meats
Taco, hard or soft shell ✎	1 (3–3½ oz)	1 carbohydrate, 1 medium-fat meat, 1 fat

*Ask at your fast-food restaurant for nutrition information about your favorite fast foods or check Web sites.

Source: *Exchange Lists for Meal Planning. The American Diabetes Association, Alexandria, VA, and The American Dietetic Association, Chicago, IL, 2003.*

MyPyramid Food Intake Patterns

The suggested amounts of food to consume from the basic food groups, subgroups, and oils to meet recommended nutrient intakes at 12 different calorie levels. Nutrient and energy contributions from each group are calculated according to the nutrient-dense forms of foods in each group (e.g., lean meats and fat-free milk). The table also shows the discretionary calorie allowance that can be accommodated within each calorie level, in addition to the suggested amounts of nutrient-dense forms of foods in each group.

Daily Amount of Food from Each Group

Calorie Level[1]	1,000	1,200	1,400	1,600	1,800	2,000	2,200	2,400	2,600	2,800	3,000	3,200
Fruits[2]	1 cup	1 cup	1.5 cups	1.5 cups	1.5 cups	2 cups	2 cups	2 cups	2 cups	2.5 cups	2.5 cups	2.5 cups
Vegetables[3]	1 cup	1.5 cups	1.5 cups	2 cups	2.5 cups	2.5 cups	3 cups	3 cups	3.5 cups	3.5 cups	4 cups	4 cups
Grains[4]	3 oz-eq	4 oz-eq	5 oz-eq	5 oz-eq	6 oz-eq	6 oz-eq	7 oz-eq	8 oz-eq	9 oz-eq	10 oz-eq	10 oz-eq	10 oz-eq
Meat and beans[5]	2 oz-eq	3 oz-eq	4 oz-eq	5 oz-eq	5 oz-eq	5.5 oz-eq	6 oz-eq	6.5 oz-eq	6.5 oz-eq	7 oz-eq	7 oz-eq	7 oz-eq
Milk[6]	2 cups	2 cups	2 cups	3 cups	3 cups	3 cups	3 cups	3 cups	3 cups	3 cups	3 cups	3 cups
Oils[7]	3 tsp	4 tsp	4 tsp	5 tsp	5 tsp	6 tsp	6 tsp	7 tsp	8 tsp	8 tsp	10 tsp	11 tsp
Discretionary calorie allowance[8]	165	171	171	132	195	267	290	362	410	426	512	648

[1] *Calorie Levels* are set across a wide range to accommodate the needs of different individuals. The following table "MyPyramid Food Intake Pattern Calorie Levels" can be used to help assign individuals to the food intake pattern at a particular calorie level.

[2] *Fruit Group* includes all fresh, frozen, canned, and dried fruits and fruit juices. In general, 1 cup of fruit or 100% fruit juice, or 1/2 cup of dried fruit can be considered as 1 cup from the fruit group.

[3] *Vegetable Group* includes all fresh, frozen, canned, and dried vegetables and vegetable juices. In general, 1 cup of raw or cooked vegetables or vegetable juice, or 2 cups of raw leafy greens can be considered as 1 cup from the vegetable group.

Vegetable Subgroup Amounts Are per Week

Calorie Level	1,000	1,200	1,400	1,600	1,800	2,000	2,200	2,400	2,600	2,800	3,000	3,200
Dark green veg.	1 c/wk	1.5 c/wk	1.5 c/wk	2 c/wk	3 c/wk	3 c/wk	3 c/wk	3 c/wk	3 c/wk	3 c/wk	3 c/wk	3 c/wk
Orange veg.	.5 c/wk	1 c/wk	1 c/wk	1.5 c/wk	2 c/wk	2 c/wk	2 c/wk	2 c/wk	2.5 c/wk	2.5 c/wk	2.5 c/wk	2.5 c/wk
Legumes	.5 c/wk	1 c/wk	1 c/wk	2.5 c/wk	3 c/wk	3 c/wk	3 c/wk	3 c/wk	3.5 c/wk	3.5 c/wk	3.5 c/wk	3.5 c/wk
Starchy veg.	1.5 c/wk	2.5 c/wk	2.5 c/wk	2.5 c/wk	3 c/wk	3 c/wk	6 c/wk	6 c/wk	7 c/wk	7 c/wk	9 c/wk	9 c/wk
Other veg.	3.5 c/wk	4.5 c/wk	4.5 c/wk	5.5 c/wk	6.5 c/wk	6.5 c/wk	7 c/wk	7 c/wk	8.5 c/wk	8.5 c/wk	10 c/wk	10 c/wk

[4] *Grains Group* includes all foods made from wheat, rice, oats, cornmeal, and barley, such as bread, pasta, oatmeal, breakfast cereals, tortillas, and grits. In general, 1 slice of bread, 1 cup of ready-to-eat cereal, or 1/2 cup of cooked rice, pasta, or cooked cereal can be considered as 1 ounce equivalent from the grains group. At least half of all grains consumed should be whole grains.

[5] *Meat & Beans Group* in general, 1 ounce of lean meat, poultry, or fish, 1 egg, 1 Tbsp. peanut butter, 1/4 cup cooked dry beans, or 1/2 ounce of nuts or seeds can be considered as 1 ounce equivalent from the meat and beans group.

[6] *Milk Group* includes all fluid milk products and foods made from milk that retain their calcium content, such as yogurt and cheese. Foods made from milk that have little to no calcium, such as cream cheese, cream, and butter, are not part of the group. Most milk group choices should be fat-free or low-fat. In general, 1 cup of milk or yogurt, 1 1/2 ounces of natural cheese, or 2 ounces of processed cheese can be considered as 1 cup from the milk group.

[7] *Oils* include fats from many different plants and from fish that are liquid at room temperature, such as canola, corn, olive, soybean, and sunflower oil. Some foods are naturally high in oils, like nuts, olives, some fish, and avocados. Foods that are mainly oil include mayonnaise, certain salad dressings, and soft margarine.

[8] *Discretionary Calorie Allowance* is the remaining amount of calories in a food intake pattern after accounting for the calories needed for all food groups—using forms of foods that are fat-free or low-fat and with no added sugars.

MyPyramid Food Intake Pattern Calorie Levels

MyPyramid assigns individuals to a calorie level based on their sex, age, and activity level. The chart below identifies the calorie levels for males and females by age and activity level. Calorie levels are provided for each year of childhood, from 2–18 years, and for adults in 5-year increments.

	Males				Females		
Activity level	Sedentary*	Mod. active*	Active*	Activity level	Sedentary*	Mod. active*	Active*
Age				**Age**			
2	1,000	1,000	1,000	2	1,000	1,000	1,000
3	1,000	1,400	1,400	3	1,000	1,200	1,400
4	1,200	1,400	1,600	4	1,200	1,400	1,400
5	1,200	1,400	1,600	5	1,200	1,400	1,600
6	1,400	1,600	1,800	6	1,200	1,400	1,600
7	1,400	1,600	1,800	7	1,200	1,600	1,800
8	1,400	1,600	2,000	8	1,400	1,600	1,800
9	1,600	1,800	2,000	9	1,400	1,600	1,800
10	1,600	1,800	2,200	10	1,400	1,800	2,000
11	1,800	2,000	2,200	11	1,600	1,800	2,000
12	1,800	2,200	2,400	12	1,600	2,000	2,200
13	2,000	2,200	2,600	13	1,600	2,000	2,200
14	2,000	2,400	2,800	14	1,800	2,000	2,400
15	2,200	2,600	3,000	15	1,800	2,000	2,400
16	2,400	2,800	3,200	16	1,800	2,000	2,400
17	2,400	2,800	3,200	17	1,800	2,000	2,400
18	2,400	2,800	3,200	18	1,800	2,000	2,400
19–20	2,600	2,800	3,000	19–20	2,000	2,200	2,400
21–25	2,400	2,800	3,000	21–25	2,000	2,200	2,400
26–30	2,400	2,600	3,000	26–30	1,800	2,000	2,400
31–35	2,400	2,600	3,000	31–35	1,800	2,000	2,200
36–40	2,400	2,600	2,800	36–40	1,800	2,000	2,200
41–45	2,200	2,600	2,800	41–45	1,800	2,000	2,200
46–50	2,200	2,400	2,800	46–50	1,800	2,000	2,200
51–55	2,200	2,400	2,800	51–55	1,600	1,800	2,200
56–60	2,200	2,400	2,600	56–60	1,600	1,800	2,200
61–65	2,000	2,400	2,600	61–65	1,600	1,800	2,000
66–70	2,000	2,200	2,600	66–70	1,600	1,800	2,000
71–75	2,000	2,200	2,600	71–75	1,600	1,800	2,000
76 and up	2,000	2,200	2,400	76 and up	1,600	1,800	2,000

*Calorie levels are based on the Estimated Energy Requirements (EER) and activity levels from the Institute of Medicine Dietary Reference Intakes Macronutrients Report, 2002.

SEDENTARY = less than 30 minutes a day of moderate physical activity in addition to daily activities.

MOD. ACTIVE = at least 30 minutes up to 60 minutes a day of moderate physical activity in addition to daily activities.

ACTIVE = 60 or more minutes a day of moderate physical activity in addition to daily activities.

Source: U.S. Department of Agriculture, Center for Nutrition Policy and Promotion, April 2005.

> ➤ Nutrition Policies and Dietary Guidance in Canada
> ➤ Nutrient Intake Recommendations for Canadians
> ➤ Canada's Food Guide
> ➤ *Canada's Physical Activity Guide to Healthy Active Living*
> ➤ Canadian Recommendations for Healthy Living
> ➤ Nutrition Labeling for Canadians
> ➤ Canadian Diabetes Association's Meal Planning Guide

Nutrition Policies and Dietary Guidance in Canada

For more than 60 years, the Canadian government has worked to promote healthy and nutritious eating habits in its citizens. Health Canada is the federal department responsible for helping Canadians maintain and improve their health while respecting individual choices and circumstances. Health Canada provides leadership for ensuring a safe food supply and promoting good nutrition. Specifically, Health Canada is responsible for:

- Establishing policies, setting standards, and providing advice on the safety and nutritional value of food

- Promoting the nutritional health and well-being of Canadians by collaboratively defining, promoting, and implementing evidence-based nutrition policies and standards

- Administering the provisions of the Food and Drugs Act that relate to public health, safety, and nutrition

- Evaluating the safety, quality, and effectiveness of veterinary drugs

Nutrient Intake Recommendations for Canadians

Health Canada has reviewed and made recommendations on nutrient requirements on a periodic basis since 1938. Known as the Recommended Nutrient Intakes, or RNI, these values were last published in 1990 as part of *Nutrition Recommendations: The Report of the Scientific Review Committee*. Because of advances in science, by 1994 it was clear that it was time to initiate another review of the scientific data.

At the same time, the Food and Nutrition Board of the National Academy of Sciences was beginning a consultation process on the review of the Recommended Dietary Allowances, the nutrient recommendations used in the United States. Health Canada considered that participating in the U.S. review would offer several advantages to Canada. These were as follows:

- The science underlying nutrient requirements knows no borders, and scientists everywhere are utilizing the same knowledge produced from studies conducted all over the world.

- The knowledge base on nutrients, foods, and health is increasing rapidly in scope and complexity. This increases the need for specialized expertise. Participating in the U.S. review permits Canada to expand the base of scientific expertise that could be utilized.

- International trade considerations, including NAFTA, suggest that the harmonization of the science base underlying nutrition policy will facilitate harmonization of such trade-related matters as nutrition labeling and food composition.

Canadian and American scientists establish Dietary Reference Intakes (DRIs) through a review process overseen by the Food and Nutrition Board. DRIs have replaced the RNIs and are found printed inside the covers of this text.

The Food and Nutrition Board (FNB) is a unit of the Institute of Medicine, part of the National Academy of Sciences. The FNB is a multidisciplinary group of biomedical scientists with expertise in various aspects of nutrition, food sciences, biochemistry, medicine, public health, epidemiology, food toxicology, and food safety. The major focus of the FNB is to evaluate emerging knowledge of nutrient requirements and relationships between diet and the reduction of risk of common chronic diseases and to relate this knowledge to strategies for promoting health and preventing disease.

The National Academy of Sciences is an American private nonprofit society of distinguished scholars engaged in scientific and engineering research, dedicated to the advancement of science and technology and to their use for the general welfare. The Academy has a mandate that requires it to advise the U.S. federal government on scientific and technical matters.

Health Canada uses the DRIs in a variety of policies and programs that benefit the health and safety of Canadians. The DRIs influence the development of regulatory standards, assessment of dietary intakes, and the development of dietary guidance for the general population and for specific life stages. DRIs are used by nutrition practitioners, governments, and nongovernmental organizations to assess and plan the nutrient intakes of individuals and population groups.

Health Canada has an internal working group that brings together the individuals working with the DRIs from the Office of Nutrition Policy and Promotion, the Bureau of Nutritional Sciences, the Bureau of Biostatistics and Computer Applications, the Natural Health Products Directorate, and the Centre for Chronic Disease Prevention and Control. This working group guides the steps that Health Canada is taking to implement the DRIs to ensure consistency in their use and application throughout Health Canada.

Canada's Food Guide

Scientists have known for some time that adequate nutrition is essential for proper growth and development. More recently, healthy eating has been accepted as a significant factor in reducing the risk of developing nutrition-related problems, including heart disease, cancer, obesity, hypertension (high blood pressure), osteoporosis, anemia, dental decay, and some bowel disorders. Canada has had a food guide since 1942, when the Official Food Rules were released as part of a wartime nutrition program. The most recent *Food Guide to Healthy Eating* was released in 1992.

Canada's *Food Guide to Healthy Eating*

The *Food Guide* is intended to assist the people of Canada aged 2 years and older in making food choices that promote health (defined as social, mental, and physical well-being). The *Food Guide* is a basic nutrition education tool used to do the following:

- Help plan healthy meals for individuals or groups
- Evaluate a person's eating habits in a general way (but not to assess nutritional status)

It describes a pattern of eating consistent with national nutrition guidelines and comprises five key principles:

- Enjoy a variety of food.
- Emphasize cereals, breads, other grain products, vegetables, and fruit.
- Choose lower-fat dairy products, leaner meats, and food prepared with little or no fat.
- Achieve and maintain a healthy body weight by enjoying regular physical activity and healthy eating.
- Limit salt, alcohol, and caffeine.

The supporting material for the *Food Guide* helps individuals to understand and apply the information in the *Food Guide*. The *Food Guide* applies to a diverse population; individuals with special dietary requirements may need additional guidance.

A Revised *Food Guide*

Health Canada is updating Canada's *Food Guide*. The decision to revise the *Food Guide* was announced in 2004, after Health Canada conducted an extensive review of the current guide. The process to revise the *Food Guide* is evidence based, open, and linked to public health priorities.

The *Food Guide* has been a credible source of nutrition-related information in Canada for many years. To maintain and build on that credibility, the following set of principles was developed to guide the revision process:

1. The *Food Guide* will promote a pattern of eating that will meet nutrient needs, promote health, and minimize the risk of nutrition-related chronic disease.

2. Revisions to the *Food Guide* will be based on the most up-to-date evidence.

3. The *Food Guide* will be linked to public health priorities and initiatives.

4. The development of messages for the *Food Guide* will be based on the premise that they need to be easily understood and implemented by the public.

5. The process to revise the *Food Guide* will be conducted in an open and transparent manner.

Throughout the revision, Health Canada has consulted with Canadians from coast to coast, including nongovernment organizations, academics, health professionals, government, industry, and consumers. Health Canada is also working closely with three advisory groups: an external Food Guide Advisory Committee, an Interdepartmental Working Group, and a Dietary Reference Intake Committee. Final decisions related to the content of the *Food Guide* rest with Health Canada; the revised *Food Guide* is expected to be released in early 2007. To follow the progress of the revision of the *Food Guide*, go to http://healthcanada.gc.ca/foodguide.

Canada's Physical Activity Guide to Healthy Active Living

Canada's Physical Activity Guide to Healthy Active Living, produced by a joint effort of Health Canada and the Canadian Society for Exercise Physiology, provides a set of Canadian guidelines for physical activity. It provides information to help Canadians understand how to achieve health benefits by being physically active. The guide complements the popular *Canada's Food Guide to Healthy Eating* and provides concrete examples of how to incorporate physical activity into daily life.

Designed for adults, the guide recommends 60 minutes of physical activity every day to stay healthy or improve health. As a person progresses to more intense activity, he or she can cut down to 30 minutes, four days a week. The guide also suggests that Canadians can add up their activities in periods of at least 10 minutes each, starting slowly and building up.

Federal, provincial, and territorial governments are working to reduce the number of inactive Canadians. *Canada's Physical Activity Guide to Healthy Active Living* is a major step toward building the knowledge and awareness necessary for all Canadians to become more active. The Healthy Active Living series now also includes *Physical Activity Guide to Healthy Active Living for Older Adults, Physical Activity Guide for Youth, Physical Activity Guide for Children*, and *Active Living at Work*.

Canadian Recommendations for Healthy Living

Canadian citizens suffer from chronic diseases and conditions that are linked to poor health choices. Among the leading causes of death in Canada are cardiovascular diseases, cancer, type 2 diabetes, and respiratory diseases, all of which are linked to preventable risk factors such as poor diet, lack of exercise, and smoking. In addition, the prevalence of overweight and obesity in Canada has increased; today nearly 60 percent of adults are overweight or obese. To address these and other health concerns, the federal, provincial, and territorial ministers of health developed the Healthy Living Strategy for Canada. The Healthy Living Strategy is "a conceptual framework for sustained action based on a population health approach."[1] Its vision is a healthy nation in which all Canadians experience the conditions that support the attainment of good health. The goals of the strategy are to improve overall health outcomes and reduce health disparities.

To address these goals, the ministers have proposed pan-Canadian Healthy Living targets, seeking to obtain a 20 percent increase in the proportion of Canadians who are physically active, eat healthfully, and are at healthy body weights. Specific targets are as follows:

- By 2015, increase the proportion of Canadians who make healthy food choices according to the Canadian Community Health Survey (CCHS) and Statistics Canada (SC)/Canadian Institute for Health Information (CIHI) health indicators.

- By 2015, increase by 20 percent the proportion of Canadians who participate in regular physical activity based on 30 minutes per day of moderate to vigorous activity as measured by the CCHS and the Physical Activity Benchmarks/Monitoring Program.

- By 2015, increase by 20 percent the proportion of Canadians at a "normal" body weight based on a body mass index (BMI) of 18.5 to 24.9 kg/m^2 as measured by the National Population Health Survey (NPHS), CCHS, and SC/CIHI health indicators.

Further discussion is needed to align these targets with the public health goals, and also to set targets for specific populations (including new Canadians and minority cultural communities), along with developing indicators to reduce health disparities among Canadians by sex, race, geographic location, and socioeconomic factors. The Coordinating Committee for the Healthy Living Network will lead implementation of the strategy. For more information, visit the Public Health Agency of Canada's Healthy Living Web site: http://www.phac-aspc.gc.ca/hl-vs-strat/index.html

Healthy Living: Canada's Guide to Healthy Eating and Physical Activity

In 2004, Health Canada published *Healthy Living: Canada's Guide to Healthy Eating and Physical Activity*. This guide is one of many products that will come from the Healthy Living Strategy to help Canadians recognize the benefits of healthy eating, regular physical activity, and maintaining a healthy body weight. The guide combines key information from two previous Health Canada publications: *Canada's Food Guide to Healthy Eating* and *Canada's Physical Activity Guide for Healthy Active Living*. (See Figure D.1.)

The guide stipulates that the amount of food a person needs every day depends on body size, age, gender, and level of physical activity. A healthy body weight can be achieved and maintained by moderating both the type and the amount of food that one eats and by building physical activity into one's daily life.

Active living is accomplished by building physical activity into one's daily life: at home, at school or work, and while in transit from one activity to the next. The physical activity component of the guide is specific regarding the duration and type of physical activity required to stay healthy or to improve health.

When the revisions to *Canada's Food Guide to Healthy Eating* are completed, *Canada's Guide to Healthy Eating and Physical Activity* will need to be reviewed to determine if a revision is necessary.

Nutrition Labeling for Canadians

The nutrition label is one of the most useful tools in selecting foods for healthy eating (Figure D.2). The *Food Guide* outlines a pattern of healthy eating; the nutrition label supports the *Food Guide* by helping consumers to choose foods according to healthy eating messages. Nutrition labeling became mandatory for most prepackaged foods on December 12, 2005. The Nutrition Facts table that is required is virtually identical to the Nutrition Facts panel required by the Food and Drug Administration in the United States.

Consumers can use labels to compare products and make choices on the basis of nutrient content. For example, consumers can choose a lower-fat product based on the fat content given on the labels. Consumers also can use label information to evaluate products in relation to healthy eating. New labeling regulations updated requirements for more than 40 nutrition claims and allowed five health claims on diet and health relationships to be used on food labels or in advertisements.

Together, the Nutrition Facts table, the nutrition and health claims, and the ingredient list provide Canadians with the tools needed to make informed food choices. Health Canada has developed numerous fact sheets to help Canadians read and use food labels.

Label Claims

A claim on a food label highlights a nutritional feature of a product. It is known to influence consumers' buying habits. Manufacturers often position label claims in a bold, banner-style format on the front panel of a package or on the side panel along with the nutrition label. Because a label claim must be backed up by detailed facts relating to the claim, the consumer should look for the Nutrition Facts table for more information.

Nutrition Claims

A nutrition claim describes the amount of a nutrient in a food. For example, a food whose label carries the claim "high fibre" must contain 4 grams or more fiber per reference amount and serving of stated size. A "sodium-free" food must contain less than 5 milligrams of sodium per reference amount and serving of stated size. Common terms include "free," "low," "reduced," "light/lite," "more," and "good source of."

Health Claims

Optional health claims highlight the characteristics of a diet that reduces the chance of developing a disease such as cancer or heart disease. They also tell how the food fits into the diet.

Characteristic of the Diet	Reduced Risk of
Low in sodium and high in potassium	High blood pressure
Adequate in calcium and vitamin D	Osteoporosis
Low in saturated and *trans* fats	Heart disease
Rich in fruits and vegetables	Some types of cancer
Nonfermentable carbohydrates in gums and hard candies	Dental caries

For the latest information, visit the Nutrition Labeling area of the Health Canada Web site at http://www.hc-sc.gc.ca/fn-an/label-etiquet/index_e.html.

Healthy Eating

Regular physical activity and healthy eating are key to a healthy lifestyle.
Enjoy a variety of foods and physical activities every day.
Use this Guide to help you make wise choices.

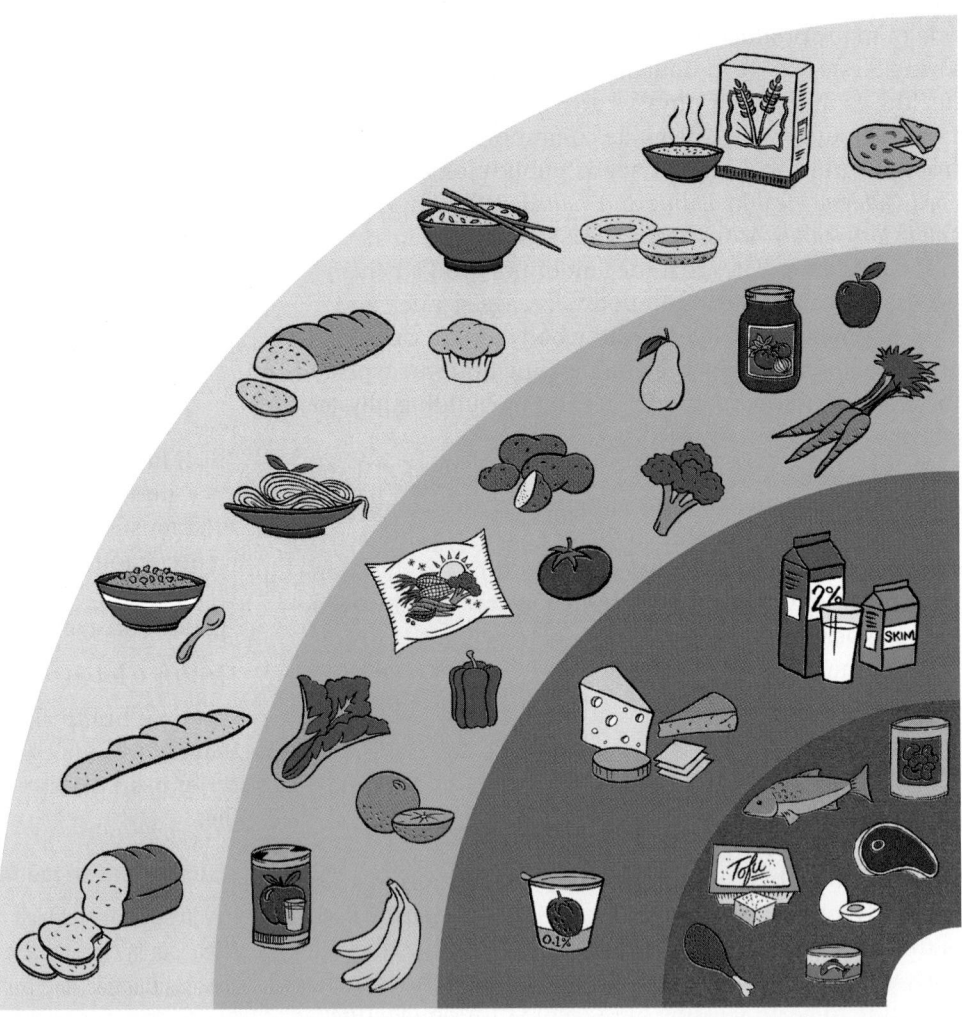

GRAIN PRODUCTS
Choose whole grain and enriched products more often.

VEGETABLES AND FRUIT
Choose dark green and orange vegetables and orange fruit more often.

MILK PRODUCTS
Choose lower-fat milk products more often.

MEAT AND ALTERNATIVES
Choose leaner meats, poultry and fish, as well as dried peas, beans and lentils more often.

Figure D.1 *Healthy Living: Canada's Guide to Healthy Eating and Physical Activity.* **Source:** Health Canada. Reprinted with permission of the Minister of Public Works and Government Services Canada.

CANADA'S GUIDE TO HEALTHY EATING AND PHYSICAL ACTIVITY

The amount of food you need every day depends on how physically active you are, as well as your body size, age and gender.

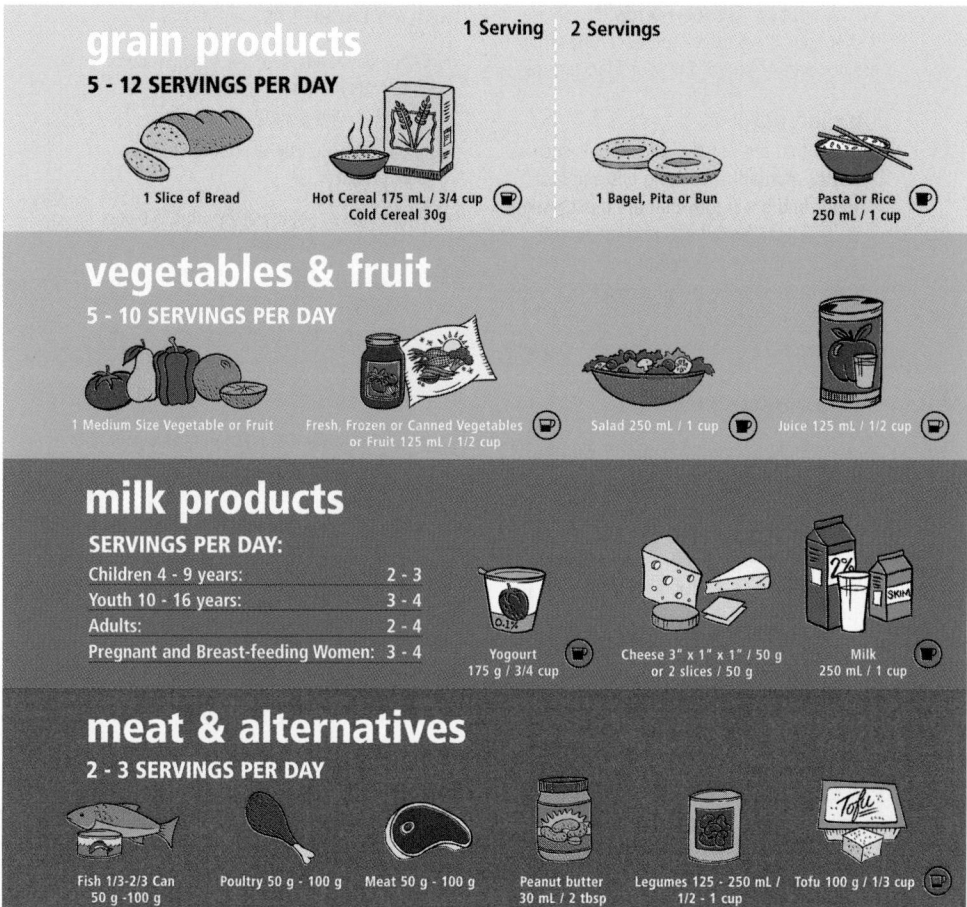

grain products
5 - 12 SERVINGS PER DAY

1 Serving | 2 Servings

1 Slice of Bread

Hot Cereal 175 mL / 3/4 cup
Cold Cereal 30g

1 Bagel, Pita or Bun

Pasta or Rice
250 mL / 1 cup

vegetables & fruit
5 - 10 SERVINGS PER DAY

1 Medium Size Vegetable or Fruit

Fresh, Frozen or Canned Vegetables or Fruit 125 mL / 1/2 cup

Salad 250 mL / 1 cup

Juice 125 mL / 1/2 cup

milk products
SERVINGS PER DAY:

Children 4 - 9 years:	2 - 3
Youth 10 - 16 years:	3 - 4
Adults:	2 - 4
Pregnant and Breast-feeding Women:	3 - 4

Yogourt
175 g / 3/4 cup

Cheese 3" x 1" x 1" / 50 g
or 2 slices / 50 g

Milk
250 mL / 1 cup

meat & alternatives
2 - 3 SERVINGS PER DAY

Fish 1/3-2/3 Can
50 g -100 g

Poultry 50 g - 100 g

Meat 50 g - 100 g

Peanut butter
30 mL / 2 tbsp

Legumes 125 - 250 mL /
1/2 - 1 cup

Tofu 100 g / 1/3 cup

If you are not physically active, consuming the number of servings from the lower-end of the ranges may be key to maintaining a healthy body weight. If you are physically active (accumulate 30-60 minutes of moderate physical activity daily), you can adjust the number of servings that you eat.

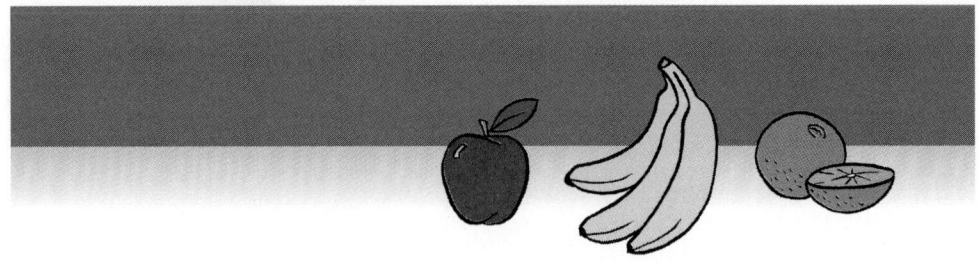

You can achieve and maintain a healthy body weight by moderating both the type and amount of food that you eat and by building physical activity into your daily life.

What About 'Other Foods'?

'Other Foods' are foods and beverages that are not part of one of the four food groups.

THEY INCLUDE:

- foods that are mostly fats and oils such as butter, margarine, cooking oils and lard
- foods and beverages that are mostly sugar such as jam, honey, syrup, candies, soft drinks and fruit-flavored drinks
- high-fat and/or high-salt snack foods such as chips (potato, corn, etc.) or pretzels
- beverages such as tea, coffee, and alcohol
- herbs, spices and condiments such as pickles, mustard and ketchup.

Some of these foods are higher in fat or sugar and contribute calories but contain few nutrients. Use these foods in moderation.

HEALTHY EATING TIPS

- Eat mainly foods from the Grain Products and Vegetables and Fruit groups. Make them the main part of your meals.

- Choose skim, partly-skim or reduced-fat milk products.

- Choose meat, poultry or fish that is baked, broiled or microwaved.

- Have peas, beans and lentils more often. Add them to soups, include them in casseroles or try baked beans.

- Have less fried foods and fewer high-fat bakery items.

- Have snacks such as chips and chocolate bars less often.

Nutrition Facts
Per 2 cookies (30g)

Amount		% Daily Value
Calories 150		
Fat 7 g		11 %
Saturated Fat 3 g + Trans Fat 1 g		20 %
Cholesterol 0 mg		
Sodium 80 mg		3 %
Carbohydrate 21 g		7 %
Fibre 1 g		4 %
Sugars 8 g		
Protein 1 g		
Vitamin A	0 % Vitamin C	0 %
Calcium	0 % Iron	8 %

PORTIONS

Portion sizes influence the number of calories and amount of fat you consume. You may be eating more than you realize.

Serve smaller portions. Offer seconds to those who want more.

Use the Nutrition Facts table on prepackaged foods to make informed food choices. Compare the amount shown in the Nutrition Facts table – two cookies in this example – to the amount you eat.

Water

Always satisfy your thirst. Choose water often and be sure to drink more in hot weather or when you are very active. Consider plain water as a calorie-free way to quench thirst.

Physical Activity

Build physical activity into your daily life…
Get active your way at home, at school, at work, at play,
and on the way...

…that's active living!

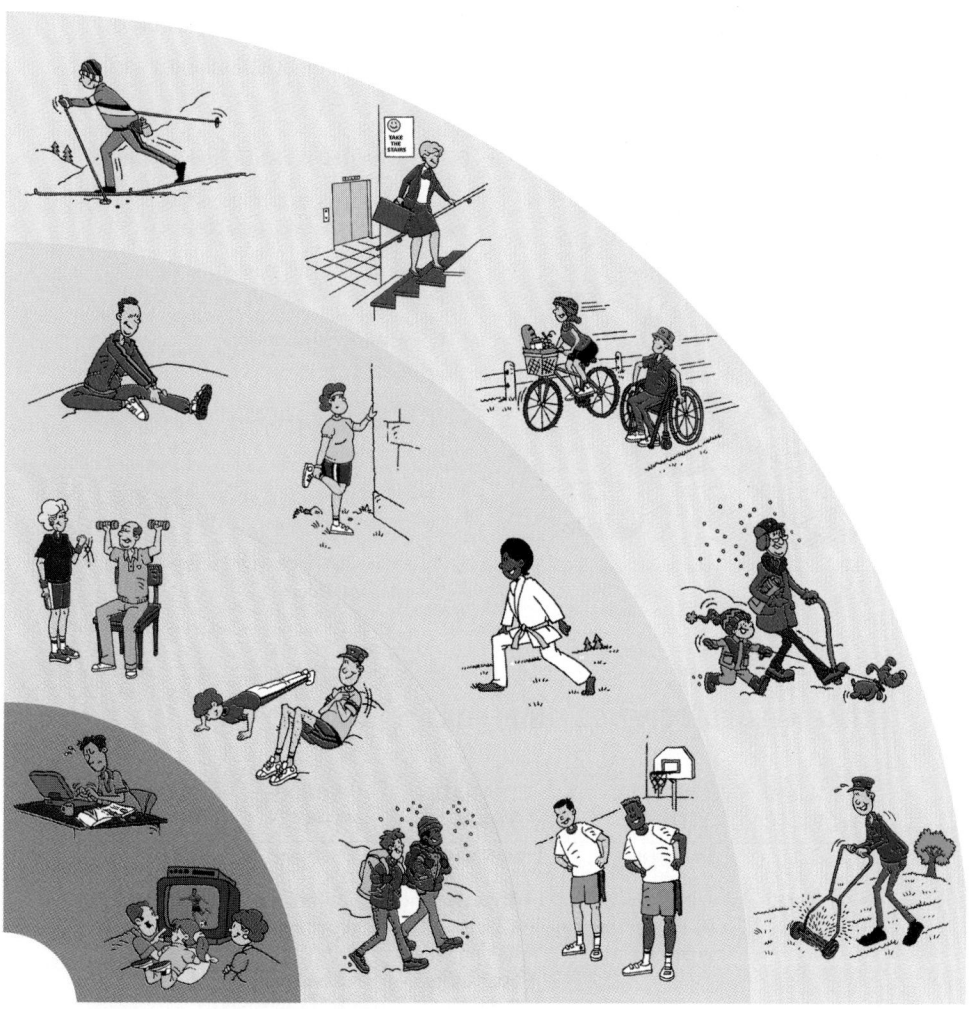

REDUCE
Sitting for Long Periods

INCREASE
Strength Activities

INCREASE
Flexibility Activities

INCREASE
Endurance Activities

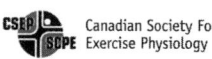
Canadian Society For
Exercise Physiology

CANADA'S GUIDE TO HEALTHY EATING AND PHYSICAL ACTIVITY

Get Active!

Your Way, Every Day – For Life!

Accumulate 30 - 60 minutes of moderate physical activity daily to stay healthy or improve your health. Add up your activities in periods of at least 10 minutes each. Start slowly… and build up.

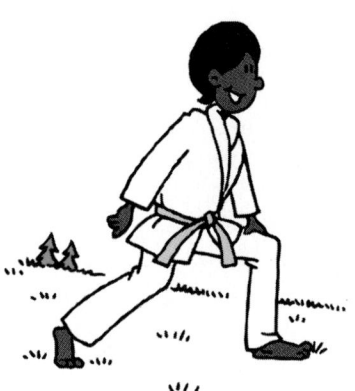

GETTING STARTED IS EASIER THAN YOU THINK

- Walk whenever you can - get off the bus early, use the stairs instead of the elevator.
- Reduce long periods of inactivity, like watching TV.
- Play actively with your kids.
- Choose to walk, wheel or cycle for short trips.
- Start with a 10 minute walk - gradually increase the time.
- Find out about walking and cycling paths nearby and use them.
- Try a new sport. Start with a lesson or join a recreational league.

TIME NEEDED DEPENDS ON EFFORT

VERY LIGHT EFFORT	LIGHT EFFORT	MODERATE EFFORT	VIGOROUS EFFORT	MAXIMUM EFFORT
	60 Minutes	30-60 Minutes	20-30 Minutes	
• Strolling	• Light walking	• Brisk walking	• Aerobics	• Sprinting
• Dusting	• Easy gardening	• Biking	• Jogging	• Racing
	• Stretching	• Raking leaves	• Hockey	
		• Swimming	• Basketball	
		• Dancing	• Fast swimming	
		• Water aerobics	• Fast dancing	

Range Needed to Stay Healthy

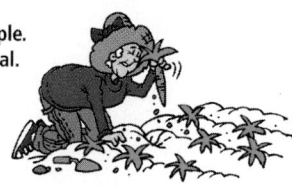

Starting slowly is very safe for most people. Not sure? Consult your health professional.

Choose a variety of activities from these groups:

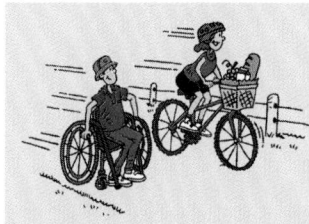

endurance

4 - 7 DAYS A WEEK
Continuous activities for your heart, lungs and circulatory system.

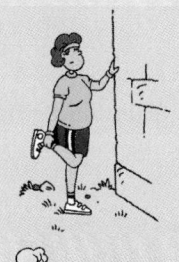

flexibility

4 - 7 DAYS A WEEK
Gentle reaching, bending and stretching activities to keep your muscles relaxed and joints mobile.

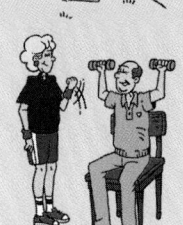

strength

2 - 4 DAYS A WEEK
Activities against resistance to strengthen muscles and bones and improve posture.

Benefits of regular physical activity and healthy eating:	Health risks of physical inactivity and unhealthy eating:
· better health · look, feel and perform better · stronger muscles and bones · weight control · better self-esteem · feeling more energetic · continued independent living in later life	· premature death and disability · heart disease · obesity · osteoporosis · high blood pressure · type 2 diabetes · stroke · some types of cancer

The Nutrition Facts Table

The Nutrition Facts table allows consumers to make informed choices.

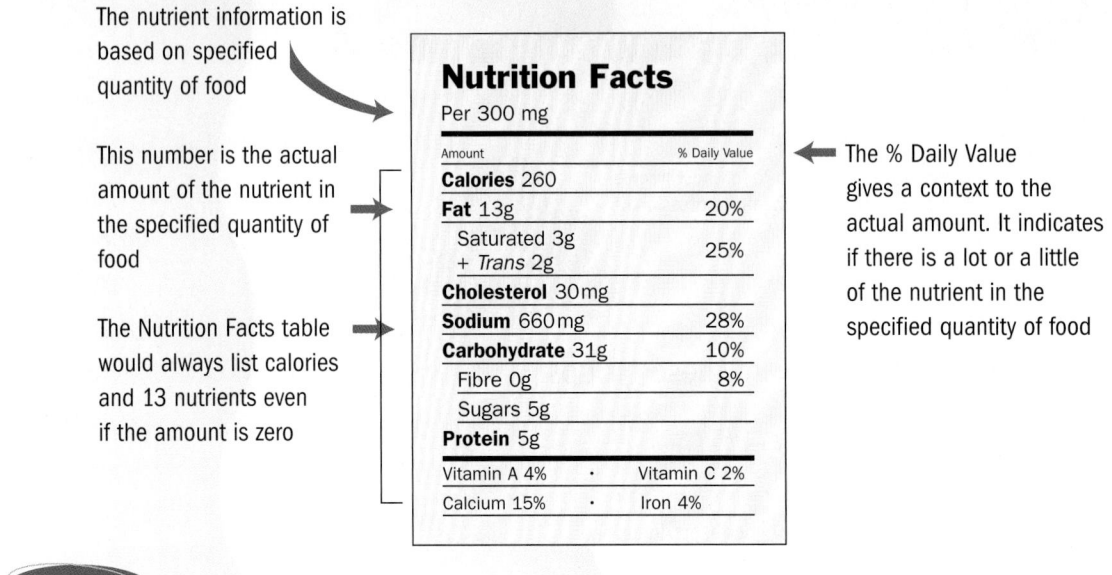

The nutrient information is based on specified quantity of food

This number is the actual amount of the nutrient in the specified quantity of food

The Nutrition Facts table would always list calories and 13 nutrients even if the amount is zero

Nutrition Facts

Per 300 mg

Amount	% Daily Value
Calories 260	
Fat 13g	20%
Saturated 3g + *Trans* 2g	25%
Cholesterol 30mg	
Sodium 660mg	28%
Carbohydrate 31g	10%
Fibre 0g	8%
Sugars 5g	
Protein 5g	

Vitamin A 4%	·	Vitamin C 2%
Calcium 15%	·	Iron 4%

The % Daily Value gives a context to the actual amount. It indicates if there is a lot or a little of the nutrient in the specified quantity of food

Figure D.2 How to read a food label.

Canadian Diabetes Association's Meal Planning Guide

The Canadian Diabetes Association (CDA) works to promote the health of Canadians through diabetes research, education, service, and advocacy. In response to the introduction of new medications and new methods for the management of diabetes, CDA has revised its meal planning guide. Like the Exchange Lists, the CDA meal planning guide was designed to make it easier for people with diabetes to eat the right amount of food for their insulin supply. The system is based on two concepts: Most foods are eaten by people with diabetes in measured amounts, and foods within each of the system's eight food groups can be interchanged.

The new guide, *Beyond the Basics: Meal Planning for Diabetes Prevention and Management*, has several features. First, food items have been modified to reflect current thinking on heart health, the glycemic index, and carbohydrate counting. A wider range of multicultural foods has been added. Portion sizes have been adjusted to be more similar to *Canada's Food Guide to Healthy Eating* and to the Quebec and U.S. meal planning systems. The guide also uses color coding to help consumers: green for "choose more often" or "everyday" foods and amber for "choose less often" or "special occasion foods." The listed portions of all carbohydrate-rich foods now contain 15 grams of available carbohydrate (total carbohydrate minus fiber and half of any sugar alcohols).

Beyond the Basics classifies foods into eight food groups:

- Grains and starches
- Fruits
- Milk and alternatives
- Other choices
- Vegetables
- Meat and alternatives
- Fats
- Extras

Within each group, food items are listed along with portions to show how much of one food is interchangeable with another food in the same group. In the past, symbols for the meal planning guide food groups were used on food labels, but this has been phased out with the new food labeling regulations. However, CDA partnered with Dietitians of Canada to develop Healthy Eating Is in Store for You, a nutrition labeling education program. For more information, visit the CDA Web site: http://www.diabetes.ca/Section_Professionals/btb.asp.

References

[1] Public Health Agency of Canada. *The Integrated Pan-Canadian Healthy Living Strategy*, 2005. http://www.phac-aspc.gc.ca/hl-vs-strat/index.html. Accessed 12/19/06.

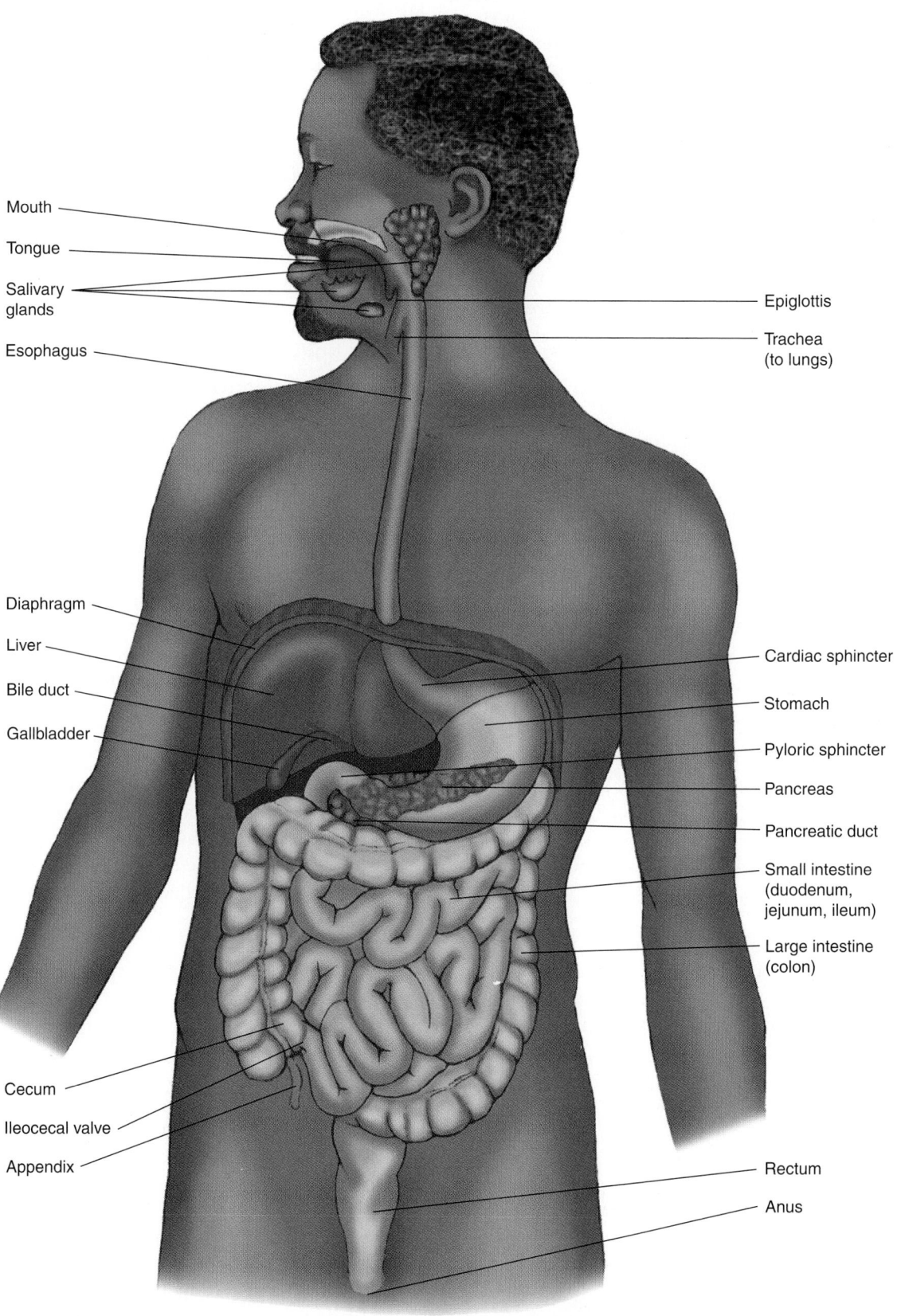

Mouth

Tongue

Salivary glands

Esophagus

Diaphragm

Liver

Bile duct

Gallbladder

Cecum

Ileocecal valve

Appendix

Epiglottis

Trachea (to lungs)

Cardiac sphincter

Stomach

Pyloric sphincter

Pancreas

Pancreatic duct

Small intestine (duodenum, jejunum, ileum)

Large intestine (colon)

Rectum

Anus

Mouth

- In the mouth, food is broken up by chewing with the teeth and tongue. Saliva lubricates food and makes swallowing easier. Salivary amylase begins the digestion of starch. The mouth warms or cools the food so that it is closer to body temperature. When the food bolus (a fairly liquid ball of food) is ready, swallowing is consciously initiated.

Tongue

- The tongue is a mobile mass of muscle that helps teeth tear food into pieces by forcing it against the bony palate. The tongue contains receptors for sweet, salty, sour, and bitter tastes. Umami, a fifth taste elicited by monosodium glutamate, is a meaty, savory sensation. Flavor is a complex combination of taste, smells (the nose has about 6 million olfactory receptor cells), physical sensations (e.g., spicy foods), and food texture.

Salivary glands

- The three pairs of salivary glands produce saliva. The water in saliva helps dissolve food particles, facilitating taste sensations. The mucus in saliva lubricates food for swallowing and transport. Digestive enzymes begin breaking down foodstuffs. Salivary amylase begins the chemical breakdown of starches into simple sugars. Lingual lipase initiates the breakdown of fat. The mineral sodium and the enzyme lysozyme in the saliva act as disinfectants, destroying bacteria and other microorganisms in food.

Epiglottis

- The epiglottis is a flap of tissue that acts as a valve during swallowing. It closes the entrance to the larynx and prevents food from entering the respiratory passages.

Trachea

- These tubes allow air to pass to and from the lungs.

Esophagus

- The esophagus is the tube that connects the mouth to the stomach. Wavelike muscle action (peristalsis) moves food through the esophagus to the stomach. The upper one-third of the muscles of the esophagus are under voluntary control, the middle third are a mixture of voluntarily controlled muscle and automatically controlled smooth muscle, while the lower third is smooth muscle alone.

Cardiac sphincter

- The cardiac sphincter is a muscular valve at the lower end of the esophagus. This control valve relaxes to allow food to pass into the stomach. When contracted, it prevents backflow (reflux) of stomach contents into the esophagus.

Named for its proximity to the heart, a malfunction can cause painful esophageal reflux (heartburn) which can be so severe that it is mistaken for a heart attack.

Stomach

- The upper bag-like portion of the stomach acts as a hopper to receive and hold the food prior to delivery to the lower two-thirds. Three layers of smooth muscle surround this lower portion of the stomach. Muscular contractions churn the food, so the solids can ferment and mix with acids, fluid and protein-splitting enzymes. The result is a sticky semi-liquid, called chyme, that is gradually released into the duodenum (the first part of the small intestine). Stomach acid halts the digestion of starch, but the stomach also produces gastric lipase, an enzyme that acts on fat.

Pyloric sphincter

- The pyloric sphincter is a muscular valve that controls passage of chyme from the stomach to the small intestine. When contracted, it prevents backflow from the small intestine into the stomach.

Liver

- The liver is the body's chemical factory and detoxification center. It has many functions in controlling metabolism and deactivating hormones, drugs, and toxins. It also produces bile—a mixture of bile salts, phospholipids, cholesterol, pigments, proteins, and inorganic ions such as sodium. The detergent-like action of bile emulsifies fat, facilitating fat digestion.

Gallbladder

- The gallbladder stores and concentrates bile. The arrival of fatty food in the duodenum stimulates the release of the duodenal hormone CCK which signals the gallbladder to contract. The bile is then released into the duodenum, where it aids fat digestion.

Bile duct

- The bile duct carries bile from the gallbladder to the duodenum.

Pancreas

- The pancreas is a complex gland that produces a pancreatic juice rich in bicarbonate and enzymes. The pancreatic juice is released into the duodenum where it does its work. Pancreatic amylase breaks down starch into maltose. Lipase splits fats into monoglycerides, fatty acids, and glycerol. The pancreatic proenzyme trypsinogen is converted to the enzyme trypsin. Trypsin splits polypeptides and proteins into amino acids. Bicarbonate produced by the pancreas neutralizes the acid chyme that enters the small intestine. In addition, the pancreas produces insulin and glucagon—hormones that have important roles in regulating carbohydrate metabolism and blood sugar.

Pancreatic duct

• The pancreatic duct carries pancreatic juice from the pancreas to the duodenum.

Small intestine

• The small intestine is a tube approximately 10 feet long that is divided into three parts: the duodenum (the first 10 to 12 inches), the jejunum (about 4 feet), and the ileum (about 5 feet). Whereas the duodenum is mainly responsible for breaking down food, the jejunum and ileum primarily deal with the absorption of food. The duodenum secretes mucus, enzymes, and hormones to aid digestion. Most digestion and absorption occur in the small intestine. Intestinal cells secrete disaccharidases and peptidases to help complete carbohydrate and protein digestion. The intestinal lining is highly folded to increase its surface area and is richly supplied with circulatory vessels, which carry away absorbed nutrients in the blood and lymph. Undigested material is passed on to the large intestine.

Ileocecal valve (sphincter)

• The ileocecal valve is the sphincter at the lower end of the small intestine. When open, it permits food residue to move from the small intestine to the large intestine. When closed, it prevents backflow from the large intestine.

Large intestine

• The large intestine is made up of the appendix, cecum, colon, rectum, and anus. The colon is about 2.5 inches in diameter and about 4 feet long. In the large intestine, bacteria break down dietary fiber and other undigested carbohydrates, releasing acids and gas. The large intestine absorbs water and minerals while dehydrating and processing the remaining undigested material into solid feces. The colon walls secrete a viscous mucus to help lubricate and mold the feces. This mucus also helps protect the colon wall from mechanical damage.

Appendix

• The appendix is a fingerlike appendage attached to the cecum, the first part of the colon. The appendix has no known function.

Cecum

• The cecum is the pouch-like beginning of the large intestine. The small intestine's ileum empties into the cecum.

Rectum

• The rectum stores waste prior to elimination.

Anus

• The anal sphincter holds the rectum closed. Either voluntary or involuntary control may open it to allow elimination.

APPENDIX F Biochemical Structures

> ➤ Nomenclature
> ➤ ATP/ADP/AMP
> ➤ Carbohydrates
> ➤ Amino Acids
> ➤ Fatty Acids
> ➤ Fat-Soluble Vitamins
> ➤ Water-Soluble Vitamins
> ➤ B Vitamins in Metabolic
> Pathways

Nomenclature

Prefixes

mono-	Means one subunit. For instance *mono*saccharide means a one-unit saccharide.
bi-, di-, and tri-	Mean two and three subunits bonded together to form a larger molecule.
poly-	Means many or a lot. A *poly*saccharide has many linked monosaccharide subunits.
oligo-	Means a structure with typically 3 to 10 subunits, but smaller than a polymer.

Suffixes

-ose	Sugars are named with *-ose* as a suffix. They are subclassified with regard to the number of carbons i.e., 3 = triose, 4 = tetrose, 5 = pentose, 6 = hexose, 7 = heptose. The suffix *-ose*, refers to monosaccharides and disaccharides: sugars like gluc*ose*, fruct*ose*, sucr*ose*, etc.
-ase	Many enzymes are named by attaching the suffix *-ase* to the substrate of the enzyme (the compound altered by enzymatic action). For instance, a lipase cleaves a lipid substrate, a disaccharidase cleaves a disaccharide, and a peptidase breaks the peptide bond between two amino acids.
-ol	Suffix for naming alcohols and phenols (e.g., ethan*ol*, glycer*ol*).
-ic, -ate, -oic, -oate	Suffixes for naming acids and acid salts.

Although the terms *lactic acid* and *lactate* often are used interchangeably, they are not identical chemical compounds. Lactic acid ($C_3H_6O_3$), as its name implies, is an acid. Lactate is any salt of lactic acid, for instance sodium lactate. When anaerobic glycolysis forms lactic acid, the acid quickly dissociates, releasing hydrogen (H^+) into solution. The lactate ion then immediately associates with sodium (Na^+) or potassium (K^+) to form a salt–sodium or potassium lactate. In substances such as pyruvate and lactate, the carboxyl group is COO^- (one oxygen has an available bond). In acids such as pyruvic acid and lactic acid, the carboxyl group is COOH (the available bond is filled with hydrogen). The suffixes -ic and -ate are used for the acid and salt forms of most carboxyl groups. For reasons of pronunciation, some carboxyl groups require the *-oic* or *-oate* suffixes, for instance butan*oic* acid, and its salt form butan*oate*.

-peptide	The suffix *peptide* refers to a molecule composed of 2 or more amino acids joined by peptide bonds. A di*peptide* is composed of 2 amino acids, a tri*peptide* of three, etc. A short string of amino acids is called a poly*peptide* and a long string is a protein.
-saccharide	The suffix *saccharide* refers to sugar. A poly*saccharide*, for example, is a large molecule composed of many sugar subunits. A polysaccharide may be composed of only one type of sugar (starch is made up of many glucose units) or of many different sugars. A lipopoly*saccharide*, for instance, is made up of a variety of sugars bonded to a lipid.
hydrogen ion	Also known as a proton, this lone hydrogen has a positive charge (H^+). It has lost its electron and associates readily with negatively charged ions, like the hydroxyl ion (OH^-).
atomic hydrogen	A hydrogen atom with a single electron. This proton-electron combination is unstable and is a short-lived intermediate in some enzymatically catalyzed reactions. During oxidation-reduction reactions it is atomic hydrogen (hydrogen + electron), not hydrogen ions (H^+), that is transferred.

Acids are substances that form hydrogen ions in solution. An acid dissociates to form a cation (H^+) and an anion (e.g., SO_4^-). When the anion ends with the suffix -*ate* its acid name is simply the anion with suffix -*ic*, followed by the word *acid*. Here are some examples:

- H_2SO_4 - hydrogen sulf*ate* becomes sulfur*ic acid*
- H_3PO_4 - hydrogen phosph*ate* becomes phosphor*ic acid*
- $HClO_3$ - hydrogen chlor*ate* becomes hydrochlor*ic acid*

Functional Group	Structural Formula	Models
Hydroxyl	–OH	
Carbonyl	$-\overset{\vert}{\underset{\vert\vert}{C}}-$ O	
Carboxyl	$-C\overset{O}{\underset{OH}{}}$	
Amino	$-N\overset{H}{\underset{H}{}}$	
Sulfhydryl	–SH	
Phosphate	$-O-\overset{H}{\underset{\vert\vert}{P}}-OH$ O	

Functional groups
These six functional groups are commonly involved in covalent and non-covalent bonding to form molecules such as proteins and DNA.

ATP and Derivatives
ATP, ADP, and AMP

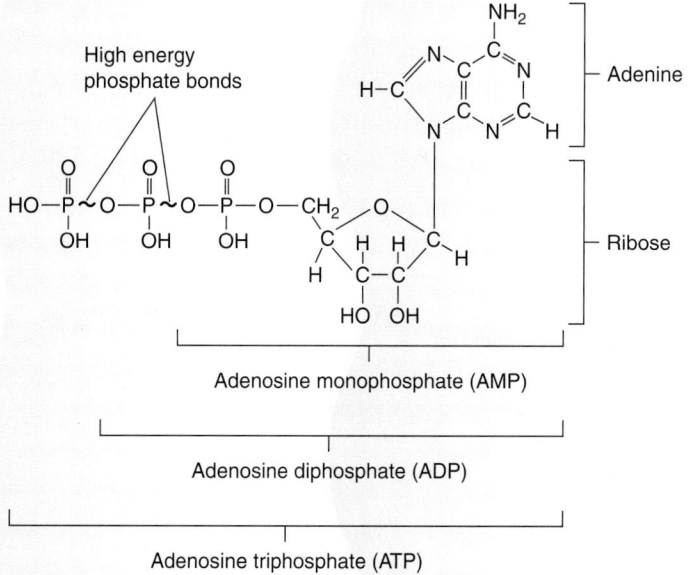

Carbohydrates

Monosaccharides

Glucose   **Galactose**   **Fructose**

The structures of glucose and galactose differ only by the location of the OH on carbon number 4.

Disaccharides

Glucose   Glucose   Glucose   Galactose   Glucose   Fructose

Maltose   **Lactose**   **Sucrose**

In maltose and sucrose, the monosaccharides are linked by alpha bonds. In lactose, a beta bond links galactose and glucose. The human digestive enzyme lactase can hydrolyze the beta bond in lactose.

Polysaccharides

Amylose
Starch molecule made of unbranched glucose chains.

Amylopectin
Starch molecule made of branched glucose chains. In amylopectin, the chain branches every thirty glucose units. Glycogen is similar, but more highly branched (every ten glucose units).

Cellulose
Cellulose is a nearly straight chain of glucose units where the glucose molecules are linked by beta bonds. Humans do not have the enzymes necessary to break the beta linkages in cellulose.

Amino Acids

Essential amino acids

Amino acids consist of a central carbon atom bonded to a carboxyl group, an amino group, a hydrogen, and a side group. The shaded areas show the structure common to all amino acids.

Valine (Val)

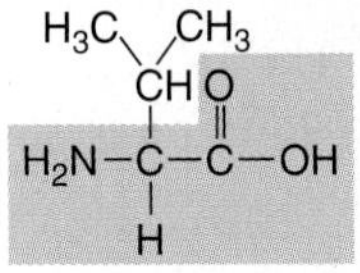

Leucine (Leu)

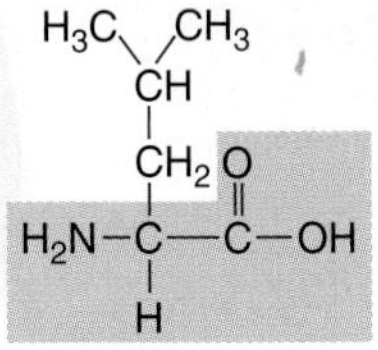

Isoleucine (Ile)

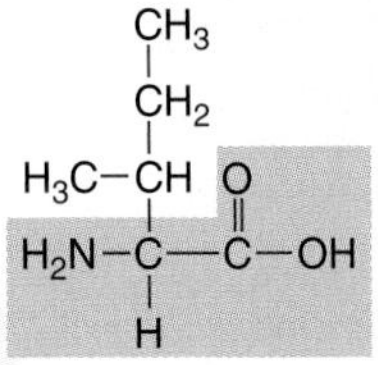

Threonine (Thr)

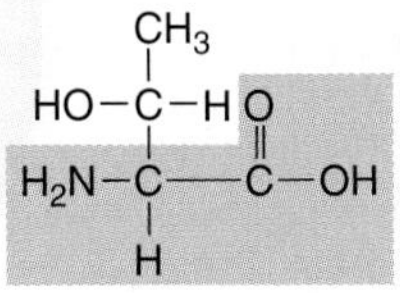

Lysine (Lys)

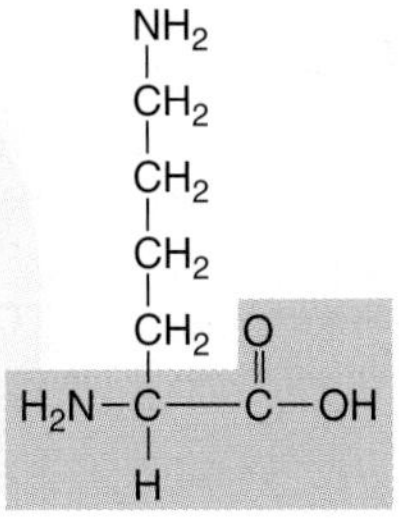

Histidine (His)

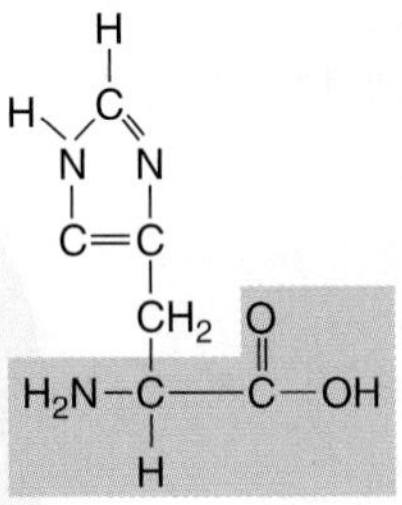

Phenylalanine (Phe)

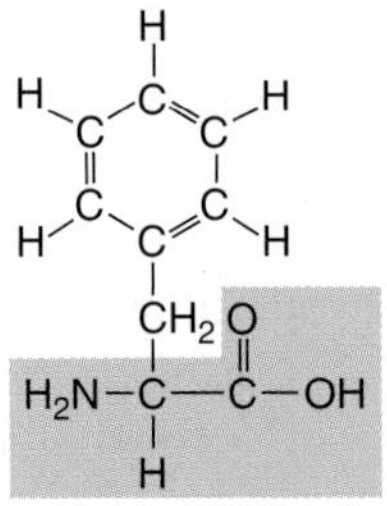

Tryptophan (Trp)

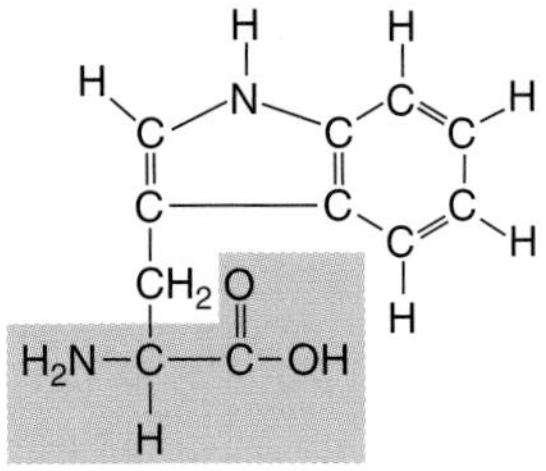

Methionine (Met)

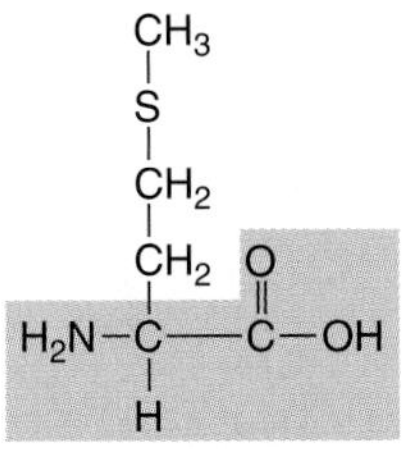

Nonessential amino acids

Glycine (Gly)

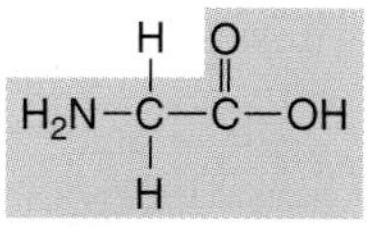

$$H_2N-\overset{\overset{\displaystyle H}{|}}{\underset{\underset{\displaystyle H}{|}}{C}}-\overset{\overset{\displaystyle O}{\|}}{C}-OH$$

Alanine (Ala)

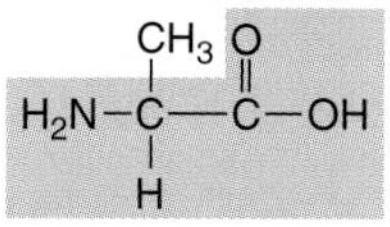

$$H_2N-\overset{\overset{\displaystyle CH_3}{|}}{\underset{\underset{\displaystyle H}{|}}{C}}-\overset{\overset{\displaystyle O}{\|}}{C}-OH$$

Serine (Ser)

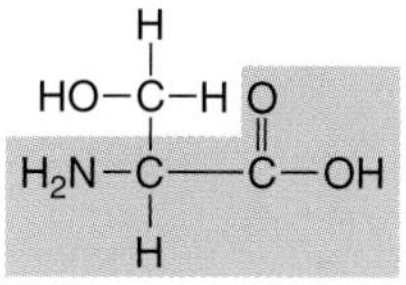

$$HO-\overset{\overset{\displaystyle H}{|}}{C}-H$$
$$H_2N-\overset{|}{\underset{\underset{\displaystyle H}{|}}{C}}-\overset{\overset{\displaystyle O}{\|}}{C}-OH$$

Aspartic acid (Asp)

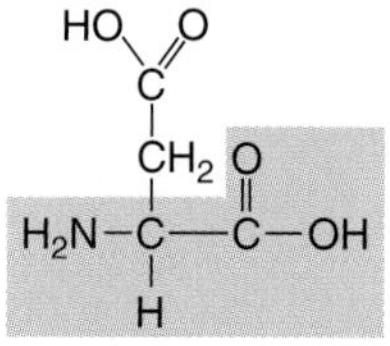

$$HO\diagdown \overset{\displaystyle O}{\underset{\displaystyle C}{\diagup}}$$
$$CH_2$$
$$H_2N-\overset{|}{\underset{\underset{\displaystyle H}{|}}{C}}-\overset{\overset{\displaystyle O}{\|}}{C}-OH$$

Glutamic acid (Glu)

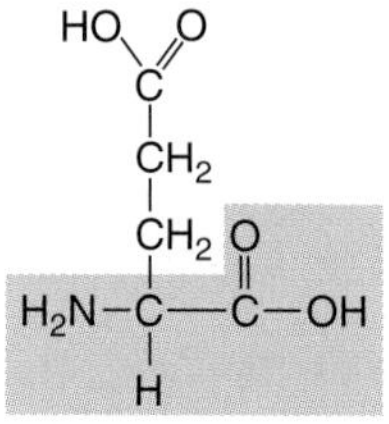

$$HO\diagdown \overset{\displaystyle O}{\underset{\displaystyle C}{\diagup}}$$
$$CH_2$$
$$CH_2$$
$$H_2N-\overset{|}{\underset{\underset{\displaystyle H}{|}}{C}}-\overset{\overset{\displaystyle O}{\|}}{C}-OH$$

Asparagine (Asn)

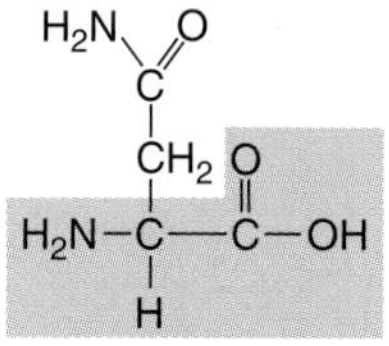

$$H_2N\diagdown \overset{\displaystyle O}{\underset{\displaystyle C}{\diagup}}$$
$$CH_2$$
$$H_2N-\overset{|}{\underset{\underset{\displaystyle H}{|}}{C}}-\overset{\overset{\displaystyle O}{\|}}{C}-OH$$

Glutamine (Gln)

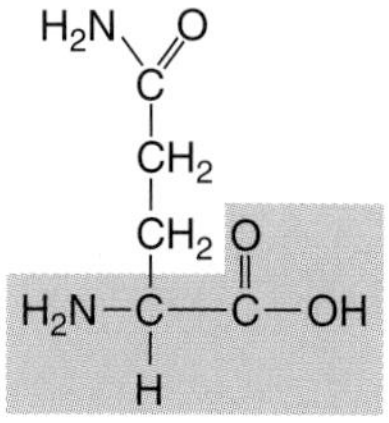

$$H_2N\diagdown \overset{\displaystyle O}{\underset{\displaystyle C}{\diagup}}$$
$$CH_2$$
$$CH_2$$
$$H_2N-\overset{|}{\underset{\underset{\displaystyle H}{|}}{C}}-\overset{\overset{\displaystyle O}{\|}}{C}-OH$$

Arginine (Arg)

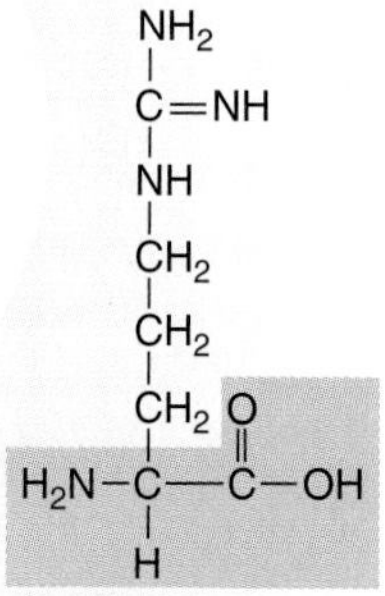

$$NH_2$$
$$C=NH$$
$$NH$$
$$CH_2$$
$$CH_2$$
$$CH_2$$
$$H_2N-\overset{|}{\underset{\underset{\displaystyle H}{|}}{C}}-\overset{\overset{\displaystyle O}{\|}}{C}-OH$$

Tyrosine (Tyr)

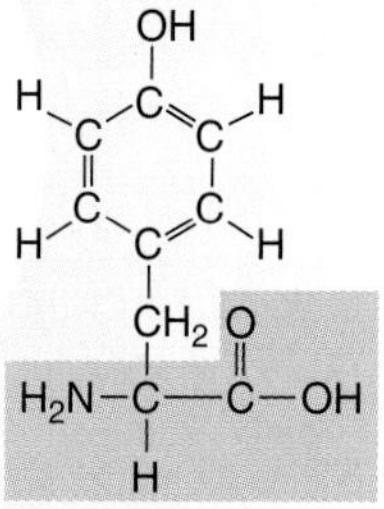

$$CH_2$$
$$H_2N-\overset{|}{\underset{\underset{\displaystyle H}{|}}{C}}-\overset{\overset{\displaystyle O}{\|}}{C}-OH$$

Cysteine (Cys)

$$SH$$
$$CH_2$$
$$H_2N-\overset{|}{\underset{\underset{\displaystyle H}{|}}{C}}-\overset{\overset{\displaystyle O}{\|}}{C}-OH$$

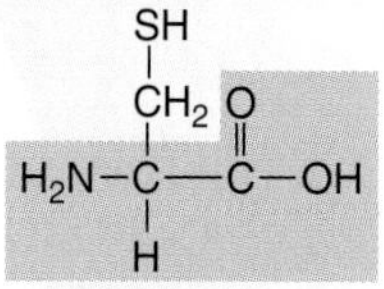

Proline (Pro)

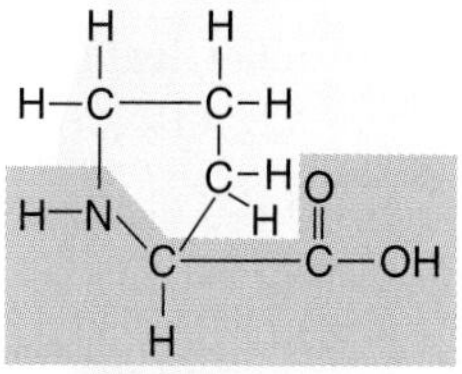

Proline is an amino acid. Its amino group has only one hydrogen and forms a ring.

Fatty Acids

Table F.1 Saturated Fatty Acids Found in Food

Saturated Fatty Acid	Chemical Formula	Number of Carbons	Major Food Sources
Butyric	$CH_3(CH_2)_2COOH$	4	Small amounts in butterfat
Caproic	$CH_3(CH_2)_4COOH$	6	Small amounts in butterfat
Caprylic	$CH_3(CH_2)_6COOH$	8	Small amounts in many fats, including butterfat. Especially found in oils of plant origin.
Capric	$CH_3(CH_2)_8COOH$	10	Small amounts in many fats, including butterfat. Especially found in oils of plant origin.
Lauric	$CH_3(CH_2)_{10}COOH$	12	Cinnamon, palm kernel, coconut oil, butter
Myristic	$CH_3(CH_2)_{12}COOH$	14	Nutmeg, palm kernel, coconut oil, butter
Palmitic	$CH_3(CH_2)_{14}COOH$	16	Common in all animal and plant fats
Stearic	$CH_3(CH_2)_{16}COOH$	18	Common in all animal and plant fats
Arachidic	$CH_3(CH_2)_{18}COOH$	20	Peanut oil
Behenic	$CH_3(CH_2)_{20}COOH$	22	Seeds
Lignoceric	$CH_3(CH_2)_{22}COOH$	24	Peanut oil

Table F.2 Unsaturated Fatty Acids Found in Food

Unsaturated Fatty Acid	Chemical Formula	Number of Carbons	Number of Double Bonds	Omega Notation*	Major Food Sources
Palmitoleic	$CH_3(CH_2)_5CH = CH(CH_2)_7COOH$	16	1	16:1ω7	Nearly all fats
Oleic	$CH_3(CH_2)_7CH = CH(CH_2)_7COOH$	18	1	18:1ω9	Perhaps the most common fatty acid in food
Linoleic	$CH_3(CH_2)_4(CH = CHCH_2)_2(CH_2)_6COOH$	18	2	18:2ω6	Corn, peanut, cottonseed, soybean, and several oils from other plants
Linolenic	$CH_3CH_2(CH = CHCH_2)_3(CH_2)_6COOH$	18	3	18:3ω3	Often in foods with linoleic acid, but particularly found in linseed oil
Arachidonic	$CH_3(CH_2)_4(CH = CHCH_2)_4(CH_2)_2COOH$	20	4	20:4ω6	Animal fats and peanut oil
Eicosapentanoic	$CH_3(CH_2)_3(CH = CHCH_2)_4(CH_2)_3COOH$	20	5	20:5ω3	Fish oils such as cod liver, mackerel, and salmon
Docosahexanoic	$CH_3(CH_2)_2(CH = CHCH_2)_6COOH$	22	6	22:6ω3	Fish oils such as cod liver, mackerel, and salmon

*Omega Notation = number of carbons: number of double bonds, the number following the omega symbol (ω) represents the location of the first double bond counting from the methyl (CH_3) end.

Fat-Soluble Vitamins

Vitamin A and Beta-carotene

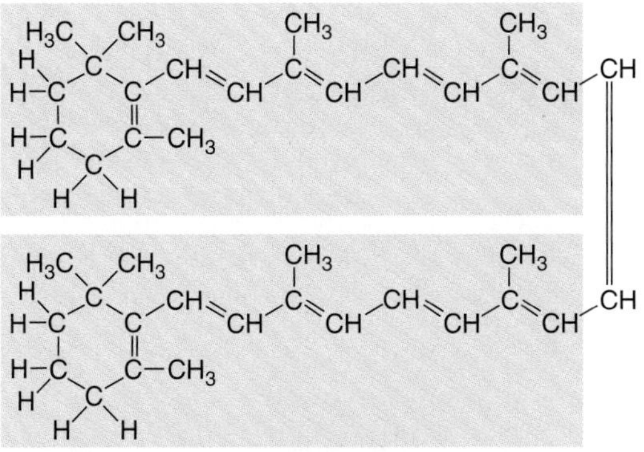

Vitamin A precursor: beta-carotene

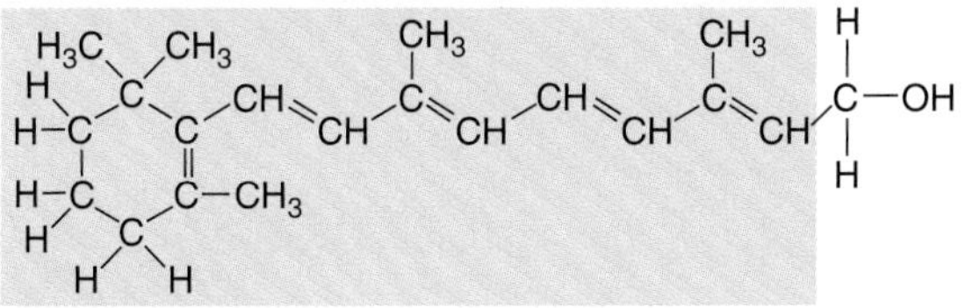

Vitamin A: retinol

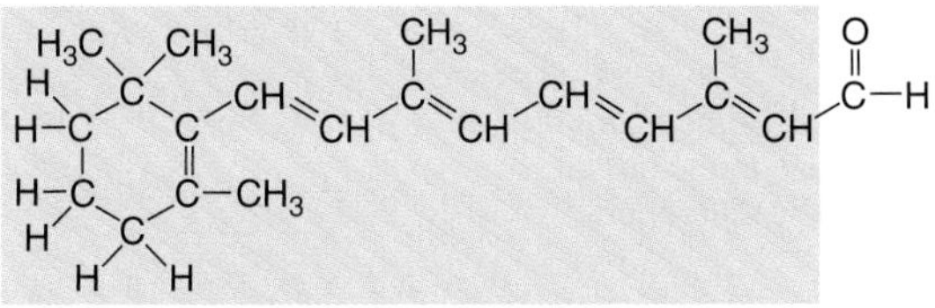

Vitamin A: retinal

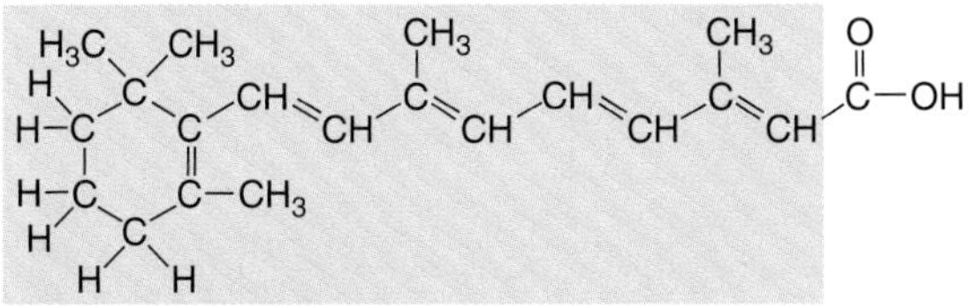

Vitamin A: retinoic acid

The shaded area highlights the structure common to all four molecules.

Vitamin D

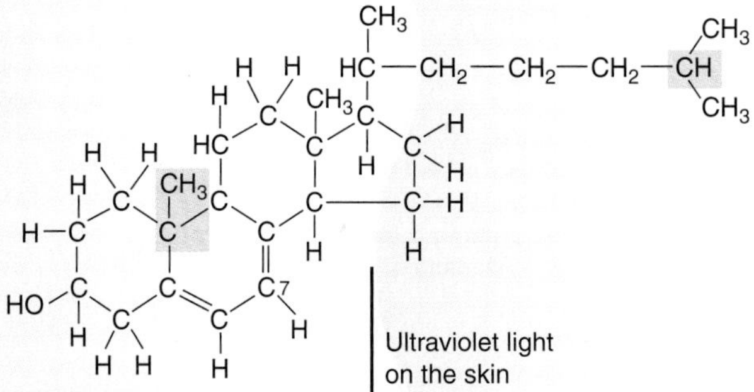

7–Dehydrocholesterol

Ultraviolet light on the skin

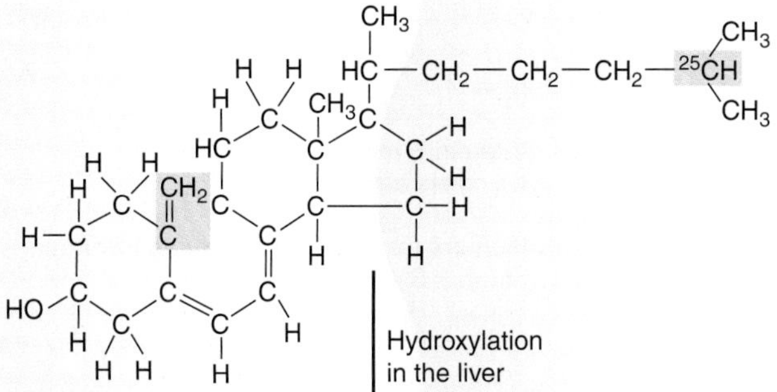

Cholecalciferol (vitamin D_3)

Hydroxylation in the liver

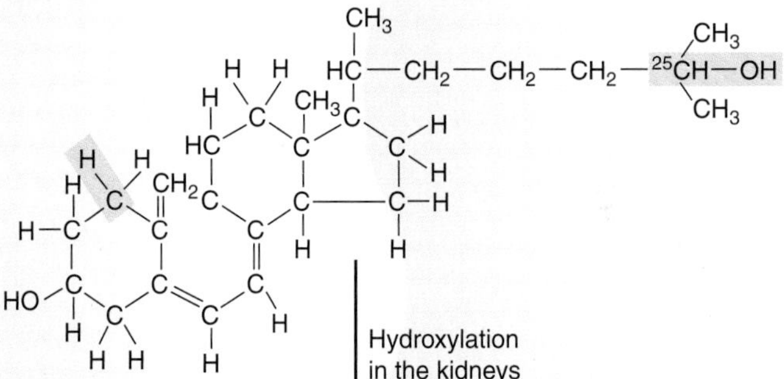

25–Hydroxycholecalciferol (25–hydroxyvitamin D_3)

Hydroxylation in the kidneys

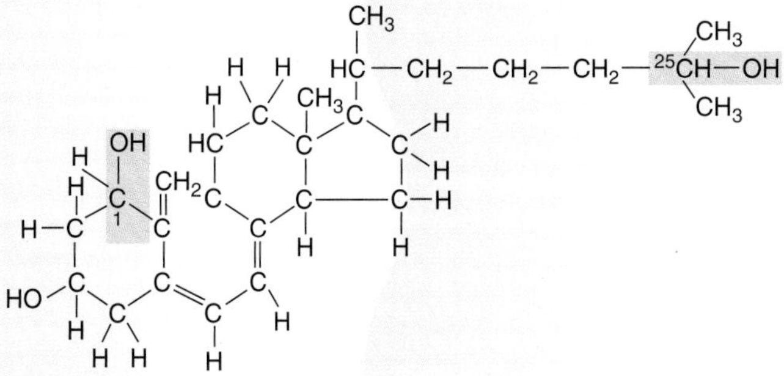

1, 25–Dihydroxycholecalciferol (1, 25–dihydroxyvitamin D_3) (calcitriol)

The shaded areas highlight the portion of the molecule that changes from stage to stage.

Vitamin E

Vitamin E (alpha-tocopherol)
4 isomers α, β, γ, δ

Vitamin E (alpha-tocotrienol)
4 isomers α, β, γ, δ

Isomers for tocopherols and tocotrienols
For α, $R_1 = CH_3$ $R_2 = CH_3$
For β, $R_1 = CH_3$ $R_2 = H$
For γ, $R_1 = H$ $R_2 = CH_3$
For δ, $R_1 = H$ $R_2 = H$

Vitamin E occurs in 8 forms but vitamin E activity is based on alpha-tocopherol. Humans do not convert β-, γ-, δ-tocopherols or the tocotrienols to alpha-tocopherol, so these forms do not contribute toward meeting the vitamin E requirement. The shading highlights the differences between tocopherols and tocotrienols.

Vitamin K

Menadione (vitamin K₃)
Synthetic form of Vitamin K

Phylloquinone (vitamin K₁)
Vitamin K naturally occurring in food

Menaquinone-n (vitamin K₂; n = 6, 7, or 9)
Vitamin K formed by bacteria in the large intestine

The shaded areas highlight the structure common to all three forms.

Water-Soluble Vitamins and Coenzymes

Thiamin and Coenzyme

Thiamin

Thiamin pyrophosphate (TPP)

Thiamin is part of the active coenzyme TPP. The shaded areas highlight the structure common to both molecules.

Water-Soluble Vitamins and Coenzymes (cont.)

Riboflavin and Coenzymes

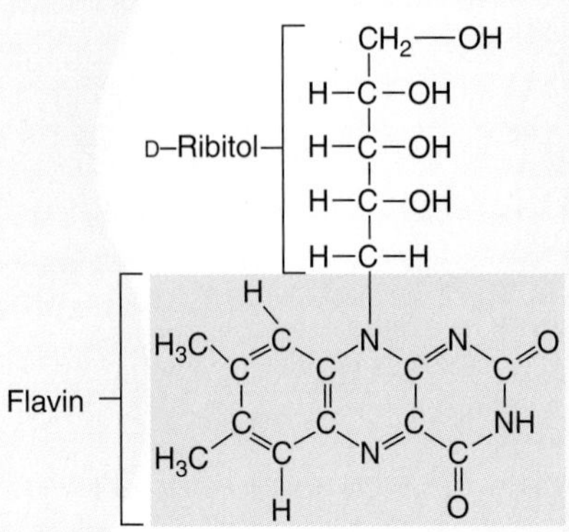
D-Ribitol
Flavin

Riboflavin

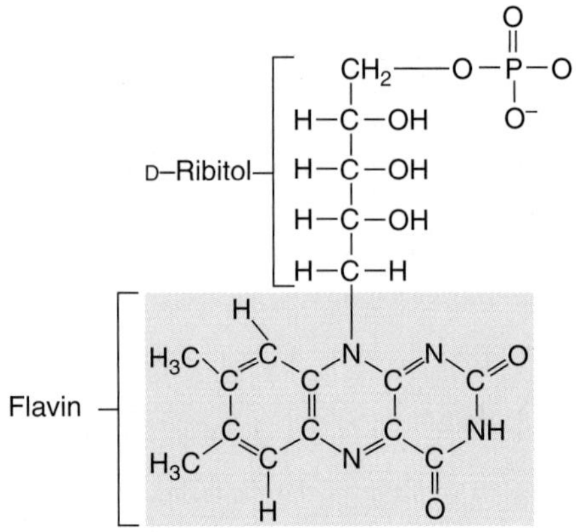
D-Ribitol
Flavin

Flavin mononucleotide (FMN)

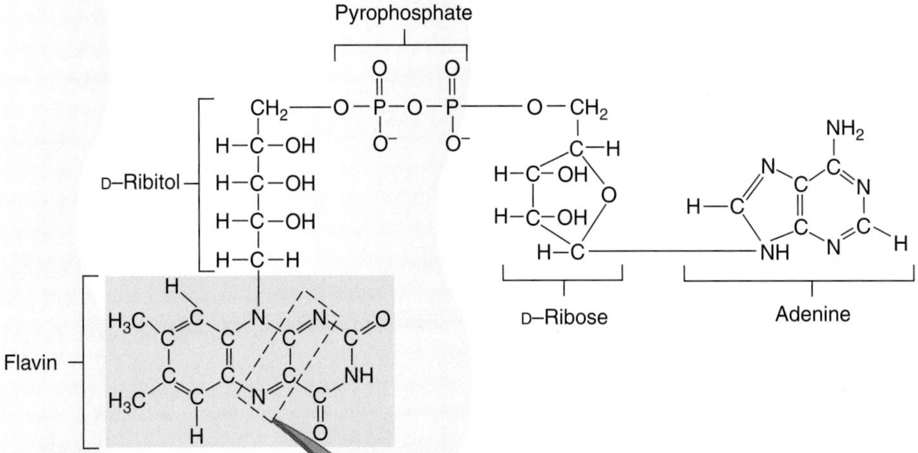
Pyrophosphate
D-Ribitol
Flavin
D-Ribose
Adenine

Flavin dinucleotide (FAD)

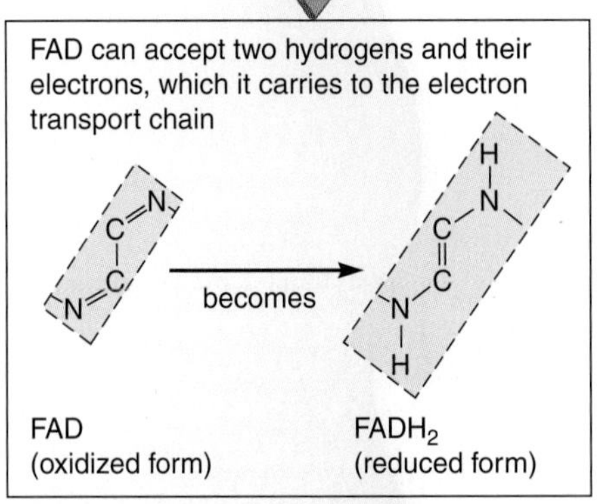
FAD can accept two hydrogens and their electrons, which it carries to the electron transport chain
becomes
FAD
(oxidized form)
$FADH_2$
(reduced form)

FAD and $FADH_2$

The flavin portion of these molecules is highlighted.

Niacin and Coenzymes

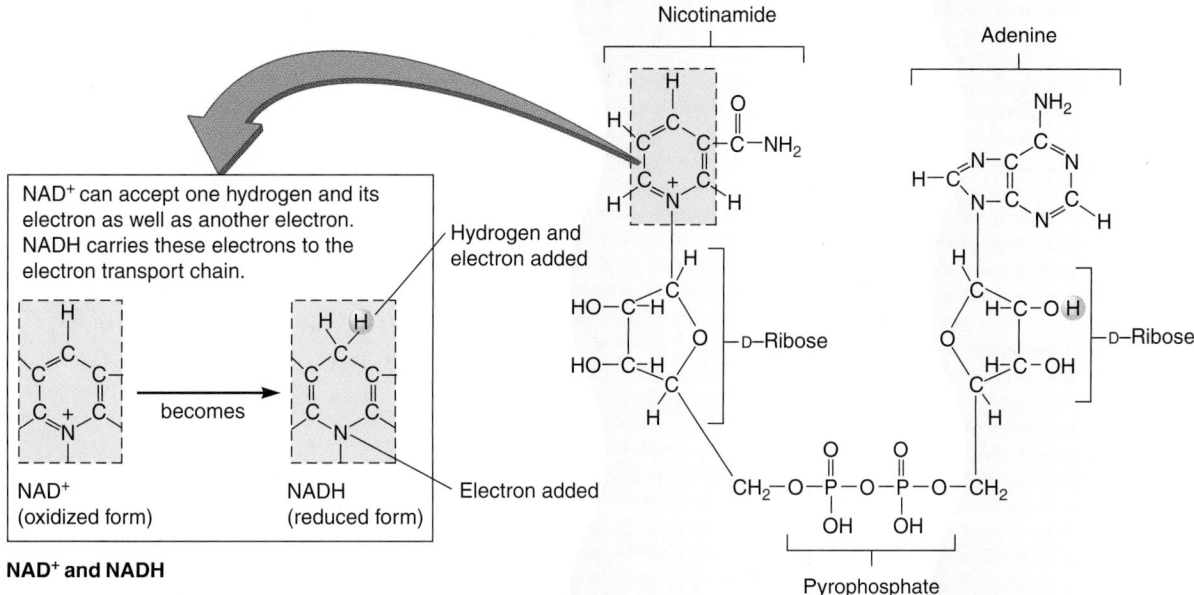

Niacin (nicotinic acid and nicotinamide)

NAD⁺ can accept one hydrogen and its electron as well as another electron. NADH carries these electrons to the electron transport chain.

becomes

NAD⁺
(oxidized form)

NADH
(reduced form)

NAD⁺ and NADH

Hydrogen and electron added

Electron added

Nicotinamide

Adenine

HO—C—H

HO—C—H

D–Ribose

D–Ribose

CH₂—O—P—O—P—O—CH₂

OH   OH

Pyrophosphate

Nicotinamide adenine dinucleotide (NAD⁺) and nicotinamide adenine dinucleotide phosphate (NADP⁺)
NADP⁺ is similar to NAD⁺ but the H attached to the O is replaced by a phosphate group.

Pantothenic Acid and Coenzyme A

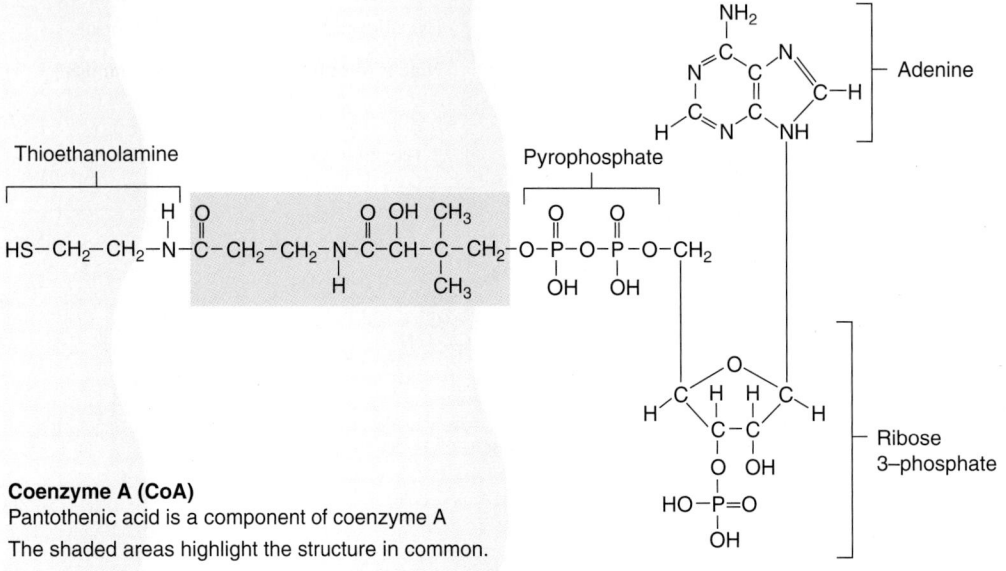

Pantothenic acid

Coenzyme A (CoA)
Pantothenic acid is a component of coenzyme A
The shaded areas highlight the structure in common.

Biotin

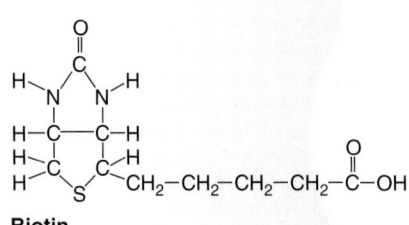

Biotin

Vitamin B₆ and Coenzymes

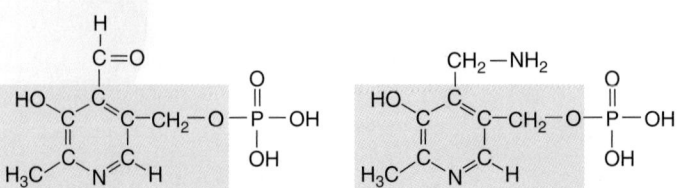

Pyridoxine   Pyridoxal   Pyridoxamine

Vitamin B₆ (pyridoxine, pyridoxal, and pyridoxamine)

Pyridoxal phosphate (PLP)   **Pyridoxamine phosphate (PMP)**

Pyridoxal phosphate (PLP) and pyridoxamine phosphate (PMP) are the two active coenzyme forms of vitamin B₆

The shaded areas highlight the structures in common.

Folate and Coenzyme

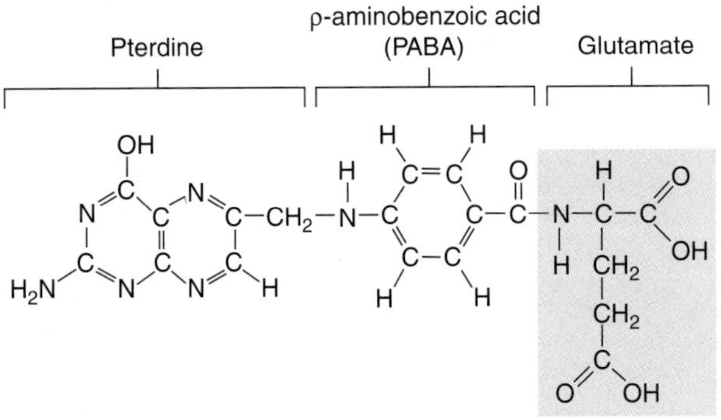

Folate

Folate contains at least one and up to 11 glutamates (see shaded area that contains a single glutamate). Folic acid contains only one glutamate.

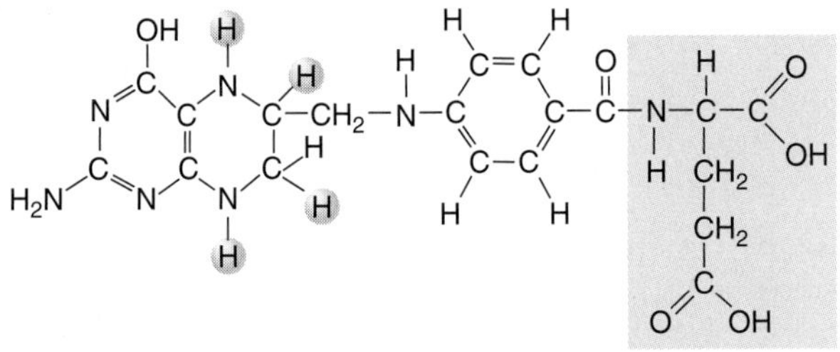

Tetrahydrofolic acid (THFA)

Adding 4 hydrogens to folate produces THFA, the active coenzyme form.

Vitamin C

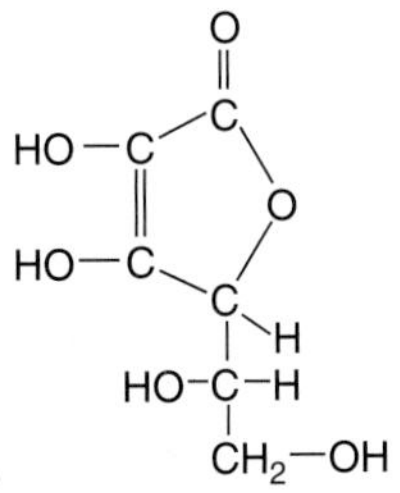

**Vitamin C
(Ascorbic acid)**

Vitamin B$_{12}$

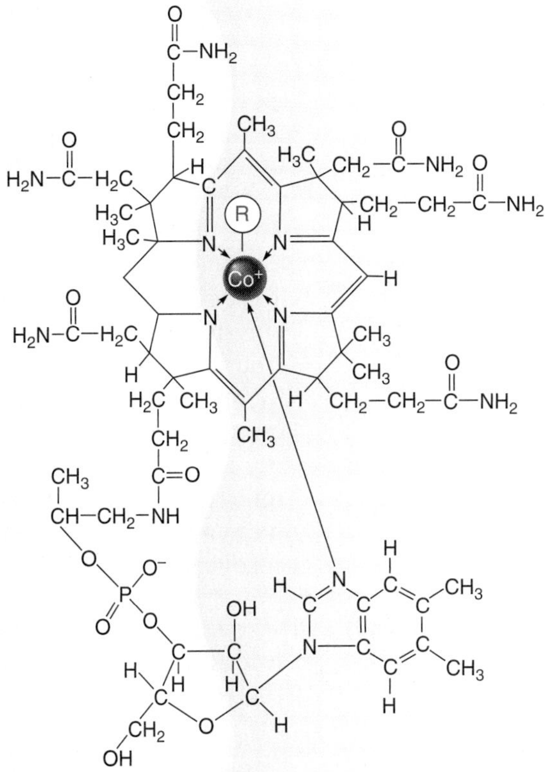

Vitamin B$_{12}$ (cobalamin)

R = CN in cyanocobalamin

R = OH in hydroxocobalamin

R = 5′–deoxyadenosyl in 5′–deoxyadenosylcobalamin

R = CH$_3$ in methylcobalamin

Arrows indicate that the free electron pairs of nitrogen are in close proximity to the positively charged cobalt.

B Vitamins in Major Metabolic Pathways

Thiamin	Pyruvate to acetyl CoA (TPP)
	Citric acid cycle (TPP)

Riboflavin	Pyruvate to acetyl CoA (FAD)
	Citric acid cycle (FAD)
	Electron transport chain (FAD, FMN)
	Beta-oxidation (fatty acids to acetyl CoA) (FAD)
	Amino acid breakdown (FAD)

Niacin	Glycolysis (NAD^+)
	Pyruvate to acetyl CoA (NAD^+)
	Citric acid cycle (NAD^+)
	Electron transport chain (NAD^+)
	Beta-oxidation (fatty acids to acetyl CoA) (NAD^+)
	Fatty acid synthesis (acetyl CoA to fatty acids) (NADPH)
	Amino acid breakdown (NAD^+)
	Amino acid synthesis (NAD^+, NADPH)
	Gluconeogenesis (NAD^+)

Pantothenic acid	Pyruvate to acetyl CoA (coenzyme A)
	Citric acid cycle (coenzyme A)
	Beta-oxidation (fatty acids to acetyl CoA) (coenzyme A)
	Fatty acid synthesis (acetyl CoA to fatty acids) (coenzyme A)

Biotin	Fatty acid synthesis (acetyl CoA to fatty acids) (biotin-enzyme)
	Gluconeogenesis (biotin-enzyme)

Vitamin B_6	Glycogen to glucose (PLP)
	Amino acid breakdown (PLP)
	Amino acid synthesis (PLP)

Folate	Amino acid synthesis (THFA)
	Synthesis of some components of DNA and RNA (THFA)

Vitamin B_{12}	Amino acid breakdown (B_{12})
	Synthesis of some components of DNA and RNA (B_{12})

Major Metabolic Pathways APPENDIX G

- Glycolysis
- Citric Acid Cycle
- Electron Transport Chain
- Urea Cycle

Glycolysis

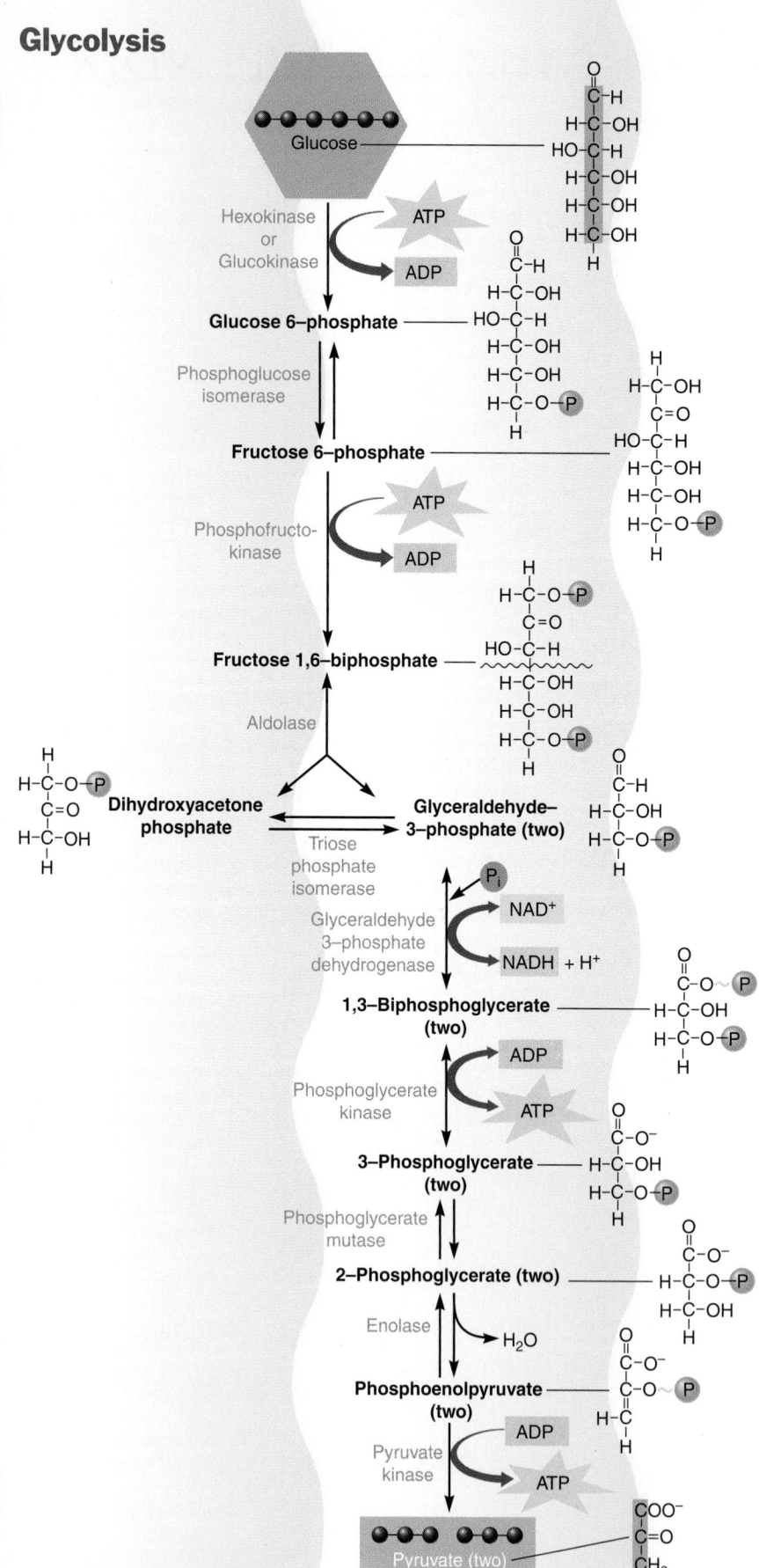

Glycolysis is the first step in metabolizing glucose and other monosaccharides for energy. Unlike the reaction that converts blood glucose to glucose 6-phosphate, the reaction that converts glucose from glycogen to glucose 6-phosphate does not require ATP. Thus the glycolysis of glucose from glycogen directly yields 3 ATP as compared to the 2 ATP from blood glucose. Additional ATP is produced from glycolytic NADH in the electron transport chain.

The reactions that convert fructose to fructose 6-phosphate require ATP so fructose produces the same amount of ATP as blood glucose. The same is true for galactose, which enters at glucose 6-phosphate.

Citric Acid Cycle

Electron Transport Chain

(site of oxidative phosphorylation)

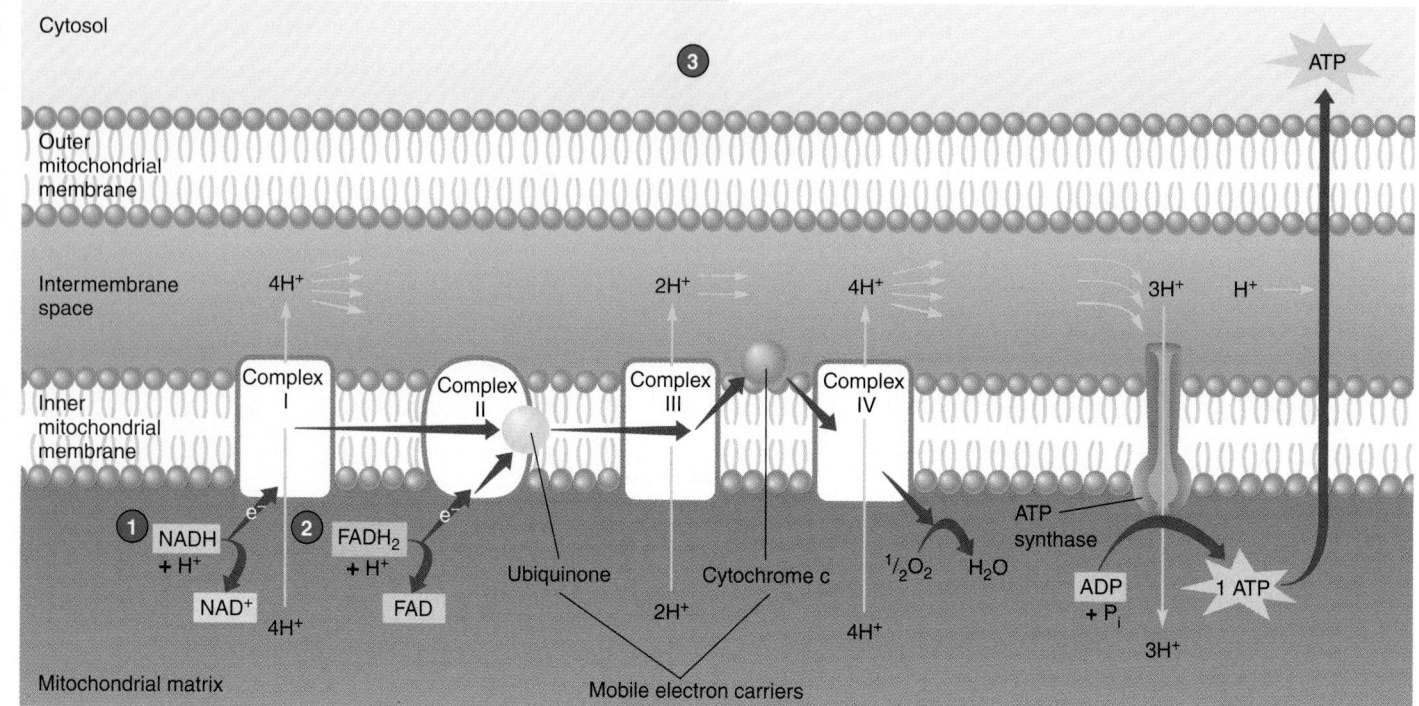

Complex I   NADH–Q reductase
Complex II   Succinate–Q reductase
Complex III Cytochrome reductase
Complex IV   Cytochrome oxidase

Complexes I, III, and IV are proton (H⁺) pumps. Complex II does not pump protons.
The three proton pumps are linked by the mobile electron carriers ubiquinone and cytochrome c.

NADH

1 A pair of electrons from NADH enters the chain at complex I (NADH-Q reductase). The flow of electrons from NADH to ubiquinone leads to the pumping of 4 H⁺ from the matrix to the intermembrane space. The flow of electrons from ubiquinone to cytochrome c through complex III (cytochrome reductase) pumps another 2 H⁺ into the intermembrane space. As complex IV (cytochrome oxidase) catalyzes the transfer of electrons from cytochrome c to O_2, it pumps another 4 H⁺. (Complex IV actually uses 4 electrons to produce 2 H_2O from a single O_2.) The transit of the NADH electron pair through the electron transport chain pumps a total of 10 H⁺ into the intermembrane space. Each 3 H⁺ returning to the matrix through the ATP synthase produces 1 ATP. Another H⁺ is consumed in transporting ATP from the matrix to the cytosol. Thus the two electrons from NADH produce about 2.5 ATP (10 pumped ÷ 4 = 2.5).

FADH₂

2 A pair of electrons from FADH₂ enter the chain at complex II (succinate-Q), which is the non-pumping complex. The flow of electrons from FADH₂ to ubiquinone does not pump any protons to the intermembrane space. The flow of electrons through complexes III and IV is the same as for NADH. Thus the transit of the two FADH₂ electrons through the electron transport chain pumps a total of 6 H⁺ into the intermembrane space and produces about 1.5 ATP (6 ÷ 4 = 1.5).

Cytosolic NADH

3 Glycolysis forms NADH in the cytosol, but the outer mitochondrial membrane is impervious to NADH. How can NADH deliver its electrons to the electron transport chain? NADH transfers its pair of electrons to special carriers that can cross the mitochondrial membrane. One carrier, glycerol 3-phosphate, shuttles the electrons to the matrix and delivers them to FAD, thereby forming FADH₂. This FADH₂ delivers the electrons to the chain where they form 1.5 ATP. In the heart and liver, malate shuttles the electrons from cytosolic NADH to the matrix. Malate crosses the mitochondrial membrane and delivers the electrons to NAD⁺, thereby forming NADH inside the mitochondrion. This NADH delivers the electron pair to the chain where they form 2.5 ATP. Depending on the carrier, cytosolic NADH may produce 1.5 or 2.5 ATP.

The Urea Cycle

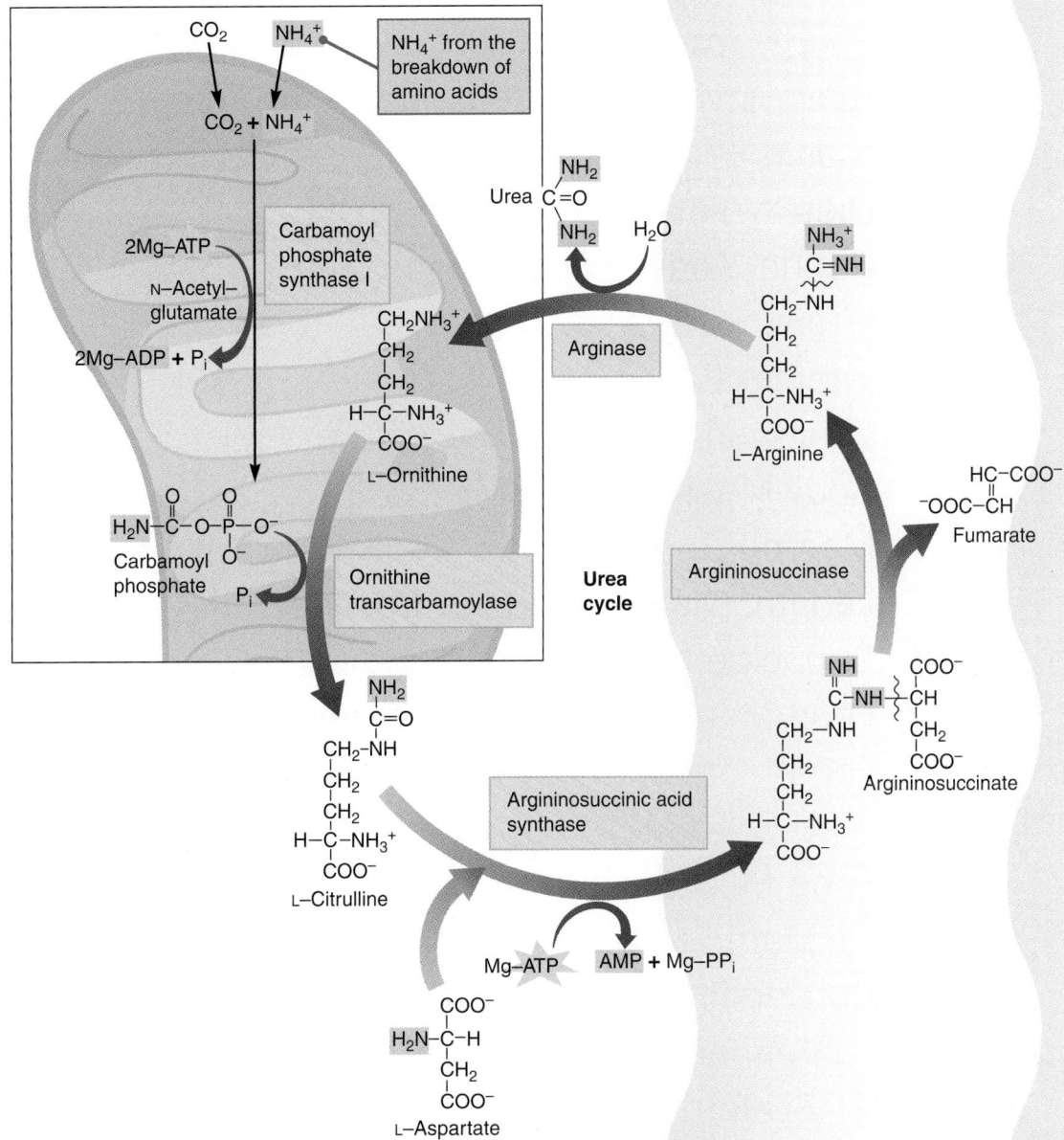

Some NH_4^+ from the breakdown of amino acids is used for biosynthesis of nitrogen compounds. Excess NH_4^+ is converted to urea and excreted.

APPENDIX H Calculations and Conversions

- Energy from Food
- Recommended Protein Intake for Adults
- Niacin Equivalents (NE)
- Dietary Folate Equivalents (DFE)
- Retinol Activity Equivalents (RAE)
- Vitamin D
- Vitamin E
- Estimating Energy Expenditure
- Body Mass Index (BMI)
- Metric Prefixes
- Length: Metric and U.S. Equivalents
- Capacities or Volumes
- Food Measurement Equivalents
- Food Measurement Conversions: U.S. to Metric
- Food Measurement Conversions: Metric to U.S.
- Conversion Factors
- Fahrenheit and Celsius (Centigrade) Scales
- Do You Speak Metric?

Energy from Food

grams carbohydrate $\times$ 4 kcal/g
grams protein $\times$ 4 kcal/g
grams fat $\times$ 9 kcal/g
grams alcohol $\times$ 7 kcal/g
total = energy from food

Example:
Carbohydrate	275 g $\times$ 4 kcal/g =	1,100 kcal
Protein	64 g $\times$ 4 kcal/g =	256 kcal
Fat	60 g $\times$ 9 kcal/g =	540 kcal
Alcohol	15 g $\times$ 7 kcal/g =	105 kcal
	TOTAL ENERGY	**2,001 kcal**

Calculating the percentage of calories for each:
Carbohydrate   (1,100 kcal $\div$ 2,001 kcal) $\times$ 100 = 54.97% (55%)
Protein   (256 kcal $\div$ 2,001 kcal) $\times$ 100 = 12.79% (13%)
Fat   (540 kcal $\div$ 2,001 kcal) $\times$ 100 = 26.99% (27%)
Alcohol   (105 kcal $\div$ 2,001 kcal) $\times$ 100 = 5.25% (5%)

1 kilocalorie = 4.184 kilojoules
1 kilojoule = 0.239 kilocalories

Recommended Protein Intake for Adults

grams of recommended protein = weight in kilograms $\times$ 0.8 g/kg

Example:
A 70-kg (154-lb) person
grams of recommended protein = 70 kg $\times$ 0.8 g/kg = 56 grams protein, or
grams of recommended protein = (154 lb $\div$ 2.2) $\times$ 0.8 g/kg = 56 grams protein

Note: Endurance athletes involved in heavy training may require 1.2 to 1.4 grams of protein per kilogram of body weight per day.

Niacin Equivalents (NE)

Determining the amount of niacin from tryptophan:

NE = milligrams niacin
NE from tryptophan = grams excess protein $\div$ 6
NE from tryptophan = (grams dietary protein − protein RDA) $\div$ 6

Example: Assume dietary protein = 86 g and protein RDA = 56 g
NE from tryptophan = (86 g − 56 g) $\div$ 6
NE from tryptophan = 5

Dietary Folate Equivalents (DFE)

Dietary folate equivalents account for differences in the absorption of food folate, synthetic folic acid in dietary supplements, and folic acid added to fortified foods. Food in the stomach also affects bioavailability. Folic acid taken as a supplement when fasting is two times more bioavailable than food folate. Folic acid taken with food and folic acid in fortified foods are 1.7 times more bioavailable than food folate.

1 μg DFE = 1 microgram of food folate
= 0.5 μg of folic acid supplement taken on an empty stomach
= 0.6 μg of folic acid supplement consumed with meals
= 0.6 μg of folic acid in fortified foods

1 μg folic acid as a fortificant = 1.7 μg DFE
1 μg folic acid as a supplement, fasting = 2.0 μg DFE

Example:
Food folate in cooked spinach   100 μg = 100 μg DFE
Ready-to-eat cereal fortified with folic acid   100 μg = 170 μg DFE
Supplemental folic acid taken without food   100 μg = 200 μg DFE

Estimating DFE from Daily Value:
DFE = %DV $\times$ DV $\times$ bioavailability factor

Example:
Assume that a serving of fortified breakfast cereal contains 10% of the Daily Value for folate
Daily Value = 400 μg folic acid

DFE = %DV $\times$ DV $\times$ bioavailability factor
DFE = 0.10 $\times$ 400 μg $\times$ 1.7
DFE = 68 μg, which can be rounded to 70 μg DFE

Retinol Activity Equivalents (RAE)

Retinol activity equivalents are a standardized measure of vitamin A activity that account for differences in the bioavailability of different sources of vitamin A. Of the provitamin A carotenoids, beta-carotene produces the most vitamin A.

1 μg RAE = 1 μg retinol
= 12 μg beta-carotene
= 24 μg of other vitamin A precursors

Although outdated, many vitamin supplements still report vitamin A content as International Units (IU).

1 μg RAE = 3.33 IU from retinol
= 10 IU from beta-carotene in supplements
= 20 IU from beta-carotene in foods

Vitamin D

Although outdated, many vitamin supplements still report vitamin D content as International Units (IU).

1 IU = 0.025 μg cholecalciferol
μg cholecalciferol = IU $\div$ 40

Example:
A vitamin supplement contains 100 IU vitamin D
μg cholecalciferol = 100 $\div$ 40 = 2.5

Vitamin E

Although outdated, many vitamin supplements still report vitamin E content as International Units (IU) rather than as milligrams of α-tocopherol. Two conversion factors are used to convert IU to milligrams of α-tocopherol. If the form of the supplement is "natural" or RRR-α-tocopherol (historically labeled as *d*-alpha-tocopherol), the conversion factor is 0.67 mg/IU. If the form of the supplement is *all rac*-α-tocopherol (historically labeled *dl*-α-tocopherol), the conversion factor is 0.45 mg/IU.

Examples:

A multivitamin supplement contains 30 IU of *d*-α-tocopherol

30 IU $\times$ 0.67 = 20 mg α-tocopherol

A multivitamin supplement contains 30 IU of *dl*-α-tocopherol

30 IU $\times$ 0.45 = 13.5 mg α-tocopherol

Estimating Energy Expenditure

The Estimated Energy Requirement (EER) is defined as the dietary energy intake (in kilocalories per day) that is predicted to maintain energy balance in a healthy adult of a defined age, gender, weight, height, and level of physical activity consistent with good health.* The EER equations predict Total Energy Expenditure (TEE).

Adult men (age 19 and older):

$$EER = 662 - 9.53 \times Age\ [yr] + PA \times (15.91 \times Weight\ [kg] + 539.6 \times Height\ [m])$$

PA is the Physical Activity coefficient that represents physical activity level

Sedentary	PA = 1.0
Low active	PA = 1.11
Active	PA = 1.25
Very active	PA = 1.48

Adult women (age 19 and older):

$$EER = 354 - 6.91 \times Age\ [yr] + PA \times (9.36 \times Weight\ [kg] + 726 \times Height\ [m])$$

PA is the Physical Activity coefficient that represents physical activity level

Sedentary	PA = 1.0
Low active	PA = 1.12
Active	PA = 1.27
Very active	PA = 1.45

Example: A 21-year-old woman, 5'4" (1.6 m) tall, who weighs 120 pounds (54.5 kilograms) and is active.

Example:
= 354 − 6.91 × 21 yr + 1.27 ×
(9.36 × 54.5 kg + 726 × 1.6 m)
= 354 − 145.11 + 1.27 × (510.12 + 1,161.6)
= 354 − 145.11 + 1.27 × 1,671.72
= 354 − 145.11 + 2,123.08
= 2,331.97
= 2,332 kcal/day

*Source: Institute of Medicine, Food and Nutrition Board. *Dietary Reference Intakes for Energy, Carbohydrate, Fiber, Fat, Fatty Acids, Cholesterol, Protein, and Amino Acids*. Washington, DC: National Academy Press; 2005.

Total energy expenditure can also be estimated by first estimating resting energy expenditure (REE) and then adding additional energy to account for physical activity and the thermic effect of food.

Resting Energy Expenditure (REE)

Harris-Benedict Equations

Adult men $\quad$ REE = 66 + 13.7W + 5.0H − 6.8A

Adult women $\quad$ REE = 655 + 9.6W + 1.8H − 4.7A

(W = weight in kilograms, H = height in centimeters, A = age)

Note: Harris-Benedict equations may overestimate resting energy expenditure, especially for obese people.

Quick Estimate

Adult men $\quad$ REE = weight (kg) × 1.0 kcal/kg × 24 hours
REE = weight (kg) × 1.0 × 24

Adult women $\quad$ REE = weight (kg) × 0.9 kcal/kg × 24 hours
REE = weight (kg) × 0.9 × 24

Physical Activity (PA)

Physical activity can be estimated as a percentage of the resting energy expenditure (REE) based on the frequency and intensity of physical activity.

Percentage of REE	Activity Level	Description
20–30%	Sedentary	Mostly resting, with little or no activity
30–45%	Light	Occasional unplanned activity (e.g., going for a stroll)
45–65%	Moderate	Daily planned activity, such as brisk walks
65–90%	Heavy	Daily workout routine requiring several hours of continuous exercise
90–120%	Exceptional	Daily vigorous workouts for extended hours; training for competition

Thermic Effect of Food (TEF)

The thermic effect of food can be estimated as 10% of the sum of REE + physical activity

Total energy expenditure (TEE) = REE + PA + TEF

Example using quick estimate of REE:

A 175-pound (79.5 kg), 30-year-old man engages in moderate activity (60% of REE).

REE = 79.5 kg × 1.0 kcal/kg/hr × 24 hr/day
= 1,908 kcal/day

PA = 60% of REE
= 0.60 × 1908 kcal/day
= 1144.8 kcal/day

TEF = 10% of REE + PA
= 0.10 × (1908 + 1144.8 kcal/day)
= 0.10 × 3052.8 kcal/day
= 305.3 kcal/day

TEE = REE + PA + TEF
= 1908 + 1144.8 + 305.3 kcal/day
= 3358 kcal/day

Body Mass Index (BMI)

U.S. Formula

BMI = [weight in pounds ÷ (height in inches)^2] × 703

Example: **A 154-pound man is 5 ft 8 inches (68 inches) tall**
BMI = [154 ÷ (68 in × 68 in)] × 703
BMI = (154 ÷ 4,624) × 703
BMI = 23.41

Metric Formula

BMI = weight in kilograms ÷ [height in meters]^2
or
BMI = [weight in kilograms ÷ (height in cm)^2] × 10,000

Example: **A 70-kg man is 1.75 meters tall**
BMI = 70 kg ÷ (1.75 m × 1.75 m)
BMI = 70 ÷ 3.0625
BMI = 22.86

Metric Prefixes

giga-	G	1,000,000,000
mega-	M	1,000,000
kilo-	k	1,000
hecto-	h.	100
deka-	da.	10
deci-	d	0.1
centi-	c	0.01
milli-	m.	0.001
micro-	μ	0.000001
nano-	n	0.000000001

Length: Metric and U.S. Equivalents

1 centimeter	0.3937 inch
1 decimeter	3.937 inches
1 foot	0.3048 meter
1 inch	2.54 centimeters
1 meter	39.37 inches
	1.094 yards
1 micron	0.001 millimeter
	0.00003937 inch
1 millimeter	0.03937 inch
1 yard	0.9144 meter

Capacities or Volumes

1 cup, measuring	8 fluid ounces
	1/2 liquid pint
1 gallon (U.S.)	231 cubic inches
	3.785 liters
	0.833 British gallon
	128 U.S. fluid ounces
1 gallon (British Imperial)	277.42 cubic inches
	1.201 U.S. gallons
	4.546 liters
	160 British fluid ounces
1 liter	1.057 liquid quarts
	0.908 dry quart
	61.024 cubic inches
1 milliliter	0.061 cubic inches
1 ounce, fluid or liquid (U.S.)	1.805 cubic inches
	29.574 milliliters
	1.041 British fluid ounces
1 pint, dry	33.600 cubic inches
	0.551 liter
1 pint, liquid	28.875 cubic inches
	0.473 liter
1 quart, dry (U.S.)	67.201 cubic inches
	1.101 liters
	0.969 British quart
1 quart, liquid (U.S.)	57.75 cubic inches
	0.946 liter
	0.833 British quart
1 quart (British)	69.354 cubic inches
	1.032 U.S. dry quarts
	1.201 U.S. liquid quarts
1 tablespoon, measuring	3 teaspoons
	1/2 fluid ounce
1 teaspoon, measuring	1/3 tablespoon
	1/6 fluid ounce
1 kilogram	2.205 pounds
1 microgram (μg)	0.000001 gram

Food Measurement Equivalents

16 tablespoons = 1 cup
12 tablespoons = 3/4 cup
10 tablespoons + 2 teaspoons = 2/3 cup
8 tablespoons = 1/2 cup
6 tablespoons = 3/8 cup
5 tablespoons + 1 teaspoon = 1/3 cup
4 tablespoons = 1/4 cup
2 tablespoons = 1/8 cup

2 tablespoons + 2 teaspoons = 1/6 cup
1 tablespoon = 1/16 cup
2 cups = 1 pint
2 pints = 1 quart
3 teaspoons = 1 tablespoon
48 teaspoons = 1 cup

Food Measurement Conversions: U.S. to Metric

Capacity

1/5 teaspoon . . . . 1 milliliter		1 cup . . . . 237 milliliters
1 teaspoon . . . . . 5 milliliters		2 cups (1 pint) . . 473 milliliters
1 tablespoon . . . . 15 milliliters		4 cups (1 quart) . . . . 0.95 liter
1 fluid ounce . . . . 30 milliliters		4 quarts (1 gal.) . . . . 3.8 liters
1/5 cup . . . . 47 milliliters		

Weight

1 ounce . . . . 28 grams
1 pound . . . . 454 grams

Food Measurement Conversions: Metric to U.S.

Capacity

	Weight
1 milliliter . . . . . 1/5 teaspoon	1 gram . . . . . . 0.035 ounce
5 milliliters . . . . 1 teaspoon	100 grams . . . . . 3.5 ounces
15 milliliters . . . 1 tablespoon	500 grams . . . . 1.10 pounds
100 milliliters . . 3.4 fluid oz	1 kilogram . . . 2.205 pounds
240 milliliters . . 1 cup	. . . . . . 35 ounces
1 liter . . . . 34 fluid oz	
. . . . 4.2 cups	
. . . . 2.1 pints	
. . . . 1.06 quarts	
. . . . 0.26 gallon	

Conversion Factors

To change	To	Multiply by
centimeters	inches	0.3937
centimeters	feet	0.03281
cubic feet	cubic meters	0.0283
cubic meters	cubic feet	35.3145
cubic meters	cubic yards	1.3079
cubic yards	cubic meters	0.7646
feet	meters	0.3048
gallons (U.S.)	liters	3.7853
grams	ounces avdp	0.0353
grams	pounds	0.002205

To change	To	Multiply by
inches	millimeters	25.4000
inches	centimeters	2.5400
inches	meters	0.0254
kilograms	pounds	2.2046
liters	gallons (U.S.)	0.2642
liters	pints (dry)	1.8162
liters	pints (liquid)	2.1134
liters	quarts (dry)	0.9081
liters	quarts (liquid)	1.0567
meters	feet	3.2808
meters	yards	1.0936
millimeters	inches	0.0394
ounces avdp	grams	28.3495
ounces	pounds	0.0625
pints (dry)	liters	0.5506
pints (liquid)	liters	0.4732
pounds	kilograms	0.4536
pounds	ounces	16
quarts (dry)	liters	1.1012
quarts (liquid)	liters	0.9463

Fahrenheit and Celsius (Centigrade) Scales

°Celsius	°Fahrenheit
−273.15	−459.67
−250	−418
−200	−328
−150	−238
−100	−148
−50	−58
−40	−40
−30	−22
−20	−4
−10	14
0	32
5	41
10	50
15	59
20	68
25	77
30	86
35	95
40	104
45	113
50	122
55	131
60	140

°Celsius		°Fahrenheit
65	....	149
70	....	158
75	....	167
80	....	176
85	....	185
90	....	194
95	....	203
100	....	212

Zero on the Fahrenheit scale represents the temperature produced by the mixing of equal weights of snow and common salt.

	°Fahrenheit	°Celsius
Boiling point of water	212°	100°
Freezing point of water	32°	0°
Normal body temperature	98.6°	37°
Comfortable room temperature	68–77°	20–25°
Absolute zero	−459.6°	−273.1°

Absolute zero is theoretically the lowest possible temperature, the point at which all molecular motion would cease.

To Convert Temperature Scales

To convert Fahrenheit to Celsius (Centigrade), subtract 32 and multiply by ⁵⁄₉.

$$°C = \tfrac{5}{9}(°F - 32)$$

To convert Celsius (Centigrade) to Fahrenheit, multiply by ⁹⁄₅ and add 32.

$$°F = (\tfrac{9}{5} \times °C) + 32$$

Do You Speak Metric?

Although the metric system isn't really a language like English or Spanish, in some sense it is the language of science. Nutritionists must be fluent in metrics. Pick up any nutrition journal and you will find units of measurement expressed in terms like kilograms and liters.

The metric system is a decimal-based system of measurement units. Like our monetary system, units are related by factors of 10. There are 10 pennies in a dime, and 10 dimes equal 1 dollar. Calculations involve the simple process of moving the decimal point to the right or to the left.

There are only seven basic units in the metric system. The most common units are the meter (m) to measure length, the gram (g) for mass, the liter (L) for volume, and degree Celsius (°C) for temperature. The metric system avoids the confusing dual use of terms, such as the current use of ounces to measure both weight and volume.

One strategy for learning metric is to find common or familiar associations. For example, when using degrees Celsius you should equate 22 degrees Celsius (22°C) with room temperature, 37 degrees Celsius (37°C) with body temperature, and 0 and 100 degrees Celsius with the freezing and boiling points of water, respectively. A millimeter (1 mm) is about the thickness of a dime, and 2 centimeters (2 cm) is about the diameter of a nickel. When you pick up a 2-pound box of sugar, you are holding about 900 grams.

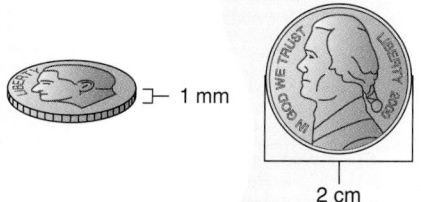

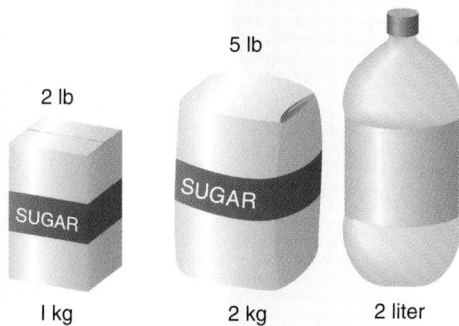

A fluid ounce can be tricky because it's a measure of liquid volume, not weight. Most people already recognize 1-liter and 2-liter soft-drink bottles. A 1-liter bottle equals 33.8 fluid ounces.

The United States is the only industrialized country in the world not officially using the metric system. Because of its many advantages (e.g., easy conversion between units of the same quantity), the metric system has become the internationally accepted system of measurement.

Many members of the international scientific community use the International System of Units (SI). The SI is the modern metric system and has adopted the joule rather than the calorie to measure food energy. Although we think of the calorie as a measure of energy, it is more accurately a measure of heat. Joules are a measure of work, not heat, and the amount of energy potential in foods is expressed best in kilojoules (kjoules). Each kilocalorie is equivalent to approximately 4.2 (4.184) kilojoules. For example, a 100-kilocalorie glass of juice provides about 420 kilojoules.

The Celsius (C) temperature scale should be used instead of the Fahrenheit (F) scale. The following are familiar points:

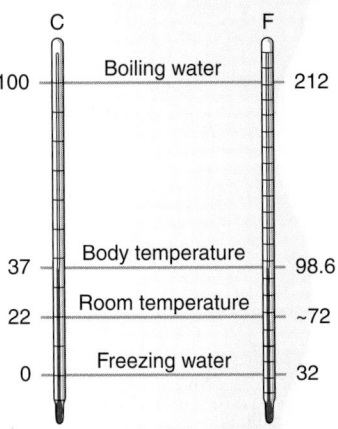

Table H.1 **Measures Commonly Used in Nutrition**

	Metric	English
Length	1 meter (m)	39.4 inches (in)
	1 centimeter (cm)	0.394 inch (in)
	2.54 centimeters (cm)	1 inch (in)
Weight (mass)	1 kilogram (kg)	2.2 pounds (lb)
	454 grams (g)	1 pound (lb)
	5 grams (g) of salt	about 1 teaspoon (tsp)
Volume	1 liter (L)	1.057 quarts (about 4 cups)
	236 milliliters (mL)	about 1 cup (c)
	15 milliliters (mL)	about 1 tablespoon (Tbsp)
	5 milliliters (mL)	about 1 teaspoon (tsp)

Note:

1 gram = 1,000 milligrams

1 milligram = 1,000 micrograms (μg or mcg)

Growth Charts APPENDIX I

A complete set of growth charts is available on the Internet at www.cdc.gov/growthcharts. There are three sets, each with a different set of percentiles. Each set includes the following charts for girls and boys:

Weight-for-age percentiles: birth to 36 months

Length-for-age percentiles: birth to 36 months

Weight-for-length percentiles: birth to 36 months

Head circumference-for-age percentiles: birth to 36 months

Weight-for-age percentiles: 2 to 20 years

Stature-for-age percentiles: 2 to 20 years

Weight-for-stature percentiles

Body mass index-for-age percentiles: 2 to 20 years

2 to 20 years: Girls
Stature-for-Age and Weight-for-Age Percentiles

NAME _____

RECORD # _____

Mother's Stature _____		Father's Stature _____		
Date	Age	Weight	Stature	BMI*

***To Calculate BMI**: Weight (kg) ÷ Stature (cm) ÷ Stature (cm) x 10,000
or Weight (lb) ÷ Stature (in) ÷ Stature (in) x 703

AGE (YEARS)

STATURE

WEIGHT

SOURCE: Developed by the National Center for Health Statistics in collaboration with
the National Center for Chronic Disease Prevention and Health Promotion (2000).
http://www.cdc.gov/growthcharts

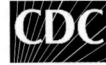

2 to 20 years: Boys
Stature-for-Age and Weight-for-Age Percentiles

NAME _____

RECORD # _____

Mother's Stature		Father's Stature		
Date	Age	Weight	Stature	BMI*

***To Calculate BMI**: Weight (kg) ÷ Stature (cm) ÷ Stature (cm) x 10,000
or Weight (lb) ÷ Stature (in) ÷ Stature (in) x 703

AGE (YEARS)

12 13 14 15 16 17 18 19 20

STATURE

WEIGHT

AGE (YEARS)

2 3 4 5 6 7 8 9 10 11 12 13 14 15 16 17 18 19 20

SOURCE: Developed by the National Center for Health Statistics in collaboration with
the National Center for Chronic Disease Prevention and Health Promotion (2000).
http://www.cdc.gov/growthcharts

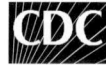

APPENDIX J Feeding Infants and Toddlers

While there is nothing complex about the nutrient needs of infants and toddlers—and the foods that are appropriate for them—it is important for caregivers to receive some education about proper feeding. The tables in this appendix summarize development stages of infants and appropriate foods at each stage, along with practical tips for feeding infants and toddlers.

Table J.1 Infant Feeding Guide (0 to 12 months)

Age (mo)	Human Milk or Iron-fortified Formula	Cereals & Breads	Vegetables	Fruits	Other Protein Foods
0–4	8–12 feedings per day 16–32 oz	None	None	None	None
4–6	4–7 feedings per day 24–32 oz	Iron-fortified baby cereal, rice, barley, oatmeal; feed by spoon; mix 2–3 tsp with human milk or formula	None	None	None
6–8	3–4 feedings per day 24–32 oz Begin to offer cup	Add mixed cereal after previous plain ones; 2 servings per day; dry toast or teething biscuit	Plain strained or mashed vegetables 2 times per day	Fresh or cooked fruits: mashed bananas, applesauce; strained plain fruits; 2 times per day	
8–10	3–4 feedings per day 16–32 oz Offer formula in cup	Infant iron-fortified cereals; Cream of Rice; dry toast, teething biscuit	Plain cooked mashed vegetables	Peeled soft fruit wedges: bananas, pears, oranges, apples, peaches	Lean meat and chicken: strained, chopped, or small tender pieces
10–12	3–4 feedings per day 16–32 oz Formula in a cup	Infant cereals, unsweetened cereals, bread, rice, noodles, and pasta	Cooked vegetable pieces	All fresh fruits peeled and seeded; canned fruit in water	Small tender pieces of meat, chicken, or fish; eggs, mild cheeses, yogurt, cooked dried beans

Table J.2 Developmental Patterns and Feeding Recommendations for Infancy

	Birth	1mo	2mo	3mo	4mo	5mo	6mo	7mo	8mo	9mo	10mo	11mo
Mouth Pattern	Suck and swallow reflex / Extrusion reflex				Transfer food from front to back / Drooling				Begin chewing / Side to side movement of tongue / Mashing food with jaws			Biting / Chewing
Hand Coordination	Random motion of hands / Hand to mouth to signal hunger				Hand to mouth purposefully		Palmar grasp	Pincer grasp	Grabs spoon		Spoon to mouth turned over	
Body Control	Minimal head control				Sits supported, loses balance when reaching		Sits unsupported and while reaching / Hand manipulation		Continued improvement of balance while sitting / Begins to stand and possibly walks			
Digestive Ability	Can digest appropriate milk				Intestinal amylase increases			Gastric acid volume increases			Can handle balanced amount of unseasoned family food	
Homeostatic Ability	Low, needs breast milk or carefully adapted formula							Increased ability to maintain hydration and chemical balance				
Nutritional Requirements	High nutrient needs for rapid growth		Iron stores depleted for preemies				Iron stores depleted for term infants		Needs gradually being met with solid diet over breast milk/formula			Move to table food and cup
Feeding Style	Nipple feeding					Begin spoon feeding	Spoon feeding	Introduce cup with meals	Begin self-feed with cup; begin proficiency with spoon			Cup and spoon self-feed
Food Selection	Breastmilk or formula					Begin solids, iron source		Semi-solid foods	Increase texture		Pieces of soft cooked foods	

Source: Adapted from Satter E. *Child of Mine: Feeding with Love and Good Sense.* 3rd ed. Palo Alto, CA: Bull Publishing Co.; 2000.

Table J.3 **Practical Feeding Tips**

4–6 months old

Avoid seasonings. Babies enjoy plain foods. Added sugar and salt are unnecessary.

Commercially prepared foods are acceptable, but so are home-prepared foods. Mash plain, cooked vegetables or fruit.

Add one new food each week.

Work up to a total of one-half cup of cereal per day.

Feed the baby from a dish, not the jar.

Throw out leftovers from the baby's dish.

Once introduced, aim for 2 tablespoons per day of vegetables and fruit.

Use baby-sized spoons, cups, and bowls.

7–9 months old

Cook fruits with a little water to soften them.

Add more finger foods to the diet. Examples include dry unsweetened oat or rice cereal, rice cakes, and cooked rice.

Grate fresh fruits and vegetables, and allow the child to pick them up and self-feed.

Offer a variety of cooked vegetables that can be either mashed or picked up in tiny pieces.

Offer a variety of protein sources: cooked fish; chicken; turkey; beef; mashed, cooked beans.

10–12 months

Allow the child to self-feed with a spoon and cup.

Have the child join the rest of the family at meals.

Feed the child both meals and healthful snacks, sometimes just smaller versions of the meal, to fulfill his or her energy needs.

Remember to offer the child water from a cup.

Table J.4 **Feeding Practices and Foods to Avoid**

Practices or Foods to Avoid	Rationale
Leaving baby alone during feeding	Infants and toddlers need to be supervised at all times. Children can accidentally choke during mealtime.
Adding salt, seasonings, and spices	Children prefer plain foods and do not need additional seasoning. Excessively salty foods can place a burden on the developing kidney system.
Egg whites and wheat	Common sources of food allergies. Neither is necessary in the diet before age 1.
Cow's milk	Neither necessary nor well tolerated until age 1. Associated with increased allergic potential and iron-deficiency anemia.
Honey and corn syrup	Both products contain spores of *Clostridium botulinum*. In infants, these spores can cause botulism, a deadly foodborne illness.
High-risk choking foods	Foods that are choking hazards for infants and toddlers include hot dogs, nuts, peanuts, raw carrots, sausage pieces, raisins, apple chunks, popcorn, hard candy, potato chips, gum, hard pretzels or pretzel nuggets, chicken bones and wings, grapes, and plain peanut butter from a spoon. Because peanuts are a common food allergen, peanut butter should not be introduced in the first year.
Heating foods on the stove/microwave	Accidental injury or burns can occur with uneven and excessive overheating of infant foods. The baby cannot tell the caregiver that the food is too hot.
Excessive amounts of breast milk or formula	During the second half of the first year, the child gradually decreases consumption of breast milk and formula in order to increase the amount of solid foods needed for energy and iron.
Excessive intake of fruit juices/drinks	Both failure to thrive and overweight have been seen from excessive consumption of juice or other drinks.
Goat's milk	Goat's milk is too low in folate, iron, vitamins C and D, and is not a suitable substitute for either human milk or formula.

Table J.5 **Common Food Habits of Toddlers**

- *Playing with food:* Toddlers frequently appear disinterested in food, merely playing with it, and refusing to let the caregiver feed them. They actually need to play with food to discover its texture, smell, and taste.

- *Food jags:* A toddler may want nothing but macaroni and cheese for dinner for a while, or refuse foods that aren't white. Nothing lasts forever, however. The caregiver should continue to offer new foods, but allow the toddler to refuse them. One day both the caregiver and the toddler may be surprised when a new food is eaten and enjoyed!

- *Food protests:* A toddler's communication skills are not as developed as his opinions or strength, which means unwanted food may end up on the floor or walls. Although this behavior is normal, it does not have to be tolerated. The toddler needs to know that the caregiver is disappointed in her. The caregiver should model positive, corrective behavior.

- *Irregular eating patterns:* Toddlers are active and need energy. However, their growth has slowed considerably by this stage, and energy requirements per unit of body weight have decreased. Toddlers will slow down their food intake and may skip meals. It is important to continue to offer both regular meals and snacks, but the caregiver should not be disappointed when the child refuses to eat. Toddlers and children do regulate their caloric intake over time: they eat when they need to and don't when they are not hungry, yet their average caloric intake remains fairly constant. Forcing children to eat only diminishes the importance of internal signals of hunger, satiation, and satiety.

Table J.6 **Survival Guidelines for Toddler Mealtimes**

- Prepare for a mess. Feed the toddler in the kitchen or a part of the home that is easy to clean.

- High chairs or booster seats help define the place and time of meals and keep the toddler focused on exploring only the meal, not the entire environment.

- Keep food for meals, not for punishment or reward. This sets a foundation for healthful food habits and associations.

- Continue to present new foods to picky eaters. Then stand back and observe. Try again if necessary.

- Try not to show frustration. Keep mealtime as positive as possible.

- Learn to trust the toddler's hunger cues. If he or she doesn't seem hungry, wait until the next meal or snack.

- Allow the toddler to choose as many foods as possible, carefully framing and limiting the choices: "Would you like a banana or applesauce?"

- Encourage self-feeding with cup and child-sized utensils.

- Remember, it is the parent's job to present a healthful nutritious diet and a safe eating environment, and it's the child's job to eat it or not!

Source: Satter E. *Child of Mine: Feeding with Love and Good Sense.* 3rd ed. Palo Alto, CA: Bull Publishing Co.; 2000; used with permission.

APPENDIX K Food Safety Tables

➤ Minimum Internal
   Cooking Temperatures
➤ Cold Storage Chart

Minimum Internal Cooking Temperatures

Fresh ground beef, veal, lamb, pork . . . . . . 160°F

Beef, veal, lamb roasts, steaks, chops

Medium . . . . 160°F

Well done . . . . 170°F

Fresh pork roasts, steaks, chops

Medium . . . . 160°F

Well done . . . . 170°F

Ham

Cook before eating . . . . 160°F

Fully cooked, to reheat . . . . 140°F

Poultry . . . . 165°F

Egg dishes, casseroles . . . . 160°F

Leftovers . . . . 165°F

Source: USDA Food Safety and Inspection Service

Cold Storage Chart

Since product dates aren't a guide for safe use of a product, consult this chart and follow these tips. These short but safe time limits will help keep refrigerated food (40°F) from spoiling or becoming dangerous.

- Purchase the product before "sell-by" or expiration dates.
- Follow handling recommendations on product.
- Keep meat and poultry in its package until just before using.
- If freezing meat and poultry in its original package longer than two months, overwrap these packages with airtight heavy-duty foil, plastic wrap, or freezer paper, or place the package inside a plastic bag.

Because freezing (0°F) keeps food safe indefinitely, recommended freezer storage times are for quality only.

Product	Refrigerator	Freezer
Eggs		
Fresh, in shell	3 weeks	Don't freeze
Raw yolks, whites	2 to 4 days	1 year
Hard cooked	1 week	Doesn't freeze well
Liquid pasteurized eggs or egg substitutes		
Opened	3 days	Don't freeze
Unopened	10 days	1 year
Cooked egg dishes	3 to 4 days	Doesn't freeze well
Dairy Products		
Swiss, brick, processed cheese	3 to 4 weeks	Can be frozen, but freezing affects texture and taste

Product	Refrigerator	Freezer
Mayonnaise, Commercial		
Refrigerate after opening	2 months	Don't freeze
TV Dinners, Frozen Casseroles		
Keep frozen until ready to heat	Keep frozen	3 to 4 months
Deli and Vacuum-Packed Products		
Store-prepared (or homemade) egg, chicken, tuna, ham, macaroni salads	3 to 5 days	Doesn't freeze well
Pre-stuffed pork and lamb chops, chicken breasts stuffed with dressing	1 day	Doesn't freeze well
Store-cooked convenience meals	3 to 4 days	Doesn't freeze well
Commercial brand vacuum-packed dinners with USDA seal, unopened	2 weeks	Doesn't freeze well
Raw Hamburger, Ground and Stew Meat		
Hamburger and stew meats	1 to 2 days	3 to 4 months
Ground turkey, veal, pork, lamb, and mixtures of them	1 to 2 days	3 to 4 months
Ham, Corned Beef		
Corned beef in pouch with pickling juices	5 to 7 days	Drained, 1 month
Ham, canned, labeled "Keep Refrigerated"		
Opened	3 to 5 days	1 to 2 months
Unopened	6 to 9 months	Don't freeze
Ham, fully cooked, whole	7 days	1 to 2 months
Ham, fully cooked, half	3 to 5 days	1 to 2 months
Ham, fully cooked, slices	3 to 4 days	1 to 2 months
Hot Dogs and Lunch Meats (in freezer wrap)		
Hot dogs		
Opened package	1 week	1 to 2 months
Unopened package	2 weeks	1 to 2 months
Lunch meats		
Opened package	3 to 5 days	1 to 2 months
Unopened package	2 weeks	1 to 2 months
Soups and Stews		
Vegetable or meat added	3 to 4 days	2 to 3 months
Bacon and Sausage		
Bacon	7 days	1 month
Sausage, raw from pork, beef, chicken, or turkey	1 to 2 days	1 to 2 months
Smoked breakfast links, patties	7 days	1 to 2 months
Summer sausage labeled "Keep Refrigerated"		
Opened	3 weeks	1 to 2 months
Unopened	3 months	1 to 2 months
Fresh Meat (Beef, Veal, Lamb, and Pork)		
Steaks	3 to 5 days	6 to 12 months
Chops	3 to 5 days	4 to 6 months
Roasts	3 to 5 days	4 to 12 months
Variety meats (tongue, kidneys, liver, heart, chitterlings)	1 to 2 days	3 to 4 months

Product	Refrigerator	Freezer
Meat Leftovers		
Cooked meat and meat dishes	3 to 4 days	2 to 3 months
Gravy and meat broth	1 to 2 days	2 to 3 months
Fresh Poultry		
Chicken or turkey, whole	1 to 2 days	1 year
Chicken or turkey, parts	1 to 2 days	9 months
Giblets	1 to 2 days	3 to 4 months
Cooked Poultry, Leftover		
Fried chicken	3 to 4 days	4 months
Cooked poultry dishes	3 to 4 days	4 to 6 months
Pieces, plain	3 to 4 days	4 months
Pieces covered with broth, gravy	1 to 2 days	6 months
Chicken nuggets, patties	1 to 2 days	1 to 3 months
Fish		
Lean (such as cod)	1 to 2 days	up to 6 months
Fatty (such as blue, perch, salmon)	1 to 2 days	2 to 3 months

Sources: Food Marketing Institute for fish and dairy products, USDA Food Safety and Inspection Service for all other foods.

Academic

www.mayoclinic.com/findinformation/healthylivingcenter/index.cfm
Mayo Clinic nutrition information

www.navigator.tufts.edu
Tufts University Nutrition Navigator

Aging

www.aoa.gov
Administration on Aging
330 Independence Avenue SW
Washington, DC 20201
(202) 619-7501

www.aarp.org
American Association of Retired Persons (AARP)
601 E Street NW
Washington, DC 20049
(800) 424-3410

www.americangeriatrics.org
American Geriatrics Society
The Empire State Building
350 Fifth Avenue, Suite 801
New York, NY 10118
(212) 308-1414

www.aoa.gov/naic
National Aging Information Center
330 Independence Avenue SW
Washington, DC 20201
(202) 619-750[1]

www.ncoa.org
National Council on the Aging
1828 L Street NW
Washington, DC 20036

www.nia.nih.gov
National Institute on Aging
Building 31, Room 5C27
31 Center Drive, MSC 2292
Bethesda, MD 20892
(301) 496-1752

www.nof.org
National Osteoporosis Foundation
1232 22nd Street NW
Washington, DC 20037-1292
(202) 223-2226

Alcohol and Drug Abuse

www.al-anon.alateen.org
Al-Anon/Alateen
1600 Corporate Landing Parkway
Virginia Beach, VA 23154-5617
(888) 425-2666; (757) 563-1600

www.aa.org
Alcoholics Anonymous (AA)
General Service Office
Grand Central Station
P.O. Box 459
New York, NY 10163
(212) 870-3400

http://prevention.samhsa.gov/
Center for Substance Abuse Prevention
Substance Abuse and Mental Health Services Administration
1 Choke Cherry Road
Room 8-1054
Rockville, MD 20857
(240) 276-2420; fax: (240) 276-2430

www.wsoinc.com
Narcotics Anonymous (NA)
P.O. Box 9999
Van Nuys, CA 91409
(818) 773-9999; fax: (818) 700-0700

www.health.org
National Clearinghouse for Alcohol and Drug
  Information (NCADI)
P.O. Box 2345
Rockville, MD 20847-2345
(800) 729-6686

www.ncadd.org
National Council on Alcoholism and Drug
  Dependence (NCADD)
20 Exchange Place
Suite 2902
New York, NY 10005
(800) 622-2255; (212) 269-7797; fax: (212) 269-7510

Canadian Government: Federal

www.agr.gc.ca
Agriculture and Agri-Food Canada
Public Information Request Services
Sir John Carling Building
930 Carling Avenue
Ottawa, ON K1A 0C7
(613) 759-1000; fax: (613) 759-6726

www.hc-sc.gc.ca/food-aliment/ns-sc/e_nutrition.html
Bureau of Nutritional Sciences
Nutrition Research Division
Sir Fredrick G. Banting Research Center
Tunney's Pasture (2203C)
Ottawa, ON K1A 0L2
(613) 957-0919; fax: (613) 941-6182

Canadian Government: Federal (continued)

www.hc-sc.gc.ca/food-aliment/ns-sc/e_nutrition.html
Bureau of Nutritional Sciences
Nutrition Evaluation Division
Sir Fredrick G. Banting Research Center
Tunney's Pasture (2203A)
Ottawa, ON K1A 0L2
(613) 957-0352; fax: (613) 941-6636

www.inspection.gc.ca
Canadian Food Inspection Agency
59 Camelot Drive
Ottowa, ON K1A 0Y9
(800) 442-2342; (613) 225-2342; fax: (613) 228-6653

www.cihi.ca
Canadian Institute for Health Information
377 Dalhousie Street
Suite 200
Ottawa, ON K1N 9N8
(613) 241-7860; fax: (613) 241-8120

www.cpha.ca
Canadian Public Health Association
400-1565 Carling Avenue
Ottawa, ON K1Z 8R1
(613) 725-3769; fax: (613) 725-9826

www.agr.gc.ca/misb/fb-ba/nutra/index_e.php?page=intro
Functional Foods and Nutraceuticals
Food Bureau
597-930 Carling Avenue
Ottawa, ON K1A 0C5

www.hc-sc.gc.ca
Health Canada

www.ccfn.ca
The Canadian Council of Food and Nutrition
3800 Steeles Avenue West, Suite 301A
Woodbridge, ON L4L 4G9
(905) 265-1349

Canadian Government: Provincial and Territorial

Consultant, Nutrition
Health and Wellness Promotion, Population Health,
    Department of Health and Social Services, Government of the
    Northwest Territories
Center Square Tower, 6th Floor
P.O. Box 1320
Yellowknife, NT X1A 2L9

Coordinator, Health Information
Resource Center
Department of Health and Social Services
1 Rochford Street, Box 2000
Charlottetown, PEI C1A 7N8

Director, Health Promotion
Department of Health, Government of Newfoundland
    and Labrador
P.O. Box 8700
Confederation Building, West Block
St. John's, NF A1B 4J6

Director, Nutrition Services
Yukon Hospital Corporation
#5 Hospital Road
Whitehorse, YT Y1A 3H7

Executive Director
Health Programs
2nd Floor 800 Portage Avenue
Winnipeg, MB R3G 0P4

Health Promotion Unit
Population Health Branch
Saskatchewan Health
3475 Albert Street
Regina, SK S4S 6X6

Nutritionist
Preventive Services Branch
Ministry of Health
1520 Blanshard Street
Victoria, BC V8W 3C8

Population Health Strategies Branch
Alberta Health
23rd Floor, TELUS Plaza, North Tower
10025 Jasper Avenue
Edmonton, AB T5J 2N3

Project Manager, Public Health Management Services
Health and Community Services
P.O. Box 5100
520 King Street
Fredericton, NB E3B 5G8

Public Health Nutritionist
Central Health Region
201 Brownlow Avenue, Unit 4
Dartmouth, NS B3B 1W2

Responsables de la santé cardiovasculaire et de la nutrition
Ministère de la Santé et des Services sociaux, Service de la
    Prévention en Santé
3e étage, 1075, chemin Sainte-Foy
Québec (Québec) G1S 2M1

Senior Consultant, Nutrition
Public Health Branch
Ministry of Health, 8th Floor
5700 Yonge St.
New York, ON M2M 4K5

Complementary and Alternative Nutrition

http://nccam.nih.gov/
National Center for Complementary and Alternative
    Medicine, NIH
Bethesda, MD 20892
(888) 644-6226

www.hc-sc.gc.ca/hpb/onhp/
Office of Natural Health Products
171 Slater Street
9th Floor
Ottawa, ON K1P 5H7
(613) 946-1615

Consumer Organizations

www.diabetes.ca
Canadian Diabetes Association
15 Toronto Street
Suite 800
Toronto, ON M5C 2E3
(800) 226-8464; (416) 363-3373

www.cspinet.org
Center for Science in the Public Interest (CSPI)
1875 Connecticut Ave NW, Suite 300
Washington, DC 20009-5728
(202) 332-9110; fax: (202) 265-4954

www.consumersunion.org
Consumers Union
101 Truman Avenue
Yonkers, NY 10703-1057
(914) 378-2000

www.pueblo.gsa.gov
Federal Consumer Information Center
Pueblo, CO 81009
(800) 688-9889; (888) 878-3256

www.ncahf.org
National Council Against Health Fraud, Inc. (NCAHF)
119 Foster Street
Peabody, MA 01960
(978) 532-9383

www.quackwatch.com
Stephen Barrett, MD
P.O. Box 1747
Allentown, PA 18105
(610) 437-1795

Eating Disorders

www.anred.com
Anorexia Nervosa and Related Eating Disorders (ANRED)
P.O. Box 5102
Eugene, OR 97405
(541) 344-1144

www.anad.org
National Association of Anorexia Nervosa and Associated
  Disorders, Inc. (ANAD)
P.O. Box 7
Highland Park, IL 60035
(847) 831-3438; fax: (847) 433-4632

www.nedic.ca
National Eating Disorder Information Centre
200 Elizabeth Street, CW 1-211
Toronto, Ontario M5G 2C4
(866) 633-4220; (416) 340-4156; fax: (416) 340-4736

www.nationaleatingdisorders.org
National Eating Disorders Association
603 Stewart Street, Suite 803
Seattle, WA 98101
(206) 382-3587

Food Safety

www.foodandfarming.info
The Alliance for Food & Farming
P.O. Box 2747
Watsonville, CA 95077
(831) 786-1666; fax: (831) 786-1668

www.cfsan.fda.gov
FDA Center for Food Safety and Applied Nutrition
5100 Paint Branch Parkway
College Park, MD 20740
(888) 723-3366

www.epa.gov/opptintr/lead/nlic.htm
National Lead Information Center
(800) 424-5323

www.npic.orst.edu/index.html
National Pesticide Information Center
Oregon State University
333 Weniger Hall
Corvallis, OR 97331-6502
(800) 858-7378

Seafood Safety Hotline
(800) 332-4010; (202) 205-4314

U.S. EPA Safe Drinking Water Hotline
(800) 426-4791

www.fsis.usda.gov
USDA Food Safety and Inspection Service
Food Safety Education Office
Room 1180-S
Washington, DC 20250
(202) 720-3333

USDA Meat and Poultry Hotline
(800) 535-4555

Infancy, Childhood, and Adolescence

www.aap.org
American Academy of Pediatrics
141 Northwest Point Boulevard
Elk Grove Village, IL 60007-1098
(847) 434-4000; fax: (847) 434-8000

www.birthdefects.org
Birth Defect Research for Children, Inc.
930 Woodcock Road
Suite 225
Orlando, FL 32803
(407) 895-0802

www.cps.ca
Canadian Paediatric Society
100-2204 Walkley Road
Ottawa, ON K1G 4G8
(613) 526-9397; fax: (613) 526-3332

Infancy, Childhood, and Adolescence (continued)

www.childrensfoundation.net
Children's Foundation
725 Fifteenth Street NW
Suite 505
Washington, DC 20005-2109
(202) 347-3300; fax: (202) 347-3382

www.KidsHealth.org
KidsHealth
The Nemours Foundation

www.ncemch.org
National Center for Education in Maternal & Child Health
2000 15th Street North
Suite 701
Arlington, VA 22201-2617
(703) 524-7802

International Agencies

www.fao.org
Food and Agriculture Organization of the United Nations (FAO)
Liaison Office for North America
2175 K Street, Suite 300
Washington, DC 20437
(202) 653-2400

www.ific.org
International Food Information Council Foundation
1100 Connecticut Avenue NW
Suite 430
Washington, DC 20036
(202) 296-6540

www.unicef.org
UNICEF
3 United Nations Plaza
New York, NY 10017
(212) 326-7000; fax: (212) 887-7465

www.who.int/home-page
World Health Organization (WHO)
Regional Office
525 23rd Street NW
Washington, DC 20037
(202) 974-3000; fax: (202) 974-3663

Pregnancy and Lactation

www.acog.org
American College of Obstetricians and Gynecologists
Resource Center
409 12th Street SW
Washington, DC 20024-2188
(202) 638-5577

www.lalecheleague.org
La Leche League International, Inc.
1400 N. Meacham Road
Schaumburg, IL 60173-4048
(847) 519-7730

www.modimes.org
March of Dimes Birth Defects Foundation
1275 Mamaroneck Avenue
White Plains, NY 10605
(888) 663-4637

Professional Nutrition Organizations

ADA, The Nutrition Line
(800) 366-1655

www.eatright.org
American Dietetic Association (ADA)
216 West Jackson Boulevard
Suite 800
Chicago, IL 60606-6995
(800) 877-1600; (312) 899-0040

www.ascn.org
American Society for Clinical Nutrition
9650 Rockville Pike
Bethesda, MD 20814-3998
(301) 530-7110; fax: (301) 634-7350

www.asns.org
American Society for Nutritional Sciences
9650 Rockville Pike
Suite 4500
Bethesda, MD 20814
(301) 634-7050; fax: (301) 634-7892

Canadian Dietetic Association
480 University Avenue
Suite 601
Toronto, ON M5G 1V2

Canadian Society for Nutritional Sciences
Department of Food and Nutrition
University of Manitoba
Winnipeg, MB R3T 2N2

www.dietitians.ca
Dietitians of Canada
480 University Avenue, Suite 604
Toronto, ON M5G 1V2
(416) 596-0857; fax: (416) 596-0603

http://hni.ilsi.org
ILSI Human Nutrition Institute (HNI)
One Thomas Circle
Washington, DC 20005
(202) 659-0524; fax: (202) 659-3617

www.ift.org
Institute of Food Technologists
525 West Van Buren
Suite 1000
Chicago, IL 60607
(312) 782-8424; fax: (312) 782-8348

www.nationalacademies.org/nrc
National Academy of Sciences/National Research
   Council (NAS/NRC)
2101 Constitution Avenue NW
Washington, DC 20418
(202) 234-2000

www.sne.org
Society for Nutrition Education
9202 North Meridian
Suite 200
Indianapolis, IN 46260
(800) 235-6690

Sports Nutrition

www.acsm.org
American College of Sports Medicine (ACSM)
401 W. Michigan Street
Indianapolis, IN 46202-3233
(317) 637-9200; fax: (317) 634-7817

www.acefitness.org
American Council on Exercise (ACE)
4851 Paramount Drive
San Diego, CA 92123
(800) 825-3636

www.cahperd.ca
Canadian Association for Health, Physical Education, Recreation,
   and Dance
403-2197 Riverside Drive
Ottawa, ON K1H 7X3
(613) 523-1348

www.csep.ca
Canadian Society for Exercise Physiology
185 Somerset St. West
Suite 202
Ottawa, ON K2P 0J2
(613) 234-3755; fax: (613) 234-3565

www.fitness.gov
President's Council on Physical Fitness and Sports
Humphrey Building, Room 738
200 Independence Avenue SW
Washington, DC 20201
(202) 690-9000; fax: (202) 690-5211

www.runnersworld.com
Runners World
Rodale, Inc.
Emmaus, PA 18098
(610) 967-8809

Sports Medicine and Science Council of Canada
1600 James Naismith Drive
Suite 306
Gloucester, Ontario K1B 5N4
(613) 748-5671; fax: (613) 748-5729

Sports Safety Board of Quebec
100 Laviolette
Bureau 306
Trois-Riveres, Quebec G9A 5S9
(819) 371-6033

www.scandpg.org
Sports, Cardiovascular and Wellness Nutritionists (SCAN)

www.ideafit.com
The International Association for Fitness Professionals (IDEA)
6190 Cornerstone Court East # 204
San Diego, CA 92121-3773
(800) 999-4332 ext 7; fax: (858) 535-8234

www.veggie.org/
Veggie Sports Association

Supplements

http://dietary-supplements.info.nih.gov/databases/ibids.html
International Bibliographic Information on Dietary Supplements
   (IBIDS)

http://dietary-supplements.info.nih.gov
Office of Dietary Supplements
National Institutes of Health
Building 31, Room 1B29
31 Center Drive, MSC 2086
Bethesda, MD 20892-2086
(301) 435-2590; fax: (301) 480-1845

Trade and Industry Organizations

www.aibonline.org
American Institute of Baking
1213 Bakers Way
P.O. Box 3999
Manhattan, KS 66505-3999
(800) 633-5137; (785) 537-4750; fax: (785) 537-1493

www.meatami.org
American Meat Institute
1700 North Moore Street
Suite 1600
Arlington, VA 22209
(703) 841-2400; fax: (703) 527-0938

www.beechnut.com
Beech-Nut Nutrition Corporation
100 S. 4th Street
St. Louis, MO 63102
(800) 233-2468

Trade and Industry Organizations (continued)

www.gssiweb.com
Gatorade Sports Science Institute
617 West Main Street
Barrington, IL 60010
(800) 616-4774

www.GeneralMills.com/corporate
General Mills, Inc.
Number One General Mills Boulevard
Minneapolis, MN 55426
(800) 328-6787

www.gerber.com
Gerber Products Co.
445 State Street
Fremont, MI 49413-0001
(800) 443-7237

www.heinz.com
H.J. Heinz Company
World Headquarters
P.O. Box 57
Pittsburgh, PA 15230-0057
(412) 456-5700

www.kelloggs.com
Kellogg Company
P.O. Box 3599
Battle Creek, MI 49016-3599
(616) 961-2000

www.kraftfoods.com
Kraft Foods
Consumer Response and Information Center
One Kraft Court
Glenview, IL 60025
(800) 323-0768

www.nationaldairycouncil.org
National Dairy Council
10255 West Higgins Road
Suite 900
Rosemont, IL 60018-5616
(847) 803-2000

www.pillsbury.com
Pillsbury Company
2866 Pillsbury Center
Minneapolis, MN 55402
(800) 775-4777

www.pg.com
Procter & Gamble Company
One Procter and Gamble Plaza
Cincinnati, OH 45202
(513) 983-1100

www.sunkist.com
Sunkist Growers
Consumer Affairs, Fresh Fruit Division
14130 Riverside Drive
Sherman Oaks, CA 91423
(800) 248-7875

www.dannon.com
The Dannon Company
120 White Plains Road
Tarrytown, NY 10591-5536
(877) 326-6668

www.nutrasweet.com
The NutraSweet Company
P.O. Box 2986
Chicago, IL 60654-0986
(800) 323-5316

www.uffva.org
United Fresh Fruit and Vegetable Association
727 North Washington Street
Alexandria, VA 22314
(703) 836-3410

www.usarice.com
USA Rice Federation
4301 North Fairfax Drive
Suite 305
Arlington, VA 22203
(703) 351-8161

www.cognis.com/veris/verisdefault.htm
VERIS Online Research Information Service

Weight Management

http://nutrition.uvm.edu/bodycomp/
Body Composition Analysis Tutorials

www.overeatersanonymous.org
Overeaters Anonymous (OA)
World Service Office
6075 Zenith Court NE
Rio Rancho, NM 87124
(505) 891-2664; fax: (505) 891-4320

www.shapeup.org
Shape Up America!
6707 Democracy Boulevard
Suite 306
Bethesda, MD 20817
(301) 493-5368

www.tops.org
TOPS (Take Off Pounds Sensibly)
4575 South Fifth Street
P.O. Box 07360
Milwaukee, WI 53207-0360
(800) 932-8677; (414) 482-4620

www.niddk.nih.gov/index.htm
Weight-control Information Network
1 WIN Way
Bethesda, MD 20892-3665
(877) 946-4627; (202) 828-1025; fax: (202) 828-1028

www.weightwatchers.com
Weight Watchers International
Consumer Affairs Department/IN
175 Crossways Park West
Woodbury, NY 11797
(516) 390-1400; fax: (516) 390-1632

World Hunger

www.bread.org
Bread for the World
50 F Street, NW
Suite 500
Washington, DC 20001
(800) 822-7323; (202) 639-9400

http://hunger.tufts.edu
Center on Hunger, Poverty and Nutrition Policy
Tufts University School of Medicine
11 Curtis Avenue
Medford, MA 02155
(617) 627-6223; fax: (617) 627-3688

www.freefromhunger.org
Freedom from Hunger
1644 DaVinci Court
Davis, CA 95616
(800) 708-2555; fax: (530) 758-6241

www.oxfamamerica.org
Oxfam America
26 West Street
Boston, MA 02111-1206
(800) 776-9326; fax: (617) 728-2594

www.worldwatch.org
Worldwatch Institute
1776 Massachusetts Avenue NW
Suite 800
Washington, DC 20036
(202) 452-1999

U.S. Government

www.nutrition.gov
Online federal government information on nutrition

www.cdc.gov
Centers for Disease Control and Prevention
1600 Clifton Road
Atlanta, GA 30333
(800) 311-3435; (404) 639-3534

FDA Consumer Information Line
(301) 827-4420

FDA Office of Nutritional Products, Labeling and
   Dietary Supplements
HFS-800
200 C Street SW
Washington, DC 20204
(202) 205-4561; fax: (202) 205-4594

FDA Office of Plant and Dairy Foods and Beverages
HFS-300
200 C Street SW
Washington, DC 20204
(202) 205-4064; fax: (202) 205-4422

www.ftc.gov
Federal Trade Commission (FTC)
CRC-240
Washington, DC 20580
(877) 382-4357

www.fda.gov
Food and Drug Administration (FDA)
Office of Consumer Affairs, HFE 1
Room 16-85
5600 Fishers Lane
Rockville, MD 20857
(888) 463-6332; (301) 443-1544

www.nal.usda.gov/fnic
Food and Nutrition Information Center
National Agricultural Library, Room 105
10301 Baltimore Avenue
Beltsville, MD 20705-2351
(301) 504-5719; fax: (301) 504-6409

www.frac.org
Food Research and Action Center (FRAC)
1875 Connecticut Avenue NW
Suite 540
Washington, DC 20009
(202) 986-2200; fax: (202) 986-2525

www.healthfinder.gov
Gateway for Health and Nutrition Information

www.nidr.nih.gov
National Institute of Dental and Craniofacial Research (NIDCR)
National Institutes of Health
Bethesda, MD 20892-2190
(301) 496-4261

www.niddk.nih.gov
National Institute of Diabetes & Digestive & Kidney Diseases
Office of Communications and Public Liaison
NIDDK, NIH
Building 31, Room 9A04 Center Drive, MSC 2560
Bethesda, MD 20892-2560

www.nih.gov/health
National Institutes of Health search engine and free access to
   MEDLINE and PubMed databases

www.usda.gov
U.S. Department of Agriculture (USDA)
14th Street SW and Independence Avenue
Washington, DC 20250
(202) 720-2791

U.S. Government (continued)

www.dhhs.gov
U.S. Department of Health and Human Services
200 Independence Avenue SW
Washington, DC 20201
(877) 696-6775; (202) 619-0257

www.epa.gov
U.S. Environmental Protection Agency (EPA)
1200 Pennsylvania Avenue NW
Washington, DC 20460
(202) 260-2090

www.pueblo.gsa.gov
U.S. General Services Administration
Federal Communication Information Center
Pueblo, CO 81009

www.bookstore.gpo.gov
U.S. Government Online Bookstore
U.S. Government Printing Office
701 N. Capitol Street, NW
Washington, DC 20401
(202) 512-0132; fax: (202) 512-1355

www.usda.gov/cnpp
USDA Center for Nutrition Policy and Promotion
3101 Park Center Drive
Room 1034
Alexandria, VA 22302-1594
(703) 305-7600; fax: (703) 305-3400

Answers to Study Questions

Chapter 1

1. Sensory, cognitive, and cultural

3. Carbohydrate, protein, fat, vitamins, minerals, and water

5. Macrominerals are found in and used by the body in the largest amounts.

   Microminerals are found in and used by the body in smaller amounts.

7. An epidemiological study observes and compares how disease rates vary among different population groups and identifies conditions related to diseases or conditions within the populations. This enables researchers to identify associations between factors within the population and the particular disease being studied.

9. A placebo is an imitation treatment that looks the same as the experimental treatment (such as a sugar pill) but has no effect. The placebo is important for reducing bias because subjects do not know if they are receiving the intervention and are less inclined to alter their responses or reported symptoms based on what they think should happen.

Chapter 2

1. Undernutrition is poor health resulting from the depletion of nutrients due to inadequate nutrient intake over time. It is most often associated with poverty, alcoholism, and some types of eating disorders.

   The most common type of overnutrition in the United States is due to the regular consumption of excess calories, fats, saturated fats, and cholesterol.

3. Grains: 6 ounce-equivalents; half should be whole grains
   Vegetable group: 2½ cups
   Fruits: 2 cups
   Milk: 3 cups
   Meat and beans: 5½ ounce equivalents

5. The Estimated Average Requirement (EAR) is the nutrient intake level that is estimated to meet the needs of 50 percent of the individuals in a life-stage and gender group.

   The Recommended Dietary Allowance (RDA) is the daily intake level that meets the needs of most (97 to 98 percent) people in a life-stage and gender group.

   An Adequate Intake (AI) level is set when an RDA has yet to be established due to a lack of knowledge and need for more scientific research.

   The Tolerable Upper Intake Level (UL) is the maximum daily intake level that is unlikely to pose health risks to almost all of the individuals in a life-stage and gender category.

7. Calories
   Calories from fat
   Total fat
   Saturated fat
   Trans fat
   Cholesterol
   Sodium
   Total carbohydrate
   Dietary fiber
   Sugars
   Protein
   Calcium, iron, vitamins A and C (all as a % Daily Value)

9. Nutrient content claims describe the level of a nutrient or dietary substance in the product using terms such as *good source, high, or free.*

   A health claim is any statement that associates a food or a substance in a food with a disease or health-related condition.

   A structure/function claim describes a benefit related to a nutrient-deficiency disease or describes the role of a nutrient or dietary ingredient intended to affect a structure or function in humans; for example, *calcium helps build strong bones.*

Spotlight on Complementary and Alternative Nutrition

1. Phytochemicals are plant chemicals, including pigments and antioxidants. They help plants resist bacteria and fungi, the destructive effects of free radicals, and high levels of UV sunlight. When we eat plants that contain phytochemicals, we receive many of the same protections.

3. Food additives may improve a food's nutritional value, maintain its palatability and consistency, provide leavening, control acidity or alkalinity, enhance flavor, or prevent spoilage.

5. The traditional macrobiotic diet is a vegetarian diet that gets progressively more restrictive, with the "highest level" consisting of little more than brown rice and water. The diet has since evolved to a simpler one-level regimen based on whole-grain cereals and vegetables, a small amount of fish, and no other animal products and no fruit.

7. • Check the label for the USP verification mark, which indicates that the manufacturer followed standards established by the U.S. Pharmacopoeia.
   • Remember that just because something is natural does not mean it is safe.
   • Consider purchasing a supplement from one of the large, nationally known manufacturers, because they generally have tighter quality controls.

9. Because herbal supplements do not have to be approved prior to sale, their safety and efficacy has not been scrutinized by the FDA. Herbal medicines have the potential to interact with drugs and with nutrients. Such interactions could affect the strength of medications and the use of nutrients in the body. In addition, because herbal medicines are not regulated as drugs, there are no standards for purity. This leaves open the possibility that contaminants in the product could cause harmful effects.

Chapter 3

1. Stomach contents have the lowest pH due to its production of hydrochloric acid. The pancreas secretes fluid that contains mostly water, bicarbonate and digestive enzymes. In the small intestine, this basic solution helps neutralize the acidic chyme entering from the stomach.

3. Small intestine

5. Any three of the following:
   - The *salivary glands* produce saliva that moistens food, lubricating it for easy swallowing. Saliva contains enzymes that begin the process of chemical digestion.
   - The *pancreas* secretes digestive enzymes that help digest nutrients.
   - The *gallbladder* stores and concentrates bile from the liver.
   - The *liver* produces and secretes bile, which emulsifies fats in the small intestine thus aiding fat digestion.

7. Gastroesophageal reflux disease (GERD) occurs when the lower esophageal sphincter (LES) is weak or relaxes inappropriately, allowing the stomach's contents to flow back up into the esophagus. The acidic stomach contents irritate the gastroesophageal lining, causing severe pain.

Chapter 4

1. Both starch and fiber are long chains of glucose molecules but we are unable to digest the bonds between the glucose units in fiber. Therefore, fiber moves through the small intestine undigested while starch is broken down into glucose and absorbed.

3. Carbohydrates provide energy (fuel) to the cells of the body. Consuming too little carbohydrate can result in the breakdown of body proteins to supply glucose and energy. Inadequate carbohydrate intake prevents fats from breaking down normally, and this results in ketosis.

5. Grains, fruits, and vegetables are the most carbohydrate-dense foods. Many dairy foods also contribute quite a bit of carbohydrate. Legumes often are rich in both carbohydrates and protein. Sweets, of course, contain carbohydrates in the form of sugars.

7. Insulin is secreted in response to meal ingestion and its job is to lower blood glucose by increasing the uptake of glucose into cells. Glucagon is released in response to low glucose sugar and is responsible for adding glucose to the blood from storage (glycogen in liver and muscle tissue).

Chapter 5

1. Oils are triglycerides. Triglycerides contain a glycerol molecule and 3 fatty acids. These fatty acids can vary in three main ways: length, saturation, and *omega* number. An oil such as corn oil has more polyunsaturated fatty acids attached to glycerol than it does monounsaturated or saturated fatty acids. Therefore corn oil is known as a mostly polyunsaturated fat but like all oils it contains a mixture of fatty acids.

3. Triglycerides

5. Provide energy (9 kilocalories per gram), provide a concentrated source of stored calories (triglycerides in fat cells), carry flavor in foods, pad and protect vital organs, provide thermal insulation (subcutaneous fat).

7. Any foods that contain ingredients derived from an animal will contain cholesterol.

Chapter 6

1. Proteins comprise muscles and organs; work as hormones, enzymes, and antibodies; help to regulate fluid and electrolyte balance; help to regulate acid-base balance; used as transporter molecules.

3. Nitrogen is part of the chemical structure of amino acids (proteins) but not in that of carbohydrates and lipids. Nitrogen is part of the amino group, $-NH_2$.

5. Two proteins that when combined, contain all of the indispensable amino acids in adequate amounts to support health. Examples include rice and beans, peanut butter on bread, corn bread and chili (beans).

7. Protein is used to make antibodies, which help fight infection. Without adequate dietary protein, synthesis of antibodies is impaired, and a person becomes more susceptible to infection.

9. Reduced blood cholesterol levels, reduced risk of some cancers, improved body weight, reduced blood pressure.

Chapter 7

1. ATP is the energy form usable by cells so it is called the universal energy currency. Most ATP is produced inside mitochondria, so they often are called the power plants of the cell.

3. NAD^+ and FAD^+ are the electron acceptors in the breakdown pathways.

   NADH and $FADH_2$ are the electron carriers. They carry these high-energy electrons to the electron transport chain where the electrons power the production of ATP.

5. Beta-oxidation, or fatty acid oxidation, is a step-by-step process that forms two-carbon molecules of acetyl CoA as it clips two carbon links from a fatty acid chain. It also produces NADH and $FADH_2$, which carry high-energy electrons to the electron transport chain for ATP production.

7. Ketone bodies refer to the three compounds (acetoacetate, acetone, and beta-hydroxybutyrate) made during incomplete fatty acid oxidation. Although some ketone bodies are always produced and used, they become a substantial alternative energy source when the body lacks carbohydrate and needs to fuel vital cells.

9. Gluconeogenesis is the making of "new" glucose. When the body has a low glucose supply, it can make glucose from the glycerol component of triglycerides and from some amino acids. Lipogenesis is the process of synthesizing long-chain fatty acids. Lipogenesis occurs when ATP is plentiful and building blocks are abundant. Precursors of fatty acid synthesis include ketogenic amino acids, alcohol, and fatty acids themselves.

Spotlight on Alcohol

1. A standard amount of beer has 12 ounces, wine has 4 to 5 ounces, and liquor has 1½ ounces of alcohol.

3. The liver is the chief location of alcohol metabolism.

5. In alcohol metabolism NAD is converted to NADH. Excess NADH blocks the entry of acetyl CoA into the citric acid cycle. The acetyl CoA is diverted and used to synthesize fatty acids. The fat is stored in the liver because that is the organ responsible for alcohol metabolism.

7. Most health officials do not encourage the consumption of alcohol; however, for people who do consume alcohol, they suggest moderation (no more than 2 drinks for males, 1 drink for females per day).

9. Alcohol can cause fetal alcohol syndrome. A safe lower limit for alcohol consumption during pregnancy is not currently known.

Chapter 8

1. Energy balance is the relationship between your energy intake and energy output. You are in energy equilibrium when your energy or caloric intake equals the amount of energy or calories you expend. People who maintain their weight over time are in energy equilibrium whether or not they are aware of their intake or expenditure. Positive energy balance (intake > output) results in weight gain while negative energy balance (intake < output) results in weight loss.

3. The amount of energy expended in physical activity depends on the activity's duration, type (e.g., walking, running, or typing), and intensity. Energy output increases the longer you perform an activity, the greater your use of large muscle groups (type of activity), and the more intensely you perform the activity.

5. Genetic, physiological, metabolic, hormonal, sociocultural, environmental, behavioral, and psychological factors.

7. Some health experts advocate the replacement of goals to attain a particular weight with the goal of *metabolic fitness,* which is the absence of metabolic or biochemical risk factors

associated with obesity. Individuals are considered metabolically fit when their blood lipids are at safe levels and their blood pressure is normal. Four suggested goals for metabolic fitness, from most to least aggressive are to (1) significantly reduce the risk factors, (2) restore abnormal risk factors to normal ranges, (3) reverse the "high normal" or "borderline" parameters, and (4) prevent risk factors in overweight individuals.

9. A balanced diet of moderate caloric intake, adequate exercise, cognitive-behavioral strategies for changing habits and behavior patterns, attention to balancing self-acceptance and the desire for change.

11. The term *underweight* is defined as a BMI of less than 18.5 kg/m^2.

Chapter 9

1. Vitamins A, D, E, and K are found in the fat and lipid components of food. Fat-soluble vitamins require bile for absorption and first travel in the lymphatic system (inside chylomicrons) before entering the blood stream. Most fat-soluble vitamins are not readily excreted and are stored in the liver and adipose tissue.

3. Vitamin A is necessary for vision, reproduction, cell differentiation, immune function, and bone health.

5. Beta-carotene

7. Cholesterol

9. Vitamin K is necessary for the production of prothrombin, a protein that when activated is responsible for the formation of a solid clot.

Chapter 10

1. Thiamin functions in energy metabolism as the coenzyme thiamin pyrophosphate (TPP).

Riboflavin functions in energy metabolism as the coenzymes flavin adenine dinucleotide (FAD) and flavin mononucleotide (FMN).

Niacin functions in energy metabolism as the coenzymes nicotinamide adenine dinucleotide (NAD) and nicotinamide adenine dinucleotide phosphate (NADP).

Biotin acts as a coenzyme critical to energy and amino acid metabolism, as well as fat and glycogen synthesis.

Pantothenic acid functions in energy metabolism as part of coenzyme A.

Vitamin B_6 functions in amino acid and fatty acid metabolism as the coenzymes pyridoxal phosphate (PLP) and pyridoxamine phosphate (PMP).

Folate functions in one-carbon transfer reactions in the synthesis of DNA and many other reactions.

Vitamin B_{12} promotes the growth and maintenance of the sheath that protects nerve fibers and activates the folate coenzyme, tetrahydrofolic acid (THFA).

Vitamin C is important in collagen synthesis, assists with absorption of iron, and is an antioxidant.

3. Thiamin: beriberi
Riboflavin: ariboflavinosis
Niacin: pellagra
Biotin: no disease name, a deficiency causes hair loss, nausea, and loss of appetite
Pantothenic acid: no disease name
Vitamin B_6: microcytic hypochromic anemia
Folate: megaloblastic anemia
Vitamin B_{12}: megaloblastic anemia and neurological damage
Vitamin C: scurvy

5. The only water-soluble vitamins with demonstrated toxicity are niacin, vitamin B_6, and vitamin C. Excessive amounts of niacin can dilate the capillaries and cause tingling sensations. When this occurs, it is called a "niacin flush." Excessive amounts of vitamin B_6 can cause irreversible nerve degeneration, and excessive doses of vitamin C can cause diarrhea, nausea, and abdominal cramps.

Chapter 11

1. The physiological state of the body (i.e., is the body in a deficient or an overload state?) and the bioavailability of the mineral affect its absorption.

3. Aldosterone helps the kidney retain sodium, which in turn causes the body to hold on to more water. When the kidneys detect dehydration, they secrete renin. Renin then causes the formation of angiotensin, which leads to the release of aldosterone.

5. The AI for sodium is 1,500 milligrams per day, a level that is substantially less than most Americans eat. The UL for sodium is 2,300 milligrams per day while the Daily Value on food labels is 2,400 milligrams per day.

7. Calcium is important for blood clotting, nerve function, muscle contractions, and cell metabolism.

9. Alcoholics are at higher risk of hypomagnesemia because their diet is poor and usually lacks magnesium. They also tend to excrete more magnesium in their urine.

Chapter 12

1. Trace minerals differ from the major minerals in terms of their dietary requirements and their amounts in the body. The daily dietary recommendations for trace elements are less than 100 milligrams and the total amount of each trace element in the body is less than 5 grams.

3. Factors that can increase or decrease a mineral's bioavailability include:
   - the type of food
   - the presence or absence of fibers and phytate
   - competition with other minerals
   - the acidity of the environment
   - a person's need for that mineral

5. The initial stage of iron deficiency is iron depletion, which causes no physiological impairment. Measuring serum ferritin, which is proportional to body iron stores, assesses iron depletion.

In the second stage of iron deficiency, there is a decrease in functional or transport iron. While hemoglobin and hematocrit remain in the normal range, other values begin to change as functional iron decreases. A new measure of this intermediate stage is the serum level of transferrin receptors (TfRs). As transport iron decreases and stores are depleted, TfR levels increase in proportion to the iron deficit. Other values used to detect this stage are transferrin saturation and protoporphyrin, the precursor of heme, which is elevated when the supply of iron is inadequate for heme synthesis.

The third and most severe stage of iron deficiency is anemia and is characterized by decreased size and number of red blood cells, reduced hemoglobin and hematocrit, and pale red blood cells. This is referred to as microcytic hypochromic anemia. Symptoms include fatigue, pallor, breathlessness with exertion, decreased cold tolerance, behavioral changes, deficits in immune function, cognitive impairment, decreased work performance, and impaired growth.

7. The primary culprits in marginal zinc deficiency are increased needs, poor intake, poor absorption, and excessive losses. Diarrhea and chronic infections like pneumonia can cause excessive zinc excretion. These diseases are commonplace in developing countries where zinc deficiency may be widespread.

9. Iodine is an essential component of the two thyroid hormones: triiodothyronine (T3) and thyroxine (T4). Although T3 is the active form of thyroid hormone, T4 is more prevalent in the body.

Thyroid hormones regulate body temperature, basal metabolic rate, reproduction, and growth.

Three selenium-dependent enzymes help convert T4 to the more active T3 form.

11. Wilson's disease is a genetic disorder of copper transport that is characterized by impaired excretion and toxic accumulation of copper in the liver, kidney, and the eye. The prevalence of Wilson's disease is higher than that of Menkes' syndrome (1 in 30,000). Patients with Wilson's disease frequently appear healthy until adolescence or early adulthood. Without treatment, patients develop serious liver and neurologic problems.

Menkes' Syndrome is a genetic copper deficiency resulting from a failure to absorb copper from the intestinal tract. The incidence is extremely rare (1 in 200,000). Menkes' syndrome results in neurological degeneration, peculiar kinky hair, and poor growth.

13. Fluoride decreases the demineralization of tooth enamel by organic acids that eat away tooth enamel. Fluoride accelerates the subsequent remineralization process. Fluoride also inhibits bacterial activity in dental plaques.

Chapter 13

1. Muscle fibers are individual muscle cells. The two primary types are slow-twitch (ST) fibers and fast-twitch (FT) fibers. ST fibers have high aerobic endurance and take twice as long to reach maximum contraction as FT fibers. FT fibers have poor aerobic endurance. They perform anaerobically, contract quickly, and tire easily due to their limited endurance.

3. It is recommended that athletes consume 60 to 70 percent of their calories from carbohydrates, 20 percent from fat, and 15 percent from protein. Compared to a nonathlete whose diet should be 55 to 60 percent carbohydrate, this diet is higher in carbohydrates and lower in fat. The nonathlete's recommended fat intake is approximately 30 percent of total calories.

5. The adult nonathlete's RDA for protein is 0.8 grams per kilogram of body weight per day. This is less than the recommended intake for endurance athletes, which is 1.2 to 1.4 grams per kilogram of body weight per day. The protein recommendation for strength athletes is 1.6 to 1.7 grams of protein per kilogram of body weight per day.

7. Increases in plasma volume (as much as 20 percent) have been observed in aerobically trained individuals as a normal consequence of training. This causes a dilution effect on blood measures. Diluted plasma yields a low hemoglobin concentration, a condition called sports anemia. Because sports anemia is a result of increased plasma volume, it is not considered a true iron-deficiency anemia. Taking extra iron supplements will do nothing for this condition.

9. Nutritional strategies that support gaining muscle mass include (1) setting realistic weight gain goals, (2) providing adequate energy intake for muscle building. and (3) determining carbohydrate and protein needs.

Spotlight on Eating Disorders

1. Social (i.e., societal pressure to be thin); Psychological (i.e., peer and family relationships); biological (i.e., neurotransmitter/ chemical balance)

3. The first goal of treatment is to stabilize the patient's physical condition. The second is to convert the patient, who is typically reluctant, into a willing participant in the treatment plan. A combination of hospitalization, psychotherapy, and pharmacotherapy is often necessary. Most experts doubt that patients with anorexia can be cured; but research suggests that with intensive therapy, most patients can increase their weight. However, they may struggle all their lives with a moderate to severe preoccupation with food and body weight, poor social relationships, and depression. The earlier a patient begins treatment, the better the prognosis.

5. During a binge, people with bulimia nervosa typically consume massive quantities of highly palatable "forbidden" foods, like pastry, ice cream, and candy. This gorging typically takes place in secret and over a relatively short time span (1 to 2 hours). Afterward, feeling physically ill from the overconsumption, sufferers use a variety of techniques to rid themselves of the food. These purging behaviors include vomiting and the use of emetics and laxatives. In addition to or instead of purging, they may follow a binge with a period of very strict fasting and increased exercise.

7. Female athletes who fall prey to the "thin-at-any-cost" philosophy are at risk of developing a condition known as the female athlete triad. This syndrome is characterized by disordered eating, amenorrhea (the loss of a consistent menstrual cycle), and abnormally low bone density.

Chapter 14

1. Both a high-fat diet and sedentary lifestyle have been shown to contribute to the onset and progression of cardiovascular disease and cancer.

3. Develop a healthy eating pattern, maintain a desirable body weight, achieve a healthy cholesterol and lipoprotein profile, and maintain a normal blood pressure level.

5. Smoking, diabetes, high-fat diet, obesity, age, heredity, gender and race.

7. Initiation occurs when something alters a cell's genetic structure and prompts it to act abnormally. Promotion occurs when a hormone, growth factors or other substance encourages initiated cells to become active.

9. Metabolic syndrome is the presence of at least three of the following signs:
   - Abdominal fat—for most men, a 40-inch waist or greater; for women, a waist of ≥ 35 inches
   - High blood glucose—at least 100 milligrams per deciliter (mg/dL) after fasting
   - High serum triglycerides—at least 150 mg/dL
   - Low HDL-cholesterol—less than 40 mg/dL for men; less than 50 mg/dL for women
   - Chronic blood pressure of at least 130 mm Hg systolic or 85 mg Hg diastolic or higher

Chapter 15

1. In the first stage of fetal growth, called the blastogenic stage, the fertilized egg rapidly divides and begins to differentiate. During the embryonic stage, the major organ systems form. The fetal stage is the longest stage of development and during this stage, the fetus grows dramatically in size.

3. • calories—increased by 340 to 450 kilocalories per day during the second and third trimesters
   • protein—increased to 71 grams per day
   • iron—increased by 9 milligrams per day (from 18 to 27 milligrams per day)
   • folate—increased by 200 micrograms per day (from 400 to 600 micrograms per day)

5. It is normal for infants to lose weight in the first few days of life. In fact, they may lose up to 6 percent of their weight. This does not necessarily mean that an infant is at nutritional risk. Infants typically regain their birth weight within 2 weeks.

7. Babies need approximately 0.7 liters of water each day in the first six months of life and 0.8 liters per day from age 7 months to 1 year. Breastfed and formula-fed infants do not need supplemental water; breast milk and properly mixed formula provide enough water for adequate hydration until significant amounts of solid foods have been added to the diet.

9. Solid foods (anything other than breast milk or infant formula) should be introduced at about 6 months of age. Then new foods should be introduced one at a time to check for any allergies or intolerances. Most parents begin with infant rice cereal, mixed to a thin consistency with water, breast milk, or infant formula. After the infant is eating cereal several times a day, strained fruits and vegetables are introduced one at a time.

Chapter 16

1. Iron, possibly zinc, vitamin D and vitamin E (if parents follow a low-fat diet).

3. Chronic nutrition problems that can affect children include overweight, lead toxicity, and early onset of indicators of heart disease. Infants and toddlers should not be given low-fat, high-fiber diets; when children reach the age of 3, dietary changes consistent with the Dietary Guidelines for Americans can gradually be made. Making sure children have regular physical activity and limiting sedentary activity such as television viewing are important factors in reducing overweight and chronic disease risk.

5. Decreased immune function can result in increased risk of respiratory infections, urinary tract infections, pressure sores, and foodborne illness.

7. Older people have less ability to produce active vitamin D from sun exposure, they typically are exposed to less sunlight, and they often do not consume enough dairy products, which are good sources of vitamin D.

9. Some nutrients in large amounts can be toxic.

   Supplements can affect the absorption of other nutrients or interfere with the absorption and metabolism of prescription medication.

   Excessive use of vitamin supplements can result in hypervitaminosis (high levels of vitamins in the blood).

   Supplements may contain more vitamin A than is needed in an elder's diet, which may lead to liver dysfunction, bone and joint pain, headaches, and other problems.

   Large amounts of vitamin C can increase the likelihood of kidney stones and gastric bleeding.

11. While inactivity increases osteoporosis risk, regular physical activity, especially weight-bearing exercise, helps prevent osteoporosis. An adequate intake of vitamin D and calcium helps slow the rate of bone loss in osteoporosis.

Chapter 17

1. Some types of pathogenic bacteria can directly infect a person who consumes contaminated food. Other may produce a toxin that can cause foodborne illness.

3. The following suggestions by the Consumers Union will help you limit your intake of pesticides:
   • Wash and peel produce.
   • Eat a wide variety of fruits and vegetables.

5. The most common food allergens are milk, eggs, peanuts, tree nuts, fish, shellfish, soy, and wheat. Symptoms of food allergies can include gastrointestinal problems, skin irritation, respiratory difficulties, shock, and death.

7. When trying to keep a kitchen safe from pathogenic microorganisms, you should
   • Make sure hands and kitchen surfaces are thoroughly clean.
   • Keep raw meats and poultry separate from other raw foods to avoid cross -contamination.
   • Use proper temperatures while cooking.
   • Chill food properly.

9. The main concerns scientists have regarding genetically engineered crops are (1) GM crops will hurt innocent creatures, (2) GM crops will lead to the emergence of superweeds, and (3) GM crops will have sudden and massive failures.

Chapter 18

1. Food insecurity is the worry that one does not have the resources to obtain adequate food. Hunger is the physical sensation of unease or pain caused by a lack of food. Food insecurity can exist with or without hunger.

3. Vitamin A, iodine, iron, protein-energy malnutrition (PEM).

5. Food Stamp Program, National School Lunch Program, School Breakfast Program, Child and Adult Care Food Program, The Food Research and Action Center (FRAC), Special Supplemental Nutrition Program for Women, Infants, and Children (WIC).

Photo Credits

Chapter openers created by Studio Montage.

All incidental and background photos and art © Photodisc, Corbis Digital Images, Digital Vision, Hemera Photo Objects, and Jones and Bartlett Publishers.

Nutrition Science in Actions, (top) © emin kuliyev/ShutterStock, Inc.; (bottom) © Leo/ShutterStock, Inc.

Chapter 1

4, Courtesy of Elizabeth Platt; 6, (left) © Mary Kate Denny/PhotoEdit, (middle) © Suza Scalora/PhotoDisc (right) © Jules Frazier/Photodisc; 7, Courtesy of Lowe Worldwide, Inc. as an agent for the National Fluid Milk Processor Promotion Board; 8, (top) © SuperStock/age footstock, (bottom) © Paul Barton/Corbis; 9, © 2005 Peter Menzel/menzelphoto.com; 10, © Natalia Bratslavsky/ShutterStock, Inc.

Chapter 2

32, © Photos.com; 35, © INGRAM Publishing/age fotostock; 46, © Photodisc; 46, © Photodisc; 50 and 51, © Hisham F. Ibrahim/Photodisc

Spotlight on Complementary and Alternative Nutrition

76, © Photodisc; 77, © Photodisc; 87, Courtesy of Jesse Geraci

Chapter 3

131, (top left) © EyeWire, (top right) © Chris Shorten/Cole Group/Photodisc, (bottom left) © PhotoLink/Photodisc, (bottom right) Courtesy of Dr. Wood/USDA; 139, (top) © A.B. Dowsett/SPL/Photo Researchers, Inc., (bottom) © Mediscan/Visuals Unlimited

Chapter 4

146, (top left) © Cn Boon/Alamy, (top right) Courtesy of David Nance/ARS Photo Library/USDA, (bottom left) Courtesy of ARS Photo Library/USDA, (bottom right), Courtesy of the USDA; 151, © Gary Gaugler/Visuals Unlimited; 153, © J.D. Litvay/Visuals Unlimited; 166, Courtesy of Julie Bolduc

Chapter 5

169, © Eric Gevaert/ShutterStock, Inc.; 187, © Steve Mason/Photodisc; 188 © Veronica Burmeister/Visuals Unlimited; 189, © Photodisc; 205, © W. Ober/Visuals Unlimited; 208, © Photodisc and (French fries) © Kirsta Mackey/ShutterStock, Inc.; 211, © Photodisc

Chapter 6

237, (left) © EyeWire, (middle) © Keith Brofsky/Photodisc/Getty Images, (right) © EyeWire; 238, (top) © Jess Alford/Photodisc, (middle) © Jules Frazier/PhotoDisc, (bottom) © PhotoLink/Photodisc; 239, © NorthGeorgiaMedia/ShutterStock, Inc.; 241, © Photodisc; 251, (top) © CDC/ Dr. Lyle Conrad, (bottom) © CDC/Dr. Edward Brink; 254, (left) © David Hernandez/ShutterStock, Inc., (middle) © Stephen Walls/ShutterStock, Inc., (right) © Photodisc

Chapter 7

296, © Losevsky Pavel/ShutterStock, Inc.

Spotlight on Alcohol

303, (top left) © Jack Star/PhotoLink/PhotoDisc, (top right) © Mitch Hrdlicka/PhotoDisc; 305, © David M. Phillips/Visuals Unlimited; 311, © PhotoDisc; 312, © Tomi/PhotoLink/Photodisc; 316, © OJ Staats/Custom Medical Stock Photo

Chapter 8

347, (left) Courtesy of Life Measurement Instruments, (right) © Photodisc; 349, © Bill Bachmann/The Medical File/Peter Arnold, Inc.; 356, (left) © ImageState/Alamy, (middle) © Visual Arts Library (London)/Alamy, (right) © Fitzroy Barrett/Landov; 357, © Photodisc; 361, © Comstock Images/Alamy Images

Index/Glossary

Key terms in the text appear here in **bold** followed by the definition.

Canada's Guidelines for Healthy Eating Key messages that are based on the 1990 *Nutrition Recommendations for Canadians* and provide positive, action-oriented, scientifically accurate eating advice to Canadians, 38

Canada's Physical Activity Guide for Older Adults, 705

Cancer A term for diseases in which abnormal cells divide without control. Cancer cells can invade nearby tissues and can spread through the bloodstream and lymphatic system to other parts of the body, 620–621

alcohol and, 316, 317, 323, 623
beta-carotene and, 86
bladder, 167
breast, 18–19, 247, 395, 441, 625
carotenoids and, 395–396, 398
colon, 401, 441, 451
colorectal, 137, 298
conjugated linoleic acid and, 193
dietary and lifestyle factors for reducing risk of, 623–625
fats and, 58, 215, 624
fiber and, 58, 78, 137
folate and, 441, 451
fruits and vegetables and, 58, 623, 624–625
legumes and, 625
liver, 317
lung, 86, 395
overweight/obesity and, 354, 355, 602, 623
physical activity and, 623
phytochemicals and, 76, 77, 80
prostate, 86, 93, 247, 395, 396
proteins and, 253
risk factors for, 605, 621–622
saccharin and, 83, 167
saw palmetto and, 86
smoking and, 316, 323
soy and, 18–19, 76, 77, 247
vitamin C and, 389
vitamin D and, 401
vitamin E and, 389, 407, 408
whole grains and, 59, 625

Cantaloupe, 395

Carbohydrate loading Changes in dietary carbohydrate intake and exercise regimen before competition to maximize glycogen stores in the muscles. It is appropriate for endurance events lasting 60 to 90 consecutive minutes or longer. Also known as glycogen loading, 546–547

Carbohydrates Compounds, including sugars, starches, and dietary fibers, that usually have the general chemical formula $(CH_2O)n$, where n represents the number of CH_2O units in the molecule. Carbohydrates are a major source of energy for body functions, 14, 146

absorption of, 154, 156–158
Acceptable Macronutrient Distribution Range for, 238
athletes and, 152, 546–551
in the body, 158–162
choosing wisely, 164–165
complex, 151–154, 165
current consumption, 163
in the diet, 162–170, 360, 362–363
Dietary Guidelines for Americans recommendations, 36–37, 163
digestion of, 154–158
elderly and, 708
energy and, 158, 269–274, 280–282
excess of, turning into fat, 285
from fat, 276, 278
foods high in, 165
health and, 170–173
high-protein, low-carbohydrate diet, 362–363
infants and, 670
metabolism and vitamin B_6, 436
Nutrition Facts label for finding, 173
pregnancy and, 655
recommended intake, 162–163, 238
simple, 147–150, 165

Carbon skeletons, 236

Carboxylation A reaction that adds a carboxyl group (–COOH) to a substrate, replacing a hydrogen atom, 435

Cardiac output The amount of blood expelled by the heart, 564

Cardiovascular disease (CVD) Any abnormal condition characterized by dysfunction of the heart and blood vessels. CVD includes atherosclerosis (especially coronary heart disease, which can lead to heart attacks), cerebrovascular disease (e.g., stroke), and hypertension (high blood pressure), 606

See also under type of
cardiovascular system and, 606–607
phytochemicals and, 77
preventing, 607, 609–610, 612–615

Carnitine [CAR-nih-teen] A compound that transports fatty acids from the cytosol into the mitochondria, where they undergo beta-oxidation, 275–276, 449

athletes and, 559

Carotenodermia A harmless yellow-orange cast to the skin due to high levels of carotenoids in the bloodstream resulting from consumption of extremely large amounts of carotenoid-rich foods, such as carrot juice, 382

Carotenoids A group of yellow, orange, and red pigments in plants, including foods. Many of these compounds are precursors of vitamin A, 78, 384, 385, 394–395

absorption and storage of, 396, 397
cancer and, 395–396, 398
functions of, 395–396
sources of, 396
supplementation, 398
vision and, 395

Carcinogens [kar-SIN-o-jins] Any substances that cause cancer, 621

Cascara, 92, 93

Case control study An investigation that uses a group of people with a particular condition, rather than a randomly selected population. These cases are compared with a control group of people who do not have the condition, 19

Catabolism [ca-TA-bol-iz-um] Any metabolic process whereby cells break down complex substances into simpler, smaller ones, 264

end products of amino acid, 278, 279
end products of glucose, 274

Catalyze To speed up a chemical reaction, 114

teins from the cell nucleus to the cytoplasm, where the ribosomes translate
mRNA into proteins, 235

Metabolic alkalosis An abnormal pH of body
fluids usually caused by significant loss of
acid from the body or increased levels of
bicarbonate, 476

Metabolic fitness The absence of all metabolic and biochemical risk factors associated with obesity, 358

Metabolic pathway(s) A series of chemical
reactions that either break down a large
compound into smaller units (catabolism)
or synthesize more complex molecules from
smaller ones (anabolism), 264

major, G-1 to G-5

Metabolic syndrome A cluster of at least three
of the following risk factors for heart disease: hypertriglyceridemia (high blood
triglycerides), low HDL cholesterol, hyperglycemia (high blood glucose), hypertension (high blood pressure), and excess
abdominal fat, 632–633

Metabolism All chemical reactions within
organisms that enable them to maintain
life. The two main categories of metabolism
are catabolism and anabolism, 263

alcohol, 307–312

biosynthesis and storage, 279–287

cells, role of, 265–266

copper, 518

energy and, 262–278

hormones of, 288

of important body parts, 292–293

iodine, 516

molybdenum, 526

physical activity and, 295

regulation of, 287–288

special states of, 288–295

water and, 459

Metabolites Any substances produced during
metabolism, 264

Metastasis [meh-TAS-ta-sis] The spread of
cancer from one part of the body to
another. Tumors formed from cells that
have spread are called "secondary tumors"
and contain cells that are like those in the

original (primary) tumor. The plural is
metastases, 621

Methanol The simplest alcohol, a one-carbon
compound with one hydroxyl group. Also
known as methyl alcohol and wood alcohol, 302, 303

Methyl alcohol. *See* **Methanol**

Methylmercury A toxic compound that results
from the chemical transformation of mercury by bacteria. Mercury is water-soluble
in trace amounts and contaminates many
bodies of water, 737–738

Metalloproteins Proteins with a mineral element as an essential part of their structure,
507

Metallothionein An abundant, nonenzymatic,
zinc-containing protein, 508, 509

Micelles Tiny emulsified fat packets that can
enter enterocytes. The complexes are composed of emulsifier molecules oriented with
their hydrophobic part facing inward and
their hydrophilic part facing outward toward
the surrounding aqueous environment,
195, 200

Microcytic hypochromic anemia Anemia characterized by small, pale red blood cells
that lack adequate hemoglobin to carry
oxygen; can be caused by deficiency of iron
or vitamin B_6, 436, 506

Microminerals. *See* **Trace minerals**

Micronutrients Nutrients, such as vitamins
and minerals, that are needed in relatively
small amounts in the diet, 13

pregnancy and, 655–656

Microsomal ethanol-oxidizing system (MEOS)
An energy-requiring enzyme system in the
liver that normally metabolizes drugs and
other foreign substances. When the blood
alcohol level is high, alcohol dehydrogenase cannot metabolize it fast enough, and
the excess alcohol is metabolized by
MEOS, 306, 307–308

Microvilli Minute, hairlike projections that
extend from the surface of absorptive cells
facing the intestinal lumen. Singular is
microvillus, 124–125

Migraine headaches, 92

Milk, cow

infants, inappropriate for, 670, 677

Nutrition Facts label for, 417

vitamin A in, 417

vitamin D in, 403, 417

vitamin K in, 417

Milk, human

See also Breastfeeding

appearance of, 673

benefits of, 665–666, 670–672

oligosaccharides in, 151

protein in, 239, 670

Milk, soy, 247

Milk thistle, 92

Mineralization The addition of minerals, such
as calcium and phosphorus, to bones and
teeth, 522

Mineralocorticoids, 197

Minerals Inorganic compounds needed
for growth and for regulation of body
processes, 15

See also **Major minerals; Trace minerals**

adolescents and, 699

alcohol and deficiencies of, 320

amount in the body, 469

athletes and, 552–554

breastfeeding and, 664

children and, 689–690

dietary supplements, 85–91, 689–690

elderly and, 709–710

infants and, 670–671

macro-, 15

micro-, 15

proteins and loss of, 252

trace, 15

Mineral water, 469

Mint, 92

Mitochondria (mitochondrion) The sites of
aerobic production of ATP, where most of
the energy from carbohydrate, protein, and
fat is captured. Called the "power plants"
of the cell, the mitochondria contain two
highly specialized membranes, an outer
membrane and a highly folded inner membrane, that separate two compartments,
the internal matrix space and the narrow
intermembrane space. A human cell contains about 2,000 mitochondria, 264, 265

Olfactory cells Nerve cells in a small patch of tissue high in the nose connected directly to the brain to transmit messages about specific smells. Also called smell cells, 110

Oligopeptide Four to 10 amino acids joined by peptide bonds, 224, 225

Oligosaccharides Short carbohydrate chains composed of 3 to 10 sugar molecules, 151

Omega-9 fatty acid Any polyunsaturated fatty acid in which the first double bond starting from the methyl (CH_3) end of the molecule lies between the ninth and tenth carbon atoms, 184, 185

Omega-6 fatty acid Any polyunsaturated fatty acid in which the first double bond starting from the methyl (CH_3) end of the molecule lies between the sixth and seventh carbon atoms, 184, 185, 186
sources of, 190–191, 208

Omega-3 fatty acids Any polyunsaturated fatty acid in which the first double bond starting from the methyl (CH_3) end of the molecule lies between the third and fourth carbon atoms, 184, 186
heart disease and, 185
sources of, 190–191, 192, 208

1,25-dihydroxyvitamin D_3 [1,25(OH)$_2$$D_3$] The active form of vitamin D. It is an important regulator of blood calcium levels, 400

Onions, crying from, 488

Opsin A protein that combines with retinal to form rhodopsin in rod cells, 388

Orexin A class of hormones in the brain that may affect food consumption, 579

Organelles Various membrane-bound structures that form part of the cytoplasm. Organelles, including mitochondria and lysosomes, perform specialized metabolic functions, 264, 265

Organic [or-GAN-ick] In chemistry, any compound that contains carbon, except carbon oxides (e.g., carbon dioxide) and sulfides and metal carbonates (e.g., potassium carbonate). The term *organic* is also used to denote crops that are grown without synthetic fertilizers or chemicals, 13

Organic foods Foods that originate from farms or handling operations that meet the standards set by the USDA National Organic Program, 732
debate over, 735
labeling requirements for, 734–735

Organogenesis The period when organ systems are developing in a growing fetus, 650

Orthomolecular medicine The preventive or therapeutic use of high-dose vitamins to treat disease, 90

Osmolarity The concentration of dissolved particles (e.g., electrolytes) in a solution expressed per unit of volume, 463

Osmoreceptors Neurons in the hypothalamus that detect changes in the fluid concentration in blood and regulate the release of antidiuretic hormone, 463

Osmosis The movement of a solvent, such as water, through a semipermeable membrane from the low-solute to the high-solute solution until the concentrations on both sides of the membrane are equal, 460, 461

Osmotic pressure The pressure exerted on a semipermeable membrane by a solvent, usually water, moving from the side of low-solute to the side of high-solute concentration, 460

Osteoarthritis, 355

Osteoblasts Bone cells that promote bone deposition and growth, 400, 477

Osteoclasts Bone cells that promote bone resorption and calcium mobilization, 400, 477

Osteomalacia A disease in adults that results from vitamin D deficiency. It is marked by softening of the bones, leading to bending of the spine, bowing of the legs, and increased risk for fractures, 404, 405

Osteoporosis A bone disease characterized by a decrease in bone mineral density and the appearance of small holes in bones due to loss of minerals, 405
alcohol and, 323
calcium and, 57, 252, 480–481, 489, 634
defined, 405, 633
dietary and lifestyle factors for reducing risk of, 634–636
fluoride and, 523

physical activity and, 57, 633, 635–636, 715–716
risk factors for, 605, 633–634
soy proteins and, 247, 252
vitamin A and, 634–635
vitamin D and, 398, 404, 634

Overnutrition The long-term consumption of an excess of nutrients. The most common type of overnutrition in the United States is due to the regular consumption of excess calories, fats, saturated fats, and cholesterol, 62

Overweight BMI at or above 25 kg/m^2 and less than 30 kg/m^2, 345
See also **Obesity; Overweight/obesity; Weight management**

Overweight/obesity
adolescents and, 694–695, 700–701
age and, 351, 353, 703
arthritis and, 355, 602, 714
behavior and, 17–18, 352–353
breathing problems and, 602
cancer and, 354, 355, 602, 623
children and, 170–171, 603, 692, 694–696
death, increased risk of premature, 602
diabetes and, 294–295, 354, 355, 602, 603, 628–629
disease and, 601–603
elderly and, 714
environment and, 17–18, 352
ethnicity and, 351, 353
factors contributing to, 357
fats and, 213
fiber and, 171
gallbladder disease and, 354, 355, 603
gender differences and, 351–353
gout and, 355
health risks of, 354–355, 602–603
heart disease and, 354, 355, 602, 603
heredity and genetic factors and, 17, 350–351
hypertension and, 354, 355, 602, 603, 617
malnutrition and, 779
physical activity and, 352–353
pregnancy and, 602–603
prevalence of, 350
proteins and, 252–253
as a public health crisis, 17–18

is attached to the rest of the molecule. Often hydrogen atoms are attached to the oxygens. Sometimes there are double bonds between the phosphorus and an oxygen, 193

Phosphocreatine. *See* **Creatine phosphate**

Phospholipids Compounds that consist of a glycerol molecule bonded to two fatty acid molecules and to a phosphate group with a nitrogen-containing component. Phospholipids have both hydrophilic and hydrophobic regions that make them good emulsifiers, 180, 181
digestion of, 199–201
as emulsifiers, 194–195
functions of, 193–195
sources of, 195
structure of, 193

Phosphorus
deficiency, 485–486
dietary recommendations for, 484
functions of, 484
sources of, 485–484
toxicity, 486

Phosphorylation The addition of phosphate to an organic (carbon-containing) compound. Oxidative phosphorylation is the formation of high-energy phosphate bonds (ADP + Pi → ATP) from the energy released by oxidation of energy-yielding nutrients, 484

Photosynthesis The process by which green plants use radiant energy from the sun to produce carbohydrates (hexoses) from carbon dioxide and water, 262, 263

Phylloquinone The form of vitamin K that comes from plant sources. Also known as vitamin K$_1$, 411

Physical activity
See also Athletes
adolescents and, 556
age and, 557, 705
bone health and, 633, 635–636
breastfeeding and, 556
cancer and, 623
children and, 556
chromium, body composition, and, 524–525
diabetes and, lack of, 629

Dietary Guidelines for Americans recommendations, 35
disease and lack of, 603
elderly and, 478, 556, 715–716
energy expenditure and, 337, 338
"fat burning," 563
gender differences and, 252–253
guidelines for, 538
hypertension and, 473, 617, 618
MyPyramid and, 41, 42
osteoporosis and, 57, 633, 635–636, 715–716
overweight/obesity and, 352–353
pregnancy and, 556
sodium and, 473
variety of, 537
weight management and, 361–362

Physical fitness
components of, 536, 538
defined, 536

Phytate (phytic acid) A phosphorous-containing compound in the outer husks of cereal grains that binds with minerals and inhibits their absorption, 470, 471

Phytochemicals Substances in plants that may possess health-protective effects, even though they are not essential for life, 13
benefits of, 77, 80
cancer and, 76, 77, 80
cardiovascular disease and, 77
functional foods and, 76–77, 80
heart disease and, 76, 77

Phytoestrogens, 79

Phytosterols Sterols found in plants. Phytosterols are poorly absorbed by humans and reduce intestinal absorption of cholesterol. They recently have been introduced as a cholesterol-lowering food ingredient, 199

Phytotherapy. *See* **Herbal therapy**

Pica The craving for and consumption of nonfood items like dirt, clay, or laundry starch, 7

Pinocytosis The process by which cells internalize fluids and macromolecules. To do so, the cell membrane invaginates and forms a pocket around the substance. From *pino*, "drinking," and *cyto*, "cell," 116

Pizza, 396
digestion and absorption of, 139–140

Placebo An inactive substance that is outwardly indistinguishable from the active substance whose effects are being studied, 20

Placebo effect A physical or emotional change that is not due to properties of an administered substance. The change reflects participants' expectations, 21, 23
athletes and, 559

Placenta The organ formed during pregnancy that produces hormones for the maintenance of pregnancy and across which oxygen and nutrients are transferred from mother to infant; it also allows waste materials to be transferred from infant to mother, 650

Plaque A flattened patch along the blood vessel wall, 607

Plasma The fluid portion of the blood that contains blood cells and other components, 460

Platelets Tiny disk-shaped components of blood that are essential for blood clotting, 607

Poisonous mushrooms Mushrooms that contain toxins that can cause stomach upset, dizziness, hallucinations, and other neurological symptoms, 738

Poisons, from puffer fish, 9

Political disruptions, malnutrition and, 772–773

Pollutants Gaseous, chemical, or organic wastes that contaminate air, soil, or water, 736, 737

Polyols. *See* **Sugar alcohols**

Polypeptide More than 10 amino acids joined by peptide bonds, 224, 225

Polyphenols Organic compounds that include an unsaturated ring containing more than one –OH group as part of their chemical structures; may produce bitterness in coffee and tea, 502

Polysaccharides Long carbohydrate chains composed of more than 10 sugar molecules. Polysaccharides can be straight or branched, 151–154